The GALE
ENCYCLOPEDIA of
MEDICINE

THIRD EDITION

The GALE ENCYCLOPEDIA *of* MEDICINE

THIRD EDITION

VOLUME

1

A-B

JACQUELINE L. LONGE, PROJECT EDITOR

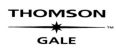

THOMSON

GALE

Detroit • New York • San Francisco • San Diego • New Haven, Conn. • Waterville, Maine • London • Munich

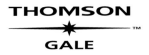

THE GALE ENCYCLOPEDIA OF MEDICINE, THIRD EDITION

Project Editor
Jacqueline L. Longe

Editorial
Shirelle Phelps, Laurie Fundukian, Jeffrey Lehman, Brigham Narins

Editorial Support Services
Luann Brennan, Grant Eldridge, Andrea Lopeman

Rights Acquisition Management
Shalice Caldwell-Shah

Imaging
Randy Bassett, Lezlie Light, Dan Newell, Christine O'Bryan, Robyn V. Young

Product Design
Tracey Rowens

Composition and Electronic Prepress
Evi Seoud, Mary Beth Trimper

Manufacturing
Wendy Blurton, Dorothy Maki

Indexing
Factiva

LIBRARY OF CONGRESS CATALOGING-IN-PUBLICATION DATA

The Gale encyclopedia of medicine / Jacqueline L. Longe, editor.– 3rd ed.
      p. ; cm.
   Includes bibliographical references and index.
   ISBN 1-4144-0368-2 (set hardcover : alk. paper) – ISBN 1-4144-0369-0 (v. 1 : hardcover
: alk. paper) – ISBN 1-4144-0370-4 (v. 2 : hardcover : alk. paper) – ISBN 1-4144-0371-2
v. 3 : hardcover : alk. paper) – ISBN 1-4144-0372-0 (v. 4 : hardcover : alk. paper) –
ISBN 1-4144-0373-9 (v. 5 : hardcover : alk. paper)
   1. Internal medicine–Encyclopedias.
   [DNLM: 1. Internal Medicine–Encyclopedias–English. 2. Complementary Therapies–
Encyclopedias–English. WB 13 G151 2005] I. Title: Encyclopedia of medicine. II. Longe,
Jacqueline L. III. Gale Group.
   RC41.G35 2006
   616'.003–dc22
                                                                      2005011418

This title is also available as an e-book
ISBN 1-4144-0485-9 (set)
Contact your Gale sales representative for ordering information.
ISBN 1-4144-0368-2 (set)
            1-4144-0369-0 (Vol. 1)
            1-4144-0370-4 (Vol. 2)
            1-4144-0371-2 (Vol. 3)
            1-4144-0372-0 (Vol. 4)
            1-4144-0373-9 (Vol. 5)

Printed in China
10 9 8 7 6 5 4 3 2 1

CONTENTS

LIST OF ENTRIES

A

Abdominal ultrasound
Abdominal wall defects
Abortion, partial birth
Abortion, selective
Abortion, therapeutic
Abscess incision & drainage
Abscess
Abuse
Acetaminophen
Achalasia
Achondroplasia
Acid phosphatase test
Acne
Acoustic neuroma
Acrocyanosis
Acromegaly and gigantism
Actinomycosis
Acupressure
Acupuncture
Acute kidney failure
Acute lymphangitis
Acute poststreptococcal
  glomerulonephritis
Acute stress disorder
Addiction
Addison's disease
Adenoid hyperplasia
Adenovirus infections
Adhesions
Adjustment disorders
Adrenal gland cancer
Adrenal gland scan
Adrenal virilism
Adrenalectomy
Adrenocorticotropic hormone test
Adrenoleukodystrophy
Adult respiratory distress syndrome
Aging

Agoraphobia
AIDS tests
AIDS
Alanine aminotransferase test
Albinism
Alcoholism
Alcohol-related neurologic disease
Aldolase test
Aldosterone assay
Alemtuzumab
Alexander technique
Alkaline phosphatase test
Allergic bronchopulmonary
  aspergillosis
Allergic purpura
Allergic rhinitis
Allergies
Allergy tests
Alopecia
Alpha$_1$-adrenergic blockers
Alpha-fetoprotein test
Alport syndrome
Altitude sickness
Alzheimer's disease
Amblyopia
Amebiasis
Amenorrhea
Amino acid disorders screening
Aminoglycosides
Amnesia
Amniocentesis
Amputation
Amylase tests
Amyloidosis
Amyotrophic lateral sclerosis
Anabolic steroid use
Anaerobic infections
Anal atresia
Anal cancer
Anal warts
Analgesics, opioid

Analgesics
Anaphylaxis
Anemias
Anesthesia, general
Anesthesia, local
Aneurysmectomy
Angina
Angiography
Angioplasty
Angiotensin-converting enzyme
  inhibitors
Angiotensin-converting enzyme
  test
Animal bite infections
Ankylosing spondylitis
Anorectal disorders
Anorexia nervosa
Anoscopy
Anosmia
Anoxia
Antacids
Antenatal testing
Antepartum testing
Anthrax
Antiacne drugs
Antiandrogen drugs
Antianemia drugs
Antiangina drugs
Antiangiogenic therapy
Antianxiety drugs
Antiarrhythmic drugs
Antiasthmatic drugs
Antibiotic-associated colitis
Antibiotics, ophthalmic
Antibiotics, topical
Antibiotics
Anticancer drugs
Anticoagulant and antiplatelet
  drugs
Anticonvulsant drugs
Antidepressant drugs, SSRI

Antidepressant drugs
Antidepressants, tricyclic
Antidiabetic drugs
Antidiarrheal drugs
Antidiuretic hormone (ADH) test
Antifungal drugs, systemic
Antifungal drugs, topical
Antigas agents
Antigastroesophageal reflux drugs
Antihelminthic drugs
Antihemorrhoid drugs
Antihistamines H-2 blockers
Antihistamines
Antihypertensive drugs
Anti-hyperuricemic drugs
Anti-insomnia drugs
Anti-itch drugs
Antimalarial drugs
Antimigraine drugs
Antimyocardial antibody test
Antinausea drugs
Antinuclear antibody test
Antiparkinson drugs
Antiprotozoal drugs
Antipsychotic drugs, atypical
Antipsychotic drugs
Anti-rejection drugs
Antiretroviral drugs
Antirheumatic drugs
Antiseptics
Antispasmodic drugs
Antituberculosis drugs
Antiulcer drugs
Antiviral drugs
Anxiety disorders
Anxiety
Aortic aneurysm
Aortic dissection
Aortic valve insufficiency
Aortic valve stenosis
Apgar testing
Aphasia
Aplastic anemia
Appendectomy
Appendicitis
Appetite-enhancing drugs
Apraxia
Arbovirus encephalitis
Aromatherapy
Arrhythmias
Art therapy
Arterial embolism
Arteriovenous fistula

Arteriovenous malformations
Arthrography
Arthroplasty
Arthroscopic surgery
Arthroscopy
Asbestosis
Ascites
Aspartate aminotransferase test
Aspergillosis
Aspirin
Asthma
Astigmatism
Aston-Patterning
Ataxia-telangiectasia
Atelectasis
Atherectomy
Atherosclerosis
Athlete's foot
Athletic heart syndrome
Atkins diet
Atopic dermatitis
Atrial ectopic beats
Atrial fibrillation and flutter
Atrial septal defect
Attention-deficit/Hyperactivity disorder (ADHD)
Audiometry
Auditory integration training
Autism
Autoimmune disorders
Autopsy
Aviation medicine
Ayurvedic medicine

B

Babesiosis
Bacillary angiomatosis
Bacteremia
Bacterial vaginosis
Bad breath
Balance and coordination tests
Balanitis
Balantidiasis
Balloon valvuloplasty
Barbiturate-induced coma
Barbiturates
Bariatric surgery
Barium enema
Bartholin's gland cyst
Bartonellosis
Battered child syndrome
Bedsores

Bed-wetting
Behcet's syndrome
Bejel
Bence Jones protein test
Bender-Gestalt test
Benzodiazepines
Bereavement
Beriberi
Berylliosis
Beta blockers
Beta$_2$-microglobulin test
Bile duct cancer
Biliary atresia
Binge-eating disorder
Biofeedback
Bipolar disorder
Bird flu
Birth defects
Birthmarks
Bites and stings
Black lung disease
Bladder cancer
Bladder stones
Bladder training
Blastomycosis
Bleeding time
Bleeding varices
Blepharoplasty
Blood clots
Blood count
Blood culture
Blood donation and registry
Blood gas analysis
Blood sugar tests
Blood typing and crossmatching
Blood urea nitrogen test
Blood-viscosity reducing drugs
Body dysmorphic disorder
Boils
Bone biopsy
Bone density test
Bone disorder drugs
Bone grafting
Bone growth stimulation
Bone marrow aspiration and biopsy
Bone marrow transplantation
Bone nuclear medicine scan
Bone x rays
Botulinum toxin injections
Botulism
Bowel preparation
Bowel resection
Bowel training

I

Insulin resistance
Intermittent claudication
Intermittent explosive disorder
Intersex states
Interstitial microwave thermal
   therapy
Intestinal obstructions
Intestinal polyps
Intrauterine growth retardation
Intravenous rehydration
Intravenous urography
Intussusception
Ipecac
Iron deficiency anemia
Iron tests
Irritable bowel syndrome
Ischemia
Isolation
Itching
IUD

J

Japanese encephalitis
Jaundice
Jaw wiring
Jet lag
Jock itch
Joint biopsy
Joint fluid analysis
Joint replacement
Juvenile arthritis

K

Kaposi's sarcoma
Kawasaki syndrome
Keloids
Keratitis
Keratosis pilaris
Kidney biopsy
Kidney cancer
Kidney disease
Kidney function tests
Kidney nuclear medicine scan
Kidney stones
Kidney transplantation
Kidney, ureter, and bladder x-ray
   study
Kinesiology, applied
Klinefelter syndrome
Knee injuries

Kneecap removal
KOH test
Korsakoff's syndrome
Kyphosis

L

Labyrinthitis
Laceration repair
Lacrimal duct obstruction
Lactate dehydrogenase isoenzymes
   test
Lactate dehydrogenase test
Lactation
Lactic acid test
Lactose intolerance
Laparoscopy
Laryngeal cancer
Laryngectomy
Laryngitis
Laryngoscopy
Laser surgery
Laxatives
Lead poisoning
Learning disorders
Leeches
Legionnaires' disease
Leishmaniasis
Leprosy
Leptospirosis
Lesch-Nyhan syndrome
Leukemia stains
Leukemias, acute
Leukemias, chronic
Leukocytosis
Leukotriene inhibitors
Lice infestation
Lichen planus
Lichen simplex chronicus
Life support
Lipase test
Lipidoses
Lipoproteins test
Liposuction
Listeriosis
Lithotripsy
Liver biopsy
Liver cancer
Liver disease
Liver encephalopathy
Liver function tests
Liver nuclear medicine scan
Liver transplantation

Low back pain
Lower esophageal ring
Lumpectomy
Lung abscess
Lung biopsy
Lung cancer, non-small cell
Lung cancer, small cell
Lung diseases due to gas or chemical
   exposure
Lung perfusion and ventilation scan
Lung surgery
Lung transplantation
Luteinizing hormone test
Lyme disease
Lymph node biopsy
Lymphadenitis
Lymphangiography
lymphedema
Lymphocyte typing
Lymphocytic choriomeningitis
Lymphocytopenia
Lymphogranuloma venereum
Lysergic acid diethylamide (LSD)

M

Macular degeneration
Magnesium imbalance
Magnetic field therapy
Magnetic resonance imaging
Malabsorption syndrome
Malaria
Malignant lymphomas
Malignant melanoma
Malingering
Mallet finger
Mallory-Weiss syndrome
Malnutrition
Malocclusion
MALT lymphoma
Mammography
Mania
Marfan syndrome
Marijuana
Marriage counseling
Marshall-Marchetti-Krantz
   procedure
Massage therapy
Mastectomy
Mastitis
Mastocytosis
Mastoidectomy
Mastoiditis

N

O

Ovarian cancer
Ovarian cysts
Ovarian torsion
Overactive bladder
Overhydration
Oxygen/ozone therapy

P

Pacemakers
Paget's disease of bone
Paget's disease of the breast
Pain management
Pain
Palpitations
Pancreas transplantation
Pancreatectomy
Pancreatic cancer, endocrine
Pancreatic cancer, exocrine
Pancreatitis
Panic disorder
Pap test
Papilledema
Paracentesis
Paralysis
Paranoia
Parathyroid hormone test
Parathyroid scan
Parathyroidectomy
Paratyphoid fever
Parkinson disease
Parotidectomy
Paroxysmal atrial tachycardia
Parrot fever
Partial thromboplastin time
Paruresis
Patau syndrome
Patent ductus arteriosus
Pellagra
Pelvic exam
Pelvic fracture
Pelvic inflammatory disease
Pelvic relaxation
Pelvic ultrasound
Penicillins
Penile cancer
Penile prostheses
Percutaneous transhepatic
  cholangiography
Perforated eardrum
Perforated septum
PericardiocentesisPericarditis
Perinatal infection

Periodic paralysis
Periodontal disease
Peripheral neuropathy
Peripheral vascular disease
Peritonitis
Pernicious anemia
Peroxisomal disorders
Personality disorders
Pervasive developmental disorders
Pet therapy
Peyronie's disease
Pharmacogenetics
Phenylketonuria
Pheochromocytoma
Phimosis
Phlebotomy
Phobias
Phosphorus imbalance
Photorefractive keratectomy and
  laser-assisted in-situ keratomileusis
Photosensitivity
Phototherapy
Physical allergy
Physical examination
Pica
Pickwickian syndrome
Piercing and tattoos
Pilates
Pinguecula and pterygium
Pinta
Pituitary dwarfism
Pituitary tumors
Pityriasis rosea
Placenta previa
Placental abruption
Plague
Plasma renin activity
Plasmapheresis
Plastic, cosmetic, and reconstructive
  surgery
Platelet aggregation test
Platelet count
Platelet function disorders
Pleural biopsy
Pleural effusion
Pleurisy
Pneumococcal pneumonia
Pneumocystis pneumonia
Pneumonia
Pneumothorax
Poison ivy and poison oak
Poisoning
Polarity therapy
Polio

Polycystic kidney disease
Polycystic ovary syndrome
Polycythemia vera
Polydactyly and syndactyly
Polyglandular deficiency syndromes
Polyhydramnios and
  oligohydramnios
Polymyalgia rheumatica
Polymyositis
Polysomnography
Porphyrias
Portal vein bypass
Positron emission tomography
  (PET)
Post-concussion syndrome
Postmenopausal bleeding
Postpartum depression
Postpolio syndrome
Post-traumatic stress disorder
Prader-Willi syndrome
Precocious puberty
Preeclampsia and eclampsia
Pregnancy
Premature ejaculation
Premature labor
Premature menopause
Premature rupture of membranes
Prematurity
Premenstrual dysphoric disorder
Premenstrual syndrome
Prenatal surgery
Prepregnancy counseling
Presbyopia
Priapism
Prickly heat
Primary biliary cirrhosis
Proctitis
Progressive multifocal
  leukoencephalopathy
Progressive supranuclear palsy
Prolactin test
Prolonged QT syndrome
Prophylaxis
Prostate biopsy
Prostate cancer
Prostate ultrasound
Prostatectomy
Prostate-specific antigen test
Prostatitis
Protease inhibitors
Protein components test
Protein electrophoresis
Protein-energy malnutrition
Prothrombin time

Proton Pump Inhibitors
Pseudogout
Pseudomonas infections
Pseudoxanthoma elasticum
Psoriasis
Psoriatic arthritis
Psychiatric confinement
Psychoanalysis
Psychological tests
Psychosis
Psychosocial disorders
Psychosurgery
Ptosis
Puberty
Puerperal infection
Pulmonary alveolar proteinosis
Pulmonary artery catheterization
Pulmonary edema
Pulmonary embolism
Pulmonary fibrosis
Pulmonary function test
Pulmonary hypertension
Pulmonary valve insufficiency
Pulmonary valve stenosis
Pyelonephritis
Pyloric stenosis
Pyloroplasty
Pyruvate kinase deficiency

Q

Q fever
Qigong

R

Rabies
Radial keratotomy
Radiation injuries
Radiation therapy
Radical neck dissection
Radioactive implants
Rape and sexual assault
Rashes
Rat-bite fever
Raynaud's disease
Recompression treatment
Rectal cancer
Rectal examination
Rectal polyps
Rectal prolapse

Recurrent miscarriage
Red blood cell indices
Reflex sympathetic dystrophy
Reflex tests
Reflexology
Rehabilitation
Reiki
Reiter's syndrome
Relapsing fever
Relapsing polychondritis
Renal artery occlusion
Renal artery stenosis
Renal tubular acidosis
Renal vein thrombosis
Renovascular hypertension
Respiratory acidosis
Respiratory alkalosis
Respiratory distress syndrome
Respiratory failure
Respiratory syncytial virus
   infection
Restless legs syndrome
Restrictive cardiomyopathy
Reticulocyte count
Retinal artery occlusion
Retinal detachment
Retinal hemorrhage
Retinal vein occlusion
Retinitis pigmentosa
Retinoblastoma
Retinopathies
Retrograde cystography
Retrograde ureteropyelography
Retrograde urethrography
Reye's syndrome
Rheumatic fever
Rheumatoid arthritis
Rhinitis
Rhinoplasty
Riboflavin deficiency
Rickets
Rickettsialpox
Ringworm
Rocky Mountain spotted fever
Rolfing
Root canal treatment
Rosacea
Roseola
Ross River Virus
Rotator cuff injury
Rotavirus infections
Roundworm infections
Rubella test
Rubella

S

Sacroiliac disease
Salivary gland scan
Salivary gland tumors
Salmonella food poisoning
Salpingectomy
Salpingo-oophorectomy
Sarcoidosis
Sarcomas
Saw palmetto
Scabies
Scarlet fever
Scars
Schistosomiasis
Schizoaffective disorder
Schizophrenia
Sciatica
Scleroderma
Sclerotherapy for esophageal varices
Scoliosis
Scrotal nuclear medicine scan
Scrotal ultrasound
Scrub typhus
Scurvy
Seasonal affective disorder
Seborrheic dermatitis
Secondary polycythemia
Sedation
Seizure disorder
Selective serotonin reuptake
   inhibitors
Self-mutilation
Semen analysis
Seniors' health
Sensory integration disorder
Sepsis
Septic shock
Septoplasty
Serum sickness
Severe acute respiratory syndrome
   (SARS)
Severe combined immunodeficiency
Sex hormones tests
Sex therapy
Sexual dysfunction
Sexual perversions
Sexually transmitted diseases
Sexually transmitted diseases cultures
Shaken baby syndrome
Shiatsu
Shigellosis
Shin splints

Traction
Traditional Chinese medicine
Trager psychophysical integration
Transcranial Doppler
    ultrasonography
Transesophageal echocardiography
Transfusion
Transhepatic biliary catheterization
Transient ischemic attack
Transposition of the great arteries
Transurethral bladder resection
Transvaginal ultrasound
Transverse myelitis
Traumatic amputations
Traveler's diarrhea
Tremors
Trench fever
Trichinosis
Trichomoniasis
Tricuspid valve insufficiency
Tricuspid valve stenosis
Trigeminal neuralgia
Trigger finger
Triglycerides test
Triple screen
Tropical spastic paraparesis
Troponins test
Tubal ligation
Tube compression of the esophagus
    and stomach
Tube feedings
Tuberculin skin test
Tuberculosis
Tularemia
Tumor markers
Tumor removal
Turner syndrome
2,3-diphosphoglycerate test
Typhoid fever
Typhus
Tzanck preparation

U

Ulcer surgery
Ulcerative colitis
Ulcers (digestive)
Ultraviolet light treatment
Umbilical cord blood banking
Undescended testes
Upper GI exam
Ureteral stenting

Urethritis
Uric acid tests
Urinalysis
Urinary anti-infectives
Urinary catheterization
Urinary diversion surgery
Urinary incontinence
Urine culture
Urine flow test
Uterine fibroid embolization
Uterine fibroids
Uveitis

V

Vaccination
Vaginal pain
Vagotomy
Valsalva maneuver
Valvular heart disease
Varicose veins
Vasculitis
Vasectomy
Vasodilators
Vegetarianism
Vegetative state
Velopharyngeal insufficiency
Vena cava filter
Venography
Venous access
Venous insufficiency
Ventricular aneurysm
Ventricular assist device
Ventricular ectopic beats
Ventricular fibrillation
Ventricular septal defect
Ventricular shunt
Ventricular tachycardia
Vesicoureteral reflux
Vibriosis
Vision training
Visual impairment
Vitamin A deficiency
Vitamin B_6 deficiency
Vitamin D deficiency
Vitamin E deficiency
Vitamin K deficiency
Vitamin tests
Vitamin toxicity
Vitamins
Vitiligo

Vitrectomy
Vocal cord nodules and polyps
Vocal cord paralysis
von Willebrand disease
Vulvar cancer
Vulvodynia
Vulvovaginitis

W

Waldenstrom's macroglobulinemia
Warts
Wechsler intelligence test
Wegener's granulomatosis
Weight loss drugs
West Nile Virus
Wheezing
Whiplash
White blood cell count and
    differential
Whooping cough
Wilderness medicine
Wilms' tumor
Wilson disease
Wiskott-Aldrich syndrome
Withdrawal syndromes
Wolff-Parkinson-White
    syndrome
Women's health
Wound culture
Wound flushing
Wounds

X

X-linked agammaglobulinemia
X rays of the orbit

Y

Yaws
Yellow fever
Yersinosis
Yoga

Z

Zoonosis

PLEASE READ—IMPORTANT INFORMATION

The *Gale Encyclopedia of Medicine* is a medical reference product designed to inform and educate readers about a wide variety of disorders, conditions, treatments, and diagnostic tests. Thomson Gale believes the product to be comprehensive, but not necessarily definitive. It is intended to supplement, not replace, consultation with a physician or other healthcare practitioner. While Thomson Gale has made substantial efforts to provide information that is accurate, comprehensive, and up-to-date, Thomson Gale makes no representations or warranties of any kind, including without limitation, warranties of merchantability or fitness for a particular purpose, nor does it guarantee the accuracy, comprehensiveness, or timeliness of the information contained in this product. Readers should be aware that the universe of medical knowledge is constantly growing and changing, and that differences of medical opinion exist among authorities. Readers are also advised to seek professional diagnosis and treatment for any medical condition, and to discuss information obtained from this book with their healthcare provider.

INTRODUCTION

The third edition of the *Gale Encyclopedia of Medicine (GEM3)* is a one-stop source for medical information on over 1,750 common medical disorders, conditions, tests, and treatments, including high-profile diseases such as AIDS, Alzheimer's disease, cancer, and heart attack. This encyclopedia avoids medical jargon and uses language that laypersons can understand, while still providing thorough coverage of each topic. The *Gale Encyclopedia of Medicine 3* fills a gap between basic consumer health resources, such as single-volume family medical guides, and highly technical professional materials.

SCOPE

More than 1,750 full-length articles are included in the *Gale Encyclopedia of Medicine 3*, including disorders/conditions, tests/procedures, and treatments/ therapies. Many common drugs are also covered, with generic drug names appearing first and brand names following in parentheses, eg. acetaminophen (Tylenol). Throughout the *Gale Encyclopedia of Medicine 3*, many prominent individuals are highlighted as sidebar biographies that accompany the main topical essays. Articles follow a standardized format that provides information at a glance. Rubrics include:

Disorders/Conditions	Tests/Treatments
Definition	Definition
Description	Purpose
Causes and symptoms	Precautions
Diagnosis	Description
Treatment	Preparation
Alternative treatment	Aftercare
Prognosis	Risks
Prevention	Normal/Abnormal results
Resources	Resources
Key terms	Key terms

In recent years there has been a resurgence of interest in holistic medicine that emphasizes the connection between mind and body. Aimed at achieving and maintaining good health rather than just eliminating disease, this approach has come to be known as alternative medicine. The *Gale Encyclopedia of Medicine 3* includes a number of essays on alternative therapies, ranging from traditional Chinese medicine to homeopathy and from meditation to aromatherapy. In addition to full essays on alternative therapies, the encyclopedia features specific **Alternative treatment** sections for diseases and conditions that may be helped by complementary therapies.

INCLUSION CRITERIA

A preliminary list of diseases, disorders, tests and treatments was compiled from a wide variety of sources, including professional medical guides and textbooks as well as consumer guides and encyclopedias. The general advisory board, made up of public librarians, medical librarians and consumer health experts, evaluated the topics and made suggestions for inclusion. The list was sorted by category and sent to *GEM3* medical advisers, for review. Final selection of topics to include was made by the medical advisors in conjunction with the Thomson Gale editor.

ABOUT THE CONTRIBUTORS

The essays were compiled by experienced medical writers, including physicians, pharmacists, nurses, and other health care professionals. *GEM3* medical advisors reviewed the completed essays to insure that they are appropriate, up-to-date, and medically accurate.

HOW TO USE THIS BOOK

The *Gale Encyclopedia of Medicine 3* has been designed with ready reference in mind.

- Straight **alphabetical arrangement** allows users to locate information quickly.

- Bold faced terms function as **print hyperlinks** that point the reader to related entries in the encyclopedia.

- **Cross-references** placed throughout the encyclopedia direct readers to where information on subjects without entries can be found. Synonyms are also cross-referenced.

- A list of **key terms** are provided where appropriate to define unfamiliar terms or concepts.

- Valuable **contact information** for organizations andsupport groups is included with each entry.

The appendix contains an extensive list of organizations arranged in alphabetical order.

- **Resources section** directs users to additional sources of medical information on a topic.

- A comprehensive **general index** allows users to easily target detailed aspects of any topic, including Latin names.

GRAPHICS

The *Gale Encyclopedia of Medicine 3* is enhanced with over 675 illustrations, including photos, charts, tables, and customized line drawings.

ADVISORS

A number of experts in the library and medical communities provided invaluable assistance in the formulation of this encyclopedia. Our advisory board performed a myriad of duties, from defining the scope of coverage to reviewing individual entries for accuracy and accessibility. The editor would like to express her appreciation to them.

MEDICAL ADVISORS

Rosalyn Carson-DeWitt, M.D.
Durham, NC

Larry I. Lutwick M.D., F.A.C.P.
Director, Infectious Diseases
VA Medical Center
Brooklyn, NY

Samuel Uretsky, Pharm.D.
Pharmacist
Wantagh, NY

CONTRIBUTORS

Margaret Alic, Ph.D.
Science Writer
Eastsound, WA

Janet Byron Anderson
Linguist/Language Consultant
Rocky River, OH

Lisa Andres, M.S., C.G.C.
Certified Genetic Counselor and Medical Writer
San Jose, CA

Greg Annussek
Medical Writer/Editor
New York, NY

Bill Asenjo, Ph.D.
Science Writer
Iowa City, IA

Sharon A. Aufox, M.S., C.G.C.
Genetic Counselor
Rockford Memorial Hospital
Rockford, IL

Sandra Bain Cushman
Massage Therapist, Alexander Technique Practitioner
Charlottesville, VA

Howard Baker
Medical Writer
North York, Ontario

Laurie Barclay, M.D.
Neurological Consulting Services
Tampa, FL

Jeanine Barone
Nutritionist, Exercise Physiologist
New York, NY

Julia R. Barrett
Science Writer
Madison, WI

Donald G. Barstow, R.N.
Clincal Nurse Specialist
Oklahoma City, OK

Carin Lea Beltz, M.S.
Genetic Counselor and Program Director
The Center for Genetic Counseling
Indianapolis, IN

Linda K. Bennington, C.N.S.
Science Writer
Virginia Beach, VA

Issac R. Berniker
Medical Writer
Vallejo, CA

Kathleen Berrisford, M.S.V.
Science Writer

Bethanne Black
Medical Writer
Atlanta, GA

Jennifer Bowjanowski, M.S., C.G.C.
Genetic Counselor
Children's Hospital Oakland
Oakland, CA

Michelle Q. Bosworth, M.S., C.G.C.
Genetic Counselor
Eugene, OR

Barbara Boughton
Health and Medical Writer
El Cerrito, CA

Cheryl Branche, M.D.
Retired General Practitioner
Jackson, MS

Michelle Lee Brandt
Medical Writer
San Francisco, CA

Maury M. Breecher, Ph.D.
Health Communicator/Journalist
Northport, AL

Ruthan Brodsky
Medical Writer
Bloomfield Hills, MI

Tom Brody, Ph.D.
Science Writer
Berkeley, CA

Leonard C. Bruno, Ph.D.
Medical Writer
Chevy Chase, MD

Diane Calbrese
Medical Sciences and Technology Writer
Silver Spring, Maryland

Richard H. Camer
Editor
International Medical News Group
Silver Spring, MD

Rosalyn Carson-DeWitt, M.D.
Medical Writer
Durham, NC

Lata Cherath, Ph.D.
Science Writing Intern
Cancer Research Institute
New York, NY

Linda Chrisman
Massage Therapist and Educator
Oakland, CA

Lisa Christenson, Ph.D.
Science Writer
Hamden, CT

Geoffrey N. Clark, D.V.M.
Editor
Canine Sports Medicine
   Update
Newmarket, NH

Rhonda Cloos, R.N.
Medical Writer
Austin, TX

Gloria Cooksey, C.N.E
Medical Writer
Sacramento, CA

Amy Cooper, M.A., M.S.I.
Medical Writer
Vermillion, SD

David A. Cramer, M.D.
Medical Writer
Chicago, IL

Esther Csapo Rastega, R.N.,
   B.S.N.
Medical Writer
Holbrook, MA

Arnold Cua, M.D.
Physician
Brooklyn, NY

Tish Davidson, A.M.
Medical Writer
Fremont, California

Dominic De Bellis, Ph.D.
Medical Writer/Editor
Mahopac, NY

Lori De Milto
Medical Writer
Sicklerville, NJ

Robert S. Dinsmoor
Medical Writer
South Hamilton, MA

Stephanie Dionne, B.S.
Medical Writer
Ann Arbor, MI

Martin W. Dodge, Ph.D.
Technical Writer/Editor
Centinela Hospital and Medical
   Center
Inglewood, CA

David Doermann
Medical Writer
Salt Lake City, UT

Stefanie B. N. Dugan, M.S.
Genetic Counselor
Milwaukee, WI

Doug Dupler, M.A.
Science Writer
Boulder, CO

Thomas Scott Eagan
Student Researcher
University of Arizona
Tucson, AZ

Altha Roberts Edgren
Medical Writer
Medical Ink
St. Paul, MN

Karen Ericson, R.N.
Medical Writer
Estes Park, CO

L. Fleming Fallon Jr., M.D.,
   Dr.PH
*Associate Professor of Public
   Health*
Bowling Green State University
Bowling Green, OH

Faye Fishman, D.O.
Physician
Randolph, NJ

Janis Flores
Medical Writer
Lexikon Communications
Sebastopol, CA

Risa Flynn
Medical Writer
Culver City, CA

Paula Ford-Martin
Medical Writer
Chaplin, MN

Janie F. Franz
Writer
Grand Forks, ND

Sallie Freeman, Ph.D., B.S.N.
Medical Writer
Atlanta, GA

Rebecca J. Frey, Ph.D.
*Research and Administrative
   Associate*
East Rock Institute
New Haven, CT

Cynthia L. Frozena, R.N.
Nurse, Medical Writer
Manitowoc, WI

Jason Fryer
Medical Writer
San Antonio, TX

Ron Gasbarro, Pharm.D.
Medical Writer
New Milford, PA

Julie A. Gelderloos
Biomedical Writer
Playa del Rey, CA

Gary Gilles, M.A.
Medical Writer
Wauconda, IL

Harry W. Golden
Medical Writer
Shoreline Medical Writers
Old Lyme, CT

Debra Gordon
Medical Writer
Nazareth, PA

Megan Gourley
Writer
Germantown, MD

Jill Granger, M.S.
Senior Research Associate
University of Michigan
Ann Arbor, MI

Alison Grant
Medical Writer
Averill Park, NY

Elliot Greene, M.A.
*former president, American
   Massage Therapy Association*
Massage Therapist
Silver Spring, MD

Peter Gregutt
Writer
Asheville, NC

Laith F. Gulli, M.D.
M.Sc., M.Sc.(MedSci), M.S.A.,
   Msc.Psych, MRSNZ
FRSH, FRIPHH, FAIC, FZS
DAPA, DABFC, DABCI
*Consultant Psychotherapist in
   Private Practice*
Lathrup Village, MI

Kapil Gupta, M.D.
Medical Writer
Winston-Salem, NC

Maureen Haggerty
Medical Writer
Ambler, PA

Clare Hanrahan
Medical Writer
Asheville, NC

Ann M. Haren
Science Writer
Madison, CT

Judy C. Hawkins, M.S.
Genetic Counselor
The University of Texas Medical
  Branch
Galveston, TX

Caroline Helwick
Medical Writer
New Orleans, LA

David Helwig
Medical Writer
London, Ontario

Lisette Hilton
Medical Writer
Boca Raton, FL

Katherine S. Hunt, M.S.
Genetic Counselor
University of New Mexico Health
  Sciences Center
Albuquerque, NM

Kevin Hwang, M.D.
Medical Writer
Morristown, NJ

Holly Ann Ishmael, M.S.,
  C.G.C.
Genetic Counselor
The Children's Mercy Hospital
Kansas City, MO

Dawn A. Jacob, M.S.
Genetic Counselor
Obstetrix Medical Group of
  Texas
Fort Worth, TX

Sally J. Jacobs, Ed.D.
Medical Writer
Los Angeles, CA

Michelle L. Johnson, M.S., J.D.
*Patent Attorney and Medical
  Writer*
Portland, OR

Paul A. Johnson, Ed.M.
Medical Writer
San Diego, CA

Cindy L. A. Jones, Ph.D.
Biomedical Writer
Sagescript Communications
Lakewood, CO

David Kaminstein, M.D.
Medical Writer
West Chester, PA

Beth A. Kapes
Medical Writer
Bay Village, OH

Janet M. Kearney
Freelance writer
Orlando, FL

Christine Kuehn Kelly
Medical Writer
Havertown, PA

Bob Kirsch
Medical Writer
Ossining, NY

Joseph Knight, P.A.
Medical Writer
Winton, CA

Melissa Knopper
Medical Writer
Chicago, IL

Karen Krajewski, M.S., C.G.C.
Genetic Counselor
Assistant Professor of Neurology
Wayne State University
Detroit, MI

Jeanne Krob, M.D., F.A.C.S.
Physician, writer
Pittsburgh, PA

Jennifer Lamb
Medical Writer
Spokane, WA

Richard H. Lampert
Senior Medical Editor
W.B. Saunders Co.
Philadelphia, PA

Jeffrey P. Larson, R.P.T.
Physical Therapist
Sabin, MN

Jill Lasker
Medical Writer
Midlothian, VA

Kristy Layman
Music Therapist
East Lansing, MI

Victor Leipzig, Ph.D.
Biological Consultant
Huntington Beach, CA

Lorraine Lica, Ph.D.
Medical Writer
San Diego, CA

John T. Lohr, Ph.D.
*Assistant Director, Biotechnology
  Center*
Utah State University
Logan, UT

Larry Lutwick, M.D., F.A.C.P.
Director, Infectious Diseases
VA Medical Center
Brooklyn, NY

Suzanne M. Lutwick
Medical Writer
Brooklyn, NY

Nicole Mallory, M.S.
Medical Student
Wayne State University
Detroit, MI

Warren Maltzman, Ph.D.
*Consultant, Molecular
  Pathology*
Demarest, NJ

Adrienne Massel, R.N.
Medical Writer
Beloit, WI

Ruth E. Mawyer, R.N.
Medical Writer
Charlottesville, VA

Richard A. McCartney M.D.
*Fellow, American College of
  Surgeons*
*Diplomat American Board of
  Surgery*
Richland, WA

Bonny McClain, Ph.D.
Medical Writer
Greensboro, NC

Sally C. McFarlane-Parrott
Medical Writer
Ann Arbor, MI

Mercedes McLaughlin
Medical Writer
Phoenixville, CA

Alison McTavish, M.Sc.
Medical Writer and Editor
Montreal, Quebec

Liz Meszaros
Medical Writer
Lakewood, OH

Betty Mishkin
Medical Writer
Skokie, IL

Barbara J. Mitchell
Medical Writer
Hallstead, PA

Mark A. Mitchell, M.D.
Medical Writer
Seattle, WA

Susan J. Montgomery
Medical Writer
Milwaukee, WI

Louann W. Murray, PhD
Medical Writer
Huntington Beach, CA

Bilal Nasser, M.Sc.
Senior Medical Student
Universidad Iberoamericana
Santo Domingo, Domincan
    Republic

Laura Ninger
Medical Writer
Weehawken, NJ

Nancy J. Nordenson
Medical Writer
Minneapolis, MN

Teresa Odle
Medical Writer
Albaquerque, NM

Lisa Papp, R.N.
Medical Writer
Cherry Hill, NJ

Lee Ann Paradise
Medical Writer
San Antonio, TX

Patience Paradox
Medical Writer
Bainbridge Island, WA

Barbara J. Pettersen
Genetic Counselor
Genetic Counseling of Central
    Oregon
Bend, OR

Genevieve Pham-Kanter, M.S.
Medical Writer
Chicago, IL

Collette Placek
Medical Writer
Wheaton, IL

J. Ricker Polsdorfer, M.D.
Medical Writer
Phoenix, AZ

Scott Polzin, M.S., C.G.C.
Medical Writer
Buffalo Grove, IL

Elizabeth J. Pulcini, M.S.
Medical Writer
Phoenix, Arizona

Nada Quercia, M.S., C.C.G.C.
Genetic Counselor
Division of Clinical and
    Metabolic Genetics
The Hospital for Sick Children
Toronto, ON, Canada

Ann Quigley
Medical Writer
New York, NY

Robert Ramirez, B.S.
Medical Student
University of Medicine &
    Dentistry of New Jersey
Stratford, NJ

Kulbir Rangi, D.O.
Medical Doctor and Writer
New York, NY

Esther Csapo Rastegari, Ed.M.,
    R.N./B.S.N.
Registered Nurse, Medical Writer
Holbrook, MA

Toni Rizzo
Medical Writer
Salt Lake City, UT

Martha Robbins
Medical Writer
Evanston, IL

Richard Robinson
Medical Writer
Tucson, AZ

Nancy Ross-Flanigan
Science Writer
Belleville, MI

Anna Rovid Spickler, D.V.M., Ph.D.
Medical Writer
Moorehead, KY

Belinda Rowland, Ph.D.
Medical Writer
Voorheesville, NY

Andrea Ruskin, M.D.
Whittingham Cancer Center
Norwalk, CT

Laura Ruth, Ph.D.
*Medical, Science, & Technology
    Writer*
Los Angeles, CA

Karen Sandrick
Medical Writer
Chicago, IL

Kausalya Santhanam, Ph.D.
Technical Writer
Branford, CT

Jason S. Schliesser, D.C.
Chiropractor
Holland Chiropractic, Inc.
Holland, OH

Joan Schonbeck
Medical Writer
Nursing
Massachusetts Department of
    Mental Health
Marlborough, MA

Laurie Heron Seaver, M.D.
Clinical Geneticist
Greenwood Genetic Center
Greenwood, SC

Catherine Seeley
Medical Writer

Kristen Mahoney Shannon, M.S., C.G.C.
Genetic Counselor
Center for Cancer Risk Analysis
Massachusetts General Hospital
Boston, MA

Kim A. Sharp, M.Ln.
Writer
Richmond, TX

Judith Sims, M.S.
Medical Writer
Logan, UT

Joyce S. Siok, R.N.
Medical Writer
South Windsor, CT

Jennifer Sisk
Medical Writer
Havertown, PA

Patricia Skinner
Medical Writer
Amman, Jordan

Genevieve Slomski, Ph.D.
Medical Writer
New Britain, CT

Stephanie Slon
Medical Writer
Portland, OR

Linda Wasmer Smith
Medical Writer
Albuquerque, NM

Java O. Solis, M.S.
Medical Writer
Decatur, GA

Elaine Souder, PhD
Medical Writer
Little Rock, AR

Jane E. Spehar
Medical Writer
Canton, OH

Lorraine Steefel, R.N.
Medical Writer
Morganville, NJ

Kurt Sternlof
Science Writer
New Rochelle, NY

Roger E. Stevenson, M.D.
Director
Greenwood Genetic Center
Greenwood, SC

Dorothy Stonely
Medical Writer
Los Gatos, CA

Liz Swain
Medical Writer
San Diego, CA

Deanna M. Swartout-Corbeil, R.N.
Medical Writer
Thompsons Station, TN

Keith Tatarelli, J.D.
Medical Writer

Mary Jane Tenerelli, M.S.
Medical Writer
East Northport, NY

Catherine L. Tesla, M.S., C.G.C.
Senior Associate, Faculty
Dept. of Pediatrics, Division of
    Medical Genetics
Emory University School of
    Medicine
Atlanta, GA

Bethany Thivierge
Biotechnical Writer/Editor
Technicality Resources
Rockland, ME

Mai Tran, Pharm.D.
Medical Writer
Troy, MI

Carol Turkington
Medical Writer
Lancaster, PA

Judith Turner, B.S.
Medical Writer
Sandy, UT

Amy B. Tuteur, M.D.
Medical Advisor
Sharon, MA

Samuel Uretsky, Pharm.D.
Medical Writer
Wantagh, NY

Amy Vance, M.S., C.G.C.
Genetic Counselor
GeneSage, Inc.
San Francisco, CA

Michael Sherwin Walston
Student Researcher
University of Arizona
Tucson, AZ

Ronald Watson, Ph.D.
Science Writer
Tucson, AZ

Ellen S. Weber, M.S.N.
Medical Writer
Fort Wayne, IN

Ken R. Wells
Freelance Writer
Laguna Hills, CA

Jennifer F. Wilson, M.S.
Science Writer
Haddonfield, NJ

Kathleen D. Wright, R.N.
Medical Writer
Delmar, DE

Jennifer Wurges
Medical Writer
Rochester Hills, MI

Mary Zoll, Ph.D.
Science Writer
Newton Center, MA

Jon Zonderman
Medical Writer
Orange, CA

Michael V. Zuck, Ph.D.
Medical Writer
Boulder, CO

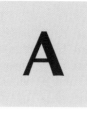

Abdominal aorta ultrasound *see* **Abdominal ultrasound**

Abdominal aortic aneurysm *see* **Aortic aneurysm**

Abdominal hernia *see* **Hernia**

Abdominal thrust *see* **Heimlich maneuver**

Abdominal ultrasound

Definition

Ultrasound technology allows doctors to "see" inside a patient without resorting to surgery. A transmitter sends high frequency sound waves into the body, where they bounce off the different tissues and organs to produce a distinctive pattern of echoes. A receiver "hears" the returning echo pattern and forwards it to a computer, which translates the data into an image on a television screen. Because ultrasound can distinguish subtle variations between soft, fluid-filled tissues, it is particularly useful in providing diagnostic images of the abdomen. Ultrasound can also be used in treatment.

Purpose

The potential medical applications of ultrasound were first recognized in the 1940s as an outgrowth of the sonar technology developed to detect submarines during World War II. The first useful medical images were produced in the early 1950s, and, by 1965, ultrasound quality had improved to the point that it came into general medical use. Improvements in the technology, application, and interpretation of ultrasound continue. Its low cost, versatility, safety and speed have brought it into the top drawer of medical imaging techniques.

While **pelvic ultrasound** is widely known and commonly used for fetal monitoring during **pregnancy**, ultrasound is also routinely used for general abdominal imaging. It has great advantage over x-ray imaging technologies in that it does not damage tissues with ionizing radiation. Ultrasound is also generally far better than plain x rays at distinguishing the subtle variations of soft tissue structures, and can be used in any of several modes, depending on the need at hand.

As an imaging tool, abdominal ultrasound generally is warranted for patients afflicted with: chronic or acute abdominal **pain**; abdominal trauma; an obvious or suspected abdominal mass; symptoms of **liver disease**, pancreatic disease, **gallstones**, spleen disease, **kidney disease** and urinary blockage; or symptoms of an abdominal **aortic aneurysm**. Specifically:

- Abdominal pain. Whether acute or chronic, pain can signal a serious problem–from organ malfunction or injury to the presence of malignant growths. Ultrasound scanning can help doctors quickly sort through potential causes when presented with general or ambiguous symptoms. All of the major abdominal organs can be studied for signs of disease that appear as changes in size, shape and internal structure.

- Abdominal trauma. After a serious accident, such as a car crash or a fall, internal bleeding from injured abdominal organs is often the most serious threat to survival. Neither the injuries nor the bleeding are immediately apparent. Ultrasound is very useful as an initial scan when abdominal trauma is suspected, and it can be used to pinpoint the location, cause, and severity of hemorrhaging. In the case of puncture **wounds**, from a bullet for example, ultrasound can locate the foreign object and provide a preliminary survey of the damage. The easy portability and versatility of ultrasound technology has brought it into common emergency room use, and even into limited ambulance service.

• Abdominal mass. Abnormal growths–tumors, cysts, abscesses, scar tissue and accessory organs–can be located and tentatively identified with ultrasound. In particular, potentially malignant solid tumors can be distinguished from benign fluid-filled cysts and abscesses. Masses and malformations in any organ or part of the abdomen can be found.

• Liver disease. The types and underlying causes of liver disease are numerous, though jaundice tends to be a general symptom. Ultrasound can differentiate between many of the types and causes of liver malfunction, and is particularly good at identifying obstruction of the bile ducts and **cirrhosis**, which is characterized by abnormal fibrous growths and reduced blood flow.

• Pancreatic disease. Inflammation and malformation of the pancreas are readily identified by ultrasound, as are pancreatic stones (calculi), which can disrupt proper functioning.

• Gallstones. Gallstones cause more hospital admissions than any other digestive malady. These calculi can cause painful inflammation of the gallbladder and also obstruct the bile ducts that carry digestive enzymes from the gallbladder and liver to the intestines. Gallstones are readily identifiable with ultrasound.

• Spleen disease. The spleen is particularly prone to injury during abdominal trauma. It may also become painfully inflamed when beset with infection or **cancer**. These conditions also lend themselves well to ultrasonic inspection and diagnosis.

• Kidney disease. The kidneys are also prone to traumatic injury and are the organs most likely to form calculi, which can block the flow of urine and cause blood **poisoning** (uremia). A variety of diseases causing distinct changes in kidney morphology can also lead to complete kidney failure. Ultrasound imaging has proven extremely useful in diagnosing kidney disorders.

• Abdominal aortic aneurysm. This is a bulging weak spot in the abdominal aorta, which supplies blood directly from the heart to the entire lower body. These aneurysms are relatively common and increase in prevalence with age. A burst aortic aneurysm is imminently life-threatening. However, they can be readily identified and monitored with ultrasound before acute complications result.

Ultrasound technology can also be used for treatment purposes, most frequently as a visual aid during surgical procedures–such as guiding needle placement to drain fluid from a cyst, or to extract tumor cells for biopsy. Increasingly, direct therapeutic applications for ultrasound are being developed.

The direct therapeutic value of ultrasonic waves lies in their mechanical nature. They are shock waves, just like audible sound, and vibrate the materials through which they pass. These vibrations are mild, virtually unnoticeable at the frequencies and intensities used for imaging. Properly focused however, high-intensity ultrasound can be used to heat and physically agitate targeted tissues.

High-intensity ultrasound is used routinely to treat soft tissue injuries, such as **strains**, tears and associated scarring. The heating and agitation are believed to promote rapid healing through increased circulation. Strongly focused, high-intensity, high-frequency ultrasound can also be used to physically destroy certain types of tumors, as well as gallstones and other types of calculi. Developing new treatment applications for ultrasound is an active area of medical research.

Precautions

Properly performed, ultrasound imaging is virtually without risk or side effects. Some patients report feeling a slight **tingling** and/or warmth while being scanned, but most feel nothing at all. Ultrasound waves of appropriate frequency and intensity are not known to cause or aggravate any medical condition, though any woman who thinks she might be pregnant should raise the issue with her doctor before undergoing an abdominal ultrasound.

The value of ultrasound imaging as a medical tool, however, depends greatly on the quality of the equipment used and the skill of the medical personnel operating it. Improperly performed and/or interpreted, ultrasound can be worse than useless if it indicates that a problem exists where there is none, or fails to detect a significant condition. Basic ultrasound equipment is relatively inexpensive to obtain, and any doctor with the equipment can perform the procedure whether qualified or not. Patients should not hesitate to verify the credentials of technicians and doctors performing ultrasounds, as well as the quality of the equipment used and the benefits of the proposed procedure.

In cases where ultrasound is used as a treatment tool, patients should educate themselves about the proposed procedure with the help of their doctors–as is appropriate before any surgical procedure. Also, any abdominal ultrasound procedure, diagnostic or therapeutic, may be hampered by a patient's body type or other factors, such as the presence of excessive bowel gas (which is opaque to ultrasound). In particular, very obese people are often not good candidates for abdominal ultrasound.

Accessory organ—A lump of tissue adjacent to an organ that is similar to it, but which serves no important purpose, if functional at all. While not necessarily harmful, such organs can cause problems if they grow too large or become cancerous. In any case, their presence points to an underlying abnormality in the parent organ.

Benign—In medical usage, benign is the opposite of malignant. It describes an abnormal growth that is stable, treatable and generally not life-threatening.

Biopsy— The surgical removal and analysis of a tissue sample for diagnostic purposes. Usually, the term refers to the collection and analysis of tissue from a suspected tumor to establish malignancy.

Calculus—Any type of hard concretion (stone) in the body, but usually found in the gallbladder, pancreas and kidneys. They are formed by the accumulation of excess mineral salts and other organic material such as blood or mucous. Calculi (pl.) can cause problems by lodging in and obstructing the proper flow of fluids, such as bile to the intestines or urine to the bladder.

Cirrhosis—A chronic liver disease characterized by the invasion of connective tissue and the degeneration of proper functioning—jaundice is often an accompanying symptom. Causes of cirrhosis include alcoholism, metabolic diseases, syphilis and congestive heart disease.

Common bile duct—The branching passage through which bile—a necessary digestive enzyme—travels from the liver and gallbladder into the small intestine. Digestive enzymes from the pancreas also enter the intestines through the common bile duct.

Computed tomography scan (CT scan)—A specialized type of x-ray imaging that uses highly focused and relatively low energy radiation to produce detailed two-dimensional images of soft tissue structures, particularly the brain. CT scans are the chief competitor to ultrasound and can yield higher quality images not disrupted by bone or gas. They are, however, more cumbersome, time consuming and expensive to perform, and they use ionizing electromagnetic radiation.

Doppler—The Doppler effect refers to the apparent change in frequency of sound wave echoes returning to a stationary source from a moving target. If the object is moving toward the source, the frequency increases; if the object is moving away, the frequency decreases. The size of this frequency shift can be used to compute the object's speed–be it a car on the road or blood in an artery. The Doppler effect holds true for all types of radiation, not just sound.

Frequency—Sound, whether traveling through air or the human body, produces vibrations–molecules bouncing into each other–as the shock wave travels along. The frequency of a sound is the number of vibrations per second. Within the audible range, frequency means pitch–the higher the frequency, the higher a sound's pitch.

Ionizing radiation—Radiation that can damage living tissue by disrupting and destroying individual cells at the molecular level. All types of nuclear radiation–x rays, gamma rays and beta rays–are potentially ionizing. Sound waves physically vibrate the material through which they pass, but do not ionize it.

Jaundice—A condition that results in a yellow tint to the skin, eyes and body fluids. Bile retention in the liver, gallbladder and pancreas is the immediate cause, but the underlying cause could be as simple as obstruction of the common bile duct by a gallstone or as serious as pancreatic cancer. Ultrasound can distinguish between these conditions.

Malignant—The term literally means growing worse and resisting treatment. It is used as a synonym for cancerous and connotes a harmful condition that generally is life-threatening.

Morphology—Literally, the study of form. In medicine, morphology refers to the size, shape and structure rather than the function of a given organ. As a diagnostic imaging technique, ultrasound facilitates the recognition of abnormal morphologies as symptoms of underlying conditions.

Description

Ultrasound includes all sound waves above the frequency of human hearing–about 20 thousand hertz, or cycles per second. Medical ultrasound generally uses frequencies between one and 10 million hertz (1-10 MHz). Higher frequency ultrasound waves produce more detailed images, but are also more readily absorbed and so cannot penetrate as deeply into the body. Abdominal ultrasound imaging is generally performed at frequencies between 2-5 MHz.

An ultrasound machine consists of two parts: the transducer and the analyzer. The transducer both produces the sound waves that penetrate the body and receives the reflected echoes. Transducers are built around piezoelectric ceramic chips. (Piezoelectric refers to electricity that is produced when you put pressure on certain crystals such as quartz). These ceramic chips react to electric pulses by producing sound waves (they are transmitting waves) and react to sound waves by producing electric pulses (receiving). Bursts of high frequency electric pulses supplied to the transducer causes it to produce the scanning sound waves. The transducer then receives the returning echoes, translates them back into electric pulses and sends them to the analyzer–a computer that organizes the data into an image on a television screen.

Because sound waves travel through all the body's tissues at nearly the same speed–about 3,400 miles per hour–the microseconds it takes for each echo to be received can be plotted on the screen as a distance into the body. The relative strength of each echo, a function of the specific tissue or organ boundary that produced it, can be plotted as a point of varying brightness. In this way, the echoes are translated into a picture. Tissues surrounded by bone or filled with gas (the stomach, intestines and bowel) cannot be imaged using ultrasound, because the waves are blocked or become randomly scattered.

Four different modes of ultrasound are used in medical imaging:

- A-mode. This is the simplest type of ultrasound in which a single transducer scans a line through the body with the echoes plotted on screen as a function of depth. This method is used to measure distances within the body and the size of internal organs. Therapeutic ultrasound aimed at a specific tumor or calculus is also A-mode, to allow for pinpoint accurate focus of the destructive wave energy.

- B-mode. In B-mode ultrasound, a linear array of transducers simultaneously scans a plane through the body that can be viewed as a two-dimensional image on screen. Ultrasound probes containing more than 100 transducers in sequence form the basis for these most commonly used scanners, which cost about $50,000.

- M-Mode. The M stands for motion. A rapid sequence of B-mode scans whose images follow each other in sequence on screen enables doctors to see and measure range of motion, as the organ boundaries that produce reflections move relative to the probe. M-mode ultrasound has been put to particular use in studying heart motion.

- Doppler mode. **Doppler ultrasonography** includes the capability of accurately measuring velocities of moving material, such as blood in arteries and veins. The principle is the same as that used in radar guns that measure the speed of a car on the highway. Doppler capability is most often combined with B-mode scanning to produce images of blood vessels from which blood flow can be directly measured. This technique is used extensively to investigate valve defects, arteriosclerosis and hypertension, particularly in the heart, but also in the abdominal aorta and the portal vein of the liver. These machines cost about $250,000.

The actual procedure for a patient undergoing an abdominal ultrasound is relatively simple, regardless of the type of scan or its purpose. **Fasting** for at least eight hours prior to the procedure ensures that the stomach is empty and as small as possible, and that the intestines and bowels are relatively inactive. Fasting also allows the gall bladder to be seen, as it contracts after eating and may not be seen if the stomach is full. In some cases, a full bladder helps to push intestinal folds out of the way so that the gas they contain does not disrupt the image. The patient's abdomen is then greased with a special gel that allows the ultrasound probe to glide easily across the skin while transmitting and receiving ultrasonic pulses.

This procedure is conducted by a doctor with the assistance of a technologist skilled in operating the equipment. The probe is moved around the abdomen to obtain different views of the target areas. The patient will likely be asked to change positions from side to side and to hold their breath as necessary to obtain the desired views. Discomfort during the procedure is minimal.

The many types and uses of ultrasound technology makes it difficult to generalize about the time and costs involved. Relatively simple imaging–scanning a suspicious abdominal mass or a suspected abdominal aortic aneurysm–will take about half an hour to perform and will cost a few hundred dollars or more, depending on the quality of the equipment, the operator and other factors. More involved techniques such as multiple M-mode and Doppler-enhanced scans, or cases where the targets not well defined in advance, generally take more time and are more expensive.

Regardless of the type of scan used and the potential difficulties encountered, ultrasound remains faster and less expensive than computed tomography scans (CT), its primary rival in abdominal imaging. Furthermore, as abdominal ultrasounds are generally undertaken as "medically necessary" procedures designed to detect the presence of suspected abnormalities, they are covered under most types of major medical insurance. As always, though, the patient would be wise to confirm that their coverage extends to the specific procedure proposed. For nonemergency situations, most underwriters stipulate prior approval as a condition of coverage.

Specific conditions for which ultrasound may be selected as a treatment option–certain types of tumors, lesions, **kidney stones** and other calculi, muscle and ligament injuries, etc.–are described in detail under the appropriate entries in this encyclopedia.

Preparation

A patient undergoing abdominal ultrasound will be advised by their physician about what to expect and how to prepare. As mentioned above, preparations generally include fasting and arriving for the procedure with a full bladder, if necessary. This preparation is particularly useful if the gallbladder, ovaries or veins are to be examined.

Aftercare

In general, no aftercare related to the abdominal ultrasound procedure itself is required.

Risks

Abdominal ultrasound carries with it no recognized risks or side effects, if properly performed using appropriate frequency and intensity ranges. Sensitive tissues, particularly those of the reproductive organs, could possibly sustain damage if violently vibrated by overly intense ultrasound waves. In general though, such damage would only result from improper use of the equipment.

Any woman who thinks she might be pregnant should raise this issue with her doctor before undergoing an abdominal ultrasound, as a fetus in the early stages of development could be injured by ultrasound meant to probe deeply recessed abdominal organs.

Normal results

As a diagnostic imaging technique, a normal abdominal ultrasound is one that indicates the absence of the suspected condition that prompted the scan. For example, symptoms such as a persistent **cough**, labored breathing, and upper abdominal pain suggest the possibility of, among other things, an abdominal aortic aneurysm. An ultrasound scan that indicates the absence of an aneurysm would rule out this life-threatening condition and point to other, less serious causes.

Abnormal results

Because abdominal ultrasound imaging is generally undertaken to confirm a suspected condition, the results of a scan often will prove abnormal–that is they will confirm the diagnosis, be it kidney stones, cirrhosis of the liver or an aortic aneurysm. At that point, appropriate medical treatment as prescribed by a patient's doctor is in order. See the relevant disease and disorder entries in this encyclopedia for more information.

Resources

PERIODICALS

Freundlich, Naomi. "Ultrasound: What's Wrong with this Picture?" *Business Week* September 15, 1997:84-5.

ORGANIZATIONS

American College of Gastroenterology. 4900 B South 31st St., Arlington, VA 22206-1656. (703) 820-7400. < http://www.acg.gi.org > .
American Institute of Ultrasound in Medicine. 14750 Sweitzer Lane, Suite 100, Laurel, MD 20707-5906. (800) 638-5352. < http://www.aium.org > .
American Society of Radiologic Technologists. 15000 Central Ave., SE, Albuquerque, NM 87123-3917. (505) 298-4500. < http://www.asrt.org > .

Kurt Richard Sternlof

Abdominal wall defects

Definition

Abdominal wall defects are birth (congenital) defects that allow the stomach or intestines to protrude.

Description

Many unexpected and fascinating events occur during the development of a fetus inside the womb. The stomach and intestines begin development outside the baby's abdomen and only later does the abdominal wall enclose them. Occasionally, either the umbilical opening is too large, or it develops improperly, allowing the bowels or stomach to remain outside or squeeze through the abdominal wall.

Causes and symptoms

There are many causes for **birth defects** that still remain unclear. Presently, the cause(s) of abdominal wall defects is unknown, and any symptoms the mother may have to indicate that the defects are present in the fetus are nondescript.

Diagnosis

At birth, the problem is obvious, because the base of the umbilical cord at the navel will bulge or, in worse cases, contain viscera (internal organs). Before birth, an ultrasound examination may detect the problem. It is always necessary in children with one birth defect to look for others, because birth defects are usually multiple.

Treatment

Abdominal wall defects are effectively treated with surgical repair. Unless there are accompanying anomalies, the surgical procedure is not overly complicated. The organs are normal, just misplaced. However, if the defect is large, it may be difficult to fit all the viscera into the small abdominal cavity.

Prognosis

If there are no other defects, the prognosis after surgical repair of this condition is relatively good. However, 10% of those with more severe or additional abnormalities die from it. The organs themselves are fully functional; the difficulty lies in fitting them inside the abdomen. The condition is, in fact, a **hernia** requiring only replacement and strengthening of the passageway through which it occurred. After surgery, increased pressure in the stretched abdomen can compromise the function of the organs inside.

Prevention

Some, but by no means all, birth defects are preventable by early and attentive prenatal care, good **nutrition**, supplemental **vitamins**, diligent avoidance of all unnecessary drugs and chemicals–especially tobacco–and other elements of a healthy lifestyle.

Resources

PERIODICALS

Dunn, J. C., and E. W. Fonkalsrud. "Improved Survival of Infantswith Omphalocele." *American Journal of Surgery* 173 (April 1997): 284-7.

J. Ricker Polsdorfer, MD

KEY TERMS

Hernia—Movement of a structure into a place it does not belong.

Umbilical—Referring to the opening in the abdominal wall where the blood vessels from the placenta enter.

Viscera—Any of the body's organs located in the chest or abdomen.

Abnormal heart rhythms *see* **Arrhythmias**

ABO blood typing *see* **Blood typing and crossmatching**

ABO incompatibility *see* **Erythroblastosis fetalis**

Abortion, habitual *see* **Recurrent miscarriage**

Abortion, partial birth

Definition

Partial birth abortion is a method of late-term (after 20 weeks) abortion that terminates a **pregnancy** and results in the **death** and intact removal of a fetus. This procedure is most commonly referred to as intact dilatation and extraction (D & X). It occurs in a rare percentage of pregnancies.

Purpose

Partial birth abortion, or D&X, is performed to end a pregnancy and results in the death of a fetus, typically in the late second or third trimester. Although D&X is highly controversial, some physicians argue that it has advantages that make it a preferable procedure in some circumstances. One perceived advantage is that the fetus is removed largely intact, allowing for better evaluation and **autopsy** of the fetus in cases of known fetal abnormalities. Intact removal of the fetus also may carry a lower risk of puncturing the uterus or damaging the cervix. Another perceived advantage is that D&X ends the pregnancy without requiring the woman to go through labor, which may be less emotionally traumatic than other methods of late-term abortion. In

---

addition, D&X may offer a lower cost and shorter procedure time.

Precautions

Women considering D&X should be aware of the highly controversial nature of this procedure. A controversy common to all late-term abortions is whether the fetus is viable, or able to survive outside of the woman's body. A specific area of controversy with D&X is that fetal death does not occur until after most of the fetal body has exited the uterus. Several states have taken legal action to limit or ban D&X and many physicians who perform abortions do not perform D&X. This may restrict the availability of this procedure to women seeking late-term abortions.

In March 2003, the United States Senate passed a bill banning partial birth abortions and implementing fines or maximum two-year jail terms for physicians who perform them. In June 2003, the House approved a ban as well. President George W. Bush signed the legislation into law, but a federal judge declared the law unconstitutional, so that the government had not been able to enforce it. One of the opponents' claims was the legislation did not provide for exceptions for cases in which the procedure was needed to protect the mother's health.

Description

Intact D&X, or partial birth abortion first involves administration of medications to cause the cervix to dilate, usually over the course of several days. Next, the physician rotates the fetus to a footling breech position. The body of the fetus is then drawn out of the uterus feet first, until only the head remains inside the uterus. Then, the physician uses an instrument to puncture the base of the skull, which collapses the fetal head. Typically, the contents of the fetal head are then partially suctioned out, which results in the death of the fetus and reduces the size of the fetal head enough to allow it to pass through the cervix. The dead and otherwise intact fetus is then removed from the woman's body.

Preparation

Medical preparation for D&X involves an outpatient visit to administer medications, such as *laminaria*, to cause the cervix to begin dilating.

In addition, preparation may involve fulfilling local legal requirements, such as a mandatory waiting period, counseling, or an informed consent procedure

---

KEY TERMS

Cervix—The narrow outer end of the uterus that separates the uterus from the vaginal canal.

Footling breech—A position of the fetus while in the uterus where the feet of the fetus are nearest the cervix and will be the first part of the fetus to exit the uterus, with the head of the fetus being the last part to exit the uterus.

Laminaria—A medical product made from a certain type of seaweed that is physically placed near the cervix to cause it to dilate.

---

reviewing stages of fetal development, **childbirth**, alternative abortion methods, and adoption.

Aftercare

D&X typically does not require an overnight hospital stay, so a follow up appointment may be scheduled to monitor the woman for any complications.

Risks

With all abortion, the later in pregnancy an abortion is performed, the more complicated the procedure and the greater the risk of injury to the woman. In addition to associated emotional reactions, D&X carries the risk of injury to the woman, including heavy bleeding, **blood clots**, damage to the cervix or uterus, pelvic infection, and anesthesia-related complications. There also is a risk of incomplete abortion, meaning that the fetus is not dead when removed from the woman's body. Possible long-term risks include difficulty becoming pregnant or carrying a future pregnancy to term.

Normal results

The expected outcome of D&X is the termination of a pregnancy with removal of a dead fetus from the woman's body.

Resources

PERIODICALS

"Court Rules Abortion Ban Unconstitutional." *Medicine & Health* (June 7, 2004): 4–6.

"House Approves Partial Birth Abortion Ban." *Medicine and Health* (June 16, 2003): 5.

"Partial-birth Abortion Ban Approved by Senate." *Medical Ethics Advisor* (April 2003): 47.

ORGANIZATIONS

Planned Parenthood Federation of America, Inc.. 810 Seventh Ave., New York, NY 10019. (800) 669-0156. < http://www.plannedparenthood.org > .

OTHER

Status of partial-birth abortion laws in the states. Othmer Institute at Planned Parenthood of NYC. 2000.

Stefanie B. N. Dugan, M.S.
Teresa G. Odle

Abortion, selective

Definition

Selective abortion, also known as selective reduction, refers to choosing to abort a fetus, typically in a multi-fetal **pregnancy**, to decrease the health risks to the mother in carrying and giving birth to more than one or two babies, and also to decrease the risk of complications to the remaining fetus(es). The term selective abortion also refers to choosing to abort a fetus for reasons such as the woman is carrying a fetus which likely will be born with some birth defect or impairment, or because the sex of the fetus is not preferred by the individual.

Purpose

A woman may decide to abort for health reasons, for example, she is at higher risk for complications during pregnancy because of a disorder or disease such as diabetes. A 2004 case reported on an embryo embedded in a **cesarean section** scar. Although rare, it can be life threatening to the mother. In this care, selective abortion was successful at saving the mother and the remaining embryos.

However, selective reduction is recommended often in cases of multi-fetal pregnancy, or the presence of more than one fetus, typically, at least three or more fetuses. In the general population, multi-fetal pregnancy happens in only about 1-2% of pregnant women. But multi-fetal pregnancies occur far more often in women using fertility drugs.

Precautions

Because women or couples who use fertility drugs have made an extra effort to become pregnant, it is possible that the individuals may be unwilling or uncomfortable with the decision to abort a fetus in cases of multi-fetal pregnancy. Individuals engaging in fertility treatment should be made aware of the risk of multi-fetal pregnancy and consider the prospect of recommended reduction before undergoing fertility treatment.

Description

Selective reduction is usually performed between nine and 12 weeks of pregnancy and is most successful when performed in early pregnancy. It is a simple procedure and can be performed on an outpatient basis. A needle is inserted into the woman's stomach or vagina and potassium chloride is injected into the fetus.

Preparation

Individuals who have chosen selective reduction to safeguard the remaining fetuses should be counseled prior to the procedure. Individuals should receive information regarding the risks of a multi-fetal pregnancy to both the fetuses and the mother compared with the risks after the reduction.

Individuals seeking an abortion for any reason should consider the ethical implications whether it be because the fetus is not the preferred sex or because the fetus would be born with a severe birth defect.

Aftercare

Counseling should continue after the abortion because it is a traumatic event. Individuals may feel guilty about choosing one fetus over another. Mental health professionals should be consulted throughout the process.

Risks

About 75% of women who undergo selective reduction will go into **premature labor**. About 4-5% of women undergoing selective reduction also miscarry one or more of the remaining fetuses. The risks associated with multi-fetal pregnancy are considered higher.

Normal results

In cases where a multi-fetal pregnancy of three or more fetuses is reduced to two fetuses, the remaining twin fetuses typically develop as they would if they had been conceived as twins.

Resources

PERIODICALS

"Multiple Pregnancy Associated With Infertility Therapy." *American Society for Reproductive Medicine, A Practice Committee Report* (November 2000): 1-8.

"Selective Reduction Eleiminates an Emryo Embedded in a Cesarean Scar." *WomenÆs Health Weekly* (April 8, 2004): 117.

ORGANIZATIONS

The Alan Guttmacher Institute. 120 Wall Street, New York, NY 10005. (212) 248-1111. <http://www.agi-usa.org>.

The American Society for Reproductive Medicine. 1209 Montgomery Highway, Birmingham, AL 35216-2809. (205) 978-5000. <http://www.asrm.org>.

Meghan M. Gourley
Teresa G. Odle

Abortion, spontaneous *see* **Miscarriage**

▌ Abortion, therapeutic

Definition

Therapeutic abortion is the intentional termination of a **pregnancy** before the fetus can live independently. Abortion has been a legal procedure in the United States since 1973.

Purpose

An abortion may be performed whenever there is some compelling reason to end a pregnancy. Women have abortions because continuing the pregnancy would cause them hardship, endanger their life or health, or because prenatal testing has shown that the fetus will be born with severe abnormalities.

Abortions are safest when performed within the first six to 10 weeks after the last menstrual period. The calculation of this date is referred to as the

gestational age and is used in determining the stage of pregnancy. For example, a woman who is two weeks late having her period is said to be six weeks pregnant, because it is six weeks since she last menstruated.

About 90% of women who have abortions do so before 13 weeks and experience few complications. Abortions performed between 13-24 weeks have a higher rate of complications. Abortions after 24 weeks are extremely rare and are usually limited to situations where the life of the mother is in danger.

Precautions

Most women are able to have abortions at clinics or outpatient facilities if the procedure is performed early in pregnancy. Women who have stable diabetes, controlled epilepsy, mild to moderate high blood pressure, or who are HIV positive can often have abortions as outpatients if precautions are taken. Women with heart disease, previous **endocarditis**, **asthma**, lupus erythematosus, uterine fibroid tumors, blood clotting disorders, poorly controlled epilepsy, or some psychological disorders usually need to be hospitalized in order to receive special monitoring and medications during the procedure.

Description

Very early abortions

Between five and seven weeks, a pregnancy can be ended by a procedure called menstrual extraction. This procedure is also sometimes called menstrual regulation, mini-suction, or preemptive abortion. The contents of the uterus are suctioned out through a thin (3-4 mm) plastic tube that is inserted through the undilated cervix. Suction is applied either by a bulb syringe or a small pump.

Another method is called the "morning after" pill, or **emergency contraception**. Basically, it involves taking high doses of birth control pills within 24 to 48 hours of having unprotected sex. The high doses of hormones causes the uterine lining to change so that it will not support a pregnancy. Thus, if the egg has been fertilized, it is simply expelled from the body.

There are two types of emergency **contraception**. One type is identical to ordinary birth control pills, and uses the hormones estrogen and progestin). This type is available with a prescription under the brand name Preven. But women can even use their regular birth control pills for emergency contraception, after they check with their doctor about the proper dose. About half of women who use birth control pills for

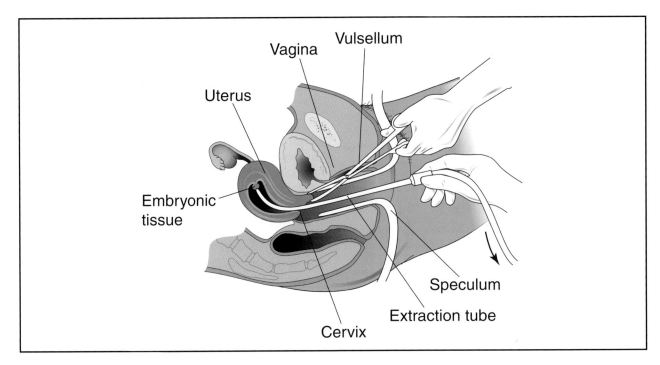

Uterus
Vagina
Vulsellum

Embryonic
tissue

Speculum
Extraction tube
Cervix

Between 5 and 7 weeks, a pregnancy can be ended by a procedure called menstrual extraction. The contents of the uterus are suctioned out through a thin extraction tube that is inserted through the undilated cervix. *(Illustration by Electronic Illustrators Group.)*

KEY TERMS

Endocarditis—An infection of the inner membrane lining of the heart.

Fibroid tumors—Fibroid tumors are non-cancerous (benign) growths in the uterus. They occur in 30-40% of women over age 40, and do not need to be removed unless they are causing symptoms that interfere with a woman's normal activities.

Lupus erythematosus—A chronic inflammatory disease in which inappropriate immune system reactions cause abnormalities in the blood vessels and connective tissue.

Prostaglandin—Oxygenated unsaturated cyclic fatty acids responsible for various hormonal reactions such as muscle contraction.

Rh negative—Lacking the Rh factor, genetically determined antigens in red blood cells that produce immune responses. If an Rh negative woman is pregnant with an Rh positive fetus, her body will produce antibodies against the fetus's blood, causing a disease known as Rh disease. Sensitization to the disease occurs when the women's blood is exposed to the fetus's blood. Rh immune globulin (RhoGAM) is a vaccine that must be given to a woman after an abortion, miscarriage, or prenatal tests in order to prevent sensitization to Rh disease.

emergency contraception get nauseated and 20 percent vomit. This method cuts the risk of pregnancy 75 percent.

The other type of morning-after pill contains only one hormone: progestin, and is available under the brand name Plan B. It is more effective than the first type with a lower risk of **nausea** and vomiting. It reduces the risk of pregnancy 89 percent.

Women should check with their physicians regarding the proper dose of pills to take, as it depends on the brand of birth control pill. Not all birth control pills will work for emergency contraception.

Menstrual extractions are safe, but because the amount of fetal material is so small at this stage of development, it is easy to miss. This results in an incomplete abortion that means the pregnancy continues.

First trimester abortions

The first trimester of pregnancy includes the first 13 weeks after the last menstrual period. In the United States, about 90% of abortions are performed during this period. It is the safest time in which to have an abortion, and the time in which women have the most choice of how the procedure is performed.

MEDICAL ABORTIONS. Medical abortions are brought about by taking medications that end the pregnancy. The advantages of a first trimester medical abortion are:

- The procedure is non-invasive; no surgical instruments are used.

- Anesthesia is not required.

- Drugs are administered either orally or by injection.

- The procedure resembles a natural **miscarriage**.

Disadvantages of a medical abortion are:

- The effectiveness decreases after the seventh week.

- The procedure may require multiple visits to the doctor.

- Bleeding after the abortion lasts longer than after a surgical abortion.

- The woman may see the contents of her womb as it is expelled.

Two different medications can be used to bring about an abortion. Methotrexate (Rheumatrex) works by stopping fetal cells from dividing which causes the fetus to die.

On the first visit to the doctor, the woman receives an injection of methotrexate. On the second visit, about a week later, she is given misoprostol (Cytotec), an oxygenated unsaturated cyclic fatty acid responsible for various hormonal reactions such as muscle contraction (prostaglandin), that stimulates contractions of the uterus. Within two weeks, the woman will expel the contents of her uterus, ending the pregnancy. A follow-up visit to the doctor is necessary to assure that the abortion is complete.

With this procedure, a woman will feel cramping and may feel nauseated from the misoprostol. This combination of drugs is 90-96% effective in ending pregnancy.

Mifepristone (RU-486), which goes by the brand name Mifeprex, works by blocking the action of progesterone, a hormone needed for pregnancy to continue, then stimulates ulerine contractions thus ending the pregnancy. It can be taken as much as 49 days after the first day of a woman's last period. On the first visit to the doctor, a woman takes a mifepristone pill. Two days later she returns and, if the miscarriage has not occurred, takes two misoprostol pills, which causes the uterus to contract. Five percent of women won't need to take misoprostol. After an observation period, she returns home.

Within four days, 90% of women have expelled the contents of their uterus and completed the abortion. Within 14 days, 95-97% of women have completed the abortion. A third follow-up visit to the doctor is necessary to confirm through observation or ultrasound that the procedure is complete. In the event that it is not, a surgical abortion is performed.

Studies show that 4.5 to 8 percent of women need surgery or a blood **transfusion** after taking mifepristone, and the pregnancy persists in about 1 percent of women. In this case, surgical abortion is recommended because the fetus may be damaged. Side effects include nausea, vaginal bleeding and heavy cramping. The bleeding is typically heavier than a normal period and may last up to 16 days.

Mifepristone is not recommended for women with ectopic pregnancy, an **IUD**, who have been taking long-term steroidal therapy, have bleeding abnormalities or on blood-thinners such as Coumadin.

Surgical abortions

First trimester surgical abortions are performed using vacuum aspiration. The procedure is also called dilation and evacuation (D & E), suction dilation, vacuum curettage, or suction curettage.

Advantages of a vacuum aspiration abortion are:

- It is usually done as a one-day outpatient procedure.

- The procedure takes only 10-15 minutes.

- Bleeding after the abortion lasts five days or less.

- The woman does not see the products of her womb being removed.

Disadvantages include:

- The procedure is invasive; surgical instruments are used.

- Infection may occur.

During a vacuum aspiration, the woman's cervix is gradually dilated by expanding rods inserted into the cervical opening. Once dilated, a tube attached to a suction pump is inserted through the cervix and the contents of the uterus are suctioned out. The procedure is 97-99% effective. The amount of discomfort a woman feels varies considerably. **Local anesthesia** is often given to numb the cervix, but it does not mask uterine cramping. After a few hours of rest, the woman may return home.

Second trimester abortions

Although it is better to have an abortion during the first trimester, some second trimester abortions may be inevitable. The results of **genetic testing** are often not available until 16 weeks. In addition, women, especially teens, may not have recognized the pregnancy or come to terms with it emotionally soon enough to have a first trimester abortion. Teens make up the largest group having second trimester abortions.

Some second trimester abortions are performed as a D & E. The procedures are similar to those used in the first trimester, but a larger suction tube must be used because more material must be removed. This increases the amount of cervical dilation necessary and increases the risk of the procedure. Many physicians are reluctant to perform a D & E this late in pregnancy, and for some women is it not a medically safe option.

The alternative to a D & E in the second trimester is an abortion by induced labor. Induced labor may require an overnight stay in a hospital. The day before the procedure, the woman visits the doctor for tests, and to either have rods inserted in her cervix to help dilate it or to receive medication that will soften the cervix and speed up labor.

On the day of the abortion, drugs, usually prostaglandins to induce contractions, and a salt water solution, are injected into the uterus. Contractions begin, and within eight to 72 hours the woman delivers the fetus.

Side effects of this procedure include nausea, **vomiting**, and **diarrhea** from the prostaglandins, and **pain** from uterine cramps. Anesthesia of the sort used in **childbirth** can be given to mask the pain. Many women are able to go home a few hours after the procedure.

Very early abortions cost between $200-$400. Later abortions cost more. The cost increases about $100 per week between the thirteenth and sixteenth week. Second trimester abortions are much more costly because they often involve more risk, more services, anesthesia, and sometimes a hospital stay. Insurance carriers and HMOs may or may not cover the procedure. Federal law prohibits federal funds including Medicaid funds, from being used to pay for an elective abortion.

Preparation

The doctor must know accurately the stage of a woman's pregnancy before an abortion is performed. The doctor will ask the woman questions about her menstrual cycle and also do a physical examination to confirm the stage of pregnancy. This may be done at an office visit before the abortion or on the day of the abortion. Some states require a waiting period before an abortion can be performed. Others require parental or court consent for a child under age 18 to receive an abortion.

Despite the fact that almost half of all women in the United States have had at least one abortion by the time they reach age 45, abortion is surrounded by controversy. Women often find themselves in emotional turmoil when deciding if an abortion is a procedure they wish to undergo. Pre-abortion counseling is important in helping a woman resolve any questions she may have about having the procedure.

Aftercare

Regardless of the method used to perform the abortion, a woman will be observed for a period of time to make sure her blood pressure is stable and that bleeding is controlled. The doctor may prescribe **antibiotics** to reduce the chance of infection. Women who are Rh negative (lacking genetically determined antigens in their red blood cells that produce immune responses) should be given a human Rh immune globulin (RhoGAM) after the procedure unless the father of the fetus is also Rh negative. This prevents blood incompatibility complications in future pregnancies.

Bleeding will continue for about five days in a surgical abortion and longer in a medical abortion. To decrease the risk of infection, a woman should avoid intercourse and not use tampons and douches for two weeks after the abortion.

A follow-up visit is a necessary part of the woman's aftercare. Contraception will be offered to women who wish to avoid future pregnancies, because menstrual periods normally resume within a few weeks.

Risks

Serious complications resulting from abortions performed before 13 weeks are rare. Of the 90% of women who have abortions in this time period, 2.5% have minor complications that can be handled without hospitalization. Less than 0.5% have complications that require a hospital stay. The rate of complications increases as the pregnancy progresses.

Complications from abortions can include:

- uncontrolled bleeding
- infection
- blood clots accumulating in the uterus
- a tear in the cervix or uterus
- missed abortion where the pregnancy continues
- incomplete abortion where some material from the pregnancy remains in the uterus

Women who experience any of the following symptoms of post-abortion complications should call the clinic or doctor who performed the abortion immediately.

- severe pain

- fever over 100.4 °F (38.2 °C)

- heavy bleeding that soaks through more than one sanitary pad per hour

- foul-smelling discharge from the vagina

- continuing symptoms of pregnancy

Normal results

Usually the pregnancy is ended without complication and without altering future fertility.

Resources

BOOKS

Carlson, Karen J., Stephanie A. Eisenstat, and Terra Ziporyn. "Abortion." In *The Harvard Guide to Women's Health.* Cambridge, MA: Harvard University Press, 1996.

Debra Gordon

Abrasions *see* **Wounds**

Abruptio placentae *see* **Placental abruption**

Abscess

Definition

An abscess is an enclosed collection of liquefied tissue, known as pus, somewhere in the body. It is the result of the body's defensive reaction to foreign material.

Description

There are two types of abscesses, septic and sterile. Most abscesses are septic, which means that they are the result of an infection. Septic abscesses can occur anywhere in the body. Only a germ and the body's immune response are required. In response to the invading germ, white blood cells gather at the infected site and begin producing chemicals called enzymes that attack the germ by digesting it. These enzymes act like acid, killing the germs and breaking them down into small pieces that can be picked up by the circulation and eliminated from the body. Unfortunately, these chemicals also digest body tissues. In most cases, the germ produces similar chemicals. The result is a thick, yellow liquid–pus–

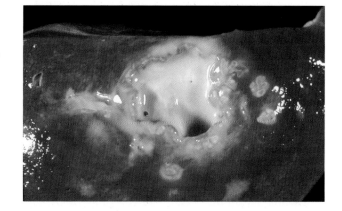

An amoebic abscess caused by *Entameoba histolytica.* *(Phototake NYC. Reproduced by permission.)*

containing digested germs, digested tissue, white blood cells, and enzymes.

An abscess is the last stage of a tissue infection that begins with a process called inflammation. Initially, as the invading germ activates the body's immune system, several events occur:

- Blood flow to the area increases.

- The temperature of the area increases due to the increased blood supply.

- The area swells due to the accumulation of water, blood, and other liquids.

- It turns red.

- It hurts, because of the irritation from the swelling and the chemical activity.

These four signs–heat, swelling, redness, and pain–characterize inflammation.

As the process progresses, the tissue begins to turn to liquid, and an abscess forms. It is the nature of an abscess to spread as the chemical digestion liquefies more and more tissue. Furthermore, the spreading follows the path of least resistance–the tissues most easily digested. A good example is an abscess just beneath the skin. It most easily continues along beneath the skin rather than working its way through the skin where it could drain its toxic contents. The contents of the abscess also leak into the general circulation and produce symptoms just like any other infection. These include chills, **fever**, aching, and general discomfort.

Sterile abscesses are sometimes a milder form of the same process caused not by germs but by non-living irritants such as drugs. If an injected drug like penicillin is not absorbed, it stays where it was injected and may cause enough irritation to generate a sterile abscess–sterile because there is no infection involved. Sterile abscesses are quite likely to turn into hard, solid lumps as they scar, rather than remaining pockets of pus.

Causes and symptoms

Many different agents cause abscesses. The most common are the pus-forming (pyogenic) bacteria like *Staphylococcus aureus*, which is nearly always the cause of abscesses under the skin. Abscesses near the large bowel, particularly around the anus, may be caused by any of the numerous bacteria found within the large bowel. Brain abscesses and liver abscesses can be caused by any organism that can travel there through the circulation. Bacteria, amoeba, and certain fungi can travel in this fashion. Abscesses in other parts of the body are caused by organisms that normally inhabit nearby structures or that infect them. Some common causes of specific abscesses are:

- skin abscesses by normal skin flora

- dental and throat abscesses by mouth flora

- lung abscesses by normal airway flora, **pneumonia** germs, or tuberculosis

- abdominal and anal abscesses by normal bowel flora

Specific types of abscesses

Listed below are some of the more common and important abscesses.

- Carbuncles and other **boils**. Skin oil glands (sebaceous glands) on the back or the back of the neck are the ones usually infected. The most common germ involved is *Staphylococcus aureus*. **Acne** is a similar condition of sebaceous glands on the face and back.

- Pilonidal abscess. Many people have as a birth defect a tiny opening in the skin just above the anus. Fecal bacteria can enter this opening, causing an infection and subsequent abscess.

- Retropharyngeal, parapharyngeal, peritonsillar abscess. As a result of throat infections like strep throat and **tonsillitis**, bacteria can invade the deeper tissues of the throat and cause an abscess. These abscesses can compromise swallowing and even breathing.

- Lung abscess. During or after pneumonia, whether it's due to bacteria [common pneumonia], tuberculosis, fungi, parasites, or other germs, abscesses can develop as a complication.

- Liver abscess. Bacteria or amoeba from the intestines can spread through the blood to the liver and cause abscesses.

- Psoas abscess. Deep in the back of the abdomen on either side of the lumbar spine lie the psoas muscles. They flex the hips. An abscess can develop in one of these muscles, usually when it spreads from the appendix, the large bowel, or the fallopian tubes.

Diagnosis

The common findings of inflammation–heat, redness, swelling, and pain–easily identify superficial abscesses. Abscesses in other places may produce only generalized symptoms such as fever and discomfort. If the patient's symptoms and physical examination do not help, a physician may have to resort to a battery of tests to locate the site of an abscess, but usually something in the initial evaluation directs the search. Recent or chronic disease in an organ suggests it may be the site of an abscess. Dysfunction of an organ or system–for instance, seizures or altered bowel function–may provide the clue. **Pain** and tenderness on **physical examination** are common findings. Sometimes a deep abscess will eat a small channel (sinus) to the surface and begin leaking pus. A sterile abscess may cause only a painful lump deep in the buttock where a shot was given.

Treatment

Since skin is very resistant to the spread of infection, it acts as a barrier, often keeping the toxic chemicals of an abscess from escaping the body on their own. Thus, the pus must be drained from the abscess by a physician. The surgeon determines when the abscess is ready for drainage and opens a path to the outside, allowing the pus to escape. Ordinarily, the body handles the remaining infection, sometimes with the help of **antibiotics** or other drugs. The surgeon may leave a drain (a piece of cloth or rubber) in the abscess cavity to prevent it from closing before all the pus has drained out.

Alternative treatment

If an abscess is directly beneath the skin, it will be slowly working its way through the skin as it is more rapidly working its way elsewhere. Since chemicals work faster at higher temperatures, applications of hot compresses to the skin over the abscess will hasten the digestion of the skin and eventually result in its breaking down, releasing the pus spontaneously. This treatment is best reserved for smaller abscesses in relatively less dangerous areas of the body–limbs, trunk, back of the neck. It is also useful for all superficial abscesses in their very early stages. It will "ripen" them.

Contrast **hydrotherapy**, alternating hot and cold compresses, can also help assist the body in resorption of the abscess. There are two homeopathic remedies that work to rebalance the body in relation to abscess formation, *Silica* and *Hepar sulphuris*. In cases of septic abscesses, bentonite clay packs (bentonite clay and a small amount of *Hydrastis* powder) can be used to draw the infection from the area.

Prognosis

Once the abscess is properly drained, the prognosis is excellent for the condition itself. The reason for the abscess (other diseases the patient has) will determine the overall outcome. If, on the other hand, the abscess ruptures into neighboring areas or permits the infectious agent to spill into the bloodstream, serious or fatal consequences are likely. Abscesses in and around the nasal sinuses, face, ears, and scalp may work their way into the brain. Abscesses within an abdominal organ such as the liver may rupture into the abdominal cavity. In either case, the result is life threatening. Blood **poisoning** is a term commonly used to describe an infection that has spilled into the blood stream and spread throughout the body from a localized origin. Blood poisoning, known to physicians as septicemia, is also life threatening.

Of special note, abscesses in the hand are more serious than they might appear. Due to the intricate structure and the overriding importance of the hand, any hand infection must be treated promptly and competently.

Prevention

Infections that are treated early with heat (if superficial) or antibiotics will often resolve without the formation of an abscess. It is even better to avoid infections altogether by taking prompt care of open injuries, particularly puncture **wounds**. Bites are the most dangerous of all, even more so because they often occur on the hand.

Resources

BOOKS

Fauci, Anthony S., et al., editors. *Harrison's Principles of Internal Medicine*. New York: McGraw-Hill, 1997.

J. Ricker Polsdorfer, MD

Abscess drainage *see* **Abscess incision and drainage**

Abscess incision & drainage

Definition

An infected skin nodule that contains pus may need to be drained via a cut if it does not respond to **antibiotics**. This allows the pus to escape, and the infection to heal.

Purpose

An **abscess** is a pus-filled sore, usually caused by a bacterial infection. The pus is made up of both live and dead organisms and destroyed tissue from the white blood cells that were carried to the area to fight the infection. Abscesses are often found in the soft tissue under the skin, such as the armpit or the groin.

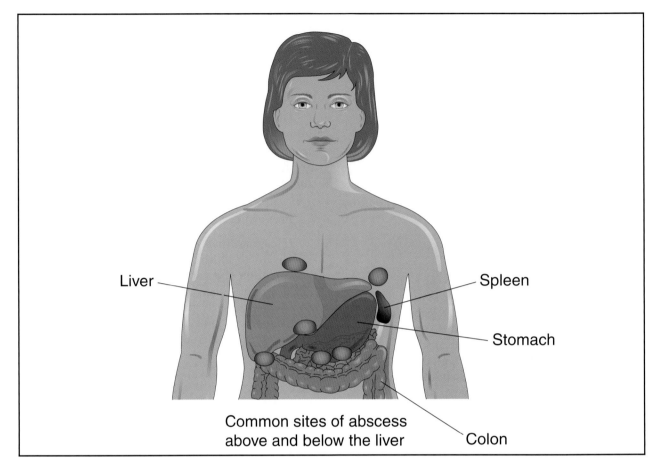

Liver

Spleen

Stomach

Common sites of abscess
above and below the liver

Colon

Although abscesses are often found in the soft tissue under the skin, such as the armpit or the groin, they may develop in any organ, such as the liver. *(Illustration by Electronic Illustrators Group.)*

However, they may develop in any organ, and are commonly found in the breast and gums. Abscesses are far more serious and call for more specific treatment if they are located in deep organs such as the lung, liver or brain.

Because the lining of the abscess cavity tends to interfere with the amount of the drug that can penetrate the source of infection from the blood, the cavity itself may require draining. Once an abscess has fully formed, it often does not respond to antibiotics. Even if the antibiotic does penetrate into the abscess, it doesn't function as well in that environment.

Precautions

An abscess can usually be diagnosed visually, although an imaging technique such as a computed tomography scan may be used to confirm the extent of the abscess before drainage. Such procedures may also be needed to localize internal abscesses, such as those in the abdominal cavity or brain.

Description

A doctor will cut into the lining of the abscess, allowing the pus to escape either through a drainage tube or by leaving the cavity open to the skin. How big the incision is depends on how quickly the pus is encountered.

Once the abscess is opened, the doctor will clean and irrigate the wound thoroughly with saline. If it is not too large or deep, the doctor may simply pack the abscess wound with gauze for 24–48 hours to absorb the pus and discharge.

If it is a deeper abscess, the doctor may insert a drainage tube after cleaning out the wound. Once the tube is in place, the surgeon closes the incision with simple stitches, and applies a sterile dressing. Drainage is maintained for several days to help prevent the abscess from reforming.

Preparation

The skin over the abscess will be cleansed by swabbing gently with an antiseptic solution.

Aftercare

Much of the **pain** around the abscess will be gone after the surgery. Healing is usually very fast. After the tube is taken out, antibiotics may be continued for several days. Applying heat and keeping the affected area elevated may help relieve inflammation.

Risks

If there is any scarring, it is likely to become much less noticeable as time goes on, and eventually almost invisible. Occasionally, an abscess within a vital organ (such as the brain) damages enough surrounding tissue that there is some permanent loss of normal function.

Normal results

Most abscesses heal after drainage alone; others require drainage and antibiotic drug treatment.

Resources

BOOKS

Turkington, Carol A., and Jeffrey S. Dover. *Skin Deep*. New York: Facts on File, 1998.

ORGANIZATIONS

National Institute of Arthritis and Musculoskeletal and Skin Diseases. 9000 Rockville Pike, Bldg. 31, Rm 9A04, Bethesda, MD 20892.

Carol A. Turkington

Abuse

Definition

Abuse is defined as anything that is harmful, injurious, or offensive. Abuse also includes excessive and wrongful misuse of a substance. There are several major types of abuse: physical and sexual abuse of a child or an adult, **substance abuse**, elderly abuse, and emotional abuse.

Description

Physical abuse of a child is the infliction of injury by another person. The injuries can include punching, kicking, biting, burning, beating, or pulling the victim's hair. The physical abuse inflicted on a child can result in **bruises**, **burns**, **poisoning**, broken bones, and internal hemorrhages. Physical assault against an adult primarily occurs with women, usually in the form of domestic violence. It is estimated that approximately three million children witness domestic violence every year.

Sexual abuse of a child refers to sexual behavior between an adult and child or between two children, one of whom is dominant or significantly older. The sexual behaviors can include touching breasts, genitals, and buttocks; either dressed or undressed. The behavior also can include exhibitionism, cunnilingus, fellatio, or penetration of the vagina or anus with sexual organs or objects.

Pornographic photography also is used in sexual abuse with children. Reported sex offenders are 97% male. Reports of child pornography have increased since with the popularity of the Internet. Females more often are perpetrators in child-care settings, since children may confuse sexual abuse by a female with normal hygiene care. The 1990s and early 2000s were rocked by reports of sexual abuse of children committed by Catholic priests. Most of the abuse appeared to have occurred during the 1970s and a prominent report released early in 2004 stated that as many as 10.667 children were sexually abused by more than 4,300 priests. Sexual abuse by stepfathers is five times more common than with biological fathers. Sexual abuse of daughters by stepfathers or fathers is the most common form of incest.

Sexual abuse also can take the form of **rape**. The legal definition of rape includes only slight penile penetration in the victim's outer vulva area. Complete erection and ejaculation are not necessary. Rape is the perpetration of an act of sexual intercourse whether:

- will is overcome by force or fear (from threats or by use of drugs).
- mental impairment renders the victim incapable of rational judgment.
- if the victim is below the legal age established for consent.

Substance abuse is an abnormal pattern of substance usage leading to significant distress or impairment. The criteria include one or more of the following occurring within a 12-month period:

- recurrent substance use resulting in failure to fulfill obligations at home, work, or school.

- using substance in situations that are physically dangerous (i.e., while driving).

- recurrent substance-related legal problems.

- continued usage despite recurrent social and interpersonal problems (i.e., arguments and fights with significant other).

Abuse of the elderly is common and occurs mostly as a result of caretaker burnout, due to the high level of dependency frail, elderly patients usually require. Abuse can be manifested by physical signs, fear, and delaying or not reporting the need for advanced medical care. Elderly patients also may exhibit financial abuse (money or possessions taken away) and abandonment.

Emotional abuse generally continues even after physical assaults have stopped. In most cases it is a personally tailored form of verbal or gesture abuse expressed to illicit a provoked response.

Causes and symptoms

Children who have been abused usually have a variety of symptoms that encompass behavioral, emotional, and psychosomatic problems (body problems caused by emotional or mental disturbance). Children who have been physically abused tend to be more aggressive, angry, hostile, depressed, and have low self-esteem. Additionally, they exhibit fear, **anxiety**, and nightmares. Severe psychological problems may result in suicidal behavior or posttraumatic stress disorder. Physically abused children may complain of physical illness even in the absence of a cause. They also may suffer from eating disorders and **encopresis**, or involuntary defecation caused or psychic origin. Children who are sexually abused may exhibit abnormal sexual behavior in the form of aggressiveness and hyperarousal. Adolescents may display promiscuity, sexual acting out, and—in some situations—homosexual contact.

Physical abuse directed towards adults can ultimately lead to **death**. Approximately 50% of women murdered in the United States were killed by a former or current male partner. Approximately one-third of emergency room consultations by women were prompted due to domestic violence. Female victims who are married also have a higher rate of internal injuries and unconsciousness than victims of stranger assault (mugging, robbery). Physical abuse or rape also can occur between married persons and persons of the same gender. Perpetrators usually sexually assault their victims to dominate, hurt, and debase them. It is common for physical and sexual violence to occur at the same time. A large percentage of sexually assaulted persons were also physically abused in the form of punching, beating, or threatening the victim with a weapon such as a gun or knife. Usually males who are hurt and humiliated tend to physically assault people whom they are intimately involved with, such as spouses and/or children. Males who assault a female tend to have experienced or witnessed violence during childhood. They also tend to abuse alcohol, to be sexually assaultive, and are at increased risk for assaultive behavior directed against children. Jealous males tend to monitor a women's movements and whereabouts and to isolate other sources of protection and support. They interpret their behavior as betrayal of trust and this causes resentment and explosive anger outbursts during periods of losing control. Males also may use aggression against females in an effort to control and intimidate partners.

Abuse in the elderly usually occurs in the frail, elderly community. The caretaker is usually the perpetrator. Caretaker abuse can be suspected if there is evidence suggesting behavioral changes in the elderly person when the caretaker is present. Additionally, elderly abuse can be possible if there are delays between injuries and treatment, inconsistencies between injury and explanations, lack of hygiene or clothing, and prescriptions not being filled.

Diagnosis

Children who are victims of domestic violence frequently are injured attempting to protect their mother from an abusive partner. Injuries are visible by inspection or self-report. Physical abuse of an adult may also be evident by inspection with visible cuts and/or bruises or self-report.

Sexual abuse of both a child and an adult can be diagnosed with a history from the victim. Victims can be assessed for signs of ejaculatory evidence from the perpetrator. Ejaculatory specimens can be retrieved from the mouth, rectum, and clothing. Tests for sexually transmitted diseases may be performed.

Elderly abuse can be suspected if the elderly patient demonstrates a fear of the caretaker. Additionally, elderly abuse can be suspected if there are signs indicating intentional delay of required medical care or a change in medical status.

Substance abuse can be suspected in a person who continues to indulge in their drug of choice despite recurrent negative consequences. The diagnosis can be made after administration of a comprehensive exam and standardized chemical abuse assessments by a therapist.

Treatment

Children who are victims of physical or sexual abuse typically require psychological support and medical attention. A complaint may be filed with the local family social services agency that will initiate investigations. The authorities usually will follow up the allegation or offense. Children may also be referred for psychological evaluation and/or treatment. The victim also may be placed in foster care pending the investigation outcome. The police also may investigate physical and sexual abuse of an adult. The victim may require immediate medical care and long-term psychological treatment. It is common for children to be adversely affected by domestic violence situations and the local family services agency may be involved.

Substance abusers should elect treatment, either inpatient or outpatient, depending on severity of **addiction**. Long term treatment and/or medications may be utilized to assist in abstinence. The patient should be encouraged to participate in community centered support groups.

Prognosis

The prognosis depends on the diagnosis. Usually victims of physical and sexual abuse require therapy to deal with emotional distress associated with the incident. Perpetrators require further psychological evaluation and treatment. Victims of abuse may have a variety of emotional problems including depression, acts of **suicide**, or anxiety. Children of sexual abuse may enter abusive relationships or have problems with intimacy as adults. The substance abuser may experience relapses, since the cardinal feature of all addictive disorders is a tendency to return to symptoms. Elderly patients may suffer from further medical problems and/or anxiety, and in some cases neglect may precipitate death.

Prevention

Prevention programs are geared to education and awareness. Detection of initial symptoms or characteristic behaviors may assist in some situations. In some cases treatment may be sought before incident. The professional treating the abused persons must develop a clear sense of the relationship dynamics and the chances for continued harm.

Resources

BOOKS

Behrman, Richard E., et al, editors. *Nelson Textbook of Pediatrics.* 16th ed. W. B. Saunders Company, 2000.

PERIODICALS

Plante, Thomas G. "Another Aftershock: What Have We Learned from the John Jay Report?." *America* (March 22, 2004): 10.

ORGANIZATIONS

National Clearinghouse on Child Abuse and Neglect Information. 330 C Street SW, Washington, DC 20447. (800) 392-3366.

OTHER

Elder Abuse Prevention. < http://www.oaktrees.org/ elder > .

National Institute on Drug Abuse. < http:// www.nida.nih.gov > .

Laith Farid Gulli, M.D.
Bilal Nasser, M.Sc.
Teresa G. Odle

Acceleration-deceleration cervical injury *see* **Whiplash**

ACE inhibitors *see* **Angiotensin-converting enzyme inhibitors**

Acetaminophen

Definition

Acetaminophen is a medicine used to relieve **pain** and reduce **fever**.

Purpose

Acetaminophen is used to relieve many kinds of minor aches and pains—headaches, muscle aches, backaches, toothaches, menstrual cramps, arthritis, and the aches and pains that often accompany colds.

Description

This drug is available without a prescription. Acetaminophen is sold under various brand names, including Tylenol, Panadol, **Aspirin** Free Anacin, and Bayer Select Maximum Strength **Headache** Pain Relief Formula. Many multi-symptom cold, flu, and sinus medicines also contain acetaminophen. The ingredients listing on the container should state if acetaminophen is included in the product.

Studies have shown that acetaminophen relieves pain and reduces fever about as well as aspirin. But differences between these two common drugs exist. Acetaminophen is less likely than aspirin to irritate the stomach. However, unlike aspirin, acetaminophen does not reduce the redness, stiffness, or swelling that accompany arthritis.

Recommended dosage

The usual dosage for adults and children age 12 and over is 325-650 mg every four to six hours as needed. No more than 4 grams (4000 mg) should be taken in 24 hours. Because the drug can potentially harm the liver, people who drink alcohol in large quantities should take considerably less acetaminophen and possibly should avoid the drug completely.

For children ages 6-11 years, the usual dose is 150-300 mg, three to four times a day. A physician should recommend doses for children under age 6 years.

Precautions

In 2004, the U.S. Food and Drug Administration (FDA) launched an advertising campaign aimed at educating consumers about proper use of acetaminophen and other over-the-counter pain killers. Often, acetaminophen is hidden in many cold and flu products and people unexpectedly overdose on the medicine. Some cases have led to **liver transplantation** or **death**. More than the recommended dosage of acetaminophen should not be taken unless told to do so by a physician or dentist.

Patients should not use acetaminophen for more than 10 days to relieve pain (five days for children) or for more than three days to reduce fever, unless directed to do so by a physician. If symptoms do not go away—or if they get worse— a physician should be contacted. Anyone who drinks three or more alcoholic beverages a day should check with a physician before using this drug and should never take more than the recommended dosage. A risk of liver damage exists from combining large amounts of alcohol and

acetaminophen. People who already have kidney or **liver disease** or liver infections should also consult with a physician before using the drug. So should women who are pregnant or breastfeeding.

Many drugs can interact with one another. A physician or pharmacist should be consulted before combining acetaminophen with any other medicine. Two different acetaminophen-containing products should not be used at the same time.

Acetaminophen interferes with the results of some medical tests. Avoiding the drug for a few days before the tests may be necessary.

Side effects

Acetaminophen causes few side effects. The most common one is lightheadedness. Some people may experience trembling and pain in the side or the lower back. Allergic reactions occur in some people, but are rare. Anyone who develops symptoms such as a rash, swelling, or difficulty breathing after taking acetaminophen should stop taking the drug and get immediate medical attention. Other rare side effects include yellow skin or eyes, unusual bleeding or bruising, weakness, **fatigue**, bloody or black stools, bloody or cloudy urine, and a sudden decrease in the amount of urine.

Overdoses of acetaminophen may cause **nausea**, **vomiting**, sweating, and exhaustion. Very large overdoses can cause liver damage. In case of an overdose, immediate medical attention should be sought. In 2004, researchers announced that an injection to counteract the liver injury caused by acetaminophen overdose has been approved by the FDA.

Interactions

Acetaminophen may interact with a variety of other medicines. When this happens, the effects of one or both of the drugs may change or the risk of side effects may be greater. Among the drugs that may interact with acetaminophen are alcohol, nonsteroidal anti-inflammatory drugs (NSAIDs) such as Motrin, oral contraceptives, the antiseizure drug phenytoin (Dilantin), the blood-thinning drug warfarin (Coumadin), the cholesterol-lowering drug cholestyramine (Questran), the antibiotic Isoniazid, and zidovudine (Retrovir, AZT). A physician or pharmacist should be consulted before combining acetaminophen with any other prescription or nonprescription (over-the-counter) medicine.

Resources

PERIODICALS

"Antidote Cleared for Acetiminophen Overdose." *Drug Topics* February 23, 2004: 12.

Mechcatie, Elizabeth. "FDA Launches Campaign About OTC Drug Risks: NSAIDs, Acetaminophen." *Family Practice News* March 15, 2004: 81

Nancy Ross-Flanigan
Teresa G. Odle

Acetylsalicylic acid *see* **Aspirin**

Achalasia

Definition

Achalasia is a disorder of the esophagus that prevents normal swallowing.

Description

Achalasia affects the esophagus, the tube that carries swallowed food from the back of the throat down into the stomach. A ring of muscle called the lower esophageal sphincter encircles the esophagus just above the entrance to the stomach. This sphincter muscle is normally contracted to close the esophagus. When the sphincter is closed, the contents of the stomach cannot flow back into the esophagus. Backward flow of stomach contents (reflux) can irritate and inflame the esophagus, causing symptoms such as **heartburn**. The act of swallowing causes a wave of esophageal contraction called peristalsis. Peristalsis pushes food along the esophagus. Normally, peristalsis causes the esophageal sphincter to relax and allow food into the stomach. In achalasia, which means "failure to relax," the esophageal sphincter remains contracted. Normal peristalsis is interrupted and food cannot enter the stomach.

Causes and symptoms

Causes

Achalasia is caused by degeneration of the nerve cells that normally signal the brain to relax the esophageal sphincter. The ultimate cause of this degeneration is unknown. Autoimmune disease or hidden infection is suspected.

Symptoms

Dysphagia, or difficulty swallowing, is the most common symptom of achalasia. The person with achalasia usually has trouble swallowing both liquid and solid foods, often feeling that food "gets stuck" on the way down. The person has chest **pain** that is often mistaken for **angina** pectoris (cardiac pain). Heartburn and difficulty belching are common. Symptoms usually get steadily worse. Other symptoms may include nighttime **cough** or recurrent **pneumonia** caused by food passing into the lower airways.

Diagnosis

Diagnosis of achalasia begins with a careful medical history. The history should focus on the timing of symptoms and on eliminating other medical conditions that may cause similar symptoms. Tests used to diagnose achalasia include:

- Esophageal manometry. In this test, a thin tube is passed into the esophagus to measure the pressure exerted by the esophageal sphincter.

- X ray of the esophagus. Barium may be swallowed to act as a contrast agent. Barium reveals the outlines of the esophagus in greater detail and makes it easier to see its constriction at the sphincter.

- Endoscopy. In this test, a tube containing a lens and a light source is passed into the esophagus. Endoscopy is used to look directly at the surface of the esophagus. This test can also detect tumors that cause symptoms like those of achalasia. Cancer of the esophagus occurs as a complication of achalasia in 2-7% of patients.

Treatment

The first-line treatment for achalasia is balloon dilation. In this procedure, an inflatable membrane or balloon is passed down the esophagus to the sphincter and inflated to force the sphincter open. Dilation is effective in about 70% of patients.

Three other treatments are used for achalasia when balloon dilation is inappropriate or unacceptable.

KEY TERMS

Botulinum toxin—Any of a group of potent bacterial toxins or poisons produced by different strains of the bacterium *Clostridium botulinum*. The toxins cause muscle paralysis.

Dysphagia—Difficulty in swallowing.

Endoscopy—A test in which a viewing device and a light source are introduced into the esophagus by means of a flexible tube. Endoscopy permits visual inspection of the esophagus for abnormalities.

Esophageal manometry—A test in which a thin tube is passed into the esophagus to measure the degree of pressure exerted by the muscles of the esophageal wall.

Esophageal sphincter—A circular band of muscle that closes the last few centimeters of the esophagus and prevents the backward flow of stomach contents.

Esophagomyotomy—A surgical incision through the muscular tissue of the esophagus.

Esophagus—The muscular tube that leads from the back of the throat to the entrance of the stomach.

Peristalsis—The coordinated, rhythmic wave of smooth muscle contraction that forces food through the digestive tract.

Reflux—An abnormal backward or return flow of a fluid.

- Botulinum toxin injection. Injected into the sphincter, botulinum toxin paralyzes the muscle and allows it to relax. Symptoms usually return within one to two years.

- Esophagomyotomy. This surgical procedure cuts the sphincter muscle to allow the esophagus to open. Esophagomyotomy is becoming more popular with the development of techniques allowing very small abdominal incisions.

- Drug therapy. Nifedipine, a calcium-channel blocker, reduces muscle contraction. Taken daily, this drug provides relief for about two-thirds of patients for as long as two years.

Prognosis

Most patients with achalasia can be treated effectively. Achalasia does not reduce life expectancy unless esophageal carcinoma develops.

Prevention

There is no known way to prevent achalasia.

Resources

BOOKS

Grendell, James H., Kenneth R. McQuaid, and Scott L. Friedman, editors. *Current Diagnosis and Treatment in Gastroenterology.* Stamford: Appleton& Lange, 1996.

Richard Robinson

Achondroplasia

Definition

Achondroplasia is the most common cause of dwarfism, or significantly abnormal short stature.

Description

Achondroplasia is one of a number of chondodystrophies, in which the development of cartilage, and therefore, bone is disturbed. The disorder appears in approximately one in every 10,000 births. Achondroplasia is usually diagnosed at birth, owing to the characteristic appearance of the newborn.

Normal bone growth depends on the production of cartilage (a fibrous connective tissue). Over time, calcium is deposited within the cartilage, causing it to harden and become bone. In achondroplasia, abnormalities of this process prevent the bones (especially those in the limbs) from growing as long as they normally should, at the same time allowing the bones to become abnormally thickened. The bones in the trunk of the body and the skull are mostly not affected, although the opening from the skull through which the spinal cord passes (foramen magnum) is often narrower than normal, and the opening (spinal canal) through which the spinal cord runs in the back bones (vertebrae) becomes increasingly and abnormally small down the length of the spine.

Causes and symptoms

Achondroplasia is caused by a genetic defect. It is a dominant trait, meaning that anybody with the genetic defect will display all the symptoms of the disorder. A parent with the disorder has a 50%

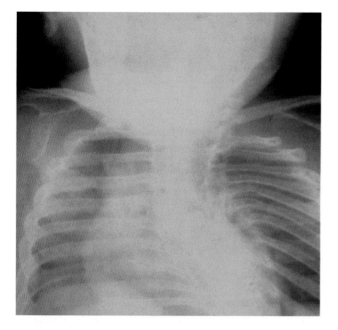

An x-ray image of an achondroplastic person's head and chest. *(Custom Medical Stock Photo. Reproduced by permission.)*

chance of passing it on to the offspring. Although achondroplasia can be passed on to subsequent offspring, the majority of cases occur due to a new mutation (change) in a gene. Interestingly enough, the defect seen in achondroplasia is one of only a few defects known to increase in frequency with increasing age of the father (many genetic defects are linked to increased age of the mother).

People with achondroplasia have abnormally short arms and legs. Their trunk is usually of normal size, as is their head. The appearance of short limbs and normal head size actually makes the head appear to be oversized. The bridge of the nose often has a scooped out appearance termed "saddle nose." The lower back has an abnormal curvature, or sway back. The face often displays an overly prominent forehead, and a relative lack of development of the face in the area of the upper jaw. Because the foramen magnum and spinal canal are abnormally narrowed, nerve damage may occur if the spinal cord or nerves become compressed. The narrowed foramen magnum may disrupt the normal flow of fluid between the brain and the spinal cord, resulting in the accumulation of too much fluid in the brain (**hydrocephalus**). Children with achondroplasia have a very high risk of serious and repeated middle ear infections, which can result in **hearing loss**. The disease does not affect either mental capacity, or reproductive ability.

Cartilage—A flexible, fibrous type of connective tissue which serves as a base on which bone is built.

Foramen magnum—The opening at the base of the skull, through which the spinal cord and the brainstem pass.

Hydrocephalus—An abnormal accumulation of fluid within the brain. This accumulation can be destructive by pressing on brain structures, and damaging them.

Mutation—A new, permanent change in the structure of a gene, which can result in abnormal structure or function somewhere in the body.

Spinal canal—The opening that runs through the center of the column of spinal bones (vertebrae), and through which the spinal cord passes.

Vertebrae—The individual bones of the spinal column which are stacked on top of each other. There is a hole in the center of each bone, through which the spinal cord passes.

Diagnosis

Diagnosis is often made at birth due to the characteristically short limbs, and the appearance of a large head. X-ray examination will reveal a characteristic appearance to the bones, with the bones of the limbs appearing short in length, yet broad in width. A number of measurements of the bones in x-ray images will reveal abnormal proportions.

Treatment

No treatment will reverse the defect present in achondroplasia. All patients with the disease will be short, with abnormally proportioned limbs, trunk, and head. Treatment of achondroplasia primarily addresses some of the complications of the disorder, including problems due to nerve compression, hydrocephalus, bowed legs, and abnormal curves in the spine. Children with achondroplasia who develop middle ear infections (acute **otitis media**) will require quick treatment with **antibiotics** and careful monitoring in order to avoid hearing loss.

Prognosis

Achondroplasia is a disease which causes considerable deformity. However, with careful attention

GALE ENCYCLOPEDIA OF MEDICINE   23 paid to the development of dangerous complications (nerve compression, hydrocephalus), most people are in good health, and can live a normal lifespan.

Prevention

The only form of prevention is through **genetic counseling**, which could help parents assess their risk of having a child with achondroplasia.

Resources

BOOKS

Krane, Stephen M., and Alan L. Schiller. "Achondroplasia." In *Harrison's Principles of Internal Medicine*, edited by Anthony S. Fauci, et al. New York: McGraw-Hill, 1997.

ORGANIZATIONS

Little People of America, c/o Mary Carten. 7238 Piedmont Drive, Dallas, TX 75227-9324. (800) 243-9273.

Rosalyn Carson-DeWitt, MD

Achromatopsia *see* **Color blindness**

Acid indigestion *see* **Heartburn**

Acid phosphatase test

Definition

Acid phosphatase is an enzyme found throughout the body, but primarily in the prostate gland. Like all enzymes, it is needed to trigger specific chemical reactions. Acid phosphatase testing is done to diagnose whether **prostate cancer** has spread to other parts of the body (metastasized), and to check the effectiveness of treatment. The test has been largely supplanted by the prostate specific antigen test (PSA).

Purpose

The male prostate gland has 100 times more acid phosphatase than any other body tissue. When prostate **cancer** spreads to other parts of the body, acid phosphatase levels rise, particularly if the cancer spreads to the bone. One-half to three-fourths of persons who have metastasized prostate cancer have high acid phosphatase levels. Levels fall after the tumor is removed or reduced through treatment.

KEY TERMS

Enzyme—A substance needed to trigger specific chemical reactions.

Metastasize—Spread to other parts of the body; usually refers to cancer.

Prostate gland—A gland of the male reproductive system.

Tissues other than prostate have small amounts of acid phosphatase, including bone, liver, spleen, kidney, and red blood cells and platelets. Damage to these tissues causes a moderate increase in acid phosphatase levels.

Acid phosphatase is very concentrated in semen. **Rape** investigations will often include testing for the presence of acid phosphatase in vaginal fluid.

Precautions

This is not a screening test for prostate cancer. Acid phosphatase levels rise only after prostate cancer has metastasized.

Description

Laboratory testing measures the amount of acid phosphatase in a person's blood, and can determine from what tissue the enzyme is coming. For example, it is important to know if the increased acid phosphatase is from the prostate or red blood cells. Acid phosphatase from the prostate, called prostatic acid phosphatase (PAP), is the most medically significant type of acid phosphatase.

Subtle differences between prostatic acid phosphatase and acid phosphatases from other tissues cause them to react differently in the laboratory when mixed with certain chemicals. For example, adding the chemical tartrate to the test mixture inhibits the activity of prostatic acid phosphatase but not red blood cell acid phosphatase. Laboratory test methods based on these differences reveal how much of a person's total acid phosphatase is derived from the prostate. Results are usually available the next day.

Preparation

This test requires drawing about 5-10 mL of blood. The patient should not have a rectal exam or prostate massage for two to three days prior to the test.

Aftercare

Discomfort or bruising may occur at the puncture site, and the person may feel dizzy or faint. Applying pressure to the puncture site until the bleeding stops will reduce bruising. Warm packs to the puncture site will relieve discomfort.

Normal results

Normal results vary based on the laboratory and the method used.

Abnormal results

The highest levels of acid phosphatase are found in metastasized prostate cancer. Diseases of the bone, such as Paget's disease or **hyperparathyroidism**; diseases of blood cells, such as **sickle cell disease** or **multiple myeloma**; or lysosomal disorders, such as Gaucher's disease, will show moderately increased levels.

Certain medications can cause temporary increases or decreases in acid phosphatase levels. Manipulation of the prostate gland through massage, biopsy, or rectal exam before a test can increase the level.

Resources

PERIODICALS

Moul, Judd W., et al. "The Contemporary Value of Pretreatment Prostatic Acid Phosphatase to Predict Pathological Stage and Recurrence in Radical Prostatectomy Cases." *Journal of Urology* (March 1998): 935-940.

Nancy J. Nordenson

Acid reflux *see* **Heartburn**

Acidosis *see* **Respiratory acidosis; Renal tubular acidosis; Metabolic acidosis**

Acne

Definition

Acne is a common skin disease characterized by pimples on the face, chest, and back. It occurs when the pores of the skin become clogged with oil, dead skin cells, and bacteria.

Description

Acne vulgaris, the medical term for common acne, is the most common skin disease. It affects nearly 17 million people in the United States. While acne can arise at any age, it usually begins at **puberty** and worsens during adolescence. Nearly 85% of people develop acne at some time between the ages of 12-25 years. Up to 20% of women develop mild acne. It is also found in some newborns.

The sebaceous glands lie just beneath the skin's surface. They produce an oil called sebum, the skin's natural moisturizer. These glands and the hair follicles within which they are found are called sebaceous follicles. These follicles open onto the skin through pores. At puberty, increased levels of androgens (male hormones) cause the glands to produce too much sebum. When excess sebum combines with dead, sticky skin cells, a hard plug, or comedo, forms that blocks the pore. Mild noninflammatory acne consists of the two types of comedones, whiteheads and blackheads.

Moderate and severe inflammatory types of acne result after the plugged follicle is invaded by *Propionibacterium acnes*, a bacteria that normally lives on the skin. A pimple forms when the damaged follicle weakens and bursts open, releasing sebum, bacteria, and skin and white blood cells into the surrounding tissues. Inflamed pimples near the skin's surface are called papules; when deeper, they are called pustules. The most severe type of acne consists of cysts (closed sacs) and nodules (hard swellings). Scarring occurs when new skin cells are laid down to replace damaged cells.

The most common sites of acne are the face, chest, shoulders, and back since these are the parts of the body where the most sebaceous follicles are found.

Causes and symptoms

The exact cause of acne is unknown. Several risk factors have been identified:

- Age. Due to the hormonal changes they experience, teenagers are more likely to develop acne.
- Gender. Boys have more severe acne and develop it more often than girls.
- Disease. Hormonal disorders can complicate acne in girls.
- Heredity. Individuals with a family history of acne have greater susceptibility to the disease.
- Hormonal changes. Acne can flare up before menstruation, during **pregnancy**, and **menopause**.

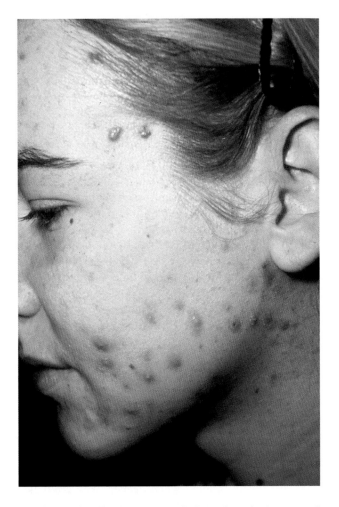

Acne vulgaris affecting a woman's face. Acne is the general name given to a skin disorder in which the sebaceous glands become inflamed. *(Photograph by Biophoto Associates, Photo Researchers, Inc. Reproduced by permission.)*

- Diet. No foods cause acne, but certain foods may cause flare-ups.

- Drugs. Acne can be a side effect of drugs including tranquilizers, antidepressants, antibiotics, **oral contraceptives**, and anabolic steroids.

- Personal hygiene. Abrasive soaps, hard scrubbing, or picking at pimples will make them worse.

- Cosmetics. Oil-based makeup and hair sprays worsen acne.

- Environment. Exposure to oils and greases, polluted air, and sweating in hot weather aggravate acne.

- **Stress**. Emotional stress may contribute to acne.

Acne is usually not conspicuous, although inflamed lesions may cause **pain**, tenderness, **itching**, or swelling. The most troubling aspects of these lesions are the negative cosmetic effects and potential for scarring. Some people, especially teenagers, become emotionally upset about their condition, and have problems forming relationships or keeping jobs.

Diagnosis

Acne patients are often treated by family doctors. Complicated cases are referred to a dermatologist, a skin disease specialist, or an endocrinologist, a specialist who treats diseases of the body's endocrine (hormones and glands) system.

Acne has a characteristic appearance and is not difficult to diagnose. The doctor takes a complete medical history, including questions about skin care, diet, factors causing flare-ups, medication use, and prior treatment. **Physical examination** includes the face, upper neck, chest, shoulders, back, and other affected areas. Under good lighting, the doctor determines what types and how many blemishes are present, whether they are inflamed, whether they are deep or superficial, and whether there is scarring or skin discoloration.

In teenagers, acne is often found on the forehead, nose, and chin. As people get older, acne tends to appear towards the outer part of the face. Adult women may have acne on their chins and around their mouths. The elderly may develop whiteheads and blackheads on the upper cheeks and skin around the eyes.

Laboratory tests are not done unless the patient appears to have a hormonal disorder or other medical problem. In this case, blood analyses or other tests may be ordered. Most insurance plans cover the costs of diagnosing and treating acne.

Treatment

Acne treatment consists of reducing sebum production, removing dead skin cells, and killing bacteria with topical drugs and oral medications. Treatment choice depends upon whether the acne is mild, moderate, or severe.

Drugs

TOPICAL DRUGS. Treatment for mild noninflammatory acne consists of reducing the formation of new comedones with topical tretinoin, benzoyl peroxide, adapalene, or salicylic acid. Tretinoin is especially effective because it increases turnover (death and replacement) of skin cells. When complicated by inflammation, **topical antibiotics** may be added to the treatment regimen. Improvement is usually seen in two to four weeks.

Topical medications are available as cream, gel, lotion, or pad preparations of varying strengths. They include **antibiotics** (agents that kill bacteria), such as erythromycin, clindamycin (Cleocin-T), and meclocycline (Meclan); comedolytics (agents that loosen hard plugs and open pores) such as the vitamin A acid tretinoin (Retin-A), salicylic acid, adapalene (Differin), resorcinol, and sulfur. Drugs that act as both comedolytics and antibiotics, such as benzoyl peroxide, azelaic acid (Azelex), or benzoyl peroxide plus erythromycin (Benzamycin), are also used. These drugs may be used for months to years to achieve disease control.

After washing with mild soap, the drugs are applied alone or in combination, once or twice a day over the entire affected area of skin. Possible side effects include mild redness, peeling, irritation, dryness, and an increased sensitivity to sunlight that requires use of a sunscreen.

ORAL DRUGS. Oral antibiotics are taken daily for two to four months. The drugs used include tetracycline, erythromycin, minocycline (Minocin), doxycycline, clindamycin (Cleocin), and trimethoprim-sulfamethoxazole (Bactrim, Septra). Possible side effects include allergic reactions, stomach upset, vaginal yeast infections, **dizziness**, and tooth discoloration.

The goal of treating moderate acne is to decrease inflammation and prevent new comedone formation. One effective treatment is topical tretinoin along with a topical or oral antibiotic. A combination of topical benzoyl peroxide and erythromycin is also very effective. Improvement is normally seen within four to six weeks, but treatment is maintained for at least two to four months.

A drug reserved for the treatment of severe acne, oral isotretinoin (Accutane), reduces sebum production and cell stickiness. It is the treatment of choice for severe acne with cysts and nodules, and is used with or without topical or oral antibiotics. Taken for four to five months, it provides long-term disease control in up to 60% of patients. If the acne reappears, another course of isotretinoin may be needed by about 20% of patients, while another 20% may do well with topical drugs or oral antibiotics. Side effects include temporary worsening of the acne, dry skin, nosebleeds, vision disorders, and elevated liver enzymes, blood fats and cholesterol. This drug must not be taken during pregnancy since it causes **birth defects**.

Anti-androgens, drugs that inhibit androgen production, are used to treat women who are unresponsive to other therapies. Certain types of oral contraceptives (for example, Ortho-Tri-Cyclen) and female sex hormones (estrogens) reduce hormone activity in the ovaries. Other drugs, for example, spironolactone and corticosteroids, reduce hormone activity in the adrenal glands. Improvement may take up to four months.

Oral **corticosteroids**, or anti-inflammatory drugs, are the treatment of choice for an extremely severe, but rare type of destructive inflammatory acne called acne fulminans, found mostly in adolescent males. Acne conglobata, a more common form of severe inflammation, is characterized by numerous, deep, inflammatory nodules that heal with scarring. It is treated with oral isotretinoin and corticosteroids.

Other treatments

Several surgical or medical treatments are available to alleviate acne or the resulting scars:

- Comedone extraction. The comedo is removed from the pore with a special tool.

- Chemical peels. Glycolic acid is applied to peel off the top layer of skin to reduce scarring.

- Dermabrasion. The affected skin is frozen with a chemical spray, and removed by brushing or planing.

- Punch grafting. Deep **scars** are excised and the area repaired with small skin grafts.

- Intralesional injection. Corticosteroids are injected directly into inflamed pimples.

- Collagen injection. Shallow scars are elevated by collagen (protein) injections.

Alternative treatment

Alternative treatments for acne focus on proper cleansing to keep the skin oil-free; eating a well-balanced diet high in fiber, zinc, and raw foods; and avoiding alcohol, dairy products, smoking, **caffeine**, sugar, processed foods, and foods high in iodine, such as salt. Supplementation with herbs such as burdock root (*Arctium lappa*), red clover (*Trifolium pratense*), and milk thistle (*Silybum marianum*), and with nutrients such as essential fatty acids, vitamin B complex, zinc, vitamin A, and chromium is also recommended. Chinese herbal remedies used for acne include cnidium seed (*Cnidium monnieri*) and honeysuckle flower (*Lonicera japonica*). Wholistic physicians or nutritionists can recommend the proper amounts of these herbs.

Prognosis

Acne is not curable, although long-term control is achieved in up to 60% of patients treated with isotretinoin. It can be controlled by proper treatment, with improvement taking two or more months. Acne tends to reappear when treatment stops, but spontaneously improves over time. Inflammatory acne may leave scars that require further treatment.

Prevention

There are no sure ways to prevent acne, but the following steps may be taken to minimize flare-ups:

- gentle washing of affected areas once or twice every day

- avoid abrasive cleansers

- use noncomedogenic makeup and moisturizers

- shampoo often and wear hair off face

- eat a well-balanced diet, avoiding foods that trigger flare-ups

- unless told otherwise, give dry pimples a limited amount of sun exposure

- do not pick or squeeze blemishes

- reduce stress

Resources

PERIODICALS

Billings, Laura. "Getting Clear." *Health Magazine* (April 1997): 48-52.

ORGANIZATIONS

American Academy of Dermatology. 930 N. Meacham Road, P.O. Box 4014, Schaumburg, IL 60168-4014. (847) 330-0230. Fax: (847) 330-0050. < http:// www.aad.org >.

Mercedes McLaughlin

Acne rosacea *see* **Rosacea**

Acoustic neurinoma *see* **Acoustic neuroma**

Acoustic neuroma

Definition

An acoustic neuroma is a benign tumor involving cells of the myelin sheath that surrounds the vestibulocochlear nerve (eighth cranial nerve).

Description

The vestibulocochlear nerve extends from the inner ear to the brain and is made up of a vestibular branch, often called the vestibular nerve, and a cochlear branch, called the cochlear nerve. The vestibular and cochlear nerves lie next to one another. They also run along side other cranial nerves. People possess two of each type of vestibulocochlear nerve, one that extends from the left ear and one that extends from the right ear.

The vestibular nerve transmits information concerning balance from the inner ear to the brain and the cochlear nerve transmits information about hearing. The vestibular nerve, like many nerves, is surrounded by a cover called a myelin sheath. A tumor, called a schwannoma, can sometimes develop from the cells of the myelin sheath. A tumor is an abnormal growth of tissue that results from the uncontrolled growth of cells. Acoustic neuromas are often called vestibular schwannomas because they are tumors that arise from the myelin sheath that surrounds the vestibular nerve. Acoustic neuromas are considered benign (non-cancerous) tumors since they do not spread to other parts of the body. They can occur anywhere along the vestibular nerve but are most likely to occur where the vestibulocochlear nerve passes through the tiny bony canal that connects the brain and the inner ear.

An acoustic neuroma can arise from the left vestibular nerve or the right vestibular nerve. A unilateral tumor is a tumor arising from one nerve and a bilateral tumor arises from both vestibular nerves. Unilateral acoustic neuromas usually occur spontaneously (by chance). Bilateral acoustic neuromas occur as part of a hereditary condition called **Neurofibromatosis** Type 2 (NF2). A person with NF2 has inherited a predisposition for developing acoustic neuromas and other tumors of the nerve cells.

Acoustic neuromas usually grow slowly and can take years to develop. Some acoustic neuromas remain so small that they do not cause any symptoms. As the acoustic neuroma grows it can interfere with the functioning of the vestibular nerve and can cause vertigo and balance difficulties. If the acoustic nerve grows large enough to press against the cochlear nerve, then hearing loss and a ringing (tinnitus) in the affected ear will usually occur. If untreated and the acoustic neuroma continues to grow it can press against other nerves in the region and cause other symptoms. This tumor can be life threatening if it becomes large enough to press against and interfere with the functioning of the brain.

Causes and symptoms

Causes

An acoustic neuroma is caused by a change or absence of both of the NF2 tumor suppressor genes in a nerve cell. Every person possesses a pair of NF2 genes in every cell of their body including their nerve cells. One NF2 gene is inherited from the egg cell of the mother and one NF2 gene is inherited from the sperm cell of the father. The NF2 gene is responsible for helping to prevent the formation of tumors in the nerve cells. In particular the NF2 gene helps to prevent acoustic neuromas.

Only one unchanged and functioning NF2 gene is necessary to prevent the formation of an acoustic neuroma. If both NF2 genes become changed or missing in one of the myelin sheath cells of the

vestibular nerve then an acoustic neuroma will usually develop. Most unilateral acoustic neuromas result when the NF2 genes become spontaneously changed or missing. Someone with a unilateral acoustic neuroma that has developed spontaneously is not at increased risk for having children with an acoustic neuroma. Some unilateral acoustic neuromas result from the hereditary condition NF2. It is also possible that some unilateral acoustic neuromas may be caused by changes in other genes responsible for preventing the formation of tumors.

Bilateral acoustic neuromas result when someone is affected with the hereditary condition NF2. A person with NF2 is typically born with one unchanged and one changed or missing NF2 gene in every cell of their body. Sometimes they inherit this change from their mother or father. Sometimes the change occurs spontaneously when the egg and sperm come together to form the first cell of the baby. The children of a person with NF2 have a 50% chance of inheriting the changed or missing NF2 gene.

A person with NF2 will develop an acoustic neuroma if the remaining unchanged NF2 gene becomes spontaneously changed or missing in one of the myelin sheath cells of their vestibular nerve. People with NF2 often develop acoustic neuromas at a younger age. The mean age of onset of acoustic neuroma in NF2 is 31 years of age versus 50 years of age for sporadic acoustic neuromas. Not all people with NF2, however, develop acoustic neuromas. People with NF2 are at increased risk for developing **cataracts** and tumors in other nerve cells.

Most people with a unilateral acoustic neuroma are not affected with NF2. Some people with NF2, however, only develop a tumor in one of the vestibulocochlear nerves. Others may initially be diagnosed with a unilateral tumor but may develop a tumor in the other nerve a number of years later. NF2 should be considered in someone under the age of 40 who has a unilateral acoustic neuroma. Someone with a unilateral acoustic neuroma and other family members diagnosed with NF2 probably is affected with NF2. Someone with a unilateral acoustic neuroma and other symptoms of NF2 such as cataracts and other tumors may also be affected with NF2. On the other hand, someone over the age of 50 with a unilateral acoustic neuroma, no other tumors and no family history of NF2 is very unlikely to be affected with NF2.

Recent studies in Europe have suggested a possible connection between the widespread use of mobile phones and an increased risk of developing acoustic neuromas. Some observers, however, question whether mobile phones have been in use long enough to be an identifiable risk factor.

Symptoms

Small acoustic neuromas usually only interfere with the functioning of the vestibulocochlear nerve. The most common first symptom of an acoustic neuroma is **hearing loss**, which is often accompanied by a ringing sound (tinnitis). People with acoustic neuromas sometimes report difficulties in using the phone and difficulties in perceiving the tone of a musical instrument or sound even when their hearing appears to be otherwise normal. In most cases the hearing loss is initially subtle and worsens gradually over time until deafness occurs in the affected ear. In approximately 10% of cases the hearing loss is sudden and severe.

Acoustic neuromas can also affect the functioning of the vestibular branch of the vestibulocochlear nerve and van cause vertigo and dysequilibrium. Twenty percent of small tumors are associated with periodic vertigo, which is characterized by **dizziness** or a whirling sensation. Larger acoustic neuromas are less likely to cause vertigo but more likely to cause dysequilibrium. Dysequilibrium, which is characterized by minor clumsiness and a general feeling of instability, occurs in nearly 50% of people with an acoustic neuroma.

As the tumor grows larger it can press on the surrounding cranial nerves. Compression of the fifth cranial nerve can result in facial **pain** and or numbness. Compression of the seventh cranial nerve can cause spasms, weakness or **paralysis** of the facial muscles. Double vision is a rare symptom but can result when the 6th cranial nerve is affected. Swallowing and/or speaking difficulties can occur if the tumor presses against the 9th, 10th, or 12th cranial nerves.

If left untreated, the tumor can become large enough to press against and affect the functioning of the brain stem. The brain stem is the stalk like portion of the brain that joins the spinal cord to the cerebrum, the thinking and reasoning part of the brain. Different parts of the brainstem have different functions such as the control of breathing and muscle coordination. Large tumors that impact the brain stem can result in headaches, walking difficulties (gait ataxia) and involuntary shaking movements of the muscles (**tremors**). In rare cases when an acoustic neuroma remains undiagnosed and untreated it can cause **nausea**, vomiting, lethargy and eventually **coma**, respiratory difficulties and death. In the vast majority of cases, however, the tumor is discovered and treated long before it is large enough to cause such serious manifestations.

Diagnosis

Anyone with symptoms of hearing loss should undergo hearing evaluations. Pure tone and speech **audiometry** are two screening tests that are often used to evaluate hearing. Pure tone audiometry tests to see how well someone can hear tones of different volume and pitch and speech audiometry tests to see how well someone can hear and recognize speech. An acoustic neuroma is suspected in someone with unilateral hearing loss or hearing loss that is less severe in one ear than the other ear (asymmetrical).

Sometimes an auditory brainstem response (ABR, BAER) test is performed to help establish whether someone is likely to have an acoustic neuroma. During the ABR examination, a harmless electrical impulse is passed from the inner ear to the brainstem. An acoustic neuroma can interfere with the passage of this electrical impulse and this interference can, sometimes be identified through the ABR evaluation. A normal ABR examination does not rule out the possibility of an acoustic neuroma. An abnormal ABR examination increases the likelihood that an acoustic neuroma is present but other tests are necessary to confirm the presence of a tumor.

If an acoustic neuroma is strongly suspected then magnetic resonance imaging (MRI) is usually performed. The MRI is a very accurate evaluation that is able to detect nearly 100% of acoustic neuromas. Computerized tomography (CT scan, CAT scan)is unable to identify smaller tumors; but it can be used when an acoustic neuroma is suspected and an MRI evaluation cannot be performed.

Once an acoustic neuroma is diagnosed, an evaluation by genetic specialists such as a geneticist and genetic counselor may be recommended. The purpose of this evaluation is to obtain a detailed family history and check for signs of NF2. If NF2 is strongly suspected then DNA testing may be recommended. DNA testing involves checking the blood cells obtained from a routine blood draw for the common gene changes associated with NF2.

Treatment

The three treatment options for acoustic neuroma are surgery, radiation, and observation. The physician and patient should discuss the pros and cons of the different options prior to making a decision about treatment. The patient's, physical health, age, symptoms, tumor size, and tumor location should be considered.

Microsurgery

The surgical removal of the tumor or tumors is the most common treatment for acoustic neuroma. In most cases the entire tumor is removed during the surgery. If the tumor is large and causing significant symptoms, yet there is a need to preserve hearing in that ear, then only part of the tumor may be removed. During the procedure the tumor is removed under microscopic guidance and general anesthetic. Monitoring of the neighboring cranial nerves is done during the procedure so that damage to these nerves can be prevented. If preservation of hearing is a possibility, then monitoring of hearing will also take place during the surgery.

Most people stay in the hospital four to seven days following the surgery. Total recovery usually takes four to six weeks. Most people experience **fatigue** and head discomfort following the surgery. Problems with balance and head and neck stiffness are also common. The mortality rate of this type of surgery is less than 2% at most major centers. Approximately 20% of patients experience some degree of post-surgical complications. In most cases these complications can be managed successfully and do not result in long term medical problems. Surgery brings with it a risk of **stroke**, damage to the brain stem, infection, leakage of spinal fluid and damage to the cranial nerves. Hearing loss and/or tinnitus often result from the surgery. A follow-up MRI is recommended one to five years following the surgery because of possible regrowth of the tumor.

Stereotactic radiation therapy

During stereotactic **radiation therapy**, also called radiosurgery or radiotherapy, many small beams of radiation are aimed directly at the acoustic neuroma. The radiation is administered in a single large dose, under local anesthetic and is performed on an outpatient basis. This results in a high dose of radiation to the tumor but little radiation exposure to the surrounding area. This treatment approach is limited to small or medium tumors. The goal of the surgery is to cause tumor shrinkage or at least limit the growth of the tumor. The long-term efficacy and risks of this treatment approach are not known; however, as of the early 2000s, more and more patients diagnosed with acoustic neuromas are choosing this form of therapy. Periodic MRI monitoring throughout the life of the patient is therefore recommended.

Radiation therapy can cause hearing loss which can sometimes occurs even years later. Radiation therapy can also cause damage to neighboring cranial nerves, which can result in symptoms such as **numbness**, pain or paralysis of the facial muscles. In many cases these symptoms are temporary. Radiation treatment can also induce the formation of other benign or malignant schwannomas. This type of treatment may therefore be contraindicated in the treatment of acoustic neuromas in those with NF2 who are predisposed to developing schwannomas and other tumors.

Observation

Acoustic neuromas are usually slow growing and in some cases they will stop growing and even become smaller or disappear entirely. It may therefore be appropriate in some cases to hold off on treatment and to periodically monitor the tumor through MRI evaluations. Long-term observation may be appropriate for example in an elderly person with a small acoustic neuroma and few symptoms. Periodic observation may also be indicated for someone with a small and asymptomatic acoustic neuroma that was detected through an evaluation for another medical problem. Observation may also be suggested for someone with an acoustic neuroma in the only hearing ear or in the ear that has better hearing. The danger of an observational approach is that as the tumor grows larger it can become more difficult to treat.

Prognosis

The prognosis for someone with a unilateral acoustic neuroma is usually quite good provided the tumor is diagnosed early and appropriate treatment is instituted. Long term-hearing loss and tinnitis in the affected ear are common, even if appropriate treatment is provided. Many patients also experience facial weakness, balance problems, and headaches. Regrowth of the tumor is also a possibility following surgery or radiation therapy and repeat treatment may be necessary. The prognosis can be poorer for those with NF2 who have an increased risk of bilateral acoustic neuromas and other tumors.

Resources

BOOKS

Beers, Mark H., MD, and Robert Berkow, MD., editors. "Acoustic Neuroma." Section 7, Chapter 85 In *The Merck Manual of Diagnosis and Therapy*. Whitehouse Station, NJ: Merck Research Laboratories, 2002.

PERIODICALS

Kondziolka, D., L. D. Lundsford, and J. C. Flickinger. "Acoustic Neuroma Radiosurgery. Origins, Contemporary Use and Future Expectations." *Neurochirurgie* 50 (June 2004): 427–435.

Kundi, M., K. Mild, L. Hardell, and M. O. Mattsson. "Mobile Telephones and Cancer—A Review of Epidemiological Evidence." *Journal of Toxicology and Environmental Health, Part B, Critical Reviews* 7 (September-October 2004): 351–384.

Ryzenman, J. M., M. L. Pensak, and J. M. Tew, Jr. "Patient Perception of Comorbid Conditions After Acoustic Neuroma Management: Survey Results from the Acoustic Neuroma Association." *Laryngoscope* 114 (May 2004): 814–820.

ORGANIZATIONS

Acoustic Neuroma Association. 600 Peachtree Pkwy, Suite 108, Cumming, GA 30041-6899. (770) 205-8211. Fax: (770) 205-0239. ANAusa@aol.com. [cited June 28, 2001]. < http://anausa.org > .

Acoustic Neuroma Association of Canada Box 369, Edmonton, AB T5J 2J6. 1-800-561-ANAC(2622). (780)428-3384. anac@compusmart.ab.ca. [cited June 28, 2001]. < http://www.anac.ca > .

Seattle Acoustic Neuroma Group. Emcityland@aol.com. [cited June 28, 2001]. < http://acousticneuromaseattle.org/entryenglish.html > .

OTHER

National Institute of Health Consensus Statement Online. *Acoustic Neuroma* 9, no. 4 (December 11-13, 1991). [cited June 28, 2001]. < http://text.nlm.nih.gov/nih/cdc/www/87txt.html > .

University of California at San Francisco (UCSF). *Information on Acoustic Neuromas*. March 18, 1998. [cited June 28, 2001]. < http://itsa.ucsf.edu/~rkj/IndexAN.html > .

Lisa Andres, MS, CGC
Rebecca J. Frey, PhD

Acquired hypogammaglobulinemia *see* **Common variable immunodeficiency**

Acquired immunodeficiency syndrome *see* **AIDS**

Acrocyanosis

Definition

Acrocyanosis is a decrease in the amount of oxygen delivered to the extremities. The hands and feet turn blue because of the lack of oxygen. Decreased blood supply to the affected areas is caused by constriction or spasm of small blood vessels.

Description

Acrocyanosis is a painless disorder caused by constriction or narrowing of small blood vessels in the skin of affected patients. The spasm of the blood vessels decreases the amount of blood that passes through them, resulting in less blood being delivered to the hands and feet. The hands may be the main area affected. The affected areas turn blue and become cold and sweaty. Localized swelling may also occur. Emotion and cold temperatures can worsen the symptoms, while warmth can decrease symptoms. The disease is seen mainly in women and the effect of the disorder is mainly cosmetic. People with the disease tend to be uncomfortable, with sweaty, cold, bluish colored hands and feet.

Causes and symptoms

The sympathetic nerves cause constriction or spasms in the peripheral blood vessels that supply blood to the extremities. The spasms are a contraction of the muscles in the walls of the blood vessels. The contraction decreases the internal diameter of the blood vessels, thereby decreasing the amount of blood flow through the affected area. The spasms occur on a persistent basis, resulting in long term reduction of blood supply to the hands and feet. Sufficient blood still passes through the blood vessels so that the tissue in the affected areas does not starve for oxygen or die. Mainly, blood vessels near the surface of the skin are affected.

Diagnosis

Diagnosis is made by observation of the main clinical symptoms, including persistently blue and sweaty hands and/or feet and a lack of **pain**. Cooling the hands increases the blueness, while warming the hands decreases the blue color. The acrocyanosis patient's pulse is normal, which rules out obstructive diseases. **Raynaud's disease** differs from acrocyanosis in that it causes white and red skin coloration phases, not just bluish discoloration.

Treatment

Acrocyanosis usually isn't treated. Drugs that block the uptake of calcium (**calcium channel blockers**) and alpha-one antagonists reduce the symptoms in most cases. Drugs that dilate blood vessels are only effective some of the time. Sweating from the affected areas can be profuse and require treatment. Surgery to cut the sympathetic nerves is performed rarely.

Prognosis

Acrocyanosis is a benign and persistent disease. The main concern of patients is cosmetic. Left untreated, the disease does not worsen.

Resources

BOOKS

Alexander, R. W., R. C. Schlant, and V. Fuster, editors. *The Heart*. 9th ed. New York: McGraw-Hill, 1998.

John T. Lohr, PhD

Acromegaly and gigantism

Definition

Acromegaly is a disorder in which the abnormal release of a particular chemical from the pituitary gland in the brain causes increased growth in bone and soft tissue, as well as a variety of other disturbances throughout the body. This chemical released from the pituitary gland is called growth hormone (GH). The body's ability to process and use nutrients like fats and sugars is also altered. In children whose bony growth plates have not closed, the chemical changes of acromegaly result in exceptional growth of long bones. This variant is called gigantism, with the additional bone growth causing unusual height. When the abnormality occurs after bone growth stops, the disorder is called acromegaly.

Description

Acromegaly is a relatively rare disorder, occurring in approximately 50 out of every one million people (50/1,000,000). Both men and women are affected. Because the symptoms of acromegaly occur so gradually, diagnosis is often delayed. The majority of patients are not identified until they are middle aged.

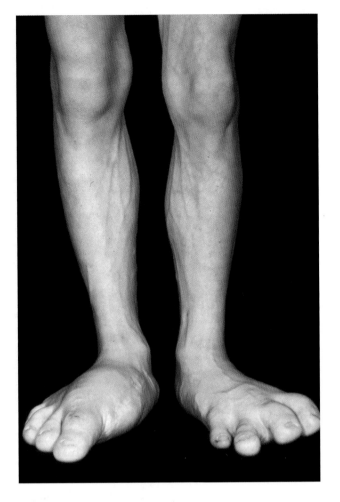

Enlarged feet is one deformity caused by acromegaly.
(Custom Medical Stock Photo. Reproduced by permission.)

Causes and symptoms

The pituitary is a small gland located at the base of the brain. A gland is a collection of cells that releases certain chemicals, or hormones, which are important to the functioning of other organs or body systems. The pituitary hormones travel throughout the body and are involved in a large number of activities, including the regulation of growth and reproductive functions. The cause of acromegaly can be traced to the pituitary's production of GH.

Under normal conditions, the pituitary receives input from another brain structure, the hypothalamus, located at the base of the brain. This input from the hypothalamus regulates the pituitary's release of hormones. For example, the hypothalamus produces growth hormone-releasing hormone (GHRH), which directs the pituitary to release GH. Input from the hypothalamus should also direct the pituitary to stop releasing hormones.

In acromegaly, the pituitary continues to release GH and ignores signals from the hypothalamus. In the liver, GH causes production of a hormone called insulin-like growth factor 1 (IGF-1), which is responsible for growth throughout the body. When the pituitary refuses to stop producing GH, the levels of IGF-1 also reach abnormal peaks. Bones, soft tissue, and organs throughout the body begin to enlarge, and the body changes its ability to process and use nutrients like sugars and fats.

In acromegaly, an individual's hands and feet begin to grow, becoming thick and doughy. The jaw line, nose, and forehead also grow, and facial features are described as "coarsening". The tongue grows larger, and because the jaw is larger, the teeth become more widely spaced. Due to swelling within the structures of the throat and sinuses, the voice becomes deeper and sounds more hollow, and patients may develop loud **snoring**. Various hormonal changes cause symptoms such as:

- heavy sweating
- oily skin
- increased coarse body hair
- improper processing of sugars in the diet (and sometimes actual diabetes)

- high blood pressure
- increased calcium in the urine (sometimes leading to kidney stones)
- increased risk of **gallstones**; and
- swelling of the thyroid gland

People with acromegaly have more skin tags, or outgrowths of tissue, than normal. This increase in skin tags is also associated with the development of growths, called polyps, within the large intestine that may eventually become cancerous. Patients with acromegaly often suffer from headaches and arthritis. The various swellings and enlargements throughout the body may press on nerves, causing sensations of local **tingling** or burning, and sometimes result in muscle weakness.

The most common cause of this disorder (in 90% of patients) is the development of a noncancerous tumor within the pituitary, called a pituitary adenoma. These tumors are the source of the abnormal release of GH. As these tumors grow, they may press on nearby structures within the brain, causing headaches and changes in vision. As the adenoma grows, it may disrupt other pituitary tissue, interfering with the release of other hormones. These disruptions may be responsible for changes in the menstrual cycle of women, decreases in the sexual drive in men and women, and the abnormal production of breast milk in women. In rare cases, acromegaly is caused by the abnormal production of GHRH, which leads to the increased production of GH. Certain tumors in the pancreas, lungs, adrenal glands, thyroid, and intestine produce GHRH, which in turn triggers production of an abnormal quantity of GH.

Diagnosis

Because acromegaly produces slow changes over time, diagnosis is often significantly delayed. In fact, the characteristic coarsening of the facial features is often not recognized by family members, friends, or long-time family physicians. Often, the diagnosis is suspected by a new physician who sees the patient for the first time and is struck by the patient's characteristic facial appearance. Comparing old photographs from a number of different time periods will often increase suspicion of the disease.

Because the quantity of GH produced varies widely under normal conditions, demonstrating high levels of GH in the blood is not sufficient to merit a diagnosis of acromegaly. Instead, laboratory tests measuring an increase of IGF-1 (3-10 times above the normal level) are useful. These results, however, must

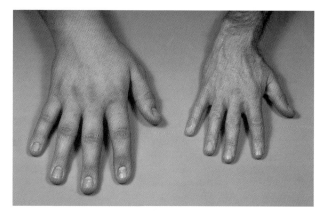

A comparison of the right hand of a person afflicted with acromegaly (left) and the hand of a normal sized person. *(Custom Medical Stock Photo. Reproduced by permission.)*

be carefully interpreted because normal laboratory values for IGF-1 vary when the patient is pregnant, undergoing puberty, elderly, or severely malnourished. Normal patients will show a decrease in GH production when given a large dose of sugar (glucose). Patients with acromegaly will not show this decrease, and will often show an increase in GH production. Magnetic resonance imaging (MRI) is useful for viewing the pituitary, and for identifying and locating an adenoma. When no adenoma can be located, the search for a GHRH-producing tumor in another location begins.

Treatment

The first step in treatment of acromegaly is removal of all or part of the pituitary adenoma. Removal requires surgery, usually performed by entering the skull through the nose. While this surgery can cause rapid improvement of many acromegaly symptoms, most patients will also require additional treatment with medication. Bromocriptine (Parlodel) is a medication that can be taken by mouth, while octreotide (Sandostatin) must be injected every eight hours. Both of these medications are helpful in reducing GH production, but must often be taken for life and produce their own unique side effects. Some patients who cannot undergo surgery are treated with radiation therapy to the pituitary in an attempt to shrink the adenoma. Radiating the pituitary may take up to 10 years, however, and may also injure/ destroy other normal parts of the pituitary.

Prognosis

Without treatment, patients with acromegaly will most likely die early because of the disease's effects on the heart, lungs, brain, or due to the development of **cancer** in the large intestine. With treatment, however, a patient with acromegaly may be able to live a normal lifespan.

Resources

BOOKS

Biller, Beverly M. K., and Gilbert H. Daniels. "Growth Hormone Excess: Acromegaly and Gigantism." In *Harrison's Principles of Internal Medicine,* edited by Anthony S. Fauci, et al. New York: McGraw-Hill, 1997.

ORGANIZATIONS

Pituitary Tumor Network Association. 16350 Ventura Blvd., #231, Encino, CA 91436. (805) 499-9973.

Rosalyn Carson-DeWitt, MD

ACT *see* **Alanine aminotransferase test**

ACTH test *see* **Adrenocorticotropic hormone test**

Actinomyces israelii infection *see* **Actinomycosis**

Actinomycosis

Definition

Actinomycosis is an infection primarily caused by the bacterium *Actinomyces israelii.* Infection most often occurs in the face and neck region and is characterized by the presence of a slowly enlarging, hard, red lump.

Description

Actinomycosis is a relatively rare infection occurring in one out of 300,000(1/300,000) people per year. It is characterized by the presence of a lump or mass that often forms, draining sinus tracts to the skin surface. Fifty percent of actinomycosis cases are of the head and neck region (also called "lumpy jaw" and "cervicofacial actinomycosis"), 15% are in the chest, 20% are in the abdomen, and the rest are in the pelvis, heart, and brain. Men are three times more likely to develop actinomycosis than women.

Causes and symptoms

Actinomycosis is usually caused by the bacterium *Actinomyces israelii.* This bacterium is normally present in the mouth but can cause disease if it enters tissues following an injury. *Actinomyces israelii* is an anaerobic bacterium which means it dislikes oxygen but grows very well in deep tissues where oxygen levels are low. **Tooth extraction**, tooth disease, **root canal treatment**, jaw surgery, or poor dental hygiene can allow *Actinomyces israelii* to cause an infection in the head and neck region.

The main symptom of cervicofacial actinomycosis is the presence of a hard lump on the face or neck. The lump may or may not be red. **Fever** occurs in some cases.

Diagnosis

Cervicofacial actinomycosis can be diagnosed by a family doctor or dentist and the patient may be referred to an oral surgeon or infectious disease specialist. The diagnosis of actinomycosis is based upon several things. The presence of a red lump with draining sinuses on the head or neck is strongly suggestive of cervicofacial actinomycosis. A recent history of tooth extraction or signs of **tooth decay** or poor dental hygiene aid in the diagnosis. Microscopic examination of the fluid draining from the sinuses shows the characteristic "sulfur Granules" (small yellow colored material in the fluid) produced by *Actinomyces israelii.* A biopsy may be performed to remove a sample of the infected tissue. This procedure can be performed under **local anesthesia** in the doctor's office. Occasionally the bacteria can be cultured from the sinus tract fluid or from samples of the infected tissue.

Actinomycosis in the lungs, abdomen, pelvis, or brain can be very hard to diagnose since the symptoms often mimic those of other diseases. Actinomycosis

---

of the lungs or abdomen can resemble **tuberculosis** or cancer. Diagnostic x-ray results, the presence of draining sinus tracts, and microscopic analysis and culturing of infected tissue assist in the diagnosis.

Treatment

Actinomycosis is difficult to treat because of its dense tissue location. Surgery is often required to drain the lesion and/or to remove the site of infection. To kill the bacteria, standard therapy has included large doses of penicillin given through a vein daily for two to six weeks followed by six to twelve months of penicillin taken by mouth. Tetracycline, clindamycin, or erythromycin may be used instead of penicillin. The antibiotic therapy must be completed to ensure that the infection does not return. However, a report in 2004 on several cases of actinomycosis said that therapy depends on the individual case and that many patients today will be diagnosed in earlier stages of the disease. Sometimes, shorter courses of antibiotic treatment are effective, with close diagnostic x-ray monitoring. Hyperbaric oxygen (oxygen under high pressure) therapy in combination with the antibiotic therapy has been successful.

Prognosis

Complete recovery is achieved following treatment. If left untreated, the infection may cause localized bone destruction.

Prevention

The best prevention is to maintain good dental hygiene.

Resources

PERIODICALS

Sudhaker, Selvin S., and John J. Rose. "Short-term Treatment of Actinomycosis: two Cases and a Review." *Clinical Infectious Diseases* (February 1, 2004): 444–448.

Belinda Rowland, PhD
Teresa G. Odle

Activated charcoal *see* **Charcoal, activated**

Activated partial thromboplastin time *see* **Partial thromboplastin time**

Acupressure

Definition

Acupressure is a form of touch therapy that utilizes the principles of **acupuncture** and Chinese medicine. In acupressure, the same points on the body are used as in acupuncture, but are stimulated with finger pressure instead of with the insertion of needles. Acupressure is used to relieve a variety of symptoms and **pain**.

Purpose

Acupressure massage performed by a therapist can be very effective both as prevention and as a treatment for many health conditions, including headaches, general aches and pains, colds and flu, arthritis, **allergies**, asthma, nervous tension, menstrual cramps, sinus problems, **sprains**, tennis elbow, and toothaches, among others. Unlike acupuncture which requires a visit to a professional, acupressure can be performed by a layperson. Acupressure techniques are fairly easy to learn, and have been used to provide quick, cost-free, and effective relief from many symptoms. Acupressure points can also be stimulated to increase energy and feelings of well-being, reduce stress, stimulate the immune system, and alleviate **sexual dysfunction**.

Description

Origins

One of the oldest text of Chinese medicine is the *Huang Di*, The Yellow Emperor's Classic of Internal Medicine, which may be at least 2,000 years old. Chinese medicine has developed acupuncture, acupressure, herbal remedies, diet, **exercise**, lifestyle changes, and other remedies as part of its healing methods. Nearly all of the forms of Oriental medicine that are used in the West today, including acupuncture, acupressure, **shiatsu**, and Chinese herbal medicine, have their roots in Chinese medicine. One legend has it that acupuncture and acupressure evolved as early Chinese healers studied the puncture **wounds** of Chinese warriors, noting that certain points on the body created interesting results when stimulated. The oldest known text specifically on acupuncture points, the *Systematic Classic of Acupuncture*, dates back to 282 A.D. Acupressure is the non-invasive form of acupuncture, as Chinese physicians determined that stimulating points on the body with massage and pressure could be effective for treating certain problems.

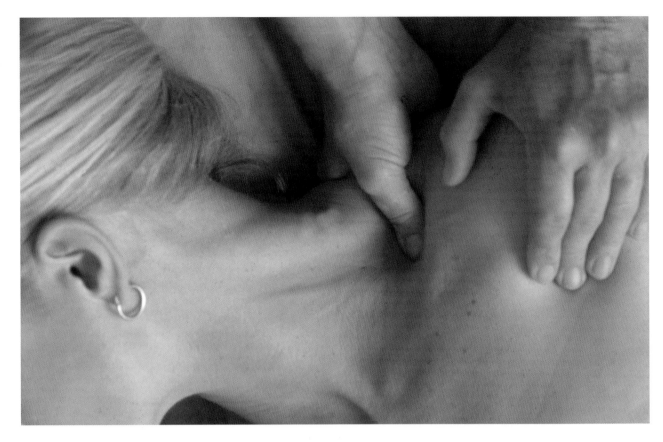

Therapist working acupressure points on a woman's shoulder. *(Photo Researchers, Inc. Reproduced by permission.)*

Outside of Asian-American communities, Chinese medicine remained virtually unknown in the United States until the 1970s, when Richard Nixon became the first U.S. president to visit China. On Nixon's trip, journalists were amazed to observe major operations being performed on patients without the use of anesthetics. Instead, wide-awake patients were being operated on, with only acupuncture needles inserted into them to control pain. At that time, a famous columnist for the *New York Times*, James Reston, had to undergo surgery and elected to use acupuncture for anesthesia. Later, he wrote some convincing stories on its effectiveness. Despite being neglected by mainstream medicine and the American Medical Association (AMA), acupuncture and Chinese medicine became a central to alternative medicine practitioners in the United States. Today, there are millions of patients who attest to its effectiveness, and nearly 9,000 practitioners in all 50 states.

Acupressure is practiced as a treatment by Chinese medicine practitioners and acupuncturists, as well as by massage therapists. Most massage schools in American include acupressure techniques as part of

their bodywork programs. Shiatsu massage is very closely related to acupressure, working with the same points on the body and the same general principles, although it was developed over centuries in Japan rather than in China. **Reflexology** is a form of bodywork based on acupressure concepts. Jin Shin Do is a bodywork technique with an increasing number of practitioners in America that combines acupressure and shiatsu principles with **qigong**, Reichian theory, and **meditation**.

Acupressure and Chinese medicine

Chinese medicine views the body as a small part of the universe, subject to laws and principles of harmony and balance. Chinese medicine does not make as sharp a destinction as Western medicine does between mind and body. The Chinese system believes that emotions and mental states are every bit as influential on disease as purely physical mechanisms, and considers factors like work, environment, and relationships as fundamental to a patient's health. Chinese medicine also uses very different symbols and ideas to discuss the body and

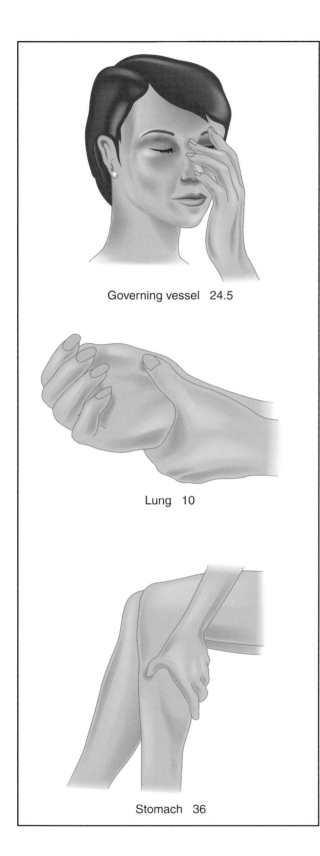

Governing vessel 24.5

Lung 10

Stomach 36

health. While Western medicine typically describes health as mainly physical processes composed of chemical equations and reactions, the Chinese use ideas like yin and yang, chi, and the organ system to describe health and the body.

Everything in the universe has properties of yin and yang. Yin is associated with cold, female, passive, downward, inward, dark, wet. Yang can be described as hot, male, active, upward, outward, light, dry, and so on. Nothing is either completely yin or yang. These two principles always interact and affect each other, although the body and its organs can become imbalanced by having either too much or too little of either.

Chi (pronounced *chee*, also spelled *qi* or *ki* in Japanese shiatsu) is the fundamental life energy. It is found in food, air, water, and sunlight, and it travels through the body in channels called *meridians*. There are 12 major meridians in the body that transport chi, corresponding to the 12 main organs categorized by Chinese medicine.

Disease is viewed as an imbalance of the organs and chi in the body. Chinese medicine has developed intricate systems of how organs are related to physical and mental symptoms, and it has devised corresponding treatments using the meridian and pressure point networks that are classified and numbered. The goal

Press on point governing vessel 24.5, the top of the bridge of the nose, lightly for two minutes to relieve hay fever symptoms. Press on lung 10, the center of the thumb pad, for one minute to alleviate a sore throat. To ease heartburn, apply pressure to stomach 36, four finger-widths below the kneecap outside the shinbone. Use on both legs. *(Illustration by Electronic Illustrators Group.)*

of acupressure, and acupuncture, is to stimulate and unblock the circulation of chi, by activating very specific points, called pressure points or *acupoints*. Acupressure seeks to stimulate the points on the chi meridians that pass close to the skin, as these are easiest to unblock and manipulate with finger pressure.

Acupressure can be used as part of a Chinese physician's prescription, as a session of massage therapy, or as a self-treatment for common aches and illnesses. A Chinese medicine practitioner examines a patient very thoroughly, looking at physical, mental and emotional activity, taking the pulse usually at the wrists, examining the tongue and complexion, and observing the patient's demeanor and attitude, to get a complete diagnosis of which organs and meridian points are out of balance. When the imbalance is located, the physician will recommend specific pressure points for acupuncture or acupressure. If acupressure is recommended, the patient might opt for a series of treatments from a massage therapist.

In **massage therapy**, acupressurists will evaluate a patient's symptoms and overall health, but a massage therapist's diagnostic training isn't as extensive as a Chinese physician's. In a massage therapy treatment, a person usually lies down on a table or mat, with thin clothing on. The acupressurist will gently feel and palpate the abdomen and other parts of the body to determine energy imbalances. Then, the therapist will work with different meridians throughout the body, depending on which organs are imbalanced in the abdomen. The therapist will use different types of finger movements and pressure on different acupoints, depending on whether the chi needs to be increased or dispersed at different points. The therapist observes and guides the energy flow through the patient's body throughout the session. Sometimes, special herbs (*Artemesia vulgaris* or moxa) may be placed on a point to warm it, a process called *moxibustion*. A session of acupressure is generally a very pleasant experience, and some people experience great benefit immediately. For more chronic conditions, several sessions may be necessary to relieve and improve conditions.

Acupressure massage usually costs from $30–70 per hour session. A visit to a Chinese medicine physician or acupuncturist can be more expensive, comparable to a visit to an allopathic physician if the practitioner is an MD. Insurance reimbursement varies widely, and consumers should be aware if their policies cover alternative treatment, acupuncture, or massage therapy.

Self-treatment

Acupressure is easy to learn, and there are many good books that illustrate the position of acupoints and meridians on the body. It is also very versatile, as it can be done anywhere, and it's a good form of treatment for spouses and partners to give to each other and for parents to perform on children for minor conditions.

While giving self-treatment or performing acupressure on another, a mental attitude of calmness and attention is important, as one person's energy can be used to help another's. Loose, thin clothing is recommended. There are three general techniques for stimulating a pressure point.

- Tonifying is meant to strengthen weak chi, and is done by pressing the thumb or finger into an acupoint with a firm, steady pressure, holding it for up to two minutes.

- Dispersing is meant to move stagnant or blocked chi, and the finger or thumb is moved in a circular motion or slightly in and out of the point for two minutes.

- Calming the chi in a pressure point utilizes the palm to cover the point and gently **stroke** the area for about two minutes.

There are many pressure points that are easily found and memorized to treat common ailments from headaches to colds.

- For headaches, toothaches, sinus problems, and pain in the upper body, the "LI4" point is recommended. It is located in the web between the thumb and index finger, on the back of the hand. Using the thumb and index finger of the other hand, apply a pinching pressure until the point is felt, and hold it for two minutes. Pregnant women should never press this point.

- To calm the nerves and stimulate digestion, find the "CV12" point that is four thumb widths above the navel in the center of the abdomen. Calm the point with the palm, using gentle stroking for several minutes.

- To stimulate the immune system, find the "TH5" point on the back of the forearm two thumb widths above the wrist. Use a dispersing technique, or circular pressure with the thumb or finger, for two minutes on each arm.

- For headaches, sinus congestion, and tension, locate the "GB20" points at the base of the skull in the back of the head, just behind the bones in back of the ears. Disperse these points for two minutes with the fingers or thumbs. Also find the "yintang" point, which is in the middle of the forehead between the eyebrows. Disperse it with gentle pressure for two minutes to clear the mind and to relieve headaches.

Precautions

Acupressure is a safe technique, but it is not meant to replace professional health care. A physician should always be consulted when there are doubts about medical conditions. If a condition is chronic, a professional should be consulted; purely symptomatic treatment can exacerbate chronic conditions. Acupressure should not be applied to open wounds, or where there is swelling and inflammation. Areas of scar tissue, blisters, boils, rashes, or **varicose veins** should be avoided. Finally, certain acupressure points should not be stimulated on people with high or low blood pressure and on pregnant women.

Research and general acceptance

In general, Chinese medicine has been slow to gain acceptance in the West, mainly because it rests on ideas very foreign to the scientific model. For instance, Western scientists have trouble with the idea of chi, the invisible energy of the body, and the idea that pressing on certain points can alleviate certain conditions seems sometimes too simple for scientists to believe.

Western scientists, in trying to account for the action of acupressure, have theorized that chi is actually part of the neuroendocrine system of the body. Celebrated orthopedic surgeon Robert O. Becker, who was twice nominated for the Nobel Prize, wrote a book on the subject called *Cross Currents: The Promise of Electromedicine; The Perils of Electropollution.* By using precise electrical measuring devices, Becker and his colleagues showed that the body has a complex web of electromagnetic energy, and that traditional acupressure meridians and points contained amounts of energy that non-acupressure points did not.

The mechanisms of acupuncture and acupressure remain difficult to document in terms of the biochemical processes involved; numerous testimonials are the primary evidence backing up the effectiveness of acupressure and acupuncture. However, a body of research is growing that verifies the effectiveness in acupressure and acupuncture techniques in treating many problems and in controlling pain.

Resources

PERIODICALS

Massage Therapy Journal. 820 Davis Street, Suite100, Evanston, IL 60201-4444.

OTHER

American Association of Oriental Medicine.December 28, 2000. < http://www.aaom.org > .

National Acupuncture and Oriental Medicine Alliance. December 28, 2000. < http://www.acuall.org > .

Douglas Dupler, MA

Acupressure, foot *see* **Reflexology**

Acupuncture

Definition

Acupuncture is one of the main forms of treatment in traditional Chinese medicine. It involves the use of sharp, thin needles that are inserted in the body at very specific points. This process is believed to adjust and alter the body's energy flow into healthier patterns, and is used to treat a wide variety of illnesses and health conditions.

Purpose

The World Health Organization (WHO) recommends acupuncture as an effective treatment for over forty medical problems, including **allergies**, respiratory conditions, gastrointestinal disorders, gynecological problems, nervous conditions, and disorders of the eyes, nose and throat, and childhood illnesses, among others. Acupuncture has been used in the treatment of **alcoholism** and **substance abuse**. It is an effective and low-cost treatment for headaches and chronic **pain**, associated with problems like back injuries and arthritis. It has also been used to supplement invasive Western treatments like **chemotherapy** and surgery. Acupuncture is generally most effective when used as prevention or before a health condition becomes acute, but it has been used to help patients suffering from **cancer** and AIDS. Acupuncture is limited in treating conditions or traumas that require surgery or emergency care (such as for broken bones).

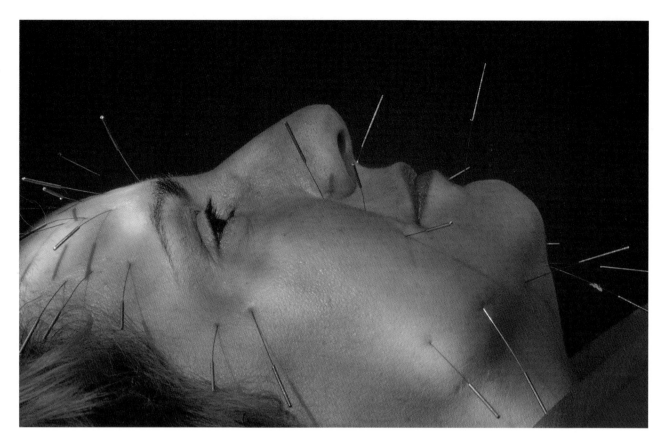

Woman undergoing facial acupuncture. *(Photograph by Yoav Levy. Phototake NYC. Reproduced by permission.)*

Description

Origins

The original text of Chinese medicine is the *Nei Ching, The Yellow Emperor's Classic of Internal Medicine*, which is estimated to be at least 2,500 years old. Thousands of books since then have been written on the subject of Chinese healing, and its basic philosophies spread long ago to other Asian civilizations. Nearly all of the forms of Oriental medicine which are used in the West today, including acupuncture, **shiatsu**, **acupressure** massage, and macrobiotics, are part of or have their roots in Chinese medicine. Legend has it that acupuncture developed when early Chinese physicians observed unpredicted effects of puncture **wounds** in Chinese warriors. The oldest known text on acupuncture, the *Systematic Classic of Acupuncture*, dates back to 282 A.D. Although acupuncture is its best known technique, Chinese medicine traditionally utilizes herbal remedies, dietary therapy, lifestyle changes and other means to treat patients.

In the early 1900s, only a few Western physicians who had visited China were fascinated by acupuncture, but outside of Asian-American communities it remained virtually unknown until the 1970s, when Richard Nixon became the first U.S. president to visit China. On Nixon's trip, journalists were amazed to observe major operations being performed on patients without the use of anesthetics. Instead, wide-awake patients were being operated on with only acupuncture needles inserted into them to control pain. During that time, a famous columnist for the *New York Times*, James Reston, had to undergo surgery and elected to use acupuncture instead of pain medication, and he wrote some convincing stories on its effectiveness.

Today, acupuncture is being practiced in all 50 states by over 9,000 practitioners, with over 4,000 MDs including it in their practices. Acupuncture has shown notable success in treating many conditions, and over 15 million Americans have used it as a therapy. Acupuncture, however, remains largely unsupported by the medical establishment. The American Medical Association has been resistant to researching it, as it is based on concepts very different from the Western scientific model.

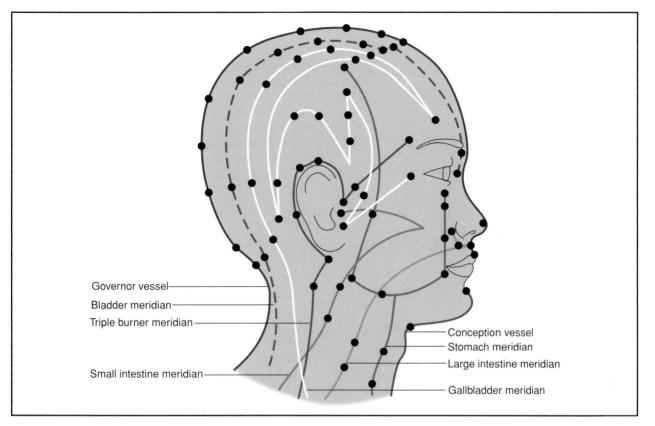

Governor vessel
Bladder meridian
Triple burner meridian

Conception vessel
Stomach meridian
Large intestine meridian

Small intestine meridian

Gallbladder meridian

Acupuncture sites and meridians on the face and neck. *(Illustration by Hans & Cassady.)*

Several forms of acupuncture are being used today in America. Japanese acupuncture uses extremely thin needles and does not incorporate herbal medicine in its practice. Auricular acupuncture uses acupuncture points only on the ear, which are believed to stimulate and balance internal organs. In France, where acupuncture is very popular and more accepted by the medical establishment, neurologist Paul Nogier developed a system of acupuncture based on neuroendocrine theory rather than on traditional Chinese concepts, which is gaining some use in America.

Basic ideas of Chinese medicine

Chinese medicine views the body as a small part of the universe, and subject to universal laws and principles of harmony and balance. Chinese medicine does not draw a sharp line, as Western medicine does, between mind and body. The Chinese system believes that emotions and mental states are every bit as influential on disease as purely physical mechanisms, and considers factors like work, environment, lifestyle and relationships as fundamental to the overall picture of a patient's health. Chinese medicine also uses very different symbols and ideas to discuss the body and health. While Western medicine typically describes health in terms of measurable physical processes made up of chemical reactions, the Chinese use ideas like yin and yang, chi, the organ system, and the five elements to describe health and the body. To understand the ideas behind acupuncture, it is worthwhile to introduce some of these basic terms.

YIN AND YANG. According to Chinese philosophy, the universe and the body can be described by two separate but complementary principles, that of yin and yang. For example, in temperature, yin is cold and yang is hot. In gender, yin is female and yang is male. In activity, yin is passive and yang is active. In light, yin is dark and yang is bright; in direction yin is inward and downward and yang is outward and up, and so on. Nothing is ever completely yin or yang, but a combination of the two. These two principles are always interacting, opposing, and influencing each other. The goal of Chinese medicine is not to eliminate either yin or yang, but to allow the two to balance each other and exist harmoniously together. For instance, if a person suffers from symptoms of high blood pressure, the Chinese system would say that the heart organ might have too much yang, and would recommend methods either to reduce the yang or to increase the yin of the heart, depending on the other symptoms and organs in the body. Thus, acupuncture therapies seek to either increase or reduce yang, or increase or reduce yin in particular regions of the body.

CHI. Another fundamental concept of Chinese medicine is that of chi (pronounced *chee*, also spelled *qi*). Chi is the fundamental life energy of the universe. It is invisible and is found in the environment in the air, water, food and sunlight. In the body, it is the invisible vital force that creates and animates life. We are all born with inherited amounts of chi, and we also get acquired chi from the food we eat and the air we breathe. The level and quality of a person's chi also depends on the state of physical, mental and emotional balance. Chi travels through the body along channels called *meridians*.

THE ORGAN SYSTEM. In the Chinese system, there are twelve main organs: the lung, large intestine, stomach, spleen, heart, small intestine, urinary bladder, kidney, liver, gallbladder, pericardium, and the "triple warmer," which represents the entire torso region. Each organ has chi energy associated with it, and each organ interacts with particular emotions on the mental level. As there are twelve organs, there are twelve types of chi which can move through the body, and these move through twelve main channels or meridians. Chinese doctors connect symptoms to organs. That is, symptoms are caused by yin/yang imbalances in one or more organs, or by an unhealthy flow of chi to or from one organ to another. Each organ has a different profile of symptoms it can manifest.

THE FIVE ELEMENTS. Another basis of Chinese theory is that the world and body are made up of five main elements: wood, fire, earth, metal, and water. These elements are all interconnected, and each element either generates or controls another element. For instance, water controls fire and earth generates metal. Each organ is associated with one of the five elements. The Chinese system uses elements and organs to describe and treat conditions. For instance, the kidney is associated with water and the heart is associated with fire, and the two organs are related as water and fire are related. If the kidney is weak, then there might be a corresponding fire problem in the heart, so treatment might be made by acupuncture or herbs to cool the heart system and/or increase energy in the kidney system.

The Chinese have developed an intricate system of how organs and elements are related to physical and mental symptoms, and the above example is a very simple one. Although this system sounds suspect to Western scientists, some interesting parallels have been observed. For instance, Western medicine has observed that with severe heart problems, kidney failure often follows, but it still does not know exactly why. In Chinese medicine, this connection between the two organs has long been established.

MEDICAL PROBLEMS AND ACUPUNCTURE. In Chinese medicine, disease as seen as imbalances in the organ system or chi meridians, and the goal of any remedy or treatment is to assist the body in reestablishing its innate harmony. Disease can be caused by internal factors like emotions, external factors like the environment and weather, and other factors like injuries, trauma, diet, and germs. However, infection is seen not as primarily a problem with germs and viruses, but as a weakness in the energy of the body which is allowing a sickness to occur. In Chinese medicine, no two illnesses are ever the same, as each body has its own characteristics of symptoms and balance. Acupuncture is used to open or adjust the flow of chi throughout the organ system, which will strengthen the body and prompt it to heal itself.

A VISIT TO THE ACUPUNCTURIST. The first thing an acupuncturist will do is get a thorough idea of a patient's medical history and symptoms, both physical and emotional. This is done with a long questionnaire and interview. Then the acupuncturist will examine the patient to find further symptoms, looking closely at the tongue, the pulse at various points in the body, the complexion, general behavior, and other signs like coughs or pains. From this, the practitioner will be able to determine patterns of symptoms which indicate which organs and areas are imbalanced. Depending on the problem, the acupuncturist will insert needles to manipulate chi on one or more of the twelve organ meridians. On these twelve meridians, there are nearly 2,000 points which can be used in acupuncture, with around 200 points being most frequently used by traditional acupuncturists. During an individual treatment, one to twenty needles may be used, depending on which meridian points are chosen.

Acupuncture needles are always sterilized and acupuncture is a very safe procedure. The depth of insertion of needles varies, depending on which chi channels are being treated. Some points barely go beyond superficial layers of skin, while some acupuncture points require a depth of 1-3 in (2.5-7.5 cm) of needle. The needles generally do not cause pain. Patients sometimes report pinching sensations and often pleasant sensations, as the body experiences healing. Depending on the problem, the acupuncturist might spin or move the needles, or even pass a slight electrical current through some of them. *Moxibustion* may be sometimes used, in which an herbal mixture (moxa or mugwort) is either burned like incense on the acupuncture point or on the end of the needle, which is believed to stimulate chi in a particular way. Also, acupuncturists sometimes use *cupping*, during which small suction cups are placed on meridian points to stimulate them.

How long the needles are inserted also varies. Some patients only require a quick in and out insertion to clear problems and provide *tonification* (strengthening of health), while some other conditions might require needles inserted up to an hour or more. The average visit to an acupuncturist takes about thirty minutes. The number of visits to the acupuncturist varies as well, with some conditions improved in one or two sessions and others requiring a series of six or more visits over the course of weeks or months.

Costs for acupuncture can vary, depending on whether the practitioner is an MD. Initial visits with non-MD acupuncturists can run from $50-$100, with follow-up visits usually costing less. Insurance reimbursement also varies widely, depending on the company and state. Regulations have been changing often. Some states authorize Medicaid to cover acupuncture for certain conditions, and some states have mandated that general coverage pay for acupuncture. Consumers should be aware of the provisions for acupuncture in their individual policies.

Precautions

Acupuncture is generally a very safe procedure. If a patient is in doubt about a medical condition, more than one physician should be consulted. Also, a patient should always feel comfortable and confident that their acupuncturist is knowledgable and properly trained.

Research and general acceptance

Mainstream medicine has been slow to accept acupuncture; although more MDs are using it, the American Medical Association does not recognize it as a specialty. The reason for this is that the mechanism of acupuncture is difficult to scientifically understand or measure, such as the invisible energy of chi in the body. Western medicine, admitting that acupuncture works in many cases, has theorized that the energy meridians are actually part of the nervous system and that acupuncture relieves pain by releasing endorphins, or natural pain killers, into the bloodstream. Despite the ambiguity in the biochemistry involved, acupuncture continues to show effectiveness in clinical tests, from reducing pain to alleviating the symptoms of chronic illnesses, and research in acupuncture is currently growing. The Office of Alternative Medicine of the National Institute of Health is currently funding research in the use of acupuncture for treating depression and attention-deficit disorder.

Resources

PERIODICALS

American Journal of Acupuncture. 1840 41st Ave., Suite 102, P.O. Box 610, Capitola, CA 95010.

OTHER

American Association of Oriental Medicine. December 28, 2000. < http://www.aaom.org > .

North American Society of Acupuncture and Alternative Medicine. December 28, 2000. < http://www.nasa-altmed.com > .

Douglas Dupler, MA

Acute glomerulonephritis *see* **Acute post-streptococcal glomerulonephritis**

Acute homeopathic remedies *see* **Homeopathic remedies, acute prescribing**

Acute kidney failure

Definition

Acute kidney failure occurs when illness, infection, or injury damages the kidneys. Temporarily, the kidneys cannot adequately remove fluids and wastes from the body or maintain the proper level of certain kidney-regulated chemicals in the bloodstream.

Description

The kidneys are the body's natural filtration system. They perform the critical task of processing approximately 200 quarts of fluid in the bloodstream every 24 hours. Waste products like urea and toxins, along with excess fluids, are removed from the bloodstream in the form of urine. Kidney (or renal) failure occurs when kidney functioning becomes impaired. Fluids and toxins begin to accumulate in the bloodstream. As fluids build up in the bloodstream, the patient with acute kidney failure may become puffy and swollen (edematous) in the face, hands, and feet. Their blood pressure typically begins to rise, and they may experience **fatigue** and **nausea**.

Unlike **chronic kidney failure**, which is long term and irreversible, acute kidney failure is a temporary condition. With proper and timely treatment, it can typically be reversed. Often there is no permanent damage to the kidneys. Acute kidney failure appears most frequently as a complication of serious illness, like heart failure, liver failure, **dehydration**, severe **burns**, and excessive bleeding (hemorrhage). It may also be caused by an obstruction to the urinary tract or as a direct result of **kidney disease**, injury, or an adverse reaction to a medicine.

Causes and symptoms

Acute kidney failure can be caused by many different illnesses, injuries, and infections. These conditions fall into three main categories: *prerenal*, *postrenal*, and *intrarenal* conditions.

Prerenal conditions do not damage the kidney, but can cause diminished kidney function. They are the most common cause of acute renal failure, and include:

- dehydration
- hemorrhage
- septicemia, or **sepsis**

- heart failure
- liver failure
- burns

Postrenal conditions cause kidney failure by obstructing the urinary tract. These conditions include:

- inflammation of the prostate gland in men (prostatitis)
- enlargement of the prostate gland (benign prostatic hypertrophy)
- bladder or pelvic tumors
- **kidney stones** (calculi)

Intrarenal conditions involve kidney disease or direct injury to the kidneys. These conditions include:

- lack of blood supply to the kidneys (ischemia)
- use of radiocontrast agents in patients with kidney problems
- drug **abuse** or overdose
- long-term use of nephrotoxic medications, like certain pain medicines
- acute inflammation of the glomeruli, or filters, of the kidney (**glomerulonephritis**)
- kidney infections (pyelitis or pyelonephritis).

Common symptoms of acute kidney failure include:

- anemia. The kidneys are responsible for producing erythropoietin (EPO), a hormone that stimulates red blood cell production. If kidney disease causes shrinking of the kidney, red blood cell production is reduced, leading to anemia.

- bad breath or bad taste in mouth. Urea in the saliva may cause an ammonia-like taste in the mouth.

- bone and joint problems. The kidneys produce vitamin D, which helps the body absorb calcium and keeps bones strong. For patients with kidney failure, bones may become brittle. In children, normal growth may be stunted. Joint **pain** may also occur as a result of high phosphate levels in the blood. Retention of uric acid may cause **gout**.

- edema. Puffiness or swelling in the arms, hands, feet, and around the eyes.

- frequent urination.

- foamy or bloody urine. Protein in the urine may cause it to foam significantly. Blood in the urine may indicate bleeding from diseased or obstructed kidneys, bladder, or ureters.

- headaches. High blood pressure may trigger headaches.

- hypertension, or high blood pressure. The retention of fluids and wastes causes blood volume to increase. This makes blood pressure rise.

- increased fatigue. Toxic substances in the blood and the presence of anemia may cause the patient to feel exhausted.

- itching. Phosphorus, normally eliminated in the urine, accumulates in the blood of patients with kidney failure. An increased phosphorus level may cause the skin to itch.

- lower back pain. Patients suffering from certain kidney problems (like kidney stones and other obstructions) may have pain where the kidneys are located, in the small of the back below the ribs.

- nausea. Urea in the gastric juices may cause upset stomach.

Diagnosis

Kidney failure is diagnosed by a doctor. A nephrologist, a doctor that specializes in the kidney, may be consulted to confirm the diagnosis and recommend treatment options. The patient that is suspected of having acute kidney failure will have blood and urine tests to determine the level of kidney function. A blood test will assess the levels of creatinine, blood urea nitrogen (BUN), uric acid, phosphate, sodium, and potassium. The kidney regulates these agents in the blood. Urine samples will also be collected, usually over a 24-hour period, to assess protein loss and/or creatinine clearance.

Determining the cause of kidney failure is critical to proper treatment. A full assessment of the kidneys is necessary to determine if the underlying disease is treatable and if the kidney failure is chronic or acute. X rays, **magnetic resonance imaging** (MRI), computed tomography scan (CT), ultrasound, renal biopsy, and/or arteriogram of the kidneys may be used to determine the cause of kidney failure and level of remaining kidney function. X rays and ultrasound of the bladder and/or ureters may also be needed.

Treatment

Treatment for acute kidney failure varies. Treatment is directed to the underlying, primary medical condition that has triggered kidney failure. Prerenal conditions may be treated with replacement fluids given through a vein, **diuretics**, blood transfusion, or medications. Postrenal conditions and intrarenal conditions may require surgery and/or medication.

Frequently, patients in acute kidney failure require *hemodialysis*, *hemofiltration*, or *peritoneal dialysis* to filter fluids and wastes from the bloodstream until the primary medical condition can be controlled.

Hemodialysis

Hemodialysis involves circulating the patient's blood outside of the body through an extracorporeal circuit (ECC), or dialysis circuit. The ECC is made up of plastic blood tubing, a filter known as a dialyzer (or artificial kidney), and a dialysis machine that monitors and maintains blood flow and administers dialysate. Dialysate is a sterile chemical solution that is used to draw waste products out of the blood. The patient's blood leaves the body through the vein and travels through the ECC and the dialyzer, where fluid removal takes place.

During dialysis, waste products in the bloodstream are carried out of the body. At the same time, electrolytes and other chemicals are added to the blood. The purified, chemically-balanced blood is then returned to the body.

A dialysis "run" typically lasts three to four hours, depending on the type of dialyzer used and the physical condition of the patient. Dialysis is used several times a week until acute kidney failure is reversed.

Blood pressure changes associated with hemodialysis may pose a risk for patients with heart problems. Peritoneal dialysis may be the preferred treatment option in these cases.

Hemofiltration

Hemofiltration, also called continuous renal replacement therapy (CRRT), is a slow, continuous blood filtration therapy used to control acute kidney failure in critically ill patients. These patients are typically very sick and may have heart problems or circulatory problems. They cannot handle the rapid filtration rates of hemodialysis. They also frequently need **antibiotics**, **nutrition**, vasopressors, and other fluids given through a vein to treat their primary condition. Because hemofiltration is continuous, prescription fluids can be given to patients in kidney failure without the risk of fluid overload.

Like hemodialysis, hemofiltration uses an ECC. A hollow fiber hemofilter is used instead of a dialyzer to remove fluids and toxins. Instead of a dialysis machine, a blood pump makes the blood flow through the ECC. The volume of blood circulating through the ECC in hemofiltration is less than that in hemodialysis. Filtration rates are slower and gentler on the circulatory system. Hemofiltration treatment will generally be used until kidney failure is reversed.

Peritoneal dialysis

Peritoneal dialysis may be used if an acute kidney failure patient is stable and not in immediate crisis. In peritoneal dialysis (PD), the lining of the patient's abdomen, the peritoneum, acts as a blood filter. A flexible tube-like instrument (catheter) is surgically inserted into the patient's abdomen. During treatment, the catheter is used to fill the abdominal cavity with dialysate. Waste products and excess fluids move from the patient's bloodstream into the dialysate solution. After a certain time period, the waste-filled dialysate is drained from the abdomen, and replaced with clean dialysate. There are three type of peritoneal dialysis, which vary according to treatment time and administration method.

Peritoneal dialysis is often the best treatment option for infants and children. Their small size can make vein access difficult to maintain. It is not recommended for patients with abdominal adhesions or other abdominal defects (like a **hernia**) that might reduce the efficiency of the treatment. It is also not recommended for patients who suffer frequent bouts of an inflammation of the small pouches in the intestinal tract (**diverticulitis**).

Prognosis

Because many of the illnesses and underlying conditions that often trigger acute kidney failure are critical, the prognosis for these patients many times is not good. Studies have estimated overall **death** rates for acute kidney failure at 42-88%. Many people, however, die because of the primary disease that has caused the kidney failure. These figures may also be misleading because patients who experience kidney failure as a result of less serious illnesses (like kidney stones or dehydration) have an excellent chance of complete recovery. Early recognition and prompt, appropriate treatment are key to patient recovery.

Up to 10% of patients who experience acute kidney failure will suffer irreversible kidney damage. They will eventually go on to develop chronic kidney failure or end-stage renal disease. These patients will require long-term dialysis or kidney transplantation to replace their lost renal functioning.

Prevention

Since acute kidney failure can be caused by many things, prevention is difficult. Medications that may impair kidney function should be given cautiously. Patients with pre-existing kidney conditions who are hospitalized for other illnesses or injuries should be carefully monitored for kidney failure complications. Treatments and procedures that may put them at risk for kidney failure (like diagnostic tests requiring radiocontrast agents or dyes) should be used with extreme caution.

Resources

PERIODICALS

Stark, June. "Dialysis Choices: Turning the Tide in Acute Renal Failure." *Nursing* 27, no. 2 (February 1997): 41-8.

ORGANIZATIONS

National Kidney Foundation. 30 East 33rd St., New York, NY 10016. (800) 622-9010. < http://www.kidney.org > .

Paula Anne Ford-Martin

Acute leukemias *see* **Leukemias, acute**

Acute lymphangitis

Definition

Acute lymphangitis is a bacterial infection in the lymphatic vessels which is characterized by painful, red streaks below the skin surface. This is a potentially serious infection which can rapidly spread to the bloodstream and be fatal.

Description

Acute lymphangitis affects a critical member of the immune system–the lymphatic system. Waste materials from nearly every organ in the body drain into the lymphatic vessels and are filtered in small organs called lymph nodes. Foreign bodies, such as bacteria or viruses, are processed in the lymph nodes to generate an immune response to fight an infection.

In acute lymphangitis, bacteria enter the body through a cut, scratch, insect bite, surgical wound, or other skin injury. Once the bacteria enter the lymphatic system, they multiply rapidly and follow the lymphatic vessel like a highway. The infected lymphatic vessel becomes inflamed, causing red streaks that are visible below the skin surface. The growth of the bacteria occurs so rapidly that the immune system does not respond fast enough to stop the infection.

If left untreated, the bacteria can cause tissue destruction in the area of the infection. A pus-filled, painful lump called an **abscess** may be formed in the infected area. **Cellulitis**, a generalized infection of the lower skin layers, may also occur. In addition, the bacteria may invade the bloodstream and cause septicemia. Lay people, for that reason, often call the red streaks seen in the skin "blood poisoning." Septicemia is a very serious illness and may be fatal.

Causes and symptoms

Acute lymphangitis is most often caused by the bacterium *Streptococcus pyogenes*. This potentially dangerous bacterium also causes strep throat, infections of the heart, spinal cord, and lungs, and in the 1990s has been called the "flesh-eating bacterium." Staphylococci bacteria may also cause lymphangitis.

Although anyone can develop lymphangitis, some people are more at risk. People who have had radical **mastectomy** (removal of a breast and nearby lymph nodes), a leg vein removed for coronary bypass surgery, or recurrent lymphangitis caused by tinea pedis (a fungal infection on the foot) are at an increased risk for lymphangitis.

The characteristic symptoms of acute lymphangitis are the wide, red streaks which travel from the site of infection to the armpit or groin. The affected areas are red, swollen, and painful. Blistering of the affected skin may occur. The bacterial infection causes a **fever** of 100-104 °F (38-40 °C). In addition, a general ill feeling, muscle aches, **headache**, chills, and loss of appetite may be felt.

Diagnosis

If lymphangitis is suspected, the person should call his or her doctor immediately or go to an emergency room. Acute lymphangitis could be diagnosed by the family doctor, infectious disease specialist, or an emergency room doctor. The painful, red streaks just below the skin surface and the high fever are diagnostic of acute lymphangitis. A sample of blood would be taken for culture to determine whether the bacteria have entered the bloodstream. A biopsy (removal of a piece of infected tissue) sample may be taken for culture to identify which type of bacteria is causing the infection. Diagnosis is immediate because it is based primarily on the symptoms. Most insurance policies should cover the expenses for the diagnosis and treatment of acute lymphangitis.

Treatment

Because of the serious nature of this infection, treatment would begin immediately even before the bacterial culture results were available. The only treatment for acute lymphangitis is to give very large doses of an antibiotic, usually penicillin, through the vein. Growing streptococcal bacteria are usually eliminated rapidly and easily by penicillin. The antibiotic clindamycin may be included in the treatment to kill any streptococci which are not growing and are in a resting state.

Alternatively, a "broad spectrum" antibiotic may be used which would kill many different kinds of bacteria.

Prognosis

Complete recovery is expected if antibiotic treatment is begun at an early stage of the infection. However, if untreated, acute lymphangitis can be a very serious and even deadly disease. Acute lymphangitis that goes untreated can spread, causing tissue damage. Extensive tissue damage would need to be repaired by **plastic surgery**. Spread of the infection into the bloodstream could be fatal.

Prevention

Although acute lymphangitis can occur in anyone, good hygiene and general health may help to prevent infections.

Resources

PERIODICALS

Dajer, Tony. "A Lethal Scratch." *Discover* (February 1998): 34-7.

Belinda Rowland, PhD

Acute pericarditis *see* **Pericarditis**

Acute poststreptococcal glomerulonephritis

Definition

Acute poststreptococcal **glomerulonephritis** (APSGN) is an inflammation of the kidney tubules (glomeruli) that filter waste products from the blood, following a streptococcal infection such as **strep throat**. APSGN is also called postinfectious glomerulonephritis.

Description

APSGN develops after certain streptococcal bacteria (group A beta-hemolytic streptococci) have infected the skin or throat. Antigens from the dead streptococci clump together with the antibodies that killed them. These clumps are trapped in the kidney tubules, cause the tubules to become inflamed, and impair that organs' ability to filter and eliminate body wastes. The onset of APSGN usually occurs

one to six weeks (average two weeks) after the streptococcal infection.

APSGN is a relatively uncommon disease affecting about one of every 10,000 people, although four or five times that many may actually be affected by it but show no symptoms. APSGN is most prevalent among boys between the ages of 3 and 7, but it can occur at any age.

Causes and symptoms

Frequent sore throats and a history of streptococcal infection increase the risk of acquiring APSGN. Symptoms of APSGN include:

- fluid accumulation and tissue swelling (**edema**) initially in the face and around the eyes, later in the legs
- low urine output (oliguria)
- blood in the urine (hematuria)
- protein in the urine (proteinuria)
- high blood pressure
- joint **pain** or stiffness

Diagnosis

Diagnosis of APSGN is made by taking the patient's history, assessing his/her symptoms, and performing certain laboratory tests. **Urinalysis** usually shows blood and protein in the urine. Concentrations of urea and creatinine (two waste products normally filtered out of the blood by the kidneys) in the blood are often high, indicating impaired kidney function. A reliable, inexpensive blood test called the anti-streptolysin-O test can confirm that a patient has or has had a streptococcal infection. A throat culture may also show the presence of group A beta-hemolytic streptococci.

Treatment

Treatment of ASPGN is designed to relieve the symptoms and prevent complications. Some patients are advised to stay in bed until they feel better and to restrict fluid and salt intake. Antibiotics may be prescribed to kill any lingering streptococcal bacteria, if their presence is confirmed. Antihypertensives may be given to help control high blood pressure and **diuretics** may be used to reduce fluid retention and swelling. **Kidney dialysis** is rarely needed.

Prognosis

Most children (up to 95%) fully recover from APSGN in a matter of weeks or months. Most adults (up to 70%) also recover fully. In those who do not recover fully, chronic or progressive problems of kidney function may occur. Kidney failure may result in some patients.

Prevention

Receiving prompt treatment for **streptococcal infections** may prevent APSGN.

Resources

BOOKS

Fauci, Anthony S., et al., editors. *Harrison's Principles of Internal Medicine.* New York: McGraw-Hill, 1997.

ORGANIZATIONS

American Kidney Fund (AKF). Suite 1010, 6110 Executive Boulevard, Rockville, MD 20852. (800) 638-8299. < http://216.248.130.102/Default.htm > .

National Kidney Foundation. 30 East 33rd St., New York, NY 10016. (800) 622-9010. < http://www.kidney.org > .

Maureen Haggerty

Acute respiratory distress syndrome *see* **Adult respiratory distress syndrome**

Acute stress disorder

Definition

Acute **stress** disorder (ASD) is an **anxiety** disorder characterized by a cluster of dissociative and anxiety symptoms occurring within one month of a traumatic event. (Dissociation is a psychological reaction to trauma in which the mind tries to cope by "sealing off" some features of the trauma from conscious awareness).

KEY TERMS

Depersonalization—A dissociative symptom in which the patient feels that his or her body is unreal, is changing, or is dissolving.

Derealization—A dissociative symptom in which the external environment is perceived as unreal.

Dissociation—A reaction to trauma in which the mind splits off certain aspects of the trauma from conscious awareness. Dissociation can affect the patient's memory, sense of reality, and sense of identity.

Trauma—In the context of ASD, a disastrous or life-threatening event.

Description

Acute stress disorder is a new diagnostic category that was introduced in 1994 to differentiate time-limited reactions to trauma from **post-traumatic stress disorder** (PTSD).

Causes and symptoms

Acute stress disorder is caused by exposure to trauma, which is defined as a stressor that causes intense fear and, usually, involves threats to life or serious injury to oneself or others. Examples are **rape**, mugging, combat, natural disasters, etc.

The symptoms of stress disorder include a combining of one or more dissociative and anxiety symptoms with the avoidance of reminders of the traumatic event. Dissociative symptoms include emotional detachment, temporary loss of memory, depersonalization, and derealization.

Anxiety symptoms connected with acute stress disorder include irritability, physical restlessness, sleep problems, inability to concentrate, and being easily startled.

Diagnosis

Diagnosis of acute stress disorder is based on a combination of the patient's history and a **physical examination** to rule out diseases that can cause anxiety. The essential feature is a traumatic event within one month of the onset of symptoms. Other diagnostic criteria include:

- The symptoms significantly interfere with normal social or vocational functioning

- The symptoms last between two days and four weeks.

Treatment

Treatment for acute stress disorder usually includes a combination of antidepressant medications and short-term psychotherapy.

Prognosis

The prognosis for recovery is influenced by the severity and duration of the trauma, the patient's closeness to it, and the patient's previous level of functioning. Favorable signs include a short time period between the trauma and onset of symptoms, immediate treatment, and appropriate social support. If the patient's symptoms are severe enough to interfere with normal life and have lasted longer than one month, the diagnosis may be changed to PTSD. If the symptoms have lasted longer than one month but are not severe enough to meet the definition of PTSD, the diagnosis may be changed to adjustment disorder.

Patients who do not receive treatment for acute stress disorder are at increased risk for **substance abuse** or major **depressive disorders**.

Prevention

Traumatic events cannot usually be foreseen and, thus, cannot be prevented. However, in theory, professional intervention soon after a major trauma might reduce the likelihood or severity of ASD. In addition, some symptoms of acute stress disorder result from biochemical changes in the central nervous system, muscles, and digestive tract that are not subject to conscious control.

Resources

BOOKS

Corbman, Gene R. "Anxiety Disorders." In *Current Diagnosis*, edited by Rex B. Conn, et al. Vol. 9. Philadelphia: W. B. Saunders Co., 1997.

Eisendrath, Stuart J. "Psychiatric Disorders." In *Current Medical Diagnosis and Treatment, 1998*, edited by Stephen McPhee, et al., 37th ed. Stamford: Appleton & Lange, 1997.

Rebecca J. Frey, PhD

Acute stress gastritis *see* **Gastritis**

Acute transverse myelitis *see* **Transverse myelitis**

Acyclovir *see* **Antiviral drugs**

Addiction

Definition

Addiction is a persistent, compulsive dependence on a behavior or substance. The term has been partially replaced by the word *dependence* for **substance abuse**. Addiction has been extended, however, to include mood-altering behaviors or activities. Some researchers speak of two types of addictions: substance addictions (for example, **alcoholism**, drug **abuse**, and **smoking**); and process addictions (for example, gambling, spending, shopping, eating, and sexual activity). There is a growing recognition that many addicts, such as polydrug abusers, are addicted to more than one substance or process.

Description

Addiction is one of the most costly public health problems in the United States. It is a progressive syndrome, which means that it increases in severity over time unless it is treated. Substance abuse is characterized by frequent relapse, or return to the abused substance. Substance abusers often make repeated attempts to quit before they are successful.

The economic cost of substance abuse in the United States exceeds $414 billion, with health care costs attributed to substance abuse estimated at more than $114 billion.

By eighth grade, 52% of adolescents have consumed alcohol, 41% have smoked tobacco, and 20% have smoked **marijuana**. Compared to females, males are almost four times as likely to be heavy drinkers, nearly one and a half more likely to smoke a pack or more of cigarettes daily, and twice as likely to smoke marijuana weekly. However, among adolescents these gender differences are not as pronounced and girls are almost as likely to abuse substances such as alcohol and cigarettes. Although frequent use of tobacco, **cocaine** and heavy drinking appears to remain stable in the 1990s, marijuana use has increased.

An estimated four million Americans over the age of 12 used prescription **pain** relievers, sedatives, and stimulants for "nonmedical" reasons during one month.

In the United States, 25% of the population regularly uses tobacco. Tobacco use reportedly kills 2.5 times as many people each year as alcohol and drug abuse combined. According to data from the World

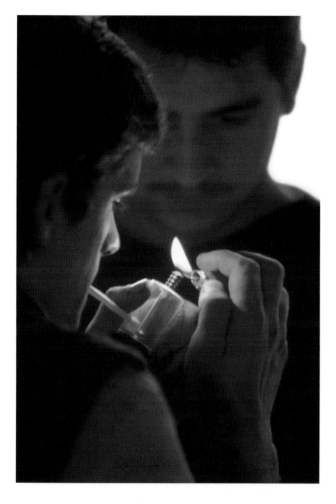

Crack users. Crack, a form of cocaine, is one of the most addictive drugs. *(Photograph by Roy Marsch, The Stock Market. Reproduced by permission.)*

Health Organization, there were 1.1 billion smokers worldwide and 10,000 tobacco-related deaths per day. Furthermore, in the United States, 43% of children aged 2-11 years are exposed to environmental tobacco smoke, which has been implicated in **sudden infant death syndrome**, low birth weight, **asthma**, middle ear disease, **pneumonia**, **cough**, and upper respiratory infection.

Eating disorders, such as **anorexia nervosa**, **bulimia nervosa**, and binge eating, affect more than five million American women and men. Fifteen percent of young women have substantially disordered attitudes toward eating and eating behaviors. More than 1,000 women die each year from anorexia nervosa.

A Harvard study found that an estimated 15.4 million Americans suffered from a gambling addiction. More than one-half (7.9 million) were adolescents.

Causes and symptoms

Addiction to substances results from the interaction of several factors:

Drug chemistry

Some substances are more addictive than others, either because they produce a rapid and intense change in mood; or because they produce painful withdrawal symptoms when stopped suddenly.

Genetic factor

Some people appear to be more vulnerable to addiction because their body chemistry increases their sensitivity to drugs. Some forms of **substance abuse and dependence** seem to run in families; and this may be the result of a genetic predisposition, environmental influences, or a combination of both.

Brain structure and function

Using drugs repeatedly over time changes brain structure and function in fundamental and long-lasting ways. Addiction comes about through an array of changes in the brain and the strengthening of new memory connections. Evidence suggests that those long-lasting brain changes are responsible for the distortions of cognitive and emotional functioning that characterize addicts, particularly the compulsion to use drugs. Although the causes of addiction remain the subject of ongoing debate and research, many experts now consider addiction to be a brain disease: a condition caused by persistent changes in brain structure and function. However, having this brain disease does not absolve the addict of responsibility for his or her behavior, but it does explain why many addicts cannot stop using drugs by sheer force of will alone.

Scientists may have come closer to solving the brain's specific involvement in addiction in 2004. Psychiatrists say they have found the craving center of the brain that triggers relapse in addicts. The anterior cingulated cortex in the frontal lobe of the brain is the area responsible for long-term craving in addicts. Knowing the area of the brain from which long-term cravings come may help scientists pinpoint therapies.

Social learning

Social learning is considered the most important single factor in addiction. It includes patterns of use in the addict's family or subculture, peer pressure, and advertising or media influence.

Availability

Inexpensive or readily available tobacco, alcohol, or drugs produce marked increases in rates of addiction.

Individual development

Before the 1980s, the so-called addictive personality was used to explain the development of addiction. The addictive personality was described as escapist, impulsive, dependent, devious, manipulative, and self-centered. Many doctors now believe that these character traits develop in addicts as a result of the addiction, rather than the traits being a cause of the addiction.

Diagnosis

In addition to a preoccupation with using and acquiring the abused substance, the diagnosis of addiction is based on five criteria:

- loss of willpower
- harmful consequences
- unmanageable lifestyle
- tolerance or escalation of use
- withdrawal symptoms upon quitting

Treatment

Treatment requires both medical and social approaches. Substance addicts may need hospital treatment to manage withdrawal symptoms. Individual or group psychotherapy is often helpful, but only after substance use has stopped. Anti-addiction medications, such as **methadone** and naltrexone, are also commonly used. A new treatment option has been developed that allows family physicians to treat heroine addiction from their offices rather than sending patients to methadone clinics. The drug is called buprenorphine (Suboxone).

Researchers continue to work to identify workable pharmacological treatments for various addictions. In 2004, clinical trials were testing a number of drugs currently in use for other diseases and conditions to see if they could be used to treat addiction. This would speed up their approval by the U.S. Food and Drug Administration (FDA). For example, cocaine withdrawal is eased by boosting dopamine levels in the brain, so scientists are studying drugs that boost dopamine, such as Ritalin, which is used to treat attention-deficit hyperactivity disorder, and amantadine, a drug used for flu and Parkinson's diease.

The most frequently recommended social form of outpatient treatment is the twelve-step program. Such programs are also frequently combined with psychotherapy. According to a recent study reported by the American Psychological Association (APA), anyone, regardless of his or her religious beliefs or lack of religious beliefs, can benefit from participation in 12-step programs such as Alcoholics Anonymous (AA) or **Narcotics** Anonymous (NA). The number of visits to 12-step self-help groups exceeds the number of visits to all mental health professionals combined. There are twelve-step groups for all major substance and process addictions.

The Twelve Steps are:

- Admit powerlessness over the addiction.
- Believe that a Power greater than oneself could restore sanity.
- Make a decision to turn your will and your life over to the care of God, as you understand him.
- Make a searching and fearless moral inventory of self.
- Admit to God, yourself, and another human being the exact nature of your wrongs.
- Become willing to have God remove all these defects from your character.
- Humbly ask God to remove shortcomings.
- Make a list of all persons harmed by your wrongs and become willing to make amends to them all.

- Make direct amends to such people, whenever possible except when to do so would injure them or others.

- Continue to take personal inventory and promptly admit any future wrongdoings.

- Seek to improve contact with a God of the individual's understanding through **meditation** and prayer.

- Carry the message of spiritual awakening to others and practice these principles in all your affairs.

Prognosis

The prognosis for recovery from any addiction depends on the substance or process, the individual's circumstances, and underlying personality structure. Polydrug users have the worst prognosis for recovery.

Prevention

The most effective form of prevention appears to be a stable family that models responsible attitudes toward mood-altering substances and behaviors. Prevention education programs are also widely used to inform the public of the harmfulness of substance abuse.

Resources

BOOKS

Robert Wood Johnson Foundation. *Substance Abuse: The Nation's #1 Problem.* Princeton, N.J., 2001.

PERIODICALS

Kalivas, Peter. "Drug Addiction: To the Cortex . . . and Beyond." *The American Journal of Psychiatry* 158, no. 3 (March 2001).

Kelly, Timothy. "Addiction: A Booming $800 Billion Industry." *The World and I* (July 1, 2000).

Leshner, Alan. "Addiction is a Brain Disease." *Issues in Science and Technology* 17, no. 3 (April 1, 2001).

"A New Office-based Treatment for Prescription Drug and Heroin Addiction." *Biotech Week* (August 4, 2004): 219.

"Research Brief: Source of Addiction Identified." *GP* (July 19, 2004): 4.

"Scientists May Use Existing Drugs to Stop Addiction." *Life Science Weekly* (Sepember 21, 2004): 1184.

ORGANIZATIONS

Al-Anon Family Groups. Box 182, Madison Square Station, New York, NY 10159. < http://www.Al-Anon Alateen.org > .

Alcoholics Anonymous World Services, Inc. Box 459, Grand Central Station, New York, NY 10163. < http://www.alcoholics-anonymous.org > .

American Anorexia Bulimina Association. < http://www.aabainc.org > .

American Psychiatric Association. < http://www.pscyh.org > .

Center for On-Line Addiction. < http://www.netaddiction.com > .

eGambling: Electronic Journal of Gambling Issues. < http://www.camh.net/egambling/main.html > .

National Alliance on Alcoholism and Drug Dependence, Inc. 12 West 21st St., New York, NY 10010. (212) 206-6770.

National Center on Addiction and Substance Abuse at Columbia University. < http://www.casacolumbia.org > .

National Clearinghouse for Alcohol and Drug Information. < http://www.health.org > .

National Institute on Alcohol Abuse and Alcoholism (NIAAA). 6000 Executive Boulevard, Bethesda, Maryland 20892-7003. < http://www.niaaa.nih.gov > .

Bill Asenjo, MS, CRC
Teresa G. Odle

Addison's disease

Definition

Addison's disease is a disorder involving disrupted functioning of the part of the adrenal gland called the cortex. This results in decreased production of two important chemicals (hormones) normally released by the adrenal cortex: cortisol and aldosterone.

Description

The adrenals are two glands, each perched on the upper part of the two kidneys. The outer part of the gland is known as the cortex; the inner part is known as the medulla. Each of these parts of the adrenal gland is responsible for producing different types of hormones.

Cortisol is a very potent hormone produced by the adrenal cortex. It is involved in regulating the functioning of nearly every type of organ and tissue throughout the body, and is considered to be one of the few hormones absolutely necessary for life. Cortisol is involved in:

- the very complex processing and utilization of many nutrients, including sugars (carbohydrates), fats, and proteins

- the normal functioning of the circulatory system and the heart

- the functioning of muscles
- normal kidney function
- production of blood cells
- the normal processes involved in maintaining the skeletal system
- proper functioning of the brain and nerves
- the normal responses of the immune system

Aldosterone, also produced by the adrenal cortex, plays a central role in maintaining the appropriate proportions of water and salts in the body. When this balance is upset, the volume of blood circulating throughout the body will fall dangerously low, accompanied by a drop in blood pressure.

Addison's disease is also called primary adrenocortical insufficiency. In other words, some process interferes directly with the ability of the adrenal cortex to produce its hormones. Levels of both cortisol and aldosterone drop, and numerous functions throughout the body are disrupted.

Addison's disease occurs in about four in every 100,000 people. It strikes both men and women of all ages.

Causes and symptoms

The most common cause of Addison's disease is the destruction and/or shrinking (atrophy) of the adrenal cortex. In about 70% of all cases, this atrophy is believed to occur due to an autoimmune disorder. In an autoimmune disorder, the immune system of the body, responsible for identifying foreign invaders such as viruses or bacteria and killing them, accidentally begins to identify the cells of the adrenal cortex as foreign, and destroy them. In about 20% of all cases, destruction of the adrenal cortex is caused by **tuberculosis**. The remaining cases of Addison's disease may be caused by fungal infections, such as **histoplasmosis**, coccidiomycosis, and **cryptococcosis**, which affect the adrenal gland by producing destructive, tumor-like masses called granulomas; a disease called **amyloidosis**, in which a starchy substance called amyloid is deposited in abnormal places throughout the body, interfering with the function of whatever structure it is present within; or invasion of the adrenal glands by **cancer**.

In about 75% of all patients, Addison's disease tends to be a very gradual, slowly developing disease. Significant symptoms are not noted until about 90% of the adrenal cortex has been destroyed. The most common symptoms include **fatigue** and loss of energy, decreased appetite, **nausea**, **vomiting**, diarrhea, abdominal **pain**, weight loss, muscle weakness,

dizziness when standing, **dehydration**, unusual areas of darkened (pigmented) skin, and dark freckling. As the disease progresses, the patient may appear to have very tanned, or bronzed skin, with darkening of the lining of the mouth, vagina, and rectum, and dark pigmentation of the area around the nipples (aereola). As dehydration becomes more severe, the blood pressure will continue to drop and the patient will feel increasingly weak and light-headed. Some patients have psychiatric symptoms, including depression and irritability. Women lose pubic and underarm hair, and stop having normal menstrual periods.

When a patient becomes ill with an infection, or stressed by an injury, the disease may suddenly and rapidly progress, becoming life-threatening. Symptoms of this "Addisonian crisis" include abnormal heart rhythms, severe pain in the back and abdomen, uncontrollable **nausea and vomiting**, a drastic drop in blood pressure, kidney failure, and unconsciousness. About 25% of all Addison's disease patients are identified due to the development of Addisonian crisis.

Diagnosis

Many patients do not recognize the slow progression of symptoms and the disease is ultimately identified when a physician notices the areas of increased pigmentation of the skin. Once suspected, a number of blood tests can lead to the diagnosis of Addison's disease. It is not sufficient to demonstrate low blood cortisol levels, as normal levels of cortisol vary quite widely. Instead, patients are given a testing dose of another hormone called corticotropin (ACTH). ACTH is produced in the body by the pituitary gland, and normally acts by promoting growth within the adrenal cortex and stimulating the production and release of cortisol. In Addison's disease, even a dose of synthetic ACTH does not increase cortisol levels.

To distinguish between primary adrenocortical insufficiency (Addison's disease) and secondary adrenocortical insufficiency (caused by failure of the pituitary to produce enough ACTH), levels of ACTH in the blood are examined. Normal or high levels of ACTH indicate that the pituitary is working properly, but the adrenal cortex is not responding normally to the presence of ACTH. This confirms the diagnosis of Addison's disease.

Treatment

Treatment of Addison's disease involves replacing the missing or low levels of cortisol. In the case of Addisonian crisis, this will be achieved by injecting a potent form of steroid preparation through a needle placed in a vein (intravenous or IV). Dehydration and salt loss will also be treated by administering carefully balanced solutions through the IV. Dangerously low blood pressure may require special medications to safely elevate it until the steroids take effect.

Patients with Addison's disease will need to take a steroid preparation (hydrocortisone) and a replacement for aldosterone (fludrocortisone) by mouth for the rest of their lives. When a patient has an illness which causes nausea and vomiting (such that they cannot hold down their medications), he or she will need to enter a medical facility where IV medications can be administered. When a patient has any kind of infection or injury, the normal dose of hydrocortisone will need to be doubled.

Prognosis

Prognosis for patients appropriately treated with hydrocortisone and aldosterone is excellent. These patients can expect to enjoy a normal lifespan. Without treatment, or with substandard treatment, patients are always at risk of developing Addisonian crisis.

Resources

BOOKS

Williams, Gordon H., and Robert G. Dluhy. "Hypofunction of the Adrenal Cortex." In *Harrison's Principles of Internal Medicine*, edited by Anthony S. Fauci, et al. New York: McGraw-Hill, 1997.

ORGANIZATIONS

National Adrenal Disease Foundation. 505 Northern Boulevard, Suite 200, Great Neck, NY 11021. (516) 487-4992.

Rosalyn Carson-DeWitt, MD

Adenoid hyperplasia

Definition

Adenoid hyperplasia is the overenlargement of the lymph glands located above the back of the mouth.

Description

Located at the back of the mouth above and below the soft palate are two pairs of lymph glands. The tonsils below are clearly visible behind the back teeth; the adenoids lie just above them and are hidden from view by the palate. Together these four arsenals of immune defense guard the major entrance to the body from foreign invaders–the germs we breathe and eat. In contrast to the rest of the body's tissues, lymphoid tissue reaches its greatest size in mid-childhood and recedes thereafter. In this way children are best able to develop the immunities they need to survive in a world full of infectious diseases.

Beyond its normal growth pattern, lymphoid tissue grows excessively (hypertrophies) during an acute infection, as it suddenly increases its immune activity to fight off the invaders. Often it does not completely return to its former size. Each subsequent infection leaves behind a larger set of tonsils and adenoids. To make matters worse, the sponge-like structure of these hypertrophied glands can produce safe havens for germs where the body cannot reach and eliminate them. Before **antibiotics** and the reduction in infectious childhood diseases over the past few generations, tonsils and adenoids caused greater health problems.

Causes and symptoms

Most tonsil and adenoid hypertrophy is simply caused by the normal growth pattern for that type of tissue. Less often, the hypertrophy is due to repeated throat infections by cold viruses, strep throat, mononucleosis, and in times gone by, **diphtheria**. The acute infections are usually referred to as **tonsillitis**, the adenoids getting little recognition because they cannot be seen without special instruments. Symptoms include painful, bright red, often ulcerated tonsils, enlargement of lymph nodes (glands) beneath the jaw, **fever**, and general discomfort.

After the acute infection subsides, symptoms are generated simply by the size of the glands. Extremely large tonsils can impair breathing and swallowing, although that is quite rare. Large adenoids can impair nose breathing and require a child to breathe through the mouth. Because they encircle the only connection

KEY TERMS

Eustacian tube—A tube connecting the middle ear with the back of the nose, allowing air pressure to equalize within the ear whenever it opens, such as with yawning.

Hyperplastic—Overgrown.

Hypertrophy—Overgrowth.

Strep throat—An infection of the throat caused by bacteria of the *Streptococcus* family, which causes tonsillitis.

Ulcerated—Damaged so that the surface tissue is lost and/or necrotic (dead).

between the middle ear and the eustachian tube, hypertrophied adenoids can also obstruct it and cause middle ear infections.

Diagnosis

A simple tongue blade depressing the tongue allows an adequate view of the tonsils. Enlarged tonsils may have deep pockets (crypts) containing dead tissue (necrotic debris). Viewing adenoids requires a small mirror or fiberoptic scope. A child with recurring middle ear infections may well have large adenoids. A **throat culture** or mononucleosis test will usually reveal the identity of the germ.

Treatment

It used to be standard practice to remove tonsils and/or adenoids after a few episodes of acute throat or ear infection. The surgery is called **tonsillectomy** and adenoidectomy (T and A). Opinion changed as it was realized that this tissue is beneficial to the development of immunity. For instance, children without tonsils and adenoids produce only half the immunity to oral **polio** vaccine. In addition, treatment of ear and throat infections with antibiotics and of recurring ear infections with surgical drainage through the ear drum (tympanostomy) has greatly reduced the incidence of surgical removal of these lymph glands.

Alternative treatment

There are many botanical/herbal remedies that can be used alone or in formulas to locally assist the tonsils and adenoids in their immune function at the opening of the oral cavity and to tone these glands. Keeping the Eustachian tubes open is an important

contribution to optimal function in the tonsils and adenoids. **Food allergies** are often the culprits for recurring ear infections, as well as tonsilitis and adenoiditis. Identification and removal of the allergic food(s) can greatly assist in alleviating the cause of the problem. Acute tonsillitis also benefits from warm saline gargles.

Prognosis

Hypertrophied adenoids are a normal part of growing up and should be respected for their important role in the development of immunity. Only when their size causes problems by obstructing breathing or middle ear drainage do they demand intervention.

Prevention

Prevention can be directed toward prompt evaluation and appropriate treatment of sore throats to prevent overgrowth of adenoid tissue. Avoiding other children with acute respiratory illness will also reduce the spread of these common illnesses.

Resources

BOOKS

Behman, Richard E., editor. "Tonsils and Adenoids." In *Nelson Textbook of Pediatrics*. Philadelphia: W. B. Saunders Co., 1996.

J. Ricker Polsdorfer, MD

Adenoid hypertrophy *see* **Adenoid hyperplasia**

Adenoid removal *see* **Tonsillectomy and adenoidectomy**

Adenoidectomy *see* **Tonsillectomy and adenoidectomy**

Adenovirus infections

Definition

Adenoviruses are DNA viruses (small infectious agents) that cause upper respiratory tract infections, **conjunctivitis**, and other infections in humans.

Description

Adenoviruses were discovered in 1953. About 47 different types have been identified since then, and

KEY TERMS

Conjunctivitis—Inflammation of the conjunctiva, the mucous membrane lining the inner surfaces of the eyelid and the front of the eyeball.

Virus—A small infectious agent consisting of a core of genetic material (DNA or RNA) surrounded by a shell of protein.

about half of them are believed to cause human diseases. Infants and children are most commonly affected by adenoviruses. Adenovirus infections can occur throughout the year, but seem to be most common from fall to spring.

Adenoviruses are responsible for 3-5% of acute respiratory infections in children and 2% of respiratory illnesses in civilian adults. They are more apt to cause infection among military recruits and other young people who live in institutional environments. Outbreaks among children are frequently reported at boarding schools and summer camps. Another example includes an increased outbreak of **gastroenteritis** among cruise passengers in 2002.

Acquired immunity

Most children have been infected by at least one adenovirus by the time they reach school age. Most adults have acquired immunity to multiple adenovirus types due to infections they had as children.

In one mode of adenovirus infection (called lytic infection because it destroys large numbers of cells), adenoviruses kill healthy cells and replicate up to one million new viruses per cell killed (of which 1-5% are infectious). People with this kind of infection feel sick. In chronic or latent infection, a much smaller number of viruses are released and healthy cells can multiply more rapidly than they are destroyed. People who have this kind of infection don't seem to be sick. This is probably why many adults have immunity to adenoviruses without realizing they have been infected.

Childhood infections

In children, adenoviruses most often cause acute upper respiratory infections with fever and runny nose. Adenovirus types 1, 2, 3, 5, and 6 are responsible for most of these infections. Occasionally more serious lower respiratory diseases, such as **pneumonia**, may occur.

Adenoviruses also cause acute pharyngoconjunctival **fever** in children. This disease is most often caused

by types 3 and 7. Symptoms, which appear suddenly and usually disappear in less than a week, include:

- inflammation of the lining of the eyelid (conjunctivitis)
- fever
- sore throat (pharyngitis)
- runny nose
- inflammation of lymph glands in the neck (cervical adenitis)

Adenoviruses also cause acute **diarrhea** in young children, characterized by fever and watery stools. This condition is caused by adenovirus types 40 and 41 and can last as long as two weeks.

As much as 51% of all hemorrhagic **cystitis** (inflammation of the bladder and of the tubes that carry urine to the bladder from the kidneys) in American and Japanese children can be attributed to adenovirus infection. A child who has hemorrhagic cystitis has bloody urine for about three days, and invisible traces of blood can be found in the urine a few days longer. The child will feel the urge to urinate frequently–but find it difficult to do so–for about the same length of time.

Adult infections

In adults, the most frequently reported adenovirus infection is acute respiratory disease (ARD, caused by types 4 and 7) in military recruits. Influenza-like symptoms including fever, sore throat, runny nose, and **cough** are almost always present; weakness, chills, **headache**, and swollen lymph glands in the neck also may occur. The symptoms typically last three to five days.

Epidemic keratoconjunctivitis (EKC, caused by adenovirus types 8, 19, and 37) was first seen in shipyard workers whose eyes had been slightly injured by chips of rust or paint. This inflammation of tissues lining the eyelid and covering the front of the eyeball also can be caused by using contaminated contact lens solutions or by drying the hands or face with a towel used by someone who has this infection.

The inflamed, sticky eyelids characteristic of conjunctivitis develop 4-24 days after exposure and last between one and four weeks. Only 5-8% of patients with epidemic keratoconjunctivitis experience respiratory symptoms. One or both eyes may be affected. As symptoms of conjunctivitis subside, eye **pain** and watering and blurred vision develop. These symptoms of **keratitis** may last for several months, and about 10% of these infections spread to at least one other member of the patient's household.

Other illnesses associated with adenovirus include:

- encephalitis (inflammation of the brain) and other infections of the central nervous system (CNS)
- gastroenteritis (inflammation of the stomach and intestines)
- acute mesenteric **lymphadenitis** (inflammation of lymph glands in the abdomen)
- chronic interstitial fibrosis (abnormal growth of connective tissue between cells)
- intussusception (a type of intestinal obstruction)
- pneumonia that doesn't respond to antibiotic therapy
- **whooping cough** syndrome when *Bordetella pertussis* (the bacterium that causes classic whooping cough) is not found

Causes and symptoms

Specific adenovirus infections can be traced to particular sources and produce distinctive symptoms. In general, however, adenovirus infection is caused by:

- inhaling airborne viruses
- getting the virus in the eyes by swimming in contaminated water, using contaminated eye solutions or instruments, wiping the eyes with contaminated towels, or rubbing the eyes with contaminated fingers.
- not washing the hands after using the bathroom, and then touching the mouth or eyes

Symptoms common to most types of adenovirus infections include:

- cough
- fever
- runny nose
- sore throat
- watery eyes

Diagnosis

Although symptoms may suggest the presence of adenovirus, distinguishing these infections from other viruses can be difficult. A definitive diagnosis is based on culture or detection of the virus in eye secretions, sputum, urine, or stool.

The extent of infection can be estimated from the results of blood tests that measure increases in the quantity of antibodies the immune system produces to fight it. Antibody levels begin to rise about a week after infection occurs and remain elevated for about a year.

Treatment

Treatment of adenovirus infections is usually supportive and aimed at relieving symptoms of the illness. Bed rest may be recommended along with medications to reduce fever and/or pain. (Aspirin should not be given to children because of concerns about Reye's syndrome.) Eye infections may benefit from topical **corticosteroids** to relieve symptoms and shorten the course of the disease. Hospitalization is usually required for severe pneumonia in infants and for EKC (to prevent blindness). No effective **antiviral drugs** have been developed.

Prognosis

Adenovirus infections are rarely fatal. Most patients recover fully.

Prevention

Practicing good personal hygiene and avoiding people with infectious illnesses can reduce the risk of developing adenovirus infection. Proper handwashing can prevent the spread of the virus by oral-fecal transmission. Sterilization of instruments and solutions used in the eye can prevent the spread of EKC, as can adequate chlorination of swimming pools.

A vaccine for pertussis has been developed and is in use in combination with **diphtheria** and **tetanus** vaccines for infants. It is shown to have nearly 90% efficacy. A vaccine containing live adenovirus types 4 and 7 is used to control disease in military recruits, but it is not recommended or available for civilian use. A recent resurgence of the adenovirus was found in a military population as soon as the **vaccination** program was halted. Vaccines prepared from purified subunits of adenovirus are under investigation.

Resources

PERIODICALS

Evans, Jeff. "Viral Gastroenteritis On Board." *Internal Medicine News* (January 15, 2003): 44.

"Guard Against Pertussis." *Contemporary Pediatrics* (February 2003): 87.

Kolavic-Gray, Shellie A., et al. "Large Epidemic of Adenovirus Type 4 Infection Among Military Trainees: Epidemiological, Clinical, and Laboratory Studies." *Clinical Infectious Diseases* (October 1, 2002): 808–811.

Maureen Haggerty
Teresa G. Odle

Adhesions

Definition

Adhesions are fibrous bands of scar tissue that form between internal organs and tissues, joining them together abnormally.

Description

Adhesions are made up of blood vessels and fibroblasts—connective tissue cells. They form as a normal part of the body's healing process and help to limit the spread of infection. However when adhesions cause the wrong tissues to grow into each other, many different complex inflammatory disorders can arise. Worldwide millions of people suffer **pain** and dysfunction due to adhesion disease.

Depending on their location, the most common types of adhesions may called:

- abdominal adhesions
- intestinal adhesions
- intraperitoneal adhesions
- pelvic adhesions
- intrauterine adhesions or Asherman's syndrome.

Adhesions can form between various tissues in the body including:

- loops of the intestines
- the intestines and other abdominal organs or the abdominal wall
- abdominal organs such as the liver or bladder and the abdominal wall
- tissues of the uterus.

Although adhesions can be congenital (present at birth) or result from inflammation, injury, or infection, the vast majority of adhesions form following surgery. Adhesions are a major complication of many common surgical procedures and may occur in 55% to more than 90% of patients, depending on the type of surgery.

All abdominal surgeries carry the risk of adhesion formation. Abdominal adhesions are rare in people who have not had abdominal surgery and very common in people who have had multiple abdominal surgeries. Adhesions are more common following procedures involving the intestines, colon, appendix, or uterus. They are less common following surgeries involving the stomach, gall bladder, or pancreas.

KEY TERMS

Asherman's syndrome—The cessation of menstruation and/or infertility caused by intrauterine adhesions.

Computed axial tomography; CT or CAT scan—A computer reconstruction of scanned x rays used to diagnose intestinal obstructions.

Endometriosis—A condition in which the endometrial tissue that lines the uterus begins to invade other parts of the body.

Endoscope—A device with a light that is used to look into a body cavity or organ.

Fibroblast—A connective-tissue cell.

Glaucoma—A group of eye diseases characterized by increased pressure within the eye that can damage the optic nerve and cause gradual loss of vision.

Hysteroscopy—A procedure in which an endoscope is inserted through the cervix to view the cervix and uterus.

Hysterosalpingography; HSG—X raying of the uterus and fallopian tubes following the injection of a contrast dye.

Irido corneal endothelial syndrome; ICE—A type of glaucoma in which cells from the back of the cornea spread over the surface of the iris and tissue that drains the eye, forming adhesions that bind the iris to the cornea.

Laparoscopic surgery; keyhole surgery—Surgery that utilizes a laparoscope with a video camera and surgical instruments inserted through small incisions.

Laparoscopy—A procedure that utilizes an endoscope to view contents of the abdominal cavity.

Pelvic inflammatory disease; PID—Inflammation of the female reproductive organs and associated structures.

Peritoneum—The membrane lining the walls of the abdominal and pelvic cavities and enclosing their organs.

Small bowel obstruction; SBO—An obstruction of the small intestine that prevents the free passage of material; sometimes caused by postoperative adhesions.

Although most abdominal adhesions do not cause problems, they can be painful when stretched or pulled because the scar tissue is not elastic.

Postoperative intestinal adhesions are a major cause of intestinal or small bowel obstruction (SBO). In a small number of people the scar tissue pulls sections of the small or large intestines out of place and partially or completely blocks the passage of food and fluids. Thus SBOs can result from abdominal surgery and also are one of the most common reasons for abdominal surgery. Although intestinal obstruction is fatal in about 5% of patients, the mortality rate associated with SBO has decreased dramatically over the past century.

Intrauterine adhesions are relatively common in women and the majority of women undergoing gynecological surgery develop postoperative adhesions. Sometimes these pelvic adhesions cause chronic pelvic pain and/or **infertility**.

Adhesions can cause a rare form of **glaucoma** called irido corneal endothelial (ICE) syndrome. In this disorder cells from the back surface of the cornea of the eye spread over the surface of the iris and the tissue that drains the eye, forming adhesions that bind the iris to the cornea and causing further blockage of the drainage channels. This blockage increases the pressure inside the eye, which may damage the optic nerve. ICE syndrome occurs most often in light-skinned females.

Causes and symptoms

Post-surgical adhesions

Common causes of postoperative adhesions include:

- abdominal surgery
- gynecological surgery
- thoracic surgery
- orthopedic surgery
- plastic surgery.

Abdominal adhesions most often result from surgeries in which the organs are handled or temporarily moved. Intrauterine adhesions form after surgeries involving the uterus, particularly curettage—the scraping of the uterine contents. Surgery to control uterine bleeding after giving birth also can lead to intrauterine adhesions. Such adhesions can cause Asherman's syndrome, closing the uterus and preventing menstruation.

Other causes of adhesions

Any inflammation or infection of the membranes that line the abdominal and pelvic walls and enclose the organs—the peritoneum—can cause adhesions. An example **peritonitis**, a severe infection that can result from **appendicitis**, may lead to adhesions. In addition to surgery or injury, pelvic adhesions can be caused by inflammation resulting from an infection such as **pelvic inflammatory disease** (PID).

Symptoms

In the majority of people adhesions do not cause symptoms or serious problems. However in some people adhesions can lead to a variety of disorders. The symptoms depend on the type of adhesion and the tissues that are involved. Adhesions may cause pain and/or **fever** in some people.

ABDOMINAL OBSTRUCTION. If a loop of intestine becomes trapped under an adhesion, the intestine may become partially or completely blocked. The symptoms of intestinal obstruction or SBOs due to adhesions depend on the degree and location of the obstruction. Partial or off-and-on intestinal obstruction due to adhesions may result in intermittent periods of painful abdominal cramping and other symptoms, including **diarrhea**.

Symptoms of significant intestinal obstruction due to adhesions include:

- severe abdominal pain and cramping
- **nausea** and vomiting
- abdominal distension (swelling)
- constipation and the inability to pass gas
- symptoms of **dehydration**.

Symptoms of dehydration include:

- dry mouth and tongue
- severe thirst
- infrequent urination
- dry skin
- fast heart rate
- low blood pressure.

In about 10% of SBOs, part of the intestine twists tightly and repeatedly around a band of adhesions, cutting off the blood supply to the intestine and resulting in strangulation and death of the twisted bowel. The mortality rate for strangulation of the bowel may be as high as 37%.

Symptoms of bowel strangulation due to adhesions include:

- severe abdominal pain, either cramping or constant

- abdominal distension due to the inability to pass stool and gas

- an extremely tender abdomen

- signs of systemic (body-wide) illness, including fever, fast heart rate, and low blood pressure.

When a portion of the obstructed bowel begins to die from lack of blood flow, fluids and bacteria that help digest food can leak out of the intestinal wall and into the abdominal cavity causing peritonitis.

PELVIC ADHESIONS. Pelvic adhesions can interfere with the functioning of the ovaries and fallopian tubes and are among the common causes of female infertility. Adhesions on the ovaries or fallopian tubes can prevent **pregnancy** by trapping the released egg. Adhesions resulting from endometriosis can cause pelvic pain, particularly during menstruation, as well as fertility problems.

Diagnosis

Adhesions are diagnosed based on the symptoms, surgical history, and a **physical examination**. The physician examines the abdomen and rectum and performs a pelvic examination on women. Blood tests and chest and abdominal x rays are taken. Sometimes exploratory surgery is used to locate the adhesions and sources of pain.

Abdominal computed axial tomography—a CT or CAT scan—is the most common diagnostic tool for SBO and intestinal strangulation due to adhesions. In this procedure a computer reconstructs a portion of the abdomen from x-ray scans. Barium contrast x-ray studies also may be used to locate an obstruction. The ingestion of a barium solution provides better visualization of the abdominal organs. However sometimes intestinal obstruction or strangulation cannot be confirmed without abdominal surgery.

Exploratory **laparoscopy** may be used to detect either abdominal or pelvic adhesions. This procedure usually is performed in a hospital under local or **general anesthesia**. A small incision is made near the naval and carbon dioxide gas is injected to raise the abdominal wall. A tube called a trocar is inserted into the abdomen. The laparascope, equipped with a light and a small video camera, is passed through the trocar for visualization of the peritoneal cavity and the abdominal or pelvic organs.

Pelvic adhesions also may be detected by **hysteroscopy**. In this procedure a uterine endoscope is inserted through the cervix to visualize the cervix and uterine cavity. With **hysterosalpingography** (HSG) a radiopaque or contrast dye is injected through a catheter in the cervix and x rays are taken of the uterus and fallopian tubes.

Treatment

Although the symptoms of adhesion disease sometimes disappear on their own, adhesions are permanent without a surgical procedure called adhesion lysis to disrupt or remove the tissue.

Abdominal adhesions

Sometimes an adhesion-trapped intestine frees itself spontaneously. Surgery may be used to reposition the intestine to relieve symptoms. Various other techniques include using suction to decompress the intestine; however untreated intestinal adhesions may lead to bowel obstruction.

Although dilation with an endoscope may be used to widen the region around an intestinal obstruction to relieve symptoms, SBOs caused almost always require immediate surgery. In cases of a partial obstruction or a complete obstruction without severe symptoms, surgery may be delayed for 12–24 hours so that a dehydrated patient can be treated with intravenous fluids. A small suction tube may be placed through the nose into the stomach to remove the stomach contents to relieve pain and nausea and prevent further bloating.

If an adhesion-related SBO disrupts the blood supply to part of the intestine, gangrene—tissue death—can occur. Strangulation of the bowel usually requires emergency abdominal surgery to remove the adhesions and restore blood flow to the intestine. Intestinal obstruction repair is performed under general anesthesia. An incision is made in the abdomen, the obstruction is located, and the adhesions are cut away, releasing the intestine. The bowel is examined for injury or tissue death. If possible, injured and dead sections are removed and the healthy ends of the intestine are stitched together (resectioned). If resectioning is not possible, the ends of the intestine are brought through an opening in the abdomen called an **ostomy**.

In some cases laparoscopic surgery can be used to removed damaged portions of the intestines. Five or six small incisions—0.2–0.4 in. (5–10 mm) in length—are made in the abdomen. The laparoscope, equipped with its light and camera, and surgical instruments are inserted through the incisions. The laparoscope guides the surgeon by projecting images of the abdominal organs on a video monitor. However the existence of multiple adhesions may preclude the use of laparoscopic surgery.

Other types of adhesions

Adhesions caused by endometriosis may be removed by either traditional open abdominal or pelvic surgery or by laparoscopic surgery. In the latter technique the laparoscope includes a laser for destroying the tissue with heat. Although untreated gynecological adhesions can lead to infertility, both types of surgeries also can result in adhesion formation.

ICE-type glaucoma caused by adhesions is difficult to treat; however untreated ICE syndrome can lead to blindness. Treatment usually includes medication and/or filtering surgery. Filtering microsurgery involves cutting a tiny hole in the white of the eye (the sclera) to allow fluid to drain, thereby lowering the pressure in the eye and preventing or reducing damage to the optic nerve.

Alternative treatment

In cases where the intestines are partially blocked by adhesions, a diet low in fiber—called a low-residue diet—may enable food to move more easily through the obstruction.

Prognosis

Intestinal obstruction surgery usually has a favorable outcome if the surgery is performed before tissue damage or death occurs. Surgery to remove adhesions and to free or reconnect the intestine often is sufficient for reducing symptoms and returning normal function to the intestine or other organ. However the risk of new adhesion formation increases with each additional surgery. Thus abdominal adhesions can become a recurring problem. Adhesions reform in 11–21% of patients who have surgery to remove an adhesion-related intestinal obstruction. The risk of recurrence is particularly high among survivors of bowel strangulation.

Prevention

Abdominal and gynecological laparoscopic surgeries—also known as "keyhole" surgeries—reduce the size of the incision and the amount of contact with the organs, thereby lowering the risk of adhesion formation. Sometimes the intestines are fixed in place during surgery so as to promote benign adhesions that will not cause obstructions.

Within five days after surgery the disturbed tissue surfaces have formed a new lining of mesothelial cells that prevent adhesions from forming. Therefore biodegradable barrier membranes, films, gels, or sprays can be used to physically separate the tissues after surgery to prevent the formation of postoperative adhesions. However these gels and other barrier agents may:

- suppress the immune system
- cause infection
- impair healing

Systemic anti-inflammatory medications may be used to help prevent adhesion formation. Recent studies suggest that the common oral arthritis drug, Celebrex, an anti-inflammatory COX-2 inhibitor, taken before and immediately after surgery, may help prevent abdominal adhesions. Celebrex is known to inhibit both the formation of blood vessels and fibroblast activity, which are necessary for the formation of scar tissue.

Recent research has focused on the incorporation of anti-inflammatory and anti-proliferation drugs into polymeric films used for preventing and treating post-surgical adhesions. New types of gels to prevent postoperative adhesions also are under development.

Resources

BOOKS

Baerga-Varela, Y. "Small Bowel Obstruction." *Mayo Clinic Gastrointestinal Surgery,* edited by K. A. Kelly, et al. St. Louis, MO: Elsevier Science, 2004.

PERIODICALS

"Surgical Complications; Celebrex Prevents Adhesions After Surgery." *Science Letter* (February 15, 2005): 1443.

ORGANIZATIONS

National Digestive Diseases Information Clearinghouse. 2 Information Way, Bethesda, MD 20892-3570. 800-891-5389. 301-654-3810. < http://digestive.niddk.nih.gov/ >.

OTHER

Abdominal Adhesions. Aetna InteliHealth. February 17, 2004 [cited March 2, 2005]. < http://www.intelihealth. com/IH/ihtIH/WSIHW000/9339/9394.html >.
Endometriosis. MayoClinic.com. September 11, 2003 [cited March 2, 2005]. < http://www.mayoclinic.com >.
Infertility. MayoClinic.com. September 21, 2004 [cited March 2, 2005]. < http://www.mayoclinic.com/ invoke.cfm?id=DS00289 >.
"Intestinal Adhesions." *Digestive Diseases.* National Digestive Diseases Information Clearinghouse. February 2004 [cited February 21, 2005]. < http:// digestive.niddk.nih.gov/ddiseases/pubs/intestinaladhe sions/index.htm >.
What is Glaucoma? Glaucoma Research Foundation. [Cited March 4, 2005]. < http://www.glaucoma.org/learn/ >.

Margaret Alic, Ph.D.

Adjustment disorders

Definition

An adjustment disorder is a debilitating reaction, usually lasting less than six months, to a stressful event or situation. It is not the same thing as post-traumatic stress disorder (PTSD), which usually occurs in reaction to a life-threatening event and can be longer lasting.

Description

An adjustment disorder usually begins within three months of a stressful event, and ends within six months after the stressor stops. There are many different subtypes of adjustment disorders, including adjustment disorder with:

- depression
- **anxiety**
- mixed anxiety and depression
- conduct disturbances
- mixed disturbance of emotions and conduct
- unspecified

Adjustment disorders are very common and can affect anyone, regardless of gender, age, race, or lifestyle. By definition, an adjustment disorder is short-lived, unless a person is faced with a chronic recurring crisis (such as a child who is repeatedly abused). In such cases, the adjustment disorder may last more than six months.

Causes and symptoms

An adjustment disorder occurs when a person can't cope with a stressful event and develops emotional or behavioral symptoms. The stressful event can be anything: it might be just one isolated incident, or a string of problems that wears the person down. The **stress** might be anything from a car accident or illness, to a divorce, or even a certain time of year (such as Christmas or summer).

People with adjustment disorder may have a wide variety of symptoms. How those symptoms combine depend on the particular subtype of adjustment disorder and on the individual's personality and psychological defenses. Symptoms normally include some (but not all) of the following:

- hopelessness
- sadness

- crying
- anxiety
- worry
- headaches or stomachaches
- withdrawal
- inhibition
- truancy
- vandalism
- reckless driving
- fighting
- other destructive acts

Diagnosis

It is extremely important that a thorough evaluation rule out other more serious mental disorders, since the treatment for adjustment disorder may be very different than for other mental problems.

In order to be diagnosed as a true adjustment disorder, the level of distress must be more severe than what would normally be expected in response to the stressor, or the symptoms must significantly interfere with a person's social, job, or school functioning. Normal expression of grief, in **bereavement** for instance, is not considered an adjustment disorder.

Treatment

Psychotherapy (counseling) is the treatment of choice for adjustment disorders, since the symptoms are an understandable reaction to a specific stress. The type of therapy depends on the mental health expert, but it usually is short-term treatment that focuses on resolving the immediate problem.

Therapy usually will help clients:

- develop coping skills
- understand how the stressor has affected their lives
- develop alternate social or recreational activities

Family or couples therapy may be helpful in some cases. Medications are not usually used to treat adjustment disorders, although sometimes a few days or weeks of an anti-anxiety drug can control anxiety or sleeping problems.

Self-help groups aimed at a specific problem (such as recovering from divorce or job loss) can be extremely helpful to people suffering from an adjustment disorder. Social support, which is usually an important part of self-help groups, can lead to a quicker recovery.

Prognosis

Most people recover completely from adjustment disorders, especially if they had no previous history of mental problems, and have a stable home life with strong social support. People with progressive or cyclic disorders (such as multiple sclerosis) may experience an adjustment disorder with each exacerbation period.

Resources

BOOKS

Luther, Suniya G., Jacob A. Burack, and Dante Cicchetti. *Developmental Psychopathology: Perspectives on Adjustment, Risk, and Disorder.* London: Cambridge University Press, 1997.

Carol A. Turkington

Adrenal gland cancer

Definition

Adrenal gland cancers are rare cancers occuring in the endocrine tissue of the adrenals. They are characterized by overproduction of adrenal gland hormones.

Description

Cancers of the adrenal gland are very rare. The adrenal gland is a hormone producing endocrine gland with two main parts, the cortex and the medulla. The main hormone of the adrenal cortex is cortisol and the main hormone of the adrenal medulla is epinephrine.

When tumors develop in the adrenal gland, they secrete excess amounts of these hormones. A **cancer** that arises in the adrenal cortex is called an adrenocortical carcinoma and can produce high blood pressure, weight gain, excess body hair, weakening of the bones and diabetes. A cancer in the adrenal medulla is called a **pheochromocytoma** and can cause high blood pressure, **headache**, **palpitations**, and excessive perspiration. Although these cancers can happen at any age, most occur in young adults.

Causes and symptoms

It is not known what causes adrenal gland cancer, but some cases are associated with hereditary diseases. Symptoms of adrenal cancer are related to the specific hormones produced by that tumor. An adrenocortical carcinoma typically secretes high amounts of cortisol, producing **Cushing's Syndrome**. This syndrome produces progressive weight gain, rounding of the face, and increased blood pressure. Women can experience menstrual cycle alterations and men can experience feminization. The symptoms for pheochromocytoma include **hypertension**, acidosis, unexplained **fever** and weight loss. Because of the hormones produced by this type of tumor, **anxiety** is often a feature also.

Diagnosis

Diagnosis for adrenal cancer usually begins with blood tests to evaluate the hormone levels. These hormones include epinephrine, cortisol, and testosterone. It also includes **magnetic resonance imaging**, and **computed tomography scans** to determine the extent of the disease. Urine and blood tests can be done to detect the high levels of hormone secreted by the tumor.

Treatment

Treatment is aimed at removing the tumor by surgery. In some cases, this can be done by **laparoscopy**. Surgery is sometimes followed by **chemotherapy** and/or **radiation therapy**. Because the surgery removes the source of many important hormones, hormones must be supplemented following surgery. If adrenocortical cancer recurs or has spread to other parts of the body (metastasized), additional surgery may be done followed by chemotherapy using the drug mitotane.

Alternative treatment

As with any form of cancer, all conventional treatment options should be considered and applied as

KEY TERMS

Cortisol—A hormone produced by the adrenal cortex. It is partially responsible for regulating blood sugar levels.

Diabetes—A disease characterized by low blood sugar.

Epinephrine—A hormone produced by the adrenal medulla. It is important in the response to stress and partially regulates heart rate and metabolism. It is also called adrenaline.

Laparoscopy—The insertion of a tube through the abdominal wall. It can be used to visualize the inside of the abdomen and for surgical procedures.

appropriate. Nutritional support, as well as supporting the functioning of the entire person diagnosed with adrenal gland cancer through **homeopathic medicine**, **acupuncture**, vitamin and mineral supplementation, and herbal medicine, can benefit recovery and enhance quality of life.

Prognosis

The prognosis for adrenal gland cancer is variable. For localized pheochromocytomas the 5-year survival rate is 95%. This rate decreases with aggressive tumors that have metastasized. The prognosis for adrenal cortical cancer is not as good with a 5-year survival rate of 10-35%.

Prevention

Since so little is known about the cause of adrenal gland cancer, it is not known if it can be prevented.

Resources

BOOKS

Norton, J. A. "Adrenal Tumors." In *Cancer, Principles and Practice of Oncology*, edited by V. T. DeVita, S. Hellman, and S. A. Rosenberg. Philadelphia: Lippincott-Raven, 1997.

OTHER

Endocrine Web. < http://www.endocrineweb.com >.

Cindy L. A. Jones, PhD

Adrenal gland removal *see* **Adrenalectomy**

Adrenal gland scan

Definition

The adrenal gland scan is a nuclear medicine evaluation of the medulla (inner tissue) of the adrenal gland.

Purpose

The adrenal glands are a pair of small organs located just above the kidney, which contain two types of tissue. The adrenal cortex produces hormones that affect water balance and metabolism in the body. The adrenal medulla produces adrenaline and noradrenaline (also called epinepherine and norepinepherine).

An adrenal gland scan is done when too much adrenaline and noradrenaline is produced in the body and a tumor in the adrenal gland is suspected. One such situation in which a tumor might be suspected is when high blood pressure (**hypertension**) does not respond to medication. Tumors that secrete adrenaline and noradrenaline can also be found outside the adrenal gland. An adrenal gland scan usually covers the abdomen, chest, and head.

Precautions

Adrenal gland scans are not recommended for pregnant women because of the potential harm to the developing fetus. A pregnant woman should discuss with her doctor the risks of the procedure against the benefits of the information it can provide in evaluating her individual medical situation.

People who have recently undergone tests that use barium must wait until the barium has been eliminated from their system in order to obtain accurate results from the adrenal gland scan.

Description

The adrenal gland scan takes several days. On the first day, a radiopharmaceutical is injected intravenously into the patient. On the second, third, and fourth day the patient is positioned under the camera for imaging. The scanning time each day takes approximately 30 minutes. It is essential that the patient remain still during imaging.

Occasionally, the scanning process may involve fewer than three days, or it may continue several days longer. The area scanned extends from the pelvis and lower abdomen to the lower chest. Sometimes the upper legs, thighs, and head are also included.

KEY TERMS

Adrenal cortex—The outer tissue of the adrenal gland. It produces a group of chemically related hormones called corticosteroids that control mineral and water balance in the body and include aldosterone and cortisol.

Adrenal medulla—The inner tissue of the adrenal gland. It produces the hormones adrenaline and noradrenaline.

Lugol's solution—A strong iodine solution.

Preparation

For two days before and ten days after the injection of the radiopharmaceutical, patients are given either Lugol's solution or potassium iodine. This prevents the thyroid from taking up radioactive iodine and interfering with the scan.

Aftercare

The patient should not feel any adverse effects of the test and can resume normal activity immediately. Follow-up tests that might be ordered include a nuclear scan of the bones or kidney, a computed tomography scan (CT) of the adrenals, or an ultrasound of the pelvic area.

Risks

The main risk associated with this test is to the fetus of a pregnant woman.

Normal results

Normal results will show no unusual areas of hormone secretion and no tumors.

Abnormal results

Abnormal results will show evidence of a tumor where there is excessive secretion of adrenaline or noradrenaline. Over 90% of these tumors are in the abdomen.

Resources

BOOKS

Fishback, Francis, editor. *A Manual of Laboratory and Diagnostic Tests.* 5th ed. Philadelphia: Lippincott, 1996.

Tish Davidson, A.M.

Adrenal hypofunction *see* **Addison's disease**
Adrenal insufficiency *see* **Addison's disease**

Adrenal virilism

Definition

Adrenal virilism is the development or premature development of male secondary sexual characteristics caused by male sex hormones (androgens) excessively produced by the adrenal gland. This disorder can occur before birth and can lead to sexual abnormalities in newborns. It can also occur in girls and women later in life.

Description

In the normal human body, there are two adrenal glands. They are small structures that lie on top of the kidneys. The adrenal glands produce many hormones that regulate body functions. These hormones include androgens, or male hormones. Androgens are produced in normal girls and women. Sometimes, one or both of the adrenal glands becomes enlarged or overactive, producing more than the usual amount of androgens. The excess androgens create masculine characteristics.

Causes and symptoms

In infants and children, adrenal virilism is usually the result of adrenal gland enlargement that is present at birth. This is called congenital adrenal hyperplasia. The cause is usually a genetic problem that leads to severe enzyme deficiencies. In rare cases, adrenal virilism is caused by an adrenal gland tumor. The tumor can be benign (adrenal adenoma) or cancerous (adrenal carcinoma). Sometimes virilism is caused by a type of tumor on a woman's ovary (arrhenoblastoma).

Newborn girls with adrenal virilism have external sex organs that seem to be a mixture of male and female organs (called female pseudohermaphrodism). Newborn boys with the disorder have enlarged external sex organs, and these organs develop at an abnormally rapid pace.

Children with **congenital adrenal hyperplasia** begin growing abnormally fast, but they stop growing earlier than normal. Later in childhood, they are typically shorter than normal but have well-developed trunks.

Women with adrenal virilization may develop facial hair. Typically, their menstrual cycles are infrequent or absent. They may also develop a deeper voice, a more prominent Adam's apple, and other masculine signs.

Diagnosis

Endocrinologists, doctors who specialize in the diagnosis and treatment of glandular disorders, have the most expertise to deal with adrenal virilization. Some doctors who treat disorders of the internal organs (internists) and doctors who specialize in treating the reproductive system of women (gynecologists) may also be able to help patients with this disorder.

Diagnosis involves performing many laboratory tests on blood samples from the patient. These tests measure the concentration of different hormones. Different abnormalities of the adrenal gland produce a different pattern of hormonal abnormalities. These tests can also help determine if the problem is adrenal or ovarian. If a tumor is suspected, special x rays may be done to visualize the tumor in the body. Final diagnosis may depend on obtaining a tissue sample from the tumor (biopsy), and examining it under a microscope in order to verify its characteristics.

Treatment

Adrenal virilism caused by adrenal hyperplasia is treated with daily doses of a glucocorticoid. Usually prednisone is the drug of choice, but in infants hydrocortisone is usually given. Laboratory tests are usually needed from time to time to adjust the dosage. Girls with pseudohermaphrodism may require surgery to make their external sex organs appear more normal. If a tumor is causing the disorder, the treatment will depend on the type and location of the tumor. Information about the tumor cell type and the spread of the tumor is used to decide the best kind of treatment for a particular patient. If the tumor is cancerous, the patient will require special treatment depending on how far the **cancer** has advanced. Treatment can be a combination of surgery, medications used to kill cancer cells (**chemotherapy**), and x rays or other high energy rays used to kill cancer cells (radiation therapy). Sometimes the doctor must remove the adrenal gland and the surrounding tissues. If the tumor is benign, then surgically removing the tumor may be the best option.

Prognosis

Ongoing glucocorticoid treatment usually controls adrenal virilism in cases of adrenal hyperplasia,

---

but there is no cure. If a cancerous tumor has caused the disorder, patients have a better prognosis if they have an early stage of cancer that is diagnosed quickly and has not spread.

Resources

PERIODICALS

Willensy, D. "The Endocrine System." *AmericanHealth* April 1996: 92-3.

Richard H. Lampert

Adrenalectomy

Definition

Adrenalectomy is the surgical removal of one or both of the adrenal glands. The adrenal glands are paired endocrine glands, one located above each kidney, that produce hormones such as epinephrine, norepinephrine, androgens, estrogens, aldosterone, and cortisol. Adrenalectomy is usually performed by conventional (open) surgery, but in selected patients surgeons may use laparoscopy. With **laparoscopy**, adrenalectomy can be accomplished through four very small incisions.

Purpose

Adrenalectomy is usually advised for patients with tumors of the adrenal glands. Adrenal gland tumors may be malignant or benign, but all typically excrete excessive amounts of one or more hormones. A successful procedure will aid in correcting hormone imbalances, and may also remove cancerous tumors that can invade other parts of the body. Occasionally, adrenalectomy may be recommended when hormones produced by the adrenal glands aggravate another condition such as **breast cancer**.

Precautions

The adrenal glands are fed by numerous blood vessels, so surgeons need to be alert to extensive bleeding during surgery. In addition, the adrenal glands lie close to one of the body's major blood vessels (the vena cava), and to the spleen and the pancreas. The surgeon needs to remove the gland(s) without damaging any of these important and delicate organs.

Description

Open adrenalectomy

The surgeon may operate from any of four directions, depending on the exact problem and the patient's body type.

In the anterior approach, the surgeon cuts into the abdominal wall. Usually the incision will be horizontal, just under the rib cage. If the surgeon intends to operate on only one of the adrenal glands, the incision will run under just the right or the left side of the rib cage. Sometimes a vertical incision in the middle of the abdomen provides a better approach, especially if both adrenal glands are involved.

In the posterior approach, the surgeon cuts into the back, just beneath the rib cage. If both glands are to be removed, an incision is made on each side of the body. This approach is the most direct route to the adrenal glands, but it does not provide quite as clear a view of the surrounding structures as the anterior approach.

In the flank approach, the surgeon cuts into the patient's side. This is particularly useful in massively obese patients. If both glands need to be removed, the surgeon must remove one gland, repair the surgical wound, turn the patient onto the other side, and repeat the entire process.

The last approach involves an incision into the chest cavity, either with or without part of the incision into the abdominal cavity. It is used when the surgeon anticipates a very large tumor, or if the surgeon needs to examine or remove nearby structures as well.

Laparoscopic adrenalectomy

This technique does not require the surgeon to open the body cavity. Instead, four small incisions (about 1/2 in diameter each) are made into a patient's flank, just under the rib cage. A laparoscope, which enables the surgeon to visualize the inside of the

---

---

abdominal cavity on a television monitor, is placed through one of the incisions. The other incisions are for tubes that carry miniaturized versions of surgical tools. These tools are designed to be operated by manipulations that the surgeon makes outside the body.

Preparation

Most aspects of preparation are the same as in other major operations. In addition, hormone imbalances are often a major challenge. Whenever possible, physicians will try to correct hormone imbalances through medication in the days or weeks before surgery. Adrenal tumors may cause other problems such as **hypertension** or inadequate potassium in the blood, and these problems also should be resolved if possible before surgery is performed. Therefore, a patient may take specific medicines for days or weeks before surgery.

Most adrenal tumors can be imaged very well with a CT scan or MRI, and benign tumors tend to look different on these tests than do cancerous tumors. Surgeons may order a CT scan, MRI, or scintigraphy (viewing of the location of a tiny amount of radioactive agent) to help locate exactly where the tumor is.

The day before surgery, patients will probably have an enema to clear the bowels. In patients with lung problems or clotting problems, physicians may advise special preparations.

Aftercare

Patients stay in the hospital for various lengths of time after adrenalectomy. The longest hospital stays are required for open surgery using an anterior approach; hospital stays of about three days are indicated for open surgery using the posterior approach or for laparoscopic adrenalectomy.

The special concern after adrenalectomy is the patient's hormone balance. There may be several sets of lab tests to define hormone problems and monitor the results of drug treatment. In addition, blood pressure problems and infections are more common after removal of certain types of adrenal tumors.

As with most open surgery, surgeons are also concerned about **blood clots** forming in the legs and traveling to the lungs (venous thromboembolism), bowel problems, and postoperative pain. With laparoscopic adrenalectomy, these problems are somewhat less difficult, but they are still present.

Risks

The special risks of adrenalectomy involve major hormone imbalances, caused by the underlying disease, the surgery, or both. These can include problems with wound healing itself, blood pressure fluctuations, and other metabolic problems.

Other risks are typical of many operations. These include:

- bleeding
- damage to adjacent organs (spleen, pancreas)
- loss of bowel function
- blood clots in the lungs
- lung problems
- surgical infections
- pain
- extensive scarring

Resources

BOOKS

Fauci, Anthony S., et al., editors. *Harrison's Principles of Internal Medicine.* New York: McGraw-Hill, 1997.

Richard H. Lampert

Adrenocortical insufficiency *see* **Addison's disease**

Adrenocorticotropic hormone test

Definition

Adrenocorticotropic hormone test (also known as an ACTH test or a corticotropin test) measures pituitary gland function.

Purpose

The pituitary gland produces the hormone ACTH, which stimulates the outer layer of the adrenal gland (the adrenal cortex). ACTH causes the release of the hormones hydrocortisone (cortisol), aldosterone, and androgen. The most important of these hormones released is cortisol. The ACTH test is used to determine if too much cortisol is being produced (**Cushing's syndrome**) or if not enough cortisol is being produced (**Addison's disease**).

Precautions

ACTH has diurnal variation, meaning that the levels of this hormone vary according to the time of day. The highest levels occur in the morning hours. Testing for normal secretion, as well as for Cushing's disease, may require multiple samples. For sequential follow-up, a blood sample analyzed for ACTH should always be drawn at the same time each day.

ACTH can be directly measured by an analyzing method (immunoassay) in many large laboratories. However, smaller laboratories are usually not equipped to perform this test and they may need to send the blood sample to a larger laboratory. Because of this delay, results may take several days to obtain.

Description

ACTH production is partly controlled by an area in the center of the brain (the hypothalamus) and partly controlled by the level of cortisol in the blood. When ACTH levels are too high, cortisol production increases to suppress ACTH release from the pituitary gland. If ACTH levels are too low, the hypothalamus produces corticotropin-releasing hormone (CRH) to stimulate the pituitary gland to make more ACTH. ACTH levels rise in response to **stress**, emotions, injury, infection, burns, surgery, and decreased blood pressure.

Cushing's syndrome

Cushing's syndrome is caused by an abnormally high level of circulating hydrocortisone. The high level may be the result of an adrenal gland tumor or enlargement of both adrenal glands due to a pituitary tumor. The high level of hydrocortisone may be the result of taking corticosteroid drugs for a long time. Corticosteroid drugs are widely used for inflammation in disorders like rheumatoid arthritis, inflammatory bowel disease, and **asthma**.

Addison's disease

Addison's disease is a rare disorder in which symptoms are caused by a deficiency of hydrocortisone and aldosterone. The most common cause of this disease is an autoimmune disorder. The immune system normally fights foreign invaders in the body like bacteria. In an autoimmune disorder, the immune systems attacks the body. In this case, the immune system produces antibodies that attack the adrenal glands. Addison's disease generally progresses slowly, with symptoms developing gradually over months or years. However, acute episodes, called Addisonian crises, are brought on by infection, injury, or other stresses. Diagnosis is generally made if the patient fails to respond to an injection of ACTH, which normally stimulates the secretion of hydrocortisone.

Preparation

A person's ACTH level is determined from a blood sample. The patient must fast from midnight until the test the next morning. This means that the patient cannot eat or drink anything after midnight except water. The patient must also avoid radioisotope scanning tests or recently administered radioisotopes prior to the blood test.

Risks

The risks associated with this test are minimal. They may include slight bleeding from the location where the blood was drawn. The patient may feel faint or lightheaded after the blood is drawn. Sometimes the patient may have an accumulation of blood under the puncture site (hematoma) after the test.

Normal results

Each laboratory will have its own set of normal values for this test. The normal values can range from: Morning (4-8 A.M.) 8-100 pg/mL or 10-80 ng/L (SI units) Evening (8-10 P.M.) less than 50 pg/mL or less than 50 ng/L (SI units)

Abnormal results

In Cushing's syndrome, high levels of ACTH may be caused by ACTH-producing tumors. These tumors may be either in the pituitary or in another area (like tumors from lung **cancer** or **ovarian cancer**). Low ACTH levels may be caused by adrenal enlargement due to high levels of cortisol and feedback to the pituitary.

In Addison's disease, high levels of ACTH may be caused by adrenal gland diseases. These diseases decrease adrenal hormones and the pituitary attempts to increase functioning. Low levels of ACTH may occur because of decreased pituitary function.

Resources

BOOKS

Pagana, Kathleen Deska. *Mosby's Manual of Diagnosticand Laboratory Tests*. St. Louis: Mosby, Inc., 1998.

Janis O. Flores

Adrenogenital syndrome *see* **Adrenal virilism**

Adrenoleukodystrophy

Definition

Adrenoleukodystrophy is a rare genetic disease characterized by a loss of myelin surrounding nerve cells in the brain and progressive adrenal gland dysfunction.

Description

Adrenoleukodystrophy (ALD) is a member of a group of diseases, leukodystrophies, that cause damage to the myelin sheath of nerve cells. Approximately one in 100,000 people is affected by ALD. There are three basic forms of ALD: childhood, adult-onset, and neonatal. The childhood form of the disease is the classical form and is the most severe. Childhood ALD is progressive and usually leads to total disability or **death**. It affects only boys because the genetic defect is sex-linked (carried on the X chromosome). Onset usually occurs between ages four and ten and can include many different symptoms, not all of which appear together. The most common symptoms are behavioral problems and poor memory. Other symptoms frequently seen are loss of vision, seizures, poorly articulated speech, difficulty swallowing, deafness, problems with gait and coordination, **fatigue**, increased skin pigmentation, and progressive **dementia**.

The adult-onset form of the disease, also called adrenomyeloneuropathy, is milder, progresses slowly, is usually associated with a normal life span, and usually appears between ages 21-35. Symptoms may include progressive stiffness, weakness, or **paralysis** of the lower limbs and loss of coordination. Brain function deterioration may also been seen. Women who are carriers of the disease occasionally experience the same symptoms, as well as others, including ataxia, hypertonia (excessive muscle tone), mild **peripheral neuropathy**, and urinary problems. The neonatal form affects both male and female infants and may produce **mental retardation**, facial abnormalities, seizures, retinal degeneration, poor muscle tone, enlarged liver, and adrenal dysfunction. Neonatal ALD usually progresses rapidly.

Causes and symptoms

The genetic defect in ALD causes a decrease in the ability to degrade very long chain fatty acids. These build up in the adrenal glands, brain, plasma, and fibroblasts. The build-up of very long chain fatty acids interferes with the ability of the adrenal gland to convert cholesterol into steroids and causes demyelination of nerves in the white matter of the brain. Demyelinated nerve cells are unable to function properly.

Diagnosis

Diagnosis is made based on observed symptoms, a biochemical test, and a family history. The biochemical test detects elevated levels of very long chain fatty acids in samples from **amniocentesis**, chorionic villi, plasma, red blood cells, or fibroblasts. A family history may indicate the likelihood of ALD because the disease is carried on the X-chromosome by the female lineage of families.

KEY TERMS

Amniocentesis—The collection of amniotic fluid through a needle inserted through the abdomen. Used to collect fetal cells for genetic analysis.

Ataxia—Loss of coordination of muscular movement.

Hypertonia—Having excessive muscular tone.

Myelin—A layer that encloses nerve cells and some axons and is made largely of lipids and lipoproteins.

Neuropathy—A disease or abnormality of the peripheral nerves.

Treatment

Treatment for all forms of ALD consists of treating the symptoms and supporting the patient with physical therapy, psychological counseling, and special education in some cases. There is no cure for this disease, and there are no drugs that can reverse demyelination of nerve and brain cells. Dietary measures consist of reducing the intake of foods high in fat, which are a source of very long chain fatty acids. A mixture called Lorenzo's Oil has been shown to reduce the level of long chain fatty acids if used long term; however, the rate of myelin loss is unaffected. Experimental **bone marrow transplantation** has not been very effective.

Prognosis

Prognosis for childhood and neonatal ALD patients is poor because of the progressive myelin degeneration. Death usually occurs between one and ten years after onset of symptoms.

Prevention

Since ALD is a genetic disease, prevention is largely limited to **genetic counseling** and fetal monitoring through amniocentesis or **chorionic villus sampling**.

Resources

BOOKS

Berkow, Robert. *Merck Manual of Medical Information.* Whitehouse Station, NJ: Merck Research Laboratories, 1997.

John T. Lohr, PhD

Adrenomyeloneuropathy *see* **Adrenoleukodystrophy**

Adult respiratory distress syndrome

Definition

Adult **respiratory distress syndrome** (ARDS), also called acute respiratory distress syndrome, is a type of lung (pulmonary) failure that may result from any disease that causes large amounts of fluid to collect in the lungs. ARDS is not itself a specific disease, but a syndrome, a group of symptoms and signs that make up one of the most important forms of lung or **respiratory failure**. It can develop quite suddenly in persons whose lungs have been perfectly normal. Very often ARDS is a true medical emergency. The basic fault is a breakdown of the barrier, or membrane, that normally keeps fluid from leaking out of the small blood vessels of the lung into the breathing sacs (the alveoli).

Description

Another name for ARDS is shock lung. Its formal name is misleading, because children, as well as adults, may be affected. In the lungs the smallest blood vessels, or capillaries, make contact with the alveoli, tiny air sacs at the tips of the smallest breathing tubes (the bronchi). This is the all-important site where oxygen passes from air that is inhaled to the blood, which carries it to all parts of the body. Any form of lung injury that damages this point of contact, called the alveolo-capillary junction, will allow blood and tissue fluid to leak into the alveoli, eventually filling them so that air cannot enter. The result is the type of breathing distress called ARDS. ARDS is one of the major causes of excess fluid in the lungs, the other being **heart failure**.

Along with fluid there is a marked increase in inflamed cells in the lungs. There also is debris left over from damaged lung cells, and fibrin, a semi-solid material derived from blood in the tissues. Typically these materials join together with large molecules in the blood (proteins), to form hyaline membranes. (These membranes are very prominent in premature infants who develop respiratory distress syndrome; it is often called hyaline membrane disease.) If ARDS is very severe or lasts a long time, the lungs do not heal, but rather become scarred, a process known as fibrosis. The lack of a normal amount of oxygen causes the blood vessels of the lung to become narrower, and in time they, too, may become scarred and filled with clotted blood. The lungs as a whole become very "stiff," and it becomes much harder for the patient to breathe.

KEY TERMS

Alveoli—The tiny air sacs at the ends of the breathing tubes of the lung where oxygen normally is taken up by the capillaries to enter the circulation.

Aspiration—The process in which solid food, liquids, or secretions that normally are swallowed are, instead, breathed into the lungs.

Capillaries—The smallest arteries which, in the lung, are located next to the alveoli so that they can pick up oxygen from inhaled air.

Face mask—The simplest way of delivering a high level of oxygen to patients with ARDS or other low-oxygen conditions.

Steroids—A class of drugs resembling normal body substances that often help control inflammation in the body tissues.

Ventilator—A mechanical device that can take over the work of breathing for a patient whose lungs are injured or are starting to heal.

Causes and symptoms

A very wide range of diseases or toxic substances, including some drugs, can cause ARDS. They include:

- Breathing in (aspiration) of the stomach contents when regurgitated, or salt water or fresh water from nearly drowning.

- Inhaling smoke, as in a fire; toxic materials in the air, such as ammonia or hydrocarbons; or too much oxygen, which itself can injure the lungs.

- Infection by a virus or bacterium, or **sepsis**, a widespread infection that gets into the blood.

- Massive trauma, with severe injury to any part of the body.

- Shock with persistently low blood pressure may not in itself cause ARDS, but it can be an important factor.

- A blood clotting disorder called disseminated intravascular coagulation, in which blood clots form in vessels throughout the body, including the lungs.

- A large amount of fat entering the circulation and traveling to the lungs, where it lodges in small blood vessels, injuring the cells lining the vessel walls.

- An overdose of a narcotic drug, a sedative, or, rarely, **aspirin**.

- Inflammation of the pancreas (**pancreatitis**), when blood proteins, called enzymes, pass to the lungs and injure lung cells.

- Severe burn injury.

- Injury of the brain, or bleeding into the brain, from any cause may be a factor in ARDS for reasons that are not clear. Convulsions also may cause some cases.

Usually ARDS develops within one to two days of the original illness or injury. The person begins to take rapid but shallow breaths. The doctor who listens to the patient's chest with a stethoscope may hear "crackling" or **wheezing** sounds. The low blood oxygen content may cause the skin to appear mottled or even blue. As fluid continues to fill the breathing sacs, the patient may have great trouble breathing, take very rapid breaths, and gasp for air.

Diagnosis

A simple test using a device applied to the ear will show whether the blood is carrying too little oxygen, and this can be confirmed by analyzing blood taken from an artery. The **chest x ray** may be normal in the early stages, but, in a short time, fluid will be seen where it does not belong. The two lungs are about equally affected. A heart of normal size indicates that the problem actually is ARDS and not heart failure. Another way a physician can distinguish between these two possibilities is to place a catheter into a vein and advance it into the main artery of the lung. In this way, the pressure within the pulmonary capillaries can be measured. Pressure within the pulmonary capillaries is elevated in heart failure, but normal in ARDS.

Treatment

The three main goals in treating patients with ARDS are:

- To treat whatever injury or disease has caused ARDS. Examples are: to treat septic infection with the proper **antibiotics**, and to reduce the level of oxygen therapy if ARDS has resulted from a toxic level of oxygen.

- To control the process in the lungs that allows fluid to leak out of the blood vessels. At present there is no certain way to achieve this. Certain steroid hormones have been tried because they can combat inflammation, but the actual results have been disappointing.

- To make sure the patient gets enough oxygen until the lung injury has had time to heal. If oxygen delivered by a face mask is not enough, the patient is placed on a ventilator, which takes over breathing, and, through a tube placed in the nose or mouth (or an incision in the windpipe), forces oxygen into the lungs. This treatment must be closely supervised, and the pressure adjusted so that too much oxygen is not delivered.

Patients with ARDS should be cared for in an intensive care unit, where experienced staff and all needed equipment are available. Enough fluid must be provided, by vein if necessary, to prevent **dehydration**. Also, the patient's nutritional state must be maintained, again by vein, if oral intake is not sufficient.

Prognosis

If the patient's lung injury does not soon begin to heal, the lack of sufficient oxygen can injure other organs, such as the kidneys. There always is a risk that bacterial **pneumonia** will develop at some point. Without prompt treatment, as many as 90% of patients with ARDS can be expected to die. With modern treatment, however, about half of all patients will survive. Those who do live usually recover completely, with little or no long-term breathing difficulty. Lung scarring is a risk after a long period on a ventilator, but it may improve in the months after the patient is taken off ventilation. Whether a particular patient will recover depends to a great extent on whether the primary disease that caused ARDS to develop in the first place can be effectively treated.

Prevention

The only way to prevent ARDS is to avoid those diseases and harmful conditions that damage the lung. For instance, the danger of aspirating stomach contents into the lungs can be avoided by making sure a patient does not eat shortly before receiving **general anesthesia**. If a patient needs **oxygen therapy**, as low a level as possible should be given. Any form of lung infection, or infection anywhere in the body that gets into the blood, must be treated promptly to avoid the lung injury that causes ARDS.

Resources

BOOKS

Smolley, Lawrence A., and Debra F. Bryse. *Breathe RightNow: A Comprehensive Guide to Understanding and Treating the Most Common Breathing Disorders.* New York: W. W. Norton & Co., 1998.

ORGANIZATIONS
National Heart, Lung and Blood Institute. P.O. Box 30105, Bethesda, MD 20824-0105. (301) 251-1222. < http:// www.nhlbi.nih.gov > .
National Respiratory Distress Syndrome Foundation. P.O. Box 723, Montgomeryville, PA 18936.

David A. Cramer, MD

AFP test *see* **Alpha-fetoprotein test**

African American health *see* **Minority health**

African sleeping sickness *see* **Sleeping sickness**

African trypanosomiasis *see* **Sleeping sickness**

Agammaglobulinemia *see* **Common variable immunodeficiency**

Aggression *see* **Conduct disorder**

Aging

Definition

Starting at what is commonly called middle age, operations of the human body begin to be more vulnerable to daily wear and tear; there is a general decline in physical, and possibly mental, functioning. In the Western countries, the length of life is often into the 70s. The upward limit of the life span, however, can be as high as 120 years. During the latter half of life, an individual is more prone to have problems with the various functions of the body and to develop any number of chronic or fatal diseases. The cardiovascular, digestive, excretory, nervous, reproductive and urinary systems are particularly affected. The most common diseases of aging include Alzheimer's, arthritis, **cancer**, diabetes, depression, and heart disease.

Description

Human beings reach a peak of growth and development around the time of their mid 20s. Aging is the normal transition time after that flurry of activity. Although there are quite a few age-related changes that tax the body, disability is not necessarily a part of aging. Health and lifestyle factors together with the genetic makeup of the individual, and determines the response to these changes. Body functions that are most often affected by age include:

- Hearing, which declines especially in relation to the highest pitched tones.

- The proportion of fat to muscle, which may increase by as much as 30%. Typically, the total padding of body fat directly under the skin thins out and accumulates around the stomach. The ability to excrete fats is impaired, and therefore the storage of fats increases, including cholesterol and fat-soluble nutrients.

- The amount of water in the body decreases, which therefore decreases the absorption of water-soluble nutrients. Also, there is less saliva and other lubricating fluids.

- The liver and the kidneys cannot function as efficiently, thus affecting the elimination of wastes.

- A decrease in the ease of digestion, with a decrease in stomach acid production.

- A loss of muscle strength and coordination, with an accompanying loss of mobility, agility, and flexibility.

- A decline in sexual hormones and sexual functioning.

- A decrease in the sensations of taste and smell.

- Changes in the cardiovascular and respiratory systems, leading to decreased oxygen and nutrients throughout the body.

- Decreased functioning of the nervous system so that nerve impulses are not transmitted as efficiently, reflexes are not as sharp, and memory and learning are diminished.

- A decrease in bone strength and density.

- Hormone levels, which gradually decline. The thyroid and sexual hormones are particularly affected.

- Declining visual abilities. Age-related changes may lead to diseases such as **macular degeneration**.

- A compromised ability to produce vitamin D from sunlight.

- A reduction in protein formation leading to shrinkage in muscle mass and decreased bone formation, possibly leading to osteoporosis.

Causes and symptoms

There are several theories as to why the aging body loses functioning. It may be that several factors work together or that one particular factor is at work more than others in a given individual.

- Programmed senescence, or aging clock, theory. The aging of the cells of each individual is programmed into the genes, and there is a preset number of possible rejuvenations in the life of a given cell. When cells die at a rate faster than they are replaced, organs do not function properly, and they are soon unable to maintain the functions necessary for life.

- Genetic theory. Human cells maintain their own seed of destruction at the level of the chromosomes.

- Connective tissue, or cross-linking theory. Changes in the make-up of the connective tissue alter the stability of body structures, causing a loss of elasticity and functioning, and leading to symptoms of aging.

- Free-radical theory. The most commonly held theory of aging, it is based on the fact that ongoing chemical reactions of the cells produce free radicals. In the presence of oxygen, these free radicals cause the cells of the body to break down. As time goes on, more cells die or lose the ability to function, and the body soon ceases to function as a whole.

- Immunological theory. There are changes in the immune system as it begins to wear out, and the body is more prone to infections and tissue damage, which may finally cause **death**. Also, as the system breaks down, the body is more apt to have autoimmune reactions, in which the body's own cells are mistaken for foreign material and are destroyed or damaged by the immune system.

Diagnosis

Many problems can arise due to age-related changes in the body. Although there is no one test to be given, a thorough physical exam and a basic blood screening and blood chemistry panel can point to areas in need of further attention. When older people become ill, the first signs of disease are often nonspecific. Further exams should be conducted if any of the following occur:

- diminished or lack of desire for food
- increasing confusion
- failure to thrive
- urinary incontinence
- dizziness
- weight loss
- falling

Treatment

For the most part, doctors prescribe medications to control the symptoms and diseases of aging. In the United States, about two-thirds of people 65 and over

take medications for various complaints. More women than men use these medications. The most common drugs used by the elderly are painkillers, **diuretics** or water pills, sedatives, cardiac drugs, **antibiotics**, and mental health drugs.

Estrogen replacement therapy (ERT) is commonly prescribed to postmenopausal women for symptoms of aging. It is often used in conjunction with progesterone. ERT functions to help keep bones strong, reduce risk of heart disease, restore vaginal lubrication, and to improve skin elasticity. Evidence suggests that it may also help maintain mental functions.

Expected results

Aging is unavoidable, but major physical impairment is not. People can lead a healthy, disability-free life well through their later years. A well established support system of family, friends, and health care providers, together with focus on good **nutrition** and lifestyle habits and good stress management, can prevent disease and lessen the impact of chronic conditions.

Alternative treatment

Nutritional supplements

Consumption of a high–quality multivitamin is recommended. Common nutritional deficiencies connected with aging include B **vitamins**, vitamins A and C, **folic acid**, calcium, magnesium, zinc, iron, chromium, and trace **minerals**. Since stomach acids may be decreased, it is suggested that the use of a powdered multivitamin formula in gelatin capsules be used, as this form is the easiest to digest. Such formulas may also contain enzymes for further help with digestion.

Antioxidants can help to neutralize damage by the free radical actions thought to contribute to problems of aging. They are also helpful in preventing and treating cancer and in treating cataracts and glaucoma. Supplements that serve as antioxidants include:

- Vitamin E, 400–1,000 IUs daily. Protects cell membranes against damage. It shows promise in prevention against heart disease, and Alzheimer's and Parkinson's diseases.

- Selenium, 50 mg taken twice daily. Research suggests that selenium may play a role in reducing the risk of cancer.

- Beta-carotene, 25,000–40,000 IUs daily. May help in treating cancer, colds and flu, arthritis, and immune support.

- Vitamin C, 1,000–2,000 mg per day. It may cause **diarrhea** in large doses. If this occurs, however, all that is needed is a decrease in the dosage.

Other supplements that are helpful in treating age-related problems including:

- B_{12}/B-complex vitamins, studies show that B_{12} may help reduce mental symptoms, such as confusion, memory loss, and depression.

- Coenzyme Q10 may be helpful in treating heart disease, as up to three-quarters cardiac patients have been found to be lacking in this heart enzyme.

Hormones

The following hormone supplements may be taken to prevent or to treat various age-related problems. However, caution should be taken before beginning treatment, and the patient should consult his or her health care professional.

DHEA improves brain functioning and serves as a building block for many other important hormones in the body. It may be helpful in restoring declining hormone levels and in building up muscle mass, strengthening the bones, and maintaining a healthy heart.

Melatonin may be helpful for **insomnia**. It has also been used to help fight viruses and bacterial infections, reduce the risk of heart disease, improve sexual functioning, and to protect against cancer.

Human growth hormone (hGH) has been shown to regulate blood sugar levels and to stimulate bone, cartilage, and muscle growth while reducing fat.

Herbs

Garlic (*Allium sativa*) is helpful in preventing heart disease, as well as improving the tone and texture of skin. Garlic stimulates liver and digestive system functions, and also helps in dealing with heart disease and high blood pressure.

Siberian ginseng (*Eleutherococcus senticosus*) supports the adrenal glands and immune functions. It is believed to be helpful in treating problems related to stress. Siberian ginseng also increases mental and physical performance, and may be useful in treating memory loss, chronic **fatigue**, and immune dysfunction.

Proanthocyanidins, or PCO, are Pycnogenol, derived from grape seeds and skin, and from pine tree bark, and may help in the prevention of cancer and poor vision.

In **Ayurvedic medicine**, aging is described as a process of increased vata, in which there is a tendency to become thinner, drier, more nervous, more restless, and more fearful, while having a loss of appetite as well as sleep. Bananas, almonds, avocados, and coconuts are some of the foods used in correcting such conditions. One of the main herbs used for such conditions is gotu kola (*Centella asiatica*), which is used to revitalize the nervous system and brain cells and to fortify the immune system. Gotu kola is also used to treat memory loss, **anxiety**, and insomnia.

In Chinese medicine, most symptoms of aging are regarded as symptoms of a yin deficiency. Moistening foods such as millet, barley soup, tofu, mung beans, wheat germ, spirulina, potatoes, black sesame seeds, walnuts, and flax seeds are recommended. Jing tonics may also be used. These include deer antler, dodder seeds, processed rehmannia, longevity soup, mussels, and chicken.

Prevention

Preventive health practices such as healthy diet, daily **exercise**, **stress** management, and control of lifestyle habits such as **smoking** and drinking, can lengthen the life span and improve the quality of life as people age. Exercise can improve the appetite, the health of the bones, the emotional and mental outlook, and the digestion and circulation.

Drinking plenty of fluids aids in maintaining healthy skin, good digestion, and proper elimination of wastes. Up to eight glasses of water should be consumed daily, along with plenty of herbal teas, diluted fruit and vegetable juices, and fresh fruits and vegetables with high water content.

Because of a decrease in the sense of taste, older people often increase their intake of salt, which can contribute to high blood pressure and nutrient loss. Use of sugar is also increased. Seaweeds and small amounts of honey can be used as replacements.

Alcohol, nicotine, and **caffeine** all have potential damaging effects, and should be limited or completely eliminated from consumption.

A diet high in fiber and low in fat is recommended. Processed foods should be replaced by complex carbohydrates, such as whole grains. If chewing becomes a problem, there should be an increased intake of protein drinks, freshly juiced fruits and vegetables, and creamed cereals.

Resources

OTHER

"Anti-Aging-Nutritional Program." December 28, 2000. < http:// www.healthy.net/hwlibrarybooks/haas/ perform/antiagin.htm > .

"Effects of Hormone in the Body." December 28, 2000. < http://www.anti-aging.org/Effects_hGH.html > .

"The Elderly-Nutritional Programs." December 28, 2000. < http://www.healthy.net/hwlibrarybooks/haas/ lifestage/elderly.htm > .

"Evaluating the Elderly Patient: the Case for Assessment Technology." December 28, 2000. < http://text.nlm. nih.gov/nih/ta/www/01.html > .

"Herbal Phytotherapy and the Elderly." December 28, 2000. < http://www.healthy.net/hwlibrarybooks/hoffman/ elders/elders.htm > .

"Pharmacokinetics." Merck & Co., Inc. (1995-2000). December 28, 2000. < http://www.merck.com/pubs/ mmanual/section22/chapter304/304a.htm > .

"To a Long and Healthy Life." December 28, 2000. < http:// www.healthy.net/hwlibraryarticles/aesoph/ longandhealthy.htm > .

Patience Paradox

Agoraphobia

Definition

The word agoraphobia is derived from Greek words literally meaning "fear of the marketplace." The term is used to describe an irrational and often disabling fear of being out in public.

Description

Agoraphobia is just one type of phobia, or irrational fear. People with **phobias** feel dread or panic when they face certain objects, situations, or activities. People with agoraphobia frequently also experience panic attacks, but panic attacks, or panic disorder, are not a requirement for a diagnosis of agoraphobia. The defining feature of agoraphobia is **anxiety** about being in places from which escape might be embarrassing or difficult, or in which help might be unavailable. The person suffering from agoraphobia usually avoids the anxiety-provoking situation and may become totally housebound.

Causes and symptoms

Agoraphobia is the most common type of phobia, and it is estimated to affect between 5-12% of Americans within their lifetime. Agoraphobia is twice as common in women as in men and usually strikes between the ages of 15-35.

The symptoms of the panic attacks which may accompany agoraphobia vary from person to person, and may include trembling, sweating, heart **palpitations** (a feeling of the heart pounding against the chest), jitters, fatigue, tingling in the hands and feet, **nausea**, a rapid pulse or breathing rate, and a sense of impending doom.

Agoraphobia and other phobias are thought to be the result of a number of physical and environmental factors. For instance, they have been associated with biochemical imbalances, especially related to certain neurotransmitters (chemical nerve messengers) in the brain. People who have a panic attack in a given situation (e.g., a shopping mall) may begin to associate the panic with that situation and learn to avoid it. According to some theories, irrational anxiety results from unresolved emotional conflicts. All of these factors may play a role to varying extents in different cases of agoraphobia.

Diagnosis

People who suffer from panic attacks should discuss the problem with a physician. The doctor can diagnose the underlying panic or anxiety disorder and make sure the symptoms aren't related to some other underlying medical condition.

The doctor makes the diagnosis of agoraphobia based primarily on the patient's description of his or her symptoms. The person with agoraphobia experiences anxiety in situations where escape is difficult or help is unavailable–or in certain situations, such as being alone. While many people are somewhat apprehensive in these situations, the hallmark of agoraphobia is that a person's active avoidance of the feared situation impairs his or her ability to work, socialize, or otherwise function.

Treatment

Treatment for agoraphobia usually consists of both medication and psychotherapy. Usually, patients can benefit from certain antidepressants, such as amitriptyline (Elavil), or **selective serotonin reuptake inhibitors**, such as paroxetine (Paxil), fluoxetine (Prozac), or sertraline (Zoloft). In addition, patients may manage panic attacks in progress with certain tranquilizers called **benzodiazepines**, such as alprazolam (Xanax) or clonazepam (Klonipin).

The mainstay of treatment for agoraphobia and other phobias is cognitive behavioral therapy. A specific technique that is often employed is called desensitization. The patient is gradually exposed to the situation that usually triggers fear and avoidance, and, with the help of breathing or relaxation techniques, learns to cope with the situation. This helps break the mental connection between the situation and the fear, anxiety, or panic. Patients may also benefit from psychodynamically oriented psychotherapy, discussing underlying emotional conflicts with a therapist or support group.

Prognosis

With proper medication and psychotherapy, 90% of patients will find significant improvement in their symptoms.

Resources

PERIODICALS

Forsyth, Sondra. "I Panic When I'm Alone." *Mademoiselle* April 1998: 119-24.

ORGANIZATIONS

American Psychiatric Association. 1400 K Street NW, Washington DC 20005. (888) 357-7924. < http:// www.psych.org > .

Anxiety Disorders Association of America. 11900 Park Lawn Drive, Ste. 100, Rockville, MD 20852. (800) 545-7367. < http://www.adaa.org > .

National Institute of Mental Health. Mental Health Public Inquiries, 5600 Fishers Lane, Room 15C-05, Rockville, MD 20857. (888) 826-9438. < http:// www.nimh.nih.gov > .

Robert Scott Dinsmoor

Agranulocytosis *see* **Neutropenia**

AIDS

Definition

Acquired immune deficiency syndrome (AIDS) is an infectious disease caused by the human **immunodeficiency** virus (HIV). It was first recognized in the United States in 1981. AIDS is the advanced form of infection with the HIV virus, which may not cause recognizable disease for a long period after the initial exposure (latency). No vaccine is currently available to prevent HIV infection. At present, all forms of AIDS therapy are focused on improving the quality and length of life for AIDS patients by slowing or halting the replication of the virus and treating or preventing infections and cancers that take advantage of a person's weakened immune system.

Description

AIDS is considered one of the most devastating public health problems in recent history. In June 2000, the Centers for Disease Control and Prevention (CDC) reported that 120,223 (includes only those cases in areas that have confidential HIV reporting) in the United States are HIV-positive, and 311,701 are living with AIDS (includes only those cases where vital status is known). Of these patients, 44% are gay or bisexual men, 20% are heterosexual intravenous drug users, and 17% are women. In addition, approximately 1,000-2,000 children are born each year with HIV infection. The World Health Organization (WHO) estimates that 33 million adults and 1.3 million children worldwide were living with HIV/AIDS as of 1999 with 5.4 million being newly infected that year. Most of these cases are in the developing countries of Asia and Africa.

Risk of acquiring HIV infection by entry site			
Entry site	Risk virus reaches entry site	Risk virus enters	Risk inoculated
Conjuntiva	Moderate	Moderate	Very low
Oral mucosa	Moderate	Moderate	Low
Nasal mucosa	Low	Low	Very low
Lower respiratory	Very low	Very low	Very low
Anus	Very high	Very high	Very high
Skin, intact	Very low	Very low	Very low
Skin, broken	Low	High	High
Sexual:			
Vagina	Low	Low	Medium
Penis	High	Low	Low
Ulcers (STD)	High	High	Very high
Blood:			
Products	High	High	High
Shared needles	High	High	Very High
Accidental needle	Low	High	Low
Traumatic wound	Modest	High	High
Perinatal	High	High	High

Risk factors

AIDS can be transmitted in several ways. The risk factors for HIV transmission vary according to category:

- Sexual contact. Persons at greatest risk are those who do not practice safe sex, those who are not monogamous, those who participate in anal intercourse, and those who have sex with a partner with symptoms of advanced HIV infection and/or other sexually transmitted diseases (STDs). In the United States and Europe, most cases of sexually transmitted HIV infection have resulted from homosexual contact, whereas in Africa, the disease is spread primarily through sexual intercourse among heterosexuals.

- Transmission in **pregnancy**. High-risk mothers include women married to bisexual men or men who have an abnormal blood condition called **hemophilia** and require blood transfusions, intravenous drug users, and women living in neighborhoods with a high rate of HIV infection among heterosexuals. The chances of transmitting the disease to the child are higher in women in advanced stages of the disease. Breast feeding increases the risk of transmission by 10-20%. The use of zidovudine (AZT) during pregnancy, however, can decrease the risk of transmission to the baby.

- Exposure to contaminated blood or blood products. With the introduction of blood product screening in the mid-1980s, the incidence of HIV transmission in blood transfusions has dropped to one in every 100,000

transfused. With respect to HIV transmission among drug abusers, risk increases with the duration of using injections, the frequency of needle sharing, the number of persons who share a needle, and the number of AIDS cases in the local population.

- Needle sticks among health care professionals. Present studies indicate that the risk of HIV transmission by a needle stick is about one in 250. This rate can be decreased if the injured worker is given AZT, an anti-retroviral medication, in combination with other medication.

HIV is not transmitted by handshakes or other casual non-sexual contact, coughing or sneezing, or by bloodsucking insects such as mosquitoes.

AIDS in women

AIDS in women is a serious public health concern. Women exposed to HIV infection through heterosexual contact are the most rapidly growing risk group in the United States population. The percentage of AIDS cases diagnosed in women has risen from 7% in 1985 to 23% in 1999. Women diagnosed with AIDS may not live as long as men, although the reasons for this finding are unclear.

AIDS in children

Since AIDS can be transmitted from an infected mother to the child during pregnancy, during the birth process, or through breast milk, all infants born to HIV-positive mothers are a high-risk group. As of 2000, it was estimated that 87% of HIV-positive women are of childbearing age; 41% of them are drug abusers. Between 15-30% of children born to HIV-positive women will be infected with the virus.

AIDS is one of the 10 leading causes of **death** in children between one and four years of age. The interval between exposure to HIV and the development of AIDS is shorter in children than in adults. Infants infected with HIV have a 20-30% chance of developing AIDS within a year and dying before age three. In the remainder, AIDS progresses more slowly; the average child patient survives to seven years of age. Some survive into early adolescence.

Causes and symptoms

Because HIV destroys immune system cells, AIDS is a disease that can affect any of the body's major organ systems. HIV attacks the body through three disease processes: immunodeficiency, autoimmunity, and nervous system dysfunction.

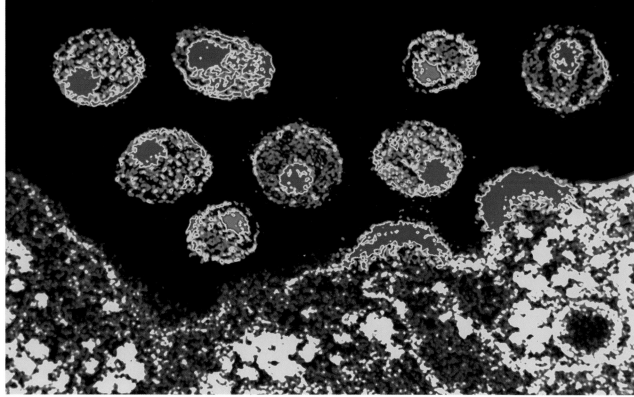

Mature HIV-1 viruses (above) and the lymphocyte from which they emerged (below). Two immature viruses can be seen budding on the surface of the lymphocyte (right of center). *(Photograph by Scott Camazir, Photo Researchers, Inc. Reproduced by permission.)*

Immunodeficiency describes the condition in which the body's immune response is damaged, weakened, or is not functioning properly. In AIDS, immunodeficiency results from the way that the virus binds to a protein called CD4, which is primarily found on the surface of certain subtypes of white blood cells called helper T cells or CD4 cells. After the virus has attached to the CD4 receptor, the virus-CD4 complex refolds to uncover another receptor called a chemokine receptor that helps to mediate entry of the virus into the cell. One chemokine receptor in particular, CCR5, has gotten recent attention after studies showed that defects in its structure (caused by genetic mutations) cause the progression of AIDS to be prevented or slowed. Scientists hope that this discovery will lead to the development of drugs that trigger an artificial mutation of the CCR5 gene or target the CCR5 receptor.

Once HIV has entered the cell, it can replicate intracellularly and kill the cell in ways that are still not completely understood. In addition to killing some lymphocytes directly, the AIDS virus disrupts the functioning of the remaining CD4 cells. Because the immune system cells are destroyed, many different types of infections and cancers that take advantage of a person's weakened immune system (opportunistic) can develop.

Autoimmunity is a condition in which the body's immune system produces antibodies that work against its own cells. Antibodies are specific proteins produced in response to exposure to a specific, usually foreign, protein or particle called an antigen. In this case, the body produces antibodies that bind to blood platelets that are necessary for proper blood clotting and tissue repair. Once bound, the antibodies mark the platelets for removal from the body, and they are filtered out by the spleen. Some AIDS patients develop a disorder, called immune-related thrombocytopenia purpura (ITP), in which the number of blood platelets drops to abnormally low levels.

Researchers do not know precisely how HIV attacks the nervous system since the virus can cause damage without infecting nerve cells directly. One theory is that, once infected with HIV, one type of

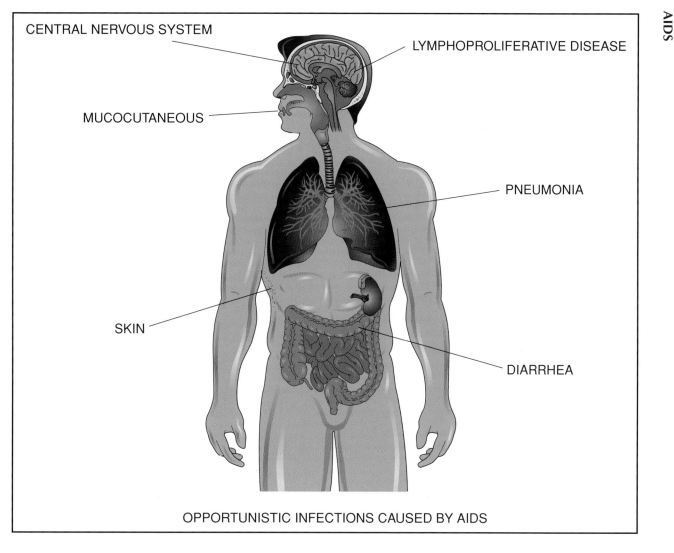

CENTRAL NERVOUS SYSTEM

LYMPHOPROLIFERATIVE DISEASE

MUCOCUTANEOUS

PNEUMONIA

SKIN

DIARRHEA

OPPORTUNISTIC INFECTIONS CAUSED BY AIDS

Because the immune system cells are destroyed by the AIDS virus, many different types of infections and cancers can develop, taking advantage of a person's weakened immune system. *(Illustration by Electronic Illustrators Group.)*

KEY TERMS

Acute retroviral syndrome—A group of symptoms resembling mononucleosis that often are the first sign of HIV infection in 50-70% of all patients and 45-90% of women.

AIDS dementia complex—A type of brain dysfunction caused by HIV infection that causes difficulty thinking, confusion, and loss of muscular coordination.

Antibody—A specific protein produced by the immune system in response to a specific foreign protein or particle called an antigen.

Antigen—Any substance that stimulates the body to produce antibody.

Autoimmunity—A condition in which the body's immune system produces antibodies in response to its own tissues or blood components instead of foreign particles or microorganisms.

CCR5—A chemokine receptor; defects in its structure caused by genetic mutation cause the progression of AIDS to be prevented or slowed.

CD4—A type of protein molecule in human blood, sometimes called the T4 antigen, that is present on the surface of 65% of immune cells. The HIV virus infects cells with CD4 surface proteins, and as a result, depletes the number of T cells, B cells, natural killer cells, and monocytes in the patient's blood.

Most of the damage to an AIDS patient's immune system is done by the virus' destruction of CD4+ lymphocytes.

Chemokine receptor—A receptor on the surface of some types of immune cells that helps to mediate entry of HIV into the cell.

Hairy leukoplakia of the tongue—A white area of diseased tissue on the tongue that may be flat or slightly raised. It is caused by the Epstein-Barr virus and is an important diagnostic sign of AIDS.

Hemophilia—Any of several hereditary blood coagulation disorders occurring almost exclusively in males. Because blood does not clot properly, even minor injuries can cause significant blood loss that may require a blood transfusion, with its associated minor risk of infection.

Human immunodeficiency virus (HIV)—A transmissible retrovirus that causes AIDS in humans. Two forms of HIV are now recognized: HIV-1, which causes most cases of AIDS in Europe, North and South America, and most parts of Africa; and HIV-2, which is chiefly found in West African patients. HIV-2, discovered in 1986, appears to be less virulent than HIV-1 and may also have a longer latency period.

Immunodeficient—A condition in which the body's immune response is damaged, weakened, or is not functioning properly.

Kaposi's sarcoma—A cancer of the connective tissue that produces painless purplish red (in people with light skin) or brown (in people with dark skin) blotches on the skin. It is a major diagnostic marker of AIDS.

Latent period—Also called incubation period, the time between infection with a disease-causing agent and the development of disease.

Lymphocyte—A type of white blood cell that is important in the formation of antibodies and that can be used to monitor the health of AIDS patients.

Lymphoma—A cancerous tumor in the lymphatic system that is associated with a poor prognosis in AIDS patients.

Macrophage—A large white blood cell, found primarily in the bloodstream and connective tissue, that helps the body fight off infections by ingesting the disease-causing organism. HIV can infect and kill macrophages.

Monocyte—A large white blood cell that is formed in the bone marrow and spleen. About 4% of the white blood cells in normal adults are monocytes.

***Mycobacterium avium* (MAC) infection**—A type of opportunistic infection that occurs in about 40% of AIDS patients and is regarded as an AIDS-defining disease.

Non-nucleoside reverse transcriptase inhibitors—The newest class of antiretroviral drugs that work by inhibiting the reverse transcriptase enzyme necessary for HIV replication.

Nucleoside analogues—The first group of effective anti-retroviral medications. They work by interfering with the AIDS virus' synthesis of DNA.

Opportunistic infection—An infection by organisms that usually don't cause infection in people whose immune systems are working normally.

Persistent generalized lymphadenopathy (PGL)—A condition in which HIV continues to produce chronic painless swellings in the lymph nodes during the latency period.

***Pneumocystis carinii* pneumonia (PCP)**—An opportunistic infection caused by a fungus that is a major cause of death in patients with late-stage AIDS.

Progressive multifocal leukoencephalopathy (PML)—A disease caused by a virus that destroys white matter in localized areas of the brain. It is regarded as an AIDS-defining illness.

Protease inhibitors—The second major category of drug used to treat AIDS that works by suppressing the replication of the HIV virus.

Protozoan—A single-celled, usually microscopic organism that is eukaryotic and, therefore, different from bacteria (prokaryotic).

Retrovirus—A virus that contains a unique enzyme called reverse transcriptase that allows it to replicate within new host cells.

T cells—Lymphocytes that originate in the thymus gland. T cells regulate the immune system's response to infections, including HIV. CD4 lymphocytes are a subset of T lymphocytes.

Thrush—A yeast infection of the mouth characterized by white patches on the inside of the mouth and cheeks.

Viremia—The measurable presence of virus in the bloodstream that is a characteristic of acute retroviral syndrome.

Wasting syndrome—A progressive loss of weight and muscle tissue caused by the AIDS virus.

immune system cell, called a macrophage, begins to release a toxin that harms the nervous system.

The course of AIDS generally progresses through three stages, although not all patients will follow this progression precisely:

Acute retroviral syndrome

Acute retroviral syndrome is a term used to describe a group of symptoms that can resemble mononucleosis and that may be the first sign of HIV infection in 50-70% of all patients and 45-90% of women. Most patients are not recognized as infected during this phase and may not seek medical attention. The symptoms may include fever, fatigue, muscle aches, loss of appetite, digestive disturbances, weight loss, skin **rashes**, headache, and chronically swollen lymph nodes (lymphadenopathy). Approximately 25-33% of patients will experience a form of **meningitis** during this phase in which the membranes that cover the brain and spinal cord become inflamed. Acute retroviral syndrome develops between one and six weeks after infection and lasts for two to three weeks. Blood tests during this period will indicate the presence of virus (viremia) and the appearance of the viral p24 antigen in the blood.

Latency period

After the HIV virus enters a patient's lymph nodes during the acute retroviral syndrome stage, the disease becomes latent for as many as 10 years or more before symptoms of advanced disease develop. During latency, the virus continues to replicate in the lymph nodes, where it may cause one or more of the following conditions:

PERSISTENT GENERALIZED LYMPHADENOPATHY (PGL). Persistent generalized lymphadenopathy, or PGL, is a condition in which HIV continues to produce chronic painless swellings in the lymph nodes during the latency period. The lymph nodes that are most frequently affected by PGL are those in the areas of the neck, jaw, groin, and armpits. PGL affects between 50-70% of patients during latency.

CONSTITUTIONAL SYMPTOMS. Many patients will develop low-grade fevers, chronic **fatigue**, and general weakness. HIV may also cause a combination of food malabsorption, loss of appetite, and increased metabolism that contribute to the so-called AIDS wasting or wasting syndrome.

OTHER ORGAN SYSTEMS. At any time during the course of HIV infection, patients may suffer from a yeast infection in the mouth called thrush, open sores or ulcers, or other infections of the mouth; **diarrhea** and other gastrointestinal symptoms that cause **malnutrition** and weight loss; diseases of the lungs and kidneys; and degeneration of the nerve fibers in the arms and legs. HIV infection of the nervous system leads to general loss of strength, loss of reflexes, and feelings of **numbness** or burning sensations in the feet or lower legs.

Late-stage disease (AIDS)

AIDS is usually marked by a very low number of CD4+ lymphocytes, followed by a rise in the frequency of opportunistic infections and cancers. Doctors monitor the number and proportion of CD4+ lymphocytes in the patient's blood in order to assess the progression of the disease and the effectiveness of different medications. About 10% of infected individuals never progress to this overt stage of the disease and are referred to as nonprogressors.

OPPORTUNISTIC INFECTIONS. Once the patient's CD4+ lymphocyte count falls below 200 cells/mm^3, he or she is at risk for a variety of opportunistic infections. The infectious organisms may include the following:

- Fungi. The most common fungal disease associated with AIDS is *Pneumocystis carinii* **pneumonia** (PCP). PCP is the immediate cause of death in 15-20% of AIDS patients. It is an important measure of a patient's prognosis. Other fungal infections include a yeast infection of the mouth (**candidiasis** or thrush) and cryptococcal meningitis.

- Protozoa. **Toxoplasmosis** is a common opportunistic infection in AIDS patients that is caused by a protozoan. Other diseases in this category include isoporiasis and cryptosporidiosis.

- Mycobacteria. AIDS patients may develop **tuberculosis** or MAC infections. MAC infections are caused by *Mycobacterium avium-intracellulare*, and occur in about 40% of AIDS patients. It is rare until CD4+ counts falls below 50 cells/mm^3.

- Bacteria. AIDS patients are likely to develop bacterial infections of the skin and digestive tract.

- Viruses. AIDS patients are highly vulnerable to cytomegalovirus (CMV), herpes simplex virus (HSV), varicella zoster virus (VZV), and Epstein-Barr virus (EBV) infections. Another virus, JC virus, causes progressive destruction of brain tissue in the brain stem, cerebrum, and cerebellum (multifocal leukoencephalopathy or PML), which is regarded as an AIDS-defining illness by the Centers for Disease Control and Prevention.

AIDS DEMENTIA COMPLEX AND NEUROLOGIC COMPLICATIONS. AIDS **dementia** complex is usually a late complication of the disease. It is unclear whether it is caused by the direct effects of the virus on the brain or by intermediate causes. AIDS dementia complex is marked by loss of reasoning ability, loss of memory, inability to concentrate, apathy and loss of initiative, and unsteadiness or weakness in walking. Some patients also develop seizures. There are no specific treatments for AIDS dementia complex.

MUSCULOSKELETAL COMPLICATIONS. Patients in late-stage AIDS may develop inflammations of the muscles, particularly in the hip area, and may have arthritis-like pains in the joints.

ORAL SYMPTOMS. In addition to thrush and painful ulcers in the mouth, patients may develop a condition called hairy leukoplakia of the tongue. This condition is also regarded by the CDC as an indicator of AIDS. Hairy leukoplakia is a white area of diseased tissue on the tongue that may be flat or slightly raised. It is caused by the Epstein-Barr virus.

AIDS-RELATED CANCERS. Patients with late-stage AIDS may develop Kaposi's sarcoma (KS), a skin tumor that primarily affects homosexual men. KS is the most common AIDS-related malignancy. It is characterized by reddish-purple blotches or patches (brownish in African-Americans) on the skin or in the mouth. About 40% of patients with KS develop symptoms in the digestive tract or lungs. KS may be caused by a herpes virus-like sexually transmitted disease agent rather than HIV.

The second most common form of **cancer** in AIDS patients is a tumor of the lymphatic system (lymphoma). AIDS-related lymphomas often affect the central nervous system and develop very aggressively.

Invasive cancer of the cervix (related to certain types of human papilloma virus [HPV]) is an important diagnostic marker of AIDS in women.

While incidence of AIDS-defining cancers such as Kaposi's sarcoma and **cervical cancer** have decreased since increase use of antiretroviral therapy, other cancers has increased in AIDS patients. People with HIV has shown higher incidence of lung cancer, head and neck cancers, Hodgkin's lymphoma, melanoma, and anorectal cancer from 1992 to 2002.

Diagnosis

Because HIV infection produces such a wide range of symptoms, the CDC has drawn up a list of 34 conditions regarded as defining AIDS. The physician will use the CDC list to decide whether the patient falls into one of these three groups:

- definitive diagnoses with or without laboratory evidence of HIV infection
- definitive diagnoses with laboratory evidence of HIV infection
- presumptive diagnoses with laboratory evidence of HIV infection.

Physical findings

Almost all the symptoms of AIDS can occur with other diseases. The general **physical examination** may range from normal findings to symptoms that are closely associated with AIDS. These symptoms are hairy leukoplakia of the tongue and Kaposi's sarcoma. When the doctor examines the patient, he or she will look for the overall pattern of symptoms rather than any one finding.

Laboratory tests for HIV infection

BLOOD TESTS (SEROLOGY). The first blood test for AIDS was developed in 1985. At present, patients who are being tested for HIV infection are usually given an enzyme-linked immunosorbent assay (ELISA) test for the presence of HIV antibody in their blood. Positive ELISA results are then tested with a Western blot or immunofluorescence (IFA) assay for confirmation. The combination of the ELISA and Western blot tests is more than 99.9% accurate in detecting HIV infection within four to eight weeks following exposure. The polymerase chain reaction (PCR) test can be used to detect the presence of viral nucleic acids in the very small number of HIV patients who have false-negative results on the ELISA and Western blot tests. These tests are also used to detect viruses and bacterium other than HIV and AIDS.

OTHER LABORATORY TESTS. In addition to diagnostic blood tests, there are other blood tests that are used to track the course of AIDS in patients that have already been diagnosed. These include blood counts, viral load tests, p24 antigen assays, and measurements of β_2-microglobulin (β_{2M}).

Doctors will use a wide variety of tests to diagnose the presence of opportunistic infections, cancers, or other disease conditions in AIDS patients. Tissue biopsies, samples of cerebrospinal fluid, and sophisticated imaging techniques, such as magnetic resonance imaging (MRI) and computed tomography scans (CT) are used to diagnose AIDS-related cancers, some opportunistic infections, damage to the central nervous system, and wasting of the muscles. Urine and stool samples are used to diagnose infections caused by parasites. AIDS patients are also given blood tests for syphilis and other **sexually transmitted diseases**.

Diagnosis in children

Diagnostic blood testing in children older than 18 months is similar to adult testing, with ELISA screening confirmed by Western blot. Younger infants can be diagnosed by direct culture of the HIV virus, PCR testing, and p24 antigen testing.

In terms of symptoms, children are less likely than adults to have an early acute syndrome. They are, however, likely to have delayed growth, a history of frequent illness, recurrent ear infections, a low blood cell count, failure to gain weight, and unexplained fevers. Children with AIDS are more likely to develop bacterial infections, inflammation of the lungs, and AIDS-related brain disorders than are HIV-positive adults.

Treatment

Treatment for AIDS covers four considerations:

TREATMENT OF OPPORTUNISTIC INFECTIONS AND MALIGNANCIES. Most AIDS patients require complex long-term treatment with medications for infectious diseases. This treatment is often complicated by the development of resistance in the disease organisms. AIDS-related malignancies in the central nervous system are usually treated with radiation therapy. Cancers elsewhere in the body are treated with chemotherapy.

PROPHYLACTIC TREATMENT FOR OPPORTUNISTIC INFECTIONS. Prophylactic treatment is treatment that is given to prevent disease. AIDS patients with a history of *Pneumocystis* pneumonia; with CD4+ counts below 200 cells/mm^3 or 14% of lymphocytes; weight loss; or thrush should be given prophylactic medications. The three drugs given are trimethoprim-sulfamethoxazole, dapsone, or pentamidine in aerosol form.

ANTI-RETROVIRAL TREATMENT. In recent years researchers have developed drugs that suppress HIV replication, as distinct from treating its effects on the body. These drugs fall into four classes:

- Nucleotide analogues. These drugs work by interfering with the action of HIV reverse transcriptase inside infected cells, thus ending the virus' replication process. These drugs include zidovudine (sometimes called azidothymidine or AZT), didanosine (ddI),

zalcitabine (ddC), stavudine (d4T), lamivudine (3TC), and abacavir (ABC).

- **Protease inhibitors**. Protease inhibitors can be effective against HIV strains that have developed resistance to nucleoside analogues, and are often used in combination with them. These compounds include saquinavir, ritonavir, indinavir, nelfinavir, amprenavir, and lopinavir..

- Non-nucleoside reverse transcriptase inhibitors. This is a new class of antiretroviral agents. Three are available, nevirapine, which was approved first, delavirdine and efavirin.

- Fusion inhibitors, the newest class of antiretrovirals. They block specific proteins on the surface of the virus or the CD4 cell. These proteins help the virus gain entry into the cell.The only FDA approved fusion inhibitor as of spring 2004 was enfuvirtide.

Treatment guidelines for these agents are in constant change as new medications are developed and introduced. Two principles currently guide doctors in working out drug regimens for AIDS patients: using combinations of drugs rather than one medication alone; and basing treatment decisions on the results of the patient's viral load tests.

STIMULATION OF BLOOD CELL PRODUCTION. Because many patients with AIDS suffer from abnormally low levels of both red and white blood cells, they may be given medications to stimulate blood cell production. Epoetin alfa (erythropoietin) may be given to anemic patients. Patients with low white blood cell counts may be given filgrastim or sargramostim.

Treatment in women

Treatment of pregnant women with HIV is particularly important in that anti-retroviral therapy has been shown to reduce transmission to the infant by 65%.

Alternative treatment

Alternative treatments for AIDS can be grouped into two categories: those intended to help the immune system and those aimed at **pain** control. Treatments that may enhance the function of the immune system include Chinese herbal medicine and western herbal medicine, macrobiotic and other special **diets, guided imagery** and creative visualization, homeopathy, and vitamin therapy. Pain control therapies include **hydrotherapy, reiki, acupuncture, meditation, chiropractic** treatments, and therapeutic massage. Alternative therapies can also be used to help with side effects of the medications used in the treatment of AIDS.

Prognosis

At the present time, there is no cure for AIDS.

Treatment stresses aggressive combination drug therapy for those patients with access to the expensive medications and who tolerate them adequately. The use of these multi-drug therapies has significantly reduced the numbers of deaths, in this country, resulting from AIDS. The data is still inconclusive, but the potential exists to possibly prolong life indefinitely using these and other drug therapies to boost the immune system, keep the virus from replicating, and ward off opportunistic infections and malignancies.

Prognosis after the latency period depends on the patient's specific symptoms and the organ systems affected by the disease. Patients with AIDS-related lymphomas of the central nervous system die within two to three months of diagnosis; those with systemic lymphomas may survive for eight to ten months.

Prevention

As of 2005, there was no vaccine effective against AIDS. Several vaccines are currently being investigated, however, both to prevent initial HIV infection and as a therapeutic treatment to prevent HIV from progressing to full-blown AIDS.

In the meantime, there are many things that can be done to prevent the spread of AIDS:

- Being monogamous and practice safe sex. Individuals must be instructed in the proper use of condoms and urged to practice safe sex. Besides avoiding the risk of HIV infection, condoms are successful in preventing other sexually transmitted diseases and unwanted pregnancies. Before engaging in a sexual relationship with someone, getting tested for HIV infection is recommended.

- Avoiding needle sharing among intravenous drug users.

- Although blood and blood products are carefully monitored, those individuals who are planning to undergo major surgery may wish to donate blood ahead of time to prevent a risk of infection from a blood **transfusion**.

- Healthcare professionals must take all necessary precautions by wearing gloves and masks when handling body fluids and preventing needle-stick injuries.

- If someone suspects HIV infection, he or she should be tested for HIV. If treated aggressively and early, the development of AIDS may be postponed indefinitely. If HIV infection is confirmed, it is also vital to let sexual partners know so that they can be tested and, if necessary, receive medical attention.

Resources

PERIODICALS

Boschert, Sherry. "Some Ca Increasing in Post-HAART Era." *Clinical Psychiatry News* June 2004: 75.

Godwin, Catherine. "WhatÆs New in the Fight Against AIDS." *RN* April 2004: 46–54.

ORGANIZATIONS

Gay Men's Health Crisis, Inc., 129 West 20th Street, New York, NY 10011-0022. (212) 807-6655.

National AIDS Hot Line. (800) 342-AIDS (English). (800) 344-SIDA (Spanish). (800) AIDS-TTY (hearing-impaired).

OTHER

"FDA Approved Drugs for HIV Infection and AIDS-RelatedConditions." *HIV/AIDS Treatment Information Service website*. January 2001. < http://hivatis.org >.

Rebecca J. Frey, PhD
Teresa G. Odle

AIDS serology *see* **AIDS tests**

AIDS tests

Definition

AIDS tests, short for acquired **immunodeficiency** syndrome tests, cover a number of different procedures used in the diagnosis and treatment of HIV patients. These tests sometimes are called AIDS serology tests. Serology is the branch of immunology that deals with the contents and characteristics of blood serum. Serum is the clear light yellow part of blood that remains liquid when blood cells form a clot. AIDS serology evaluates the presence of human immunodeficiency virus (HIV) infection in blood serum and its effects on each patient's immune system.

Purpose

AIDS serology serves several different purposes. Some AIDS tests are used to diagnose patients or confirm a diagnosis; others are used to measure the progression of the disease or the effectiveness of specific treatment regimens. Some AIDS tests also can be used to screen blood donations for safe use in transfusions.

In order to understand the different purposes of the blood tests used with AIDS patients, it is helpful to understand how HIV infection affects human blood and the immune system. HIV is a retrovirus that enters the blood stream of a new host in the following ways:

- by sexual contact
- by contact with infected body fluids (such as blood and urine)
- by transmission during **pregnancy**, or
- through **transfusion** of infected blood products

A retrovirus is a virus that contains a unique enzyme called reverse transcriptase that allows it to replicate within new host cells. The virus binds to a protein called CD4, which is found on the surface of certain subtypes of white blood cells, including helper T cells, macrophages, and monocytes. Once HIV enters the cell, it can replicate and kill the cell in ways that are still not completely understood. In addition to killing some lymphocytes directly, the AIDS virus disrupts the functioning of the remaining CD4 cells. CD4 cells ordinarily produce a substance called interleukin-2 (IL-2), which stimulates other cells (T cells and B cells) in the human immune system to respond to infections. Without the IL-2, T cells do not reproduce as they normally would in response to the HIV virus, and B cells are not stimulated to respond to the infection.

Precautions

In some states such as New York, a signed consent form is needed in order to administer an AIDS test. As with all blood tests, healthcare professionals should always wear latex gloves and avoid being pricked by the needle used in drawing blood for the tests. It may be difficult to get blood from a habitual intravenous drug user due to collapsed veins.

Description

Diagnostic tests

Diagnostic blood tests for AIDS usually are given to persons in high-risk populations who may have been exposed to HIV or who have the early symptoms of AIDS. Most persons infected with HIV will develop

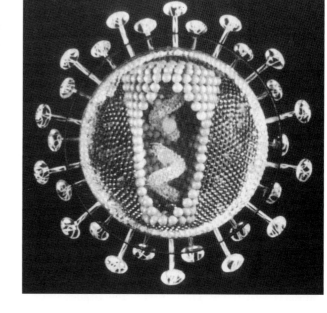

A three-dimensional model of the HIV virus. (*Corbis Corporation (New York). Reproduced by permission.*)

a detectable level of antibody within three months of infection. The condition of testing positive for HIV antibody in the blood is called seroconversion, and persons who have become HIV-positive are called seroconverters.

It is possible to diagnose HIV infection by isolating the virus itself from a blood sample or by demonstrating the presence of HIV antigen in the blood. Viral culture, however, is expensive, not widely available, and slow—it takes 28 days to complete the viral culture test. More common are blood tests that work by detecting the presence of antibodies to the HIV virus. These tests are inexpensive, widely available, and accurate in detecting 99.9% of AIDS infections when used in combination to screen patients and confirm diagnoses.

ENZYME-LINKED IMMUNOSORBENT ASSAY (ELISA). This type of blood test is used to screen blood for transfusions as well as diagnose patients. An ELISA test for HIV works by attaching HIV antigens to a plastic well or beads. A sample of the patient's blood serum is added, and excess proteins are removed. A second antibody coupled to an enzyme is added, followed by addition of a substance that will cause the enzyme to react by forming a color. An instrument called a spectrophotometer can measure the color. The name of the test is derived from the use of the enzyme that is coupled or linked to the second antibody.

Antibody—A protein in the blood that identifies and helps remove disease organisms or their toxins. Antibodies are secreted by B cells. AIDS diagnostic tests work by demonstrating the presence of HIV antibody in the patient's blood.

Antigen—Any substance that stimulates the body to produce antibodies.

B cell—A type of white blood cell derived from bone marrow. B cells are sometimes called B lymphocytes. They secrete antibody and have a number of other complex functions within the human immune system.

CD4—A type of protein molecule in human blood that is present on the surface of 65% of human T cells. CD4 is a receptor for the HIV virus. When the HIV virus infects cells with CD4 surface proteins, it depletes the number of T cells, B cells, natural killer cells, and monocytes in the patient's blood. Most of the damage to an AIDS patient's immune system is done by the virus' destruction of CD4+ lymphocytes. CD4 is sometimes called the T4 antigen.

Complete blood count (CBC)—A routine analysis performed on a sample of blood taken from the patient's vein with a needle and vacuum tube. The measurements taken in a CBC include a white blood cell count, a red blood cell count, the red cell distribution width, the hematocrit (ratio of the volume of the red blood cells to the blood volume), and the amount of hemoglobin (the blood protein that carries oxygen). CBCs are a routine blood test used for many medical reasons, not only for AIDS patients. They can help the doctor determine if a patient is in advanced stages of the disease.

Electrophoresis—A method of separating complex protein molecules suspended in a gel by running an electric current through the gel.

Enzyme-linked immunosorbent assay (ELISA)—A diagnostic blood test used to screen patients for AIDS or other viruses. The patient's blood is mixed with antigen attached to a plastic tube or bead surface. A sample of the patient's blood serum is added, and excess proteins are removed. A second antibody coupled to an enzyme is added, followed by a chemical that will cause a color reaction that can be measured by a special instrument.

Human immunodeficiency virus (HIV)—A transmissible retrovirus that causes AIDS in humans. Two forms of HIV are now recognized: HIV-1, which causes most cases of AIDS in Europe, North and South America, and most parts of Africa; and HIV-2, which is chiefly found in West African patients. HIV-2, discovered in 1986, appears to be less virulent than HIV-1, but also may have a longer latency period.

Immunofluorescent assay (IFA)—A blood test sometimes used to confirm ELISA results instead of using the Western blotting. In an IFA test, HIV antigen is mixed with a fluorescent compound and then with a sample of the patient's blood. If HIV antibody is present, the mixture will fluoresce when examined under ultraviolet light.

Lymphocyte—A type of white blood cell that is important in the formation of antibodies. Doctors can monitor the health of AIDS patients by measuring the number or proportion of certain types of lymphocytes in the patient's blood.

Macrophage—A large white blood cell, found primarily in the bloodstream and connective tissue, that helps the body fight off infections by ingesting the disease organism. HIV can infect and kill macrophages.

Monocyte—A large white blood cell that is formed in the bone marrow and spleen. About 4% of the white blood cells in normal adults are monocytes.

Opportunistic infection—An infection that develops only when a person's immune system is weakened, as happens to AIDS patients.

Polymerase chain reaction (PCR)—A test performed to evaluate false-negative results to the ELISA and Western blot tests. In PCR testing, numerous copies of a gene are made by separating the two strands of DNA containing the gene segment, marking its location, using DNA polymerase to make a copy, and then continuously replicating the copies. The amplification of gene sequences that are associated with HIV allows for detection of the virus by this method.

Retrovirus—A virus that contains a unique enzyme called reverse transcriptase that allows it to replicate within new host cells.

Seroconversion—The change from HIV- negative to HIV-positive status during blood testing. Persons who are HIV-positive are called seroconverters.

Serology—The analysis of the contents and properties of blood serum.

Serum—The part of human blood that remains liquid when blood cells form a clot. Human blood serum is clear light yellow in color.

T cells—Lymphocytes that originate in the thymus gland. T cells regulate the immune system's response to infections, including HIV. CD4 lymphocytes are a subset of T lymphocytes.

Viral load test—A new blood test for monitoring the speed of HIV replication in AIDS patients. The viral load test is based on PCR techniques and supplements the CD4+ cell count tests.

Western blot—A technique developed in 1979 that is used to confirm ELISA results. HIV antigen is purified by electrophoresis and attached by blotting to a nylon or nitrocellulose filter. The patient's serum is reacted against the filter, followed by treatment with developing chemicals that allow HIV antibody to show up as a colored patch or blot. If the patient is HIV-positive, there will be stripes at specific locations for two or more viral proteins. A negative result is blank.

WBC differential—A white blood cell count in which the technician classifies the different white blood cells by type as well as calculating the number of each type. A WBC differential is necessary to calculate the absolute CD4+ lymphocyte count.

The latest generation of ELISA tests are 99.5% sensitive to HIV. Occasionally, the ELISA test will be positive for a patient without symptoms of AIDS from a low-risk group. Because this result is likely to be a false-positive, the ELISA must be repeated *on the same sample of the patient's blood*. If the second ELISA is positive, the result should be confirmed by the Western blot test.

WESTERN BLOT (IMMUNOBLOT). The Western blot or immunoblot test is used as a reference procedure to confirm the diagnosis of AIDS. In Western blot testing, HIV antigen is purified by electrophoresis (large protein molecules are suspended in a gel and separated from one another by running an electric current through the gel). The HIV antigens are attached by blotting to a nylon or nitrocellulose filter. The patient's serum is reacted against the filter, followed by treatment with developing chemicals that allow HIV antibody to show up as a colored patch or blot. A commercially produced Western blot test for HIV-1 is now available. It consists of a prefabricated strip that is incubated with a sample of the patient's blood serum and the developing chemicals. About nine different HIV-1 proteins can be detected in the blots.

When used in combination with ELISA testing, Western blot testing is 99.9% specific. It can, however, yield false negatives in patients with very early HIV infection and in those infected by HIV-2. In some patients the Western blot yields indeterminate results.

IMMUNOFLUORESCENCE ASSAY (IFA). This method is sometimes used to confirm ELISA results instead of Western blotting. An IFA test detects the presence of HIV antibody in a sample of the patient's serum by mixing HIV antigen with a fluorescent chemical, adding the blood sample, and observing the reaction under a microscope with ultraviolet light.

POLYMERASE CHAIN REACTION (PCR). This test is used to evaluate the very small number of AIDS patients with false-negative ELISA and Western blot tests. These patients are sometimes called antibody-negative asymptomatic (without symptoms) carriers, because they do not have any symptoms of AIDS and there is no detectable quantity of antibody in the blood serum. Antibody-negative asymptomatic carriers may be responsible for the very low ongoing risk of HIV infection transmitted by blood transfusions. It is estimated that the risk is between 1 in 10,000 and 1 in 100,000 units of transfused blood.

The polymerase chain reaction (PCR) test can measure the presence of viral nucleic acids in the patient's blood even when there is no detectable antibody to HIV. This test works by amplifying the presence of HIV nucleic acids in a blood sample. Numerous copies of a gene are made by separating the two strands of DNA containing the gene segment, marking its location, using DNA polymerase to make a copy, and then continuously replicating the copies. It is questionable whether PCR will replace Western blotting as the method of confirming AIDS diagnoses. Although PCR can detect the low number of persons (1%) with HIV infections that have not yet generated an antibody response to the virus, the overwhelming majority of infected persons will be detected by ELISA screening within one to three months of infection. In addition, PCR testing is based on present knowledge of the genetic sequences in HIV. Since the virus is continually generating new variants, PCR testing could yield a false negative in patients with these new variants. In 2004, researchers reported on a new test that was more sensitive to HIV, detecting the infection in as little as 12 days after infection. However, the manufacturer was still seeking FDA approval for the test, which would cost about the same as PCR testing.

In 1999, the U.S. Food and Drug Administration (FDA) approved an HIV home testing kit. The kit contained multiple components, including material for specimen collection, a mailing envelope to send the specimen to a laboratory for analysis, and provides pre- and post-test counseling. It uses a finger prick process for blood collection. Other tests have been in development that would allow patients to monitor their own therapy in the home without sending out for results.

Prognostic tests

Blood tests to evaluate patients already diagnosed with HIV infection are as important as the diagnostic tests. Because AIDS has a long latency period, some persons may be infected with the virus for 10 years or longer before they develop symptoms of AIDS. These patients are sometimes called antibody-positive asymptomatic carriers. Prognostic tests also help drug researchers evaluate the usefulness of new medications in treating AIDS.

BLOOD CELL COUNTS. Doctors can measure the number or proportion of certain types of cells in an AIDS patient's blood to see whether and how rapidly the disease is progressing, or whether certain treatments are helping the patient. These cell count tests include:

• Complete **blood count** (CBC). A CBC is a routine analysis performed on a sample of blood taken from the patient's vein with a needle and vacuum tube. The measurements taken in a CBC include a white blood cell count (WBC), a red blood cell count (RBC), the red cell distribution width, the **hematocrit** (ratio of the volume of the red blood cells to the blood volume), and the amount of hemoglobin (the blood protein that carries oxygen). Although CBCs are used on more than just AIDS patients, they can help the doctor determine if an AIDS patient has an advanced form of the disease. Specific AIDS-related signs in a CBC include a low hematocrit, a sharp decrease in the number of blood platelets, and a low level of a certain type of white blood cell called neutrophils.

• Absolute CD4+ lymphocytes. A lymphocyte is a type of white blood cell that is important in the formation of an immune response. Because HIV targets CD4+ lymphocytes, their number in the patient's blood can be used to track the course of the infection. This blood cell count is considered the most accurate indicator for the presence of an opportunistic infection in an AIDS patient. The absolute CD4+ lymphocyte count is obtained by multiplying the patient's white blood cell count (WBC) by the percentage of lymphocytes among the white blood cells, and multiplying the result by the percentage of lymphocytes bearing the CD4+ marker. An absolute count below 200-300 CD+4 lymphocytes in 1 cubic millimeter (mm^3) of blood indicates that the patient is vulnerable to some opportunistic infections.

• CD4+ lymphocyte percentage. Some doctors think that this is a more accurate test than the absolute count because the percentage does not depend on a manual calculation of the number of types of different white blood cells. A white blood cell count that is broken down into categories in this way is called a WBC differential.

It is important for doctors treating AIDS patients to measure the lymphocyte count on a regular basis. Experts consulted by the United States Public Health Service recommend the following frequency of serum testing based on the patient's CD4+ level:

• CD4+ count more than 600 cells/mm^3: Every six months.

• CD4+ count between 200-600 cells/mm^3: Every three months.

• CD4+ count less than 200 cells/mm^3: Every three months.

When the CD4+ count falls below 200 cells/mm^3, the doctor will put the patient on a medication regimen to protect him or her against opportunistic infections.

HIV VIRAL LOAD TESTS. Another type of blood test for monitoring AIDS patients is the viral load test. It supplements the CD4+ count, which can tell the doctor the extent of the patient's loss of immune function, but not the speed of HIV replication in the body. The viral load test is based on PCR techniques and can measure the number of copies of HIV nucleic acids. Successive test results for a given patient's viral load are calculated on a base 10 logarithmic scale.

ORAL HIV TESTS. Scientists have developed oral HIV tests that can be conducted with saliva samples. One of the unintented effects of these tests is the misperception that HIV can be transmitted through saliva. Still, they present an excellent alternative to blood sample testing.

RAPID HIV TESTS. Researchers constantly work on more rapid tests for HIV that can be done in physician offices or by less skilled people and more convenient locations in developing countries. A finger-stick test that can be read quickly from a whole blood sample had shown promising results in the fall of 2003.

Another test, called the VScan test kit, requires no refrigeration or electricity and can safely be stored at room temperature. Even if the positive results must be confirmed by ELISA or Western blotting, an accurate initial rapid test can help screen populations for HIV antibodies.

In 2004, a new three-minute test for HIV was lunched in the United States under FDA approval. The hope of this test is that health care providers such as family practice physician offices can quickly test a patient in the office and provide results while the patient waits, rather than sending results to a lab.

BETA₂-MICROGLOBULIN (BETA₂M). Beta-microglobulin is a protein found on the surface of all human cells with a nucleus. It is released into the blood when a cell dies. Although rising blood levels of β_{2M} are found in patients with **cancer** and other serious diseases, a rising β_{2M} blood level can be used to measure the progression of AIDS.

P24 ANTIGEN CAPTURE ASSAY. Found in the viral core of HIV, p24 is a protein that can be measured by the ELISA technique. Doctors can use p24 assays to measure the antiviral activity of the patient's medications. In addition, the p24 assay is sometimes useful in detecting HIV infection before seroconversion. However, p24 is consistently present in only 25% of persons infected with HIV.

GENOTYPIC DRUG RESISTANCE TEST. Genotypic testing can help determine whether specific gene mutations, common in people with HIV, are causing drug resistance and drug failure. The test looks for specific genetic mutations within the virus that are known to cause resistance to certain drugs used in HIV treatment. For example the drug 3TC, also known as lamivudine (Epivir), is not effective against strains of HIV that have a mutation at a particular position on the reverse transcriptase protein—amino acid 184—known as M184V (M→V, methionine to valine). So if the genotypic resistance test shows a mutation at position M184V, it is likely the person is resistant to 3TC and not likely to respond to 3TC treatment. Genotypic tests are only effective if the person is already taking antiviral medication and if the viral load is greater than 1,000 copies per milliliter (mL) of blood. The cost of the test, usually between $300 and $500, is usually now covered by many insurance plans.

PHENOTYPIC DRUG RESISTANCE TESTING. Phenotypic testing directly measures the sensitivity of a patient's HIV to particular drugs and drug combinations. To do this, it measures the concentration of a drug required to inhibit viral replication in the test tube. This is the same method used by researchers to determine whether a drug might be effective against HIV before using it in human clinical trials. Phenotypic testing is a more direct measurement of resistance than genotypic testing. Also, unlike genotypic testing, phenotypic testing does not require a high viral load but it is recommended that persons already be taking **antiretroviral drugs**. The cost is between $700 and $900 and is now covered by many insurance plans.

AIDS serology in children

Children born to HIV-infected mothers may acquire the infection through the mother's placenta or during the birth process. Public health experts recommend the testing and monitoring of all children born to mothers with HIV. Diagnostic testing in children older than 18 months is similar to adult testing, with ELISA screening confirmed by Western blot. Younger infants can be diagnosed by direct culture of the HIV virus, PCR testing, and p24 antigen testing. These techniques allow a pediatrician to identify 50% of infected children at or near birth, and 95% of cases in infants three to six months of age.

Preparation

Preparation and aftercare are important parts of AIDS diagnostic testing. Doctors are now advised to take the patient's emotional, social, economic, and other circumstances into account and to provide counseling before and after testing. Patients are generally better able to cope with the results if the doctor has spent some time with them before the blood test explaining the basic facts about HIV infection and testing. Many doctors now offer this type of informational counseling before performing the tests.

Aftercare

If the test results indicate that the patient is HIV-positive, he or she will need counseling, information, referral for treatment, and support. Doctors can either counsel the patient themselves or invite an experienced HIV counselor to discuss the results of the blood tests with the patient. They also will assess the patient's emotional and psychological status, including the possibility of violent behavior and the availability of a support network.

Risks

The risks of AIDS testing are primarily related to disclosure of the patient's HIV status rather than to any physical risks connected with blood testing. Some patients are better prepared to cope with a positive diagnosis than others, depending on their age, sex, health, resources, belief system, and similar factors.

Normal results

Normal results for ELISA, Western blot, IFA, and PCR testing are negative for HIV antibody.

Normal results for blood cell counts:

- WBC differential: Total lymphocytes 24-44% of the white blood cells.

- Hematocrit: 40-54% in men; 37-47% in women.

- T cell lymphocytes: 644-2200/mm^3, 60-88% of all lymphocytes.

- B cell lymphocytes: 82-392/mm^3, 3-20% of all lymphocytes.

- CD4+ lymphocytes: 500-1200/mm^3, 34-67% of all lymphocytes.

Abnormal results

The following results in AIDS tests indicate progression of the disease:

- Percentage of CD4+ lymphocytes: less than 20% of all lymphocytes.

- CD4+ lymphocyte count: less than 200 cells/mm^3.

- Viral load test: Levels more than 5000 copies/mL.

- β:-2-microglobulin: Levels more than 3.5 mg/dL.

- P24 antigen: Measurable amounts in blood serum.

Resources

BOOKS

Bennett, Rebecca, and Erin, Charles A., editors. *HIV and AIDS Testing, Screening, and Confidentiality: Ethics, Law, and Social Policy*. Oxford, England: Oxford University Press, 2001.

PERIODICALS

"Finger-stick Test is Accurate and Acceptable to Women in Thailand." *Drug Week* (September 5, 2003): 168.

Kaplan, Edward H., and Glen A. Satten. "Repeat Screening for HIV: When to Test and Why." *The Journal of the American Medical Association.*

Medical Devices & Surgical Technology Week (September 12, 2004): 102.

"Researcher Developing Home Test Kit for HIV Therapies." *Medical Devices & Surgical Technology Week* (December 23, 2001): 2.

"Researchers Report New Ultra-sensitive AIDS Test." *Biotech Week* (July 14, 2004): 246.

Weinhardt, Lance S., et al. "Human Immunodeficiency Virus Testing and Behavior Change." *Archives of Internal Medicine* (May 22, 2000): 1538.

Ken R. Wells
Teresa G. Odle

Air embolism *see* **Gas embolism**

Alanine aminotransferase test

Definition

The alanine aminotransferase test, also known as ALT, is one of a group of tests known as **liver function tests** (or LFTs) and is used to monitor damage to the liver.

Purpose

ALT levels are used to detect liver abnormalities. Since the alanine aminotransferase enzyme is also found in muscle, tests indicating elevated AST levels might also indicate muscle damage. However, other tests, such as the levels of the MB fraction of creatine kinase should indicate whether the abnormal test levels are because of muscle or liver damage.

Description

The alanine aminotransferase test (ALT) can reveal liver damage. It is probably the most specific test for liver damage. However, the severity of the liver damage is not necessarily shown by the ALT test, since the amount of dead liver tissue does not correspond to higher ALT levels. Also, patients with normal, or declining, ALT levels may experience serious liver damage without an increase in ALT.

Nevertheless, ALT is widely used, and useful, because ALT levels are elevated in most patients with **liver disease**. Although ALT levels do not necessarily indicate the severity of the damage to the liver, they may indicate how much of the liver has been damaged. ALT levels, when compared to the levels of a similar enzyme, aspartate aminotransferase (AST), may provide important clues to the nature of the liver disease. For example, within a certain range of values, a ratio of 2:1 or greater for AST: ALT might indicate that a patient suffers from alcoholic liver disease. Other diagnostic data may be gleaned from ALT tests to indicate abnormal results.

Preparation

No special preparations are necessary for this test.

Aftercare

This test involves blood being drawn, probably from a vein in the patient's elbow. The patient should keep the wound from the needle puncture covered (with a bandage) until the bleeding stops. Patients should report any unusual symptoms to their physician.

Normal results

Normal values vary from laboratory to laboratory, and should be available to your physician at the time of the test. An informal survey of some laboratories indicates many laboratories find values from approximately seven to 50 IU/L to be normal.

Abnormal results

Low levels of ALT (generally below 300 IU/L) may indicate any kind of liver disease. Levels above 1,000 IU/L generally indicate extensive liver damage from toxins or drugs, viral hepatitis, or a lack of oxygen (usually resulting from very low blood pressure or a **heart attack**). A briefly elevated ALT above 1,000 IU/L that resolves in 24-48 hours may indicate a blockage of the bile duct. More moderate levels of ALT (300-1,000IU/L) may support a diagnosis of acute or chronic hepatitis.

It is important to note that persons with normal livers may have slightly elevated levels of ALT. This is a normal finding.

Michael V. Zuck, PhD

Albers-Schönberg disease *see* **Osteopetroses**

Albinism

Definition

Albinism is an inherited condition present at birth, characterized by a lack of pigment that normally gives color to the skin, hair, and eyes. Many types of albinism exist, all of which involve lack of pigment in varying degrees. The condition, which is found in all races, may be accompanied by eye problems and may lead to skin **cancer** later in life.

Description

Albinism is a rare disorder found in fewer than five people per 100,000 in the United States and Europe. Other parts of the world have a much higher rate; for example, albinism is found in about 20 out of every 100,000 people in southern Nigeria.

There are 10 types of the most common form of the condition, known as "oculocutaneous albinism," which affects the eyes, hair, and skin. In its most severe form, hair and skin remain pure white throughout life. People with a less severe form are born with white hair and skin, which turn slightly darker as they age. Everyone with oculocutaneous albinism experiences abnormal flickering eye movements (**nystagmus**) and sensitivity to bright light. There may be other eye problems as well, including poor vision and crossed or "lazy" eyes (strabismus).

The second most common type of the condition is known as "ocular" albinism, in which only the eyes lack color; skin and hair are normal. There are five forms of ocular albinism; some types cause more problems–especially eye problems–than others.

Causes and symptoms

Every cell in the body contains a matched pair of genes, one inherited from each parent. These genes act as a sort of "blueprint" that guides the development of a fetus.

Albinism is an inherited problem caused by a flaw in one or more of the genes that are responsible for directing the eyes and skin to make melanin (pigment). As a result, little or no pigment is made, and the child's skin, eyes and hair may be colorless.

In most types of albinism, a recessive trait, the child inherits flawed genes for making melanin from both parents. Because the task of making melanin is complex, there are many different types of albinism, involving a number of different genes.

It's also possible to inherit one normal gene and one albinism gene. In this case, the one normal gene provides enough information in its cellular blueprint to make some pigment, and the child will have normal skin and eye color. They "carry" one gene for albinism. About one in 70 people are albinism carriers, with one flawed gene but no symptoms; they have a 50% chance of passing the albinism gene to their child. However, if both parents are carriers with one flawed gene each, they have a 1 in 4 chance of passing on both copies of the flawed gene to the child, who will have albinism. (There is also a type of ocular albinism that is carried on the X chromosome and occurs almost exclusively in males because they have only one X

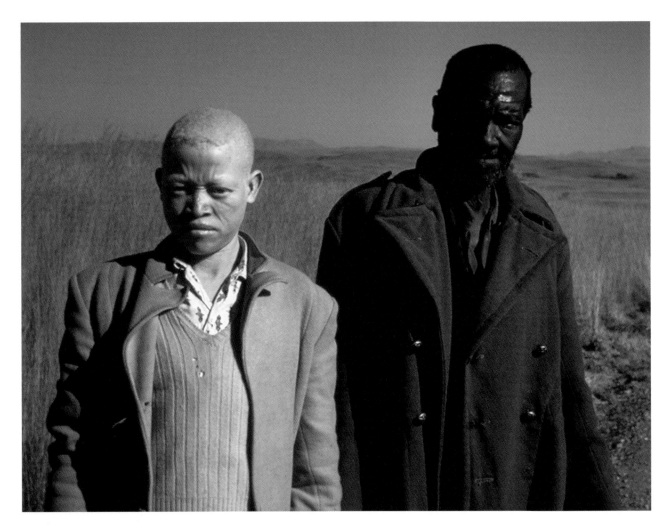

A man with albinism stands with his normally pigmented father. *(Photograph by Norman Lightfoot, Photo Researchers, Inc. Reproduced by permission.)*

chromosome and, therefore, no other gene for the trait to override the flawed one.)

Symptoms of albinism can involve the skin, hair, and eyes. The skin, because it contains little pigment, appears very light, as does the hair.

Although people with albinism may experience a variety of eye problems, one of the myths about albinism is that it causes people to have pink or red eyes. In fact, people with albinism can have irises varying from light gray or blue to brown. (The iris is the colored portion of the eye that controls the size of the pupil, the opening that lets light into the eye.) If people with albinism seem to have reddish eyes, it's because light is being reflected from the back of the eye (retina) in much the same way as happens when people are photographed with an electronic flash.

People with albinism may have one or more of the following eye problems:

- They may be very far-sighted or near-sighted, and may have other defects in the curvature of the lens of the eye (**astigmatism**) that cause images to appear unfocused.

- They may have a constant, involuntary movement of the eyeball called nystagmus.

- They may have problems in coordinating the eyes in fixing and tracking objects (strabismus), which may lead to an appearance of having "crossed eyes" at times. **Strabismus** may cause some problems with depth perception, especially at close distances.

- They may be very sensitive to light (photophobia) because their irises allow "stray" light to enter their eyes. It's a common misconception that people with albinism shouldn't go out on sunny days, but wearing sunglasses can make it possible to go outside quite comfortably.

KEY TERMS

Amino acids—Natural substances that are the building blocks of protein. The body breaks down the protein in food into amino acids, and then uses these amino acids to create other proteins. The body also changes amino acids into melanin pigment.

Astigmatism—An eye condition in which the lens doesn't focus light evenly on the retina, leading to problems with visual sharpness.

Carrier—A person with one normal gene and one faulty gene, who can pass on a condition to others without actually having symptoms.

DNA—The abbreviation for "deoxyribonucleic acid," the primary carrier of genetic information found in the chromosomes of almost all organisms. The entwined double structure allows the chromosomes to be copied exactly during cell division.

DOPA—The common name for a natural chemical (3, 4-dihydroxyphenylalanine) made by the body during the process of making melanin.

Enzyme—A protein that helps the body convert one chemical substance to another.

Gene—The basic unit of genetic material carried in a particular place on a chromosome. Genes are passed on from parents to child when the sperm and egg unite during conception.

Hairbulb—The root of a strand of hair from which the color develops.

Hermansky-Pudlak Syndrome (HPS)—A rare type of albinism characterized by a problem with blood clotting and a buildup of waxy material in lungs and intestines.

Melanin—Pigment made in the hair, skin and eyes.

Nystagmus—An involuntary back-and-forth movement of the eyes that is often found in albinism.

Strabismus—Crossed or "lazy" eyes, often found in albinism.

Tyrosine—A protein building block found in a wide variety of foods that is used by the body to make melanin.

Tyrosinase—An enzyme in a pigment cell which helps change tyrosine to DOPA during the process of making melanin.

In addition to the characteristically light skin and eye problems, people with a rare form of albinism called Hermansky-Pudlak Syndrome (HPS) also have a greater tendency to have bleeding disorders, inflammation of the large bowel (colitis), lung (pulmonary) disease, and kidney (renal) problems.

Diagnosis

It's not always easy to diagnose the exact type of albinism a person has; there are two tests available that can identify only two types of the condition. Recently, a blood test has been developed that can identify carriers of the gene for some types of albinism; a similar test during amniocentesis can diagnose some types of albinism in an unborn child. A **chorionic villus sampling** test during the fifth week of pregnancy may also reveal some types of albinism.

The specific type of albinism a person has can be determined by taking a good family history and examining the patient and several close relatives.

The "hairbulb pigmentation test" is used to identify carriers by incubating a piece of the person's hair in a solution of tyrosine, a substance in food which the body uses to make melanin. If the hair turns dark, it means the hair is making melanin (a "positive" test); light hair means there is no melanin. This test is the source of the names of two types of albinism: "ty-pos" and "ty-neg."

The tyrosinase test is more precise than the hairbulb pigmentation test. It measures the rate at which hair converts tyrosine into another chemical (DOPA), which is then made into pigment. The hair converts tyrosine with the help of a substance called "tyrosinase." In some types of albinism, tyrosinase doesn't do its job, and melanin production breaks down.

Treatment

There is no treatment that can replace the lack of melanin that causes the symptoms of albinism. Doctors can only treat, not cure, the eye problems that often accompany the lack of skin color. Glasses are usually needed and can be tinted to ease pain from too much sunlight. There is no cure for involuntary eye movements (nystagmus), and treatments for focusing problems (surgery or contact lenses) are not effective in all cases.

Crossed eyes (strabismus) can be treated during infancy, using eye patches, surgery or medicine injections. Treatment may improve the appearance of the eye, but it can do nothing to cure the underlying condition.

Patients with albinism should avoid excessive exposure to the sun, especially between 10 a.m. and 2 p.m. If exposure can't be avoided, they should use UVA-UVB sunblocks with an SPF of at least 20. Taking beta- carotene may help provide some skin color, although it doesn't protect against sun exposure.

Prognosis

In the United States, people with this condition can expect to have a normal lifespan. People with albinism may experience some social problems because of a lack of understanding on the part of others. When a member of a normally dark-skinned ethnic group has albinism, he or she may face some very complex social challenges.

One of the greatest health hazards for people with albinism is excessive exposure to sun without protection, which could lead to skin cancer. Wearing opaque clothes and sunscreen rated SPF 20, people with albinism can safely work and play outdoors safely even during the summer.

Prevention

Genetic counseling is very important to prevent further occurrences of the conditon.

Resources

BOOKS

National Association for the Visually Handicapped. *Larry: A Book for Children with Albinism Going to School.* New York: National Association for the Visually Handicapped.

ORGANIZATIONS

Albinism World Alliance. < http://www.albinism.org/awa. html >.

American Foundation for the Blind. 15 W. 16th St., New York, NY 10011. (800) AFB-LIND.

Hermansky-Pudlak Syndrome Network, Inc. One South Road, Oyster Bay, NY 11771-1905. (800) 789-9477. < appell@theonramp.net >.

National Organization for Albinism and Hypopigmentation (NOAH). 1530 Locust St., #29, Philadelphia, PA 19102-4415. (800) 473-2310. < http://www.albinism.org >.

Carol A. Turkington

Albuterol *see* **Bronchodilators**

Alcohol abuse *see* **Alcoholism**

Alcohol dependence *see* **Alcoholism**

Alcohol-related neurologic disease

Definition

Alcohol, or ethanol, is a poison with direct toxic effects on nerve and muscle cells. Depending on which nerve and muscle pathways are involved, alcohol can have far-reaching effects on different parts of the brain, peripheral nerves, and muscles, with symptoms of memory loss, incoordination, seizures, weakness, and sensory deficits. These different effects can be grouped into three main categories: (1) intoxication due to the acute effects of ethanol, (2) withdrawal syndrome from suddenly stopping drinking, and (3) disorders related to long-term or chronic alcohol **abuse**. Alcohol-related neurologic disease includes Wernicke-Korsakoff disease, alcoholic cerebellar degeneration, alcoholic myopathy, alcoholic neuropathy, alcohol withdrawal syndrome with seizures and **delirium** tremens, and **fetal alcohol syndrome**.

Description

Acute excess intake of alcohol can cause drunkenness (intoxication) or even **death**, and chronic or long-term abuse leads to potentially irreversible damage to virtually any level of the nervous system. Any given patient with long-term alcohol abuse may have no neurologic complications, a single alcohol-related disease, or multiple conditions, depending on the genes they have inherited, how well nourished they are, and other environmental factors, such as exposure to other drugs or toxins.

Neurologic complications of alcohol abuse may also result from nutritional deficiency, because alcoholics tend to eat poorly and may become depleted of thiamine or other **vitamins** important for nervous system function. Persons who are intoxicated are also at higher risk for **head injury** or for compression injuries of the peripheral nerves. Sudden changes in blood chemistry, especially sodium, related to alcohol abuse may cause central pontine myelinolysis, a condition of the brainstem in which nerves lose their myelin coating. **Liver disease** complicating alcoholic **cirrhosis** may cause **dementia**, delirium, and movement disorder.

Causes and symptoms

When a person drinks alcohol, it is absorbed by blood vessels in the stomach lining and flows rapidly throughout the body and brain, as ethanol freely crosses the blood-brain barrier that ordinarily keeps

KEY TERMS

Abstinence—Refraining from the use of alcoholic beverages.

Atrophy—A wasting or decrease in size of a muscle or other tissue.

Cerebellum—The part of the brain involved in coordination of movement, walking, and balance.

Degeneration—Gradual, progressive loss of nerve cells.

Delirium—Sudden confusion with decreased or fluctuating level of consciousness.

Delirium tremens— A complication that may accompany alcohol withdrawal. The symptoms include body shaking (tremulousness), insomnia, agitation, confusion, hearing voices or seeing images that are not really there (hallucinations), seizures, rapid heart beat, profuse sweating, high blood pressure, and fever.

Dementia—Loss of memory and other higher functions, such as thinking or speech, lasting six months or more.

Myoglobinuria—Reddish urine caused by excretion of myoglobin, a breakdown product of muscle.

Myopathy—A disorder that causes weakening of muscles.

Neuropathy—A condition affecting the nerves supplying the arms and legs. Typically, the feet and hands are involved first. If sensory nerves are involved, numbness, tingling, and pain are prominent, and if motor nerves are involved, the patient experiences weakness.

Thiamine—A B vitamin essential for the body to process carbohydrates and fats. Alcoholics may suffer complications (including Wernike-Korsakoff syndrome) from a deficiency of this vitamin.

Wernicke-Korsakoff syndrome—A combination of symptoms, including eye-movement problems, tremors, and confusion, that is caused by a lack of the B vitamin thiamine and may be seen in alcoholics.

large molecules from escaping from the blood vessel to the brain tissue. Drunkenness, or intoxication, may occur at blood ethanol concentrations of as low as 50-150 mg per dL in people who don't drink. Sleepiness, stupor, **coma**, or even death from respiratory depression and low blood pressure occur at progressively higher concentrations.

Although alcohol is broken down by the liver, the toxic effects from a high dose of alcohol are most likely a direct result of alcohol itself rather than of its breakdown products. The fatal dose varies widely because people who drink heavily develop a tolerance to the effects of alcohol with repeated use. In addition, alcohol tolerance results in the need for higher levels of blood alcohol to achieve intoxicating effects, which increases the likelihood that habitual drinkers will be exposed to high and potentially toxic levels of ethanol. This is particularly true when binge drinkers fail to eat, because **fasting** decreases the rate of alcohol clearance and causes even higher blood alcohol levels.

When a chronic alcoholic suddenly stops drinking, withdrawal of alcohol leads to a syndrome of increased excitability of the central nervous system, called delirium tremens or "DTs." Symptoms begin six to eight hours after abstinence, and are most pronounced 24-72 hours after abstinence. They include body shaking (tremulousness), **insomnia**, agitation, confusion, hearing voices or seeing images that are not really there (such as crawling bugs), seizures, rapid heart beat, profuse sweating, high blood pressure, and **fever**. Alcohol-related seizures may also occur without withdrawal, such as during active heavy drinking or after more than a week without alcohol.

Wernicke-Korsakoff syndrome is caused by deficiency of the B-vitamin thiamine, and can also be seen in people who don't drink but have some other cause of thiamine deficiency, such as chronic **vomiting** that prevents the absorption of this vitamin. A 2004 study demonstrated that alcohol-dependent patients admitted to a **detoxification** facility had consumed significantly less thiamine than a comparison group of healthy volunteers. Patients with this condition have the sudden onset of Wernicke encephalopathy; the symptoms include marked confusion, delirium, disorientation, inattention, memory loss, and drowsiness. Examination reveals abnormalities of eye movement, including jerking of the eyes (**nystagmus**) and double vision. Problems with balance make walking difficult. People may have trouble coordinating their leg movements, but usually not their arms. If thiamine is not given promptly, Wernicke encephalopathy may progress to stupor, coma, and death.

If thiamine is given and death averted, **Korsakoff's syndrome** may develop in some patients, who suffer from memory impairment that leaves them unable to remember events for a period of a few years before the onset of illness (retrograde **amnesia**) and unable to learn new information (anterograde amnesia). Most patients have very limited insight into their memory dysfunction and have a tendency to make up explanations for events they have forgotten (confabulation).

Severe **alcoholism** can cause cerebellar degeneration, a slowly progressive condition affecting portions of the brain called the anterior and superior cerebellar vermis, causing a wide-based gait, leg incoordination, and an inability to walk heel-to-toe in tightrope fashion. The gait disturbance usually develops over several weeks, but may be relatively mild for some time, and then suddenly worsen after binge drinking or an unrelated illness.

Fetal alcohol syndrome occurs in infants born to alcoholic mothers when prenatal exposure to ethanol retards fetal growth and development. Affected infants often have a distinctive appearance with a thin upper lip, flat nose and mid-face, short stature and small head size. Almost half are mentally retarded, and most others are mildly impaired intellectually or have problems with speech, learning, and behavior. Fetal alcohol syndrome is the leading cause of **mental retardation** and many physicians warn that there is no safe level of alcohol for a pregnant mother to consume.

Alcoholic myopathy, or weakness secondary to breakdown of muscle tissue, is also known as alcoholic rhabdomyolysis or alcoholic myoglobinuria. Males are affected by acute (sudden onset) alcoholic myopathy four times as often as females. Breakdown of muscle tissue (myonecrosis), can come on suddenly during binge drinking or in the first days of alcohol withdrawal. In its mildest form, this breakdown may cause no noticeable symptoms, but may be detected by a temporary elevation in blood levels of an enzyme found predominantly in muscle, the MM fraction of creatine kinase.

The severe form of acute alcoholic myopathy is associated with the sudden onset of muscle **pain**, swelling, and weakness; a reddish tinge in the urine caused by myoglobin, a breakdown product of muscle excreted in the urine; and a rapid rise in muscle enzymes in the blood. Symptoms usually worsen over hours to a few days, and then improve over the next week to 10 days as the patient is withdrawn from alcohol. Muscle symptoms are usually generalized, but pain and swelling may selectively involve the calves or other muscle groups. The muscle breakdown of acute alcoholic myopathy may be worsened by crush injuries, which may occur when people drink so much that they compress a muscle group with their body weight for a long time without moving, or

by withdrawal seizures with generalized muscle activity.

In patients who abuse alcohol over many years, chronic alcoholic myopathy may develop. Males and females are equally affected. Symptoms include painless weakness of the limb muscles closest to the trunk and the girdle muscles, including the thighs, hips, shoulders, and upper arms. This weakness develops gradually, over weeks or months, without symptoms of acute muscle injury. Muscle atrophy, or decreased bulk, may be striking. The nerves of the extremities may also begin to break down, a condition known as alcoholic **peripheral neuropathy**, which can add to the person's difficulty in moving.

The way in which alcohol destroys muscle tissue is still not well understood. Proposed mechanisms include muscle membrane changes affecting the transport of calcium, potassium, or other **minerals**; impaired muscle energy metabolism; and impaired protein synthesis. Alcohol is metabolized or broken down primarily by the liver, with a series of chemical reactions in which ethanol is converted to acetate. Acetate is metabolized by skeletal muscle, and alcohol-related changes in liver function may affect skeletal muscle metabolism, decreasing the amount of blood sugar available to muscles during prolonged activity. Because not enough sugar is available to supply needed energy, muscle protein may be broken down as an alternate energy source. However, toxic effects on muscle may be a direct result of alcohol itself rather than of its breakdown products.

Although alcoholic peripheral neuropathy may contribute to muscle weakness and atrophy by injuring the motor nerves controlling muscle movement, alcoholic neuropathy more commonly affects sensory fibers. Injury to these fibers can cause **tingling** or burning pain in the feet, which may be severe enough to interfere with walking. As the condition worsens, pain decreases but **numbness** increases.

Diagnosis

The diagnosis of alcohol-related neurologic disease depends largely on finding characteristic symptoms and signs in patients who abuse alcohol. Other possible causes should be excluded by the appropriate tests, which may include blood chemistry, **thyroid function tests**, brain MRI (**magnetic resonance imaging**) or CT (computed tomography scan), and/or cerebrospinal fluid analysis.

Acute alcoholic myopathy can be diagnosed by finding myoglobin in the urine and increased creatine kinase and other blood enzymes released from injured muscle. The surgical removal of a small piece of muscle for microscopic analysis (muscle biopsy) shows the scattered breakdown and repair of muscle fibers. Doctors must rule out other acquired causes of muscle breakdown, which include the abuse of drugs such as heroin, **cocaine**, or amphetamines; trauma with crush injury; the depletion of phosphate or potassium; or an underlying defect in the metabolism of carbohydrates or lipids. In chronic alcoholic myopathy, serum creatine kinase often is normal, and muscle biopsy shows atrophy, or loss of muscle fibers. **Electromyography** (EMG) may show features characteristic of alcoholic myopathy or neuropathy.

Treatment

Acute management of alcohol intoxication, delirium tremens, and withdrawal is primarily supportive, to monitor and treat any cardiovascular or **respiratory failure** that may develop. In delirium tremens, fever and sweating may necessitate treatment of fluid loss and secondary low blood pressure. Agitation may be treated with **benzodiazepines** such as chlordiazepoxide, beta-adrenergic antagonists such as atenolol, or alpha 2-adrenergic agonists such as clonidine. Because Wernicke's syndrome is rapidly reversible with thiamine, and because death may intervene if thiamine is not given promptly, all patients admitted for acute complications of alcohol, as well as all patients with unexplained encephalopathy, should be given intravenous thiamine.

Withdrawal seizures typically resolve without specific anti-epileptic drug treatment, although status epilepticus (continual seizures occurring without interruption) should be treated vigorously. Acute alcoholic myopathy with myoglobinuria requires monitoring and maintenance of kidney function, and correction of imbalances in blood chemistry including potassium, phosphate, and magnesium levels.

Chronic alcoholic myopathy and other chronic conditions are treated by correcting associated nutritional deficiencies and maintaining a diet adequate in protein and carbohydrate. The key to treating any alcohol-related disease is helping the patient overcome alcohol **addiction**. Behavioral measures and social supports may be needed in patients who develop broad problems in their thinking abilities (dementia) or remain in a state of confusion and disorientation (delirium). People with walking disturbances may benefit from physical therapy and assistive devices. Doctors may also prescribe drugs to treat the pain associated with peripheral neuropathy.

Prognosis

Complete recovery from Wernicke's syndrome may follow prompt administration of thiamine. However, repeated episodes of encephalopathy or prolonged alcohol abuse may cause persistent dementia or Korsakoff **psychosis**. Most patients recover fully from acute alcoholic myopathy within days to weeks, but severe cases may be fatal from **acute kidney failure** and disturbances in heart rhythm secondary to increased potassium levels. Recovery from chronic alcoholic myopathy may occur over weeks to months of abstinence from alcohol and correction of **malnutrition**. Cerebellar degeneration and alcoholic neuropathy may also improve to some extent with abstinence and balanced diet, depending on the severity and duration of the condition.

Prevention

Prevention requires abstinence from alcohol. Persons who consume small or moderate amounts of alcohol might theoretically help prevent nutritional complications of alcohol use with dietary supplements including B vitamins. However, proper **nutrition** cannot protect against the direct toxic effect of alcohol or of its breakdown products. Patients with any alcohol-related symptoms or conditions, pregnant women, and patients with liver or neurologic disease should abstain completely. Persons with family history of alcoholism or alcohol-related conditions may also be at increased risk for neurologic complications of alcohol use.

Resources

PERIODICALS

"Missouri Clinics Will Diagnose and Treat Fetal Alcohol Syndrome." *Mental Health Weekly Digeste* (June 7, 2004): 33.

Stacey, Philip S. "Preliminary Investigation of Thiamine and Alcohol Intake in Clinical and Healthy Samples." *Psychological Reports* (June 2004): 845–849.

ORGANIZATIONS

National Institute on Alcohol Abuse and Alcoholism. 6000 Executive Boulevard, Willco Building, Bethesda, MD 20892-7003. < http://silk.nih.gov/silk/niaaa1 > .

Laurie Barclay, MD
Teresa G. Odle

Alcohol withdrawal *see* **Withdrawal syndromes**

Alcoholic cerebellar disease *see* **Alcohol-related neurologic disease**

Alcoholic hepatitis *see* **Hepatitis, alcoholic**

Alcoholic rose gardener's disease *see*
Sporotrichosis

Alcoholism

Definition

Alcoholism is the popular term for alcohol **abuse** and alcohol dependence. These disorders involve repeated life problems that can be directly attributed to the use of alcohol. Both disorders can have serious consequences, affecting an individual's health and personal life, as well as having an impact on society at large.

Description

The effects of alcoholism are far reaching. Alcohol affects every body system, causing a wide range of health problems. Problems include poor **nutrition**, memory disorders, difficulty with balance and walking, liver disease (including **cirrhosis** and hepatitis), high blood pressure, muscle weakness (including the heart), heart rhythm disturbances, anemia, clotting disorders, decreased immunity to infections, gastrointestinal inflammation and irritation, acute and chronic problems with the pancreas, low blood sugar, high blood fat content, interference with reproductive fertility, and weakened bones.

On a personal level, alcoholism results in marital and other relationship difficulties, depression, unemployment, **child abuse**, and general family dysfunction.

Alcoholism causes or contributes to a variety of severe social problems including homelessness, murder, **suicide**, injury, and violent crime. Alcohol is a contributing factor in at least 50% of all deaths from motor vehicle accidents. In fact, about 100,000 deaths occur each year due to the effects of alcohol, of which 50% are due to injuries of some sort. According to a special report prepared for the U.S. Congress by the National Institute on Alcohol Abuse and Alcoholism, the impact of alcohol on society, including violence, traffic accidents, lost work productivity, and premature **death**, costs our nation an estimated $185 billion annually. In addition, it is estimated that approximately one in four children (19 million children or 29% of children up to 17 years of age) is exposed at some time to familial alcohol abuse, alcohol dependence, or both. Furthermore, it has been estimated that approximately 18% of adults experience an

episode of alcohol abuse or dependence a some time during their lives.

Causes and symptoms

There are probably a number of factors that work together to cause a person to become an alcoholic. Recent genetic studies have demonstrated that close relatives of an alcoholic are four times more likely to become alcoholics themselves. Furthermore, this risk holds true even for children who were adopted away from their biological families at birth and raised in a non-alcoholic adoptive family, with no knowledge of their biological family's difficulties with alcohol. More research is being conducted to determine if genetic factors could account for differences in alcohol metabolism that may increase the risk of an individual becoming an alcoholic.

The symptoms of alcoholism can be broken down into two major categories: symptoms of acute alcohol use and symptoms of long-term alcohol use.

Immediate (acute) effects of alcohol use

Alcohol exerts a depressive effect on the brain. The blood-brain barrier does not prevent alcohol from entering the brain, so the brain alcohol level will quickly become equivalent to the blood alcohol level. Alcohol's depressive effects result in difficulty walking, poor balance, slurring of speech, and generally poor coordination (accounting in part for the increased likelihood of injury). The affected person also may have impairment of peripheral vision. At higher alcohol levels, a person's breathing and heart rates will be slowed, and **vomiting** may occur (with a high risk of the vomit being breathed into the lungs, resulting in severe problems, including the possibility of **pneumonia**). Still higher alcohol levels may result in coma and death.

Effects of long-term (chronic) alcoholism

Long-term use of alcohol affects virtually every organ system of the body:

KEY TERMS

Blood-brain barrier— A network of blood vessels characterized by closely spaced cells that prevents many potentially toxic substances from penetrating the blood vessel walls to enter the brain. Alcohol is able to cross this barrier.

Detoxification—The phase of treatment during which a patient stops drinking and is monitored and cared for while he or she experiences withdrawal from alcohol.

Relapse—A return to a disease state, after recovery appeared to be occurring. In alcoholism, relapse refers to a patient beginning to drink alcohol again after a period of avoiding alcohol.

Tolerance—A phenomenon during which a drinker becomes physically accustomed to a particular quantity of alcohol, and requires ever-increasing quantities in order to obtain the same effects.

Withdrawal—Those signs and symptoms experienced by a person who has become physically dependent on a drug, experienced upon decreasing the drug's dosage or discontinuing its use.

- Nervous system. An estimated 30-40% of all men in their teens and twenties have experienced alcoholic blackout, which occurs when drinking a large quantity of alcohol results in the loss of memory of the time surrounding the episode of drinking. Alcohol is well-known to cause sleep disturbances, so that overall sleep quality is affected. Numbness and **tingling** may occur in the arms and legs. Two syndromes, which can occur together or separately, are known as Wernicke's and Korsakoff's syndromes. Both are due to the low thiamine (a form of vitamin B complex) levels found in alcoholics. Wernicke's syndrome results in disordered eye movements, very poor balance and difficulty walking, while **Korsakoff's syndrome** severely affects one's memory, preventing new learning from taking place.

- Gastrointestinal system. Alcohol causes loosening of the muscular ring that prevents the stomach's contents from re-entering the esophagus. Therefore, the acid from the stomach flows backward into the esophagus, burning those tissues, and causing **pain** and bleeding. Inflammation of the stomach also can result in bleeding and pain, and decreased desire to eat. A major cause of severe, uncontrollable bleeding (hemorrhage) in an alcoholic is the development of enlarged (dilated) blood vessels within the esophagus, which are called esophageal varices. These varices actually are developed in response to liver disease, and are extremely prone to bursting and hemorrhaging. **Diarrhea** is a common symptom, due to alcohol's effect on the pancreas. In addition, inflammation of the pancreas (**pancreatitis**) is a serious and painful problem in alcoholics. Throughout the intestinal tract, alcohol interferes with the absorption of nutrients, creating a malnourished state. Because alcohol is broken down (metabolized) within the liver, the organ is severely affected by constant levels of alcohol. Alcohol interferes with a number of important chemical processes that also occur in the liver. The liver begins to enlarge and fill with fat (**fatty liver**), fibrous scar tissue interferes with the liver's normal structure and function (cirrhosis), and the liver may become inflamed (hepatitis).

- Blood. Alcohol can cause changes to all the types of blood cells. Red blood cells become abnormally large. White blood cells (important for fighting infections) decrease in number, resulting in a weakened immune system. This places alcoholics at increased risk for infections, and is thought to account in part for the increased risk of cancer faced by alcoholics (10 times the risk for nonalcoholics). Platelets and blood clotting factors are affected, causing an increased risk of bleeding.

- Heart. Small amounts of alcohol cause a drop in blood pressure, but with increased use, alcohol begins to increase blood pressure into a dangerous range. High levels of fats circulating in the bloodstream increase the risk of heart disease. Heavy drinking results in an increase in heart size, weakening of the heart muscle, abnormal heart rhythms, a risk of **blood clots** forming within the chambers of the heart, and a greatly increased risk of stroke (due to a blood clot from the heart entering the circulatory system, going to the brain, and blocking a brain blood vessel).

- Reproductive system. Heavy drinking has a negative effect on fertility in both men and women, by decreasing testicle and ovary size, and interfering with both sperm and egg production. When **pregnancy** is achieved in an alcoholic woman, the baby has a great risk of being born with **fetal alcohol syndrome**, which causes distinctive facial defects, lowered IQ, and behavioral problems.

Diagnosis

Two different types of alcohol-related difficulties have been identified. The first is called *alcohol dependence*, which refers to a person who literally depends on the use of alcohol. Three of the following traits must be present to diagnose alcohol dependence:

- tolerance, meaning that a person becomes accustomed to a particular dose of alcohol, and must increase the dose in order to obtain the desired effect

- withdrawal, meaning that a person experiences unpleasant physical and psychological symptoms when he or she does not drink alcohol

- the tendency to drink more alcohol than one intends (once an alcoholic starts to drink, he or she finds it difficult to stop)

- being unable to avoid drinking or stop drinking once started

- having large blocks of time taken up by alcohol use

- choosing to drink at the expense of other important tasks or activities

- drinking despite evidence of negative effects on one's health, relationships, education, or job

Diagnosis is sometimes brought about when family members call an alcoholic's difficulties to the attention of a physician. A clinician may begin to be suspicious when a patient suffers repeated injuries or begins to experience medical problems related to the use of alcohol. In fact, some estimates suggest that about 20% of a physician's patients will be alcoholics.

Diagnosis is aided by administering specific psychological assessments that try to determine what aspects of a person's life may be affected by his or her use of alcohol. Determining the exact quantity of alcohol that a person drinks is of much less importance than determining how his or her drinking affects relationships, jobs, educational goals, and family life. In fact, because the metabolism (how the body breaks down and processes) of alcohol is so individual, the quantity of alcohol consumed is not part of the criteria list for diagnosing either alcohol dependence or alcohol abuse.

One simple tool for beginning the diagnosis of alcoholism is called the CAGE questionnaire. It consists of four questions, with the first letters of each key word spelling out the word CAGE:

- Have you ever tried to *Cut* down on your drinking?

- Have you ever been *Annoyed* by anyone's comments about your drinking?

- Have you ever felt *Guilty* about your drinking?

- Do you ever need an *Eye-opener* (a morning drink of alcohol) to start the day)?

Other, longer lists of questions exist to help determine the severity and effects of a person's alcohol use. Given the recent research pointing to a genetic basis for alcoholism, it is important to ascertain whether anyone else in the person's family has ever suffered from alcoholism.

Treatment

Treatment of alcoholism has two parts. The first step in the treatment of alcoholism, called detoxification, involves helping the person stop drinking and ridding his or her body of the harmful (toxic) effects of alcohol. Because the person's body has become accustomed to alcohol, the person will need to be supported through withdrawal. Withdrawal will be different for different patients, depending on the severity of the alcoholism, as measured by the quantity of alcohol ingested daily and the length of time the patient has been an alcoholic. Withdrawal symptoms can range from mild to life-threatening. Mild withdrawal symptoms include **nausea**, achiness, diarrhea, difficulty sleeping, sweatiness, **anxiety**, and trembling. This phase is usually over in about three to five days. More severe effects of withdrawal can include **hallucinations** (in which a patient sees, hears, or feels something that is not actually real), seizures, an unbearable craving for more alcohol, confusion, **fever**, fast heart rate, high blood pressure, and **delirium** (a fluctuating level of consciousness). Patients at highest risk for the most severe symptoms of withdrawal (referred to as delirium tremens) are those with other medical problems, including **malnutrition**, **liver disease**, or Wernicke's syndrome. Delirium tremens usually begin about three to five days after the patient's last drink, progressing from the more mild symptoms to the more severe, and may last a number of days.

Patients going through only mild withdrawal are simply monitored carefully to make sure that more severe symptoms do not develop. No medications are necessary, however. Treatment of a patient suffering the more severe effects of withdrawal may require the use of sedative medications to relieve the discomfort of withdrawal and to avoid the potentially life-threatening complications of high blood pressure, fast heart rate, and seizures. Drugs called benzodiazapines are helpful in those patients suffering from hallucinations. Because of the patient's nausea, fluids may need to be given through a vein (intravenously), along with some necessary sugars and salts. It is crucial that thiamine be included in the fluids, because thiamine is usually quite low in alcoholic patients, and deficiency of thiamine is responsible for the Wernicke-Korsakoff syndrome.

After cessation of drinking has been accomplished, the next steps involve helping the patient avoid ever taking another drink. This phase of treatment is referred to as **rehabilitation**. The best programs incorporate the family into the therapy, because the family has undoubtedly been severely affected by the patient's drinking. Some therapists believe that family members, in an effort to deal with their loved one's drinking problem, sometimes develop patterns of behavior that accidentally support or "enable" the patient's drinking. This situation is referred to as "co-dependence," and must be addressed in order to successfully treat a person's alcoholism.

Sessions led by peers, where recovering alcoholics meet regularly and provide support for each other's recoveries, are considered among the best methods of preventing a return to drinking (relapse). Perhaps the most well-known such group is called Alcoholics Anonymous, which uses a "12-step" model to help people avoid drinking. These steps involve recognizing the destructive power that alcohol has held over the alcoholic's life, looking to a higher power for help in overcoming the problem, and reflecting on the ways in which the use of alcohol has hurt others and, if possible, making amends to those people. According to a recent study reported by the American Psychological Association (APA), anyone, regardless of his or her religious beliefs or lack of religious beliefs, can benefit from participation in 12-step programs such as Alcoholics Anonymous (AA) or **Narcotics** Anonymous (NA). The number of visits to 12-step self-help groups exceeds the number of visits to all mental health professionals combined.

There are also medications that may help an alcoholic avoid returning to drinking. These have been used with variable success. Disulfiram (Antabuse) is a drug which, when mixed with alcohol, causes unpleasant reactions including nausea, vomiting, diarrhea, and trembling. Naltrexone, along with a similar compound, Nalmefene, can be helpful in limiting the effects of a relapse. Acamprosate is helpful in preventing relapse. None of these medications would be helpful unless the patient was also willing to work very hard to change his or her behavior. In 2004, a new compound was discovered that blocks actions of chemicals in the brain that may lead to relapses. Clinical tests were still underway, but development of such a drug could have great potential in the medical management of alcoholism. Another study that year found that topiramate (Topamax), an antiseizure medication, was effective in treating alcohol dependence in 150 participants in a clinical trial. The authors called for further study of this possible treatment.

Alternative treatment

Alternative treatments can be a helpful adjunct for the alcoholic patient, once the medical danger of withdrawal has passed. Because many alcoholics have very stressful lives (whether because of or leading to the alcoholism is sometimes a matter of debate), many of the treatments for alcoholism involve dealing with and relieving **stress**. These include massage, **meditation**, and **hypnotherapy**. The malnutrition of long-term alcohol use is addressed by nutrition-oriented practitioners with careful attention to a healthy diet and the use of nutritional supplements such as **vitamins** A, B complex, and C, as well as certain fatty acids, amino acids, zinc, magnesium, and selenium. Herbal treatments include milk thistle (*Silybum marianum*), which is thought to protect the liver against damage. Other herbs are thought to be helpful for the patient suffering through withdrawal. Some of these include lavender (*Lavandula officinalis*), skullcap (*Scutellaria lateriflora*), chamomile (*Matricaria recutita*), peppermint (*Mentha piperita*) yarrow (*Achillea millefolium*), and valerian (*Valeriana officinalis*). **Acupuncture** is believed to both decrease withdrawal symptoms and to help improve a patient's chances for continued recovery from alcoholism.

Prognosis

Recovery from alcoholism is a life-long process. In fact, people who have suffered from alcoholism are encouraged to refer to themselves ever after as "a recovering alcoholic," never a recovered alcoholic. This is because most researchers in the field believe that since the potential for alcoholism is still part of the individual's biological and psychological makeup, one can never fully recover from alcoholism. The potential for relapse (returning to illness) is always there, and must be acknowledged and respected. Statistics suggest that, among middle-class alcoholics in stable financial and family situations who have undergone treatment, 60% or more can be successful at an attempt to stop drinking for at least a year, and many for a lifetime.

Prevention

Prevention must begin at a relatively young age since the first instance of intoxication (drunkenness) usually occurs during the teenage years. In fact, a 2004 study found that girls experimented with alcohol and cigarettes at a younger age — 20% by seventh grage — than boys. It is particularly important that teenagers who are at high risk for alcoholism—those with a family history of alcoholism, an early or frequent use of alcohol, a tendency to drink to drunkenness, alcohol use that interferes with school work, a poor family environment, or a history of domestic violence — receive education about alcohol and its long-term effects. How this is best achieved, without irritating the youngsters and thus losing their attention, is the subject of continuing debate and study.

Resources

BOOKS

National Institute on Alcohol Abuse and Alcoholism. *10th Special Report to the U.S. Congress on Alcohol and Health.* National Institute of Health, 2000.

PERIODICALS

Koch Kubetin, Sally. "Girls Before Boys in Cigarette and Alcohol Use: Longitudinal Study." *Pediatric News* (March 2004): 29.

"Research Findings Suggest Compound Might Help in Fight Against Alcoholism." *Drug Week* (January 9, 2004): 18.

Walling, Anne D. "Topiramate in the Treatment of Alcohol Dependence." *American Family Physician* (January 1, 2004): 195.

ORGANIZATIONS

Al-Anon, Alanon Family Group, Inc. P.O. Box 862, Midtown Station, New York, NY 10018-0862. (800) 356-9996. < http://www.recovery.org/aa > .

Alcoholics Anonymous. Grand Central Station, Box 459, New York, NY 10163. < http://www.alcoholics-anonymous.org/ > .

National Alliance on Alcoholism and Drug Dependence, Inc. 12 West 21st St., New York, NY 10010. (212) 206-6770.

National Clearinghouse for Alcohol and Drug Information. 11426 Rockville Pike, Suite 200, Rockville, MD. 20852. (800) 729-6686. < http:\\www.health.org > .

National Institute on Alcohol Abuse and Alcoholism (NIAAA). 6000 Executive Boulevard, Bethesda, Maryland 20892-7003. < http://www.niaaa.nih.gov > .

Bill Asenjo, MS, CRC
Teresa G. Odle

ALD *see* **Adrenoleukodystrophy**

❚ Aldolase test

Definition

Aldolase is an enzyme found throughout the body, particularly in muscles. Like all enzymes, it is needed to trigger specific chemical reactions. Aldolase

helps muscle turn sugar into energy. Testing for aldolase is done to diagnose and monitor skeletal muscle diseases.

Purpose

Skeletal muscle diseases increase the aldolase level found in a person's blood. Skeletal muscles are those muscles attached to bones and whose contractions make those bones move. When the muscles are diseased or damaged, such as in **muscular dystrophy**, the cells deteriorate and break open. The contents of the cells, including aldolase, spill into the bloodstream. Measuring the amount of aldolase in the blood indicates the degree of muscle damage.

As muscles continue to deteriorate, aldolase levels decrease and eventually fall below normal. Less muscle means fewer cells and less aldolase.

Muscle weakness may be caused by neurologic as well as muscular problems. The measurement of aldolase levels can help pinpoint the cause. Aldolase levels will be normal where muscle weakness is caused by neurological disease, such as poliomyelitis or **multiple sclerosis**, but aldolase levels will be elevated in cases of muscular disease, such as muscular dystrophy.

Aldolase is also found in the liver and cardiac muscle of the heart. Damage or disease to these organs, such as chronic hepatitis or a **heart attack**, will also increase aldolase levels in the blood, but to a lesser degree.

Description

Aldolase is measured by mixing a person's serum with a substance with which aldolase is known to trigger a reaction. The end product of this reaction is measured, and, from that measurement, the amount of aldolase in the person's serum is determined.

The test is covered by insurance when medically necessary. Results are usually available the next day.

Preparation

To collect the 5-10 ml of blood needed for this test, a healthcare worker ties a tourniquet on the patient's upper arm, locates a vein in the inner elbow region, and inserts a needle into that vein. Vacuum action draws the blood through the needle into an attached tube. Collection of the sample takes only a few minutes.

The patient should avoid strenuous **exercise** and have nothing to eat or drink, except water, for eight to ten hours before this test.

Aftercare

Discomfort or bruising may occur at the puncture site and the person may feel dizzy or faint. Pressure to the puncture site until the bleeding stops will reduce bruising. Warm packs to the puncture site will relieve discomfort.

Normal results

Newborns have the highest normal aldolase levels and adults the lowest. Normal values will vary based on the laboratory and the method used.

Abnormal results

As noted, aldolase is elevated in skeletal muscle diseases, such as muscular dystrophies. Duchenne's muscular dystrophy, the most common type of muscular dystrophy, will increase the aldolase level more than any other disease.

Nondisease conditions that affect the muscle, such as injury, **gangrene**, or an infection, can also increase the aldolase level. Also, strenuous exercise can temporarily increase a person's aldolase level.

Certain medications can increase the aldolase level, while others can decrease it. To interpret what the results of the aldolase test mean, a physician will evaluate the result, the person's clinical symptoms, and other tests that are more specific for muscle damage and disease.

Resources

BOOKS

Mayo Medical Laboratories. *Interpretive Handbook*. Rochester, MN: Mayo Medical Laboratories, 1997.

Nancy J. Nordenson

Aldosterone assay

Definition

This test measures the levels of aldosterone, a hormone produced by the outer part (cortex) of the two adrenal glands, organs which sit one on top of each of the kidneys. Aldosterone regulates the amounts of sodium and potassium in the blood. This helps maintain water balance and blood volume, which, in turn, affects blood pressure.

Purpose

Aldosterone measurement is useful in detecting a condition called aldosteronism, which is caused by excess secretion of the hormone from the adrenal glands. There are two types of aldosteronism: primary and secondary. Primary aldosteronism is most commonly caused by an adrenal tumor, as in Conn's syndrome. Idiopathic (of unknown cause) **hyperaldosteronism** is another type of primary aldosteronism. Secondary aldosteronism is more common and may occur with congestive heart failure, **cirrhosis** with fluid in the abdominal cavity (ascites), certain kidney diseases, excess potassium, sodium-depleted diet, and toxemia of **pregnancy**.

To differentiate primary aldosteronism from secondary aldosteronism, a plasma renin test should be performed at the same time as the aldosterone assay. Renin, an enzyme produced in the kidneys, is high in secondary aldosteronism and low in primary aldosteronism.

Description

Aldosterone testing can be performed on a blood sample or on a 24-hour urine specimen. Several factors, including diet, posture (upright or lying down), and time of day that the sample is obtained can cause aldosterone levels to fluctuate. Blood samples are affected by short-term fluctuations. A urine specimen collected over an entire 24-hour period lessens the effects of those interfering factors and provides a more reliable aldosterone measurement.

Preparation

Fasting is not required for either the blood sample or urine collection, but the patient should maintain a normal sodium diet (approximately 0.1 oz [3g]/day) for at least two weeks before either test. The doctor should decide if drugs that alter sodium, potassium, and fluid balance (e.g., **diuretics**, antihypertensives, steroids, **oral contraceptives**) should be withheld. The test will be more accurate if these are suspended at at least two weeks before the test. Renin inhibitors (e.g., propranolol) should not be taken one week before the test, unless permitted by the physician. The patient should avoid licorice for at least two weeks before the test, because of its aldosterone-like effect. Strenuous **exercise** and stress can increase aldosterone levels as well. Because the test is usually performed by a method called radioimmunoassay, recently administered radioactive medications will affect test results.

Since posture and body position affect aldosterone, hospitalized patients should remain in an upright position (at least sitting) for two hours before blood is drawn. Occasionally blood will be drawn again before the patient gets out of bed. Nonhospitalized patients should arrive at the laboratory in time to maintain an upright position for at least two hours.

Risks

Risks for this test are minimal, but may include slight bleeding from the blood-drawing site, fainting or feeling lightheaded after venipuncture, or hematoma (blood accumulating under the puncture site).

Normal results

Normal results are laboratory-specific and also vary with sodium intake, with time of day, source of specimen (e.g., peripheral vein, adrenal vein, 24-hour urine), age, sex, and posture.

Reference ranges for blood include:

- supine (lying down): 3-10 ng/dL
- upright (sitting for at least two hours): Female: 5-30ng/dL; Male: 6-22 ng/dL.

Reference ranges for urine: 2-80 mg/24 hr.

Abnormal results

Increased levels of aldosterone are found in Conn's disease (aldosterone-producing adrenal tumor), and in cases of Bartter's syndrome (a condition in which the kidneys overexcrete potassium, sodium and chloride, resulting in low blood levels of potassium and high blood levels of aldosterone and renin). Among other conditions, elevated levels are also seen in secondary aldosteronism, **stress**, and malignant **hypertension**.

Decreased levels of aldosterone are found in aldosterone deficiency, steroid therapy, high-sodium **diets**, certain antihypertensive therapies, and Addison's disease (an autoimmune disorder).

Resources

BOOKS

Pagana, Kathleen Deska. *Mosby's Manual of Diagnostic and Laboratory Tests*. St. Louis: Mosby, Inc., 1998.

Janis O. Flores

Alemtuzumab

Definition

Alemtuzumab is sold as Campath in the United States. Alemtuzumab is a humanized monoclonal antibody that selectively binds to CD52, a protein found on the surface of normal and malignant B and T cells, that is used to reduce the numbers of circulating malignant cells of patients who have B-cell chronic lymphocytic leukemia (B-CLL).

Purpose

Alemtuzumab is a monoclonal antibody used to treat B-CLL, one of the most prevalent forms of adult chronic leukemia. It specifically binds CD52, a protein found on the surface of essentially all B and T cells of the immune system. By binding the CD52 protein on the malignant B cells, the antibody targets it for removal from the circulation. Scientists believe that alemtuzumab triggers antibody-mediated lysis of the B cells, a method that the immune system uses to eliminate foreign cells.

Alemtuzumab has been approved by the FDA for treatment of refractory B-CLL. For a patient's disease to be classified as refractory, both alkylating agents and fludarabine treatment must have been tried and failed. Thus, this drug gives patients who have tried all

KEY TERMS

Alkylating agent—A chemical that alters the composition of the genetic material of rapidly dividing cells, such as cancer cells, causing selective cell death; used as a chemotherapeutic agent to treat B-CLL.

Antibody—A protective protein made by the immune system in response to an antigen, also called an immunoglobulin.

Autoimmune—An immune reaction of a patient against their own cells.

Humanization—Fusing the constant and variable framework region of one or more human immunoglobulins with the binding region of an animal immunoglobulin, done to reduce human reaction against the fusion antibody.

Monoclonal—Genetically engineered antibodies specific for one antigen.

Tumor lysis syndrome—A side effect of some immunotherapies, like monoclonal antibodies, that lyse the tumor cells, due to the toxicity of flooding the bloodstream with such a quantity of cellular contents.

approved treatments for B-CLL another option. As most patients with B-CLL are in stage III or IV by the time both alkylating agents and fludarabine have been tried, the experience with alemtuzumab treatment are primarily with those stages of the disease. In clinical trials, about 30% of patients had a partial response to the drug, with 2% of these being complete responses.

This antibody has been tested with limited success in the treatment of non-Hodgkin's lymphoma (NHL) and for the preparation of patients with various immune cell malignancies for bone marrow transplantation. There is also a clinical trial ongoing to test the ability of this antibody to prevent rejection in **kidney transplantation**.

Description

Alemtuzumab is produced in the laboratory using genetically engineered single clones of B-cells. Like all antibodies, it is a Y-shaped molecule can bind one particular substance, the antigen for that monoclonal antibody. For alemtuzumab, the antigen is CD52, a protein found on the surface of normal and malignant B and T cells as well as other cells of the immune and male reproductive systems. Alemtuzumab is a humanized antibody, meaning that the regions that bind CD52, located on the tips of the Y branches, are

derived from rat antibodies, but the rest of the antibody is human sequence. The presence of the human sequences helps to reduce the immune response by the patient against the antibody itself, a problem seen when complete mouse antibodies are used for **cancer** therapies. The human sequences also help to ensure that the various cell-destroying mechanisms of the human immune system are properly triggered with binding of the antibody.

Alemtuzumab was approved in May of 2001 for the treatment of refractory B-CLL. It is approved for use alone but clinical trials have tested the ability of the antibody to be used in combination with the purine analogs pentostatin, fludarabine, and cladribine, and rituximab, a monoclonal antibody specific for the CD20 antigen, another protein found on the surface of B cells.

Recommended dosage

This antibody should be administered in a gradually escalating pattern at the start of treatment and any time administration is interrupted for seven or more days. The recommended beginning dosage for B-CLL patients is a daily dose of 3 mg of Campath administered as a two-hour IV infusion. Once this amount is tolerated, the dose is increased to 10 mg per day. After tolerating this dose, it can be increased to 30 mg, administered three days a week. Acetaminophen and diphenhydramine hydrochoride are given thirty to sixty minutes before the infusion to help reduce side effects.

Additionally, patients generally receive anti-infective medication before treatment to help minimize the serious opportunistic infections that can result from this treatment. Specifically, trimethoprim/sulfamethoxazole (to prevent bacterial infections) and famciclovir (to prevent viral infections) were used during the clinical trial to decrease infections, although they were not eliminated.

Precautions

Blood studies should be done on a weekly basis while patients are receiving the alemtuzumab treatment. **Vaccination** during the treatment session is not recommended, given the T cell depletion that occurs during treatment. Furthermore, given that antibodies like alemtuzumab can pass through the placenta to the developing fetus and in breast milk, use during **pregnancy** and breast-feeding is not recommended unless clearly needed.

Side effects

A severe side effect of alemtuzumab treatment is the possible depletion of one or more types of blood cells. Because CD52 is expressed on a patient's normal B and T cells, as well as on the surface of the abnormal B cells, the treatment eliminates both normal and cancerous cells. The treatment also seems to trigger autoimmune reactions against various other blood cells. This results in severe reduction of the many circulating blood cells including red blood cells (anemia), white blood cells (**neutropenia**), and clotting cells (thrombopenia). These conditions are treated with blood transfusions. The great majority of patients treated exhibit some type of blood cell depletion.

A second serious side effect of this drug is the prevalence of opportunistic infections that occurs during the treatment. Serious, and sometimes fatal bacterial, viral, fungal, and protozoan infections have been reported. Treatments to prevent **pneumonia** and herpes infections reduce, but do not eliminate these infections.

The majority of other side effects occur after or during the first infusion of the drug. Some common side effects of this drug include **fever** and chills, **nausea and vomiting**, **diarrhea**, shortness of breath, skin rash, and unusual **fatigue**. This drug can also cause low blood pressure (hypotension).

In patients with high tumor burden (a large number of circulating malignant B cells) this drug can cause a side effect called tumor lysis syndrome. Thought to be due to the release of the lysed cells' contents into the blood stream, it can cause a misbalance of urea, uric acid, phosphate, potassium, and calcium in the urine and blood. Patients at risk for this side effect must keep hydrated and can be given allopurinol before infusion.

Interactions

There have been no formal drug interaction studies done for alemtuzumab.

Michelle Johnson, MS, JD

Alendronate *see* **Bone disorder drugs**

Alexander technique

Definition

The Alexander technique is a somatic method for improving physical and mental functioning. Excessive tension, which Frederick Alexander, the originator, recognized as both physical and mental, restricts movement and creates pressure in the joints, the spine, the breathing mechanism, and other organs. The goal of the technique is to restore freedom and expression to the body and clear thinking to the mind.

Purpose

Because the Alexander technique helps students improve overall functioning, both mental and physical, it offers a wide range of benefits. Nikolaas Tinbergen, in his 1973 Nobel lecture, hailed the "striking improvements in such diverse things as high blood pressure, breathing, depth of sleep, overall cheerfulness and mental alertness, resilience against outside pressures, and the refined skill of playing a musical instrument." He went on to quote a list of other conditions helped by the Alexander technique: "rheumatism, including various forms of arthritis, then respiratory troubles, and even potentially lethal **asthma**; following in their wake, circulation defects, which may lead to high blood pressure and also to some dangerous heart conditions; gastrointestinal disorders of many types, various gynecological conditions, sexual failures, migraines and depressive states."

Literature in the 1980s and 1990s went on to include improvements in back **pain**, chronic pain, postural problems, repetitive strain injury, benefits during pregnancy and **childbirth**, help in applying physical therapy and rehabilitative exercises, improvements in strain caused by computer use, improvements in the posture and performance of school children, and improvements in vocal and dramatic performance among the benefits offered by the technique.

Description

Origins

Frederick Matthias Alexander was born in 1869 in Tasmania, Australia. He became an actor and Shakespearean reciter, and early in his career he began to suffer from strain on his vocal chords. He sought medical attention for chronic hoarseness, but after treatment with a recommended prescription and extensive periods of rest, his problem persisted.

Alexander realized that his hoarseness began about an hour into a dramatic performance and reasoned that it was something he did in the process of reciting that caused him to lose his voice. Returning to his medical doctor, Alexander told him of his observation. When the doctor admitted that he didn't know what Alexander was doing to injure his vocal chords, Alexander decided to try and find out for himself.

KEY TERMS

Direction—Bringing about the free balance of the head on the spine and the resulting release of the erector muscles of the back and legs which establish improved coordination.

Habit—Referring to the particular set of physical and mental tensions present in any individual.

Inhibition—Referring to the moment in an Alexander lesson when the student refrains from beginning a movement in order to avoid tensing of the muscles.

Sensory awareness—Bringing attention to the sensations of tension and/or release in the muscles.

Thus began a decade of self-observation and discovery. Using as many as three mirrors to observe himself in the act of reciting, normal speaking, and later standing, walking, and sitting, Alexander managed to improve his coordination and to overcome his vocal problems. One of his most startling discoveries was that in order to change the way he used his body he had to change the way he was thinking, redirecting his thoughts in such a way that he did not produce unnecessary tension when he attempted speech or movement. After making this discovery at the end of the nineteenth century, Alexander became a pioneer in body-mind medicine.

At first, performers and dancers sought guidance from Alexander to overcome physical complaints and to improve the expression and spontaneity of their performances. Soon a great number of people sought help from his teaching for a variety of physical and mental disorders.

The Alexander technique is primarily taught one-on-one in private lessons. Introductory workshops or workshops for special applications of the technique (e.g.,workshops for musicians) are also common. Private lessons range from a half-hour to an hour in length, and are taught in a series. The number of lessons varies according to the severity of the student's difficulties with coordination or to the extent of the student's interest in pursuing the improvements made possible by continued study. The cost of lessons ranges from $40-80 per hour. Insurance coverage is not widely available, but discounts are available for participants in some complementary care insurance plans. Pre-tax Flexible Spending Accounts for health care cover Alexander technique lessons if they are prescribed by a physician.

In lessons teachers guide students through simple movements (while students are dressed in comfortable clothing) and use their hands to help students identify and stop destructive patterns of tension. Tensing arises from mental processes as well as physical, so discussions of personal reactions or behavior are likely to arise in the course of a lesson.

The technique helps students move with ease and improved coordination. At the beginning of a movement (the lessons are a series of movements), most people pull back their heads, raise their shoulders toward their ears, over-arch their lower backs, tighten their legs, and otherwise produce excessive tension in their bodies. Alexander referred to this as misuse of the body.

At any point in a movement, proper use can be established. If the neck muscles are not over-tensed, the head will carry slightly forward of the spine, simply because it is heavier in the front. When the head is out of balance in the forward direction, it sets off a series of stretch reflexes in the extensor muscles of the back. It is skillful use of these reflexes, along with reflex activity in the feet and legs, the arms and hands, the breathing mechanism, and other parts of the body, that lessons in the technique aim to develop.

Alexander found that optimal functioning of the body was very hard to maintain, even for the short period of time it took to complete a single movement. People, especially adults, have very strong tension habits associated with movement. Chronic misuse of the muscles is common. It may be caused by slouching in front of televisions or video monitors, too much sitting or driving and too little walking, or by tension associated with past traumas and injuries. Stiffening the neck after a **whiplash** injury or favoring a broken or sprained leg long after it has healed are examples of habitual tension caused by injury.

The first thing a teacher of the Alexander technique does is to increase a student's sensory awareness of this excessive habitual tension, particularly that in the neck and spine. Next the student is taught to inhibit the tension. If the student prepares to sit down, for example, he will tense his muscles in his habitual way. If he is asked to put aside the intention to sit and instead to free his neck and allow less constriction in his muscles, he can begin to change his tense habitual response to sitting.

By leaving the head resting on the spine in its natural free balance, by keeping eyes open and focused, not held in a tense stare, by allowing the shoulders to release, the knees to unlock and the back to lengthen and widen, a student greatly reduces strain. In Alexander lessons students learn to direct themselves this way in activity and become skilled in fluid, coordinated movement.

Precautions

Side effects

The focus of the Alexander technique is educational. Teachers use their hands simply to gently guide students in movement. Therefore, both contraindications and potential physiological side effects are kept to a minimum. No forceful treatment of soft tissue or bony structure is attempted, so damage to tissues, even in the case of errors in teaching, is unlikely.

As students' sensory awareness develops in the course of Alexander lessons, they become more acutely aware of chronic tension patterns. As students learn to release excessive tension in their muscles and to sustain this release in daily activity, they may experience tightness or soreness in the connective tissue. This is caused by the connective tissue adapting to the lengthened and released muscles and the expanded range of movement in the joints.

Occasionally students may get light-headed during a lesson as contracted muscles release and effect the circulatory or respiratory functioning.

Forceful contraction of muscles and rigid postures often indicate suppression of emotion. As muscles release during or after an Alexander lesson, students may experience strong surges of emotion or sudden changes in mood. In some cases, somatic memories surface, bringing to consciousness past injury or trauma. This can cause extreme **anxiety**, and referrals may be made by the teacher for counseling.

Research and general acceptance

Alexander became well known among the intellectual, artistic, and medical communities in London, England, during the first half of the twentieth century. Among Alexander's supporters were John Dewey, Aldous Huxley, Bernard Shaw, and renowned scientists Raymond Dart, G.E. Coghill, Charles Sherrington, and Nikolaas Tinbergen.

Researchers continue to study the effects and applications of the technique in the fields of education, preventive medicine, and **rehabilitation**. The Alexander technique has proven an effective treatment for reducing **stress**, for improving posture and performance in schoolchildren, for relieving chronic pain, and for improving psychological functioning. The technique has been found to be as effective as beta-blocker medications in controlling stress responses in professional musicians, to enhance respiratory function in normal adults, and to mediate the effects of **scoliosis** in adolescents and adults.

Resources

BOOKS

Dimon, Theodore. *THE UNDIVIDED SELF: Alexander Technique and the Control of Stress.* North Atlantic Books: 1999.

ORGANIZATIONS

Alexander Technique International, 1692 Massachusetts Ave., 3rd Floor, Cambridge, MA 02138 USA. (888) 321-0856. Fax: 617-497-2615. ati@ati-net.com. < http://www.ati-net.com >.

OTHER

Alexander Technique Resource Guide. (Includes list of teachers) AmSAT Books. (800) 473-0620 or (804) 295-2840.

Sandra Bain Cushman

Alkali-resistant hemoglobin test *see* **Fetal hemoglobin test**

Alkaline phosphatase test

Definition

Alkaline phosphatase is an enzyme found throughout the body. Like all enzymes, it is needed, in small amounts, to trigger specific chemical reactions. When it is present in large amounts, it may signify bone or **liver disease** or a tumor.

Purpose

Medical testing of alkaline phosphatase is concerned with the enzyme that is found in liver, bone, placenta, and intestine. In a healthy liver, fluid containing alkaline phosphate and other substances is continually drained away through the bile duct. In a diseased liver, this bile duct is often blocked, keeping fluid within the liver. Alkaline phosphatase accumulates and eventually escapes into the bloodstream.

The alkaline phosphatase of the liver is produced by the cells lining the small bile ducts (ductoles) in the liver. Its origin differs from that of other enzymes called aminotransferases. If the liver disease is primarily of an obstructive nature (cholestatic), i.e. involving the biliary drainage system, the alkaline phosphatase will be the first and foremost enzyme elevation. If, on the other hand, the disease is primarily of the liver cells (hepatocytes), the aminotransferases will rise prominently. Thus, these enzymes are very useful in distinguishing the type of liver disease–cholestatic or hepatocellular.

Growing bones need alkaline phosphatase. Any condition of bone growth will cause alkaline phosphatase levels to rise. The condition may be normal, such as a childhood growth spurt or the healing of a broken bone; or the condition may be a disease, such as bone **cancer**, Paget's disease, or **rickets**.

During **pregnancy**, alkaline phosphatase is made by the placenta and leaks into the mother's bloodstream. This is normal. Some tumors, however, start production of the same kind of alkaline phosphatase produced by the placenta. These tumors are called germ cell tumors and include **testicular cancer** and certain brain tumors.

Alkaline phosphatase from the intestine is increased in a person with inflammatory bowel disease, such as **ulcerative colitis**.

Description

Alkaline phosphatase is measured by combining the person's serum with specific substances with which alkaline phosphatase is known to react. The end product of this reaction is measured; and from that measurement, the amount of alkaline phosphatase in the person's serum is determined.

Each tissue–liver, bone, placenta, and intestine–produces a slightly different alkaline phosphatase. These variations are called isoenzymes. In the laboratory, alkaline phosphatase is measured as the total amount or the amount of each of the the four isoenzymes. The isoenzymes react differently to heat, certain chemicals, and other processes in the laboratory. Methods to measure them separately are based on these differences.

The test is covered by insurance when medically necessary. Results are usually available the next day.

Preparation

To collect the 5-10 ml blood needed for this test, a healthcare worker ties a tourniquet on the person's upper arm, locates a vein in the inner elbow region, and inserts a needle into that vein. Vacuum action draws the blood through the needle into an attached tube. Collection of the sample takes only a few minutes.

A person being tested for alkaline phosphatase should not have anything to eat or drink, except water, for eight to ten hours before the test. Some people release alkaline phosphatase from the intestine into the bloodstream after eating. This will temporarily increase the result of the test.

Aftercare

Discomfort or bruising may occur at the puncture site or the person may feel dizzy or faint. Pressure to the puncture site until the bleeding stops will reduce bruising. Warm packs to the puncture site will relieve discomfort.

Normal results

Normal results vary by age and by sex. They also vary based on the laboratory and the method used.

Abnormal results

Bone and liver disease increase alkaline phosphatase more than any other disease, up to five times the normal level. Irritable bowel disease, germ cell tumors, and infections involving the liver, such as viral hepatitis and **infectious mononucleosis**, increase the enzyme also, but to a lesser degree. Healing bones, pregnancy, and normal growth in children also increase levels.

Resources

BOOKS

Lehmann, Craig A., editor. *Saunders Manual of Clinical Laboratory Science*. Philadelphia: W. B. Saunders Co., 1998.

Nancy J. Nordenson

Alkalosis *see* **Metabolic alkalosis; Respiratory alkalosis**

Allergic alveolitis *see* **Hypersensitivity pneumonitis**

Allergic bronchopulmonary aspergillosis

Definition

Allergic bronchopulmonary **aspergillosis**, or ABPA, is one of four major types of infections in humans caused by *Aspergillus* fungi. ABPA is a hypersensitivity reaction that occurs in asthma patients who are allergic to this specific fungus.

Description

ABPA is an allergic reaction to a species of *Aspergillus* called *Aspergillus fumigatus*. It is sometimes grouped together with other lung disorders characterized by eosinophilia–an abnormal increase of a certain type of white blood cell in the blood–under the heading of eosinophilic pneumonia. These disorders are also called hypersensitivity lung diseases.

ABPA appears to be increasing in frequency in the United States, although the reasons for the increase are not clear. The disorder is most likely to occur in adult asthmatics aged 20-40. It affects males and females equally.

Causes and symptoms

ABPA develops when the patient breathes air containing *Aspergillus* spores. These spores are found worldwide, especially around riverbanks, marshes, bogs, forests, and wherever there is wet or decaying vegetation. They are also found on wet paint, construction materials, and in air conditioning systems. ABPA is a nosocomial infection, which means that a patient can get it in a hospital. When *Aspergillus* spores reach the bronchi, which are the branches of the windpipe that lead into the lungs, the bronchi react by contracting spasmodically. So the patient has difficulty breathing and usually wheezes or coughs. Many patients with ABPA also run a low-grade fever and lose their appetites.

Complications

Patients with ABPA sometimes **cough** up large amounts of blood, a condition that is called **hemoptysis**. They may also develop a serious long-term form of **bronchiectasis**, the formation of fibrous tissue in the lungs. Bronchiectasis is a chronic bronchial disorder caused by repeated inflammation of the airway, and

marked by the abnormal enlargement of, or damage to, the bronchial walls. ABPA sometimes occurs as a complication of cystic fibrosis.

KEY TERMS

Antifungal—A medicine used to treat infections caused by a fungus.

Antigen—A substance that stimulates the production of antibodies.

Bronchiectasis—A disorder of the bronchial tubes marked by abnormal stretching, enlargement, or destruction of the walls. Bronchiectasis is usually caused by recurrent inflammation of the airway and is a diagnostic criterion of ABPA.

Bronchodilator— A medicine used to open up the bronchial tubes (air passages) of the lungs.

Eosinophil—A type of white blood cell containing granules that can be stained by eosin (a chemical that produces a red stain).

Eosinophilia—An abnormal increase in the number of eosinophils in the blood.

Hemoptysis—The coughing up of large amounts of blood. Hemoptysis can occur as a complication of ABPA.

Hypersensitivity—An excessive response by the body to a foreign substance.

Immunoglobulin E (IgE)—A type of protein in blood plasma that acts as an antibody to activate allergic reactions. About 50% of patients with allergic disorders have increased IgE levels in their blood serum.

Nosocomial infection—An infection that can be acquired in a hospital. ABPA is a nosocomial infection.

Precipitin—An antibody in blood that combines with an antigen to form a solid that separates from the rest of the blood.

Spirometer—An instrument used to test a patient's lung capacity.

"Wheal and flare" reaction—A rapid response to a skin allergy test characterized by the development of a red, itching spot in the area where the allergen was injected.

Wheezing—A whistling or musical sound caused by tightening of the air passages inside the patient's chest.

Diagnosis

The diagnosis of ABPA is based on a combination of the patient's history and the results of blood tests, sputum tests, skin tests, and diagnostic imaging. The doctor will be concerned to distinguish between ABPA and a worsening of the patient's **asthma**, **cystic fibrosis**, or other lung disorders. There are seven major criteria for a diagnosis of allergic bronchopulmonary aspergillosis:

- a history of asthma.

- an accumulation of fluid in the lung that is visible on a chest x ray.

- bronchiectasis (abnormal stretching, enlarging, or destruction of the walls of the bronchial tubes).

- skin reaction to *Aspergillus* antigen.

- eosinophilia in the patient's blood and sputum.

- *Aspergillus* precipitins in the patient's blood. Precipitins are antibodies that react with the antigen to form a solid that separates from the rest of the solution in the test tube.

- a high level of IgE in the patient's blood. IgE refers to a class of antibodies in blood plasma that activate allergic reactions to foreign particles.

Other criteria that may be used to support the diagnosis include the presence of *Aspergillus* in samples of the patient's sputum, the coughing up of plugs of brown mucus, or a late skin reaction to the *Aspergillus* antigen.

Laboratory tests

The laboratory tests that are done to obtain this information include a complete **blood count** (CBC), a **sputum culture**, a blood serum test of IgE levels, and a skin test for the *Aspergillus* antigen. In the skin test, a small amount of antigen is injected into the upper layer of skin on the patient's forearm about four inches below the elbow. If the patient has a high level of IgE antibodies in the tissue, he or she will develop what is called a "wheal and flare" reaction in about 15-20 minutes. A "wheal and flare" reaction is characterized by the eruption of a reddened, **itching** spot on the skin. Some patients with ABPA will develop the so-called late reaction to the skin test, in which a red, sore, swollen area develops about six to eight hours after the initial reaction.

Diagnostic imaging

Chest x rays and CT scans are used to check for the presence of fluid accumulation in the lungs and signs of bronchiectasis.

Treatment

ABPA is usually treated with prednisone (Meticorten) or other **corticosteroids** taken by mouth, and with **bronchodilators**.

Antifungal drugs are *not* used to treat ABPA because it is caused by an allergic reaction to *Aspergillus* rather than by direct infection of tissue.

Follow-up care

Patients with ABPA should be given periodic check-ups with chest x rays and a spirometer test. A spirometer is an instrument that evaluates the patient's lung capacity.

Prognosis

Most patients with ABPA respond well to corticosteroid treatment. Others have a chronic course with gradual improvement over time. The best indicator of a good prognosis is a long-term fall in the patient's IgE level. Patients with lung complications from ABPA may develop severe airway obstruction.

Prevention

ABPA is difficult to prevent because *Aspergillus* is a common fungus; it can be found in the saliva and sputum of most healthy individuals. Patients with ABPA can protect themselves somewhat by avoiding haystacks, compost piles, bogs, marshes, and other locations with wet or rotting vegetation; by avoiding construction sites or newly painted surfaces; and by having their air conditioners cleaned regularly. Some patients may be helped by air filtration systems for their bedrooms or offices.

Resources

BOOKS

Stauffer, John L. "Lung." In *Current Medical Diagnosis and Treatment, 1998*, edited by Stephen McPhee, et al., 37th ed. Stamford: Appleton & Lange, 1997.

ORGANIZATIONS

Centers for Disease Control and Prevention. 1600 Clifton Rd., NE, Atlanta, GA 30333. (800) 311-3435, (404) 639-3311. < http://www.cdc.gov > .

National Institute of Allergy and Infectious Disease. Building 31, Room 7A-50, 31 Center Drive MSC 2520, Bethesda, MD 20892-2520. (301) 496-5717. < http://www.niaid.nih.gov/default.htm > .

National Organization for Rare Disorders. P.O. Box 8923, New Fairfield, CT 06812-8923. (800) 999-6673. < http://www.rarediseases.org > .

Rebecca J. Frey, PhD

Allergic purpura

Definition

Allergic purpura (AP) is an allergic reaction of unknown origin causing red patches on the skin and other symptoms. AP is also called Henoch-Schonlein purpura, named after the two doctors who first described it.

Description

"Purpura" is a bleeding disorder that occurs when capillaries rupture, allowing small amounts of blood to accumulate in the surrounding tissues. In AP, this occurs because the capillaries are blocked by protein complexes formed during an abnormal immune reaction. The skin is the most obvious site of reaction, but the joints, gastrointestinal tract, and kidneys are also often affected.

AP affects approximately 35,000 people in the United States each year. Most cases are children between the ages of two and seven. Boys are affected more often than girls, and most cases occur from late fall to winter.

Causes and symptoms

Causes

AP is caused by a reaction involving antibodies, special proteins of the immune system. Antibodies are designed to bind with foreign proteins, called antigens. In some situations, antigen-antibody complexes can become too large to remain suspended in the bloodstream. When this occurs, they precipitate out and become lodged in the capillaries. This can cause the capillary to burst, allowing a local hemorrhage.

The source of the antigen causing AP is unknown. Antigens may be introduced by bacterial or viral infection. More than 75% of patients report having had an infection of the throat, upper respiratory tract, or gastrointestinal system several weeks before the onset of AP. Other complex molecules can act as antigens as well, including drugs such as **antibiotics** or vaccines. Otherwise harmless substances that stimulate an immune reaction are known as allergens. Drug allergens that may cause AP include penicillin, ampicillin, erythromycin, and quinine. Vaccines possibly linked to AP include those for typhoid, measles, **cholera**, and **yellow fever**.

Symptoms

The onset of AP may be preceded by a **headache**, **fever**, and loss of appetite. Most patients first develop

an itchy skin rash. The rash is red, either flat or raised, and may be small and freckle-like. The rash may also be larger, resembling a bruise. **Rashes** become purple and then rust colored over the course of a day, and fade after several weeks. Rashes are most common on the buttocks, abdomen, and lower extremities. Rashes higher on the body may also occur, especially in younger children.

Joint **pain** and swelling is common, especially in the knees and ankles. Abdominal pain occurs in almost all patients, along with blood in the body waste (feces). About half of all patients show blood in the urine, low urine volume, or other signs of kidney involvement. Kidney failure may occur due to widespread obstruction of the capillaries in the filtering structures called glomeruli. Kidney failure develops in about 5% of all patients, and in 15% of those with elevated blood or protein in the urine.

Less common symptoms include prolonged headache, fever, and pain and swelling of the scrotum. Involvement of other organ systems may lead to heart attack (myocardial infarction), inflammation of the pancreas (**pancreatitis**), intestinal obstruction, or bowel perforation.

Diagnosis

Diagnosis of AP is based on the symptoms and their development, a careful medical history, and blood and urine tests. X rays or computed tomography scans (CT) may be performed to assess complications in the bowel or other internal organs.

Treatment

Most cases of AP resolve completely without treatment. Nonetheless, a hospital stay is required because of the possibility of serious complications. Non-aspirin pain relievers may be given for joint pain. **Corticosteroids** (like prednisone) are sometimes used, although not all specialists agree on their utility. Kidney involvement requires monitoring and correction of blood fluids and electrolytes.

Patients with severe kidney complications may require a kidney biopsy so that tissue can be analyzed. Even after all other symptoms subside, elevated levels of blood or protein in the urine may persist for months and require regular monitoring. Hypertension or kidney failure may develop months or even years after the acute phase of the disease. Kidney failure requires dialysis or transplantation.

Prognosis

Most people who develop AP become better on their own after several weeks. About half of all patients have at least one recurrence. Cases that do not have kidney complications usually have the best prognosis.

Resources

PERIODICALS

Andreoli, S. P. "Chronic Glomerulonephritis in Childhood. Membranoproliferative Glomerulonephritis, Henoch-Schonlein PurpuraNnephritis, and IgA Nephropathy." *Pediatric Clinics of North America* 42, no. 6 (December 1995): 1487-1503.

OTHER

"Henoch-Schonlein Purpura." Vanderbilt University Medical Center. < http://www.mc.vanderbilt.edu/peds/pidl/nephro/henoch.html > .

Richard Robinson

Allergic rhinitis

Definition

Allergic **rhinitis**, more commonly referred to as hay fever, is an inflammation of the nasal passages caused by allergic reaction to airborne substances.

Description

Allergic rhinitis (AR) is the most common allergic condition and one of the most common of all minor afflictions. It affects between 10-20% of all people in the United States, and is responsible for 2.5% of all doctor visits. **Antihistamines** and other drugs used to treat allergic rhinitis make up a significant fraction of both prescription and over-the-counter drug sales each year.

There are two types of allergic rhinitis: seasonal and perennial. Seasonal AR occurs in the spring, summer, and early fall, when airborne plant pollens are at their highest levels. In fact, the term hay **fever** is really a misnomer, since allergy to grass pollen is only one cause of symptoms for most people. Perennial AR

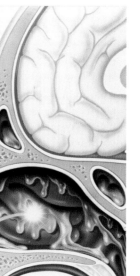

This illustration depicts excessive mucus production in the nose after inhalation of airborne pollen. *(Photo Researchers, Inc. Reproduced by permission.)*

occurs all year and is usually caused by home or workplace airborne pollutants. A person can be affected by one or both types. Symptoms of seasonal AR are worst after being outdoors, while symptoms of perennial AR are worst after spending time indoors.

Both types of **allergies** can develop at any age, although onset in childhood through early adulthood is most common. Although allergy to a particular substance is not inherited, increased allergic sensitivity may "run in the family." While allergies can improve on their own over time, they can also become worse over time.

Causes and symptoms

Causes

Allergic rhinitis is a type of immune reaction. Normally, the immune system responds to foreign

KEY TERMS

Allergen—A substance that provokes an allergic response.

Anaphylaxis—Increased sensitivity caused by previous exposure to an allergen1 that can result in blood vessel dilation (swelling) and smooth muscle contraction. Anaphylaxis can result in sharp blood pressure drops and difficulty breathing.

Antibody—A specific protein produced by the immune system in response to a specific foreign protein or particle called an antigen.

Antigen—A foreign protein to which the body reacts by making antibodies.

Granules—Small packets of reactive chemicals stored within cells.

Histamine—A chemical released by mast cells that activates pain receptors and causes cells to become leaky.

Mast cells—A type of immune system cell that is found in the lining of the nasal passages and eyelids, displays a type of antibody called immunoglobulin type E (IgE) on its cell surface, and participates in the allergic response by releasing histamine from intracellular granules.

microorganisms, or particles, like pollen or dust, by producing specific proteins, called antibodies, that are capable of binding to identifying molecules, or antigens, on the foreign particle. This reaction between antibody and antigen sets off a series of reactions designed to protect the body from infection. Sometimes, this same series of reactions is triggered by harmless, everyday substances. This is the condition known as allergy, and the offending substance is called an allergen.

Like all allergic reactions, AR involves a special set of cells in the immune system known as mast cells. Mast cells, found in the lining of the nasal passages and eyelids, display a special type of antibody, called immunoglobulin type E (IgE), on their surface. Inside, mast cells store reactive chemicals in small packets, called granules. When the antibodies encounter allergens, they trigger release of the granules, which spill out their chemicals onto neighboring cells, including blood vessels and nerve cells. One of these chemicals, histamine, binds to the surfaces of these other cells, through special proteins called histamine receptors. Interaction of histamine with receptors on blood vessels causes neighboring cells to become leaky, leading to the fluid collection, swelling, and

increased redness characteristic of a runny nose and red, irritated eyes. Histamine also stimulates **pain** receptors, causing the itchy, scratchy nose, eyes, and throat common in allergic rhinitis.

The number of possible airborne allergens is enormous. Seasonal AR is most commonly caused by grass and tree pollens, since their pollen is produced in large amounts and is dispersed by the wind. Showy flowers, like roses or lilacs, that attract insects produce a sticky pollen that is less likely to become airborne. Different plants release their pollen at different times of the year, so seasonal AR sufferers may be most affected in spring, summer, or fall, depending on which plants provoke a response. The amount of pollen in the air is reflected in the pollen count, often broadcast on the daily news during allergy season. Pollen counts tend to be lower after a good rain that washes the pollen out of the air and higher on warm, dry, windy days.

Virtually any type of tree or grass may cause AR. A few types of weeds that tend to cause the most trouble for people include the following:

- ragweed
- sagebrush
- lamb's-quarters
- plantain
- pigweed
- dock/sorrel
- tumbleweed

Perennial AR is often triggered by house dust, a complicated mixture of airborne particles, many of which are potent allergens. House dust contains some or all of the following:

- house mite body parts. All houses contain large numbers of microscopic insects called house mites. These harmless insects feed on fibers, fur, and skin shed by the house's larger occupants. Their tiny body parts easily become airborne.

- animal dander. Animals constantly shed fur, skin flakes, and dried saliva. Carried in the air, or transferred from pet to owner by direct contact, dander can cause allergy in many sensitive people.

- mold spores. Molds live in damp spots throughout the house, including basements, bathrooms, air ducts, air conditioners, refrigerator drains, damp windowsills, mattresses, and stuffed furniture. Mildew and other molds release airborne spores that circulate throughout the house.

Other potential causes of perennial allergic rhinitis include the following:

- cigarette smoke
- perfume
- cosmetics
- cleansers
- copier chemicals
- industrial chemicals
- construction material gases

Symptoms

Inflammation of the nose, or rhinitis, is the major symptom of AR. Inflammation causes itching, sneezing, runny nose, redness, and tenderness. Sinus swelling can constrict the eustachian tube that connects the inner ear to the throat, causing a congested feeling and "ear popping." The drip of mucus from the sinuses down the back of the throat, combined with increased sensitivity, can also lead to throat irritation and redness. AR usually also causes redness, **itching**, and watery eyes. **Fatigue** and headache are also common.

Diagnosis

Diagnosing seasonal AR is usually easy and can often be done without a medical specialist. When symptoms appear in spring or summer and disappear with the onset of cold weather, seasonal AR is almost certainly the culprit. Other causes of rhinitis, including infection, can usually be ruled out by a **physical examination** and a nasal smear, in which a sample of mucus is taken on a swab for examination.

Allergy tests, including skin testing and provocation testing, can help identify the precise culprit, but may not be done unless a single source is suspected and subsequent avoidance is possible. Skin testing involves placing a small amount of liquid containing a specific allergen on the skin and then either poking, scratching, or injecting it into the skin surface to observe whether redness and swellings occurs. Provocation testing involves challenging an individual with either a small amount of an inhalable or ingestable allergen to see if a response is elicited.

Perennial AR can also usually be diagnosed by careful questioning about the timing of exposure and the onset of symptoms. Specific allergens can be identified through allergy skin testing.

Treatment

Avoidance of the allergens is the best treatment, but this is often not possible. When it is not possible to avoid one or more allergens, there are two major forms of medical treatment, drugs and immunotherapy.

Drugs

ANTIHISTAMINES. Antihistamines block the histamine receptors on nasal tissue, decreasing the effect of histamine release by mast cells. They may be used after symptoms appear, though they may be even more effective when used preventively, before symptoms appear. A wide variety of antihistamines are available.

Older antihistamines often produce drowsiness as a major side effect. Such antihistamines include the following:

- diphenhydramine (Benadryl and generics)
- chlorpheniramine (Chlor-trimeton and generics)
- brompheniramine (Dimetane and generics)
- clemastine (Tavist and generics).

Newer antihistamines that do not cause drowsiness are available by prescription and include the following:

- astemizole (Hismanal)
- fexofenadine (Allegra)
- cetirizine (Zyrtec)
- azelastin HCl (Astelin).

Loratidine (Claritin) was available only by prescription but was released to over-the-counter status by the FDA.

Hismanal has the potential to cause serious heart **arrhythmias** when taken with the antibiotic erythromycin, the antifungal drugs ketoconazole and itraconazole, or the antimalarial drug quinine. Taking more than the recommended dose of Hismanal can also cause arrhythimas. Seldane (terfenadine), the original nondrowsy antihistamine, was voluntarily withdrawn from the market by its manufacturers in early 1998 because of this potential and because of the availability of an equally effective, safer alternative drug, fexofenadine.

LEUKOTRIENE RECEPTOR ANTAGONISTS. Leukotriene receptor antagonists (montelukast or Singulair and zafirlukast or Accolate) are a newer class of drugs used daily to help prevent **asthma**. They've also become approved in the United States to treat allergic rhinitis.

DECONGESTANTS. **Decongestants** constrict blood vessels to counteract the effects of histamine. This decreases the amount of blood in the nasopahryngeal and sinus mucosa and reduces swelling. Nasal sprays are available that can be applied directly to the nasal lining and oral systemic preparations are available. Decongestants are stimulants and may cause increased heart rate and blood pressure, headaches, isomnia, agitation and difficulty emptying the bladder. Use of topical decongestants for longer than several days can cause loss of effectiveness and rebound congestion, in which nasal passages become more severely swollen than before treatment.

TOPICAL CORTICOSTEROIDS. Topical **corticosteroids** reduce mucous membrane inflammation and are available by prescription. Allergies tend to become worse as the season progresses because the immune system becomes sensitized to particular antigens and can produce a faster, stronger response. Topical corticosteroids are especially effective at reducing this seasonal sensitization because they work more slowly and last longer than most other medication types. As a result, they are best started before allergy season begins. Side effects are usually mild, but may include headaches, nosebleeds, and unpleasant taste sensations.

MAST CELL STABILIZERS. Cromolyn sodium prevents the release of mast cell granules, thereby preventing release of histamine and the other chemicals contained in them. It acts as a preventive treatment if it is begun several weeks before the onset of the allergy season. It can be used for perennial AR as well.

Immunotherapy

Immunotherapy, also known as desensitization or allergy shots, alters the balance of antibody types in the body, thereby reducing the ability of IgE to cause allergic reactions. Immunotherapy is preceded by allergy testing to determine the precise allergens responsible. Injections involve very small but gradually increasing amounts of allergen, over several weeks or months, with periodic boosters. Full benefits may take up to several years to achieve and are not seen at all in about one in five patients. Individuals receiving all shots will be monitored closely following each shot because of the small risk of **anaphylaxis**, a condition that can result in difficulty breathing and a sharp drop in blood pressure.

Alternative treatment

Alternative treatments for AR often focus on modulation of the body's immune response, and frequently center around diet and lifestyle adjustments. Chinese herbal medicine can help rebalance a person's system, as can both acute and constitutional homeopathic treatment. Vitamin C in substantial amounts can help stabilize the mucous membrane response. For symptom relief, western herbal remedies including eyebright (*Euphrasia officinalis*) and nettle (*Urtica dioica*) may be helpful. Bee pollen may also be effective in alleviating or eliminating AR symptoms. A 2004 report said that **phototherapy** (treatment with a combination of ultraviolet and visible light) decreased the symptoms of allergic rhinitis in a majority of patients who did not respond well to traditional drug treatment.

Prognosis

Most people with AR can achieve adequate relief with a combination of preventive strategies and treatment. While allergies may improve over time, they may also get worse or expand to include new allergens. Early treatment can help prevent an increased sensitization to other allergens.

Prevention

Reducing exposure to pollen may improve symptoms of seasonal AR. Strategies include the following:

- stay indoors with windows closed during the morning hours, when pollen levels are highest
- keep car windows up while driving
- use a surgical face mask when outside
- avoid uncut fields
- learn which trees are producing pollen in which seasons, and avoid forests at the height of pollen season
- wash clothes and hair after being outside
- clean air conditioner filters in the home regularly
- use electrostatic filters for central air conditioning

Moving to a region with lower pollen levels is rarely effective, since new allergies often develop

Preventing perennial AR requires identification of the responsible allergens.

Mold spores:

- keep the house dry through ventilation and use of dehumidifiers
- use a disinfectant such as dilute bleach to clean surfaces such as bathroom floors and walls
- have ducts cleaned and disinfected
- clean and disinfect air conditioners and coolers
- throw out moldy or mildewed books, shoes, pillows, or furniture

House dust:

- vacuum frequently, and change the bag regularly. Use a bag with small pores to catch extra-fine particles

• clean floors and walls with a damp mop

• install electrostatic filters in heating and cooling ducts, and change all filters regularly

Animal dander:

• avoid contact if possible

• wash hands after contact

• vacuum frequently

• keep pets out of the bedroom, and off furniture, rugs, and other dander-catching surfaces

• have your pets bathed and groomed frequently

Resources

PERIODICALS

Finn, Robert. "Rhinoohototherapy Targets Allergic Rhinitis." *Skin & Allergy News* (July 2004): 62.
"What's New in: Asthma and Allergic Rhinitis." *Pulse* (September 20, 2004): 50.

Richard Robinson
Teresa G. Odle

Allergies

Definition

Allergies are abnormal reactions of the immune system that occur in response to otherwise harmless substances.

Description

Allergies are among the most common of medical disorders. It is estimated that 60 million Americans, or more than one in every five people, suffer from some form of allergy, with similar proportions throughout much of the rest of the world. Allergy is the single largest reason for school absence and is a major source of lost productivity in the workplace.

An allergy is a type of immune reaction. Normally, the immune system responds to foreign microorganisms or particles by producing specific proteins called antibodies. These antibodies are capable of binding to identifying molecules, or antigens, on the foreign particle. This reaction between antibody and antigen sets off a series of chemical reactions designed to protect the body from infection. Sometimes, this same series of reactions is triggered by harmless, everyday substances such as pollen, dust, and animal danders.

When this occurs, an allergy develops against the offending substance (an allergen.)

Mast cells, one of the major players in allergic reactions, capture and display a particular type of antibody, called immunoglobulin type E (IgE) that binds to allergens. Inside mast cells are small chemical-filled packets called granules. Granules contain a variety of potent chemicals, including histamine.

Immunologists separate allergic reactions into two main types: immediate hypersensitivity reactions, which are predominantly mast cell-mediated and occur within minutes of contact with allergen; and delayed hypersensitivity reactions, mediated by T cells (a type of white blood cells) and occurring hours to days after exposure.

Inhaled or ingested allergens usually cause immediate hypersensitivity reactions. Allergens bind to IgE antibodies on the surface of mast cells, which spill the contents of their granules out onto neighboring cells, including blood vessels and nerve cells. Histamine binds to the surfaces of these other cells through special proteins called histamine receptors. Interaction of histamine with receptors on blood vessels causes increased leakiness, leading to the fluid collection, swelling and increased redness. Histamine also stimulates **pain** receptors, making tissue more sensitive and irritable. Symptoms last from one to several hours following contact.

In the upper airways and eyes, immediate hypersensitivity reactions cause the runny nose and itchy, bloodshot eyes typical of **allergic rhinitis**. In the gastrointestinal tract, these reactions lead to swelling and irritation of the intestinal lining, which causes the cramping and **diarrhea** typical of food allergy. Allergens that enter the circulation may cause **hives**, angioedema, **anaphylaxis**, or **atopic dermatitis**.

Allergens on the skin usually cause delayed hypersensitivity reaction. Roving T cells contact the allergen, setting in motion a more prolonged immune response. This type of allergic response may develop over several days following contact with the allergen, and symptoms may persist for a week or more.

Causes and symptoms

Allergens enter the body through four main routes: the airways, the skin, the gastrointestinal tract, and the circulatory system.

• Airborne allergens cause the sneezing, runny nose, and itchy, bloodshot eyes of hay fever (allergic **rhinitis**). Airborne allergens can also affect the lining of the lungs, causing **asthma**, or conjunctivitis (pink

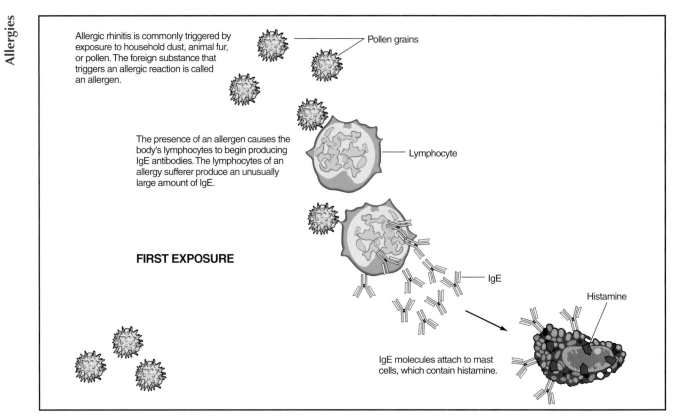

Allergic rhinitis is commonly triggered by exposure to household dust, animal fur, or pollen. The foreign substance that triggers an allergic reaction is called an allergen.

Pollen grains

The presence of an allergen causes the body's lymphocytes to begin producing IgE antibodies. The lymphocytes of an allergy sufferer produce an unusually large amount of IgE.

Lymphocyte

FIRST EXPOSURE

IgE

Histamine

IgE molecules attach to mast cells, which contain histamine.

The allergic response. *(Illustration by Hans & Cassady.)*

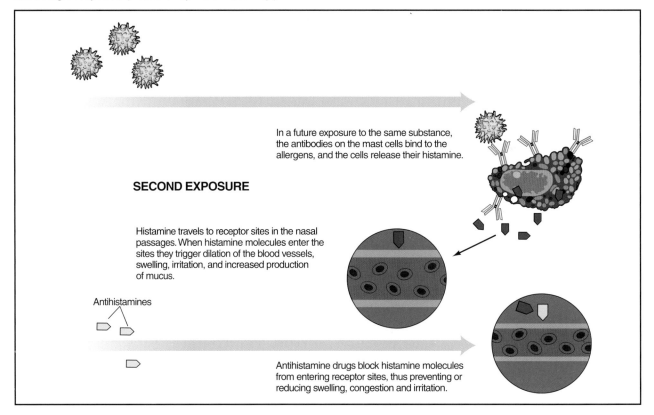

In a future exposure to the same substance, the antibodies on the mast cells bind to the allergens, and the cells release their histamine.

SECOND EXPOSURE

Histamine travels to receptor sites in the nasal passages. When histamine molecules enter the sites they trigger dilation of the blood vessels, swelling, irritation, and increased production of mucus.

Antihistamines

Antihistamine drugs block histamine molecules from entering receptor sites, thus preventing or reducing swelling, congestion and irritation.

Second and subsequent exposure to allergen. *(Illustration by Hans & Cassady.)*

KEY TERMS

Allergen—A substance that provokes an allergic response.

Allergic rhinitis—Inflammation of the mucous membranes of the nose and eyes in response to an allergen.

Anaphylaxis—Increased sensitivity caused by previous exposure to an allergen that can result in blood vessel dilation and smooth muscle contraction. Anaphylaxis can result in sharp blood pressure drops and difficulty breathing.

Angioedema—Severe non-inflammatory swelling of the skin, organs, and brain that can also be accompanied by fever and muscle pain.

Antibody—A specific protein produced by the immune system in response to a specific foreign protein or particle called an antigen.

Antigen—A foreign protein to which the body reacts by making antibodies.

Asthma—A lung condition in which the airways become narrow due to smooth muscle contraction, causing wheezing, coughing, and shortness of breath.

Atopic dermatitis—Infection of the skin as a result of exposure to airborne or food allergens.

Conjunctivitis—Inflammation of the thin lining of the eye called the conjunctiva.

Contact dermatitis—Inflammation of the skin as a result of contact with a substance.

Delayed hypersensitivity reactions—Allergic reactions mediated by T cells that occur hours to days after exposure.

Granules—Small packets of reactive chemicals stored within cells.

Histamine—A chemical released by mast cells that activates pain receptors and causes cells to become leaky.

Immune hypersensitivity reaction—Allergic reactions that are mediated by mast cells and occur within minutes of allergen contact.

Mast cells—A type of immune system cell that is found in the lining of the nasal passages and eyelids, displays a type of antibody called immunoglobulin type E (IgE) on its cell surface, and participates in the allergic response by releasing histamine from intracellular granules.

T cells—Immune system cells or more specifically, white blood cells, that stimulate cells to create and release antibodies.

eye). Exposure to cockroach allergens has been associated with the development of asthma. Airborne allergens from household pets are another common source of environmental exposure.

- Allergens in food can cause **itching** and swelling of the lips and throat, cramps, and diarrhea. When absorbed into the bloodstream, they may cause hives (urticaria) or more severe reactions involving recurrent, non-inflammatory swelling of the skin, mucous membranes, organs, and brain (angioedema). Some food allergens may cause anaphylaxis, a potentially life-threatening condition marked by tissue swelling, airway constriction, and drop in blood pressure. Allergies to foods such as cow's milk, eggs, nuts, fish, and legumes (peanuts and soybeans) are common. Allergies to fruits and vegetables may also occur.

- In contact with the skin, allergens can cause reddening, itching, and blistering, called contact **dermatitis**. Skin reactions can also occur from allergens introduced through the airways or gastrointestinal tract. This type of reaction is known as atopic dermatitis.

Dermatitis may arise from an allergic response (such as from poison ivy), or exposure to an irritant causing nonimmune damage to skin cells (such as soap, cold, and chemical agents).

- Injection of allergens, from insect **bites and stings** or drug administration, can introduce allergens directly into the circulation, where they may cause system-wide responses (including anaphylaxis), as well as the local ones of swelling and irritation at the injection site.

People with allergies are not equally sensitive to all allergens. Some may have severe allergic rhinitis but no **food allergies**, for instance, or be extremely sensitive to nuts but not to any other food. Allergies may get worse over time. For example, childhood ragweed allergy may progress to year-round dust and pollen allergy. On the other hand, a person may lose allergic sensitivity. Infant or childhood atopic dermatitis disappears in almost all people. More commonly, what seems to be loss of sensitivity is instead a reduced exposure to allergens or an increased tolerance for the same level of symptoms.

While allergy to specific allergens is not inherited, the likelihood of developing some type of allergy seems to be, at least for many people. If neither parent has allergies, the chances of a child developing allergy is approximately 10-20%; if one parent has allergies, it is 30-50%; and if both have allergies, it is 40-75%. One source of this genetic predisposition is in the ability to produce higher levels of IgE in response to allergens. Those who produce more IgE will develop a stronger allergic sensitivity.

COMMON ALLERGENS. The most common airborne allergens are the following:

- plant pollens
- animal fur and dander
- body parts from house mites (microscopic creatures found in all houses)
- house dust
- mold spores
- cigarette smoke
- solvents
- cleaners

Common food allergens include the following:

The following types of drugs commonly cause allergic reactions:

- penicillin or other **antibiotics**
- flu vaccines
- tetanus toxoid vaccine
- gamma globulin

Common causes of **contact dermatitis** include the following:

- poison ivy, oak, and sumac
- nickel or nickel alloys
- latex

Insects and other arthropods whose bites or stings typically cause allergy include the following:

- bees, wasps, and hornets
- mosquitoes
- fleas
- scabies

Symptoms depend on the specific type of allergic reaction. Allergic rhinitis is characterized by an itchy, runny nose, often with a scratchy or irritated throat due to post-nasal drip. Inflammation of the thin membrane covering the eye (allergic **conjunctivitis**) causes redness, irritation, and increased tearing in the eyes. Asthma causes **wheezing**, coughing, and shortness of breath. Symptoms of food allergies depend on the tissues most sensitive to the allergen and whether the allergen was spread systemically by the circulatory system. Gastrointestinal symptoms may include swelling and **tingling** in the lips, tongue, palate or throat; **nausea**; cramping; diarrhea; and gas. Contact dermatitis is marked by reddened, itchy, weepy skin blisters, and an eczema that is slow to heal. It sometimes has a characteritic man-made pattern, such as a glove allergy with clear demarcation on the hands, wrist, and arms where the gloves are worn, or on the earlobes by wearing earrings.

Whole body or systemic reactions may occur from any type of allergen, but are more common following ingestion or injection of an allergen. Skin reactions include the raised, reddened, and itchy patches called hives that characteristically blanch with pressure and resolve within twenty-four hours. A deeper and more extensive skin reaction, involving more extensive fluid collection and pain, is called angioedema. This usually occurs on the extremities, fingers, toes, and parts of the head, neck, and face. Anaphylaxis is marked by airway constriction, blood pressure drop, widespread tissue swelling, heart rhythm abnormalities, and in some cases, loss of consciousness. Other syptoms may include, **dizziness**, weakness, seizures, coughing, flushing, or cramping. The symptoms may begin within five minutes after exposure to the allergen up to one hour or more later. Mast cells in the tissues and basophils in the blood release mediators that give rise to the clinical symptoms of this IgE-mediated hypersensitivity reaction. Commonly, this is associated with allergies to medications, foods, and insect venoms. In some individuals, anaphylaxis can occur with **exercise**, plasma exchange, hemodialysis, reaction to insulin, contrast media used in certain types of medical tests, and rarely during the administration of local anesthetics.

Diagnosis

Allergies can often be diagnosed by a careful medical history, matching the onset of symptoms to the exposure to possible allergens. Allergy is suspected if the symptoms presented are characteristic of an allergic reaction and this occurs repeatedly upon exposure to the suspected allergen. **Allergy tests** can be used to identify potential allergens, but these must be supported by eveidence of allergic responses in the patient's clinical history.

Skin tests

Skin tests are performed by administering a tiny dose of the suspected allergen by pricking, scratching, puncturing or injecting the skin. The allergen is applied to the skin as an auqeous extract, usually on the back, forearms, or top of the thighs. Once in the skin, the allergen may produce a classic immune wheal and flare response (a skin lesion with a raised, white, compressible area surrounded by a red flare). The tests usually begin with prick tests or patch tests that expose the skin to small amounts of allergen to observe the response. A positive reaction will occur on the skin even if the allergen is at levels normally encountered in food or in the airways. Reactions are usually evaluated approximately fifteen minutes after exposure. Intradermal skin tests involved injection of the allergen into the dermis of the skin. These tests are more sensitive and are used for allergies associated with risk of **death**, such as allergies to antibiotics.

Allergen-Specific IgE Measurement

Tests that measure allergen-specific IgE antibodies generally follow a basic method. The allergen is bound to a solid support, either in the form of a cellulose sponge, microtiter plate, or paper disk. The patient's serum is prepared from a blood sample and is incubated with the solid phase. If allergen specific IgE antibodies are present, they will bind to the solid phase and be retained there when the rest of the serum is washed away. Next, an labeled antibody against the IgE is added and will bind to any IgE on the solid phase. The excess is washed away and the levels of IgE are determined. The commonly used RAST test (radio allergo sorbent test) employed radio-labeled Anti-IgE antibodies. Updated methods now incorporate the use of enyzme-labeled antibodies in ELISA assays (enzyme-linked immunosorbent assays).

Total Serum IgE

The total level of IgE in the serum is commonly measured with a two-site immunometric assay. Some research indicates that there is a higher level of total serum IgE in allergic as compared to non-allergic people. However, this may not always be the case as there is considerable overlap between the two groups. This test is useful for the diagnosis of allergic fungal sinusitis and bronchopulmonary **aspergillosis**. Other conditions that are not allergic in nature may give rise to higher IgE levels such as **smoking**, **AIDS**, infection with parasites, and IgE myeloma.

Provocation tests

These tests involve the administration of allergen to elicit an immune response. Provocation tests, most commonly done with airborne allergens, present the allergen directly through the route normally involved. Delayed allergic contact dermatitis diagnosis involves similar methods by application of a skin patch with allergen to induce an allergic skin reaction. Food allergen provocation tests require abstinence from the suspect allergen for two weeks or more, followed by ingestion of a measured amount of the test substance administered as an opaque capsule along with a placebo control. Provocation tests arc not used if anaphylaxis is is a concern due to the patient's medical history.

Future diagnostic methods

Attempts have been made for direct measurement of immune mediators such as histamine, eosinophil cationic protein (ECP), and mast cell tryptase. Another, somewhat controversial, test is electrodermal testing or electro-acupuncture allergy testing. This test has been used in Europe and is under investigation in the United States, though not approved by the Food and Drug Administration. An electric potential is applied to the skin, the allergen presented, and the electrical resistance observed for changes. This method has not been verified.

Treatment

Avoiding allergens is the first line of defense to reduce the possibility of an allergic attack. It is helpful to avoid environmental irritants such as tobacco smoke, perfumes, household cleaning agents, paints, glues, air fresheners, and potpourri. Nitrogen dioxide from poorly vented gas stoves, woodburning stoves, and artificial fireplaces has also been linked to poor asthma control. Dust mite control is particularly important in the bedroom areas by use of allergen-impermeable covers on mattress and pillows, frequent washing of bedding in hot water, and removal of items that collect dust such as stuffed toys. Mold growth may be reduced by lowering indoor humidity, repair of house foundations to reduce indoor leaks and seepage, and installing exhaust systems to ventilate areas where steam is generated such as the bathroom or kitchen. Allergic individuals should avoid pet allergens such as saliva, body excretions, pelts, urine, or feces. For those who insist on keeping a pet, restriction of the animal's activity to certain areas of the home may be beneficial.

Complete environmental control is often difficult to accomplish, hence therapuetic interventions may become necessary. A large number of prescription and over-the-counter drugs are available for treatment of immediate hypersensitivity reactions. Most of these work by decreasing the ability of histamine to provoke symptoms. Other drugs counteract the effects of histamine by stimulating other systems or reducing immune responses in general.

Antihistamines

Antihistamines block the histamine receptors on nasal tissue, decreasing the effect of histamine released by mast cells. They may be used after symptoms appear, though they may be even more effective when used preventively, before symptoms appear. Antihistamines help reduce sneezing, itching, and rhinorrhea. A wide variety of antihistamines are available.

Older, first generation antihistamines often produce drowsiness as a major side effect, as well as **dry mouth**, tachycardia, blurred vision, **constipation**, and lower the threshold for seizures. These medications also have similar effects to a alcohol and care should be taken when operating motor vehicles, as individuals may not be aware that they are impaired. Such antihistamines include the following:

- diphenhydramine (Benadryl and generics)
- chlorpheniramine (Chlor-trimeton and generics)
- brompheniramine (Dimetane and generics)
- clemastine (Tavist and generics)

Newer antihistamines that do not cause drowsiness or pass the blood-brain barrier are available by prescription and include the following:

- loratidine (Claritin)
- cetirizine (Zyrtec)
- fexofenadine (Allegra)

Desloratadine (Clarinex) was approved in 2004 in syrup form for children two years and older for seasonal allergies and for hives of unknown cause in children as young as six months. It is the only nonsedating antihistamine approved as of 2004 for children as young as six months.

Hismanal has the potential to cause serious heart **arrhythmias** when taken with the antibiotic erythromycin, the antifungal drugs ketoconazole and itraconazole, or the antimalarial drug quinine. Taking more than the recommended dose of Hismanal can also cause arrhythimas. Seldane (terfenadine), the original nondrowsy antihistamine, was voluntarily withdrawn from the market by its manufacturers in early 1998 because of this potential and because of the availability of an equally effective, safer alternative drug, fexofenadine.

Decongestants

Decongestants constrict blood vessels to the mucosa to counteract the effects of histamine. This decreases the amount of blood in the nasopahryngeal and sinus mucosa and reduces swelling. Nasal sprays are available that can be applied directly to the nasal lining and oral systematic preparations are available. Decongestants are stimulants and may cause increased heart rate and blood pressure, headaches, **insomnia**, agitation, and difficulty emptying the bladder. Use of topical decongestants for longer than several days can cause loss of effectiveness and rebound congestion, in which nasal passages become more severely swollen than before treatment.

Topical corticosteroids

Topical **corticosteroids** reduce mucous membrane inflammation by decreasing the amount of fluid moved from the vascular spaces into the tissues. These medications reduce the recruitment of inflammatory cells as well as the synthesis of cytokines. They are available by prescription. Allergies tend to become worse as the season progresses because the immune system becomes sensitized to particular antigens and can produce a faster, stronger response. Topical corticosteroids are especially effective at reducing this seasonal sensitization because they work more slowly and last longer than most other medication types. As a result, they are best started before allergy season begins. Side effects are usually mild, but may include headaches, nosebleeds, and unpleasant taste sensations.

Bronchodilators or metered-dose inhalers (MDI)

Because allergic reactions involving the lungs cause the airways or bronchial tubes to narrow, as in asthma, **bronchodilators**, which cause the smooth muscle lining the airways to open or dilate, can be very effective. When inhalers are used, it is important that the patient be educated in the proper use of these medications. The inhaler should be shaken, and the patient should breathe out to expel air from the lungs. The inhaler should be placed at least two fingerbreadths in front of the mouth. The medication should be aimed at the back of the throat, and the inhaler activated while breathing in quite slowly 3-4 seconds. The breath should be held for at least ten seconds, and then expelled. At least thirty to sixty seconds should pass before the inhaler is used again. Care should be taken to properly wash out the mouth and brush the teeth following use, as residual medication remains in this area with only a small amount actually reaching the lungs. Some bronchodilators used to treat acute asthma attacks include adrenaline, albuterol, Maxair, Proventil, or other "adrenoceptor stimulants," most often administered as aerosols. Successfully managing asthma and allergies can reduce the use of inhalers.

This is done through good communication between the physician and patient, self-management with written action plans, avoiding allergy triggers, and through the use of preventive medications such as montelukast.

Anticholinergics

Ipratropium bromide (atrovent) and atropine sulfate are achticholinergic drugs used for the treatment of asthma. Ipratropium is used for treating asthmatics in emergency situations with a nebulizer.

Nonsteroidal drugs

MAST CELL STABILIZERS. Cromolyn sodium prevents the release of mast cell granules, thereby preventing the release of histamine and other chemicals contained in them. It acts as a preventive treatment if it is begun several weeks before the onset of the allergy season. It can also be used for year round allergy prevention. Cromolyn sodium is available as a nasal spray for allergic rhinitis and in aerosol (a suspension of particles in gas) form for asthma.

LEUKOTRIENE MODIFIERS. These medications are useful for individuals with aspirin sensitivity, **sinusitis**, polposis, urticaria. Examples include zafirlukast (Accolate), montelukast (Singulair), and zileuton (Zyflo). When zileuton is used, care must be taken to measure liver enzymes.

Immunotherapy

In this form of therapy, allergen is injected into the skin in increasing doses over a specific period of time. This may be helpful for patients who do not respond to medications or avoidance of allergens in the environment. This type of therapy may reduce the need for medications. A 2004 study recommended that children who have severe reactions to insect sting receive immunotherapy to protect them against future stings.

Treatment of contact dermatitis

An individual suffering from contact dermatitis should initially take steps to avoid possible sources of exposure to the offending agent. Calamine lotion applied to affected skin can reduce irritation somewhat, as can cold water compresses. Side effects of topical agents may include over-drying of the skin. In the case of acute contact dermatitis, short-term oral corticosteroid therapy may be appropriate. Moderately strong coricosteroids can also be applied as a wrap for twenty-four hours. Health care workers are especially at risk for hand eruptions due to glove use.

Treatment of anaphylaxis

The emergency condition of anaphylaxis is treated with injection of adrenaline, also known as epinephrine. People who are prone to anaphylaxis because of food or insect allergies often carry an "Epi-pen" containing adrenaline in a hypodermic needle. Other medications may be given to aid the action of the epi-pen. Prompt injection can prevent a more serious reaction from developing. Particular care should be taken to assess the affected individual's airway status, and he or she should be placed in a recumbent pose and vital signs determined. If a reaction resulted from insect sting or an injection, a tourniquet may need to be placed proximal to the area where the agent penetrated the skin. This should then be released at intervals of ten minutes at a time, for one to two minutes duration. If the individual does not respond to such interventions, then emergency treatment is appropriate.

Alternative treatment

Any alternative treatment for allergies begins with finding the cause and then helping the patient to avoid or eliminate the allergen, although this is not always possible. As with any alternative therapy, a physician should be consulted before initiating a new form of treatment. Education on the use of alternative agents is critical, as they are still "drugs" even though they are derived from natural sources. Various categories of alternative remedies may be helpful in allergy treatment, including:

- antihistamines: vitamin C and the bioflavonoid hesperidin act as natural anithistamines.
- decongestants: vitamin C, the homeopathic remedies *Ferrum phosphoricum* and *Kali muriaticum* (used alternately), and the dietary supplement N-acetylcysteine are believed to have decongestant effects.
- mast cell stabilizers: the bioflavonoids quercetin and hesperidin may help stabilize mast cells.
- immunotherapy: the herbs **echinacea** (*Echinacea* spp.) and astragalus or milk-vetch root (*Astragalus membranaceus*) may possibly help to strengthen the immune system.
- bronchodilators: the herbal remedies ephedra (*Ephedra sinica*, also known as ma huang in traditional Chinese medicine), khellin (*Ammi visnaga*) and cramp bark (*Viburnum opulus*) are believed to help open the airways.

Treatment of contact dermatitis

A variety of herbal remedies, either applied topically or taken internally, may possibly assist in the treatment of contact dermatitis. A poultice (crushed herbs applied directly to the affected area) made of jewelweed (*Impatiens* spp.) or chickweed (*Stellaria media*) may soothe the skin. A cream or wash containing calendula (*Calendula officinalis*), a natural antiseptic and anti-inflammatory agent, may help heal the rash when applied topically. Homeopathic treatment may include such remedies as *Rhus toxicodendron*, *Apis mellifica*, or *Anacardium* taken internally. A qualified homeopathic practitioner should be consulted to match the symptoms with the correct remedy. Care should be taken with any agent taken internally.

Prognosis

Allergies can improve over time, although they often worsen. While anaphylaxis and severe asthma are life-threatening, other allergic reactions are not. Learning to recognize and avoid allergy-provoking situations allows most people with allergies to lead normal lives.

Prevention

Avoiding allergens is the best means of limiting allergic reactions. For food allergies, there is no effective treatment except avoidance. By determining the allergens that are causing reactions, most people can learn to avoid allergic reactions from food, drugs, and contact allergens such as poison ivy or latex. The government will help now, since passing the Food Allergen Labeling and Consumer Protection Act in 2004. Beginning January 1, 2006, food manufacturers will be required to clearly state if a product contains any of the eight major food allergens that are responsible for more than 90% of allergic reactions to foods. These are milk, eggs, peanuts, tree nuts, fish, shellfish, wheat, and soy.

Airborne allergens are more difficult to avoid, although keeping dust and animal dander from collecting in the house may limit exposure. Cromolyn sodium can prevent mast cell degranulation, thereby limiting the allergic response.

Immunotherapy, also known as desensitization or allergy shots, alters the balance of antibody types in the body, thereby reducing the ability of IgE to cause allergic reactions. Immunotherapy is preceded by allergy testing to determine the precise allergens responsible. Injections involve very small but gradually increasing amounts of allergen, over several weeks or months, with periodic boosters. Full benefits may

take up to several years to achieve and are not seen at all in about one in five patients. Individuals receiving all shots will be monitored closely following each shot because of the small risk of anaphylaxis, a condition that can result in difficulty breathing and a sharp drop in blood pressure.

Other drugs, such as leukotriene modifiers, are used to prevent asthma attacks and in the long-term management of allergies and asthma.

Resources

BOOKS

Hans-Uwe, Simon, editor. *CRC Desk Reference for Allergy and Asthma*. Boca Raton: CRC Press, 2000.

Kemp, Stephen F., and Richard Lockey, editors. *Diagnostic Testing of Allergic Disease*. New York: Marcel Dekker, Inc., 2000.

Lieberman, Phil, and Johh Anderson, editors. *Allergic Diseases: Diagnosis and Treatment*. 2nd ed. Totowa: Humana Press, Inc., 2000.

PERIODICALS

"Children With Serious Insect-sting Allergies Should Get Shots." *Drug Week* (September 3, 2004): 19.

"FDA Approves Clarinex Syrup for Allergies and Hives in Children." *Biotech Week* (September 29, 2004): 617.

"President Bush Signs Bill that Will Benefit Millions With Food Allergies." *Immunotherapy Weekly* (September 1, 2004): 50.

"What's New in: Asthma and Allergic Rhinitis." *Pulse* (September 20, 2004): 50.

Richard Robinson
Jill Granger, MS
Teresa G. Odle

Allergy tests

Definition

Allergy tests indicate a person's allergic sensitivity to commonly encountered environmental substances.

Purpose

Allergy is a reaction of the immune system. Normally, the immune system responds to foreign microorganisms and particles, like pollen or dust, by producing specific proteins called antibodies that are capable of binding to identifying molecules, or antigens, on the foreign organisms. This reaction between antibody and antigen sets off a series of reactions designed to protect the body from infection. Sometimes, this same series of reactions is

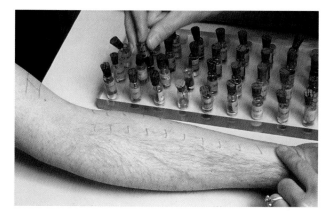

This patient is being exposed to certain allergens as part of an allergy test. *(Custom Medical Stock Photo. Reproduced by permission.)*

triggered by harmless, everyday substances. This is the condition known as allergy, and the offending substance is called an allergen. Common inhaled allergens include pollen, dust, and insect parts from tiny house mites. Common food allergens include nuts, fish, and milk.

Allergic reactions involve a special set of cells in the immune system known as mast cells. Mast cells serve as guards in the tissues where the body meets the outside world: the skin, the mucous membranes of the eyes and other areas, and the linings of the respiratory and digestive systems. Mast cells display a special type of antibody, called immunoglobulin type E (IgE), on their surface. Inside, mast cells store reactive chemicals in small packets, called granules. When the antibodies encounter allergens, they trigger the release of granules, which spill out their chemicals onto neighboring cells, including blood vessels and nerve cells. One of these chemicals, histamine, binds to the surfaces of these other cells, through special proteins called histamine receptors. Interaction of histamine with receptors on blood vessels causes neighboring cells to become leaky, leading to the fluid collection, swelling, and increased redness characteristic of a runny nose and red, irritated eyes. Histamine also stimulates **pain** receptors, causing the itchy, scratchy nose, eyes, and throat common in **allergic rhinitis**.

The particular allergens to which a person is sensitive can be determined through allergy testing. Allergy tests may be performed on the skin or using blood serum in a test tube. During skin tests, potential allergens are placed on the skin and the reaction is observed. In radio-allergosorbent allergy testing (RAST), a patient's blood serum is combined with allergen in a test tube to determine if serum antibodies react with the allergen. Provocation testing involves direct exposure to a likely allergen, either through inhalation or ingestion. Positive reactions from any of these tests may be used to narrow the candidates for the actual allergen causing the allergy.

Identification of the allergenic substance may allow the patient to avoid the substance and reduce allergic reactions. In addition, allergy testing may be done in those with **asthma** that is difficult to manage, eczema, or skin **rashes** to determine if an allergy is causing the condition or making it worse. Allergy tests may also be done before allergen desensitization to ensure the safety of more extensive exposure.

Skin testing is the most common type of allergy test. There are two forms: percutaneous and intradermal. In percutaneous or prick testing, allergen solutions are placed on the skin, and the skin is then pricked with a needle, allowing the allergen to enter the skin and become exposed to mast cells. Scratch testing, in which the skin is scratched instead of punctured, is used less often. Intradermal testing involves directly injecting allergen solutions into the skin. In both tests, a reddened, swollen spot develops at the injection site for each substance to which the person is sensitive. Skin reactivity is seen for allergens regardless of whether they usually affect the skin. In other words, airborne and food allergens cause skin reactions equally well.

The range of allergens used for testing is chosen to reflect possible sources in the environment and may include the following:

- pollen from a variety of trees, common grasses, and weeds
- mold and fungus spores
- house dust
- house mites
- animal skin cells (dander) and saliva
- food extracts
- antibiotics
- insect venoms

Radio-allergosorbent testing (RAST) is a laboratory test performed when a person may be too sensitive to risk skin testing or when medications or skin conditions prevent it.

Provocation testing is done to positively identify suspected allergens after preliminary skin testing. A purified preparation of the allergen is inhaled or ingested in increasing concentrations to determine if it will provoke a response. In 2004, scientists introduced an optical method to continuously measure the changes in nasal mucosa (lining) changes with an infrared light to help improve the accuracy of provocation testing. Food testing is much more tedious than inhalation testing, since full passage through the digestive system may take a day or more.

Precautions

While allergy tests are quite safe for most people, the possibility of a condition known as **anaphylaxis** exists. Anaphylaxis is a potentially dangerous condition that can result in difficulty breathing and a sharp drop in blood pressure. People with a known history of anaphylaxis should inform the testing clinician. Skin tests should never include a substance known to cause anaphylaxis in the person being tested.

Provocation tests may cause an allergic reaction. Therefore, treatment medications should be available following the tests, to be administered, if needed.

Description

In prick testing, a drop of each allergen to be tested is placed on the skin, usually on the forearm or the back.

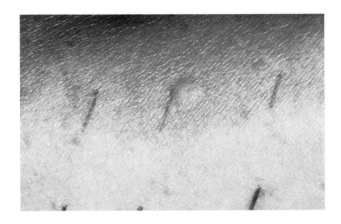

A close-up of a patient's arm after allergy testing. *(Custom Medical Stock Photo. Reproduced by permission.)*

A typical battery of tests may involve two dozen allergen drops, including a drop of saline solution that should not provoke a reaction (negative control) and a drop of histamine that should provoke a reaction (positive control). A small needle is inserted through the drop, and used to prick the skin below. A new needle is used for each prick. The sites are examined over the next 20 minutes for evidence of swelling and redness, indicating a positive reaction. In some instances, a tracing of the set of reactions may be made by placing paper over the tested area. Similarly, in intradermal testing, separate injections are made for each allergen tested. Observations are made over the next 20 minutes.

In RAST testing, a blood sample is taken for use in the laboratory, where the antibody-containing serum is separated from the blood cells. The serum is then exposed to allergens bound to a solid medium. If a person has antibodies to a particular allergen, those antibodies will bind to the solid medium and remain behind after a rinse. Location of allergen-antibody combinations is done by adding antibody-reactive antibodies, so called anti-antibodies, that are chemically linked with a radioactive dye. By locating radioactive spots on the solid medium, the reactive allergens are discovered.

Provocation testing may be performed to identify airborne or food allergens. Inhalation testing is performed only after a patient's lung capacity and response to the medium used to dilute the allergen has been determined. Once this has been determined, the patient inhales increasingly concentrated samples of a particular allergen, followed each time by measurement of the exhalation capacity. Only one allergen is tested per day. Testing for **food allergies** is usually done by removing the suspect food from the diet for two weeks, followed by eating a single portion of the suspect food and follow-up monitoring.

Preparation

Skin testing is preceded by a brief examination of the skin. The patient should refrain from using anti-allergy drugs for at least 48 hours before testing. Prior to inhalation testing, patients with asthma who can tolerate it may be asked to stop any asthma medications. Testing for food **allergies** requires the person to avoid all suspect food for at least two weeks before testing.

Aftercare

Skin testing does not usually require any aftercare. A generalized redness and swelling may occur in the test area, but it will usually resolve within a day or two.

Inhalation tests may cause delayed asthma attacks, even if the antigen administered in the test initially produced no response. Severe initial reactions may justify close professional observation for at least 12 hours after testing.

Risks

Intradermal testing may inadvertently result in the injection of the allergen into the circulation, with an increased risk of adverse reactions. Inhalation tests may provoke an asthma attack. Exposure to new or unsuspected allergens in any test carries the risk of anaphylaxis. Because patients are monitored following allergy testing, an anaphylactic reaction is usually recognized and treated promptly. Occasionally, a delayed anaphylactic response can occur that will require immediate care. Proper patient education regarding how to recognize anaphylaxis is vital.

Normal results

Lack of redness or swelling on a skin test indicates no allergic response. In an inhalation test, the exhalation capacity should remain unchanged. In a food challenge, no symptoms should occur.

Abnormal results

Presence of redness or swelling, especially over 5 mm (1/4 inch) in diameter, indicates an allergic response. This does not mean the substance actually causes the patient's symptoms, however, since he or she may have no regular exposure to the allergen. In fact, the actual allergen may not have been included in the test array.

Following allergen inhalation, reduction in exhalation capacity of more than 20%, and for at least 10-20 minutes, indicates a positive reaction to the allergen.

Gastrointestinal symptoms within 24 hours following the ingestion of a suspected food allergen indicates a positive response.

Resources

PERIODICALS

Hampel, U., et al. "Optical Measurements of Nasal Swellings." *IEEE Transactions on Biomedical Engineering* (September 2004): 1673–1680.

Richard Robinson
Teresa G. Odle

Allogenic transplant *see* **Bone marrow transplantation**

Allopurino *see* **Gout drugs**

Alopecia

Definition

Alopecia simply means hair loss (baldness).

Description

Hair loss occurs for a great many reasons, from conditions that make people literally pull it out to complete hair loss caused by the toxicity of cancer **chemotherapy**. Some causes are considered natural, while others signal serious health problems. Some conditions are confined to the scalp. Others reflect disease throughout the body. Being plainly visible, the skin and its components can provide early signs of disease elsewhere in the body.

Oftentimes, conditions affecting the skin of the scalp will result in hair loss. The first clue to the specific cause is the pattern of hair loss, whether it be complete baldness (alopecia totalis), patchy bald spots, thinning, or hair loss confined to certain areas. Also a factor is the condition of the hair and the scalp beneath it. Sometimes only the hair is affected; sometimes the skin is visibly diseased as well.

Causes and symptoms

- Male pattern baldness (androgenic alopecia) is considered normal in adult males. It is easily recognized by the distribution of hair loss over the top and front of the head and by the healthy condition of the scalp.

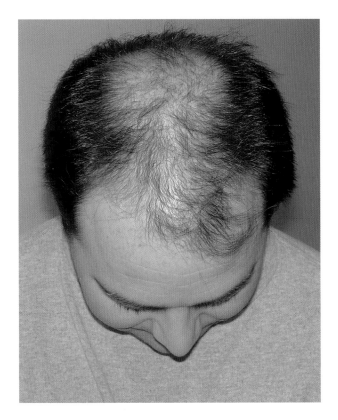

Top of balding male's head. *(Photograph by Kelly A. Quin. Reproduced by permission.)*

- Alopecia areata is a hair loss condition of unknown cause that can be patchy or extend to complete baldness.

- Fungal infections of the scalp usually cause patchy hair loss. The fungus, similar to the ones that cause **athlete's foot** and **ringworm**, often glows under ultraviolet light.

- Trichotillomania is the name of a mental disorder that causes a person to pull out his or her own hair.

- Complete hair loss is a common result of **cancer** chemotherapy, due to the toxicity of the drugs used.

- Systemic diseases often affect hair growth either selectively or by altering the skin of the scalp. One example is thyroid disorders. Hyperthyroidism (too much thyroid hormone) causes hair to become thin and fine. **Hypothyroidism** (too little thyroid hormone) thickens both hair and skin.

- Several autoimmune diseases (when protective cells begin to attack self cells within the body) affect the skin, notably lupus erythememous.

- In 2004, a report a the annual meeting of the American Academy of Dermatology said that alopecia was becoming nearly epidemic among black

women as a result of some hairstyles that pull too tightly on the scalp and harsh chemical treatments that damage the hair shaft and follicles.

Diagnosis

Dermatologists are skilled in diagnosis by sight alone. For more obscure diseases, they may have to resort to a **skin biopsy**, removing a tiny bit of skin using a local anesthetic so that it can be examined under a microscope. Systemic diseases will require a complete evaluation by a physician, including specific tests to identify and characterize the problem.

Treatment

Successful treatment of underlying causes is most likely to restore hair growth, be it the completion of chemotherapy, effective cure of a scalp fungus, or control of a systemic disease. Two relatively new drugs–minoxidil (Rogaine) and **finasteride** (Proscar)–promote hair growth in a significant minority of patients, especially those with male pattern baldness and alopecia areata. While both drugs have so far proved to be quite safe when used for this purpose, **minoxidil** is a liquid that is applied to the scalp and finasteride is the first and only approved treatment in a pill form.

Minoxidil was approved for over-the-counter sales in 1996. When used continuously for long periods of time, minoxidil produces satisfactory results in about one-fourth of patients with androgenic alopecia and as many as half the patients with alopecia areata. There is also an over-the-counter extra-strength version of minoxidil (5% concentration) approved for use by men only. The treatment often results in new hair that is thinner and lighter in color. It is important to note that new hair stops growing soon after the use of minoxidil is discontinued.

Over the past few decades a multitude of hair replacement methods have been performed by physicians and non-physicians. They range from simply weaving someone else's hair in with the remains of one's own to surgically transplanting thousands of hair follicles one at a time.

Hair transplantation is completed by taking tiny plugs of skin, each containing one to several hairs, from the back side of the scalp. The bald sections are then implanted with the plugs. Research completed in 2000 looked at the new technique of hair grafting, and found that micrografts (one or two hairs transplanted per follicle) resulted in fewer complications and the best results.

Another surgical procedure used to treat androgenic alopecia is scalp reduction. By stretching skin, the hairless scalp can be removed and the area of bald skin decreased by closing the space with hair-covered scalp. Hair-bearing skin can also be folded over an area of bald skin with a technique called a flap.

Stem cell research is generating new hope for baldness. Scientists know that a part of the hair follicle called the bulge contains stem cells that can give rise to new hair and help heal skin **wounds**. Early research with mice in 2004 showed promise for identifying the genes that cause baldness and to identify drugs that can reverse the process.

Prognosis

The prognosis varies with the cause. It is generally much easier to lose hair than to regrow it. Even when it returns, it is often thin and less attractive than the original.

Resources

PERIODICALS

Cohen, Philip. "Stem Cells Generate Hair and Hope for the Bald." *New Scientist* (March 20, 2004): 17.

Lohr, Elizabeth. "Alopecia Nearly Epidemic Among Black Women." *Clinical Psychiatry News* (March 2004): 96.

Nielsen, Timothy A., and Martin Reichel. "Alopecia: Diagnosis and Management." *American Family Physician*.

OTHER

Androgenetic Alopecia.com. "How can minoxidil be used to treat baldness?" May1, 2001. < http://androgenetic-alopecia.com/baldnesstreatments/minoxidil/002minoxidilbaldnessusee.shtml > .

Mayo Clinic. "Alopecia" January 26, 2001. [cited May 1, 2001]. < http://www.mayohealth.org > .

WebMD Medical News. "Hair Today, Gone Tomorrow, Hair Again" 2000. [cited May 1, 2001]. < http://my.webmd.com/content/article/1728.53923 > .

Beth A. Kapes
Teresa G. Odle

Alpha-fetoprotein test

Definition

The alpha-fetoprotein (AFP) test is a blood test that is performed during **pregnancy**. This screening test measures the level of AFP in the mother's blood and indicates the probability that the fetus has one of several serious birth defects. The level of AFP can also be determined by analyzing a sample of amniotic fluid. This screening test cannot diagnose a specific condition; it only indicates increased risk for several **birth defects**. Outside pregnancy, the AFP test is used to detect **liver disease**, certain cancerous tumors, and to monitor the progress of cancer treatment.

Purpose

Alpha-fetoprotein is a substance produced by the liver of a fetus. The exact function of this protein is unknown. After birth, the infant's liver stops producing AFP, and an adult liver contains only trace amounts. During pregnancy, the fetus excretes AFP in urine and some of the protein crosses the fetal membranes to enter the mother's blood. The level of AFP can then be determined by analyzing a sample of the mother's blood. By analyzing the amount of AFP found in a blood or amniotic fluid sample, doctors can determine the probability that the fetus is at risk for certain birth defects. It is very important that the doctor know precisely how old the fetus is when the test is performed since the AFP level changes over the length of the pregnancy. Alone, AFP screening cannot diagnose a birth defect. The test is used as an indicator of risk and then an appropriate line of testing (such as **amniocentesis** or ultrasound) follows, based on the results.

Abnormally high AFP may indicate that the fetus has an increased risk of a neural tube defect, the most common and severe type of disorder associated with increased AFP. These types of defects include spinal column defects (**spina bifida**) and anencephaly (a severe and usually fatal brain abnormality). If the tube that becomes the brain

KEY TERMS

Amniotic fluid—Fluid within the uterine sac in which the fetus lives until born.

Fetus—The stage in human development from the second month of pregnancy until birth.

and spinal cord does not close correctly during fetal development, AFP may leak through this abnormal opening and enter the amniotic fluid. This leakage creates abnormally high levels of AFP in amniotic fluid and in maternal blood. If the screening test indicates abnormally high AFP, ultrasound is used to diagnose the problem.

Other fetal conditions that can raise AFP levels above normal include:

- cysts at the end of the spine
- blockage in the esophagus or intestines
- liver disease causing liver cells to die
- defects in the abdominal wall
- kidney or urinary tract defects or disease
- brittle bone disease

Levels may also be high if there is too little fluid in the amniotic sac around the fetus, more than one developing fetus, or a pregnancy that is farther along than estimated.

For unknown reasons, abnormally low AFP may indicate that the fetus has an increased risk of **Down syndrome**. Down syndrome is a condition that includes mental retardation and a distinctive physical appearance linked to an abnormality of chromosome 21 (called trisomy 21). If the screening test indicates an abnormally low AFP, amniocentesis is used to diagnose the problem. Abnormally low levels of AFP can also occur when the fetus has died or when the mother is overweight.

AFP is often part of a "triple check" blood test that analyzes three substances as risk indicators of possible birth defects: AFP, estriol, and human chorionic gonadotropin (HCG). When all three substances are measured in the mother's blood, the accuracy of the test results increases.

In 2004, a new study showed that the risk of an infant's **death** from **sudden infant death syndrome** (SIDS) increased if levels of AFP were higher during the second trimester of the mother's pregnancy.

Although AFP in human blood gradually disappears after birth, it never disappears entirely. It may reappear in liver disease, or tumors of the liver, ovaries, or testicles. The AFP test is used to screen people at high risk for these conditions. After a cancerous tumor is removed, an AFP test can monitor the progress of treatment. Continued high AFP levels suggest the **cancer** is growing.

Precautions

It is very important that the doctor know precisely how old the fetus is when the test is performed since the AFP level considered normal changes over the length of the pregnancy. Errors in determining the age of the fetus lead to errors when interpreting the test results. Since an AFP test is only a screening tool, more specific tests must follow to make an accurate diagnosis. An abnormal test result does not necessarily mean that the fetus has a birth defect. The test has a high rate of abnormal results (either high or low) to prevent missing a fetus that has a serious condition.

Description

The AFP test is usually performed at week 16 of pregnancy. Blood is drawn from the patient's (mother's) vein, usually on the inside of the elbow. AFP can also be measured in the sample of amniotic fluid taken at the time of amniocentesis. Test results are usually available after about one week.

Preparation

There is no specific physical preparation for the AFP test.

Aftercare

There is no specific aftercare involved with this screening test.

Risks

The risks associated with drawing blood are minimal, but may include bleeding from the puncture site, feeling faint or lightheaded after the blood is drawn, or blood accumulating under the puncture site (hematoma).

Normal results

Alpha-fetoprotein is measured in nanograms per milliliter (ng/mL) and is expressed as a probability. The probability (1:100, for example) translates into the chance that the fetus has a defect (a one in 100 chance, for example).

When testing for cancer or liver diseases, AFP results are reported as nanograms per milliliter. An AFP level less than or equal to 50 ng/mL is considered normal.

Abnormal results

The doctor will inform the woman of her specific increased risk as compared to the "normal" risk of a standard case. If the risk of Down syndrome is greater than the standard risk for women who are 35 years old or older (one in 270), amniocentesis is recommended. Again, the test has a high rate of showing an abnormal AFP level in order to prevent missing a fetus that has Down's syndrome. This screening test only predicts risk; appropriate diagnostic testing will follow after an abnormal screening result.

In tumor or liver disease testing, an AFP level greater than 50 ng/mL is considered abnormal.

Resources

PERIODICALS

Smith, Gordon C.S., et al. "Second-trimester Maternal Serum Levels of Alpha-fetoprotein and the Subsequent Risk of Sudden Infant Death Syndrome." *New England Journal of Medicine* (September 2, 2004): 978.

ORGANIZATIONS

March of Dimes Birth Defects Foundation. 1275 Mamaroneck Ave., White Plains, NY 10605. (914) 428-7100. resourcecenter@modimes.org. <http://www.modimes.org>.

National Cancer Institute. Building 31, Room 10A31, 31 Center Drive, MSC 2580, Bethesda, MD 20892-2580. (800) 422-6237. <http://www.nci.nih.gov>.

Adrienne Massel, RN
Teresa G. Odle

Alpha-thalassemia *see* **Thalassemia**

Alpha₁-adrenergic blockers

Definition

Alpha₁-adrenergic blockers are drugs that work by blocking the alpha₁-receptors of vascular smooth muscle, thus preventing the uptake of catecholamines by the smooth muscle cells. This causes vasodilation and allows blood to flow more easily.

Purpose

These drugs, called alpha blockers for short, are used for two main purposes: to treat high blood pressure (**hypertension**) and to treat benign prostatic hyperplasia (BPH), a condition that affects men and is characterized by an **enlarged prostate** gland.

High blood pressure

High blood pressure puts a strain on the heart and the arteries. Over time, hypertension can damage the blood vessels to the point of causing **stroke**, **heart failure** or kidney failure. People with high blood pressure may also be at higher risk for heart attacks. Controlling high blood pressure makes these problems less likely. Alpha blockers help lower blood pressure by causing vasodilation, meaning an increase in the diameter of the blood vessels, which allows blood to flow more easily.

Benign prostatic hyperplasia (BPH)

This condition particularly affects older men. Over time, the prostate, a donut-shaped gland below the bladder, enlarges. When this happens, it may interfere with the passage of urine from the bladder out of the body. Men who are diagnosed with BPH may have to urinate more often. Or they may feel that they can not completely empty their bladders. Alpha blockers inhibit the contraction of prostatic smooth muscle and thus relax muscles in the prostate and the bladder, allowing urine to flow more freely.

Description

Commonly prescribed alpha blockers for hypertension and BPH include doxazosin (Cardura, prazosin (Minipress) and terazosin (Hytrin). Prazosin is also used in the treatment of heart failure. All are available only with a physician's prescription and are sold in tablet form.

Recommended dosage

The recommended dose depends on the patient and the type of alpha blocker and may change over the course of treatment. The prescribing physician will gradually increase the dosage, if necessary. Some patients may need as much as 15-20 mg per day of terazosin, 16 mg per day of doxazosin, or as much as 40 mg per day of prazosin, but most people benefit from lower doses. As the dosage increases, so does the possibility of unwanted side effects.

KEY TERMS

Adrenergic—Refers to neurons (nerve cells) that use catecholamines as neurotransmitters at a synapse.

Adrenergic receptor—There are three families of adrenergic receptors, alpha₁, alpha₂ and beta, and each family contains three distinct subtypes. Each of the nine subtypes are coded by separate genes, and display specific drug specificities and regulatory properties.

Alpha blockers—Medications that bind alpha adrenergic receptors and decrease the workload of the heart and lower blood pressure. They are commonly used to treat hypertension, peripheral vascular disease, and hyperplasia.

Arteries—Blood vessels that carry oxygenated blood away from the heart to the cells, tissues, and organs of the body.

Catecholamines—Family of neurotransmitters containing dopamine, norepinephrine and epinephrine, produced and secreted by cells of the adrenal medulla in the brain. Catecholamines have excitatory effects on smooth muscle cells of the vessels that supply blood to the skin and mucous membranes and have inhibitory effects on smooth muscle cells located in the wall of the gut, the bronchial tree of the lungs, and the vessels that supply blood to skeletal

muscle. There are two different main types of receptors for these neurotransmitters, called alpha and beta adrenergic receptors. The catecholamines are therefore are also known as adrenergic neurotransmitters.

Hyperplasia—The abnormal increase in the number of normal cells in a given tissue.

Hypertension—Persistently high arterial blood pressure.

Neurotransmitter—Substance released from neurons of the peripheral nervous system that travels across the synaptic clefts (gaps) of other neurons to excite or inhibit the target cell.

Palpitation—Rapid, forceful, throbbing, or fluttering heartbeat.

Receptor—A molecular structure in a cell or on the surface of a cell that allows binding of a specific substance that causes a specific physiologic response.

Synapse—A connection between nerve cells, by which nervous excitation is transferred from one cell to the other.

Vasodilation—The increase in the internal diameter of a blood vessel that results from relaxation of smooth muscle within the wall of the vessel thus causing an increase in blood flow.

Alpha blockers should be taken exactly as directed, even if the medication does not seem to be working at first. It should not be stopped even if symptoms improve because it needs to be taken regularly to be effective. Patients should avoid missing any doses, and should not take larger or more frequent doses to make up for missed doses.

Precautions

Alpha blockers may lower blood pressure to a greater extent than desired. This can cause dizziness, lightheadedness, heart **palpitations**, and **fainting**. Activities such as driving, using machines, or doing anything else that might be dangerous for 24 hours after taking the first dose should be avoided. Patients should be reminded to be especially careful not to fall when getting up in the middle of the night. The same precautions are recommended if the dosage is increased or if the drug has been stopped and then started again. Anyone whose safety on the job could be affected by taking alpha blockers should

inform his or her physician, so that the physician can take this factor into account when increasing dosage.

Some people may feel drowsy or less alert when using these drugs. They should accordingly avoid driving or performing activities that require full attention.

People diagnosed with **kidney disease** or **liver disease** may also be more sensitive to alpha blockers. They should inform their physicians about these conditions if alpha blockers are prescribed. Older people may also be more sensitive and may be more likely to have unwanted side effects, such as fainting, dizziness, and lightheadedness.

It should be noted that alpha blockers do not cure high blood pressure. They simply help to keep the condition under control. Similarly, these drugs will not shrink an enlarged prostate gland. Although they will help relieve the symptoms of prostate enlargement, the prostate may continue to grow, and it eventually may be necessary to have prostate surgery.

Alpha blockers may lower blood counts. Patients may need to have their blood checked regularly while taking this medicine.

Anyone who has had unusual reactions to alpha blockers in the past should let his or her physician know before taking the drugs again. The physician should also be told about any allergies to foods, dyes, preservatives, or other substances.

The effects of taking alpha blockers during **pregnancy** are not fully understood. Women who are pregnant or planning to become pregnant should inform their physicians. Breastfeeding mothers who need to take alpha blockers should also talk to their physicians. These drugs can pass into breast milk and may affect nursing babies. It may be necessary to stop breastfeeding while being treated with alpha blockers.

Side effects

The most common side effects are dizziness, drowsiness, tiredness, **headache**, nervousness, irritability, stuffy or runny nose, **nausea**, **pain** in the arms and legs, and weakness. These problems usually go away as the body adjusts to the drug and do not require medical treatment. If they do not subside or if they interfere with normal activities, the physician should be informed.

If any of the following side effects occur, the prescribing physician should be notified as soon as possible:

- fainting
- shortness of breath or difficulty breathing
- fast, pounding, or irregular heartbeat
- swollen feet, ankles, wrists

Other side effects may occur. Anyone who has unusual symptoms after taking alpha blockers should contact his or her physician.

Interactions

Doxazosin (Cardura) is not known to interact with any other drugs. Terazosin (Hytrin) may interact with **nonsteroidal anti-inflammatory drugs**, such as ibuprofen (Motrin), and with other blood pressure drugs, such as enalapril (Vasotec), and verapamil (Calan,Verelan). Prazosin (Minipress) may interact with beta adrenergic blocking agents such as propranolol (Inderal) and others, and with verapamil (Calan, Isoptin.) When drugs interact, the effects of one or both of the drugs may change or the risk of side effects may be greater.

Nancy Ross-Flanigan

Alport syndrome

Definition

A hereditary disease of the kidneys that primarily affects men, causing blood in the urine, hearing loss and eye problems. Eventually, **kidney dialysis** or transplant may be necessary.

Description

Alport syndrome affects about one in 5,000 Americans, striking men more often and severely than women. There are several varieties of the syndrome, some occurring in childhood and others not causing symptoms until men reach their 20s or 30s. All varieties of the syndrome are characterized by **kidney disease** that usually progresses to chronic kidney failure and by uremia (the presence of excessive amounts of urea and other waste products in the blood).

Causes and symptoms

Alport syndrome in most cases is caused by a defect in one or more genes located on the X chromosome. It is usually inherited from the mother, who is a normal carrier. However, in up to 20% of cases there is no family history of the disorder. In these cases, there appears to be a spontaneous genetic mutation causing Alport syndrome.

Blood in the urine (hematuria) is a hallmark of Alport syndrome. Other symptoms that may appear in varying combinations include:

- protein in the urine (proteinuria)
- sensorineural **hearing loss**
- eye problems [involuntary, rhythmic eye movements (**nystagmus**), **cataracts**, or cornea problems]
- skin problems
- platelet disorders
- abnormal white blood cells
- smooth muscle tumors

Not all patients with Alport syndrome have hearing problems. In general, those with normal hearing have less severe cases of Alport syndrome.

Diagnosis

Alport syndrome is diagnosed with a medical evaluation and family history, together with a kidney biopsy that can detect changes in the kidney typical of

KEY TERMS

Albumin—A protein that is important in maintaining blood volume. Low albumin levels is one sign of Alport syndrome.

Dialysis—A technique of removing waste material from the blood. It is used with patients whose kidneys have stopped functioning and can no longer cleanse the blood on their own.

Diuretic—A drug that increases the amount of urine a person produces.

Hematuria—Blood in the urine, Hematuria is a hallmark of Alport syndrome.

Pulmonary edema—Excess fluid in the air spaces of the lungs.

Uremia—The presence of excessive amounts of urea and other waste products in the blood.

the condition. **Urinalysis** may reveal blood or protein in the urine. Blood tests can reveal a low platelet level.

In addition, tests for the Alport gene are now available. Although testing is fairly expensive, it is covered by many types of health insurance. DNA tests can diagnose affected children even before birth, and genetic linkage tests tracing all family members at risk for Alport syndrome are also available.

Treatment

There is no specific treatment that can "cure" Alport syndrome. Instead, care is aimed at easing the problems related to kidney failure, such as the presence of too many waste products in the blood (uremia).

To control kidney inflammation (**nephritis**), patients should:

- restrict fluids
- control high blood pressure
- manage **pulmonary edema**
- control high blood levels of potassium

Rarely patients with Alport syndrome may develop nephrotic syndrome, a group of symptoms including too much protein in the urine, low albumin levels, and swelling. To ease these symptoms, patients should:

- drink less
- eat a salt-free diet
- use **diuretics**
- have albumin transfusions

The treatment for **chronic kidney failure** is dialysis or a kidney transplant.

Prognosis

Women with this condition can lead a normal life, although they may have slight hearing loss. An affected woman may notice blood in her urine only when under **stress** or pregnant.

Men generally have a much more serious problem with the disease. Most will experience kidney disease in their 20s or 30s, which may eventually require dialysis or transplantation, and many develop significant hearing loss. Men with Alport syndrome often die of complications by middle age.

Prevention

Alport syndrome is a genetic disease and prevention efforts are aimed at providing affected individuals and their families with information concerning the genetic mechanisms responsible for the disease. Since it is possible to determine if a woman is a carrier, or if an unborn child has the condition, **genetic counseling** can provide helpful information and support for the decisions that affected individuals and their families may have to make.

Resources

ORGANIZATIONS

American Association of Kidney Patients. 100 S. Ashley Dr., #280, Tampa, FL 33602. (800) 749-2257. < http://www.aakp.org > .

American Kidney Fund (AKF). Suite 1010, 6110 Executive Boulevard, Rockville, MD 20852. (800) 638-8299. < http://216.248.130.102/Default.htm > .

National Kidney and Urologic Disease Information Clearinghouse. 3 Information Way, Bethesda, MD 20892. (301) 654-4415. < http://www.niddk.nih.gov > .

National Kidney Foundation. 30 East 33rd St., New York, NY 10016. (800) 622-9010. < http://www.kidney.org > .

National Organization for Rare Diseases. P.O. Box 8923, Fairfield, CT 06812. (213) 745-6518. < http://www.w2.com > .

OTHER

Alport Syndrome Home Page. < http://www.cc.utah.edu/~cla6202/ASHP.htm > .

"Alport Syndrome." Pediatric Database Home Page. < http://www.icondata.com/health/pedbase/files/ALPORTSY.HTM > .

The Hereditary Nephritis Foundation (HNF) Home Page. < http://www.cc.utah.edu/~cla6202/HNF.htm > .

Carol A. Turkington

Alprazolam *see* **Benzodiazepines**

ALS *see* **Amyotrophic lateral sclerosis**

Alteplase *see* **Thrombolytic therapy**

Altitude sickness

Definition

Altitude sickness is a general term encompassing a spectrum of disorders that occur at higher altitudes. Since the severity of symptoms varies with altitude, it is important to understand the range of the different altitudes that may be involved. High altitude is defined as height greater than 8,000 feet (2,438m); medium altitude is defined as height between 5,000 and 8,000 feet (1,524-2,438m); and extreme altitude is defined as height greater than 19,000 feet (5,791 m). The majority of healthy individuals suffer from altitude sickness when they reach very high altitudes. In addition, about 20% of people ascending above 9,000 feet (2,743m) in one day will develop altitude sickness. Children under six years and women in the premenstrual part of their cycles may be more vulnerable. Individuals with preexisting medical conditions–even a minor respiratory infection– may become sick at more moderate altitudes.

Description

There are three major clinical syndromes that fall under the heading of altitude sickness: acute mountain sickness (AMS), high-altitude pulmonary edema (HAPE), and high-altitude cerebral **edema** (HACE). These syndromes are not separate, individual syndromes as much as they are a continuum of severity, all resulting from a decrease in oxygen in the air. AMS is the mildest, and the other two represent severe, life-threatening forms of altitude sickness.

Altitude sickness occurs because the partial pressure of oxygen decreases with altitude. (Partial pressure is a term applied to gases that is similar to the way the term concentration is applied to liquid solutions.) For instance, at 18,000 feet (5,486 m) the partial pressure of oxygen drops to one-half its value at sea level and, therefore, there is a substantially lower amount of oxygen available for the individual to inhale. This is known as hypoxia. Furthermore, since there is less oxygen to inhale, less oxygen reaches the blood. This is known as hypoxemia. These two conditions are the major factors that form the basis for all the medical problems associated with altitude sickness.

> ### KEY TERMS
>
> **Cerebral**—Pertaining to the brain.
>
> **Edema**—Accumulation of excess fluid in the tissues of the body.
>
> **Hypoxemia**—Insufficient oxygenation of the blood.
>
> **Hypoxia**—A deficiency in the amount of oxygen required for effective ventilation.
>
> **Pulmonary**—Pertaining to the lungs.

As a person becomes hypoxemic, his natural response is to breathe more rapidly (hyperventilate). This is the body's attempt to bring in more oxygen at a rapid rate. This attempt at alleviating the effects of the hypoxia at higher altitudes is known as acclimatization, and it occurs during the first few days. Acclimatization is a response that occurs in individuals who travel from lower to higher altitudes. There are groups of people who have lived at high altitudes (for example, in the Himalayan and Andes mountains) for generations, and they are simply accustomed to living at such altitudes, perhaps through a genetic ability.

Causes and symptoms

Acute mountain sickness (AMS) is a mild form of altitude sickness that results from ascent to altitudes higher greater than 8,000 feet (2,438m)–even 6,500 feet (1,981 m) in some susceptible individuals. Although hypoxia is associated with the development of AMS, the exact mechanism by which this condition develops has yet to be confirmed. It is important to realize that some individuals acclimatize to higher altitudes more efficiently than others. As a result, under similar conditions some will suffer from AMS while others will not. At present, the susceptibility of otherwise healthy individuals to contracting AMS cannot be accurately predicted. Of those who do suffer from AMS, the condition tends to be most severe on the second or third day after reaching the high altitude, and it usually abates after three to five days if they remain at the same altitude. However, it can recur if the individuals travel to an even higher altitude. Symptoms usually appear a few hours to a few days following ascent, and they include **dizziness, headache, shortness of breath, nausea, vomiting**, loss of appetite, and **insomnia**.

High-altitude **pulmonary edema** (HAPE) is a life-threatening condition that afflicts a small percentage of those who suffer from AMS. In this condition, fluid leaks from within the pulmonary blood vessels into the lung tissue. As this fluid begins to accumulate within the lung tissue (pulmonary edema), the individual begins to become more and more short of breath. HAPE is known to afflict all types of individuals, regardless of their level of physical fitness.

Typically, the individual who suffers from HAPE ascends quickly to a high altitude and almost immediately develops shortness of breath, a rapid heart rate, a **cough** productive of a large amount of sometimes bloody sputum, and a rapid rate of breathing. If no medical assistance is provided by this point, the patient goes into a coma and dies within a few hours.

High-altitude cerebral edema (HACE), the rarest and most severe form of altitude sickness, involves cerebral edema, and its mechanism of development is also poorly understood. The symptoms often begin with those of AMS, but neurologic symptoms such as an altered level of consciousness, speech abnormalities, severe headache, loss of coordination, **hallucinations**, and even seizures. If no intervention is implemented, death is the result.

Diagnosis

The diagnosis for altitude sickness may be made from the observation of the individual's symptoms during travel to higher altitudes.

Treatment

Mild AMS requires no treatment other than an **aspirin** or ibuprofen for headache, and avoidance of further ascent. **Narcotics** should be avoided because they may blunt the respiratory response, making it even more difficult for the person to breathe deeply and rapidly enough to compensate for the lower levels of oxygen in the environment. Oxygen may also be used to alleviate symptoms of mild AMS.

As for HAPE and HACE, the most important course of action is descent to a lower altitude as soon as possible. Even a 1,000-2,000-foot (305-610 m) descent can dramatically improve one's symptoms. If descent is not possible, **oxygen therapy** should be started. In addition, dexamethasone (a steroid) has been suggested in order to reduce cerebral edema.

Prognosis

The prognosis for mild AMS is good, if appropriate measures are taken. As for HAPE and HACE, the prognosis depends upon the rapidity and distance of descent and the availability of medical intervention. Descent often leads to improvement of symptoms, however, recovery times vary among individuals.

Prevention

When individuals ascend from sea level, it is recommended that they spend at least one night at an intermediate altitude prior to ascending to higher elevations. In general, climbers should take at least two days to go from sea level to 8,000 feet (2,438m). After reaching that point, healthy climbers should generally allow one day for each additional 2,000 feet (610m), and one day of rest should be taken every two or three days. Should mild symptoms begin to surface, further ascent should be avoided. If the symptoms are severe, the individual should return to a lower altitude. Some reports indicate that acetazolamide (a diuretic) may be taken before ascent as a preventative measure for AMS.

Paying attention to diet can also help prevent altitude sickness. Water loss is a problem at higher altitudes, so climbers should drink ample water (enough to produce copious amounts of relatively light-colored or clear urine). Alcohol and large amounts of salt should be avoided. Eating frequent small, high-carbohydrate snacks (for example, fruits, jams and starchy foods) can help, especially in the first few days of climbing.

Resources

BOOKS

Crystal, R. G., et al., editors. *The Lung: Scientific Foundations*. Lippincott-Raven Publishers, 1997.

Kapil Gupta, MD

Aluminum hydroxide *see* **Antacids**

Alzheimer's disease

Definition

Alzheimer's disease (AD) is the most common form of **dementia**, a neurologic disease characterized by loss of mental ability severe enough to interfere with normal activities of daily living, lasting at least six months, and not present from birth. AD usually occurs in old age, and is marked by a decline in cognitive functions such as remembering, reasoning, and planning.

Description

A person with AD usually has a gradual decline in mental functions, often beginning with slight memory loss, followed by losses in the ability to maintain employment, to plan and execute familiar tasks, and to reason and **exercise** judgment. Communication ability,

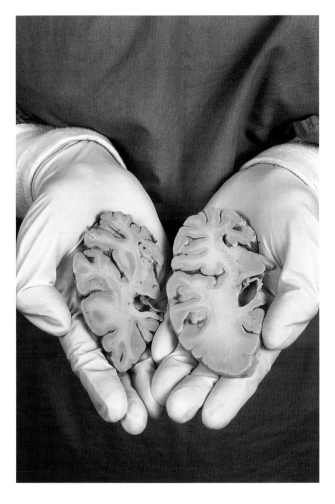

A brain segment affected by Alzheimer's disease on the right compared with a healthy brain segment (left). The diseased brain appears shrunken, and the fissures are noticeably larger. *(Simon Fraser/MRC Unit, Newcastle General Hospital/ Science Photo Library. Photo Researchers, Inc. Reproduced by permission.)*

mood, and personality also may be affected. Most people who have AD die within eight years of their diagnosis, although the interval may be as short as one year or as long as 20 years. AD is the fourth leading cause of **death** in adults after heart disease, **cancer**, and **stroke**.

Between two and four million Americans have AD; that number is expected to grow to as many as 14 million by the middle of the 21st century as the population ages. While a small number of people in their 40s and 50s develop the disease (called early-onset AD), AD predominantly affects the elderly. AD affects about 3% of all people between ages 65 and 74, about 19% of those between 75 and 84, and about 47% of those over 85. Slightly more women than men are affected with AD, but this may be

because women tend to live longer, leaving a higher proportion of women in the most affected age groups.

The cost of caring for a person with AD is considerable. The annual cost of caring for one AD patient in 1998 was estimated as about $18,400 for a patient with mild AD, $30,100 for a patient with moderate AD, and $36,100 for a patient with severe AD. The annual direct and indirect costs of caring for AD patients in the United States was estimated to be as much as $100 billion. Slightly more than half of people with AD are cared for at home, while the remainder are cared for in a variety of health care institutions.

Causes and symptoms

Causes

The cause or causes of Alzheimer's disease are largely unknown, though some forms have genetic links. Some strong leads have been found through recent research, however, and these have given some theoretical support to several new experimental treatments.

At first AD destroys neurons (nerve cells) in parts of the brain that control memory, including the hippocampus, which is a structure deep in the deep that controls short-term memory. As these neurons in the hippocampus stop functioning, the person's short-term memory fails, and the ability to perform familiar tasks decreases. Later AD affects the cerebral cortex, particularly the areas responsible for language and reasoning. Many language skills are lost and the ability to make judgments is affected. Personality changes occur, which may include emotional outbursts, wandering, and agitation. The severity of these changes increases with disease progression. Eventually many other areas of the brain become involved, the brain regions affected atrophy (shrink and lose function), and the person with AD becomes bedridden, incontinent, helpless, and non-responsive.

Autopsy of a person with AD shows that the regions of the brain affected by the disease become clogged with two abnormal structures, called neurofibrillary tangles and amyloid plaques. Neurofibrillary tangles are twisted masses of protein fibers inside nerve cells, or neurons. In AD, tau proteins, which normally help bind and stabilize parts of neurons, are changed chemically, become twisted and tangled, and no longer can stabilize the neurons. Amyloid plaques consist of insoluble deposits of beta-amyloid, (a protein fragment from a larger protein called amyloid precursor protein (APP), mixed with parts of neurons and non-nerve cells. Plaques are found in the spaces between the nerve cells of the brain. While it is not clear exactly

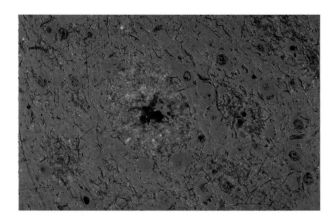

Diseased tissue from the brain of an Alzheimer's patient showing senile plaques within the brain's gray matter. *(Photograph by Cecil Fox, Photo Researchers, Inc. Reproduced by permission.)*

KEY TERMS

Acetylcholine—One of the substances in the body that helps transmit nerve impulses.

Dementia—Impaired intellectual function that interferes with normal social and work activities.

Ginkgo—An herb from the *Ginkgo biloba* tree that some alternative practitioners recommend for the prevention and treatment of AD.

Neurofibrillary tangle—Twisted masses of protein inside nerve cells that develop in the brains of people with AD.

Senile plaque—Structures composed of parts of neurons surrounding brain proteins called beta-amyloid deposits found in the brains of people with AD.

how these structures cause problems, many researchers believe that their formation is responsible for the mental changes of AD, presumably by interfering with the normal communication between neurons in the brain and later leading to the death of neurons. By 2000, three drugs for the treatment of AD symptoms were approved by the U.S. Food and Drug Administration (FDA). They act by increasing the level of chemical signaling molecules in the brain, known as neurotransmitters, to make up for this decreased communication ability. All act by inhibiting the activity of acetylcholinesterase, which is an enzyme that breaks down acetylcholine, an important neurotransmitter released by neurons that is necessary for cognitive function. These drugs modestly increase cognition and improve one's ability to perform normal activities of daily living.

Exactly what triggers the formation of plaques and tangles and the development of AD is unknown. AD likely results from many interrelated factors, including genetic, environmental, and others not yet identified. Two types of AD exist: familial AD (FAD), which is a rare autosomal dominant inherited disease, and sporadic AD, with no obvious inheritance pattern. AD also is described in terms of age at onset, with early onset AD occurring in people younger than 65, and late-onset occurring in those 65 and older. Early onset AD comprises about 5-10 % of AD cases and affects people aged 30 to 60. Some cases of early onset AD are inherited and are common in some families. Early-onset AD often progresses faster than the more common late-onset type.

All cases of FAD, which is relatively uncommon, that have been identified to date are the early onset type. As many as 50% of FAD cases are known to be caused by three genes located on three different chromosomes. Some families have mutations in the APP gene located on chromosome 21, which causes the production of abnormal APP protein. Others have mutations in a gene called presenilin 1 located on chromosome 14, which causes the production of abnormal presenilin 1 protein, and others have mutations in a similar gene called presenilin 2 located on chromosome 1, which causes production of abnormal presenilin 2. Presenilin 1 may be one of the enzymes that clips APP into beta-amyloid; it also may be important in the synaptic connections between brain cells.

There is no evidence that the mutated genes that cause early onset FAD also cause late onset AD, but genetics appears to play a role in this more common form of AD. Discovered by researchers at Duke University in the early 1990s, potentially the most important genetic link to AD was on chromosome 19. A gene on this chromosome, called APOE (apolipoprotein E), codes for a protein involved in transporting lipids into neurons. APOE occurs in at least three forms (alleles), called APOE e2, APOE e3, and APOE e4. Each person inherits one APOE from each parent, and therefore can either have one copy of two different forms, or two copies of one. The relatively rare APOE e2 appears to protect some people from AD, as it seems to be associated with a lower risk of AD and a later age of onset if AD develops. APOE e3 is the most common version found in the general population, and only appears to have a neutral role in AD. However, APOE e4 appears to increase the risk of developing late onset AD with the inheritance of one or two copies of APOE e4. Compared to those without APOE e4, people with one copy are about three times as likely to develop late-onset AD, and those with two copies are almost four times as likely to do so. Having APOE e4 also can lower the age of onset by as much as 17 years. However, APOE e4 only increases the risk of developing AD and does not cause it, as not everyone with APOE e4 develops AD, and people without it can still have the disease. Why APOE e4 increases the chances of developing AD is not known with certainty. However, one theory is that APOE e4 facilitates beta-amyloid buildup in plaques, thus contributing to the lowering of the age of onset of AD; other theories involve interactions with cholesterol levels and effects on nerve cell death independent of its effects on plaque buildup. In 2000, four new AD-related regions in the human genome were identified, where one out of several hundred genes in each of these regions may be a risk factor gene for AD. These genes, which are not yet identified, appear to make a contribution to the risk of developing late-onset AD that is at least as important as APOE e4.

Other non-genetic factors have been studied in relation to the causes of AD. Inflammation of the brain may play a role in development of AD, and use of **nonsteroidal anti-inflammatory drugs** (NSAIDs) were once thought to reduce the risk of developing AD. Other agents once thought to reduce chances of dementia are now thought to increase its risk. In 2002, **hormone replacement therapy** (HRT), which combines estrogen and progestogen, was found to double the risk of developing dementia in postmenopausal women. Highly reactive molecular fragments called free radicals damage cells of all kinds, especially brain cells, which have smaller supplies of protective antioxidants thought to protect against free radical damage. Vitamin E is one such antioxidant, and its use in AD may be of possible theoretical benefit.

While the ultimate cause or causes of Alzheimer's disease still are unknown, there are several risk factors that increase a person's likelihood of developing the disease. The most significant one is, of course, age; older people develop AD at much higher rates than younger ones. There is some evidence that strokes and AD may be linked, with small strokes that go undetected clinically contributing to the injury of neurons. A 2003 Dutch study reported that symptomless, unnoticed strokes could double the risk of AD and other dementias. Blood cholesterol levels also may be important. Scientists have shown that high blood cholesterol levels in special breeds of genetically engineered (transgenic) mice may increase the rate of plaque deposition. There are also parallels between AD and other progressive neurodegenerative disorders that cause dementia, including prion diseases, Parkinson's disease, and Huntington's disease.

Numerous epidemiological studies of populations also are being conducted to learn more about whether and to what extent early life events, socioeconomic factors, and ethnicity have an impact on the development of AD. For example, a 2003 report showed that the more formal education a person has, the better his or her memory is, despite presence of AD. Other studies have related education level or participation in leisure activities such as playing cards or doing crossword puzzles to delayed onset of AD.

Many environmental factors have been suspected of contributing to AD, but epidemiological population studies have not borne out these links. Among these have been pollutants in drinking water, aluminum from commercial products, and metal dental fillings. To date, none of these factors has been shown to cause AD or increase its likelihood. Further research may yet turn up links to other environmental factors.

Symptoms

The symptoms of Alzheimer's disease begin gradually, usually with memory lapses. Occasional memory lapses are of course common to everyone, and do not by themselves signify any change in cognitive function. The person with AD may begin with only the routine sort of memory lapse — forgetting where the car keys are — but progress to more profound or disturbing losses, such as forgetting that he or she can even drive a car. Becoming lost or disoriented on a walk around the neighborhood becomes more likely as the disease progresses. A person with AD may forget the names of family members, or forget what was said at the beginning of a sentence by the time he hears the end.

As AD progresses, other symptoms appear, including inability to perform routine tasks, loss of judgment, and personality or behavior changes. Some people with AD have trouble sleeping and may suffer from confusion or agitation in the evening ("sunsetting" or Sundowner's Syndrome). In some cases, people with AD repeat the same ideas, movements, words, or thoughts. In the final stages people may have severe problems with eating, communicating, and controlling their bladder and bowel functions.

The Alzheimer's Association has developed a list of 10 warning signs of AD. A person with several of these symptoms should see a physician for a thorough evaluation:

- memory loss that affects job skills
- difficulty performing familiar tasks
- problems with language
- disorientation of time and place

- poor or decreased judgment
- problems with abstract thinking
- misplacing things
- changes in mood or behavior
- changes in personality
- loss of initiative

Other types of dementia, including some that are reversible, can cause similar symptoms. It is important for the person with these symptoms to be evaluated by a professional who can weigh the possibility that his or her symptoms may have another cause. Approximately 20% of those originally suspected of having AD turn out to have some other disorder; about half of these cases are treatable.

Diagnosis

Diagnosis of Alzheimer's disease is complex, and may require office visits to several different specialists over several months before a diagnosis can be made. While a confident provisional diagnosis may be made in most cases after thorough testing, AD cannot be diagnosed definitively until autopsy examination of the brain for plaques and neurofibrillary tangles.

The diagnosis of AD begins with a thorough physical exam and complete medical history. Except in the disease's earliest stages, accurate history from family members or caregivers is essential. Since there are both prescription and over-the-counter drugs that can cause the same mental changes as AD, a careful review of the patient's drug, medicine, and alcohol use is important. AD-like symptoms also can be provoked by other medical conditions, including tumors, infection, and dementia caused by mild strokes (multi-infarct dementia). These possibilities must be ruled out as well through appropriate blood and urine tests, brain magnetic resonance imaging (MRI), positron emission tomography (**PET**) or single photon emission computed tomography (SPECT) scans, tests of the brain's electrical activity (electroencephalographs or EEGs), or other tests. Several types of oral and written tests are used to aid in the AD diagnosis and to follow its progression, including tests of mental status, functional abilities, memory, and concentration. Still, the **neurologic exam** is normal in most patients in early stages.

One of the most important parts of the diagnostic process is to evaluate the patient for depression and **delirium**, since each of these can be present with AD, or may be mistaken for it. (Delirium involves a decreased consciousness or awareness of one's environment.)

Depression and memory loss both are common in the elderly, and the combination of the often can be mistaken for AD. On the other hand, depression can be a risk factor for AD. A 2003 study showed that a history of depressive symptoms can be associated with nearly twice the risk of eventually developing AD. Depression can be treated with drugs, although some antidepressants can worsen dementia if it is present, further complicating both diagnosis and treatment.

An early and accurate diagnosis of AD is important in developing strategies for managing symptoms and for helping patients and their families planning for the future and pursuing care options while the patient can still take part in the decision-making process.

A genetic test for the APOE e4 gene is available, but is not used for diagnosis, since possessing even two copies does not ensure that a person will develop AD. In addition, access to genetic information could affect the insurability of a patient if disclosed, and also affect employment status and legal rights.

Treatment

Alzheimer's disease is presently incurable. Recent reports show that prompt intervention can slow decline from AD. The use of medications mentioned below as early as possible in the course of AD can help people with the disease maintain independent function as long as possible. The remaining treatment for a person with AD is good nursing care, providing both physical and emotional support for a person who is gradually able to do less and less for himself, and whose behavior is becoming more and more erratic. Modifications of the home to increase safety and security often are necessary. The caregiver also needs support to prevent anger, despair, and burnout from becoming overwhelming. Becoming familiar with the issues likely to lie ahead, and considering the appropriate financial and legal issues early on, can help both the patient and family cope with the difficult process of the disease. Regular medical care by a practitioner with a non-defeatist attitude toward AD is important so that illnesses such as urinary or respiratory infections can be diagnosed and treated properly, rather than being incorrectly attributed to the inevitable decline seen in AD.

People with AD often are depressed or anxious, and may suffer from sleeplessness, poor **nutrition**, and general poor health. Each of these conditions is treatable to some degree. It is important for the person with AD to eat well and continue to exercise. Professional advice from a nutritionist may be useful to provide healthy, easy-to-prepare meals. Finger foods may be preferable to those requiring utensils to be eaten. Regular exercise (supervised if necessary for safety) promotes overall health. A calm, structured environment with simple orientation aids (such as calendars and clocks) may reduce **anxiety** and increase safety. Other psychiatric symptoms, such as depression, anxiety, **hallucinations** (seeing or hearing things that aren't there), and **delusions** (false beliefs) may be treated with drugs if necessary.

Drugs

As of 2003, four drugs—tacrine (Cognex), donepezil hydrochloride (Aricept), and rivastigmine (Exelon)—have been approved by the FDA for its treatment. Tacrine has been shown to be effective for improving memory skills, but only in patients with mild-to-moderate AD, and even then in less than half of those who take it. Its beneficial effects are usually mild and temporary, but it may delay the need for nursing home admission. The most significant side effect is an increase in a liver enzyme known as alanine aminotransferase, or ALT. Patients taking tacrine must have a weekly blood test to monitor their ALT levels. Other frequent side effects include **nausea**, **vomiting**, **diarrhea**, abdominal pain, **indigestion**, and skin rash. The cost of tacrine was about $125 per month in early 1998, with additional costs for the weekly blood monitoring. Despite its high cost, tacrine appears to be cost-effective for those who respond to it, since it may decrease the number of months a patient needs nursing care. Donepezil is the drug most commonly used to treat mild to moderate symptoms of AD, although it only helps some patients for periods of time ranging from months to about two years. Donepezil has two advantages over tacrine: it has fewer side effects, and it can be given once daily rather than three times daily. Donepezil does not appear to affect liver enzymes, and therefore does not require weekly blood tests. The frequency of abdominal side effects is also lower. The monthly cost is approximately the same. Rivastigmine, approved for use in April of 2000, has been shown to improve the ability of patients to carry out daily activities, such as eating and dressing, decrease behavioral symptoms such as delusions and agitation, and improve cognitive functions such as thinking, memory, and speaking. The cost is similar to those of the other two drugs. However, none of these three drugs stops or reverses the progression of AD. Galantamine (Reminyl) works in the early and moderates stages of AD. It has fewer side effects than other drugs, with the exception of donepezil and must be taken

twice a day. Three other drugs were being tested for AD treatment in mid-2003.

Estrogen, the female sex hormone, is widely prescribed for post-menopausal women to prevent **osteoporosis**. Studies once showed that estrogen was beneficial to women with AD, but in 2003, a large clinical trial called the Women's Health Initiative showed dementia among other negative effects of combined estrogen therapy.

Preliminary studies once suggested a reduced risk for developing AD in elderly people who regularly used nonsteroidal anti-inflammatory drugs (NSAIDs), including **aspirin**, ibuprofen, and naproxen, although not **acetaminophen**. However, an important study published in 2003 showed that NSAIDs were not effective in preventing or slowing the progression of AD. The study authors recommended that people stop taking NSAIDs to slow dementia.

Antioxidants, which act to inhibit and protect against oxidative damage caused by free radicals, have been shown to inhibit toxic effects of beta-amyloid in tissue culture. Therefore, research is being conducted to see whether antioxidants may delay or prevent AD.

Another antioxidant, vitamin E, is also thought to delay AD onset. Hoever, it is not yet clear whether this is due to the specific action of vitamin E on brain cells, or to an increase in the overall health of those taking it.

Drugs such as antidepressants, anti-psychotics, and sedatives are used to treat the behavioral symptoms (agitation, aggression, wandering, and sleep disorders) of AD. Research is being conducted to search for better treatments, including non-drug approaches for AD patients.

Nursing care and safety

The person with Alzheimer's disease will gradually lose the ability to dress, groom, feed, bathe, or use the toilet by himself; in the later stages of the disease, he may be unable to move or speak. In addition, the person's behavior becomes increasingly erratic. A tendency to wander may make it difficult to leave him unattended for even a few minutes and make even the home a potentially dangerous place. In addition, some people with AD may exhibit inappropriate sexual behaviors.

The nursing care required for a person with AD is well within the abilities of most people to learn. The difficulty for many caregivers comes in the constant but unpredictable nature of the demands put on them. In addition, the personality changes undergone by a person with AD can be heartbreaking for family members as a loved one deteriorates, seeming to become a different person. Not all people with AD develop negative behaviors. Some become quite gentle, and spend increasing amounts of time in dreamlike states.

A loss of good grooming may be one of the early symptoms of AD. Mismatched clothing, unkempt hair, and decreased interest in personal hygiene become more common. Caregivers, especially spouses, may find these changes socially embarrassing and difficult to cope with. The caregiver usually will need to spend increasing amounts of time on grooming to compensate for the loss of attention from the patient, although some adjustment of expectations (while maintaining cleanliness) is often needed as the disease progresses.

Proper nutrition is important for a person with AD, and may require assisted feeding early on, to make sure the person is taking in enough nutrients. Later on, as movement and swallowing become difficult, a feeding tube may be placed into the stomach through the abdominal wall. A feeding tube requires more attention, but is generally easy to care for if the patient is not resistant to its use.

For many caregivers, incontinence becomes the most difficult problem to deal with at home, and is a principal reason for pursuing nursing home care. In the early stages, limiting fluid intake and increasing the frequency of toileting can help. Careful attention to hygiene is important to prevent skin irritation and infection from soiled clothing.

Persons with dementia must deal with six basic safety concerns: injury from falls, injury from ingesting dangerous substances, leaving the home and getting lost, injury to self or others from sharp objects, fire or **burns**, and the inability to respond rapidly to crisis situations. In all cases, a person diagnosed with AD should no longer be allowed to drive, because of the increased potential for accidents and the increased likelihood of wandering very far from home while disoriented. In the home, simple measures such as grab bars in the bathroom, bed rails on the bed, and easily negotiable passageways can greatly increase safety. Electrical appliances should be unplugged and put away when not in use, and matches, lighters, knives, or weapons should be stored safely out of reach. The hot water heater temperature may be set lower to prevent accidental scalding. A list of emergency numbers, including the poison control center and the hospital emergency room, should be posted by the phone. As the disease progresses, caregivers need to periodically reevaluate the physical safety of the home and introduce new strategies for continued safety.

Care for the caregiver

Family members or others caring for a person with AD have an extremely difficult and stressful job, which becomes harder as the disease progresses. Dementia caregivers spend significantly more time on caregiving than do people providing care for those with other types of illnesses. This type of caregiving also has a greater impact in terms of employment complications, caregiver strain, mental and physical health problems, time for leisure and other family members, and family conflict than do other types of caregiving. It is common for AD caregivers to develop feelings of anger, resentment, guilt, and hopelessness, in addition to the sorrow they feel for their loved one and for themselves. Depression is an extremely common consequence of being a full-time caregiver for a person with AD. Support groups are an important way to deal with the stress of caregiving. Becoming a member of an AD caregivers' support group can be one of the most important things a family member does, not only for him or herself, but for the person with AD as well. The location and contact numbers for AD caregiver support groups are available from the Alzheimer's Association; they also may be available through a local social service agency, the patient's physician, or pharmaceutical companies that manufacture the drugs used to treat AD. Medical treatment for depression may be an important adjunct to group support.

Outside help, nursing homes, and governmental assistance

Most families eventually need outside help to relieve some of the burden of around-the-clock care for a person with AD. Personal care assistants, either volunteer or paid, may be available through local social service agencies. Adult daycare facilities are becoming increasingly common. Meal delivery, shopping assistance, or respite care may be available as well.

Providing the total care required by a person with late-stage AD can become an overwhelming burden for a family, even with outside help. At this stage, many families consider nursing home care. This decision often is one of the most difficult for the family, since it is often seen as an abandonment of the loved one and a failure of the family. Careful counseling with a sympathetic physician, clergy, or other trusted adviser may ease the difficulties of this transition. Selecting a nursing home may require a difficult balancing of cost, services, location, and availability. Keeping the entire family involved in the decision may help prevent further stress from developing later on.

Several federal government programs may ease the cost of caring for a person with AD, including Social Security Disability, Medicare, and Supplemental Security Income. Each of these programs may provide some assistance for care, medication, or other costs, but none of them will pay for nursing home care indefinitely. Medicaid is a state-funded program that may provide for some or all of the cost of nursing home care, although there are important restrictions. Details of the benefits and eligibility requirements of these programs are available through the local Social Security or Medicaid office, or from local social service agencies.

Private long-term care insurance, special "reverse mortgages," viatical insurance, and other financial devices are other ways of paying for care for those with the appropriate financial situations. Further information on these options may be available through resources listed below.

Alternative treatment

Several substances are currently being tested for their ability to slow the progress of Alzheimer's disease. These include acetylcarnitine, a supplement that acts on the cellular energy structures known as mitochondria. Ginkgo extract, derived from the leaves of the *Ginkgo biloba* tree, appears to have antioxidant as well as anti-inflammatory and anticoagulant properties. Ginkgo extract has been used for many years in China and is widely prescribed in Europe for treatment of circulatory problems. A 1997 study of patients with dementia seemed to show that ginkgo extract could improve their symptoms, though the study was criticized for certain flaws in its method. Large scale follow-up studies are being conducted to determine whether Ginkgo extract can prevent or delay the development of AD. Ginkgo extract is available in many health food or nutritional supplement stores. Some alternative practitioners also advise people with AD to take supplements of phosphatidylcholine, vitamin B$_{12}$, gotu kola, ginseng, St. Johnõs Wort, rosemary, saiko-keishi-to-shakuyaku (A Japanese herbal mixture), and folic acid.

Prognosis

While Alzheimer's disease may not be the direct cause of death, the generally poorer health of a person with AD increases the risk of life-threatening infection, including **pneumonia**. In addition, other diseases common in old age–cancer, stroke, and heart disease– may lead to more severe consequences in a person with AD. On average, people with AD live eight years past their diagnosis, with a range from one to 20 years.

Prevention

Currently, there is no sure way to prevent Alzheimer's disease. treatments discussed above may eventually be proven to reduce the risk of developing the disease. Avoiding risks such as hormone replacement therapy may help prevent development of AD.

Research on the prevention of AD is focusing on blocking the production of amyloid in the brain as well as breaking down beta-amyloid once it is released from cells but before it has a chance to aggregate into insoluble plaques. There also are promising studies being conducted to develop an AD vaccine, where immune responses may result in the elimination of the formation of amyloid plaques.

The Alzheimer's Disease Research Centers (ADCs) program promotes research, training and education, technology transfer, and multicenter and cooperative studies in AD, other dementias, and normal brain **aging**. Each ADC enrolls and performs studies on AD patients and healthy older people. Persons can participate in research protocols and clinical drug trials at these centers. Data from the ADCs as well as from other sources are coordinated and made available for use by researchers at the National Alzheimer's Coordinating Center, established in 1999.

Resources

BOOKS

Cohen, Donna, and Carl Eisdorfer. *The Loss of Self: A Family Resource for the Care of Alzheimer's Disease and Related Disorders*. Revised. NewYork: W.W. Norton & Company, 2001.

Geldmacher, David S. *Contemporary Diagnosis and Management ofAlzheimer's Disease*. Newtown, PA: Associates in Medical Marketing Co., Inc., 2001.

Gruetzner, Howard. *Alzheimer's: A Caregiverõs Guideand Sourcebook*. 3rd ed. New York: John Wiley & Sons, 2001.

Mace, Nancy L., and Peter V. Rabins. *The 36-Hour Day: A Family Guide for Caring with Persons with Alzheimer Disease, Related Dementing Illnesses, and MemoryLoss in Later Life*. New York: Warner Books, 2001.

Teitel, Rosette, and Marc L. Gordon. *The Handholderõs Handbook: A Guide for Caregivers of Alzheimerõs and other Dementias*. NewBrunswick, NJ: Rutgers University Press, 2001.

PERIODICALS

"Alzheimer's Could be Linked to Depression." *GP* (May 26, 2003): 4.

"Alzheimer's Could Reduced by Education." *The Lancet* (June 28, 2003): 2215.

"Contrary to Some Earlier Results, New Study Shows NSAIDs Do Not Slow Progression of Alzheimer's Disease." *The Brown University Geriatric Psychopharmacology Update* (July 2003): 1.

Gitlin, L.N., and M. Corcoran. "Making Homes Safer: Environmental Adaptations for People with Dementia." *Alzheimer's Care Quarterly* 1 (2000): 50-58.

Helmuth, L. "Alzheimer's Congress: Further Progress on aB-Amyloid Vaccine." *Science* 289, no. 5476 (2000): 375.

Josefson, Deborah. "Latests HRT Trial Results Show Risk of Dementia." *British Medical Journal* (June 7, 2003): 1232.

McReady, Norah. "Prompt Intervention May Slow Alzheimer's Decline." *Family Practice News* (May 1, 2003): 32-41.

Naditz, Alan. "Deeply Affected: As the Nation Ages, Alzheimer's Will Strike More People Close to Us." *Contemporary Long Term Care* (July 2003): 20-23.

"Researchers Believe "Silent" Strokes Boost Risk." *GP* (April 14, 2003): 9.

OTHER

Alzheimer's Disease Books and Videotapes. <http://www.alzheimersbooks.com>.

National Institute on Aging, National Institutes of Health. *2000: Progress Report on Alzheimer's Disease - Taking the Next Steps.* NIH Publication No. 4859 (2000). <http://www.alzheimers.org/pubs/prog00.htm#References>.

Judith Sims
Teresa G. Odle

Ambiguous genitals *see* **Intersex states**

Amblyopia

Definition

Amblyopia is an uncorrectable decrease in vision in one or both eyes with no apparent structural abnormality seen to explain it. It is a diagnosis of exclusion, meaning that when a decrease in vision is detected, other causes must be ruled out. Once no other cause is found, amblyopia is the diagnosis. Generally, a difference of two lines or more (on an eye-chart test of visual acuity) between the two eyes or a best corrected vision of 20/30 or worse would be defined as amblyopia. For example, if someone has 20/20 vision with the right eye and only 20/40 with the left, and the left eye cannot achieve better vision with corrective lenses, the left eye is said to be amblyopic.

Description

Lazy eye is a common non-medical term used to describe amblyopia because the eye with poorer vision doesn't seem to be doing its job of seeing. Amblyopia is the most common cause of impaired vision in children, affecting nearly three out of every 100 people or 2-4% of the population. Vision is a combination of the clarity of the images of the eyes (visual acuity) and the processing of those images by the brain. If the images produced by the two eyes are substantially different, the brain may not be able to fuse the images. Instead of seeing two different images or double vision (diplopia), the brain suppresses the blurrier image. This suppression can lead to amblyopia. During the first few years of life, preferring one eye over the other may lead to poor visual development in the blurrier eye.

Causes and symptoms

Some of the major causes of amblyopia are as follows:

- **Strabismus.** A misalignment of the eyes (strabismus) is the most common cause of functional amblyopia. The two eyes are looking in two different directions at the same time. The brain is sent two different images and this causes confusion. Images from the misaligned or "crossed" eye are turned off to avoid double vision.

- Anisometropia. This is another type of functional amblyopia. In this case, there is a difference of refractive states between the two eyes (in other words, a difference of prescriptions between the two eyes). For example, one eye may be more nearsighted than the other eye, or one eye may be farsighted and the other eye nearsighted. Because the brain cannot fuse the two dissimilar images, the brain will suppress the blurrier image, causing the eye to become amblyopic.

- Cataract. Clouding of the lens of the eye will cause the image to be blurrier than the other eye. The brain "prefers" the clearer image. The eye with the cataract may become amblyopic.

- **Ptosis.** This is the drooping of the upper eyelid. If light cannot enter the eye because of the drooping lid, the eye is essentially not being used. This can lead to amblyopia.

- **Nutrition.** A type of organic amblyopia in which nutritional deficiencies or chemical toxicity may result in amblyopia. Alcohol, tobacco, or a deficiency in the B **vitamins** may result in toxic amblyopia.

- Heredity. Amblyopia can run in families.

Barring the presence of strabismus or ptosis, children may or may not show signs of amblyopia.

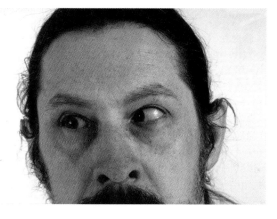

Man with a lazy eye. *(Custom Medical Stock Photo. Reproduced by permission.)*

Children may hold their heads at an angle while trying to favor the eye with normal vision. They may have trouble seeing or reaching for things when approached from the side of the amblyopic eye. Parents should see if one side of approach is preferred by the child or infant. If an infant's good eye is covered, the child may cry.

Diagnosis

Because children with outwardly normal eyes may have amblyopia, it is important to have regular vision screenings performed for all children. While there is some controversy regarding the age children should have their first vision examination, their eyes can, in actuality, be examined at any age, even at one day of life.

Some recommend that children have their vision checked by their pediatrician, family physician, ophthalmologist, or optometrist at or before six months of age. Others recommend testing by at least the child's fourth birthday. There may be a "critical period" in the development of vision, and amblyopia may not be treatable after age eight or nine. The earlier amblyopia is found, the better the possible outcome. Most physicians test vision as part of a child's medical examination. If there is any sign of an eye problem, they may refer a child to an eye specialist.

There are objective methods, such as retinoscopy, to measure the refractive status of the eyes. This can help determine anisometropia. In retinoscopy, a hand-held instrument is used to shine a light in the child's (or infant's) eyes. Using hand-held lenses, a rough prescription can be obtained. Visual acuity can be determined using a variety of methods. Many different eye charts are available (e.g., tumbling E, pictures, or letters). In amblyopia, single letters are easier to

recognize than when a whole line is shown. This is called the "crowding effect" and helps in diagnosing amblyopia. Neutral density filters may also be held over the eye to aid in the diagnosis. Sometimes visual fields to determine defects in the area of vision will be performed. Color vision testing may also be performed. Again, it must be emphasized that amblyopia is a diagnosis of exclusion. Visual or life-threatening problems can also cause a decrease in vision. An examination of the eyes and visual system is very important when there is an unexplained decrease in vision.

Treatment

The primary treatment for amblyopia is occlusion therapy. It is important to alternate patching the good eye (forcing the amblyopic eye to work) and the amblyopic eye. If the good eye is constantly patched, it too may become amblyopic because of disuse. The treatment plan should be discussed with the doctor to fully understand how long the patch will be on. When patched, eye exercises may be prescribed to force the amblyopic eye to focus and work. This is called vision therapy or **vision training** (eye exercises). Even after vision has been restored in the weak eye, part-time patching may be required over a period of years to maintain the improvement.

While patching is necessary to get the amblyopic eye to work, it is just as important to correct the reason for the amblyopia. Glasses may also be worn if there are errors in refraction. Surgery or vision training may be necessary in the case of strabismus. Better nutrition is indicated in some toxic amblyopias. Occasionally, amblyopia is treated by blurring the vision in the good eye with eye drops or lenses to force the child to use the amblyopic eye.

Prognosis

The younger the person, the better the chance for improvement with occlusion and vision therapy. However, treatment may be successful in older children–even adults. Success in the treatment of amblyopia also depends upon how severe the amblyopia is, the specific type of amblyopia, and patient compliance. It is important to diagnose and treat amblyopia early because significant vision loss can occur if left untreated. The best outcomes result from early diagnosis and treatment.

Prevention

To protect their child's vision, parents must be aware of amblyopia as a potential problem. This awareness may encourage parents to take young children for vision exams early on in life–certainly before school age. Proper nutrition is important in the avoidance of toxic amblyopia.

Resources

ORGANIZATIONS

American Academy of Ophthalmology. 655 Beach Street, P.O. Box 7424, San Francisco, CA 94120-7424. < http://www.eyenet.org > .

American Optometric Association. 243 North Lindbergh Blvd., St. Louis, MO 63141. (314) 991-4100. < http://www.aoanet.org > .

Lorraine Steefel, RN

Amebiasis

Definition

Amebiasis is an infectious disease caused by a parasitic one-celled microorganism (protozoan) called *Entamoeba histolytica*. Persons with amebiasis may experience a wide range of symptoms, including **diarrhea**, **fever**, and cramps. The disease may also affect the intestines, liver, or other parts of the body.

Description

Amebiasis, also known as amebic **dysentery**, is one of the most common parasitic diseases occurring in humans, with an estimated 500 million new cases each year. It occurs most frequently in tropical and subtropical areas where living conditions are crowded, with inadequate sanitation. Although most cases of amebiasis occur in persons who carry the disease but do not exhibit any symptoms (asymptomatic), as many as 100,000 people die of amebiasis each year. In the United States, between 1 and 5% of the general population will develop amebiasis in any given year, while male homosexuals, migrant workers, institutionalized people, and recent immigrants develop amebiasis at a higher rate.

Human beings are the only known host of the amebiasis organism, and all groups of people, regardless of age or sex, can become affected. Amebiasis is primarily spread in food and water that has been contaminated by human feces but is also spread by person-to-person contact. The number of cases is typically limited, but regional outbreaks can occur in areas where human feces are used as fertilizer for crops, or in cities with water supplies contaminated with human feces.

Causes and symptoms

Recently, it has been discovered that persons with symptom-causing amebiasis are infected with *Entamoeba histolytica*, and those individuals who exhibit no symptoms are actually infected with an almost identical-looking ameba called *Entamoeba dispar*. During their life cycles, the amebas exist in two very different forms: the infective cyst or capsuled form, which cannot move but can survive outside the human body because of its protective covering, and the disease-producing form, the trophozoite, which although capable of moving, cannot survive once excreted in the feces and, therefore, cannot infect others. The disease is most commonly transmitted when a person eats food or drinks water containing *E. histolytica* cysts from human feces. In the digestive tract the cysts are transported to the intestine where the walls of the cysts are broken open by digestive secretions, releasing the mobile trophozoites. Once released within the intestine, the trophozoites multiply by feeding on intestinal bacteria or by invading the lining of the large intestine. Within the lining of the large intestine, the trophozoites secrete a substance that destroys intestinal tissue and creates a distinctive bottle-shaped sore (ulcer). The trophozoites may remain inside the intestine, in the intestinal wall, or may break through

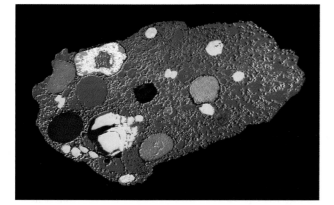

A micrograph of Entameoba histolytica, a parasitic amoeba which invades and destroys the tissues of the intestines, causing amebiasis and ulceration to the intestinal wall. *(Photo Researchers, Inc. Reproduced by permission.)*

the intestinal wall and be carried by the blood to the liver, lungs, brain, or other organs. Trophozoites that remain in the intestines eventually form new cysts that are carried through the digestive tract and excreted in the feces. Under favorable temperature and humidity conditions, the cysts can survive in soil or water for weeks to months, ready to begin the cycle again.

Although 90% of cases of amebiasis in the United States are mild, pregnant women, children under two years of age, the elderly, malnourished individuals, and people whose immune systems may be compressed, such as **cancer** or **AIDS** patients and those individuals taking prescription medications that suppress the immune system, are at a greater risk for developing a severe infection.

The signs and symptoms of amebiasis vary according to the location and severity of the infection and are classified as follows:

Intestinal amebiasis

Intestinal amebiasis can be subdivided into several categories:

ASYMPTOMATIC INFECTION. Most persons with amebiasis have no noticeable symptoms. Even though these individuals may not feel ill, they are still capable of infecting others by person-to-person contact or by contaminating food or water with cysts that others may ingest, for example, by preparing food with unwashed hands.

CHRONIC NON-DYSENTERIC INFECTION. Individuals may experience symptoms over a long period of time during a chronic amebiasis infection and

experience recurrent episodes of diarrhea that last from one to four weeks and recur over a period of years. These patients may also suffer from abdominal cramps, **fatigue**, and weight loss.

AMEBIC DYSENTERY. In severe cases of intestinal amebiasis, the organism invades the lining of the intestine, producing sores (ulcers), bloody diarrhea, severe abdominal cramps, **vomiting**, chills, and fevers as high as 104-105°F (40-40.6°C). In addition, a case of acute amebic dysentery may cause complications, including inflammation of the appendix (**appendicitis**), a tear in the intestinal wall (perforation), or a sudden, severe inflammation of the colon (fulminating colitis).

AMEBOMA. An ameboma is a mass of tissue in the bowel that is formed by the amebiasis organism. It can result from either chronic intestinal infection or acute amebic dysentery. Amebomas may produce symptoms that mimic cancer or other intestinal diseases.

PERIANAL ULCERS. Intestinal amebiasis may produce skin infections in the area around the patient's anus (perianal). These ulcerated areas have a "punched-out" appearance and are painful to the touch.

Extraintestinal amebiasis

Extraintestinal amebiasis accounts for approximately 10% of all reported amebiasis cases and includes all forms of the disease that affect other organs.

The most common form of extraintestinal amebiasis is amebic **abscess** of the liver. In the United States, amebic liver abscesses occur most frequently in young Hispanic adults. An amebic liver abscess can result from direct infection of the liver by *E. histolytica* or as a complication of intestinal amebiasis. Patients with an amebic abscess of the liver complain of **pain** in the chest or abdomen, fever, **nausea**, and tenderness on the right side directly above the liver.

Other forms of extraintestinal amebiasis, though rare, include infections of the lungs, chest cavity, brain, or genitals. These are extremely serious and have a relatively high mortality rate.

Diagnosis

Diagnosis of amebiasis is complicated, partly because the disease can affect several areas of the body and can range from exhibiting few, if any, symptoms to being severe, or even life-threatening. In most cases, a physician will consider a diagnosis of amebiasis when a patient has a combination of symptoms, in particular, diarrhea and a possible history of recent exposure to amebiasis through travel, contact with infected persons, or anal intercourse.

It is vital to distinguish between amebiasis and another disease, inflammatory bowel disease (IBD) that produces similar symptoms because, if diagnosed incorrectly, drugs that are given to treat IBD can encourage the growth and spread of the amebiasis organism. Because of the serious consequences of misdiagnosis, potential cases of IBD must be confirmed with multiple stool samples and blood tests, and a procedure involving a visual inspection of the intestinal wall using a thin lighted, tubular instrument (**sigmoidoscopy**) to rule out amebiasis.

A diagnosis of amebiasis may be confirmed by one or more tests, depending on the location of the disease.

Stool examination

This test involves microscopically examining a stool sample for the presence of cysts and/or trophozoites of *E. histolytica* and not one of the many other intestinal amebas that are often found but that do not cause disease. A series of three stool tests is approximately 90% accurate in confirming a diagnosis of amebic dysentery. Unfortunately, however, the stool test is not useful in diagnosing amebomas or extraintestinal infections.

Sigmoidoscopy

Sigmoidoscopy is a useful diagnostic procedure in which a thin, flexible, lighted instrument, called a sigmoidoscope, is used to visually examine the lower part of the large intestine for amebic ulcers and take tissue or fluid samples from the intestinal lining.

Blood tests

Although tests designed to detect a specific protein produced in response to amebiasis infection (antibody) are capable of detecting only about 10% of cases of mild amebiasis, these tests are extremely useful in confirming 95% of dysentery diagnoses and 98% of liver abscess diagnoses. Blood serum will usually test positive for antibody within a week of symptom onset. Blood testing, however, cannot always distinguish between a current or past infection since the antibodies may be detectable in the blood for as long as 10 years following initial infection.

Imaging studies

A number of sophisticated imaging techniques, such as **computed tomography scans** (CT), **magnetic resonance imaging** (MRI), and ultrasound, can be used to determine whether a liver abscess is present. Once located, a physician may then use a fine needle to withdraw a sample of tissue to determine whether the abscess is indeed caused by an amebic infection.

Treatment

Asymptomatic or mild cases of amebiasis may require no treatment. However, because of the potential for disease spread, amebiasis is generally treated with a medication to kill the disease-causing amebas. More severe cases of amebic dysentery are additionally treated by replacing lost fluid and blood. Patients with an amebic liver abscess will also require hospitalization and bed rest. For those cases of extraintestinal amebiasis, treatment can be complicated because different drugs may be required to eliminate the parasite, based on the location of the infection within the body. Drugs used to treat amebiasis, called amebicides, are divided into two categories:

Luminal amebicides

These drugs get their name because they act on organisms within the inner cavity (lumen) of the bowel. They include diloxanide furoate, iodoquinol, metronidazole, and paromomycin.

Tissue amebicides

Tissue amebicides are used to treat infections in the liver and other body tissues and include emetine, dehydroemetine, metronidazole, and chloroquine. Because these drugs have potentially serious side effects, patients given emetine or dehydroemetine require bed rest and heart monitoring. Chloroquine has been found to be the most useful drug for treating amebic liver abscess. Patients taking metronidazole must avoid alcohol because the drug-alcohol combination causes nausea, vomiting, and **headache**.

Most patients are given a combination of luminal and tissue amebicides over a treatment period of seven to ten days. Follow-up care includes periodic stool examinations beginning two to four weeks after the end of medication treatment to check the effectiveness of drug therapy.

Prognosis

The prognosis depends on the location of the infection and the patient's general health prior to infection. The prognosis is generally good, although the mortality rate is higher for patients with ameboma, perforation of the bowel, and liver infection. Patients who develop fulminant colitis have the most serious prognosis, with over 50% mortality.

Prevention

There are no immunization procedures or medications that can be taken prior to potential exposure to prevent amebiasis. Moreover, people who have had the disease can become reinfected. Prevention requires effective personal and community hygiene.

Specific safeguards include the following:

- Purification of drinking water. Water can be purified by filtering, boiling, or treatment with iodine.
- Proper food handling. Measures include protecting food from contamination by flies, cooking food properly, washing one's hands after using the bathroom and before cooking or eating, and avoiding foods that cannot be cooked or peeled when traveling in countries with high rates of amebiasis.
- Careful disposal of human feces.

- Monitoring the contacts of amebiasis patients. The stools of family members and sexual partners of infected persons should be tested for the presence of cysts or trophozoites.

Resources

BOOKS

Friedman, Lawrence S. "Liver, Biliary Tract, & Pancreas." In *Current Medical Diagnosis and Treatment, 1998,* edited by Stephen McPhee, et al., 37th ed. Stamford: Appleton & Lange, 1997.

Rebecca J. Frey, PhD

Amebic dysentery *see* **Amebiasis**

Amenorrhea

Definition

The absence of menstrual periods is called amenorrhea. Primary amenorrhea is the failure to start having a period by the age of 16. Secondary amenorrhea is more common and refers to either the temporary or permanent ending of periods in a woman who has menstruated normally in the past. Many women miss a period occasionally. Amenorrhea occurs if a woman misses three or more periods in a row.

Description

The absence of menstrual periods is a symptom, not a disease. While the average age that menstruation begins is 12, the range varies. The incidence of primary amenorrhea in the United States is just 2.5%.

Some female athletes who participate in rowing, long distance running, and cycling, may notice a few missed periods. Women athletes at a particular risk for developing amenorrhea include ballerinas and gymnasts, who typically exercise strenuously and eat poorly.

Causes and symptoms

Amenorrhea can have many causes. Primary amenorrhea can be the result of hormonal imbalances, psychiatric disorders, eating disorders, malnutrition, excessive thinness or fatness, rapid weight loss, body fat content too low, and excessive physical conditioning. Intense physical training prior to **puberty** can delay menarche (the onset of menstruation). Every year of training can delay menarche for up to five months.

KEY TERMS

Hymen—Membrane that stretches across the opening of the vagina.

Hypothyroidism—Underactive thyroid gland.

Hysterectomy—Surgical removal of the uterus.

Turner's syndrome—A condition in which one female sex chromosome is missing.

Some medications such as anti-depressants, tranquilizers, steroids, and heroin can induce amenorrhea.

Primary amenorrhea

However, the main cause is a delay in the beginning of puberty either from natural reasons (such as heredity or poor **nutrition**) or because of a problem in the endocrine system, such as a pituitary tumor or **hypothyroidism**. An obstructed flow tract or inflammation in the uterus may be the presenting indications of an underlying metabolic, endocrine, congenital or gynecological disorder.

Typical causes of primary amenorrhea include:

- excessive physical activity
- drastic weight loss (such as occurs in anorexia or bulimia)
- extreme **obesity**
- drugs (antidepressants or tranquilizers)
- chronic illness
- turner's syndrome. (A chromosomal problem in place at birth, relevant only in cases of primary amenorrhea)
- the absence of a vagina or a uterus
- imperforate hymen (lack of an opening to allow the menstrual blood through)

Secondary amenorrhea

Some of the causes of primary amenorrhea can also cause secondary amenorrhea – strenuous physical activity, excessive weight loss, use of antidepressants or tranquilizers, in particular. In adolescents, **pregnancy** and **stress** are two major causes. Missed periods are usually caused in adolescents by stress and changes in environment. Adolescents are especially prone to irregular periods with fevers, weight loss, changes in environment, or increased physical or athletic activity. However, any cessation of periods for four months should be evaluated.

The most common cause of seconardy amenorrhea is pregnancy. Also, a woman's periods may halt temporarily after she stops taking birth control pills. This temporary halt usually lasts only for a month or two, though in some cases it can last for a year or more. Secondary amenorrhea may also be related to hormonal problems related to stress, depression, **anorexia nervosa** or drugs, or it may be caused by any condition affecting the ovaries, such as a tumor. The cessation of menstruation also occurs permanently after **menopause** or a **hysterectomy**.

Diagnosis

It may be difficult to find the cause of amenorrhea, but the exam should start with a pregnancy test; pregnancy needs to be ruled out whenever a woman's period is two to three weeks overdue. Androgen excess, estrogen deficiency, or other problems with the endocrine system need to be checked. Prolactin in the blood and the thyroid stimulating hormone (TSH) should also be checked.

The diagnosis usually includes a patient history and a physical exam (including a pelvic exam). If a woman has missed three or more periods in a row, a physician may recommend blood tests to measure hormone levels, a scan of the skull to rule out the possibility of a pituitary tumor, and ultrasound scans of the abdomen and pelvis to rule out a tumor of the adrenal gland or ovary.

Treatment

Treatment of amenorrhea depends on the cause. Primary amenorrhea often requires no treatment, but it's always important to discover the cause of the problem in any case. Not all conditions can be treated, but any underlying condition that is treatable should be treated.

If a hormonal imbalance is the problem, progesterone for one to two weeks every month or two may correct the problem. With polycystic ovary syndrome, birth control pills are often prescribed. A pituitary tumor is treated with bromocriptine, a drug that reduces certain hormone (prolactin) secretions. Weight loss may bring on a period in an obese woman. Easing up on excessive **exercise** and eating a proper diet may bring on periods in teen athletes. In very rare cases, surgery may be needed for women with ovarian or uterine cysts.

Prognosis

Prolonged amenorrhea can lead to **infertility** and other medical problems such as **osteoporosis** (thinning of the bones). If the halt in the normal period is caused by stress or illness, periods should begin again when the stress passes or the illness is treated. Amenorrhea that occurs with discontinuing birth control pills usually go away within six to eight weeks, although it may take up to a year.

The prognosis for polycystic ovary disease depends on the severity of the symptoms and the treatment plan. Spironolactone, a drug that blocks the production of male hormones, can help in reducing body hair. If a woman wishes to become pregnant, treatment with clomiphene may be required or, on rare occasions, surgery on the ovaries.

Prevention

Primary amenorrhea caused by a congenital condition cannot be prevented. In general, however, women should maintain a healthy diet, with plenty of exercise, rest, and not too much stress, avoiding **smoking** and **substance abuse**. Female athletes should be sure to eat a balanced diet and rest and exercise normally. However, many cases of amenorrhea cannot be prevented.

Resources

PERIODICALS

Hogg, Anne Cahill. "Breaking the Cycle: Often Confused and Frustrated, Sufferers of Amenorrhea Now have Better Treatment Options." *American Fitness* 15, no. 4 (July-August 1997): 30-4.

ORGANIZATIONS

American College of Obstetricians and Gynecologists. 409 12th St., S.W., P.O. Box 96920, Washington, DC 20090-6920. <http://www.acog.org>.
Federation of Feminist Women's Health Centers.1469 Humboldt Rd, Suite 200, Chico, CA 96928. (530) 891-1911.
National Women's Health Network. 514 10th St. NW, Suite 400, Washington, DC 20004. (202) 628-7814. <http://www.womenshealthnetwork.org>.

Carol A. Turkington

Amikiacin *see* **Aminoglycosides**

Amiloride *see* **Diuretics**

Amino acid disorders screening

Definition

Amino acid disorder screening checks for inherited disorders in amino acid metabolism. Tests are most commonly done on newborns. Two tests are available, one using a blood sample and the other a urine sample.

Purpose

Amino acid disorder screening is done in newborns, and sometimes children and adults, to detect inborn errors in metabolism of amino acids. Twenty of the 100 known amino acids are the main building blocks for human proteins. Proteins regulate every aspect of cellular function. Of these 20 amino acids, ten are not made by the body and must be acquired through diet. Congenital (present at birth) enzyme deficiencies that affect amino acid metabolism or congenital abnormalities in the amino acid transport system of the kidneys creates a condition called aminoaciduria.

Screening is especially important in newborns. Some congenital amino acid metabolic defects cause **mental retardation** that can prevented with prompt treatment of the newborn. One of the best known examples of this is **phenylketonuria** (PKU). This is an genetic error in metabolism of phenylalanine, an amino acid found in milk. Individuals with PKU do not produce the enzyme necessary to break down phenylalanine.

PKU occurs in about one out of 16,000 live births in the United States, but is more prevalent in caucasians and less prevalent in Ashkenazi Jews and African Americans. Newborns in the United States are routinely screened for PKU by a blood test.

There are two types of aminoacidurias. Primary or overflow aminoaciduria results from deficiencies in the enzymes necessary to metabolize amino acids. Overflow aminoaciduria is best detected by a blood plasma test.

Secondary or renal aminoaciduria occurs because of a congenital defect in the amino acid transport system in the tubules of the kidneys. This produces increased amino acids in the urine. Blood and urine test in combination are used to determine if the aminoaciduria is of the overflow or renal type. Urine tests are also used to monitor specific amino acid disorders.

Newborns are screened for amino acid disorders. Young children with acidosis (accumulation of acid in the body), severe **vomiting** and diarrhea, or urine with an abnormal color or odor, are also screened with a urine test for specific amino acid levels.

Precautions

Both blood and urine tests are simple tests that can be done in a doctor's office or clinic. These tests can be done on even the youngest patients.

KEY TERMS

Amino acid—An organic compound composed of both an amino group and an acidic carboxyl group; amino acids are the basic building blocks of proteins.

Aminoaciduria—The abnormal presence of amino acids in the urine.

Chromatography—A family of laboratory techniques that separate mixtures of chemicals into their individual components.

Enzyme—A biological catalyst that increases the rate of a chemical reaction without being used up in the reaction.

Metabolism—The sum of all the chemical and energy reactions that take place in the human body.

Description

Two types of amino acid screening tests are used together to diagnose amino acid disorders.

Blood plasma screening

In the blood test, a medical technician draws a small amount of blood from a baby's heel. The procedure is rapid and relatively painless. Total time for the test is less than ten minutes. The blood is sent to a laboratory where results will be available in about two days.

Urine test

In the urine test, the patient is asked to urinate into a collecting cup. For an infant, the urine is collected in a pediatric urine collector. The process is painless. The length of time the test takes is determined by how long it takes the patient to urinate. Results also take about two days.

Both these tests use thin layer chromatography to separate the amino acids present. Using this technique, the amino acids form a characteristic patterns on a glass plate coated with a thin layer of silica gel. This pattern is then compared to the normal pattern to determine if there are abnormalities.

Preparation

Before the blood test, the patient must not eat or drink for four hours. Failure to fast will alter the results of the test.

The patient should eat and drink normally before the urine test. Some drugs may affect the results of the urine test. The technician handling the urine sample should be informed of any medications the patient is taking. Mothers of breastfeeding infants should report any medications they are taking, since these can pass from mother to child in breast milk.

Aftercare

The blood screening is normally done first. Depending on the results, it is followed by the urine test. It takes both tests to distinguish between overflow and renal aminoaciduria. Also, if the results are abnormal, a 24-hour urine test is performed along with other tests to determine the levels of specific amino acids. In the event of abnormal results, there are many other tests that will be performed to determine the specific amino acid involved in the abnormality.

Risks

There are no particular risks associated with either of these tests. Occasionally minor bruising may occur at the site where the blood was taken.

Normal results

The pattern of amino acid banding on the thin layer chromatography plates will be normal.

Abnormal results

The blood plasma amino acid pattern is abnormal in overflow aminoaciduria and is normal in renal aminoaciduria. The pattern is abnormal in the urine test, suggesting additional tests need to be done to determine which amino acids are involved. In addition to PKU, a variety of other amino acid metabolism disorders can be detected by these tests, including tyrosinosis, histidinemia, maple syrup urine disease, hypervalinemia, hyperprolinemia, and homocystinuria.

Resources

ORGANIZATIONS

Association for Neuro-Metabolic Disorders. 5223 Brookfield Lane, Sylvania, OH 43560-1809. (419) 885-1497.

Children's PKU Network (CPN). 3790 Via De La Valle, Ste 120, Del Mar, CA 92014. (800) 377-6677. < http://www.pkunetwork.org/ > .

National Phenylketonuria Foundation. 6301 Tejas Drive, Pasadena, TX 77503. (713) 487-4802.

Tish Davidson, A.M.

Aminoglycosides

Definition

Aminoglycosides are a group of **antibiotics** that are used to treat certain bacterial infections. This group of antibiotics includes at least eight drugs: amikacin, gentamicin, kanamycin, neomycin, netilmicin, paromomycin, streptomycin, and tobramycin. All of these drugs have the same basic chemical structure.

Purpose

Aminoglycosides are primarily used to combat infections due to aerobic, Gram-negative bacteria. These bacteria can be identified by their reaction to Gram's stain. In Gram's staining, a film of material containing the possible bacteria is placed on a glass slide and dried. The slide is stained with crystal violet for one minute, cleaned off with water and then placed into a solution of Gram's iodine solution for one minute. The iodine solution is rinsed off and the slide is immersed in 95% ethyl alcohol. The slide is then stained again with reddish carbolfuchsin or safranine for 30 seconds, rinsed in water, dried and examined. Gram-positive bacteria retain the violet purple stain. Gram-negative bacteria accept the red stain. Bacteria that can successfully be combated with aminoglycosides include *Pseudomonas*, *Acinetobacter*, and *Enterobacter* species, among others. Aminoglycosides are also effective against mycobacteria, the bacteria responsible for **tuberculosis**.

The aminoglycosides can be used against certain Gram-positive bacteria, but are not typically employed because other antibiotics are more effective and have fewer side effects. Aminoglycosides are ineffective against anaerobic bacteria (bacteria that cannot grow in the presence of oxygen), viruses, and fungi. And only one aminoglycoside, paromomycin, is used against parasitic infection.

Like all other antibiotics, aminoglycosides are not effective against **influenza**, the **common cold**, or other viral infections.

Precautions

Pre-existing medical conditions–such as **kidney disease**, eighth cranial nerve disease, myasthenia gravis, and Parkinson's disease–should be discussed prior to taking any aminoglycosides. Pregnant women are usually advised against taking aminoglycosides, because their infants may suffer damage to

their hearing, kidneys, or sense of balance. However, those factors need to be considered alongside the threat to the mother's health and life in cases of serious infection. Aminoglycosides do not pass into breast milk to any great extent, so nursing mothers may be prescribed aminoglycosides without injuring their infants.

Description

Streptomycin, the first aminoglycoside, was isolated from *Streptomyces griseus* in the mid-1940s. This antibiotic was very effective against tuberculosis. One of the main drawbacks to streptomycin is its toxicity, especially to cells in the inner and middle ear and the kidney. Furthermore, some strains of tuberculosis are resistant to treatment with streptomycin. Therefore, medical researchers have put considerable

---

KEY TERMS

Aerobic bacteria—Bacteria which require oxygen in order to grow and survive.

Anaerobic bacteria—Bacteria which cannot grow or reproduce in the presence of oxygen.

Eighth cranial nerve disease—A disorder affecting the eighth cranial nerve, characterized by a loss of hearing and/or balance.

Gram-negative—Referring to a bacteria that take on a pink color when exposed to Gram's stain.

Gram-positive—Referring to a bacteria that takes on a purplish- black color when exposed to Gram's stain.

Gram's stain—A stain used in microbiology to classify bacteria and help identify the species to which they belong. This identification aids in determining treatment.

Kidney disease—Any disorder which impairs the kidney's ability to remove waste and toxins from the body.

Myasthenis gravis—A neuromuscular disease characterized by muscle weakness in the limbs and face.

Parkinson's disease—A neurological disorder caused by deficiency of dopamine, a neurotransmitter, that is a chemical that assists in transmitting messages between the nerves within the brain. It is characterized by muscle tremor or palsy and rigid movements.

---

effort into identifying other antibiotics with streptomycin's efficacy, but without its toxicity.

Aminoglycosides are absorbed very poorly from the gastrointestinal tract; in fact, aminoglycosides taken orally are excreted virtually unchanged and undiminished in quantity. The route of drug administration depends on the type and location of the infection being treated. The typical routes of administration are by intramuscular (injection into a muscle) or intravenous injection (injection into a vein), irrigation, topical skin application, or inhalation. If the infection being treated involves the central nervous system, the drug can be injected into the spinal canal.

The bactericidal ability of aminoglycosides has not been fully explained. It is known that the drug attaches to a bacterial cell wall and is drawn into the cell via channels made up of the protein, porin. Once inside the cell, the aminoglycoside attaches to the cell's ribosomes. Ribosomes are the intracellular structures responsible for manufacturing proteins. This attachment either shuts down protein production or causes the cell to produce abnormal, ineffective proteins. The bacterial cell cannot survive with this impediment.

Antibiotic treatment using aminoglycosides may pair the drug with a second type of antibiotic, usually a beta-lactam or vancomycin, administered separately. Beta-lactams disrupt the integrity of the bacteria cell wall, making it more porous. The increased porosity allows more of the aminoglycoside into the bacteria cell.

Traditionally, aminoglycosides were administered at even doses given throughout the day. It was thought that a steady plasma concentration was necessary to combat infection. However, this administration schedule is time and labor intensive. Furthermore, administering a single daily dose can be as effective, or more effective, than several doses throughout the day.

Dosage depends on the patient's age, weight, gender, and general health. Since the drug is cleared by the kidneys, it is important to assess any underlying problems with kidney function. Kidney function is assessed by measuring the blood levels of creatinine, a protein normally found in the body. If these levels are high, it is an indication that the kidneys may not be functioning at an optimal rate and dosage will be lowered accordingly.

Risks

Aminoglycosides have been shown to be toxic to certain cells in the ears and in the kidneys.

Approximately 5-10% of the people who are treated with aminoglycosides experience some side effect, affecting their hearing, sense of balance, or kidneys. However, in most cases the damage is minor and reversible once medication is stopped.

If cells in the inner ear are damaged or destroyed, an individual may experience a loss of balance and feelings of **dizziness**. Damage to the middle ear may result in **hearing loss** or tinnitus. Neomycin, kanamycin, and amikacin are the most likely to cause problems with hearing, and streptomycin and gentamicin carry the greatest risk of causing vertigo and loss of balance. Kidney damage, apparent with changes in urination frequency or urine production, is most likely precipitated by neomycin, tobramycin, and gentamicin.

Young children and the elderly are at the greatest risk of suffering side effects. Excessive dosage or poor clearance of the drug from the body can be injurious at any age.

Less common side effects include skin **rashes** and itching. Very rarely, certain aminoglycosides may cause difficulty in breathing, weakness, or drowsiness. Gentamicin, when injected, may cause leg cramps, skin rash, **fever**, or seizures.

If side effects linger or become worse after medication is stopped, it is advisable to seek medical advice. Side effects that may be of concern include **tinnitus** or loss of hearing, dizziness or loss of balance, changes in urination frequency or urine production, increased thirst, appetite loss, and **nausea** or **vomiting**.

Normal results

At the proper dosage and in the presence of gram-negative enteric (intestinal) bacteria, aminoglycosides are very effective in treating an infection.

Abnormal results

In some cases, bacteria are resistant to antibiotics that would normally kill them. This resistance becomes apparent after repeated exposure to the antibiotic and arises from a mutation that alters the bacteria's susceptibility to the drug. Various degrees of resistance have been observed in bacteria that normally would be destroyed by aminoglycosides. In general, though, aminoglycoside effectiveness has held up well over time.

Resources

BOOKS

Chambers, Henry F., W. Keith Hadley, and Ernest Jawetz. "Aminoglycosides & Spectinomycin." In *Basic and*

Clinical Pharmacology, edited by Bertram G. Katzung, 7th ed. Stamford: Appleton & Lange, 1998.

Julia Barrett

Amitriptyline *see* **Antidepressants, tricyclic**

Amlodipine *see* **Calcium channel blockers**

Amnesia

Definition

Amnesia refers to the loss of memory. Memory loss may result from two-sided (bilateral) damage to parts of the brain vital for memory storage, processing, or recall (the limbic system, including the hippocampus in the medial temporal lobe).

Description

Amnesia can be a symptom of several neurodegenerative diseases; however, people whose primary symptom is memory loss (amnesiacs), typically remain lucid and retain their sense of self. They may even be aware that they suffer from a memory disorder.

People who experience amnesia have been instrumental in helping brain researchers determine how the brain processes memory. Until the early 1970s, researchers viewed memory as a single entity. Memory of new experiences, motor skills, past events, and previous conditioning were grouped together in one system that relied on a specific area of the brain.

If all memory were stored in the same way, it would be reasonable to deduce that damage to the specific brain area would cause complete memory loss. However, studies of amnesiacs counter that theory. Such research demonstrates that the brain has multiple systems for processing, storing, and drawing on memory.

Causes and symptoms

Amnesia has several root causes. Most are traceable to brain injury related to physical trauma, disease, infection, drug and alcohol **abuse**, or reduced blood flow to the brain (vascular insufficiency). In Wernicke-Korsakoff syndrome, for example, damage to the memory centers of the brain results from the use of alcohol or **malnutrition**. Infections that damage brain tissue, including **encephalitis** and herpes, can also cause amnesia. If the amnesia is thought to be of psychological origin, it is termed psychogenic.

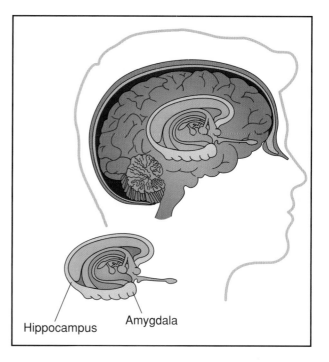

Hippocampus   Amygdala

Memory loss may result from bilateral damage to the limbic system of the brain responsible for memory storage, processing, and recall. *(Illustration by Electronic Illustrators Group).*

There are at least three general types of amnesia:

- Anterograde. This form of amnesia follows brain trauma and is characterized by the inability to remember new information. Recent experiences and short-term memory disappear, but victims can recall events prior to the trauma with clarity.

- Retrograde. In some ways, this form of amnesia is the opposite of anterograde amnesia: the victim can recall events that occurred after a trauma, but cannot remember previously familiar information or the events preceding the trauma.

- Transient global amnesia. This type of amnesia has no consistently identifiable cause, but researchers have suggested that migraines or transient ischemic attacks may be the trigger. (A **transient ischemic attack**, sometimes called "a small stroke," occurs when a blockage in an artery temporarily blocks off blood supply to part of the brain.) A victim experiences sudden confusion and forgetfulness. Attacks can be as brief as 30-60 minutes or can last up to 24 hours. In severe attacks, a person is completely disoriented and may experience retrograde amnesia that extends back several years. While very frightening for the patient, transient global amnesia generally has an excellent prognosis for recovery.

KEY TERMS

Classical conditioning—The memory system that links perceptual information to the proper motor response. For example, Ivan Pavlov conditioned a dog to salivate when a bell was rung.

Emotional conditioning—The memory system that links perceptual information to an emotional response. For example, spotting a friend in a crowd causes a person to feel happy.

Explicit memory—Conscious recall of facts and events that is classified into episodic memory (involves time and place) and semantic memory (does not involve time and place). For example, an amnesiac may remember he has a wife (semantic memory), but cannot recall his last conversation with her (episodic memory).

Limbic system—The brain structures involved in memory.

Magnetic resonance imaging (MRI)—MRI uses a large circular magnet and radio waves to generate signals from atoms in the body. These signals are used to construct images of internal structures.

Motor skill learning—This memory system is associated with physical movement and activity. For example, learning to swim is initially difficult, but once an efficient stroke is learned, it requires little conscious effort.

Neurodegenerative disease—A disease in which the nervous system progressively and irreversibly deteriorates.

Priming memory—The memory system that joins perceptual and conceptual representations.

Transient ischemic attack—A sudden and brief blockage of blood flow in the brain.

Working memory—The memory system that relates to the task at hand and coordinates recall of memories necessary to complete it.

Diagnosis

In diagnosing amnesia and its cause, doctors look at several factors. During a **physical examination**, the doctor inquires about recent traumas or illnesses, drug and medication history, and checks the patient's general health. Psychological exams may be ordered to determine the extent of amnesia and the memory system affected. The doctor may also order imaging tests such as **magnetic resonance imaging** (MRI) to reveal whether the brain has been damaged, and blood work to exclude treatable metabolic causes or chemical imbalances.

Treatment

Treatment depends on the root cause of amnesia and is handled on an individual basis. Regardless of cause, cognitive **rehabilitation** may be helpful in learning strategies to cope with memory impairment.

Prognosis

Some types of amnesia, such as transient global amnesia, are completely resolved and there is no permanent loss of memory. Others, such as Korsakoff syndrome, associated with prolonged alcohol abuse or amnesias caused by severe brain injury, may be permanent. Depending on the degree of amnesia and its cause, victims may be able to lead relatively normal lives. Amnesiacs can learn through therapy to rely on other memory systems to compensate for what is lost.

Prevention

Amnesia is only preventable in so far as brain injury can be prevented or minimized. Common sense approaches include wearing a helmet when bicycling or participating in potentially dangerous sports, using automobile seat belts, and avoiding excessive alcohol or drug use. Brain infections should be treated swiftly and aggressively to minimize the damage due to swelling. Victims of strokes, brain aneurysms, and transient ischemic attacks should seek immediate medical treatment.

Resources

PERIODICALS

Squire, Larry R., and Stuart M. Zola. "Amnesia, Memory and Brain Systems." *Philosophical Transactions of the Royal Society of London, Series B* 352 (1997): 1663.

Julia Barrett

Amniocentesis

Definition

Amniocentesis is a procedure used to diagnose fetal defects in the early second trimester of pregnancy. A sample of the amniotic fluid, which surrounds a fetus

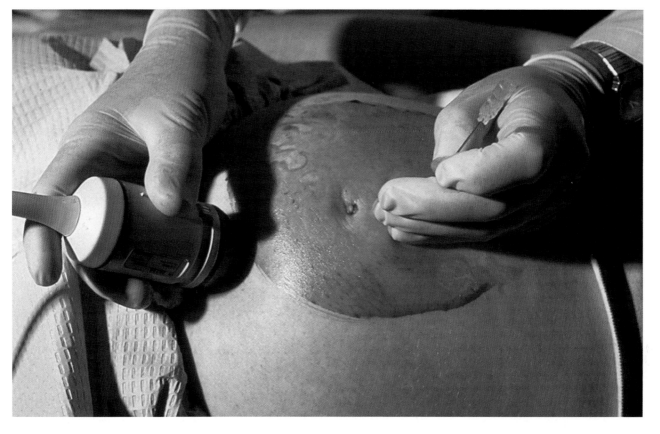

A physician uses an ultrasound monitor (left) to position the needle for insertion into the amnion when performing amniocentesis. *(Photograph by Will and Deni McIntyre, Photo Researchers, Inc. Reproduced by permission.)*

in the womb, is collected through a pregnant woman's abdomen using a needle and syringe. Tests performed on fetal cells found in the sample can reveal the presence of many types of genetic disorders, thus allowing doctors and prospective parents to make important decisions about early treatment and intervention.

Purpose

Since the mid-1970s, amniocentesis has been used routinely to test for **Down syndrome**, by far the most common, nonhereditary, genetic birth defect, afflicting about one in every 1,000 babies. By 1997, approximately 800 different diagnostic tests were available, most of them for hereditary genetic disorders such as Tay-Sachs disease, sickle cell anemia, **hemophilia**, **muscular dystrophy** and **cystic fibrosis**.

Amniocentesis, often called amnio, is recommended for women who will be older than 35 on their due-date. It is also recommended for women who have already borne children with birth defects, or when either of the parents has a family history of a birth defect for which a diagnostic test is available.

Another reason for the procedure is to confirm indications of Down syndrome and certain other defects which may have shown up previously during routine maternal blood screening.

The risk of bearing a child with a nonhereditary genetic defect such as Down syndrome is directly related to a woman's age–the older the woman, the greater the risk. Thirty-five is the recommended age to begin amnio testing because that is the age at which the risk of carrying a fetus with such a defect roughly equals the risk of miscarriage caused by the procedure–about one in 200. At age 25, the risk of giving birth to a child with this type of defect is about one in 1,400; by age 45 it increases to about one in 20. Nearly half of all pregnant women over 35 in the United States undergo amniocentesis and many younger women also decide to have the procedure. Notably, some 75% of all Down syndrome infants born in the United States each year are to women younger than 35.

One of the most common reasons for performing amniocentesis is an abnormal alpha-fetoprotein (AFP) test. Alpha-fetoprotein is a protein produced

KEY TERMS

Alpha-fetoprotein (AFP)—A protein normally produced by the liver of a fetus and detectable in maternal blood samples. AFP screening measures the amount of alpha-fetoprotein in the blood. Levels outside the norm may indicate fetal defects.

Anencephaly—A hereditary defect resulting in the partial to complete absence of a brain and spinal cord. It is fatal.

Chorionic villus sampling (CVS)—A procedure similar to amniocentesis, except that cells are taken from the chorionic membrane for testing. These cells, called chorionic villus cells, eventually become the placenta. The samples are collected either through the abdomen, as in amnio, or through the vagina. CVS can be done earlier in the pregnancy than amnio, but carries a somewhat higher risk.

Chromosome—Chromosomes are the strands of genetic material in a cell that occur in nearly identical pairs. Normal human cells contain 23 chromosome pairs—one in each pair inherited from the mother, and one from the father. Every human cell contains the exact same set of chromosomes.

Down syndrome—The most prevalent of a class of genetic defects known as trisomies, in which cells contain three copies of certain chromosomes rather than the usual two. Down syndrome, or trisomy 21, usually results from three copies of chromosome 21.

Genetic—The term refers to genes, the basic units of biological heredity, which are contained on the chromosomes, and contain chemical instructions which direct the development and functioning of an individual.

Hereditary—Something which is inherited–passed down from parents to offspring. In biology and medicine, the word pertains to inherited genetic characteristics.

Maternal blood screening—Maternal blood screening is normally done early in pregnancy to test for a variety of conditions. Abnormal amounts of certain proteins in a pregnant woman's blood raise the probability of fetal defects. Amniocentesis is recommended if such a probability occurs.

Tay-Sachs disease—An inherited disease prevalent among the Ashkenazi Jewish population of the United States. Infants with the disease are unable to process a certain type of fat which accumulates in nerve and brain cells, causing mental and physical retardation, and death by age four.

Ultrasound—A technique which uses high-frequency sound waves to create a visual image (a sonogram) of soft tissues. The technique is routinely used in prenatal care and diagnosis.

by the fetus and present in the mother's blood. A simple blood screening, usually conducted around the 15th week of pregnancy, can determine the AFP levels in the mother's blood. Levels that are too high or too low may signal possible fetal defects. Because this test has a high false-positive rate, another test such as amnio is recommended whenever the AFP levels fall outside the normal range.

Amniocentesis is generally performed during the 16th week of **pregnancy**, with results usually available within three weeks. It is possible to perform an amnio as early as the 11th week but this is not usually recommended because there appears to be an increased risk of miscarriage when done at this time. The advantage of early amnio and speedy results lies in the extra time for decision making if a problem is detected. Potential treatment of the fetus can begin earlier. Important, also, is the fact that elective abortions are safer and less controversial the earlier they are performed.

Precautions

As an invasive surgical procedure, amnio poses a real, although small, risk to the health of a fetus. Parents must weigh the potential value of the knowledge gained, or indeed the reassurance that all is well, against the small risk of damaging what is in all probability a normal fetus. The serious emotional and ethical dilemmas that adverse test results can bring must also be considered. The decision to undergo amnio is always a matter of personal choice.

Description

The word amniocentesis literally means "puncture of the amnion," the thin-walled sac of fluid in which a developing fetus is suspended during pregnancy. During the sampling procedure, the obstetrician inserts a very fine needle through the woman's abdomen into the uterus and amniotic sac and withdraws approximately one ounce of amniotic fluid for testing. The relatively painless procedure is performed on an outpatient basis, sometimes using **local anesthesia**.

The physician uses ultrasound images to guide needle placement and collect the sample, thereby minimizing the risk of fetal injury and the need for repeated needle insertions. Once the sample is collected, the woman can return home after a brief observation period. She may be instructed to rest for the first 24 hours and to avoid heavy lifting for two days.

The sample of amniotic fluid is sent to a laboratory where fetal cells contained in the fluid are isolated and grown in order to provide enough genetic material for testing. This takes about seven to 14 days. The material is then extracted and treated so that visual examination for defects can be made. For some disorders, like Tay-Sachs, the simple presence of a telltale chemical compound in the amniotic fluid is enough to confirm a diagnosis. Depending on the specific tests ordered, and the skill of the lab conducting them, all the results are available between one and four weeks after the sample is taken.

Cost of the procedure depends on the doctor, the lab, and the tests ordered. Most insurers provide coverage for women over 35, as a follow-up to positive maternal blood screening results, and when genetic disorders run in the family.

An alternative to amnio, now in general use, is chorionic villus sampling, or CVS, which can be performed as early as the eighth week of pregnancy. While this allows for the possibility of a first trimester abortion, if warranted, CVS is apparently also riskier and is more expensive. The most promising area of new research in prenatal testing involves expanding the scope and accuracy of maternal blood screening as this poses no risk to the fetus.

Preparation

It is important for a woman to fully understand the procedure and to feel confident in the obstetrician performing it. Evidence suggests that a physician's experience with the procedure reduces the chance of mishap. Almost all obstetricians are experienced in performing amniocentesis. The patient should feel free to ask questions and seek emotional support before, during and after the amnio is performed.

Aftercare

Necessary aftercare falls into two categories, physical and emotional.

Physical aftercare

During and immediately following the sampling procedure, a woman may experience dizziness, **nausea**, a rapid heartbeat, and cramping. Once past these immediate hurdles, the physician will send the woman home with instructions to rest and to report any complications requiring immediate treatment, including:

- vaginal bleeding. The appearance of blood could signal a problem.

- **premature labor**. Unusual abdominal **pain** and/or cramping may indicate the onset of premature labor. Mild cramping for the first day or two following the procedure is normal.

- signs of infection. Leaking of amniotic fluid or unusual vaginal discharge, and **fever** could signal the onset of infection.

Emotional aftercare

Once the procedure has been safely completed, the anxiety of waiting for the test results can prove to be the worst part of the process. A woman should seek and receive emotional support from family and friends, as well as from her obstetrician and family doctor. Professional counseling may also prove necessary, particularly if a fetal defect is discovered.

Risks

Most of the risks and short-term side effects associated with amniocentesis relate to the sampling procedure and have been discussed above. A successful amnio sampling results in no long-term side effects. Risks include:

- maternal/fetal hemorrhaging. While spotting in pregnancy is fairly common, bleeding following amnio should always be investigated.

- infection. Infection, although rare, can occur after amniocentesis. An unchecked infection can lead to severe complications.

- fetal injury. A very slight risk of injury to the fetus resulting from contact with the amnio needle does exist.

- **miscarriage**. The rate of miscarriage occurring during standard, second trimester amnio appears to be approximately 0.5%. This compares to a miscarriage rate of 1% for CVS. Many fetuses with severe genetic defects miscarry naturally during the first trimester.

- the trauma of difficult family-planning decisions. The threat posed to parental and family mental health from the trauma accompanying an abnormal test result can not be underestimated.

Normal results

Negative results from an amnio analysis indicate that everything about the fetus appears normal and the pregnancy can continue without undue concern. A negative result for Down syndrome means that it is 99% certain that the disease does not exist.

An overall "normal" result does not, however, guarantee that the pregnancy will come to term, or that the fetus does not suffer from some other defect. Laboratory tests are not 100% accurate at detecting targeted conditions, nor can every possible fetal condition be tested for.

Abnormal results

Positive results on an amnio analysis indicate the presence of the fetal defect being tested for, with an accuracy approaching 100%. Prospective parents are then faced with emotionally and ethically difficult choices regarding treatment options, the prospect of dealing with a severely affected newborn, and the option of elective abortion. At this point, the parents need expert medical advice and counseling.

Resources

PERIODICALS

Dreisbach, Shaun. "Amnio Alternative." *Working Mother* (March 1997): 11.

ORGANIZATIONS

American College of Obstetricians and Gynecologists. 409 12th St., S.W., P.O. Box 96920, Washington, DC 20090-6920. < http://www.acog.org >.

OTHER

Holbrook Jr., Harold R. Stanford University School of MedicineWeb Home Page. February 2001. < http://www.stanford.edu/-holbrook >.

Kurt Richard Sternlof

Amniotic fluid analysis *see* **Amniocentesis**

Amoxicillin *see* **Penicillins**

Amphetamines *see* **Central nervous system stimulants**

Amphotericin B *see* **Antifungal drugs, systemic**

Amputation

Definition

Amputation is the intentional surgical removal of a limb or body part. It is performed to remove diseased tissue or relieve **pain**.

Purpose

Arms, legs, hands, feet, fingers, and toes can be amputated. Most amputations involve small body parts such as a finger, rather than an entire limb. About 65,000 amputations are performed in the United States each year.

Amputation is performed for the following reasons:

- to remove tissue that no longer has an adequate blood supply
- to remove malignant tumors
- because of severe trauma to the body part

The blood supply to an extremity can be cut off because of injury to the blood vessel, hardening of the arteries, **arterial embolism**, impaired circulation as a complication of **diabetes mellitus**, repeated severe infection that leads to **gangrene**, severe **frostbite**, **Raynaud's disease**, or Buerger's disease.

More than 90% of amputations performed in the United States are due to circulatory complications of diabetes. Sixty to eighty percent of these operations involve the legs or feet. Although attempts have been made in the United States to better manage diabetes and the foot ulcers that can be complications of the disease, the number of resulting amputations has not decreased.

Precautions

Amputations cannot be performed on patients with uncontrolled diabetes mellitus, heart failure, or infection. Patients with blood clotting disorders are also not good candidates for amputation.

Description

Amputations can be either planned or emergency procedures. Injury and arterial embolisms are the main reasons for emergency amputations. The operation is performed under regional or general anesthesia by a general or orthopedic surgeon in a hospital operating room.

Details of the operation vary slightly depending on what part is to be removed. The goal of all

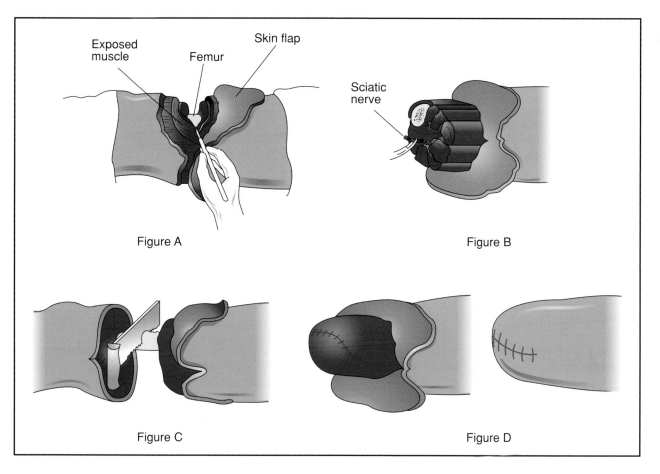

Amputation of leg. Figure A: After the surgeon creates two flaps of skin and tissue, the muscle is cut and the main artery and veins of the femur bone are exposed. Figure B: The surgeon severs the main artery and veins. New connections are formed between them, restoring blood circulation. The sciatic nerve is then pulled down, clamped and tied, and severed. Figure C: The surgeon saws through the exposed femur bone. Figure D: The muscles are closed and sutured over the bone. The remaining skin flaps are then sutured together, creating a stump. *(Illustration by Electronic Illustrators Group.)*

amputations is twofold: to remove diseased tissue so that the wound will heal cleanly, and to construct a stump that will allow the attachment of a prosthesis or artificial replacement part.

The surgeon makes an incision around the part to be amputated. The part is removed, and the bone is smoothed. A flap is constructed of muscle, connective tissue, and skin to cover the raw end of the bone. The flap is closed over the bone with sutures (surgical stitches) that remain in place for about one month. Often, a rigid dressing or cast is applied that stays in place for about two weeks.

Preparation

Before an amputation is performed, extensive testing is done to determine the proper level of amputation. The goal of the surgeon is to find the place where healing is most likely to be complete, while allowing the maximum amount of limb to remain for effective **rehabilitation**.

The greater the blood flow through an area, the more likely healing is to occur. These tests are designed to measure blood flow through the limb. Several or all of them can be done to help choose the proper level of amputation.

- measurement of blood pressure in different parts of the limb

- xenon 133 studies, which use a radiopharmaceutical to measure blood flow

- oxygen tension measurements in which an oxygen electrode is used to measure oxygen pressure under the skin. If the pressure is 0, the healing will not occur. If the

KEY TERMS

Arterial embolism—A blood clot arising from another location that blocks an artery.

Buerger's disease—An episodic disease that causes inflammation and blockage of the veins and arteries of the limbs. It tends to be present almost exclusively on men under age 40 who smoke, and may require amputation of the hand or foot.

Diabetes mellitus—A disease in which insufficient insulin is made by the body to metabolize sugars.

Raynaud's disease—A disease found mainly in young women that causes decreased circulation to the hands and feet. Its cause is unknown.

pressure reads higher than 40mm Hg (40 milliliters of mercury), healing of the area is likely to be satisfactory.

- laser Doppler measurements of the microcirculation of the skin
- skin fluorescent studies that also measure skin microcirculation
- skin perfusion measurements using a blood pressure cuff and photoelectric detector
- infrared measurements of skin temperature

No single test is highly predictive of healing, but taken together, the results give the surgeon an excellent idea of the best place to amputate.

Aftercare

After amputation, medication is prescribed for pain, and patients are treated with antibiotics to discourage infection. The stump is moved often to encourage good circulation. Physical therapy and rehabilitation are started as soon as possible, usually within 48 hours. Studies have shown that there is a positive relationship between early rehabilitation and effective functioning of the stump and prosthesis. Length of stay in the hospital depends on the severity of the amputation and the general health of the amputee, but ranges from several days to two weeks.

Rehabilitation is a long, arduous process, especially for above the knee amputees. Twice daily physical therapy is not uncommon. In addition, psychological counseling is an important part of rehabilitation.

Many people feel a sense of loss and grief when they lose a body part. Others are bothered by phantom limb syndrome, where they feel as if the amputated part is still in place. They may even feel pain in the limb that does not exist. Many amputees benefit from joining self-help groups and meeting others who are also living with amputation. Addressing the emotional aspects of amputation often speeds the physical rehabilitation process.

Risks

Amputation is major surgery. All the risks associated with the administration of anesthesia exist, along with the possibility of heavy blood loss and the development of **blood clots**. Infection is of special concern to amputees. Infection rates in amputations average 15%. If the stump becomes infected, it is necessary to remove the prosthesis and sometimes to amputate a second time at a higher level.

Failure of the stump to heal is another major complication. Nonhealing is usually due to an inadequate blood supply. The rate of nonhealing varies from 5-30% depending on the facility. Centers that specialize in amputation usually have the lowest rates of complication.

Persistent pain in the stump or pain in the phantom limb is experienced by most amputees to some degree. Treatment of phantom limb pain is difficult. Finally, many amputees give up on the rehabilitation process and discard their prosthesis. Better fitting prosthetics and earlier rehabilitation have decreased the incidence of this problem. Researchers and prosthetic manufacturers continue to refine the materials and methods used to try to improve the comfort and function of prosthetic devices for amputees. For example, a 2004 study showed that a technique called the bone bridge amputation technique helped improve comfort and stability for transtibial amputees.

Normal results

The five-year survival rate for all lower extremity amputees is less than 50%. For diabetic amputees, the rate is less than 40%. Up to 50% of people who have one leg amputated because of diabetes will lose the other within five years. Amputees who walk using a prosthesis have a less stable gait. Three to five percent of these people fall and break bones because of this instability. Although the **fractures** can be treated, about one-half of amputees who suffer them then remain wheelchair bound.

Resources

PERIODICALS

Edwards, Anthony R. "Study Helps Build Functional Bridges for Amputee Patients." *Biomechanics* (May 1, 2004): 17.

Jeffcoat, William. "Incidence of Amputation is a Poor Measure of the Quality of Ulcer Care." *The Diabetic Foot* Summer (2004): 70–74.

ORGANIZATIONS

American Diabetes Association. 1701 North Beauregard Street, Alexandria, VA 22311. (800) 342-2383. < http://www.diabetes.org >.

OTHER

Amputation Prevention Global Resource Center Page. February 2001. < http://www.diabetesresource.com >.

Tish Davidson, A.M.
Teresa G. Odle

Amylase tests

Definition

Amylase is a digestive enzyme made primarily by the pancreas and salivary glands. Enzymes are substances made and used by the body to trigger specific chemical reactions. The primary function of the enzyme amylase is to break down starches in food so that they can be used by the body. Amylase testing is usually done to determine the cause of sudden abdominal pain.

Purpose

Amylase testing is performed to diagnose a number of diseases that elevate amylase levels. Pancreatitis, for example, is the most common reason for a high amylase level. When the pancreas is inflamed, amylase escapes from the pancreas into the blood. Within six to 48 hours after the **pain** begins, amylase levels in the blood start to rise. Levels will stay high for several days before gradually returning to normal.

There are other causes of increased amylase. An ulcer that erodes tissue from the stomach and goes into the pancreas will cause amylase to spill into the blood. During a **mumps** infection, amylase from the inflamed salivary glands increases. Amylase is also found in the liver, fallopian tubes, and small intestine; inflammation of these tissues also increases levels. Gall bladder disease, tumors of the lung or ovaries, alcohol poisoning, ruptured aortic aneurysm, and intestinal

KEY TERMS

Amylase—A digestive enzyme made primarily by the pancreas and salivary glands.

Enzyme—A substance made and used by the body to trigger specific chemical reactions.

Pancreatitis—Inflammation of the pancreas.

strangulation or perforation can also cause unusually high amylase levels.

Precautions

This is not a screening test for future pancreatic disease.

Description

Amylase testing is done on both blood and urine. The laboratory may use any of several testing methods that involve mixing the blood or urine sample with a substance with which amylase is known to react. By measuring the end-product or the reaction time, technicians can calculate the amount of amylase present in the sample. More sophisticated methods separately measure the amylase made by the pancreas and the amylase made by the salivary glands.

Urine testing is a better long-term monitor of amylase levels. The kidneys quickly move extra amylase from the blood into the urine. Urine levels rise six to 10 hours after blood levels and stay high longer. Urine is usually collected throughout a 2- or 24-hour time period. Results are usually available the same day.

Preparation

In most cases, no special preparation is necessary for a person undergoing an amylase blood test. Patients taking longer term urine amylase tests will be given a container and instructions for collecting the urine at home. The urine should be refrigerated until it is brought to the laboratory.

Aftercare

Discomfort or bruising may occur at the puncture site or the person may feel dizzy or faint. Pressure to the puncture site until the bleeding stops reduces bruising. Applying warm packs to the puncture site relieves discomfort.

Normal results

Normal results vary based on the laboratory and the method used.

Abnormal results

Eight out of ten persons with acute **pancreatitis** will have high amylase levels, up to four times the normal level. Other causes of increased amylase, such as mumps, kidney failure, pregnancy occurring in the abdomen but outside the uterus (ectopic **pregnancy**), certain tumors, a penetrating ulcer, certain complications of diabetes, and advanced pancreatic **cancer**, are further investigated based on the person's symptoms, medical history, and the results of other tests.

In **kidney disease**, the kidneys are not as efficient at removing amylase from the blood. Amylase rises in the blood, but stays at normal levels in the urine.

People with macroamylasia have large clumps of amylase in their blood. These clumps are too large to move through the kidney, so they stay in the blood. Amylase levels in the blood will be high; levels in the urine will be low.

Amylase levels may be low in severe **liver disease** (including hepatitis), conditions in which the pancreas fails to secrete enough enzyme for proper digestions (pancreatic insufficiency), when toxic materials build up in the blood during pregnancy (pre-eclampsia), following burns, in thyroid disorders, and in advanced **cystic fibrosis**. Some medications can raise or lower levels.

Resources

BOOKS

Pagana, Kathleen Deska. *Mosby's Manual of Diagnosticand Laboratory Tests.* St. Louis: Mosby, Inc., 1998.

Nancy J. Nordenson

Amyloidosis

Definition

Amyloidosis is a progressive, incurable, metabolic disease characterized by abnormal deposits of protein in one or more organs or body systems.

Description

Amyloid proteins are manufactured by malfunctioning bone marrow. Amyloidosis, which occurs when accumulated amyloid deposits impair normal body function, can cause organ failure or **death**. It is a rare disease, occurring in about eight of every 1,000,000 people. It affects males and females equally and usually develops after the age of 40. At least 15 types of amyloidosis have been identified. Each one is associated with deposits of a different kind of protein.

Types of amyloidosis

The major forms of this disease are primary systemic, secondary, and familial or hereditary amyloidosis. There is also another form of amyloidosis associated with **Alzheimer's disease**.

Primary systemic amyloidosis usually develops between the ages of 50 and 60. With about 2,000 new cases diagnosed annually, primary systemic amyloidosis is the most common form of this disease in the United States. Also known as light-chain-related amyloidosis, it may also occur in association with **multiple myeloma** (bone marrow **cancer**).

Secondary amyloidosis is a result of chronic infection or inflammatory disease. It is often associated with:

- familial Mediterranean **fever** (a bacterial infection characterized by chills, weakness, **headache**, and recurring fever)
- granulomatous ileitis (inflammation of the small intestine)
- Hodgkin's disease (cancer of the lymphatic system)
- leprosy
- osteomyelitits (bacterial infection of bone and bone marrow)
- rheumatoid arthritis

Familial or hereditary amyloidosis is the only inherited form of the disease. It occurs in members of most ethnic groups, and each family has a distinctive pattern of symptoms and organ involvement. Hereditary amyloidosis is though to be autosomal dominant, which means that only one copy of the defective gene is necessary to cause the disease. A child of a parent with familial amyloidosis has a 50-50 chance of developing the disease.

Amyloidosis can involve any organ or system in the body. The heart, kidneys, gastrointestinal system, and nervous system are affected most often. Other

KEY TERMS

Amyloid—A waxy, starch-like protein.

Peripheral nerves—Nerves that carry information to and from the spinal cord.

Stem cells—Parent cells from which other cells are made.

common sites of amyloid accumulation include the brain, joints, liver, spleen, pancreas, respiratory system, and skin.

Causes and symptoms

The cause of amyloidosis is unknown. Most patients have gastrointestinal abnormalities, but other symptoms vary according to the organ(s) or system(s) affected by the disease. Usually the affected organs are rubbery, firm, and enlarged.

Heart

Because amyloid protein deposits can limit the heart's ability to fill with blood between beats, even the slightest exertion can cause **shortness of breath**. If the heart's electrical system is affected, the heart's rhythm may become erratic. The heart may also be enlarged and **heart murmurs** may be present. Congestive heart failure may result.

Kidneys

The feet, ankles, and calves swell when amyloidosis damages the kidneys. The kidneys become small and hard, and kidney failure may result. It is not unusual for a patient to lose 20-25 pounds and develop a distaste for meat, eggs, and other protein-rich foods. Cholesterol elevations that don't respond to medication and protein in the urine (proteinuria) are common.

Nervous system

Nervous system symptoms often appear in patients with familial amyloidosis. Inflammation and degeneration of the peripheral nerves (peripheral neuropathy) may be present. One of four patients with amyloidosis has carpal tunnel syndrome, a painful disorder that causes **numbness** or **tingling** in response to pressure on nerves around the wrist. Amyloidosis that affects nerves to the feet can cause burning or numbness in the toes and soles and eventually weaken

the legs. If nerves controlling bowel function are involved, bouts of **diarrhea** alternate with periods of constipation. If the disease affects nerves that regulate blood pressure, patients may feel dizzy or faint when they stand up suddenly.

Liver and spleen

The most common symptoms are enlargement of these organs. Liver function is not usually affected until quite late in the course of the disease. Protein accumulation in the spleen can increase the risk of rupture of this organ due to trauma.

Gastrointestinal system

The tongue may be inflamed, enlarged, and stiff. Intestinal movement (motility) may be reduced. Absorption of food and other nutrients may be impaired (and may lead to **malnutrition**), and there may also be bleeding, abdominal **pain**, **constipation**, and diarrhea.

Skin

Skin symptoms occur in about half of all cases of primary and secondary amyloidosis and in all cases where there is inflammation or degeneration of the peripheral nerves. Waxy-looking raised bumps (papules) may appear on the face and neck, in the groin, armpits, or anal area, and on the tongue or in the ear canals. Swelling, hemorrhage beneath the skin (purpura), hair loss, and dry mouth may also occur.

Respiratory system

Airways may be obstructed by amyloid deposits in the nasal sinus, larynx and traches (windpipe).

Diagnosis

Blood and urine tests can reveal the presence of amyloid protein, but tissue or bone-marrow biopsy is necessary to positively diagnose amyloidosis. Once the diagnosis has been confirmed, additional laboratory tests and imaging procedures are performed to determine:

- which type of amyloid protein is involved
- which organ(s) or system(s) have been affected
- how far the disease has progressed

Treatment

The goal of treatment is to slow down or stop production of amyloid protein, eliminate existing amyloid deposits, alleviate underlying disorders (that give rise to secondary amyloidosis), and relieve symptoms caused by heart or kidney damage. Specialists in cardiology, hematology (the study of blood and the tissues that form it), nephrology (the study of kidney function and abnormalities), neurology (the study of the nervous system), and rheumatology (the study of disorders characterized by inflammation or degeneration of connective tissue) work together to assess a patient's medical status and evaluate the effects of amyloidosis on every part of the body.

Colchicine (Colebenemid, Probeneaid), prednisone, (Prodium), and other anti-inflammatory drugs can slow or stop disease progression. Bone-marrow and stem-cell transplants can enable patients to tolerate higher and more effective doses of melphalan (Alkeran) and other **chemotherapy** drugs prescribed to combat this non-malignant disease. Surgery can relieve nerve pressure and may be performed to correct other symptom-producing conditions. Localized amyloid deposits can also be removed surgically. Dialysis or **kidney transplantation** can lengthen and improve the quality of life for patients whose amyloidosis results in kidney failure. Heart transplants are rarely performed.

Supportive measures

Although no link has been established between diet and development of amyloid proteins, a patient whose heart or kidneys have been affected by the disease may be advised to use a diuretic or follow a low-salt diet.

Prognosis

Most cases of amyloidosis are diagnosed after the disease has reached an advanced stage. The course of each patient's illness is unique but death, usually a result of heart disease or kidney failure, generally occurs within a few years. Amyloidosis associated by multiple myeloma usually has a poor prognosis. Most patients with both diseases die within one to two years.

Prevention

Genetic couseling may be helpful for patients with hereditary amyloidosis and their families. Use of Cholchicine in patients with familial Mediterranean fever has successfully prevented amyloidosis.

Resources

ORGANIZATIONS

Amyloidosis Network International. 7118 Cole Creek Drive, Houston, TX 77092-1421. (888) 1AMYLOID. < http://www.health.gov/nhic/Scripts/ Entry.cfm?HRCode = HR2397 > .

National Organization for Rare Disorders. P.O. Box 8923, New Fairfield, CT 06812-8923. (800) 999-6673. < http://www.rarediseases.org > .

Maureen Haggerty

Amyotrophic lateral sclerosis

Definition

Amyotrophic lateral sclerosis (ALS) is a disease that breaks down tissues in the nervous system (a neurodegenerative disease) of unknown cause that affects the nerves responsible for movement. It is also known as motor neuron disease and Lou Gehrig's disease, after the baseball player whose career it ended.

Description

ALS is a disease of the motor neurons, those nerve cells reaching from the brain to the spinal cord (upper motor neurons) and the spinal cord to the peripheral nerves (lower motor neurons) that control muscle movement. In ALS, for unknown reasons, these neurons die, leading to a progressive loss of the ability to move virtually any of the muscles in the body. ALS affects "voluntary" muscles, those controlled by conscious thought, such as the arm, leg, and trunk muscles. ALS, in and of itself, does not affect sensation, thought processes, the heart muscle, or the "smooth" muscle of the digestive system, bladder, and other internal organs. Most people with ALS retain function of their eye muscles as well. However, various forms of ALS may be associated with a loss of intellectual function (**dementia**) or sensory symptoms.

ALS progresses rapidly in most cases. It is fatal within three years for 50% of all people affected, and within five years for 80%. Ten percent of people with ALS live beyond eight years.

Causes and symptoms

Causes

The symptoms of ALS are caused by the death of motor neurons in the spinal cord and brain. Normally,

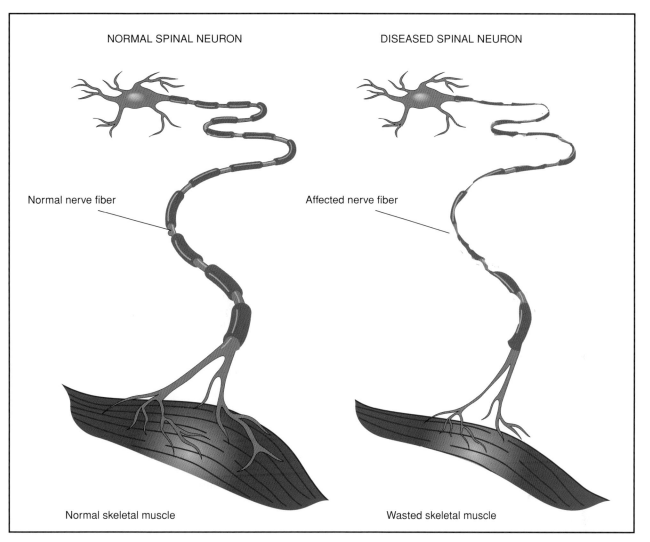

NORMAL SPINAL NEURON   DISEASED SPINAL NEURON

Normal nerve fiber   Affected nerve fiber

Normal skeletal muscle   Wasted skeletal muscle

Amyotrophic lateral sclerosis (ALS) is caused by the degeneration and death of motor neurons in the spinal cord and brain. These neurons convey electrical messages from the brain to the muscles to stimulate movement in the arms, legs, trunk, neck, and head. As motor neurons degenerate, the muscles are weakened and cannot move as effectively, leading to muscle wasting. *(Illustration by Electronic Illustrators Group.)*

these neurons convey electrical messages from the brain to the muscles to stimulate movement in the arms, legs, trunk, neck, and head. As motor neurons die, the muscles they enervate cannot be moved as effectively, and weakness results. In addition, lack of stimulation leads to muscle wasting, or loss of bulk. Involvement of the upper motor neurons causes spasms and increased tone in the limbs, and abnormal reflexes. Involvement of the lower motor neurons causes muscle wasting and twitching (fasciculations).

Although many causes of motor neuron degeneration have been suggested for ALS, none has yet been proven responsible. Results of recent research have implicated toxic molecular fragments known as free radicals. Some evidence suggests that a cascade of events leads to excess free radical production inside motor neurons, leading to their death. Why free radicals should be produced in excess amounts is unclear, as is whether this excess is the cause or the effect of other degenerative processes. Additional agents within this toxic cascade may include excessive levels of a neurotransmitter known as glutamate, which may over-stimulate motor neurons, thereby increasing free-radical production, and a faulty detoxification enzyme known as SOD-1, for superoxide dismutase type 1. The actual pathway of destruction is not

KEY TERMS

Aspiration—Inhalation of food or liquids into the lungs.

Bulbar muscles—Muscles of the mouth and throat responsible for speech and swallowing.

Fasciculations—Involuntary twitching of muscles.

Motor neuron—A nerve cell that controls a muscle.

Riluzole (Rilutek)—The first drug approved in the United States for the treatment of ALS.

Voluntary muscle—A muscle under conscious control; contrasted with smooth muscle and heart muscle which are not under voluntary control.

known, however, nor is the trigger for the rapid degeneration that marks ALS. Further research may show that other pathways are involved, perhaps ones even more important than this one. Autoimmune factors or premature **aging** may play some role, as could viral agents or environmental toxins.

Two major forms of ALS are known: familial and sporadic. Familial ALS accounts for about 10% of all ALS cases. As the name suggests, familial ALS is believed to be caused by the inheritance of one or more faulty genes. About 15% of families with this type of ALS have mutations in the gene for SOD-1. SOD-1 gene defects are dominant, meaning only one gene copy is needed to develop the disease. Therefore, a parent with the faulty gene has a 50% chance of passing the gene along to a child.

Sporadic ALS has no known cause. While many environmental toxins have been suggested as causes, to date no research has confirmed any of the candidates investigated, including aluminum and mercury and lead from dental fillings. As research progresses, it is likely that many cases of sporadic ALS will be shown to have a genetic basis as well.

A third type, called Western Pacific ALS, occurs in Guam and other Pacific islands. This form combines symptoms of both ALS and Parkinson's disease.

Symptoms

The earliest sign of ALS is most often weakness in the arms or legs, usually more pronounced on one side than the other at first. Loss of function is usually more rapid in the legs among people with familial ALS and in the arms among those with sporadic ALS. Leg weakness may first become apparent by an increased frequency of stumbling on uneven pavement, or an unexplained difficulty climbing stairs. Arm weakness may lead to difficulty grasping and holding a cup, for instance, or loss of dexterity in the fingers.

Less often, the earliest sign of ALS is weakness in the *bulbar* muscles, those muscles in the mouth and throat that control chewing, swallowing, and speaking. A person with bulbar weakness may become hoarse or tired after speaking at length, or speech may become slurred.

In addition to weakness, the other cardinal signs of ALS are muscle wasting and persistent twitching (fasciculation). These are usually seen after weakness becomes obvious. Fasciculation is quite common in people without the disease, and is virtually never the first sign of ALS.

While initial weakness may be limited to one region, ALS almost always progresses rapidly to involve virtually all the voluntary muscle groups in the body. Later symptoms include loss of the ability to walk, to use the arms and hands, to speak clearly or at all, to swallow, and to hold the head up. Weakness of the respiratory muscles makes breathing and coughing difficult, and poor swallowing control increases the likelihood of inhaling food or saliva (aspiration). Aspiration increases the likelihood of lung infection, which is often the cause of death. With a ventilator and scrupulous bronchial hygiene, a person with ALS may live much longer than the average, although weakness and wasting will continue to erode any remaining functional abilities. Most people with ALS continue to retain function of the extraocular muscles that move their eyes, allowing some communication to take place with simple blinks or through use of a computer-assisted device.

Diagnosis

The diagnosis of ALS begins with a complete medical history and physical exam, plus a neurological examination to determine the distribution and extent of weakness. An electrical test of muscle function, called an electromyogram, or EMG, is an important part of the diagnostic process. Various other tests, including blood and urine tests, x rays, and CT scans, may be done to rule out other possible causes of the symptoms, such as tumors of the skull base or high cervical spinal cord, thyroid disease, spinal arthritis, **lead poisoning**, or severe vitamin deficiency. ALS is rarely misdiagnosed following a careful review of all these factors.

Treatment

There is no cure for ALS, and no treatment that can significantly alter its course. There are many things which can be done, however, to help maintain quality of life and to retain functional ability even in the face of progressive weakness.

As of the early 2000s, only one drug had been approved for treatment of ALS. Riluzole (Rilutek) appears to provide on average a three-month increase in life expectancy when taken regularly early in the disease, and shows a significant slowing of the loss of muscle strength. Riluzole acts by decreasing glutamate release from nerve terminals. Experimental trials of nerve growth factor have not demonstrated any benefit. No other drug or vitamin currently available has been shown to have any effect on the course of ALS.

A physical therapist works with an affected person and family to implement **exercise** and stretching programs to maintain strength and range of motion, and to promote general health. Swimming may be a good choice for people with ALS, as it provides a low-impact workout to most muscle groups. One result of chronic inactivity is contracture, or muscle shortening. **Contractures** limit a person's range of motion, and are often painful. Regular stretching can prevent contracture. Several drugs are available to reduce cramping, a common complaint in ALS.

An occupational therapist can help design solutions to movement and coordination problems, and provide advice on adaptive devices and home modifications.

Speech and swallowing difficulties can be minimized or delayed through training provided by a speech-language pathologist. This specialist can also provide advice on communication aids, including computer-assisted devices and simpler word boards.

Nutritional advice can be provided by a nutritionist. A person with ALS often needs softer foods to prevent jaw exhaustion or **choking**. Later in the disease, nutrition may be provided by a **gastrostomy** tube inserted into the stomach.

Mechanical ventilation may be used when breathing becomes too difficult. Modern mechanical ventilators are small and portable, allowing a person with ALS to maintain the maximum level of function and mobility. Ventilation may be administered through a mouth or nose piece, or through a tracheostomy tube. This tube is inserted through a small hole made in the windpipe. In addition to providing direct access to the airway, the tube also decreases the risk aspiration. While many people with rapidly progressing ALS choose not to use ventilators for lengthy periods, they are increasingly being used to prolong life for a short time.

The progressive nature of ALS means that most persons will eventually require full-time nursing care. This care is often provided by a spouse or other family member. While the skills involved are not difficult to learn, the physical and emotional burden of care can be overwhelming. Caregivers need to recognize and provide for their own needs as well as those of people with ALS, to prevent depression, burnout, and bitterness.

Throughout the disease, a support group can provide important psychological aid to affected persons and their caregivers as they come to terms with the losses ALS inflicts. Support groups are sponsored by both the ALS Society and the Muscular Dystrophy Association.

Alternative treatment

Given the grave prognosis and absence of traditional medical treatments, it is not surprising that a large number of alternative treatments have been tried for ALS. Two studies published in 1988 suggested that amino-acid therapies may provide some improvement for some people with ALS. While individual reports claim benefits for megavitamin therapy, herbal medicine, and removal of dental fillings, for instance, no evidence suggests that these offer any more than a brief psychological boost, often followed by a more severe letdown when it becomes apparent the disease has continued unabated. However, once the causes of ALS are better understood, alternative therapies may be more intensively studied. For example, if damage by free radicals turns out to be the root of most of the symptoms, antioxidant **vitamins** and supplements may be used more routinely to slow the progression of ALS. Or, if environmental toxins are implicated, alternative therapies with the goal of detoxifying the body may be of some use.

Prognosis

ALS usually progresses rapidly, and leads to death from respiratory infection within three to five years in most cases. The slowest disease progression is seen in those who are young and have their first symptoms in the limbs. About 10% of people with ALS live longer than eight years.

Prevention

There is no known way to prevent ALS or to alter its course.

Resources

BOOKS

Feldman, Eva L. "Motor neuron diseases." In *Cecil Textbook of Medicine,* edited by Lee Goldman and J. Claude Bennett, 21st ed. Philadelphia: W.B. Saunders, 2000, pp. 2089-2092.

PERIODICALS

Ansevin CF. "Treatment of ALS with pleconaril." *Neurology* 56, no. 5 (2001): 691-692.

Eisen, A., and M. Weber. "The motor cortex and amyotrophiclateral sclerosis." *Muscle and Nerve* 24, no. 4 (2001): 564-573.

Gelanis DF. "Respiratory Failure or Impairment in Amyotrophic Lateral Sclerosis." *Current treatment options in neurology* 3, no. 2 (2001): 133-138.

Ludolph AC. "Treatment of amyotrophic lateral sclerosis–what is the next step?" *Journal of Neurology* 246, Supplement 6 (2000): 13-18.

Pasetti, C., and G. Zanini. "The physician-patient relationship inamyotrophic lateral sclerosis." *Neurological Science* 21, no. 5 (2000): 318-323.

Robberecht W. "Genetics of amyotrophic lateral sclerosis." *Journal of Neurology* 246, Supplement 6 (2000): 2-6.

Robbins, R.A., Z. Simmons, B.A. Bremer, S.M. Walsh, and S. Fischer. "Quality of life in ALS is maintained as physical function declines." *Neurology* 56, no. 4 (2001): 442-444.

ORGANIZATIONS

American Medical Association. 515 N. State Street, Chicago, IL 60610. (312) 464-5000. < http://www.ama-assn.org/ > .

Muscular Dystrophy Association. 3300 East Sunrise Drive, Tucson AZ 85718-3208. (520) 529-2000 or (800) 572-1717. < http://www.mdausa.org > .

OTHER

ALS Society of Canada. < http://www.als.ca/ > .

ALS Survival Guide. < http://www.lougehrigsdisease.net/ > .

American Academy of Family Physicians. < http://www.aafp.org/afp/990315ap/1489.html > .

National Institute of Neurological Disorders and Stroke. < http://www.ninds.nih.gov/health_and_medical/disorders/amyotrophiclateralsclerosis_doc.htm > .

National Library of Medicine. < http://www.nlm.nih.gov/medlineplus/amyotrophiclateralsclerosis.html > .

National Organization for Rare Diseases. < http://www.stepstn.com/cgi-win/nord.exe?proc = Redirect&type = rdb_sum&id = 57.htm > .

World Federation of Neurology. < http://www.wfnals.org/ > .

L. Fleming Fallon, Jr., MD, DrPH

▌Anabolic steroid use

Definition

Anabolic steroids are drugs containing hormones, or hormone-like substances, that are used to increase strength and promote muscle growth.

Description

Steroids are a synthetic version of the human hormone called testosterone. Testosterone stimulates and maintains the male sexual organs. It also stimulates development of bones and muscle, promotes skin and hair growth, and can influence emotions and energy levels. In males, testosterone is produced by the testicles and the adrenal gland. Women have only the amount of testosterone produced by the adrenal gland—much less than men have. This is why testosterone is often called a "male" hormone. There are more than 100 different types of anabolic steroids that have been developed, and each requires a prescription to be used legally in the United States. The average adult male naturally produces 2.5 to 11 milligrams of testosterone daily. The average steroid abuser often takes more than 100 mg a day, through "stacking" or combining several different brands of steroids.

Medical uses

Anabolic steroids were first developed in the 1930s in Europe, in part to increase the physical strength of German soldiers. Anabolic steroids were tried by physicians for many other purposes in the 1940s and 1950s with varying success. Disadvantages outweighed benefits for most purposes, and during the later decades of the twentieth century medical use in North America and Europe was restricted to a few conditions. These include:

- Bone marrow stimulation: During the second half of the twentieth century anabolic steroids were the mainstay of therapy for hypoplastic anemia not due to nutrient deficiency, especially **aplastic anemia**. Anabolic steroids were slowly replaced by synthetic protein hormones that selectively stimulate growth of blood cell precursors.

- Growth stimulation: Anabolic steroids were used heavily by pediatric endocrinologists for children with growth failure from the 1960s through the 1980s. Availability of synthetic growth hormone and increasing social stigmatization of anabolic steroids led to reduction of this use.

- Stimulation of appetite and preservation of muscle mass: Anabolic steroids have been given to people with chronic wasting conditions such as **cancer** and HIV/AIDS.

- Induction of male **puberty**: Androgens are given to many boys distressed about extreme delay of puberty. Testosterone is as of 2005 nearly the only androgen used for this purpose, but synthetic anabolic steroids were often used prior to the 1980s.

- To treat certain kinds of **breast cancer** in some women.

- To treat angioedema, which causes swelling of the face, arms, legs, throat, windpipe, bowels, or sexual organs.

Abuse of steroids

The controversy surrounding steroid **abuse** began in the 1950s during the Olympic Games when the athletic community discovered that athletes from Russia and some East European nations, which had dominated the games, had taken large doses of steroids. Many of the male athletes developed such large prostate glands (a gland located near the bladder and urethra that aids in semen production) that they needed a tube inserted in order to urinate. Some of the female athletes developed so many male characteristics chromosome tests were necessary to prove that they were still women. Competitive weightlifters also began using steroids in the 1950s as a way to increase their athletic performance. Use gradually spread throughout the world among athletes in other sports.

Concerns over the growing illicit market and the prevalence of abuse, combined with the possibility of harmful long-term effects of steroids use, led the U.S. Congress in 1991 to place anabolic steroids in Schedule III of the Controlled Substances Act (CSA). The CSA defines anabolic steroids as any drug or hormonal substance chemically and pharmacologically related to testosterone (other than estrogens, progestins, and **corticosteroids**) that promotes muscle growth. Most illicit anabolic steroids are sold at gyms, bodybuilding competitions, and through the mail and Internet. For the most part, these substances are smuggled into the United States. Anabolic steroids commonly encountered on the illicit market include: boldenone (Equipoise), ethlestrenol (Maxibolin), fluoxymesterone (Halotestin), methandriol, methandrostenolone (Dianabol), methyltestosterone, nandrolone (Durabolin, DecaDurabolin), oxandrolone (Anavar), oxymetholone (Anadrol), stanozolol (Winstrol), testosterone (including sustanon), and trenbolone (Finajet). In addition, a number of counterfeit products are sold as anabolic steroids.

KEY TERMS

Adrenal gland—An endocrine gland located above each kidney. The inner part of each gland secretes epinephrine and the outer part secretes steroids.

Androgen—A natural or artificial steroid that acts as a male sex hormone. Androgens are responsible for the development of male sex organs and secondary sexual characteristics. Testosterone and androsterone are androgens.

Androstenedione—Also called "andro," this hormone occurs naturally during the making of testosterone and estrogen.

Catabolic—A metabolic process in which energy is released through the conversion of complex molecules into simpler ones.

Corticosteroids—A steroid hormone produced by the adrenal gland and involved in metabolism and immune response.

Endocrinologist—A medical specialist who treats endocrine (glands that secrete hormones internally directly into the lymph or bloodstream) disorders.

Estrogen—Any of several steroid hormones, produced mainly in the ovaries, that stimulate estrus and the development of female secondary sexual characteristics.

Hormone—A chemical substance produced in the body's endocrine glands or certain other cells that exerts a regulatory or stimulatory effect, for example, in metabolism.

Hypoplastic anemia—Anemia that is characterized by defective function of the blood-forming organs (such as bone marrow) and is caused by toxic agents such as chemicals or x rays. Anemia is a blood condition in which there are too few red blood cells or the red blood cells are deficient in hemoglobin.

Progestins—A female steroid sex hormone.

Prohormones—A physiologically inactive precursor of a hormone.

Prostate gland—An O-shaped gland in males that secretes a fluid into the semen that acts to improve the movement and viability of sperm.

Testosterone—A male steroid hormone produced in the testicles and responsible for the development of secondary sex characteristics.

In 2004, federal health officials initiated a crackdown on companies that manufacture, market, or distribute products containing androstenedione, or "andro," due to concerns about the safety of the substance. Widely marketed to athletes and body builders, androstenedione has been advertised to promote muscle growth, improve muscular strength, reduce fat, and slow **aging**. Androstenedione acts like a steroid once it is metabolized by the body and can pose similar kinds of health risks. People produce androstenedione naturally during the making of testosterone and estrogen. When people consume androstenedione, it is converted into testosterone and estrogen. Scientific evidence shows that when androstenedione is taken over time and in sufficient quantities, it may increase the risk of serious and life-threatening diseases, including liver failure.

On January 20, 2005, the Anabolic Steroid Control Act of 2004 took effect, amending the Controlled Substance Act by placing both anabolic steroids and prohormones on a list of controlled substances, making possession of the banned substances a federal crime. Also in 2005, Major League Baseball (MLB), amid long-time rumors of anabolic steroid abuse among players, was rocked by the publication of *Juiced* by former Oakland Athletics outfielder Jose Canseco who alleged steroid abuse was wide-spread in professional baseball. In response, Congress held hearings in March 2005 on steroid abuse in the MLB, subpoenaing such baseball superstars as home run champion Mark McGwire (now retired), Sammy Sosa, and Curt Schilling to testify. In response, MLB officials promised a crackdown on anabolic steroid use among players.

It has been estimated that at least one in 15 male high school seniors in the United States—more than 500,000 boys—has used steroids. Some are athletes attempting to increase their strength and size; others are simply youths attempting to speed up their growth to keep pace with their peers. In some countries, anabolic steroids are available over the counter. In the United States, a doctor's prescription is necessary.

Causes and symptoms

While the effects of steroids can seem desirable at first, there are serious side effects. Excessive use can cause a harmful imbalance in the body's normal hormonal balance and body chemistry. Heart attacks, water retention leading to high blood pressure and **stroke**, and liver and kidney tumors all are possible. Young people may develop **acne**, sometimes severe, and a halting of bone growth. Males may experience shrinking testicles, falling sperm counts, enlarged

breasts, and **enlarged prostate** glands. Women frequently show signs of masculinity and may be at higher risk for certain types of cancer and the possibility of **birth defects** in their children. Steroids fool the body into thinking that testosterone is being produced. The body, sensing an excess of testosterone, shuts down bodily functions involving testosterone, such as bone growth. The ends of long bones fuse together and stop growing, resulting in stunted growth.

The psychological effects of steroid use are also alarming: drastic mood swings, inability to sleep, depression, and feelings of hostility. Steroids may also be psychologically addictive. Once started, users—particularly athletes—enjoy the physical so-called benefits of increased size, strength, and endurance so much that they are reluctant to stop even when told about the risks.

In addition to these dangerous side effects, steroid abuse brings other risks, some of which are connected to the way some steroids are manufactured and distributed. The drugs are often made in motel rooms and warehouses in Mexico, Europe, and other countries and then smuggled into the United States. The potency, purity, and strength of the steroids produced this way are not regulated; therefore, users cannot know how much they are taking. Counterfeit steroids are also sold as the real thing. So it is often impossible to tell exactly what some products contain.

Most data on the long-term effects of anabolic steroids on humans come from case reports rather than formal scientific studies. From the case reports, the incidence of life-threatening effects appears to be low, but serious adverse effects may be under-recognized or under-reported. Data from animal studies seem to support this possibility. One study found that exposing male mice for one-fifth of their lifespan to steroid doses comparable to those taken by human athletes caused a high percentage of premature deaths. Most effects of anabolic steroid use are reversible if the abuser stops taking the drugs, but some can be permanent.

Diagnosis

Anyone who is using anabolic steroids without a prescription and not under the direction of a physician is considered abusing the drug and should seek medical help in stopping the use.

Treatment

Few studies of treatments for anabolic steroid abuse have been conducted. Knowledge as of 2005 is based largely on the experiences of a small number of physicians who have worked with patients undergoing steroid withdrawal. The physicians have found that supportive therapy is sufficient in some cases. Patients are educated about what they may experience during withdrawal and are evaluated for suicidal thoughts. If symptoms are severe or prolonged, medications or hospitalization may be needed.

Some medications that have been used for treating steroid withdrawal restore the hormonal system after its disruption by steroid abuse. Other medications target specific withdrawal symptoms, for example, antidepressants to treat depression, and **analgesics (pain** killers, such as **aspirin** and ibuprofen) for headaches and muscle and joint pains. Some patients require assistance beyond simple treatment of withdrawal symptoms and are treated with behavioral therapies.

Alternative treatment

There is little data on alternative medicines or treatments for anabolic steroid abuse. However, anabolic steroid manufacturers recommend **saw palmetto** to be taken in conjunction with androstenedione as it can help reduce associated hair loss and is useful in controlling prostate enlargement.

Prognosis

Anabolic steroid abuse is a treatable condition and can be stopped. Teenagers and adults can overcome the problem with the help of parents and other family members, support groups, psychotherapy, medication, treatment programs, and family counseling. These programs are customized to help teens and adults lead productive and normal lives. However, heavy steroid use—even if it is stopped after a few years—may increase the risk of **liver cancer**. A steroid user who quits may suffer a side effect commonly linked to low testosterone—severe depression—which can lead to suicidal thoughts and even **suicide**. The risk of depression and suicide is highest among teens.

Some physicians recommend that athletes using steroids avoid sudden discontinuance of all steroids at the same time because their bodies may enter an immediate catabolic (sudden release of energy) phase. The cortisone receptors will be free and in combination with the low testosterone and androgen levels, a considerable loss of strength and mass, and an increase of fat and water, and often breast enlargement in males can occur. Breast enlargement is possible because the suddenly low androgen level shifts the relationship in favor of the estrogens which suddenly become the domineering hormone.

Prevention

The best prevention is education to alert young people to the dangers, both medical and legal, in the illegal use of anabolic steroids. In its effort to alert teenagers to the dangers of steroid abuse, the U.S. Food and Drug Administration (FDA) developed a series of pamphlets, posters, and public service announcements. Much of this information is available on-line at < http://www.fda.gov >. Anabolic steroids are in the same regulatory category as **cocaine**, heroin, **LSD**, and other habit-forming drugs. This means that, in addition to the FDA, the Drug Enforcement Agency (DEA) helps to enforce laws relating to their abuse.

Athletic organizations have joined the fight. The Olympic Games are now closely monitored to prevent athletes who use steroids from participating. The National Football League has a strict testing policy in its training camps; it delivers fines and suspensions to those who test positive and bans repeat offenders. The National Collegiate Athletic Association, too, has established stricter measures for testing and disciplining steroid users.

Resources

BOOKS

Aretha, David. *Steroids and Other Performance-Enhancing Drugs.* Berkeley Heights, NJ: MyReportLinks.com, 2005.

Canseco, Jose. *Juiced: Wild Times, Rampant 'Roids, Smash Hits, and How Baseball Got Big.* New York City: Regan Books, 2005.

Levert, Suzanne. *The Facts about Steroids.* New York: Benchmark Books, 2004.

Taylor, William N. *Anabolic Therapy in Modern Medicine.* Jefferson, NC: McFarland & Company, 2002.

PERIODICALS

Adler, Jerry. "Toxic Strength: The Headlines about Illegal Steroids Have Focused on Professional and Olympic Athletes. But the Most Vulnerable Users May Be Kids in Your Neighborhood, High-Schoolers Who Are Risking an Array of Frightful Side Effects that Can Lead to Death." *Newsweek* (December 20, 2004): 44.

Bates, Betsy. "Elite Athletes Not Alone in Anabolic Steroid Abuse: Missed by Drug Testing." *Internal Medicine News* (February 1, 2004): 38.

Brown, Tim. "McGwire Appears to Suffer Lasting Damage to Credibility after Refusing to Discuss Steroids, and Baseball Will Tinker with Details of Its Drug Policy." *Los Angeles Times* (March 19, 2005): D–1.

Goodlad, Terry. "Dancing with the Dark Side: So, You Think You're Ready for Your First Steroid Cycle?" *Flex* (April 2004): 90–96.

Ingram, Scott. "Buff Enough? More Teens Are Using Steroids to Look Pumped and Do Better at Sports. Do they Know the Terrible Risk They're Taking?" *Current Science* (September 24, 2004): 4–8.

Poniewozik, James. "This Is Your Nation on Steroids: Why Does a Performance-Enhanced Society Scorn Performance-Enhanced Athletes?" *Time* (December 20, 2004): 168.

ORGANIZATIONS

National Center for Drug Free Sport Inc. 810 Baltimore St., Kansas City, MO 64105. (816) 474-7329. <http://www.drugfreesport.com>.

National Institute on Drug Abuse. 6001 Executive Blvd., Bethesda, MD 20892. (301)443-1124. <information@lists.nida.nih.gov>. <http://www.drugabuse.gov>.

OTHER

Drug Enforcement Administration. *Steroid Abuse in Today's Society*, March 2004. [cited March 21, 2005]. <http://www.deadiversion.usdoj.gov/pubs/brochures/steroids/professionals/professionals.pdf>.

Focus Adolescent Service. *Teens and Anabolic Steroids*, 2005. [cited March 21, 2005]. <http://www.focusas.com/Steroids.html>.

Ken R. Wells

Anaerobic infections

Definition

An anaerobic infection is an infection caused by bacteria (called anaerobes) which cannot grow in the presence of oxygen. Anaerobic bacteria can infect deep **wounds**, deep tissues, and internal organs where there is little oxygen. These infections are characterized by **abscess** formation, foul-smelling pus, and tissue destruction.

Description

Anaerobic means "life without air." Anaerobic bacteria grow in places which completely, or almost completely, lack oxygen. They are normally found in the mouth, gastrointestinal tract, and vagina, and on the skin. Commonly known diseases caused by anaerobic bacteria include gas **gangrene**, **tetanus**, and **botulism**. Nearly all dental infections are caused by anaerobic bacteria.

Anaerobic bacteria can cause an infection when a normal barrier (such as skin, gums, or intestinal wall) is damaged due to surgery, injury, or disease. Usually, the immune system kills any invading bacteria, but sometimes the bacteria are able to grow and cause an

---

infection. Body sites that have tissue destruction (necrosis) or a poor blood supply are low in oxygen and favor the growth of anaerobic bacteria. The low oxygen condition can result from blood vessel disease, **shock**, injury, and surgery.

Anaerobic bacteria can cause infection practically anywhere in the body. For example:

- Mouth, head, and neck. Infections can occur in the root canals, gums (gingivitis), jaw, tonsils, throat, sinuses, and ears.

- Lung. Anaerobic bacteria can cause **pneumonia**, lung abscesses, infecton of the lining of the lung (**empyema**), and dilated lung bronchi (**bronchiectasis**).

- Intraabdominal. Anaerobic infections within the abdomen include abscess formation, **peritonitis**, and **appendicitis**.

- Female genital tract. Anaerobic bacteria can cause pelvic abscesses, **pelvic inflammatory disease**, inflammation of the uterine lining (endometritis), and pelvic infections following abortion, **childbirth**, and surgery.

- Skin and soft tissue. Anaerobic bacteria are common causes of diabetic skin ulcers, gangrene, destructive infection of the deep skin and tissues (necrotizing fascitis), and bite wound infections.

- Central nervous system. Anaerobic bacteria can cause brain and spinal cord abscesses.

- Bloodstream. Anaerobic bacteria can be found in the bloodstream of ill patients (a condition called bacteremia).

Causes and symptoms

People who have experienced shock, injury, or surgery, and those with blood vessel disease or tumors are at an increased risk for infection by anaerobic bacteria. There are many different kinds of anaerobic bacteria which can cause an infection. Indeed, most anaerobic infections are "mixed infections" which means that there is a mixture of different bacteria growing. The anaerobic bacteria that most frequently cause infections are *Bacteroides fragilis*, *Peptostreptococcus*, and *Clostridium* species.

The signs and symptoms of anaerobic infection can vary depending on the location of the infection. In general, anaerobic infections result in tissue destruction, an abscess which drains foul-smelling pus, and possibly **fever**. Symptoms for specific infections are as follows:

- Tooth and gum infections. Swollen, tender bleeding gums, **bad breath**, and **pain**. Severe infections may produce oozing sores.

- Throat infection. An extremely **sore throat**, bad breath, a bad taste in the mouth, fever, and a sense of **choking**.

- Lung infection. Chest pain, coughing, difficulty breathing, fever, foul-smelling sputum, and weight loss.

- Intraabdominal infection. Pain, fever, and possibly, if following surgery, foul- smelling drainage from the wound.

- Pelvic infection. Foul-smelling pus or blood draining from the uterus, general or localized pelvic pain, fever, and chills.

- Skin and soft tissue infection. Infected wounds are red, painful, swollen, and may drain a foul-smelling pus. Skin infection causes localized swelling, pain, redness, and possibly a painful, open sore (ulcer) which drains foul-smelling pus. Severe skin infections may cause extensive tissue destruction (necrosis).

- Bloodstream. Bloodstream invasion causes high fever (up to 105°F [40.6°C]), chills, a general ill feeling, and is potentially fatal.

Diagnosis

The diagnosis of anaerobic infection is based primarily on symptoms, the patient's medical history, and location of the infection. A foul-smelling infection or drainage from an abscess is diagnostic of anaerobic infection. This foul smell is produced by anaerobic bacteria and occurs in one third to one half of patients late in the infection. Other clues to anaerobic infection include tissue necrosis and gas production at the infection site. A sample from the infected site may be obtained, using a swab or a needle and syringe, to determine which bacteria is (are) causing the infection. Because these bacteria can be easily killed by oxygen, they rarely grow in the laboratory cultures of tissue or pus samples.

The recent medical history of the patient is helpful in diagnosing anaerobic infection. A patient who has or recently had surgery, dental work, tumors, blood vessel disease, or injury are susceptible to this infection. The failure to improve following treatment with **antibiotics** that aren't able to kill anaerobes is another clue that the infection is caused by anaerobes. The location and type of infection also help in the diagnosis.

Diagnostic tests may include blood tests to see if bacteria are in the bloodstream and x rays to look at internal infections.

Treatment

Serious infections may require hospitalization for treatment. Immediate antibiotic treatment of anaerobic infections is necessary. Laboratory testing may identify the bacteria causing the infection and also which antibiotic will work best. Every antibiotic does not work against all anaerobic bacteria but nearly all anaerobes are killed by chloramphenicol (Chloromycetin), metronidazole (Flagyl or Protostat), and imipenem (Primaxin). Other antibiotics which may be used are clindamycin (Cleocin) or cefoxitin (Mefoxin).

Surgical removal or drainage of the abscess is almost always required. This may involve drainage by needle and syringe to remove the pus from a skin abscess (called "aspiration"). The area would be numbed prior to the aspiration procedure. Also, some internal abscesses can be drained using this procedure with the help of ultrasound (a device which uses sound waves to visualize internal organs). This type of abscess drainage may be performed in the doctor's office.

Prognosis

Complete recovery should be achieved with the appropriate surgery and antibiotic treatment. Untreated or uncontrolled infections can cause severe tissue and bone destruction, which would require **plastic surgery** to repair. Serious infections can be life threatening.

Prevention

Although anaerobic infections can occur in anyone, good hygiene and general health may help to prevent infections.

Resources

BOOKS

Fauci, Anthony S., et al., editors. *Harrison's Principles of Internal Medicine.* New York: McGraw-Hill, 1997.

Belinda Rowland, PhD

Anaerobic myositis *see* **Gangrene**

Anal atresia

Definition

The anus is either not present or it is in the wrong place.

Description

There are basically two kinds of anal atresia. In boys with high anal atresia, there may be a channel (**fistula**) connecting the large intestine to either the urethra (which delivers urine from the bladder) or the bladder itself. In girls, the channel may connect with the vagina. Sixty percent of children with high anal atresia have other defects, including problems with the esophagus, urinary tract, and bones. In low anal atresia, the channel may open in front of the circular mass of muscles that constrict to close the anal opening (anal sphincter) or, in boys, below the scrotum. Occasionally, the intestine ends just under the skin. It is estimated that overall abnormalities of the anus and rectum occur in about one in every 5,000 births and are slightly more common among boys. A mother who has one child with these kind of conditions has a 1% chance of having another child who suffers from this ailment.

Causes and symptoms

Anal atresia is a defect in the development of the fetus. The cause is unknown, but genetics seem to play a minor role.

Diagnosis

Usually a physician can make an obvious visual diagnosis of anal atesia right after birth. Occasionally, however, anal atresia is missed until the baby is fed and signs of intestinal obstruction appear. At the end of the first or second day, the abdomen swells and there is vomiting of fecal material. To determine the type of anal atresia and the exact position, x rays will be taken which include injecting opaque dye into the opening. Magnetic resonance imaging (MRI) or **computed tomography scans** (CT), as well as ultrasound, are the imaging techniques used to determine the type and size of the anal atresia. Ultrasound uses sound waves, CT scans pass x rays through the body at different angles, and an MRI uses a magnetic field and radio waves.

Treatment

Surgery is the only treatment for anal atresia. For high anal atresia, immediately after the diagnosis is made, a surgical incision is made in the large intestine to make a temporary opening (colostomy) in the abdomen where waste is excreted. Several months later, the intestine is moved into the ring of muscle (sphincter) that is part of the anus and a hole is made in the skin. The **colostomy** is closed several weeks later. In low anal atresia, immediately after diagnosis, a hole is made in the skin to open the area where the anus should be. If the channel is in the wrong place, the intestine is moved into the correct position sometime during the child's first year. After surgery, the pediatric surgeon uses an instrument to dilate or widen the rectum and teaches the parents how to do this daily at home to prevent scar tissue from contracting.

Prognosis

With high anal atresia, many children have problems controlling bowel function. Most also become constipated. With low anal atresia, children generally have good bowel control, but they may still become constipated.

Prevention

There is no known way to prevent anal atresia.

Resources

BOOKS

Paidas, Charles N., and Alberto Pena. "Rectum and Anus." In *Surgery of Infants and Children*. Philadelphia: Lippincott-Raven, 1997.

Jeanine Barone, Physiologist

KEY TERMS

Anus—The canal at the end of the large intestine through which waste is excreted to the outside of the body.

Bowel obstruction—Anything that prevents waste from moving normally to the anal opening.

Colostomy—An operation where the large intestine is diverted through an opening in the abdomen and waste is excreted.

Feces—Bodily waste material that normally passes through the anus.

Fistula—An abnormal channel that connects two organs or connects an organ to the skin.

Anal cancer

Definition

Anal **cancer** is an uncommon form of cancer affecting the anus. The anus is the inch-and-a-half-long end portion of the large intestine, which opens to allow solid wastes to exit the body. Other parts of the large intestine include the colon and the rectum.

Description

Different cancers can develop in different parts of the anus, part of which is inside the body and part of which is outside. Sometimes abnormal changes of the anus are harmless in their early stages but may later develop into cancer. Some **anal warts**, for example, contain precancerous areas and can develop into cancer. Types of anal cancer include:

- Squamous Cell Carcinomas. Approximately half of anal cancers are squamous cell carcinomas, which arise from the cells lining the anal margin and the anal canal. The anal margin is the part of the anus that is half inside and half outside the body, and the anal canal is the part of the anus that is inside the body. The earliest form of squamous cell carcinoma is known as carcinoma in situ, or Bowen's disease.

- Cloacogenic Carcinomas. Approximately one-fourth to one-third of anal tumors are cloacogenic carcinomas. These tumors develop in the transitional zone, or cloaca, which is a ring of tissue between the anal canal and the rectum.

- Adenocarcinomas. About 15% of anal cancers are adenocarcinomas, which affect glands in the anal area. One type of adenocarcinoma that can occur in the anal area is called Paget's disease, which can also affect the vulva, breasts, and other areas of the body.

- Skin cancers. A small percentage of anal cancers are either basal cell carcinomas, or malignant melanomas, two types of skin cancer. Malignant melanomas, which develop from skin cells that produce the brown pigment called melanin, are far more common on areas of the body exposed to the sun.

Approximately 3,500 Americans will be diagnosed with anal cancer in 2001, and an estimated 500 individuals will die of the disease during this same interval, according to the American Cancer Society. Anal cancers are fairly rare: they make up only 1% to 2% of cancers affecting the digestive system. The disease affects women somewhat more often than men, although the number of cases among men, particularly homosexual men, seems to be increasing.

Causes and symptoms

The exact cause of most anal cancers is unknown, although certain individuals appear to have a higher risk of developing the disease. Smokers are at higher risk, as are individuals with certain types of the human papillomavirus (HPV), and those with long-term problems in the anal area, such as abnormal openings known as fistulas. Since it increases the risk of HPV infection, the practice of anal sex appears to increase the risk of anal cancer—male homosexuals who practice anal sex are about 33 times more likely to have anal cancers than heterosexual men. Those with weakened immune systems, such individuals with HIV, or transplant patients taking immunosuppressant drugs, are also at higher risk. Most individuals with anal cancer are over the age of 50.

Symptoms of anal cancer resemble those found in other harmless conditions. They include pain, **itching** and bleeding, straining during a bowel movement, change in bowel habits, change in the diameter of the stool, discharge from the anus, and swollen lymph nodes in the anal or groin area.

Diagnosis

Anal cancer is sometimes diagnosed during routine physicals, or during minor procedures such as hemorrhoid removal. It may also be diagnosed during a digital rectal examination (DRE), when a physician inserts a gloved, lubricated finger into the anus to feel for unusual growths. Individuals over the age of 50 who have no symptoms should have a digital **rectal examination** (DRE) every five to 10 years, according to American Cancer Society (ACS) guidelines for early detection of colorectal cancer.

Other diagnostic procedures for anal cancer include: **Anoscopy**. A procedure that involves use of a special device to examine the anus. Proctoscopy. A procedure that involves use of a lighted scope to see the anal canal. Transrectal ultrasound. A procedure in which sound waves are used to create an image of the anus and nearby tissues.

A biopsy is performed on any suspicious growths; that is, a tiny piece of the growth is examined under a microscope for cancer cells. The physician may also perform a procedure called a fine needle aspiration biopsy, in which a needle is used to withdraw fluid from lymph nodes located near the growth, to make sure the cancer has not spread to these nodes.

Anal cancer severity is categorized by the following stages:

- Stage 0 anal cancer is found only in the top layer of anal tissue.

- Stage I anal cancer has spread beyond the top layer of anal tissue, but is less than 1 inch in diameter.

- Stage II anal cancer has spread beyond the top layer of anal tissue and is larger than 1 inch in diameter, but has not spread to nearby organs or lymph nodes.

- Stage IIIA anal cancer has spread to the lymph nodes around the rectum or to nearby organs such as the vagina or bladder.

- Stage IIIB anal cancer has spread to lymph nodes in the mid-abdomen or groin, or to nearby organs and the lymph nodes around the rectum.

- Stage IV anal cancer has spread to distant lymph nodes within the abdomen or to distant organs.

Treatment

Anal cancer is treated using three methods, used either in concert or individually: surgery, radiation therapy, and **chemotherapy**.

Two types of surgery may be performed. A local resection, performed if the cancer has not spread, removes the tumor and an area of tissue around the tumor. An abdominoperineal resection is a more complex procedure in which the anus and the lower rectum are removed, and an opening called a **colostomy** is created for body wastes to exit. This procedure is fairly uncommon today because radiation and chemotherapy are just as effective.

Chemotherapy fights cancer using drugs, which may be delivered via pill or needle. Some chemotherapy types kill cancer cells directly, while others act indirectly by making cancer cells more vulnerable to radiation. The main drugs used to treat anal cancer are 5-fluorouracil (5-FU) and mitomycin or 5-FU and cisplatin. Side effects of chemotherapy, which damages normal cells in addition to cancer cells, may include **nausea and vomiting**, hair loss, loss of appetite, **diarrhea**, mouth sores, **fatigue**, **shortness of breath**, and a weakened immune system.

Alternative treatment

Research suggests **acupuncture** can help manage chemotherapy-related **nausea** and **vomiting** and control **pain** associated with surgery.

Prognosis

Anal cancer is often curable. The chance of recovery depends on the cancer stage and the patient's general health.

Prevention

Reducing the risks of the **sexually transmitted diseases** HPV and HIV also reduces the risk of anal cancer. In addition, quitting **smoking** lowers the risk of anal cancer.

Resources

PERIODICALS

Murakami, M, K. J. Gurski, and M. A. Steller "Human Papillomavirus Vaccines For Cervical Cancer." *Journal of Immunotherapy* 22, no. 3 (1999): 212-8.

ORGANIZATIONS

American Cancer Society 1599 Clifton Road, NE, Atlanta, GA 30329. (404) 320-3333 or (800) ACS-2345. Fax: (404) 329-7530. < http://www.cancer.org >.

American College of Gastroenterology. 4900 B South 31st St., Arlington, VA 22206-1656. (703) 820-7400. < http://www.acg.gi.org >.

American Gastroenterological Association. 7910 Woodmont Ave., Seventh Floor, Bethesda, MD 20814. (301) 654-2055. < http://www.gastro.org >.

American Society of Colon and Rectal Surgeons. 85 W. Algonquin Road, Suite 550, Arlington Heights, Illinois 60005. (847) 290-9184.

National Cancer Institute (National Institutes of Health). 9000 Rockville Pike, Bethesda, MD 20892. (800) 422-6237. <http://www.nci.nih.gov>.

National Coalition for Cancer Survivorship. 1010 Wayne Avenue, 5th Floor, Suite 300, Silver Spring, MD 20910. (888) 650-9127.

NCI Office of Cancer Complementary and Alternative Medicine. <http://occam.nci.nih.gov>.

NIH National Center for Complementary and Alternative Medicine. Post Office Box 8218, Silver Spring, MD 20907-8218. (888) 644-6226. <http://nccam.nih.gov>.

United Ostomy Association. (800) 826-0826. <http://www.uoa.org>.

Ann Quigley

Anal fissure *see* **Anorectal disorders**

Anal warts

Definition

Anal **warts**, also known as condyloma acuminata, are small warts that can occur in the rectum.

Description

Initially appear as tiny blemishes that can be as small as the head of a pin or grow into larger cauliflower-like protuberances. They can be yellow, pink, or light brown in color, and only rarely are painful or uncomfortable. In fact, infected individuals often are unaware that they exist. Most cases are caused by sexual transmission.

Most individuals have between one to 10 genital warts thtat range in size from roughly 0.5–1.9 cm². Some will complain of painless bumps or **itching**, but often, these warts can remain completely unnoticed.

Causes and symptoms

Condyloma acuminatum is one of the most common sexually transmitted disease (STD) in the United States. Young adults aged 17 to 33 years are at greatest risk. Risk factors include smoking, using oral contraceptives, having multiple sexual partners, and an early coital age. In addition, individuals who have a history of immunosuppression or anal intercourse are also at risk.

Roughly 90% of all anal warts are caused by the human papilloma virus (HPV) types 6 and 11, which are the least likely of over 60 types of HPV to become cancerous. Anal warts are usually transmitted through

---

> **KEY TERMS**
>
> **Electrocoagulation**—a technique using electrical energy to destroy the warts. Usually done for warts within the anus with a local anesthesia, electrocoagulation is most painful form of therapy, and can cause both bleeding and discharge from the anus.

direct sexual contact with someone who is infected with condyloma acuminata anywhere in the genital area, including the penis and vagina. Studies have shown that roughly 75% of those who engage in sexual contact with someone infected with condyloma acuminata will develop these warts within three months.

Treatment

According to guidelines from the Centers for Disease Control (CDC), the treatment of all genital warts, including anal warts, should be conducted according to the methods preferred by the patient, the medications or procedures most readily available, and the experience of the patient's physician in removing anal warts.

Treatment options include electrical cautery, surgical removal, or both. Warts that appear inside the anal canal will almost always be treated with cauterization or surgical removal. Surgical removal, also known as excision, has the highest success rates and lowest recurrence rates. Indeed, studies have shown that initial cure rates range from 63–91%.

Unfortunately, most cases require numerous treatments because the virus that causes the warts can live in the surrounding tissue. The area may seem normal and wart-free for six months or longer before another wart develops.

Electrocoagulation, a technique that uses electrical energy to destroy the warts, is usually the most painful of the procedures done to eliminate condyloma acuminata of the anus, and is usually reserved for larger warts. It is done with **local anesthesia**, and may cause discharge or bleeding from the anus.

Follow-up visits to the physician are necessary to make sure that the warts have not recurred. It is recommended that these patients see their physicians every three to six months for up to 1.5 years, which is how long the incubation period is for the HPV virus.

Carbon dioxide laser treatment and electrodesiccation are other options, but these are usually reserved for extensive warts or those that continue to recur despite numerous treatments. However, because HPV virus can be transmitted via the smoke caused by these procedures, they are usually reserved for the worst infections.

For small warts that affect only the skin around the anus, several medications are available, which can be applied directly to the surface of the warts by a physician or by the patients themselves.

Such medications include podophyllum resin (Podocon-25, Pod-Ben-25), a substance made from the cytotoxic extracts of several plants. This agent offers a cure rate of 20–50% when used alone, and is applied by the physician weekly and then washed off 6 hours later by the patient.

Podofilox (Condylox) is another agent, and is available for patients to use at home. It can be applied twice daily for up to 4 weeks. Podofilox offers a slightly higher cure rate than podophyllin, and can also be used to prevent warts.

Trichloroacetic and bichloroacetic acids are available in several concentrations up to 80% for the treatment of condyloma acuminata. These acids work to cauterize the skin, and are quite caustic. Nevertheless, they cause less irritation and overall body effects than the other agents mentioned above. Recurrence, however, is higher with these acids.

Bleomycin (Blenoxane) is another treatment option, but it has several drawbacks. First, it must be administered by a physician into each lesion via injection, but is can have a host of side effects, and patients must be followed carefully by their physician.

Imiquimod 5% cream is also available for patients to apply themselves. It is to be applied three times weekly, for up to 16 weeks, and has been shown to clear warts within eight to 10 weeks.

Finally, the interferon drugs, which are naturally occurring proteins that have antiviral and antitumor effects, are available. These include interferon alfa 2a and 2b (Roferon, Intron A), which are to be injected into each lesion twice a week for up to eight weeks.

Prognosis

Once a diagnosis of anal warts has been made, further outbreaks can be controlled or sometimes prevented with proper care. Unfortunately, many cases of anal warts either fail to respond to treatment or recur. Patients have to undergo roughly six to nine treatments over several months to assure that the warts are completely eradicated.

Recurrence rates have been estimated to be over 50% after one year and may be due to the long incubation of HPV (up to 1.5 years), deep lesions, undetected lesions, virus present in surrounding skin that is not treated.

Prevention

Sexual abstinence and monogamous relationships can be the most effective form of prevention, and condoms may also decrease the chances of transmission of condyloma acuminata. Abstinence from sexual relations with people who have anal or **genital warts** can prevent infection. Unfortunately, since many people may not be aware that they have this condition, this is not always possible.

Individuals infected with anal warts should have follow-up checkups every few weeks after their initial treatment, after which self-exams can be done.

Sexual partners of people who have anal warts should also be examined, as a precautionary preventive measure.

Finally, 5-flourouracil (Adrucil, Efudex, Fluoroplex) may be useful to prevent recurrence once the warts have been removed. Treatment must, however, be initiated within 1 month of wart removal.

Resources

PERIODICALS

Maw, Raymond, and Geo von Krogh. "The Management of Anal Warts." *British Medical Journal* no. 321 (October 14, 2000): 910-11.

ORGANIZATIONS

Centers for Disease Control and Prevention. Sexually Transmitted Diseases Hotline: (800) 227-8922.

OTHER

< http://www.arthritis-baldness-impotency-obesity.com/ medcenter/NF009.html >.
< http://www.emedicine.com >.
< http://www.mayohealth.org >.
< http://wwwmedlineplus.adam.com >.

Liz Meszaros

Analgesics

Definition

Analgesics are medicines that relieve **pain**.

Purpose

Analgesics are those drugs that mainly provide pain relief. The primary classes of analgesics are the

narcotics, including additional agents that are chemically based on the morphine molecule but have minimal **abuse** potential; **nonsteroidal anti-inflammatory drugs** (NSAIDs) including the salicylates; and **acetaminophen**. Other drugs, notably the **tricyclic antidepressants** and anti-epileptic agents such as gabapentin, have been used to relieve pain, particularly neurologic pain, but are not routinely classified as analgesics. Analgesics provide symptomatic relief, but have no effect on the cause, although clearly the NSAIDs, by virtue of their dual activity, may be beneficial in both regards.

Description

Pain has been classified as "productive" pain and "non-productive" pain. While this distinction has no physiologic meaning, it may serve as a guide to treatment. "Productive" pain has been described as a warning of injury, and so may be both an indication of need for treatment and a guide to diagnosis. "Non-productive" pain by definition serves no purpose either as a warning or diagnostic tool.

Although pain syndromes may be dissimilar, the common factor is a sensory pathway from the affected organ to the brain. Analgesics work at the level of the nerves, either by blocking the signal from the peripheral nervous system, or by distorting the interpretation by the central nervous system. Selection of an appropriate analgesic is based on consideration of the risk-benefit factors of each class of drugs, based on type of pain, severity of pain, and risk of adverse effects. Traditionally, pain has been divided into two classes, acute and chronic, although severity and projected patient survival are other factors that must be considered in drug selection.

Acute pain

Acute pain is self limiting in duration, and includes post-operative pain, pain of injury, and **childbirth**. Because pain of these types is expected to be short term, the long-term side effects of analgesic therapy may routinely be ignored. Thus, these patients may safely be treated with narcotic analgesics without concern about possible **addiction**, or NSAIDs with only limited concern for the risk of ulcers. Drugs and doses should be adjusted based on observation of healing rate, switching patients from high to low doses, and from narcotic analgesics to non-narcotics when circumstances permit.

An important consideration of **pain management** in severe pain is that patients should not be subject to the return of pain. Analgesics should be dosed adequately to ensure that the pain is at least tolerable,

KEY TERMS

Acute pain—Pain that is usually temporary and results from something specific, such as a surgery, an injury, or an infection.

Analgesic—Medicine used to relieve pain.

Chronic pain—Pain that lasts more than three months and threatens to disrupt daily life.

Inflammation—Pain, redness, swelling, and heat that usually develop in response to injury or illness.

Osteoarthritis—Joint pain resulting from damage to the cartilage.

and frequently enough to avoid the **anxiety** that accompanies the anticipated return of pain. Analgesics should never be dosed on an as needed basis, but should be administered often enough to assure constant blood levels of analgesic. This applies to both the narcotic and non-narcotic analgesics.

Chronic pain

Chronic pain, pain lasting over three months and severe enough to impair function, is more difficult to treat, since the anticipated side effects of the analgesics are more difficult to manage. In the case of narcotic analgesics this means the addiction potential, as well as respiratory depression and **constipation**. For the NSAIDs, the risk of gastric ulcers limit dose. While some classes of drugs, such as the narcotic agonist/antagonist drugs bupronophine, nalbuphine and pentazocine, and the selective **COX-2 inhibitors** celecoxib and rofecoxib represent advances in reduction of adverse effects, they are still not fully suitable for long-term management of severe pain. Generally, chronic pain management requires a combination of drug therapy, life-style modification, and other treatment modalities.

Narcotic analgesics

The narcotic analgesics, also termed opioids, are all derived from opium. The class includes morphine, codeine, and a number of semi-synthetics including meperidine (Demerol), propoxyphen (Darvon) and others. The narcotic analgesics vary in potency, but all are effective in treatment of visceral pain when used in adequate doses. Adverse effects are dose related. Because these drugs are all addictive, they are controlled under federal and state laws. A variety of dosage forms are available, including oral solids, liquids, intravenous and intrathecal injections, and transcutaneous patches.

NSAIDs are effective analgesics even at doses too low to have any anti-inflammatory effects. There are a number of chemical classes, but all have similar therapeutic effects and side effects. Most are appropriate only for oral administration; however ketorolac (Toradol) is appropriate for injection and may be used in moderate to severe pain for short periods.

Acetaminophen is a non-narcotic analgesic with no anti-inflammatory properties. It is appropriate for mild to moderate pain. Although the drug is well tolerated in normal doses, it may have significant toxicity at high doses. Because acetaminophen is largely free of side effects at therapeutic doses, it has been considered the first choice for mild pain, including that of **osteoarthritis**.

Topical analgesics (topical being those that are applied on the skin) have become much more popular in recent years. Those applied for local effect include capsaicin, methylsalicylate, and transdermal lidocaine. Transdermal fentanyl may be applied for systemic (the entire body in general) effect. In some cases, these topical agents reduce the need for drug therapy. Sales of pain relief patches have increased substantially in recent years. They are particularly useful for elderly patients who may not want to take a lot of tablets.

Recommended dosage

Appropriate dosage varies by drug, and should consider the type of pain, as well as other risks associated with patient age and condition. For example, narcotic analgesics should usually be avoided in patients with a history of **substance abuse**, but may be fully appropriate in patients with **cancer** pain. Similarly, because narcotics are more rapidly metabolized in patients who have used these drugs for a long period, higher than normal doses may be needed to provide adequate pain management. NSAIDs, although comparatively safe in adults, represent an increased risk of gastrointestinal bleeding in patients over the age of 60.

Precautions

Narcotic analgesics may be contraindicated in patients with respiratory depression. NSAIDS may be hazardous to patients with ulcers or an ulcer history. They should be used with care in patients with renal insufficiency or **coagulation disorders**. NSAIDs are contraindicated in patients allergic to **aspirin**.

Side effects

Each drug's adverse effects should be reviewed individually. Drugs within a class may vary in their frequency and severity of adverse effects.

The primary adverse effects of the narcotic analgesics are addiction, constipation, and respiratory depression. Because narcotic analgesics stimulate the production of enzymes that cause the metabolism of these drugs, patients on narcotics for a prolonged period may require increasing doses. This is not the same thing as addiction, and is not a reason for withholding medication from patients in severe pain.

NSAIDs can lead to ulcers and may cause kidney problems. Gastrointestinal discomfort is common, although in some cases, these drugs may cause ulcers without the prior warning of gastrointestinal distress. Platelet aggregation problems may occur, although not to the same extent as is seen with aspirin.

Interactions

Interactions depend on the specific type of analgesic.

Resources

PERIODICALS

"Analgesics: No Pain, No Gain." *Chemist & Druggist* (September 11, 2004): 38.

Kuritzky, Louis. "Topical Capsaicin for Chronic Pain." *Internal Medicine Alert* (September 29, 2004): 144.

"Pain Relief Patches Are Flying Off Store Shelves." *Chain Drug Review* (August 16, 2004): 15.

Samuel D. Uretsky, PharmD
Teresa G. Odle

Analgesics, opioid

Definition

Opioid **analgesics**, also known as narcotic analgesics, are **pain** relievers that act on the central nervous system. Like all **narcotics**, they may become habit-forming if used over long periods.

Purpose

Opioid analgesics are used to relieve pain from a variety of conditions. Some are used before or during surgery (including dental surgery) both to relieve pain and to make anesthetics work more effectively. They

Opioid analgesics

Drug	Route of administration	Onset of action (min)	Time to peak effect (min)	Duration of action (h)
Strong agonists				
Fentanyl (Sublimaze)	IM	7–15	20–30	1–2
	IV	1–2	3–5	0.5–1
Hydromorphone (Dilaudid)	Oral	30	90–120	4
	IM	15		
	IV	10–15	30–60	2–3
	Sub-Q	30		15–30
Levorphanol (Levo-Dromoran)	Oral	10–60	90–120	4–5
	IM			
	IV	—	60	4–5
	Sub-Q	10–60	within 20	
Meperidine (Demerol)	Oral	15	60–90	2–4
	IM	10–15		
	IV		30–50	2–4
	Sub-Q	1		
Methadone (Dolophine)	Oral	30–60	90–120	4–6
	IM			
	IV	10–20	60–120	4–5
Morphine (many trade names)	Oral	—	60–120	4–5
	IM	10–30		
	IV		30–60	4–5
	Sub-Q	—		
	Epidural	10–30	20	4–5
Oxymorphone (Numorphan)	IM	10–15	30–90	3–6
	IV			
	Sub-Q	5–10	15–30	3–4
	Rectal			
Mild-to-moderate agonists				
Codiene (many trade names)	Oral	30–40	60–120	4
	IM	10–30	30–60	4
	Sub-Q	10–30		4
Hydrocodone (Hycodan)	Oral	10–30	30–60	4–6
Oxycodone (Percodan)	Oral	—	60	3–4
Propoxyphene (Darvon, Dolene)	Oral	15–60	120	4–6
Butophanol (Stadol)	IM	10–30	30–60	3–4
	IV	2–3	30	2–4
Nalbuphine (Nubian)	IM	within 15	60	3–6
	IV	2–3	30	3–4
	Sub-Q	within 15	—	3–6
Pentazocine (Talwin)	Oral	15–30	60–90	3
	IM	15–20	30–60	2–3
	IV	2–3	15–30	2–3
	Sub-Q	15–20	30–60	2–3

may also be used for the same purposes during labor and delivery.

Opioids are also given to relieve the pain of terminal **cancer**, **diabetic neuropathy**, lower back pain, and other chronic diseases or disorders. The World Health Organization (WHO) has established a three-stage "ladder" for the use of opioids in managing cancer pain.

Description

Opioid analgesics relieve pain by acting directly on the central nervous system. However, this can also lead to unwanted side effects, such as drowsiness, **dizziness**, breathing problems, and physical or mental dependence.

Among the drugs in this category are codeine, propoxyphene (Darvon), propoxyphene and **acetaminophen** (Darvocet N), meperidine (Demerol), hydromorphone (Dilaudid), morphine, oxycodone, oxycodone and acetaminophen (Percocet, Roxicet), and hydrocodone and acetaminophen (Lortab, Anexsia). These drugs come in many forms—tablets, syrups, suppositories, and injections, and are sold only by prescription. For some, a new prescription is required for each new supply—refills are prohibited according to federal regulations.

KEY TERMS

Analgesic—Medicine used to relieve pain.

Central nervous system—The brain and spinal cord.

Colitis—Inflammation of the colon (large bowel)

Hallucination—A false or distorted perception of objects, sounds, or events that seems real. Hallucinations usually result from drugs or mental disorders.

Inflammation—Pain, redness, swelling, and heat that usually develop in response to injury or illness.

Narcotic—A drug derived from opium or compounds similar to opium. Such drugs are potent pain relievers and can affect mood and behavior. Long-term use of narcotics can lead to dependence and tolerance.

Tolerance—A decrease in sensitivity to a drug. When tolerance occurs, a person must take more and more of the drug to get the same effect.

Withdrawal symptoms—A group of physical or mental symptoms that may occur when a person suddenly stops using a drug to which he or she has become dependent.

Recommended dosage

Recommended doses vary, depending on the type of opioid analgesic and the form in which it is being used. Doses may be different for different patients. Check with the physician who prescribed the drug or the pharmacist who filled the prescription for correct dosages, and make sure to understand how to take the drug.

Always take opioid analgesics exactly as directed. Never take larger or more frequent doses, and do not take the drug for longer than directed. Do not stop taking the drug suddenly without checking with the physician or dentist who prescribed it. Gradually tapering the dose may the chance of withdrawal symptoms.

Precautions

Anyone who uses opioid analgesics—or any narcotic—over a long time may become physically or mentally dependent on the drug. Physical dependence may lead to withdrawal symptoms when the person stops taking the medicine. Building tolerance to these drugs is also possible when they are used for a long period. Over time, the body needs larger and larger doses to relieve pain.

Take these drugs exactly as directed. Never take more than the recommended dose, and do not take the drugs more often than directed. If the drugs do not seem to be working, consult your physician. Do not share these or any other prescription drugs with others because the drug may have a completely different effect on the person for whom it was not prescribed.

Children and older people are especially sensitive to opioid analgesics and may have serious breathing problems after taking them. Children may also become unusually restless or agitated when given these drugs.

Opioid analgesics increase the effects of alcohol. Anyone taking these drugs should not drink alcoholic beverages.

Some of these drugs may also contain **aspirin**, **caffeine**, or acetaminophen. Refer to the entries on each of these drugs for additional precautions.

Special conditions

People with certain medical conditions or who are taking certain other medicines can have problems if they take opioid analgesics. Before taking these drugs, be sure to let the physician know about any of these conditions.

ALLERGIES. Let the physician know about any **allergies** to foods, dyes, preservatives, or other substances and about any previous reactions to opioid analgesics.

PREGNANCY. Women who are pregnant or plan to become pregnant while taking opioid analgesics should let their physicians know. No evidence exists that these drugs cause **birth defects** in people, but some do cause birth defects and other problems when given to pregnant animals in experiments. Babies can become dependent on opioid analgesics if their mothers use too much during **pregnancy**. This can cause the baby to go through withdrawal symptoms after birth. If taken just before delivery, some opioid analgesics may cause serious breathing problems in the newborn.

BREAST FEEDING. Some opioid analgesics can pass into breast milk. Women who are breast feeding should check with their physicians about the safety of taking these drugs.

OTHER MEDICAL CONDITIONS. These conditions may influence the effects of opioid analgesics:

- head injury. The effects of some opioid analgesics may be stronger and may interfere with recovery in people with head injuries.

- history of convulsions. Some of these drugs may trigger convulsions.

- asthma, **emphysema**, or any chronic lung disease

- heart disease
- kidney disease
- liver disease
- HIV infection. Patients undergoing highly active antiretroviral therapy, or HAART, are at increased risk for adverse effects from opioid analgesics.
- underactive thyroid. The chance of side effects may be greater.
- Addison's disease (a disease of the adrenal glands)
- colitis
- gallbladder disease or **gallstones**. Side effects can be dangerous in people with these conditions.
- enlarged prostate or other urinary problems
- current or past alcohol **abuse**
- current or past drug abuse, especially narcotic abuse
- current or past emotional problems. The chance of side effects may be greater.

USE OF CERTAIN MEDICINES. Taking opioid narcotics with certain other drugs may increase the chances of serious side effects.

Side effects

Some people experience drowsiness, dizziness, lightheadedness, or a false sense of well-being after taking opioid analgesics. Anyone who takes these drugs should not drive, use machines, or do anything else that might be dangerous until they know how the drug affects them. **Nausea and vomiting** are common side effects, especially when first beginning to take the medicine. If these symptoms do not go away after the first few doses, check with the physician or dentist who prescribed the medicine.

Dry mouth is another common side effect. Dry mouth can be relieved by sucking on sugarless hard candy or ice chips or by chewing sugarless gum. Saliva substitutes, which come in liquid or tablet forms, also may help. Patients who must use opioid analgesics over long periods and who have dry mouth should see their dentists, as the problem can lead to **tooth decay** and other dental problems.

The following side effects are less common. They usually do not need medical attention and will go away after the first few doses. If they continue or interfere with normal activity, check with the physician who prescribed the medicine.

- headache
- loss of appetite

- restlessness or nervousness
- nightmares, unusual dreams, or problems sleeping
- weakness or tiredness
- mental sluggishness
- stomach pain or cramps
- blurred or double vision or other vision problems
- problems urinating, such as pain, difficulty urinating, frequent urge to urinate, or decreased amount of urine
- constipation.

Other side effects may be more serious and may require quick medical attention. These symptoms could be signs of an overdose. Get emergency medical care immediately.

- cold, clammy skin
- bluish discoloration of the skin
- extremely small pupils
- serious difficulty breathing or extremely slow breathing
- extreme sleepiness or unresponsiveness
- severe weakness
- confusion
- severe dizziness
- severe drowsiness
- slow heartbeat
- low blood pressure
- severe nervousness or restlessness

In addition, these less common side effects do not require emergency medical care, but should have medical attention as soon as possible:

- **hallucinations** or a sense of unreality
- depression or other mood changes
- ringing or buzzing in the ears
- pounding or unusually fast heartbeat
- itching, **hives**, or rash
- facial swelling
- trembling or twitching
- dark urine, pale stools, or yellow eyes or skin (after taking propoxyphene)
- increased sweating, red or flushed face (more common after taking hydrocodone and meperidine)

Interactions

Anyone taking these drugs should notify his or her physician before taking opioid analgesics:

- Central nervous system (CNS) depressants, such as **antihistamines** and other medicines for allergies, hay **fever**, or colds; tranquilizers; some other prescription pain relievers; seizure medicines; **muscle relaxants**; sleeping pills; some anesthetics (including dental anesthetics).

- Monoamine oxidase (MAO) inhibitors, such as phenelzine (Nardil) and tranylcypromine (Parnate). The combination of the opioid analgesic meperidine (Demerol) and MAO inhibitors is especially dangerous.

- Tricyclic antidepressants, such as amitriptyline (Elavil).

- Anti-seizure medicines, such as carbamazepine (Tegretol). May lead to serious side effects, including **coma**, when combined with propoxyphene and acetaminophen (Darvocet-N) or propoxyphene (Darvon).

- Muscle relaxants, such as cyclobenzaprine (Flexeril).

- Sleeping pills, such as triazolam (Halcion).

- Blood-thinning drugs, such as warfarin (Coumadin).

- Naltrexone (Trexan, Revia). Cancels the effects of opioid analgesics.

- Rifampin (Rifadin).

- Zidovudine (AZT, Retrovir). Serious side effects when combined with morphine.

Opioids may also interact with certain herbal preparations sold as dietary supplements. Among the herbs known to interact with opioids are valerian (*Valeriana officinalis*), ginseng (*Panax ginseng*), kava kava (*Piper methysticum*), and chamomile (*Matricaria chamomilla*). As of early 2004 the National Center for Complementary and Alternative Medicine (NCCAM) is beginning a study of the possible interactions between **St. John's wort** (*Hypericum perforatum*, a herb frequently used to relieve symptoms of depression, and the opioid analgesics fentanyl and oxycodone. It is just as important for patients to inform their doctor of herbal remedies that they take on a regular basis as it is to give the doctor a list of their other prescription medications.

Resources

BOOKS

Beers, Mark H., MD, and Robert Berkow, MD., editors. "Pain." Section 14, Chapter 167 In *The Merck Manual of Diagnosis and Therapy*. Whitehouse Station, NJ: Merck Research Laboratories, 2002.

Pelletier, Dr. Kenneth R. *The Best Alternative Medicine, Part I: Western Herbal Medicine.* New York: Simon and Schuster, 2002.

Wilson, Billie Ann, RN, PhD, Carolyn L. Stang, PharmD, and Margaret T. Shannon, RN, PhD. *Nurses Drug Guide 2000.* Stamford, CT: Appleton and Lange, 1999.

PERIODICALS

Campbell, D. C. "Parenteral Opioids for Labor Analgesia." *Clinical Obstetrics and Gynecology* 46 (September 2003): 616–622.

Compton, P., and P. Athanasos. "Chronic Pain, Substance Abuse and Addiction." *Nursing Clinics of North America* 38 (September 2003): 525–537.

Faragon, J. J., and P. J. Piliero. "Drug Interactions Associated with HAART: Focus on Treatments for Addiction and Recreational Drugs." *AIDS Reader* 13 (September 2003): 433–450.

Markowitz, J. S., J. L. Donovan, C. L. DeVane, et al. "Effect of St John's Wort on Drug Metabolism by Induction of Cytochrome P450 3A4 Enzyme." *Journal of the American Medical Association* 290 (September 17, 2003): 1500–1504.

Soares, L. G., M. Marins, and R. Uchoa. "Intravenous Fentanyl for Cancer Pain: A 'Fast Titration' Protocol for the Emergency Room." *Journal of Pain and Symptom Management* 26 (September 2003): 876–881.

Watson, C. P., D. Moulin, J. Watt-Watson, et al. "Controlled-Release Oxycodone Relieves Neuropathic Pain: A Randomized Controlled Trial in Painful Diabetic Neuropathy." *Pain* 105 (September 2003): 71–78.

ORGANIZATIONS

National Center for Complementary and Alternative Medicine (NCCAM) Clearinghouse. P.O. Box 7923, Gaithersburg, MD 20898-7923. (888) 644-6226. < http://nccam.nih.gov > .

U. S. Food and Drug Administration (FDA). 5600 Fishers Lane, Rockville, MD 20857. (888) 463-6332. < http://www.fda.gov > .

Nancy Ross-Flanigan
Rebecca J. Frey, PhD

Anaphylactic shock *see* **Anaphylaxis**
Anaphylactoid purpura *see* **Allergic purpura**

Anaphylaxis

Definition

Anaphylaxis is a rapidly progressing, life-threatening allergic reaction.

Description

Anaphylaxis is a type of allergic reaction, in which the immune system responds to otherwise harmless substances from the environment. Unlike other allergic reactions, however, anaphylaxis can kill. Reaction may begin within minutes or even seconds of exposure, and rapidly progress to cause airway constriction, skin and intestinal irritation, and altered heart rhythms. In severe cases, it can result in complete airway obstruction, **shock**, and **death**.

Causes and symptoms

Causes

Like the majority of other allergic reactions, anaphylaxis is caused by the release of histamine and other chemicals from mast cells. Mast cells are a type of white blood cell and they are found in large numbers in the tissues that regulate exchange with the environment: the airways, digestive system, and skin.

On their surfaces, mast cells display antibodies called IgE (immunoglobulin type E). These antibodies are designed to detect environmental substances to which the immune system is sensitive. Substances from a genuinely threatening source, such as bacteria or viruses, are called antigens. A substance that most people tolerate well, but to which others have an allergic response, is called an allergen. When IgE antibodies bind with allergens, they cause the mast cell to release histamine and other chemicals, which spill out onto neighboring cells.

The interaction of these chemicals with receptors on the surface of blood vessels causes the vessels to leak fluid into surrounding tissues, causing fluid accumulation, redness, and swelling. On the smooth muscle cells of the airways and digestive system, they cause constriction. On nerve endings, they increase sensitivity and cause **itching**.

In anaphylaxis, the dramatic response is due both to extreme hypersensivity to the allergen and its usually systemic distribution. Allergens are more likely to cause anaphylaxis if they are introduced directly into the circulatory system by injection. However, exposure by ingestion, inhalation, or skin contact can also cause anaphylaxis. In some cases, anaphylaxis may develop over time from less severe **allergies**.

Anaphylaxis is most often due to allergens in foods, drugs, and insect venom. Specific causes include:

- Fish, shellfish, and mollusks
- Nuts and seeds

- Stings of bees, wasps, or hornets
- Papain from meat tenderizers
- Vaccines, including flu and **measles** vaccines
- Penicillin
- Cephalosporins
- Streptomycin
- Gamma globulin
- Insulin
- Hormones (ACTH, thyroid-stimulating hormone)
- **Aspirin** and other NSAIDs
- Latex, from exam gloves or condoms, for example.

Exposure to cold or **exercise** can trigger anaphylaxis in some individuals.

Symptoms

Symptoms may include:

- Urticaria (**hives**)
- Swelling and irritation of the tongue or mouth
- Swelling of the sinuses
- Difficulty breathing
- Wheezing
- Cramping, **vomiting**, or **diarrhea**
- Anxiety or confusion
- Strong, very rapid heartbeat (**palpitations**)
- Loss of consciousness.

Not all symptoms may be present.

Diagnosis

Anaphylaxis is diagnosed based on the rapid development of symptoms in response to a suspect allergen. Identification of the culprit may be done with RAST testing, a blood test that identifies IgE reactions to specific allergens. Skin testing may be done for less severe anaphylactic reactions.

Treatment

Emergency treatment of anaphylaxis involves injection of adrenaline (epinephrine) which constricts blood vessels and counteracts the effects of histamine. Oxygen may be given, as well as intravenous replacement fluids. **Antihistamines** may be used for skin rash, and aminophylline for bronchial constriction. If the upper airway is obstructed, placement of a breathing tube or tracheostomy tube may be needed.

Prognosis

The rapidity of symptom development is an indication of the likely severity of reaction: the faster symptoms develop, the more severe the ultimate reaction. Prompt emergency medical attention and close monitoring reduces the likelihood of death. Nonetheless, death is possible from severe anaphylaxis. For most people who receive rapid treatment, recovery is complete.

Prevention

Avoidance of the allergic trigger is the only reliable method of preventing anaphylaxis. For insect allergies, this requires recognizing likely nest sites. Preventing **food allergies** requires knowledge of the prepared foods or dishes in which the allergen is likely to occur, and careful questioning about ingredients when dining out. Use of a Medic-Alert tag detailing drug allergies is vital to prevent inadvertent administration during a medical emergency.

People prone to anaphylaxis should carry an "Epi-pen" or "Ana-kit," which contain an adrenaline dose ready for injection.

Resources

OTHER

The Merck Page. February 20, 1998. < http://www.merck.com >.

Richard Robinson

Anemias

Definition

Anemia is a condition characterized by abnormally low levels of healthy red blood cells or hemoglobin (the component of red blood cells that delivers oxygen to tissues throughout the body).

Description

The tissues of the human body need a regular supply of oxygen to stay healthy. Red blood cells, which contain hemoglobin that allows them to deliver oxygen throughout the body, live for only about 120 days. When they die, the iron they contain is returned to the bone marrow and used to create new red blood cells. Anemia develops when heavy bleeding causes significant iron loss or when something happens to slow down the production of red blood cells or to increase the rate at which they are destroyed.

Types of anemia

Anemia can be mild, moderate, or severe enough to lead to life-threatening complications. More than 400 different types of anemia have been identified. Many of them are rare.

IRON DEFICIENCY ANEMIA. The onset of iron deficiency anemia is gradual and, at first, there may not be any symptoms. The deficiency begins when the body loses more iron than it derives from food and other sources. Because depleted iron stores cannot meet the red blood cell's needs, fewer red blood cells develop. In this early stage of anemia, the red blood cells look normal, but they are reduced in number. Then the body tries to compensate for the iron deficiency by producing more red blood cells, which are characteristically small in size. Symptoms develop at this stage.

FOLIC ACID DEFICIENCY ANEMIA. Folic acid anemia is especially common in infants and teenagers. Although this condition usually results from a dietary deficiency, it is sometimes due to inability to absorb enough folic acid from such foods as:

- cheese
- eggs
- fish
- green vegetables
- meat
- milk
- mushrooms
- yeast

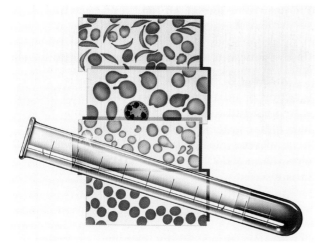

An illustration of normal red blood cells (left) and those in three different types of anemia (from left), iron-deficiency anemia, megaloblastic anemia, and sickle cell anemia. *(Illustration by John Bavosi, Custom Medical Stock Photo. Reproduced by permission.)*

Smoking raises the risk of developing this condition by interfering with the absorption of Vitamin C, which the body needs to absorb folic acid. Folic acid anemia can be a complication of **pregnancy**, when a woman's body needs eight times more folic acid than it does otherwise.

VITAMIN B$_{12}$ DEFICIENCY ANEMIA. Less common in this country than folic acid anemia, vitamin B$_{12}$ deficiency anemia is another type of megaloblastic anemia that develops when the body doesn't absorb enough of this nutrient. Necessary for the creation of red blood cells, B$_{12}$ is found in meat and vegetables.

Large amounts of B$_{12}$ are stored in the body, so this condition may not become apparent until as much as four years after B$_{12}$ absorption stops or slows down. The resulting drop in red blood cell production can cause:

- loss of muscle control
- loss of sensation in the legs, hands, and feet
- soreness or burning of the tongue
- weight loss
- yellow-blue color blindness

The most common form of B$_{12}$ deficiency is **pernicious anemia**. Since most people who eat meat or eggs get enough B$_{12}$ in their **diets**, a deficiency of this vitamin usually means that the body is not absorbing it properly. This can occur among people who have had intestinal surgery or among those who do not produce adequate amounts of intrinsic factor, a chemical secreted by the stomach lining that combines with B$_{12}$ to help its absorption in the small intestine.

Pernicious anemia usually strikes between the ages of 50–60. Eating disorders or an unbalanced diet increase the risk of developing pernicious anemia. So do:

- diabetes mellitus
- **gastritis**, **stomach cancer**, or stomach surgery
- thyroid disease
- family history of pernicious anemia

VITAMIN C DEFICIENCY ANEMIA. A rare disorder that causes the bone marrow to manufacture abnormally small red blood cells, Vitamin C deficiency anemia results from a severe, long-standing dietary deficiency.

HEMOLYTIC ANEMIA. Some people are born with **hemolytic anemia**. Some acquire this condition, in which infection or antibodies destroy red blood cells more rapidly than bone marrow can replace them.

Hemolytic anemia can enlarge the spleen, accelerating the destruction of red blood cells (hemolysis). Other complications of hemolytic anemia include:

- **pain**
- shock
- gallstones and other serious health problems

THALASSEMIAS. An inherited form of hemolytic anemia, **thalassemia** stems from the body's inability to manufacture as much normal hemoglobin as it needs. There are two categories of thalassemia, depending on which of the amino acid chains is affected. (Hemoglobin is composed of four chains of amino acids.) In alpha-thalassemia, there is an imbalance in the production of the alpha chain of amino acids; in beta-thalassemia, there is an imbalance in the beta chain. Alpha-thalassemias most commonly affect blacks (25% have at least one gene); beta-thalassemias most commonly affect people of Mediterranean ancestry and Southeast Asians.

Characterized by production of red blood cells that are unusually small and fragile, thalassemia only affects people who inherit the gene for it from each parent (autosomal recessive inheritance).

AUTOIMMUNE HEMOLYTIC ANEMIAS. Warm antibody hemolytic anemia is the most common type of this disorder. This condition occurs when the body produces autoantibodies that coat red blood cells. The coated cells are destroyed by the spleen, liver, or bone marrow.

Warm antibody hemolytic anemia is more common in women than in men. About one-third of patients who have warm antibody hemolytic anemia also have lymphoma, leukemia, lupus, or connective tissue disease.

In cold antibody hemolytic anemia, the body attacks red blood cells at or below normal body temperature. The acute form of this condition frequently develops in people who have had **pneumonia**, mononucleosis, or other acute infections. It tends to be mild and short-lived, and disappears without treatment.

Chronic cold antibody hemolytic anemia is most common in women and most often affects those who are over 40 and who have arthritis. This condition usually lasts for a lifetime, generally causing few symptoms. However, exposure to cold temperatures can accelerate red blood cell destruction, causing **fatigue**, joint aches, and discoloration of the arms and hands.

SICKLE CELL ANEMIA. Sickle cell anemia is a chronic, incurable condition that causes the body to produce defective hemoglobin, which forces red blood cells to assume an abnormal crescent shape. Unlike normal oval cells, fragile sickle cells can't hold enough hemoglobin to nourish body tissues. The deformed shape makes it hard for sickle cells to pass through narrow blood vessels. When capillaries become obstructed, a life-threatening condition called sickle cell crisis is likely to occur.

Sickle cell anemia is hereditary. It almost always affects blacks and people of Mediterranean descent. A child who inherits the sickle cell gene from each parent will have the disease. A child who inherits the sickle cell gene from only one parent carries the sickle cell trait, but does not have the disease.

APLASTIC ANEMIA. Sometimes curable by bone marrow transplant, but potentially fatal, **aplastic anemia** is characterized by decreased production of red and white blood cells and platelets (disc-shaped cells that allow the blood to clot). This disorder may be inherited or acquired as a result of:

- recent severe illness
- long-term exposure to industrial chemicals
- use of **anticancer drugs** and certain other medications

ANEMIA OF CHRONIC DISEASE. Cancer, chronic infection or inflammation, and kidney and **liver disease** often cause mild or moderate anemia. Chronic liver failure generally produces the most severe symptoms. People infected with the Human **immunodeficiency** virus (HIV) that causes **AIDS** often face severe fatigue.

Causes and symptoms

Anemia is caused by bleeding, decreased red blood cell production, or increased red blood cell destruction. Poor diet can contribute to vitamin deficiency and iron deficiency anemias in which fewer red blood cells are produced. Hereditary disorders and certain diseases can cause increased blood cell destruction. However, excessive bleeding is the most common cause of anemia, and the speed with which blood loss occurs has a significant effect on the severity of symptoms. Chronic blood loss is usually a consequence of:

- cancer
- gastrointestinal tumors
- diverticulosis
- polyposis
- heavy menstrual flow
- hemorrhoids
- nosebleeds
- stomach ulcers
- long-standing alcohol abuse

Acute blood loss is usually the result of:

- childbirth
- injury
- a ruptured blood vessel
- surgery

When a lot of blood is lost within a short time, blood pressure and the amount of oxygen in the body drop suddenly. **Heart failure** and **death** can follow.

Loss of even one-third of the body's blood volume in the space of several hours can be fatal. More gradual blood loss is less serious, because the body has time to create new red blood cells to replace those that have been lost.

Symptoms

Weakness, fatigue, and a run-down feeling may be signs of mild anemia. Skin that is pasty or sallow, or lack of color in the creases of the palm, gums, nail beds, or lining of the eyelids are other signs of anemia. Someone who is weak, tires easily, is often out of breath, and feels faint or dizzy may be severely anemic.

Other symptoms of anemia are:

- angina pectoris (chest pain, often accompanied by a **choking** sensation that provokes severe **anxiety**)
- cravings for ice, paint, or dirt
- headache
- inability to concentrate, memory loss
- inflammation of the mouth (**stomatitis**) or tongue (glossitis)
- insomnia
- irregular heartbeat
- loss of appetite
- nails that are dry, brittle, or ridged
- rapid breathing
- sores in the mouth, throat, or rectum
- sweating
- swelling of the hands and feet
- thirst
- tinnitus (ringing in the ears)
- unexplained bleeding or bruising

In pernicious anemia, the tongue feels unusually slick. A patient with pernicious anemia may have:

- problems with movement or balance
- tingling in the hands and feet
- confusion, depression, and memory loss

Pernicious anemia can damage the spinal cord. A doctor should be notified whenever symptoms of this condition occur.

A doctor should also be notified if a patient who has been taking iron supplements develops:

- diarrhea
- cramps
- vomiting

Diagnosis

Personal and family health history may suggest the presence of certain types of anemia. Laboratory tests that measure the percentage of red blood cells or the amount of hemoglobin in the blood are used to confirm diagnosis and determine which type of anemia is responsible for a patient's symptoms. X rays and examinations of bone marrow may be used to identify the source of bleeding.

Treatment

Anemia due to nutritional deficiencies can usually be treated at home with iron supplements or self administered injections of vitamin B_{12}. People with folic acid anemia should take oral folic acid replacements. Vitamin C deficiency anemia can be cured by taking one vitamin C tablet a day.

Surgery may be necessary to treat anemia caused by excessive loss of blood. Transfusions of red blood cells may be used to accelerate production of red blood cells.

Medication or surgery may also be necessary to control heavy menstrual flow, repair a bleeding ulcer, or remove polyps (growths or nodules) from the bowels.

Patients with thalassemia usually do not require treatment. However people with a severe form may require periodic hospitalization for blood transfusions and/or **bone marrow transplantation**.

SICKLE CELL ANEMIA. Treatment for sickle cell anemia involves regular eye examinations, immunizations for pneumonia and infectious diseases, and prompt treatment for sickle cell crises and infections of any kind. Psychotherapy or counseling may help patients deal with the emotional impact of this condition.

VITAMIN B_{12} DEFICIENCY ANEMIA. A life-long regimen of B_{12} shots is necessary to control symptoms of pernicious anemia. The patient may be advised to limit physical activity until treatment restores strength and balance.

APLASTIC ANEMIA. People who have aplastic anemia are especially susceptible to infection. Treatment for aplastic anemia may involve blood transfusions and bone marrow transplant to replace malfunctioning cells with healthy ones.

ANEMIA OF CHRONIC DISEASE. There is no specific treatment for anemia associated with chronic disease, but treating the underlying illness may alleviate this condition. Erythropoietin is a hormone that stimulates production of red blood cells. It is sometimes used to treat anemia from **kidney disease** or cancer **chemotherapy**. This type of anemia rarely becomes severe. If it does, transfusions or hormone treatments to stimulate red blood cell production may be prescribed. A working group met in 2004 to address the specific management of anemia in patients infected with HIV.

HEMOLYTIC ANEMIA. There is no specific treatment for cold-antibody hemolytic anemia. About one-third of patients with warm-antibody hemolytic anemia respond well to large doses of intravenous and oral **corticosteroids**, which are gradually discontinued as the patient's condition improves. Patients with this condition who don't respond to medical therapy must have the spleen surgically removed. This operation controls anemia in about one-half of the patients on whom it's performed. Immune-system suppressants are prescribed for patients whose surgery is not successful.

Self-care

Anyone who has anemia caused by poor **nutrition** should modify his or her diet to include more **vitamins**, **minerals**, and iron. Vitamin C can stimulate iron absorption. The following foods are also good sources of iron:

- almonds
- broccoli
- dried beans
- dried fruits
- enriched breads and cereals
- lean red meat
- liver
- potatoes
- poultry
- rice
- shellfish
- tomatoes

Because light and heat destroy folic acid, fruits and vegetables should be eaten raw or cooked as little as possible.

Alternative treatment

As is the case in standard medical treatment, the cause of the specific anemia will determine the alternative treatment recommended. If the cause is a deficiency, for example iron deficiency, folic acid deficiency, B_{12} deficiency, or vitamin C deficiency, supplementation is the treatment. For extensive blood loss, the cause should be identified and corrected. Other types of anemias should be addressed

on a deep healing level with crisis intervention when necessary.

Many alternative therapies for iron-deficiency anemia focus on adding iron-rich foods to the diet or on techniques to improve circulation and digestion. Iron supplementation, especially with iron citrate (less likely to cause **constipation**), is used by alternative practitioners. This can be given in combination with herbs that are rich in iron. Some examples of iron-rich herbs are dandelion (*Taraxacum officinale*), parsley (*Petroselinum crispum*), and nettle (*Urtica dioica*). The homeopathic remedy ferrum phosphoricum can also be helpful.

An iron-rich herbal tonic can also me made using the following recipe:

- soak 1/2 oz of yellow dock root and 1/2 oz dandelion root in 1 qt of boiled water for four to 8 hours
- strain and simmer until the amount of liquid is reduced to 1 cup
- remove from heat and add 1/2 cup black strap molasses, mixing well
- store in refrigerator; take 1 tsp-2 Tbsp daily

Other herbal remedies used to treat iron-deficiency anemia aim to improve the digestion. Gentian (*Gentiana lutea*) is widely used in Europe to treat anemia and other nutritionally based disorders. The bitter qualities of gentian help stimulate the digestive system, making iron and other nutrients more available for absorption. This bitter herb can be brewed into tea or purchased as an alcoholic extract (tincture).

Other herbs recommended to promote digestion include:

- anise (*Pimpinella anisum*)
- caraway (*Carum carvi*)
- cumin (*Cuminum cyminum*)
- linden (*Tilia* spp.)
- licorice (*Glycyrrhiza glabra*)

Traditional Chinese treatments for anemia include:

- acupuncture to stimulate a weakened spleen
- asian ginseng (*Panax ginseng*) to restore energy
- dong quai (*Angelica sinensis*) to control heavy menstrual bleeding
- a mixture of dong quai and Chinese foxglove (*Rehmannia glutinosa*) to clear a sallow complexion

Prognosis

Folic-acid and iron-deficiency anemias

It usually takes three to six weeks to correct folic acid or iron deficiency anemia. Patients should continue taking supplements for another six months to replenish iron reserves. They should have periodic blood tests to make sure the bleeding has stopped and the anemia has not recurred.

Pernicious anemia

Although pernicious anemia is considered incurable, regular B$_{12}$ shots will alleviate symptoms and reverse complications. Some symptoms will disappear almost as soon as treatment begins.

Aplastic anemia

Aplastic anemia can sometimes be cured by bone marrow transplantation. If the condition is due to immunosuppressive drugs, symptoms may disappear after the drugs are discontinued.

Sickle cell anemia

Although sickle cell anemia cannot be cured, effective treatments enable patients with this disease to enjoy longer, more productive lives.

Thalassemia

People with mild thalassemia (alpha thalassemia trait or beta thalassemia minor) lead normal lives and do not require treatment. Those with severe thalassemia may require bone marrow transplantation. Genetic therapy is is being investigated and may soon be available.

Hemolytic anemia

Acquired hemolytic anemia can generally be cured when the cause is removed.

Prevention

Inherited anemias cannot be prevented. **Genetic counseling** can help parents cope with questions and concerns about transmitting disease-causing genes to their children.

Avoiding excessive use of alcohol, eating a balanced diet that contains plenty of iron-rich foods, and taking a daily multivitamin can help prevent anemia.

Methods of preventing specific types of anemia include:

- avoiding lengthy exposure to industrial chemicals and drugs known to cause aplastic anemia

- not taking medication that has triggered hemolytic anemia and not eating foods that have caused hemolysis (breakdown of red blood cells)
- receiving regular B$_{12}$ shots to prevent pernicious anemia resulting from gastritis or stomach surgery

Resources

PERIODICALS

"Biopharmaceuitcal Company Announces Manufacturing Agreement for Anemia Drug." *Obesity, Wellness, & Fitness Week* (September 4, 2004): 406.
"Management Strategy for Anemia in HIV Infection Elucidated." *Immunotherapy Weekly* (July 7, 2004): 75.

Maureen Haggerty
Teresa G. Odle

Anencephaly *see* **Congenital brain defects**

Anesthesia, general

Definition

General anesthesia is the induction of a state of unconsciousness with the absence of **pain** sensation over the entire body, through the administration of anesthetic drugs. It is used during certain medical and surgical procedures.

Purpose

General anesthesia has many purposes including:

- pain relief (analgesia)
- blocking memory of the procedure (**amnesia**)
- producing unconsciousness
- inhibiting normal body reflexes to make surgery safe and easier to perform
- relaxing the muscles of the body

Description

Anesthesia performed with general anesthetics occurs in four stages which may or may not be observable because they can occur very rapidly:

- Stage One: Analgesia. The patient experiences analgesia or a loss of pain sensation but remains conscious and can carry on a conversation.
- Stage Two: Excitement. The patient may experience **delirium** or become violent. Blood pressure rises and

ANESTHETICS: HOW THEY WORK

Type	Name(s)	Administered	Affect
General	Halothane, Enflurane Isoflurane, Ketamine, Nitrous Oxide, Thiopental	Intravenously, Inhalation	Produces total unconsciousness affecting the entire body
Regional	Mepivacaine, Chloroprocaine, Lidocaine	Intravenously	Temporarily interrupts transmission of nerve impulses (temperature, touch, pain) and motor functions in a large area to be treated; does not produce unconsciousness
Local	Procaine, Lidocaine, Tetracaine, Bupivacaine	Intravenously	Temporarily blocks transmission of nerve impulses and motor functions in a specific area; does not produce unconsciousness
Topical	Benzocaine, Lidocaine Dibucaine, Pramoxine, Butamben, Tetracaine	Demal (Sprays, Drope, Ointments, Creams, Gels)	Temporarily blocks nerve endings in skin and mucous membranes; does not produce unconsciousness

KEY TERMS

Amnesia—The loss of memory.

Analgesia—A state of insensitivity to pain even though the person remains fully conscious.

Anesthesiologist—A medical specialist who administers an anesthetic to a patient before he is treated.

Anesthetic—A drug that causes unconsciousness or a loss of general sensation.

Arrhythmia—Abnormal heart beat.

Barbiturate—A drug with hypnotic and sedative effects.

Catatonia—Psychomotor disturbance characterized by muscular rigidity, excitement or stupor.

Hypnotic agent—A drug capable of inducing a hypnotic state.

Hypnotic state—A state of heightened awareness that can be used to modulate the perception of pain.

Hypoxia—Reduction of oxygen supply to the tissues.

Malignant hyperthermia—A type of reaction (probably with a genetic origin) that can occur during general anesthesia and in which the patient experiences a high fever, muscle rigidity, and irregular heart rate and blood pressure.

Medulla oblongata—The lowest section of the brainstem, located next to the spinal cord. The medulla is the site of important cardiac and respiratory regulatory centers.

Opioid—Any morphine-like synthetic narcotic that produces the same effects as drugs derived from the opium poppy (opiates), such as pain relief, sedation, constipation and respiratory depression.

Pneumothorax—A collapse of the lung.

Stenosis—A narrowing or constriction of the diameter of a passage or orifice, such as a blood vessel.

becomes irregular, and breathing rate increases. This stage is typically bypassed by administering a barbiturate, such as sodium pentothal, before the anesthesia.

- Stage Three: Surgical Anesthesia. During this stage, the skeletal muscles relax, and the patient's breathing becomes regular. Eye movements slow, then stop, and surgery can begin.

- Stage Four: Medullary **Paralysis**. This stage occurs if the respiratory centers in the medulla oblongata of the brain that control breathing and other vital functions cease to function. **Death** can result if the patient cannot be revived quickly. This stage should never be reached. Careful control of the amounts of anesthetics administered prevent this occurrence.

Agents used for general anesthesia may be either gases or volatile liquids that are vaporized and inhaled with oxygen, or drugs delivered intravenously. A combination of inhaled anesthetic gases and intravenous drugs are usually delivered during general anesthesia; this practice is called balanced anesthesia and is used because it takes advantage of the beneficial effects of each anesthetic agent to reach surgical anesthesia. If necessary, the extent of the anesthesia produced by

inhaling a general anesthetic can be rapidly modified by adjusting the concentration of the anesthetic in the oxygen that is breathed by the patient. The degree of anesthesia produced by an intravenously injected anesthesic is fixed and cannot be changed as rapidly. Most commonly, intravenous anesthetic agents are used for induction of anesthesia and then followed by inhaled anesthetic agents.

General anesthesia works by altering the flow of sodium molecules into nerve cells (neurons) through the cell membrane. Exactly how the anesthetic does this is not understood since the drug apparently does not bind to any receptor on the cell surface and does not seem to affect the release of chemicals that transmit nerve impulses (neurotransmitters) from the nerve cells. It is known, however, that when the sodium molecules do not get into the neurons, nerve impulses are not generated and the brain becomes unconscious, does not store memories, does not register pain impulses from other areas of the body, and does not control involuntary reflexes. Although anesthesia may feel like deep sleep, it is not the same. In sleep, some parts of the brain speed up while others slow down. Under anesthesia, the loss of consciousness is more widespread.

When general anesthesia was first introduced in medical practice, ether and chloroform were inhaled with the physician manually covering the patient's mouth. Since then, general anesthesia has become much more sophisticated. During most surgical procedures, anesthetic agents are now delivered and controlled by computerized equipment that includes anesthetic gas monitoring as well as patient monitoring equipment. Anesthesiologists are the physicians that specialize in the delivery of anesthetic agents. Currently used inhaled general anesthetics include halothane, enflurane, isoflurane, desflurane, sevoflurane, and nitrous oxide.

- Halothane (Fluothane) is a powerful anesthetic and can easily be overadministered. This drug causes unconsciousness but little pain relief so it is often used with other agents to control pain. Very rarely, it can be toxic to the liver in adults, causing death. It also has the potential for causing serious cardiac dysrhythmias. Halothane has a pleasant odor, and was frequently the anesthetic of choice for use with children, but since the introduction of sevoflurane in the 1990s, halothane use has declined.

- Enflurane (Ethrane) is less potent and results in a more rapid onset of anesthesia and faster awakening than halothane. In addition, it acts as an enhancer of paralyzing agents. Enflurane has been found to increase intracranial pressure and the risk of seizures; therefore, its use is contraindicated in patients with seizure disorders.

- Isoflurane (Forane) is not toxic to the liver but can cause some cardiac irregularities. Isoflurane is often used in combination with intravenous anesthetics for anesthesia induction. Awakening from anesthesia is faster than it is with halothane and enflurane.

- Desflurane (Suprane) may increase the heart rate and should not be used in patients with **aortic valve stenosis**; however, it does not usually cause heart **arrhythmias**. Desflurane may cause coughing and excitation during induction and is therefore used with intravenous anesthetics for induction. Desflurane is

rapidly eliminated and awakening is therefore faster than with other inhaled agents.

- Sevoflurane (Ultane) may also cause increased heart rate and should not be used in patients with narrowed aortic valve (stenosis); however, it does not usually cause heart arrhythmias. Unlike desflurane, sevoflurane does not cause any coughing or other related side effects, and can therefore be used without intravenous agents for rapid induction. For this reason, sevoflurane is replacing halothane for induction in pediatric patients. Like desflurane, this agent is rapidly eliminated and allows rapid awakening.

- Nitrous oxide (laughing gas) is a weak anesthetic and is used with other agents, such as thiopental, to produce surgical anesthesia. It has the fastest induction and recovery and is the safest because it does not slow breathing or blood flow to the brain. However, it diffuses rapidly into air-containing cavities and can result in a collapsed lung (**pneumothorax**) or lower the oxygen contents of tissues (hypoxia).

Commonly administered intravenous anesthetic agents include ketamine, thiopental, opioids, and propofol.

- Ketamine (Ketalar) affects the senses, and produces a dissociative anesthesia (**catatonia**, amnesia, analgesia) in which the patient may appear awake and reactive, but cannot respond to sensory stimuli. These properties make it especially useful for use in developing countries and during warfare medical treatment. Ketamine is frequently used in pediatric patients because anesthesia and analgesia can be achieved with an intramuscular injection. It is also used in high-risk geriatric patients and in **shock** cases, because it also provides cardiac stimulation.

- Thiopental (Pentothal) is a barbiturate that induces a rapid hypnotic state of short duration. Because thiopental is slowly metabolized by the liver, toxic accumulation can occur; therefore, it should not be continuously infused. Side effects include **nausea and vomiting** upon awakening.

- Opioids include fentanyl, sufentanil, and alfentanil, and are frequently used prior to anesthesia and surgery as a sedative and analgesic, as well as a continuous infusion for primary anesthesia. Because opioids rarely affect the cardiovascular system, they are particularly useful for cardiac surgery and other high-risk cases. Opioids act directly on spinal cord receptors, and are freqently used in epidurals for spinal anesthesia. Side effects may include **nausea** and **vomiting**, **itching**, and respiratory depression.

- Propofol (Diprivan) is a nonbarbiturate hypnotic agent and the most recently developed intravenous anesthetic. Its rapid induction and short duration of action are identical to thiopental, but recovery occurs more quickly and with much less nausea and vomiting. Also, propofol is rapidly metabolized in the liver and excreted in the urine, so it can be used for long durations of anesthesia, unlike thiopental. Hence, propofol is rapidly replacing thiopental as an intravenous induction agent. It is used for **general surgery**, cardiac surgery, neurosurgery, and pediatric surgery.

General anesthetics are given only by anesthesiologists, the medical professionals trained to use them. These specialists consider many factors, including a patient's age, weight, medication **allergies**, medical history, and general health, when deciding which anesthetic or combination of anesthetics to use. General anesthetics are usually inhaled through a mask or a breathing tube or injected into a vein, but are also sometimes given rectally.

General anesthesia is much safer today than it was in the past. This progress is due to faster-acting anesthetics, improved safety standards in the equipment used to deliver the drugs, and better devices to monitor breathing, heart rate, blood pressure, and brain activity during surgery. Unpleasant side effects are also less common.

Recommended dosage

The dosage depends on the type of anesthetic, the patient's age and physical condition, the type of surgery or medical procedure being done, and other medication the patient takes before, during, or after surgery.

Precautions

Although the risks of serious complications from general anesthesia are very low, they can include **heart attack**, **stroke**, brain damage, and death. Anyone scheduled to undergo general anesthesia should thoroughly discuss the benefits and risks with a physician. The risks of complications depend, in part, on a patient's age, sex, weight, allergies, general health, and history of **smoking**, drinking alcohol, or drug use. Some of these risks can be minimized by ensuring that the physician and anesthesiologist are fully informed of the detailed health condition of the patient, including any drugs that he or she may be using. Older people are especially sensitive to the effects of certain anesthetics and may be more likely to experience side effects from these drugs.

Patients who have had general anesthesia should not drink alcoholic beverages or take medication that slow down the central nervous system (such as **antihistamines**, sedatives, tranquilizers, sleep aids, certain pain relievers, **muscle relaxants**, and anti-seizure medication) for at least 24 hours, except under a doctor's care.

Special conditions

People with certain medical conditions are at greater risk of developing problems with anesthetics. Before undergoing general anesthesia, anyone with the following conditions should absolutely inform their doctor.

ALLERGIES. Anyone who has had allergic or other unusual reactions to **barbiturates** or general anesthetics in the past should notify the doctor before having general anesthesia. In particular, people who have had malignant hyperthermia or whose family members have had malignant hyperthermia during or after being given an anesthetic should inform the physician. Signs of malignant hyperthermia include rapid, irregular heartbeat, breathing problems, very high **fever**, and muscle tightness or spasms. These symptoms can occur following the administration of general anesthesia using inhaled agents, especially halothane. In addition, the doctor should also be told about any allergies to foods, dyes, preservatives, or other substances.

PREGNANCY. The effects of anesthetics on pregnant women and fetuses vary, depending on the type of drug. In general, giving large amounts of general anesthetics to the mother during labor and delivery may make the baby sluggish after delivery. Pregnant women should discuss the use of anesthetics during labor and delivery with their doctors. Pregnant women who may be given general anesthesia for other medical procedures should ensure that the treating physician is informed about the **pregnancy**.

BREASTFEEDING. Some general anesthetics pass into breast milk, but they have not been reported to cause problems in nursing babies whose mothers were given the drugs.

OTHER MEDICAL CONDITIONS. Before being given a general anesthetic, a patient who has any of the following conditions should inform his or her doctor:

- neurological conditions, such as epilepsy or stroke
- problems with the stomach or esophagus, such as ulcers or **heartburn**
- eating disorders
- loose teeth, dentures, bridgework
- heart disease or family history of heart problems
- lung diseases, such as **emphysema** or **asthma**
- history of smoking
- immune system diseases

- arthritis or any other conditions that affect movement
- diseases of the endocrine system, such as diabetes or thyroid problems

Side effects

Because general anesthetics affect the central nervous system, patients may feel drowsy, weak, or tired for as long as a few days after having general anesthesia. Fuzzy thinking, blurred vision, and coordination problems are also possible. For these reasons, anyone who has had general anesthesia should not drive, operate machinery, or perform other activities that could endanger themselves or others for at least 24 hours, or longer if necessary.

Most side effects usually disappear as the anesthetic wears off. A nurse or doctor should be notified if these or other side effects persist or cause problems, such as:

- **Headache**
- vision problems, including blurred or double vision
- shivering or trembling
- muscle pain
- dizziness, lightheadedness, or faintness
- drowsiness
- mood or mental changes
- nausea or vomiting
- sore throat
- nightmares or unusual dreams

A doctor should be notified as soon as possible if any of the following side effects occur within two weeks of having general anesthesia:

- severe headache
- pain in the stomach or abdomen
- back or leg pain
- severe nausea
- black or bloody vomit
- unusual tiredness or weakness
- weakness in the wrist and fingers
- weight loss or loss of appetite
- increase or decrease in amount of urine
- pale skin
- yellow eyes or skin

Interactions

General anesthetics may interact with other medicines. When this happens, the effects of one or both of the drugs may be altered or the risk of side effects may be greater. Anyone scheduled to undergo general anesthesia should inform the doctor about all other medication that he or she is taking. This includes prescription drugs, nonprescription medicines, and street drugs. Serious and possibly life-threatening reactions may occur when general anesthetics are given to people who use street drugs, such as **cocaine**, **marijuana**, phencyclidine (PCP or angel dust), amphetamines (uppers), barbiturates (downers), heroin, or other **narcotics**. Anyone who uses these drugs should make sure their doctor or dentist knows what they have taken.

Resources

BOOKS

Dobson, Michael B. *Anaesthesia at the District Hospital.* 2nd ed. World Health Organization, 2000.

PERIODICALS

Adachi, Y.U., K. Watanabe, H. Higuchi, and T. Satoh. "The Determinants of Propofol Induction of Anesthesia Dose." *Anesthesia and Analgesia* 92 (2001): 656-661.

OTHER

Wenker, O. "Review of Currently Used Inhalation Anesthetics Part I." "The Internet Journal of Anesthesiology." 1999. < http://www.ispub.com/journals/IJA/Vol3N2/inhal1.htm > .

Jennifer Sisk

Anesthesia, local

Definition

Local or regional anesthesia involves the injection or application of an anesthetic drug to a specific area of the body, as opposed to the entire body and brain as occurs during **general anesthesia**.

Purpose

Local anesthetics are used to prevent patients from feeling **pain** during medical, surgical, or dental procedures. Over-the-counter local anesthetics are also available to provide temporary relief from pain, irritation, and **itching** caused by various conditions,

KEY TERMS

Canker sore—A painful sore inside the mouth.

Cold sore—A small blister on the lips or face, caused by a virus. Also called a fever blister.

Epidural space—The space surrounding the spinal fluid sac.

Malignant hyperthermia—A type of reaction (probably with a genetic basis) that can occur during general anesthesia in which the patient experiences a high fever, the muscles become rigid, and the heart rate and blood pressure fluctuate.

Subarachnoid space—The space surrounding the spinal cord that is filled with cerebrospinal fluid.

Topical—Not ingested; applied to the outside of the body, for example to the skin, eye, or mouth.

such as cold sores, **canker sores**, sore throats, **sunburn**, insect bites, poison ivy, and minor cuts and scratches.

Types of surgery or medical procedures that regularly make use of local or regional anesthesia include the following:

• biopsies in which skin or tissue samples are taken for diagnostic procedures

• childbirth

• surgeries on the arms, hands, legs, or feet

• eye surgery

• surgeries involving the urinary tract or sexual organs

Surgeries involving the chest and abdomen are usually performed under general anesthesia.

Local and regional anesthesia have advantages over general anesthesia in that patients can avoid some unpleasant side effects, can receive longer lasting pain relief, have reduced blood loss, and maintain a sense of psychological comfort by not losing consciousness.

Description

Regional anesthesia typically affects a larger area than local anesthesia, for example, everything below the waist. As a result, regional anesthesia may be used for more involved or complicated surgical or medical procedures. Regional anesthetics are injected. Local anesthesia involves the injection into the skin or muscle or application to the skin of an anesthetic directly where pain will occur. Local anesthesia can be divided

Local and regional anesthesia work by altering the flow of sodium molecules into nerve cells or neurons through the cell membrane. Exactly how the anesthetic does this is not understood, since the drug apparently does not bind to any receptor on the cell surface and does not seem to affect the release of chemicals that transmit nerve impulses (neurotransmitters) from the nerve cells. It is known, however, that when the sodium molecules do not get into the neurons, nerve impulses are not generated and pain impulses are not transmitted to the brain. The duration of action of an anesthetic depends on the type and amount of anesthetic administered.

Regional anesthesia

Types of regional anesthesia include:

• Spinal anesthesia. Spinal anesthesia involves the injection of a small amount of local anesthetic directly into the cerebrospinal fluid surrounding the spinal cord (the subarachnoid space). Blood pressure drops are common but are easily treated.

• Epidural anesthesia. Epidural anesthesia involves the injection of a large volume of local anesthetic directly into the space surrounding the spinal fluid sac (the epidural space), not into the spinal fluid. Pain relief occurs more slowly but is less likely to produce blood pressure drops. Also, the block can be maintained for long periods, even days.

• Nerve blocks. Nerve blocks involve the injection of an anesthetic into the area around a nerve that supplies a particular region of the body, preventing the nerve from carrying nerve impulses to the brain.

Anesthetics may be administered with another drug, such as epinephrine (adrenaline), which decreases bleeding, and sodium bicarbonate to decrease the acidity of a drug so that it will work faster. In addition, drugs may be administered to help a patient remain calm and more comfortable or to make them sleepy.

Local anesthesia

INJECTABLE LOCAL ANESTHETICS. These medicines are given by injection to numb and provide pain relief to some part of the body during surgery, dental procedures, or other medical procedures. They are given only by a trained health care professional and only in a doctor's office or a hospital. Some commonly used injectable local anesthetics are procaine (Novocain), lidocaine (Dalcaine, Dilocaine, L-Caine, Nervocaine,

Xylocaine, and other brands), and tetracaine (Pontocaine).

TOPICAL ANESTHETICS. Topical anesthetics, such as benzocaine, lidocaine, dibucaine, pramoxine, butamben, and tetracaine, relieve pain and itching by deadening the nerve endings in the skin. They are ingredients in a variety of nonprescription products that are applied to the skin to relieve the discomfort of sunburn, insect bites or stings, poison ivy, and minor cuts, scratches, and **burns**. These products are sold as creams, ointments, sprays, lotions, and gels.

DENTAL ANESTHETICS (NON-INJECTABLE). Some local anesthetics are intended for pain relief in the mouth or throat. They may be used to relieve throat pain, teething pain, painful canker sores, toothaches, or discomfort from dentures, braces, or bridgework. Some dental anesthetics are available only with a doctor's prescription. Others may be purchased without a prescription, including products such as Num-Zit, Orajel, Chloraseptic lozenges, and Xylocaine.

OPHTHALMIC ANESTHETICS. Other local anesthetics are designed for use in the eye. The ophthalmic anesthetics proparacaine and tetracaine are used to numb the eye before certain eye examinations. Eye doctors may also use these medicines before measuring eye pressure or removing stitches or **foreign objects** from the eye. These drugs are to be given only by a trained health care professional.

Recommended dosage

The recommended dosage depends on the type of local anesthetic and the purpose for which it is being used. When using a nonprescription local anesthetic, follow the directions on the package. Questions concerning how to use a product should be referred to a medical doctor, dentist, or pharmacist.

Precautions

People who strongly feel that they cannot psychologically cope with being awake and alert during certain procedures may not be good candidates for local or regional anesthesia. Other medications may be given in conjunction with the anesthetic, however, to relieve **anxiety** and help the patient relax.

Local anesthetics should be used only for the conditions for which they are intended. For example, a topical anesthetic meant to relieve sunburn pain should not be used on cold sores. Anyone who has had an unusual reaction to any local anesthetic in the past should check with a doctor before using any type of local anesthetic again. The doctor should also be told about any **allergies** to foods, dyes, preservatives, or other substances.

Older people may be more sensitive to the effects of local anesthetics, especially lidocaine. This increased sensitivity may increase the risk of side effects. Older people who use nonprescription local anesthetics should be especially careful not to use more than the recommended amount. Children also may be especially sensitive to the effects of some local anesthetics, which may increase the chance of side effects. Anyone using these medicines on a child should be careful not to use more than the amount that is recommended for children. Certain types of local anesthetics should not be used at all young children. Follow package directions carefully and check with a doctor of pharmacist if there are any questions.

Regional anesthetics

Serious, possibly life-threatening, side effects may occur when anesthetics are given to people who use street drugs. Anyone who uses **cocaine**, **marijuana**, amphetamines, **barbiturates**, phencyclidine (PCP, or angel dust), heroin, or other street drugs should make sure their doctor or dentist knows what they have used.

Patients who have had a particular kind of reaction called malignant hyperthermia (or who have one or more family members who have had this problem) during or just after receiving a general anesthetic should inform their doctors before receiving any kind of anesthetic. Signs of malignant hyperthermia include fast and irregular heartbeat, very high **fever**, breathing problems, and **muscle spasms** or tightness.

Although problems are rare, some unwanted side effects may occur when regional anesthetics are used during labor and delivery. These anesthetics can prolong labor and increase the risk of **Cesarean section**. Pregnant women should discuss with their doctors the risks and benefits of being given these drugs.

Patients should not drive or operate other machinery immediately following a procedure involving regional anesthesia, due to **numbness** and weakness, or if local anesthesia also included drugs to make the patient sleep or strong pain medications. Injection sites should be kept clean, dry, and uncovered to prevent infection.

Injectable local anesthetics

Until the anesthetic wears off, patients should be careful not to injure the numbed area. If the anesthetic was used in the mouth, do not eat or chew gum until feeling returns.

Topical anesthetics

Unless advised by a doctor, topical anesthetics should not be used on or near any part of the body with large sores, broken or scraped skin, severe injury, or infection. They should also not be used on large areas of skin. Some topical anesthetics contain alcohol and should not be used near an open flame, or while **smoking**.

Anyone using a topical anesthetic should be careful not to get this medication in the eyes, nose, or mouth. When using a spray form of this medication, do not spray it directly on the face, but apply it to the face with a cotton swab or sterile gauze pad. After using a topical anesthetic on a child, make sure the child does not get the medicine in his or her mouth.

Topical anesthetics are intended for the temporary relief of pain and itching. They should not be used for more than a few days at a time. Check with a doctor if:

- the discomfort continues for more than seven days

- the problem gets worse

- the treated area becomes infected

- new signs of irritation, such as skin rash, burning, stinging, or swelling appear

Dental anesthetics (non-injectable)

Dental anesthetics should not be used if certain kinds of infections are present. Check package directions or check with a dentist or medical doctor if uncertain. Dental anesthetics should be used only for temporary pain relief. If problems such as **toothache**, mouth sores, or pain from dentures or braces continue, check with a dentist. Check with a doctor if **sore throat** pain is severe, lasts more than two days, or is accompanied by other symptoms such as fever, **headache**, skin rash, swelling, **nausea**, or **vomiting**.

Patients should not eat or chew gum while the mouth is numb from a dental anesthetic. There is a risk of accidently biting the tongue or the inside of the mouth. Also nothing should be eaten or drunk for one hour after applying a dental anesthetic to the back of the mouth or throat, since the medicine may interfere with swallowing and may cause **choking**. If normal feeling does not return to the mouth within a few hours after receiving a dental anesthetic or if it is difficult to open the mouth, check with a dentist.

Ophthalmic anesthetics

When anesthetics are used in the eye, it is important not to rub or wipe the eye until the effect of the anesthetic has worn off and feeling has returned. Rubbing the eye while it is numb could cause injury.

Side effects

Side effects of regional or local anesthetics vary depending on the type of anesthetic used and the way it is administered. Anyone who has unusual symptoms following the use of an anesthetic should get in touch with his or her doctor immediately.

There is a small risk of developing a severe headache called a spinal headache following a spinal or epidural block. This headache is severe when the patient is upright and hardly felt when the patient lies down. Though rare, it can occur and can be treated by performing a blood patch, in which a small amount of the patient's own blood is injected into the area in the back where the anesthetic was injected. The **blood clots** and closes up any area that may have been leaking spinal fluid. Relief is almost immediate. Finally, blood clots or **abscess** can form in the back, but these are also readily treatable and so pose little risk.

A physician should be notified immediately if any of these symptoms occur:

- large swellings that look like **hives** on the skin, in the mouth, or in the throat

- severe headache

- blurred or double vision

- dizziness or lightheadedness

- drowsiness

- confusion

- anxiety, excitement, nervousness, or restlessness

- convulsions (seizures)

- feeling hot, cold, or numb

- ringing or buzzing in the ears

- shivering or trembling

- sweating

- pale skin

- slow or irregular heartbeat

- breathing problems

- nusual weakness or tiredness

Interactions

Some anesthetic drugs may interact with other medicines. When this happens, the effects of one or both of the drugs may change or the risk of side effects may be greater. Anyone who receives a regional or local anesthetic should let the doctor know all other drugs he or she is taking including prescription drugs, nonprescription drugs, and street drugs (such as cocaine, marijuana, and heroin).

Resources

BOOKS

Harvey, Richard A., et al., editors. "Anesthetics." In *Lippincott's Illustrated Reviews: Pharmacology.* Philadelphia: J.B. Lippincott & Co., 1992.

Nancy Ross-Flanigan

▌Aneurysmectomy

Definition

Aneurysmectomy is a surgical procedure performed to repair a weak area in the aorta. The aorta is the largest artery in the body and the main blood vessel leading away from the heart.

Purpose

The purpose of aneurysmectomy is to repair an **aortic aneurysm** that is likely to rupture if left in place. Aneurysmectomy is indicated for an aortic aneurysm that grows to at least 2 in(5 cm) or for an aortic aneurysm of any size that is symptomatic, tender, or enlarging rapidly.

Precautions

Aneurysmectomy may not be appropriate for patients with severely debilitating diseases such as **cancer**, **emphysema**, and **heart failure**.

Description

An aortic aneurysm is a bulge in the wall of the aorta that is usually due to arteriosclerosis or **atherosclerosis**. People who are 50-80 years old are most likely to develop an aortic aneurysm, with men four times more likely to develop one than women.

An aortic aneurysm develops and grows slowly. It rarely produces symptoms and is usually only diagnosed by accident during a routine physical exam or on an x ray or ultrasound done for another reason. As the aneurysm grows larger, the risk of bursting with no warning, which causes catastrophic bleeding, rises. A ruptured aortic aneurysm can cause sudden loss of a fatal amount of blood within minutes or it can leak in a series of small bleeds that lead within hours or days to massive bleeding. A leaking aortic aneurysm that is not treated is always fatal.

Aneurysmectomy is performed to repair the two most common types of aortic aneurysms: abdominal aortic aneurysms that occur in the abdomen below the kidneys, and thoracic aortic aneurysms that occur in the chest. It is major surgery performed in a hospital under **general anesthesia** and involves removing debris and then implanting a flexible tube (graft) to replace the enlarged artery. Aneurysmectomy for an aneurysm of the ascending aorta (the first part of the aorta that travels upward from the heart) requires the use of a heart-lung machine that temporarily stops the heart while the aneurysm is repaired. Aneurysmectomy requires a one-week hospital stay; the recovery period is five weeks.

During surgery, the site of the aneurysm (either the abdomen or the chest) is opened with an incision to expose the aneurysm. The aorta is clamped above and below the aneurysm to stop the flow of blood. Then, an incision is made in the aneurysm. An artificial Dacron tube is sewn in place above and below the opened aneurysm, but the aneurysm is not removed. Plaque or clotted blood are cleaned from the diseased tissue. The clamps are removed and blood flow is re-established through the graft. The wall of the aneurysm is wrapped around the graft to protect it and the skin of the abdomen or chest is sewn up.

Aneurysmectomy can be performed as elective or emergency surgery. Elective aneurysmectomy takes about an hour and is far safer than emergency aneurysmectomy, with a mortality rate of 3-5% for elective abdominal aneurysmectomy and 5-10% for elective thoracic aneurysmectomy. When an aneurysm ruptures, 62% of patients die before they reach the hospital. Of those who make it into emergency aneurysmectromy, 50% die. After a successful aneurysmectomy, the patient has nearly the same life expectancy as other people of the same age.

Preparation

Before elective aneurysmectomy, blood studies, a **chest x ray**, cardiac catherization, electrocardiogram (ECG), and ultrasound are performed.

Aftercare

After aneurysmectomy, the patient is monitored in an Intensive Care Unit for the first 24–48 hours. Follow-up tests include ECG, chest x ray, and ultrasound.

Risks

Elective aneurysmectomy has a 5-10% rate of complications, such as bleeding, kidney failure, respiratory complications, **heart attack**, **stroke**, infection, limb loss, bowel **ischemia**, and **impotence**. These complications are many times more common in emergency aneurysmectomy.

Resources

PERIODICALS

Donaldson, M. C., M. Belkin, and A. D. Whittemore. "Mesenteric Revascularization During Aneurysmectomy." *Surgery Clinic of North America* 77 (April 1997): 443-459.

Lori De Milto

Aneurysms *see* **Aneurysmectomy; Cerebral aneurysm; Ventricular aneurysm**

Angina

Definition

Angina is **pain**, "discomfort," or pressure localized in the chest that is caused by an insufficient supply of blood (**ischemia**) to the heart muscle. It is also sometimes characterized by a feeling of **choking**, suffocation, or crushing heaviness. This condition is also called angina pectoris.

Description

Often described as a muscle spasm and choking sensation, the term "angina" is used primarily to describe chest (thoracic) pain originating from insufficient oxygen to the heart muscle. An episode of angina is not an actual **heart attack**, but rather pain that results from the heart muscle temporarily receiving too little blood. This temporary condition may be the result of demanding activities such as **exercise** and does not necessarily indicate that the heart muscle is experiencing permanent damage. In fact, episodes of angina seldom cause permanent damage to heart muscle.

Angina can be subdivided further into two categories: angina of effort and variant angina.

Angina of effort

Angina of effort is a common disorder caused by the narrowing of the arteries (**atherosclerosis**) that supply oxygen-rich blood to the heart muscle. In the case of angina of effort, the heart (coronary) arteries can provide the heart muscle (myocardium) adequate blood during rest but not during periods of exercise, **stress**, or excitement–any of which may precipitate pain. The pain is relieved by resting or by administering nitroglycerin, a medication that reduces ischemia of the heart. Patients with angina of effort have an increased risk of heart attack (myocardial infarction).

Variant angina

Variant angina is uncommon and occurs independently of atherosclerosis which may, however, be present as an incidental finding. Variant angina occurs at rest and is not related to excessive work by the heart muscle. Research indicates that variant angina is caused by coronary artery muscle spasm of insufficient duration or intensity to cause an actual heart attack.

Causes and symptoms

Angina causes a pressing pain or sensation of heaviness, usually in the chest area under the breast

KEY TERMS

Ischemia —Decreased blood supply to an organ or body part, often resulting in pain.

Myocardial infarction —A blockage of a coronary artery that cuts off the blood supply to part of the heart. In most cases, the blockage is caused by fatty deposits.

Myocardium —The thick middle layer of the heart that forms the bulk of the heart wall and contracts as the organ beats.

bone (sternum). It occasionally is experienced in the shoulder, arm, neck, or jaw regions. Because episodes of angina occur when the heart's need for oxygen increases beyond the oxygen available from the blood nourishing the heart, the condition is often precipitated by physical exertion. In most cases, the symptoms are relieved within a few minutes by resting or by taking prescribed angina medications. Emotional stress, extreme temperatures, heavy meals, cigarette **smoking**, and alcohol can also cause or contribute to an episode of angina.

Diagnosis

Physicians can usually diagnose angina based on the patient's symptoms and the precipitating factors. However, other diagnostic testing is often required to confirm or rule out angina, or to determine the severity of the underlying heart disease.

Electrocardiogram (ECG)

An electrocardiogram is a test that records electrical impulses from the heart. The resulting graph of electrical activity can show if the heart muscle isn't functioning properly as a result of a lack of oxygen. Electrocardiograms are also useful in investigating other possible abnormal features of the heart.

Stress test

For many individuals with angina, the results of an electrocardiogram while at rest will not show any abnormalities. Because the symptoms of angina occur during stress, the functioning of the heart may need to be evaluated under the physical stress of exercise. The **stress test** records information from the electrocardiogram before, during, and after exercise in search of stress-related abnormalities. Blood pressure is also measured during the stress test and symptoms are

noted. A more involved and complex stress test (for example, thallium scanning) may be used in some cases to picture the blood flow in the heart muscle during the most intense time of exercise and after rest.

Angiogram

The angiogram, which is basically an x ray of the coronary artery, has been noted to be the most accurate diagnostic test to indicate the presence and extent of coronary disease. In this procedure, a long, thin, flexible tube (catheter) is maneuvered into an artery located in the forearm or groin. This catheter is passed further through the artery into one of the two major coronary arteries. A dye is injected at that time to help the x rays "see" the heart and arteries more clearly. Many brief x rays are made to create a "movie" of blood flowing through the coronary arteries, which will reveal any possible narrowing that causes a decrease in blood flow to the heart muscle and associated symptoms of angina.

Treatment

Conservative treatment

Artery disease causing angina is addressed initially by controlling existing factors placing the individual at risk. These risk factors include cigarette smoking, high blood pressure, **high cholesterol** levels, and **obesity**. Angina is often controlled by medication, most commonly with nitroglycerin. This drug relieves symptoms of angina by increasing the diameter of the blood vessels carrying blood to the heart muscle. Nitroglycerin is taken whenever discomfort occurs or is expected. It may be taken by mouth by placing the tablet under the tongue or transdermally by placing a medicated patch directly on the skin. In addition, **beta blockers** or **calcium channel blockers** may be prescribed to also decrease the demand on the heart by decreasing the rate and workload of the heart.

Surgical treatment

When conservative treatments are not effective in the reduction of angina pain and the risk of heart attack remains high, physicians may recommend **angioplasty** or surgery. Coronary artery bypass surgery is an operation in which a blood vessel (often a long vein surgically removed from the leg) is grafted onto the blocked artery to bypass the blocked portion. This newly formed pathway allows blood to flow adequately to the heart muscle.

Another procedure used to improve blood flow to the heart is balloon angioplasty. In this procedure, the physician inserts a catheter with a tiny balloon at the end into a forearm or groin artery. The catheter is then threaded up into the coronary arteries and the balloon is inflated to open the vessel in narrowed sections. Other techniques using laser and mechanical devices are being developed and applied, also by means of catheters.

Alternative treatment

During an angina episode, relief has been noted by applying massage or kinesiological methods, but these techniques are not standard recommendations by physicians. For example, one technique places the palm and fingers of either hand on the forehead while simultaneously firmly massaging the sternum (breast bone) up and down its entire length using the other hand. This is followed by additional massaging by the fingertip and thumb next to the sternum, on each side.

Once the angina has subsided, the cause should be determined and treated. Atherosclerosis, a major associated cause, requires diet and lifestyle adjustments, primarily including regular exercise, reduction of dietary sugar and saturated fats, and increase of dietary fiber. Both conventional and alternative medicine agree that increasing exercise and improving diet are important steps to reduce high cholesterol levels. Alternative medicine has proposed specific cholesterol-lowering treatments, with several gaining the attention and interest of the public. One of the most recent popular treatments is garlic (*Allium sativum*). Some studies have shown that adequate dosages of garlic can reduce total cholesterol by about 10%, LDL (bad) cholesterol by 15%, and raise HDL (good) cholesterol by 10%. Other studies have not shown significant benefit. Although its effect on cholesterol is not as great as that achieved by medications, garlic may possibly be of benefit in relatively mild cases of high cholesterol, without causing the side effects associated with **cholesterol-reducing drugs**. Other herbal remedies that may help lower cholesterol include alfalfa (*Medicago sativa*), fenugreek (*Trigonella foenum-graecum*), Asian ginseng (*Panax ginseng*), and tumeric (*Curcuma longa*).

Antioxidants, including vitamin A (beta carotene), vitamin C, vitamin E, and selenium, can limit the oxidative damage to the walls of blood vessels that may be a precursor of atherosclerotic plaque formation.

Prognosis

The prognosis for a patient with angina depends on its origin, type, severity, and the general health of the individual. A person who has angina has the best prognosis if he or she seeks prompt medical attention and learns the pattern of his or her angina, such as what causes the attacks, what they feel like, how long episodes usually last, and whether medication relieves the attacks. If patterns of the symptoms change significantly, or if symptoms resemble those of a heart attack, medical help should be sought immediately.

Prevention

In most cases, the best prevention involves changing one's habits to avoid bringing on attacks of angina. If blood pressure medication has been prescribed, compliance is a necessity and should be a priority as well. Many healthcare professionals–including physicians, dietitians, and nurses–can provide valuable advice on proper diet, weight control, blood cholesterol levels, and blood pressure. These professionals also offer suggestions about current treatments and information to help stop smoking. In general, the majority of those with angina adjust their lives to minimize episodes of angina, by taking necessary precautions and using medications if recommended and necessary. **Coronary artery disease** is the underlying problem that should be addressed.

Resources

ORGANIZATIONS

National Heart, Lung and Blood Institute. P.O. Box 30105, Bethesda, MD 20824-0105. (301) 251-1222. < http://www.nhlbi.nih.gov > .

OTHER

"Angina." Healthtouch Online Page. Sepember 1997. [cited May 21, 1998]. < http://www.healthtouch.com > .

Jeffrey P. Larson, RPT

Angioedema *see* **Hives**

Angiogram *see* **Angiography**

Angiography

Definition

Angiography is the x-ray study of the blood vessels. An angiogram uses a radiopaque substance, or dye, to make the blood vessels visible under x ray. Arteriography is a type of angiography that involves the study of the arteries.

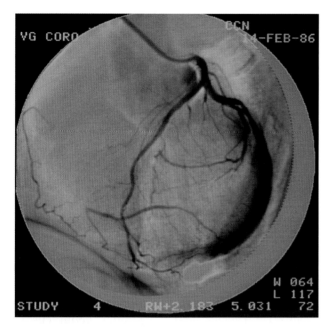

An angiogram of a coronary artery. *(Phototake NYC. Reproduced by permission.)*

Purpose

Angiography is used to detect abnormalities or blockages in the blood vessels (called occlusions) throughout the circulatory system and in some organs. The procedure is commonly used to identify **atherosclerosis**; to diagnose heart disease; to evaluate kidney function and detect kidney cysts or tumors; to detect an aneurysm (an abnormal bulge of an artery that can rupture leading to hemorrhage), tumor, blood clot, or **arteriovenous malformations** (abnormals tangles of arteries and veins) in the brain; and to diagnose problems with the retina of the eye. It is also used to give surgeons an accurate "map" of the heart prior to open-heart surgery, or of the brain prior to neurosurgery.

Precautions

Patients with **kidney disease** or injury may suffer further kidney damage from the contrast mediums used for angiography. Patients who have blood clotting problems, have a known allergy to contrast mediums, or are allergic to iodine, a component of some contrast mediums, may also not be suitable candidates for an angiography procedure. Because x rays carry

---

KEY TERMS

Arteriosclerosis—A chronic condition characterized by thickening and hardening of the arteries and the build-up of plaque on the arterial walls. Arteriosclerosis can slow or impair blood circulation.

Carotid artery—An artery located in the neck.

Catheter—A long, thin, flexible tube used in angiography to inject contrast material into the arteries.

Cirrhosis—A condition characterized by the destruction of healthy liver tissue. A cirrhotic liver is scarred and cannot break down the proteins in the bloodstream. Cirrhosis is associated with portal hypertension.

Embolism—A blood clot, air bubble, or clot of foreign material that travels and blocks the flow of blood in an artery. When blood supply to a tissue or organ is blocked by an embolism, infarction, or death of the tissue the artery feeds, occurs. Without immediate and appropriate treatment, an embolism can be fatal.

Femoral artery—An artery located in the groin area that is the most frequently accessed site for arterial puncture in angiography.

Fluorescein dye—An orange dye used to illuminate the blood vessels of the retina in fluorescein angiography.

Fluoroscopic screen—A fluorescent screen which displays "moving x-rays" of the body. Fluoroscopy allows the radiologist to visualize the guide wire and catheter he is moving through the patient's artery.

Guide wire—A wire that is inserted into an artery to guides a catheter to a certain location in the body.

Iscehmia—A lack of normal blood supply to a organ or body part because of blockages or constriction of the blood vessels.

Necrosis—Cellular or tissue death; skin necrosis may be caused by multiple, consecutive doses of radiation from fluoroscopic or x-ray procedures.

Plaque—Fatty material that is deposited on the inside of the arterial wall.

Portal hypertension—A condition caused by cirrhosis of the liver. It is characterized by impaired or reversed blood flow from the portal vein to the liver, an enlarged spleen, and dilated veins in the esophagus and stomach.

Portal vein thrombosis—The development of a blood clot in the vein that brings blood into the liver. Untreated portal vein thrombosis causes portal hypertension.

---

risks of ionizing radiation exposure to the fetus, pregnant women are also advised to avoid this procedure.

Description

Angiography is usually performed at a hospital by a trained radiologist and assisting technician or nurse. It takes place in an x-ray or fluoroscopy suite, and for most types of angiograms, the patient's vital signs will be monitored throughout the procedure.

Angiography requires the injection of a contrast dye that makes the blood vessels visible to x ray. The dye is injected through a procedure known as *arterial puncture*. The puncture is usually made in the groin area, armpit, inside elbow, or neck. The site is cleaned with an antiseptic agent and injected with a local anesthetic. First, a small incision is made in the skin to help the needle pass. A needle containing an inner wire called a stylet is inserted through the skin into the artery. When the radiologist has punctured the artery with the needle, the stylet is removed and replaced with another long wire called a guide wire. It is normal for blood to spout out of the needle before the guide wire is inserted.

The guide wire is fed through the outer needle into the artery and to the area that requires angiographic study. A fluoroscopic screen that displays a view of the patient's vascular system is used to pilot the wire to the correct location. Once it is in position, the needle is removed and a catheter is slid over the length of the guide wire until it to reaches the area of study. The guide wire is removed and the catheter is left in place in preparation for the injection of the contrast medium, or dye.

Depending on the type of angiography procedure being performed, the contrast medium is either injected by hand with a syringe or is mechanically injected with an automatic injector connected to the catheter. An automatic injector is used frequently because it is able to propel a large volume of dye very quickly to the angiogram site. The patient is warned that the injection will start, and instructed to remain very still. The injection causes some mild to moderate discomfort. Possible side effects or reactions include **headache**, **dizziness**, irregular heartbeat, **nausea**, warmth, burning sensation, and chest **pain**, but they usually last only momentarily. To view the area of study from different angles or perspectives, the patient may be asked to change positions several times, and subsequent dye injections may be administered. During any injection, the patient or the camera may move.

Throughout the dye injection procedure, x-ray pictures and/or fluoroscopic pictures (or moving x rays) will be taken. Because of the high pressure of arterial blood flow, the dye will dissipate through the patient's system quickly, so pictures must be taken in rapid succession. An automatic film changer is used because the manual changing of x-ray plates can eat up valuable time.

Once the x rays are complete, the catheter is slowly and carefully removed from the patient. Pressure is applied to the site with a sandbag or other weight for 10-20 minutes in order for clotting to take place and the arterial puncture to reseal itself. A pressure bandage is then applied.

Most angiograms follow the general procedures outlined above, but vary slightly depending on the area of the vascular system being studied. A variety of common angiography procedures are outlined below:

Cerebral angiography

Cerebral angiography is used to detect aneurysms, **blood clots**, and other vascular irregularities in the brain. The catheter is inserted into the femoral or carotid artery and the injected contrast medium travels through the blood vessels on the brain. Patients frequently experience headache, warmth, or a burning sensation in the head or neck during the injection portion of the procedure. A cerebral angiogram takes two to four hours to complete.

Coronary angiography

Coronary angiography is administered by a cardiologist with training in radiology or, occasionally, by a radiologist. The arterial puncture is typically given in the femoral artery, and the cardiologist uses a guide wire and catheter to perform a contrast injection and x-ray series on the coronary arteries. The catheter may also be placed in the left ventricle to examine the mitral and aortic valves of the heart. If the cardiologist requires a view of the right ventricle of the heart or of the tricuspid or pulmonic valves, the catheter will be inserted through a large vein and guided into the right ventricle. The catheter also serves the purpose of monitoring blood pressures in these different locations inside the heart. The angiogram procedure takes several hours, depending on the complexity of the procedure.

Pulmonary angiography

Pulmonary, or lung, angiography is performed to evaluate blood circulation to the lungs. It is also considered the most accurate diagnostic test for detecting a **pulmonary embolism**. The procedure differs from cerebral and coronary angiograms in that the guide wire and catheter are inserted into a vein instead of an artery, and are guided up through the chambers of the heart and into the pulmonary artery. Throughout the procedure, the patient's vital signs are monitored to ensure that the catheter doesn't cause **arrhythmias**, or irregular heartbeats. The contrast medium is then injected into the pulmonary artery where it circulates through the lung capillaries. The test typically takes up to 90 minutes.

Kidney angiography

Patients with chronic renal disease or injury can suffer further damage to their kidneys from the contrast medium used in a kidney angiogram, yet they often require the test to evaluate kidney function. These patients should be well-hydrated with a intravenous saline drip before the procedure, and may benefit from available medications (e.g., dopamine) that help to protect the kidney from further injury due to contrast agents. During a kidney angiogram, the guide wire and catheter are inserted into the femoral artery in the groin area and advanced through the abdominal aorta, the main artery in the abdomen, and into the renal arteries. The procedure will take approximately one hour.

Fluorescein angiography

Fluorescein angiography is used to diagnose retinal problems and circulatory disorders. It is typically conducted as an outpatient procedure. The patient's pupils are dilated with eye drops and he rests his chin and forehead against a bracing apparatus to keep it still. Sodium fluorescein dye is then injected with a syringe into a vein in the patient's arm. The dye will travel through the patient's body and into the blood vessels of the eye. The procedure does not require x rays. Instead, a rapid series of close-up photographs of the patient's eyes are taken, one set immediately after the dye is injected, and a second set approximately 20 minutes later once the dye has moved through the patient's vascular system. The entire procedure takes up to one hour.

Celiac and mesenteric angiography

Celiac and mesenteric angiography involves x-ray exploration of the celiac and mesenteric arteries, arterial branches of the abdominal aorta that supply blood to the abdomen and digestive system. The test is commonly used to detect aneurysm, thrombosis, and signs of **ischemia** in the celiac and mesenteric arteries, and to locate the source of gastrointestinal bleeding. It is also

used in the diagnosis of a number of conditions, including portal **hypertension**, and **cirrhosis**. The procedure can take up to three hours, depending on the number of blood vessels studied.

Splenoportography

A splenoportograph is a variation of an angiogram that involves the injection of contrast medium directly into the spleen to view the splenic and portal veins. It is used to diagnose blockages in the splenic vein and portal vein thrombosis and to assess the strength and location of the vascular system prior to **liver transplantation**.

Most angiography procedures are typically paid for by major medical insurance. Patients should check with their individual insurance plans to determine their coverage.

Preparation

Patients undergoing an angiogram are advised to stop eating and drinking eight hours prior to the procedure. They must remove all jewelry before the procedure and change into a hospital gown. If the arterial puncture is to be made in the armpit or groin area, shaving may be required. A sedative may be administered to relax the patient for the procedure. An IV line will also be inserted into a vein in the patient's arm before the procedure begins in case medication or blood products are required during the angiogram.

Prior to the angiography procedure, patients will be briefed on the details of the test, the benefits and risks, and the possible complications involved, and asked to sign an informed consent form.

Aftercare

Because life-threatening internal bleeding is a possible complication of an arterial puncture, an overnight stay in the hospital is sometimes recommended following an angiography procedure, particularly with cerebral and coronary angiograms. If the procedure is performed on an outpatient basis, the patient is typically kept under close observation for a period of at six to 12 hours before being released. If the arterial puncture was performed in the femoral artery, the patient will be instructed to keep his leg straight and relatively immobile during the observation period. The patient's blood pressure and vital signs will be monitored and the puncture site observed closely. Pain medication may be prescribed if the patient is experiencing discomfort from the puncture, and a cold pack is applied to the site to reduce swelling. It is normal for the puncture site to be sore and bruised for several weeks. The patient may also develop a hematoma, a hard mass created by the blood vessels broken during the procedure. Hematomas should be watched carefully, as they may indicate continued bleeding of the arterial puncture site.

Angiography patients are also advised to enjoy two to three days of rest and relaxation after the procedure in order to avoid placing any undue **stress** on the arterial puncture. Patients who experience continued bleeding or abnormal swelling of the puncture site, sudden dizziness, or chest pains in the days following an angiography procedure should seek medical attention immediately.

Patients undergoing a fluorescein angiography should not drive or expose their eyes to direct sunlight for 12 hours following the procedure.

Risks

Because angiography involves puncturing an artery, internal bleeding or hemorrhage are possible complications of the test. As with any invasive procedure, infection of the puncture site or bloodstream is also a risk, but this is rare.

A **stroke** or **heart attack** may be triggered by an angiogram if blood clots or plaque on the inside of the arterial wall are dislodged by the catheter and form a blockage in the blood vessels or artery. The heart may also become irritated by the movement of the catheter through its chambers during pulmonary and coronary angiography procedures, and arrhythmias may develop.

Patients who develop an allergic reaction to the contrast medium used in angiography may experience a variety of symptoms, including swelling, difficulty breathing, **heart failure**, or a sudden drop in blood pressure. If the patient is aware of the allergy before the test is administered, certain medications can be administered at that time to counteract the reaction.

Angiography involves minor exposure to radiation through the x rays and fluoroscopic guidance used in the procedure. Unless the patient is pregnant, or multiple radiological or fluoroscopic studies are required, the small dose of radiation incurred during a single procedure poses little risk. However, multiple studies requiring fluoroscopic exposure that are conducted in a short time period have been known to cause skin necrosis in some individuals. This risk can be minimized by careful monitoring and documentation of cumulative radiation doses administered to these patients.

Normal results

The results of an angiogram or arteriogram depend on the artery or organ system being examined. Generally, test results should display a normal and unimpeded flow of blood through the vascular system. Fluorescein angiography should result in no leakage of fluorescein dye through the retinal blood vessels.

Abnormal results

Abnormal results of an angiography may display a restricted blood vessel or arterial blood flow (ischemia) or an irregular placement or location of blood vessels. The results of an angiography vary widely by the type of procedure performed, and should be interpreted and explained to the patient by a trained radiologist.

Resources

BOOKS

Baum, Stanley, and Michael J. Pentecost, editors. *Abrams' Angiography.* 4th ed. Philadelphia: Lippincott-Raven, 1996.

Paula Anne Ford-Martin

Angiomas *see* **Birthmarks**

Angioplasty

Definition

Angioplasty is a term describing a procedure used to widen vessels narrowed by stenoses or occlusions. There are various types of these procedures and their names are associated with the type of vessel entry and equipment used. For example, percutaneous transluminal angioplasty (PTA) describes entry through the skin (percutaneous) and navigates to the area of the vessel of interest through the same vessel or one that communicates with it (transluminal). In the case of a procedure involving the coronary arteries, the point of entry could be the femoral artery in the groin and the catheter/guidewire system is passed through the aorta to the heart and the origin of the coronary arteries at the base of the aorta just outside the aortic valve.

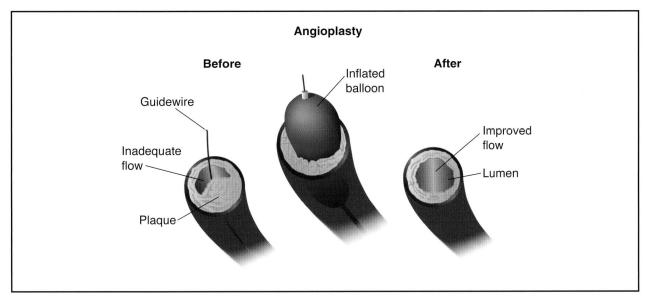

Angioplasty

Before

Guidewire

Inadequate flow

Plaque

Inflated balloon

After

Improved flow

Lumen

In balloon angioplasty, plaque is pushed out of the clogged artery by the inflation of the balloon device. *(Illustration by Argosy Inc.)*

Purpose

In individuals with an occulsive vascular disease such as **atherosclerosis**, blood flow is impaired to an organ (such as the heart) or to a distal body part (such as the lower leg) by the narrowing of the vessel's lumen due to fatty deposits or calcium accumulation. This narrowing may occur in any vessel but may occur anywhere. Once the vessel has been widened, adequate blood flow is returned. The vessel may narrow again over time at the same location and the procedure could be repeated.

Precautions

Angioplasty procedures are performed on hospital inpatients in facilities for proper monitoring and recovery. If the procedure is to be performed in a coronary artery, the patient's care is likely to be provided by specially trained physicians, nurses, and vascular specialists. Typically, patients are given anticoagulants prior to the procedure to assist in the prevention of thromboses (**blood clots**). Administration of anticoagulants, however, may impede the sealing of the vascular entry point. The procedure will be performed using fluoroscopic guidance and contrast media. Since the decision to perform angioplasty may have been made following a diagnostic angiogram, the patient's sensitivity to iodinated contrast media is likely to known. The procedure may then require the use of non-ionic contrast agents.

Description

Angioplasty was originally performed by dilating the vessel with the introduction of larger and larger stiff catheters through the narrowed space. Complications of this procedure caused researchers to develop means of widening the vessel using a minimally sized device. Today, catheters contain balloons that are inflated to widen the vessel and stents to provide structural support for the vessel. Lasers may be used to assist in the break up of the fat or calcium plaque. Catheters may also be equipped with spinning wires or drill tips to clean out the plaque.

Angioplasty may be performed while the patient is sedated or anesthetized, depending on the vessels involved. If a percutaneous transluminal coronary angioplasty (PTCA) is to be performed, the patient will be kept awake to report on discomfort and **cough** if required. PTCA procedures are performed in **cardiac catheterization** labs with sophisticated monitoring devices. If angioplasty is performed in the radiology department's angiographic suite, the patient may be sedated for the procedure and a nurse will monitor the patient's vital signs during the procedure. If performed by a vascular surgeon, the angioplasty procedure will be performed in an operating room or specially designed vascular procedure suite.

The site of the introduction of the angioplasty equipment is prepared as a sterile surgical site. Although many procedures are performed by puncturing the vessel through skin, many procedures are also performed by surgically exposing the site of entry. Direct view of the vessel's puncture site aids in monitoring damage to the vessel or excessive bleeding at the site. Once the vessel is punctured and the guidewire is introduced, fluoroscopy is used to monitor small injections of contrast media used to visualize the path through the vessel. If the fluoroscopy system has a feature called 'roadmap', the amount of contrast media injected will be greater in order to define the full route the guidewire will take. The fluoroscopy system will then superimpose subsequent images over the roadmap while the vessel is traversed, that is, the physician moves the guidewire along the map to the destination.

Having reached the area of stenosis, the physician will inflate the balloon on the catheter that has been passed along the guidewire. Balloons are inflated in size and duration depending on the size and location of the vessel. In some cases, the use of a stent (a mesh of wire that resembles a Chinese finger puzzle) may also be used. The vessel may be widened before, during, or after the deployment of the stent. Procedures for deploying stents are dependent on the type of stent used. In cases where the vessel is tortuous or at intersections of vessels, the use of a graph may be necessary to provide structural strength to the vessel. Stents, graphs, and balloon dilation may all be used together or separately.

The procedure is verified using fluoroscopy and contrast media to produce an angiogram or by using intravascular ultrasound or both. All equipment is withdrawn from the vessel and the puncture site repaired.

Risks

During the procedure there is a danger of puncturing the vessel with the guidewire. This is a very small risk. Patients must be monitored for hematoma or hemorrhage at the puncture site. There is also a small risk of **heart attack**, emboli, and although

unlikely **death**. Hospitalization will vary in length by the patient's overall condition, any complications, and availability of home care.

Resources

PERIODICALS

"The angioplasty correct follow up strategy after stent implantation." *Heart* 84, no. 4 (April, 2001): 363.
Carnall, Douglas. "Angioplasty." *The Western Journal of Medicine* 173, no. 3 (September 2000): 201.
"New Imaging Technique Could Improve Outcome of Popular Heart Procedure." *Heart Disease Weekly* May 13, 2001: 3.
"Success clearing clogged arteries." *Science News* 159, no. 5 (February 3, 2001): 72.

OTHER

"Cardiovascular System" Miami Heart Research Institute 2001. [cited July 5, 2001]. < http://www.miamiheartresearch.org/Learning Center/Your Cardiovascular.../Cardiovascular.htm >.
"Coronary angioplasty: Opening clogged arteries" MayoClinic.com, Condition Centers, Treatments and Tests. 2000. [cited July 5, 2001]. < http://www.mayoclinic.com >.
"Heart *American Heart Association online.* 2000. [cited July 5, 2001]. < http://www.americanheart.org/Heart_and_Stroke_A_Z_Guide/angiol.html >.
"STS Patient Information: What to Expect after your Heart Surgery." Society of Thoracic Surgeons online. 2000. [cited July 5, 2001]. < http://www.sts.org/doc/3563 >.
"When you need to have Angioplast: A patient guide" Heart Information Network. 2000. [cited July 5, 2001]. < http://www.heartinfo.org/news97/gdangio111897.htm >.

Elaine R. Proseus, MBA/TM, BSRT, RT(R)

Angiotensin-converting enzyme inhibitors

Definition

Angiotensin-converting enzyme inhibitors (also called ACE inhibitors) are medicines that block the conversion of the chemical angiotensin I to a substance that increases salt and water retention in the body.

Purpose

ACE inhibitors are used in the treatment of high blood pressure. They may be used alone or in combination with other medicines for high blood pressure.

KEY TERMS

Arteries—Blood vessels that carry blood away from the heart to the cells, tissues, and organs of the body.

Chronic—A word used to describe a long-lasting condition. Chronic conditions often develop gradually and involve slow changes.

Enzyme—A type of protein, produced in the body, that brings about or speeds up chemical reactions.

Fetus—A developing baby inside the womb.

Scleroderma—A disease that first affects the skin and later affects certain internal organs. The first symptoms are the hardening, thickening, and shrinking of the skin.

Systemic lupus erythematosus (SLE)—A chronic disease that affects the skin, joints, and certain internal organs.

Venom—A poisonous substance secreted by an animal, usually delivered through a bite or a sting.

They work by preventing a chemical in the blood, angiotensin I, from being converted into a substance that increases salt and water retention in the body. Increased salt and water retention lead to high blood pressure. ACE inhibitors also make blood vessels relax, which helps lower blood pressure and allows more oxygen-rich blood to reach the heart.

Treating high blood pressure is important because the condition puts a burden on the heart and the arteries, which can lead to permanent damage over time. If untreated, high blood pressure increases the risk of heart attacks, **heart failure**, **stroke**, or kidney failure.

ACE inhibitors may also be prescribed for other conditions. For example, captopril (Capoten) is used to treat kidney problems in people who take insulin to control diabetes. Captopril and lisinopril are also given to some patients after a **heart attack**. Heart attacks damage and weaken the heart muscle, and the damage continues even after a person recovers from the attack. This medicine helps slow down further damage to the heart. ACE inhibitors also may be used to treat congestive heart failure.

Description

ACE inhibitors are available only with a physician's prescription and come in tablet, capsule, and injectable forms. Some commonly used ACE inhibitors are benazepril (Lotensin), captopril (Capoten), enalapril (Vasotec), fosinopril (Monopril), lisinopril (Prinivil, Zestril), moexipril (Univasc), perindopril (Aceon), quinapril (Accupril), ramipril (Altace) and trandolapril (Mavik).

Recommended dosage

The recommended dosage depends on the type of ACE inhibitor and the medical condition for which it is being taken. Check with the physician who prescribed the drug or the pharmacist who filled the prescription for the correct dosage.

This medicine may take weeks to noticeably lower blood pressure. Take it exactly as directed.

Do not stop taking this medicine without checking with the physician who prescribed it.

Precautions

A person taking an ACE inhibitor should see a physician regularly. The physician will check the blood pressure to make sure the medicine is working as it should and will note any unwanted side effects. People who have high blood pressure often feel perfectly fine. However, they should continue to see their physicians even when they feel well so that the physician can keep a close watch on their condition. It is also important for patients to keep taking their medicine even when they feel fine.

ACE inhibitors will not cure high blood pressure, but will help control the condition. To avoid the serious health problems that high blood pressure can cause, patients may have to take medicine for the rest of their lives. Furthermore, medicine alone may not be enough. Patients with high blood pressure may also need to avoid certain foods, such as salty snacks, and keep their weight under control. The health care professional who is treating the condition can offer advice on what measures may be necessary. Patients being treated for high blood pressure should not change their **diets** without consulting their physicians.

Anyone taking this medicine for high blood pressure should not take any other prescription or over-the-counter (OTC) medicine without first checking with his or her physician. Some medicines, such as certain cold remedies, may increase blood pressure.

Some people feel dizzy or lightheaded after taking the first dose of an ACE inhibitor, especially if they have been taking a water pill (diuretic). Anyone who takes these drugs should not drive, use machines or do anything else that might be dangerous until they have found out how the drugs affect them. Such symptoms should be reported to the physician or pharmacist if they do not subside within a day or so. For the first one or two days of taking an ACE inhibitor, patients may become lightheaded when arising from bed in the morning. Patienst should rise slowly to a sitting position before standing up.

While a goal of treatment with an ACE inhibitor is to lower the blood pressure, patients must be careful not to let their blood pressure get too low. Low blood pressure can lead to **dizziness**, lightheadedness and **fainting**. To prevent the blood pressure from getting too low, observe these precautions:

- Do not drink alcohol without checking with the physician who prescribed this medicine.

- Captopril and moexipril should be taken one hour before meals. Other ACE inhinbitors may be taken with or without meals.

- Avoid overheating when exercising or in hot weather. The loss of water from the body through heavy sweating can cause low blood pressure.

- Check with a physician right away if illness occurs while taking an ACE inhibitor. This is especially true if the illness involves severe **nausea**, **vomiting**, or **diarrhea**. Vomiting and diarrhea can cause the loss of too much water from the body, which can lead to low blood pressure.

Anyone who is taking ACE inhibitors should be sure to tell the health care professional in charge before having any surgical or dental procedures or receiving emergency treatment.

Some ACE inhibitors may change the results of certain medical tests, such as blood or urine tests. Before having medical tests, anyone taking this medicine should alert the health care professional in charge.

Do not use a potassium supplement or a salt substitute that contains potassium without first checking with the physician who prescribed the ACE inhibitor.

Patients who are being treated with bee or wasp venom to prevent allergic reactions to stings may have a severe allergic reaction to certain ACE inhibitors.

Special conditions

People with certain medical conditions or who are taking certain other medicines can have problems if they take ACE inhibitors. Before taking these drugs, be sure to let the physician know about any of these conditions.

ALLERGIES. Anyone who has had unusual reactions to an ACE inhibitor in the past should let his or her physician know before taking this type of medicine again. The physician should also be told about any **allergies** to foods, dyes, preservatives, or other substances.

PREGNANCY. The use of ACE inhibitors in **pregnancy** can cause serious problems and even **death** in the fetus or newborn. Women who are pregnant or who may become pregnant should check with their physicians before using this medicine. Women who become pregnant while taking this medicine should check with their physicians immediately.

BREASTFEEDING. Some ACE inhibitors pass into breast milk. Women who are breastfeeding should check with their physicians before using ACE inhibitors.

OTHER MEDICAL CONDITIONS. Before using ACE inhibitors, people with any of these medical problems should make sure their physicians are aware of their conditions:

- diabetes
- heart or blood vessel disease
- recent heart attack or stroke
- liver disease
- kidney disease
- kidney transplant
- scleroderma
- systemic lupus erythematosus (SLE)

USE OF CERTAIN MEDICINES. Taking ACE inhibitors with certain other drugs may affect the way the drugs work or may increase the chance of side effects.

Side effects

The most common side effect is a dry, continuing **cough**. This usually does not subside unless the medication is stopped. Ask the physician if the cough can be treated. Less common side effects, such as **headache**, loss of taste, unusual tiredness, and nausea or diarrhea also may occur and do not need medical attention unless they are severe or they interfere with normal activities.

More serious side effects are rare, but may occur. If any of the following side effects occur, check with a physician immediately:

- swelling of the face, lips, tongue, throat, arms, legs, hands, or feet

- itchy skin
- sudden breathing or swallowing problems
- chest pain
- hoarseness
- sore throat
- fever and chills
- stomach pain
- yellow eyes or skin

In addition, anyone who has any of the following symptoms while taking an ACE inhibitor should check with his or her physician as soon as possible:

- dizziness, lightheadedness, fainting
- confusion
- nervousness
- fever
- joint pain
- numbness or **tingling** in hands, feet, or lips
- weak or heavy feeling in the legs
- skin rash
- irregular heartbeat
- shortness of breath or other breathing problems

Other side effects may occur. Anyone who has unusual symptoms after taking an ACE inhibitor should get in touch with his or her physician.

Interactions

ACE inhibitors may interact with certain foods and other medicines. For example, captopril (Capoten) interacts with food and should be taken one hour before meals. Anyone who takes ACE inhibitors should let the physician know all other medicines he or she is taking and should ask about foods that should be avoided. Among the foods and drugs that may interact with ACE inhibitors are:

- water pills (diuretics)
- lithium, used to treat bipolar disorder
- tetracycline, an antibiotic
- medicines or supplements that contain potassium
- salt substitutes that contain potassium

The list above may not include everything that interacts with ACE inhibitors. Be sure to check with a physician or pharmacist before combining ACE inhibitors with any other prescription or nonprescription (over-the-counter) medicine.

Nancy Ross-Flanigan

Angiotensin-converting enzyme test

Definition

This test measures blood levels of angiotensin-converting enzyme (ACE), also known as Serum Angiotensin-Converting Enzyme (SASE). The primary function of ACE is to help regulate arterial pressure by converting angiotensin I to angiotensin II.

Purpose

The ACE test is used primarily to detect and monitor the clinical course of **sarcoidosis** (a disease that affects many organs, especially the lungs), to differentiate between sarcoidosis and similar diseases, and to delineate between active and inactive sarcoid disease. Elevated ACE levels are also found in a number of other conditions, including Gaucher's disease (a rare familial disorder of fat metabolism) and **leprosy**.

Precautions

It should be noted that people under 20 years of age normally have very high ACE levels. Decreased levels may be seen in the condition of excess fat in the blood (hyperlipidemia). Drugs that may cause decreased ACE levels include ACE inhibitor antihypertensives and steroids.

Description

ACE plays an important role in the renin/aldosterone mechanism which controls blood pressure by converting angiotensin I to angiotensin II, two proteins involved in regulating blood pressure. Angiotensin I by itself is inactive, but when converted by ACE to the active form, angiotensin II, it causes narrowing of the small blood vessels in tissues, resulting in an increase in blood pressure. Angiotensin II also stimulates the hormone aldosterone, which causes an increase in blood pressure. Certain kidney disorders increase the production of angiotensin II, another cause of **hypertension**. Despite the action of ACE on blood pressure regulation, determination of this

KEY TERMS

Sarcoidosis—Sarcoidosis is a rare disease of unknown cause in which inflammation occurs in lymph nodes and other tissues throughout the body, usually the lungs, skin, liver, and eyes.

enzyme is not very helpful in the evaluation of hypertension (high blood pressure).

Preparation

Determination of ACE levels requires a blood sample. The patient need not be **fasting**.

Risks

Risks for this test are minimal, but may include slight bleeding from the puncture site, **fainting** or feeling lightheaded after venipuncture, or hematoma (blood accumulating under the puncture site).

Normal results

Normal ranges for this test are laboratory-specific but can range from 8-57 U/ml for patients over 20 years of age.

Abnormal results

Serum ACE levels are elevated in approximately 80-90% of patients with active sarcoidosis. Thyroid hormone may have an effect on ACE activity, as hypothyroid (low thyroid) patients, as well as patients with **anorexia nervosa** with associated findings of **hypothyroidism**, may have low serum ACE activity. ACE can also be decreased in lung **cancer** (bronchogenic carcinoma).

Resources

BOOKS

Pagana, Kathleen Deska. *Mosby's Manual of Diagnostic and Laboratory Tests*. St. Louis: Mosby, Inc., 1998.

Janis O. Flores

Animal bite infections

Definition

The most common problem following an animal bite is simple infection. The saliva of dogs, cats, ferrets,

and rabbits is known to contain a wide variety of bacteria. According to one recent study, bacteria or other pathogens show up in about 85 percent of bites. When an animal bites, it can then transmit pathogens into the wound. These microorganisms may grow within the wound and cause an infection. The consequences of infection range from mild discomfort to life-threatening complications.

Description

Two to 4.5 million animal bites occur each year in the United States; about 1% of these bites require hospitalization. Animal bites result in 334,000 emergency room visits per year, which represents approximately 1% of all emergency hospital visits, at an annual cost of $100 million dollars in health care expenses and lost income. Children are the most frequent victims of dog bites, with 5–9 year-old boys having the highest incidence. Men are more often bitten by dogs than are women (3:1), whereas women are more often bitten by cats (3:1).

Dog bites make up 80–85% of all reported incidents. Cats account for about 10% of reported bites, and other animals (including hamsters, ferrets, rabbits, horses, raccoons, bats, skunks, and monkeys) make up the remaining 5–10%. Cat bites become infected more frequently than dog bites. A dog's mouth is rich in bacteria, but only 15–20% of dog bites become infected. In contrast, approximately 30–50% of cat bites become infected.

Many factors contribute to the infection rates, including the type of wound inflicted, the location of the wound, pre-existing health conditions in the bitten person, the extent of delay before treatment, patient compliance and the presence of a foreign body in the wound. Dogs usually inflict crush injuries because they have rounded teeth and strong jaws; thus, the bite of an adult dog can exert up to 200 pounds per square inch of pressure. This pressure usually results in a crushing injury, causing damage to such deep structures as bones, blood vessels, tendons, muscles, and nerves. The canine teeth in a dog's mouth are also sharp and strong, often inflicting lacerations. Cats, with their needle-like incisors and carnassial teeth, typically cause puncture **wounds**. Puncture wounds appear innocuous on the surface, but the underlying injury goes deep. Cat teeth essentially inject bacteria into the bite, and the deep, narrow wound is difficult to clean. Persons with impaired immunocompetence—for example, individuals with HIV infection—are especially vulnerable to infection from cat bites. Lastly, bites or stings from marine creatures

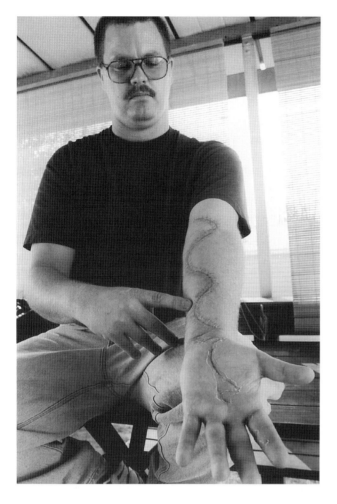

This snake breeder shows the scar from his surgery after he was bitten by a venomous West African Gabon viper. His arm was cut open in order to relieve swelling from the snake bite in his middle finger. *(Photograph by Joe Crocetta, AP/Wide World Photo. Reproduced by permission.)*

(sharks, rays, eels, etc.) require immediate medical attention as these bites may contain disease organisms unique to the ocean environment as well as causing severe loss of blood.

The bacterial species most commonly found in bite wounds include *Pasteurella multocida*, *Staphylococcus aureus*, *Pseudomonas sp*, and *Streptococcus sp*. *P. multocida*, the root cause of pasteurellosis, is especially prominent in cat bite infections. Other infectious diseases from animal bites include **cat-scratch disease**, **tetanus** and **rabies**.

Doctors are increasingly aware of the importance of checking animal bite wounds for anaerobic organisms, which are microbes that can live and multiply in the absence of air or oxygen. A study published in 2003 reported that about two-thirds of animal bite wounds contain anaerobes. These organisms can produce such

complications as septic arthritis, tenosynovitis, **meningitis**, and infections of the lymphatic system.

With regard to the most common types of domestic pets, it is useful to note that biting and other aggressive behavior has different causes in dogs and cats. To some extent these differences are rooted in divergent evolutionary pathways, but they have also been influenced by human interference through selective breeding. Dogs were first domesticated by humans as early as 10,000 B.C. for hunting and as guard or attack dogs. Many species travel in packs or groups in the wild, and many human fatalities resulting from dog bites involve a large group of dogs attacking one or two persons. In addition, dogs typically relate to humans according to a hierarchical model of dominance and submission, and many of the techniques of dog training are intended to teach the dog to respect human authority. Certain breeds of dogs are much more likely to attack humans than others; those most often involved in fatal attacks are pit bulls, Rottweilers, German shepherds, huskies, and mastiffs. According to the Centers for Disease Control (CDC), there are between 15 and 20 fatal dog attacks on humans in the United States each year. There are several assessment or evaluation scales that veterinarians or animal trainers can use to score individual or mixed-breed dogs for dominant or aggressive behavior.

Unlike dogs, cats were not domesticated until about 3000 B.C., and were important to ancient civilizations as rodent catchers and household companions rather than as protectors or hunters of wild game. Biologists classify cats as solitary predators rather than as pack or herd animals; as a result, cats do not relate to humans as authority figures in the same way that dogs do, and they do not form groups that attack humans when threatened or provoked. In addition, domestic cats have been selectively bred for appearance rather than for fierceness or aggression. Most cat bites are the result of fear on the cat's part (as when being placed in a carrier for a trip to the vet) or a phenomenon known as petting-induced aggression. Petting-induced aggression is a behavior in which a cat that has been apparently enjoying contact with a human suddenly turns on the human and bites. This behavior appears to be more common in cats that had no contact with humans during their first seven weeks of life. In other cats, this type of aggression appears to be related to a hypersensitive nervous system; petting or cuddling that was pleasurable to the cat for a few seconds or minutes becomes irritating, and the cat bites as a way of indicating that it has had enough. In older cats, petting-induced aggression is often a sign that the cat feels **pain** from touching or pressure on arthritic joints in its neck or back.

Causes and symptoms

The most common sign of infection from an animal bite is inflammation. The skin around the wound is red and feels warm, and the wound may exude pus. Nearby lymph glands may be swollen. Complications can arise if the infection is not treated and spreads into deeper structures or into the bloodstream. If the bite is deep or occurs on the hand or at a joint, complications are more likely.

Live disease-causing bacteria within the bloodstream and tissues cause complications far from the wound site. Such complications include meningitis, brain abscesses, **pneumonia** and lung abscesses, and heart infections, among others. These complications can be fatal. Deep bites or bites near joints can damage joints and bones, causing inflammation of the bone and bone marrow or septic arthritis.

Cat-scratch disease is caused by *Bartonella henselae*, a bacterium that is carried in cat saliva; infection may be transmitted by a bite or scratch. Approximately 22,000 cases are reported each year in the United States; worldwide, nine out of every 100,000 individuals become infected. More than 80% of reported cases occur in persons under the age of 21. The disease is not normally severe in individuals with healthy immune systems. Symptoms may become serious, however, in immunocompromised individuals, such as those with acquired immune deficiency syndrome (**AIDS**) or those undergoing **chemotherapy**. Common symptoms include an inflamed sore in the area of the bite or scratch, swollen lymph nodes, **fever**, **fatigue**, and rash.

Rabies is caused by a virus that is transmitted through the bite of an animal that is already infected. It is classified as a **zoonosis**, which is a term that refers to any disease of animals that can be transmitted to humans. More than 90% of animal rabies cases occur in such wild animals as skunks, bats, and raccoons, with such domestic animals as dogs and cats accounting for fewer than 10% of cases. The World Health Organization (WHO) estimates that between 35,000 and 50,000 individuals worldwide die each year as a result of rabies. The highest incidence of rabies occurs in Asia where, in 1997, over 33,000 deaths were noted, most occurring in India. Rabies is nowadays rare in the United States, as a result of good animal control practices. Onset is delayed, usually weeks to months after the person has been bitten. Early symptoms of rabies include fever, **headache**, and flu-like symptoms. These progress to **anxiety**, **hallucinations**, **muscle spasms**, partial **paralysis**, fear of water (hydrophobia), and other neurological symptoms as the virus spreads to the central nervous system. Medical treatment must be sought soon after exposure because **death** invariably follows once the infection becomes established.

Most deaths from rabies in the United States result from bat bites; the most recent victim was a 66-year-old man in California who died in September 2003 after failing to report a bat bite.

Diagnosis

A medical examination involves taking the history of the injury and assessing the wound type and damage. Tetanus immunization and general health status are checked. An x ray may be ordered to assess bone damage and to check for **foreign objects** in the wound. Wound cultures are done for infected bites if the victim is at high risk for complications or if the infection does not respond to treatment. Evaluation of possible exposure to rabies is also important. A biting animal suspected of having rabies is usually apprehended, tested, and observed for a period of time for evidence of pre-existing infection.

Treatment

Treatment depends on the wound type, its site, and risk factors for infection. All wounds are cleaned and disinfected as thoroughly as possible. Bites to the head and face usually receive sutures, as do severe lacerations elsewhere. Puncture wounds are left open. If **abscess** formation occurs, the physician may perform an incision so as to drain the abscess.

If infection occurs, **antibiotics** are prescribed. Antibiotics may also be used for infection prevention. Since a single bite wound may contain many different types of bacteria, no single antibiotic is always effective. Commonly prescribed antibiotics are penicillin or a combination of amoxicillin and clavulanate potassium. Aztreonam has been reported to be effective in treating infections caused by *P. multocida*.

Because rabies is caused by a virus, antibiotics are not effective. In addition, as of 2003, there is no known cure for the disease once symptoms become apparent. It is therefore recommended that individuals with a high risk of contracting the disease (veterinarians, animal handlers, some laboratory workers) receive preexposure **vaccination**. Individuals bitten by an unknown or potentially rapid animal should receive postexposure vaccination, also called postexposure **prophylaxis** (PEP). The PEP regimen consists of one dose of vaccine given at the initial visit as well as one dose of human immune globulin. Additional doses of vaccine are given on days 3, 7, 14, and 28.

Prognosis

Once a bacterial infection is halted, the bite victim usually recovers fully. There is no known cure for rabies once symptoms become evident and death is almost certain. WHO reports that 114 rabies deaths occurred in the Americas in 1997, with only four deaths occurring that year in the United States, thus emphasizing the importance of good animal control practice and postexposure prophylaxis.

Prevention

Preventing bites obviously prevents subsequent infections. With regard to domestic pets, parents should inform themselves about the aggression level and other characteristics of a particular breed before bringing a purebred pet dog into the family, and consider having a specific dog evaluated by a veterinarian or animal behaviorist before adopting it. In addition, parents should make sure that the dog has been neutered or spayed, since intact dogs of either sex are more likely to bite than those that have been altered. Cat bites can often be prevented by learning about a cat's body language and recognizing the signs of petting-induced aggression. These include dilating pupils, a low growl, stiffening of the body, twitching of the tail, and flattening the ears backward against the head.

Children under 12 years of age are at a higher risk for bites due to their small size and their inexperience with animals; therefore, they should be supervised with animals and taught to act appropriately around them. In particular, children should be taught not to tease a dog by pulling its fur or tail; to leave a dog alone while it is eating; and to avoid running or screaming in the presence of a dog, as the animal is more likely to chase a moving object. Direct eye contact with a threatening dog should be avoided, as the dog may interpret that as aggression. It is best to stand still if at all possible, with feet together and arms against the chest; most dogs will lose interest in an object that is not moving, and will eventually go away.

A wild animal that is unusually aggressive or behaving strangely (e.g. a raccoon or bat that is active during the daytime or is physically uncoordinated) should be avoided and reported to the local animal control authorities; it may be infected with the rabies virus. Wild animals should not be taken in as pets, and garbage or pet food that might attract wild animals should not be left outside the home or camp site. People should also avoid trying to break up fights between animals and should as a rule approach unknown cats and dogs very cautiously, especially on their territory. Finally, animals should not be trained to fight.

Domestic pets should be vaccinated against rabies; people should consult a veterinarian for advice about the frequency of booster vaccinations for the area in which they live. In addition, people who are traveling to countries where rabies is endemic should consider vaccination before leaving the United States.

Resources

BOOKS

Beers, Mark H., MD, and Robert Berkow, MD., editors. "Central Nervous System Viral Diseases: Rabies (Hydrophobia)." Section 13, Chapter 162 In *The Merck Manual of Diagnosis and Therapy*. Whitehouse Station, NJ: Merck Research Laboratories, 1999.

Beers, Mark H., MD, and Robert Berkow, MD., editors. "Infections of Bones and Joints." Section 5, Chapter 54 In *The Merck Manual of Diagnosis and Therapy*. Whitehouse Station, NJ: Merck Research Laboratories, 1999.

Dodman, Nicholas H., DVM. *If Only They Could Speak: Stories About Pets and Their People*. New York and London: W. W. Norton and Company, 2002. Contains several useful appendices about aggression in various dog breeds and a sample assessment form for evaluating a dog's potential for biting.

Garvey, Michael S., DVM, Ann E. Hohenhaus, DVM, Katherine A. Houpt, VMD, PhD, et al. *The Veterinarians' Guide to Your Cat's Symptoms*. New York: Villard, 1999.

PERIODICALS

Brook, I. "Microbiology and Management of Human and Animal Bite Wound Infections." *Primary Care* 30 (March 2003): 25–39.

Fooks, A. R., N. Johnson, S. M. Brookes, et al. "Risk Factors Associated with Travel to Rabies Endemic Countries." *Journal of Applied Microbiology* 94, Supplement (2003): 31S–36S.

Garcia Triana, M., M. A. Fernandez Echevarria, R. L. Alvaro, et al. "*Pasteurella multocida* Tenosynovitis of the Hand: Sonographic Findings." *Journal of Clinical Ultrasound* 31 (March-April 2003): 159–162.

"Human Death Associated with Bat Rabies—California, 2003." *Morbidity and Mortality Weekly Report* 53 (January 23, 2004): 33–35.

Le Moal, G., C. Landron, G. Grollier, et al. "Meningitis Due to *Capnocytophaga canimorsus* After Receipt of a Dog Bite: Case Report and Review of the Literature." *Clinical Infectious Diseases* 36 (February 1, 2003): 42–46.

Messenger, S. L., J. S. Smith, L. A. Orciari, et al. "Emerging Pattern of Rabies Deaths and Increased Viral Infectivity." *Emerging Infectious Diseases* 9 (February 2003): 151–154.

Perkins, R. A., and S. S. Morgan. "Poisoning, Envenomation, and Trauma from Marine Creatures." *American Family Physician* 69 (February 15, 2004): 885–890.

Sacks, Jeffrey J., MD, MPH, Leslie Sinclair, DVM, Julie Gilchrist, MD, et al. "Special Report: Breeds of Dogs Involved in Fatal Human Attacks in the United States Between 1979 and 1998." *Journal of the American Veterinary Medical Association* 217 (September 15, 2000): 836–840.

Weiss, R. A. "Cross-Species Infections." *Current Topics in Microbiology and Immunology* 278 (2003): 47–71.

Winner, J. S., C. A. Gentry, L. J. Machado, and P. Cornea. "Aztreonam Treatment of *Pasteurella multocida* Cellulitis and Bacteremia." *Annals of Pharmacotherapy* 37 (March 2003): 392–394.

ORGANIZATIONS

American Academy of Emergency Medicine (AAEM). 555 East Wells Street, Suite 1100, Milwaukee, WI 53202. (800) 884-2236. Fax: (414) 276-3349. < http://www.aaem.org > .

American Veterinary Medical Association (AVMA). 1931 North Meacham Road, Suite 100, Schaumburg, IL 60173-4360. < http://www.avma.org > .

Centers for Disease Control and Prevention. 1600 Clifton Rd., NE, Atlanta, GA 30333. (800) 311-3435, (404) 639-3311. < http://www.cdc.gov > .

OTHER

National Association of State Public Health Veterinarians, Inc. "Compendium of Animal Rabies Prevention and Control, 2003." *Morbidity and Mortality Weekly Report Recommendations and Reports* 52 (March 21, 2003) (RR-5): 1–6.

"Rabies Situation and Trends." Paris: World Health Organization. 2001. < http://www.who.int/emc/diseases/zoo/rabies.html > .

Julia Barrett
Rebecca J. Frey, PhD

Ankylosing spondylitis

Definition

Ankylosing spondylitis (AS) refers to inflammation of the joints in the spine. AS is also known as rheumatoid spondylitis or Marie-Strümpell disease (among other names).

Description

A form of arthritis, AS is characterized by chronic inflammation, causing **pain** and stiffness of the back,

KEY TERMS

Ankylosing—When bones of a joint are fused, stiff, or rigid.

HLA-B27—An antigen or protein marker on cells that may indicate ankylosing spondylitis.

Immune suppressing—Anything that reduces the activity of the immune system.

Inflammation—A reaction of tissues to disease or injury, often associated with pain and swelling.

Spondylitis—An inflammation of the spine.

progressing to the chest and neck. Eventually, the whole back may become curved and inflexible if the bones fuse (this is known as "bamboo spine"). AS is a systemic disorder that may involve multiple organs, such as the:

- eye (causing an inflammation of the iris, or iritis)
- heart (causing aortic valve disease)
- lungs
- skin (causing a scaly skin condition, or psoriasis)
- gastrointestinal tract (causing inflammation within the small intestine, called ileitis, or inflammation of the large intestine, called colitis)

Less than 1% of the population has AS; however, 20% of AS sufferers have a relative with the disorder.

Causes and symptoms

Genetics play an important role in the disease, but the cause of AS is still unknown. More than 90% of patients have a gene called HLA-B27, but only 10-15% of those who inherit the gene develop the disease. Symptoms of AS include:

- low back and hip pain and stiffness
- difficulty expanding the chest
- pain in the neck, shoulders, knees, and ankles
- low-grade fever
- fatigue
- weight loss

AS is seen most commonly in males 30 years old and older. Initial symptoms are uncommon after the age of 30, although the diagnosis may not be established until after that age. The incidence of AS in Afro-Americans is about 25% of the incidence in Caucasians.

Diagnosis

Doctors usually diagnose the disease simply by the patient's report of pain and stiffness. Doctors also review spinal and pelvic x rays since involvement of the hip and pelvic joints is common and may be the first abnormality seen on the x ray. The doctor may also order a blood test to determine the presence of HLA-B27 antigen. When a diagnosis is made, patients may be referred to a rheumatologist, a doctor who specializes in treating arthritis. Patients may also be referred to an orthopedic surgeon, a doctor who can surgically correct joint or bone disorders.

Treatment

Physical therapists prescribe exercises to prevent a stooped posture and breathing problems when the spine starts to fuse and ribs are affected. Back braces may be used to prevent continued deformity of the spine and ribs. Only in severe cases of deformity is surgery performed to straighten and realign the spine, or to replace knee, shoulder, or hip joints.

Alternative treatment

To reduce inflammation various herbal remedies, including white willow (*Salix alba*), yarrow (*Achillea millefolium*), and lobelia (*Lobelia inflata*), may be helpful. **Acupuncture**, performed by a trained professional, has helped some patients manage their pain. Homeopathic practitioners may prescribe such remedies as *Bryonia* and *Rhus toxicodendron* for pain relief.

Prognosis

There is no cure for AS, and the course of the disease is unpredictable. Generally, AS progresses for about 10 years and then its progression levels off. Most patients can lead normal lives with treatment to control symptoms.

Prevention

There is no known way to prevent AS.

Resources

ORGANIZATIONS

Arthritis Foundation.1300 W. Peachtree St., Atlanta, GA 30309. (800) 283-7800. < http://www.arthritis.org > .

National Institute of Arthritis and Musculoskeletal and Skin Diseases Information Clearinghouse. 1 AMS Circle, Bethesda, MD 29892-3675. (301) 495-4484.

Spondylitis Association of America. P.O. Box 5872, Sherman Oaks, CA 91413. (800) 777-8189.

OTHER

Matsen III, Frederick, ed. "Ankylosing Spondylitis." University of Washington Orthopaedics and Sports Medicine. < http://www.orthop.washington.edu/ arthritis/types/ankylosingspondylitis > .

Jeanine Barone, Physiologist

Anorectal abscess *see* **Anorectal disorders**

Anorectal disorders

Definition

Anorectal disorders are a group of medical disorders that occur at the junction of the anal canal and the rectum.

Description

The anal canal, also called the anus, is the opening at the bottom end of the digestive tract and is a combination of external skin and tissue from the digestive tract. It has many sensory nerves and is sensitive to **pain**. The rectum is the last section of the digestive tract and has a mucus layer as its inside surface. It has very few sensory nerves and is, therefore, relatively insensitive to pain. The anal canal has a ring of muscle, called the anal sphincter, which keeps the anus closed. There are a number of different anorectal disorders.

Causes and symptoms

An anal fissure is a tear in the lining of the anus that is usually caused by a hard bowel movement. Fissures are painful and bleed when the tissue is stressed during bowel movements.

Anorectal abscesses are characterized by pus-forming infections in the anorectal region. Painful abscesses form under the skin.

An anorectal **fistula** is an abnormal opening or channel from the anorectal area to another part of the body. Typically, the channel leads to pockets of skin near the anus. When seen in infants, anorectal fistulas are considered **birth defects**. These are seen more frequently in boys than in girls. Fistulas are also seen more frequently in people who have other diseases, including **Crohn's disease**, **tuberculosis**, **cancer**, and **diverticulitis**. Anorectal fistulas also occur following anorectal abscesses or other injury to the anal area. Fistulas are usually painful and discharge pus.

Diagnosis

Diagnosis is made by visual inspection of the skin around the anus. Also, the doctor may probe the rectum with a gloved finger. An anoscope is a short instrument that allows the physician to view the inside of the anus. A proctoscope is a longer, rigid viewing tube of approximately six to ten inches in length, which may be used to look for anorectal disorders. A sigmoidoscope is a longer, flexible tube, that allows the physician to view up to about two feet of the inside of the large intestine. Tissue samples and material for microbial culture may be obtained during the examination.

Treatment

Treatment usually isn't required for hemorrhoids. Most hemorrhoids will heal if the patient takes stool softeners to relieve the constipation. Enlarged blood vessels can be eliminated by surgery if they are considered a severe problem. In the case of fissures, treatment involves stool softeners that eliminate **stress** on the fissure during bowel movements, which allows the fissure to heal. If the fissure doesn't heal, surgery is required. Treatment for anorectal abscesses consists of cutting the **abscess** and draining the pus. Fistulas are treated by surgery. The usual treatment for proctitis is **antibiotics**.

Resources

BOOKS

Berkow, Robert, editor. *Merck Manual of Medical Information*. Whitehouse Station, NJ: Merck Research Laboratories, 1997.

John T. Lohr, PhD

Anorectal fistula *see* **Anorectal disorders**

Anorexia nervosa

Definition

Anorexia nervosa is an eating disorder characterized by unrealistic fear of weight gain, self-starvation, and conspicuous distortion of body image. The name comes from two Latin words that mean nervous inability to eat. In females who have begun to menstruate, anorexia nervosa is usually marked by **amenorrhea**, or skipping at least three menstrual periods in a row. The fourth edition of the *Diagnostic and Statistical Manual of Mental Disorders*, or *DSM-IV* (1994), defines two subtypes of anorexia nervosa–a restricting type, characterized by strict dieting and **exercise** without binge eating; and a binge-eating/purging type, marked by episodes of compulsive eating with or without self-induced **vomiting** and the use of **laxatives** or **enemas**. *DSM-IV* defines a binge as a time-limited (usually under two hours) episode of compulsive eating in which the individual consumes a significantly larger amount of food than most people would eat in similar circumstances.

Description

Anorexia nervosa was not officially classified as a psychiatric disorder until the third edition of *DSM* in 1980. It is, however, a growing problem among adolescent females. Its incidence in the United States has doubled since 1970. The rise in the number of reported cases reflects a genuine increase in the number of persons affected by the disorder, and not simply earlier or more accurate diagnosis. Estimates of the incidence of anorexia range between 0.5–1% of caucasian female adolescents. Over 90% of patients diagnosed with the disorder as of 1998 are female. It was originally thought that only 5% of anorexics are male, but that estimate is being revised upward. The peak age range for onset of the disorder is 14-18 years, although there are patients who develop anorexia as late as their 40s. In the 1970s and 1980s, anorexia was regarded as a disorder of upper- and middle-class women, but that generalization is also changing. More recent studies indicate that anorexia is increasingly common among women of all races and social classes in the United States.

Anorexia nervosa is a serious public health problem not only because of its rising incidence, but also because it has one of the highest mortality rates of any psychiatric disorder. Moreover, the disorder may cause serious long-term health complications, including congestive **heart failure**, sudden **death**, growth retardation, dental problems, **constipation**, stomach rupture, swelling of the salivary glands, anemia and other abnormalities of the blood, loss of kidney function, and **osteoporosis**.

Causes and symptoms

Anorexia is a disorder that results from the interaction of cultural and interpersonal as well as biological factors. While the precise cause of the disease is not known, it has been linked to the following:

KEY TERMS

Amenorrhea—Absence of the menses in a female who has begun to have menstrual periods.

Binge eating—A pattern of eating marked by episodes of rapid consumption of large amounts of food; usually food that is high in calories.

Body dysmorphic disorder—A psychiatric disorder marked by preoccupation with an imagined physical defect.

Hyperalimentation—A method of refeeding anorexics by infusing liquid nutrients and electrolytes directly into central veins through a catheter.

Lanugo—A soft, downy body hair that develops on the chest and arms of anorexic women.

Purging—The use of vomiting, diuretics, or laxatives to clear the stomach and intestines after a binge.

Russell's sign—Scraped or raw areas on the patient's knuckles, caused by self-induced vomiting.

Superior mesenteric artery syndrome—A condition in which a person vomits after meals due to blockage of the blood supply to the intestine.

Social influences

The rising incidence of anorexia is thought to reflect the present idealization of thinness as a badge of upper-class status as well as of female beauty. In addition, the increase in cases of anorexia includes "copycat" behavior, with some patients developing the disorder from imitating other girls.

The onset of anorexia in adolescence is attributed to a developmental crisis caused by girls' changing bodies coupled with society's overemphasis on women's looks. The increasing influence of the mass media in spreading and reinforcing gender stereotypes has also been noted.

Occupational goals

The risk of developing anorexia is higher among adolescents preparing for careers that require attention to weight and/or appearance. These high-risk groups include dancers, fashion models, professional athletes (including gymnasts, skaters, long-distance runners, and jockeys), and actresses.

Genetic and biological influences

Women whose biological mothers or sisters have the disorder appear to be at increased risk.

Psychological factors

A number of theories have been advanced to explain the psychological aspects of the disorder. No single explanation covers all cases. Anorexia nervosa has been interpreted as:

- A rejection of female sexual maturity. This rejection is variously interpreted as a desire to remain a child, or as a desire to resemble men as closely as possible.

- A reaction to sexual **abuse** or assault.

- A desire to appear as fragile and nonthreatening as possible. This hypothesis reflects the idea that female passivity and weakness are attractive to men.

- Overemphasis on control, autonomy, and independence. Some anorexics come from achievement-oriented families that **stress** physical fitness and dieting. Many anorexics are perfectionistic and "driven" about schoolwork and other matters in addition to weight control.

- Evidence of family dysfunction. In some families, a daughter's eating disorder serves as a distraction from marital discord or other family tensions.

- Inability to interpret the body's hunger signals accurately due to early experiences of inappropriate feeding.

Male anorexics

Although anorexia nervosa is still considered a disorder that largely affects women, its incidence in the male population is rising. Less is known about the causes of anorexia in males, but some risk factors are the same as for females. These include certain occupational goals and increasing media emphasis on external appearance in men. Moreover, homosexual males are under pressure to conform to an ideal body weight that is about 20 pounds lighter than the standard "attractive" weight for heterosexual males.

Diagnosis

Diagnosis of anorexia nervosa is complicated by a number of factors. One is that the disorder varies somewhat in severity from patient to patient. A second factor is denial, which is regarded as an early sign of the disorder. Most anorexics deny that they are ill and are usually brought to treatment by a family member.

Most anorexics are diagnosed by pediatricians or family practitioners. Anorexics develop emaciated bodies, dry or yellowish skin, and abnormally low blood pressure. There is usually a history of amenorrhea (failure to menstruate) in females, and sometimes of abdominal **pain**, constipation, or lack of energy. The patient may feel chilly or have developed lanugo, a growth of downy body hair. If the patient has been vomiting, she may have eroded tooth enamel or Russell's sign (**scars** on the back of the hand). The second step in diagnosis is measurement of the patient's weight loss. *DSM-IV* specifies a weight loss leading to a body weight 15% below normal, with some allowance for body build and weight history.

The doctor will need to rule out other physical conditions that can cause weight loss or vomiting after eating, including metabolic disorders, brain tumors (especially hypothalamus and pituitary gland lesions), diseases of the digestive tract, and a condition called superior mesenteric artery syndrome. Persons with this condition sometimes vomit after meals because the blood supply to the intestine is blocked. The doctor will usually order blood tests, an electrocardiogram, **urinalysis**, and bone densitometry (**bone density test**) in order to exclude other diseases and to assess the patient's nutritional status.

The doctor will also need to distinguish between anorexia and other psychiatric disorders, including depression, **schizophrenia**, social phobia, **obsessive-compulsive disorder**, and **body dysmorphic disorder**. Two diagnostic tests that are often used are the Eating Attitudes Test (EAT) and the Eating Disorder Inventory (EDI).

Treatment

Treatment of anorexia nervosa includes both short- and long-term measures, and requires assessment by dietitians and psychiatrists as well as medical specialists. Therapy is often complicated by the patient's resistance or failure to carry out treatment plan.

Hospital treatment

Hospitalization is recommended for anorexics with any of the following characteristics:

- weight of 40% or more below normal; or weight loss over a three-month period of more than 30 pounds

- severely disturbed metabolism

- severe binging and purging

- signs of **psychosis**

- severe depression or risk of **suicide**

- family in crisis

Hospital treatment includes individual and **group therapy** as well as refeeding and monitoring of the patient's physical condition. Treatment usually requires two to four months in the hospital. In extreme cases, hospitalized patients may be force-fed through a tube inserted in the nose (nasogastric tube) or by over-feeding (hyperalimentation techniques).

Outpatient treatment

Anorexics who are not severely malnourished can be treated by outpatient psychotherapy. The types of treatment recommended are supportive rather than insight-oriented, and include behavioral approaches as well as individual or group therapy. **Family therapy** is often recommended when the patient's eating disorder is closely tied to family dysfunction. Self-help groups are often useful in helping anorexics find social support and encouragement. Psychotherapy with anorexics is a slow and difficult process; about 50% of patients continue to have serious psychiatric problems after their weight has stabilized.

Medications

Anorexics have been treated with a variety of medications, including antidepressants, **antianxiety drugs**, **selective serotonin reuptake inhibitors**, and lithium carbonate. The effectiveness of medications in treatment regimens is still debated. However, at least one study of Prozac showed it helped the patient maintain weight gained while in the hospital.

Prognosis

Figures for long-term recovery vary from study to study, but the most reliable estimates are that 40-60% of anorexics will make a good physical and social recovery, and 75% will gain weight. The long-term mortality rate for anorexia is estimated at around 10%, although some studies give a lower figure of 3-4%. The most frequent causes of death associated with anorexia are **starvation**, electrolyte imbalance, heart failure, and suicide.

Prevention

Short of major long-term changes in the larger society, the best strategy for prevention of anorexia is the cultivation of healthy attitudes toward food, weight control, and beauty (or body image) within families.

Resources

BOOKS

Baron, Robert B. "Nutrition." In *Current Medical Diagnosis and Treatment, 1998*, edited by Stephen McPhee, et al., 37th ed. Stamford: Appleton & Lange, 1997.

ORGANIZATIONS

American Anorexia/Bulimia Association. 418 East 76th St., New York, NY 10021. (212) 734-1114.

National Institute of Mental Health Eating Disorders Program. Building 10, Room 3S231. 9000 Rockville Pike, Bethesda, MD 20892. (301) 496-1891.

Rebecca J. Frey, PhD

Anoscopy

Definition

An anoscopy is an examination of the rectum in which a small tube is inserted into the anus to screen, diagnose, and evaluate problems of the anus and anal canal.

Purpose

This test may be ordered for the evaluation of perianal or anal **pain**, **hemorrhoids**, **rectal prolapse**, digital **rectal examination** that shows a mass, perianal **abscess** and condyloma (a wart-like growth). An anoscopy may be performed to check for abnormal openings between the anus and the skin, or anal fissures. The test is also used to diagnose **rectal cancer**.

Precautions

Anoscopy should not be performed on patients with acute cardiovascular problems due to the vasovagal reaction it may cause. This test is also not recommended for patients with acute abdominal problems and those with a constricted or narrowed anal canal.

Description

Anoscopy views the anus and anal canal by using an anoscope. An anoscope is a plastic, tube-shaped speculum that is a smaller version of a sigmoidscope. Before the anoscope is used, the doctor completes a digital rectal examination with a lubricated, gloved index finger. The anoscope is then lubricated and gently inserted a few inches into the rectum. This procedure enlarges the rectum to allow the doctor to view the entire anal canal with a light. If any suspicious areas are noticed, a piece of tissue can be biopsied.

During the anoscopy procedure there may be a feeling of pressure or the need to go to the bathroom. If a biopsy is taken, the patient may feel a slight pinch.

KEY TERMS

Anal fissure—An ulcer on the margin of the anus.

Digital rectal examination—An examination where a gloved, lubricated index finger is inserted into the rectum to check for any abnormalities.

Polyps—A tumor with a small flap that attaches itself to the wall of various vascular organs such as the nose, uterus and rectum. Polyps bleed easily, and if they are suspected to be cancerous they should be surgically removed.

Vasovagal reaction—Regarding the action of stimuli from the vagus nerve on blood vessels.

The procedure is performed on an out-patient basis, and takes approximately an hour to complete.

Preparation

The patient will be instructed to clear their rectum of stool before the procedure. This may be done by taking a laxative, enema, or other preparation that may help with the evacuation.

Aftercare

If a biopsy is needed during an anoscopy, there may be slight anal bleeding for less than two days following the procedure. The patient may be instructed to sit in a bathtub of warm water for 10 to 15 minutes, three times a day, to help decrease the pain and swelling.

Risks

A simple anoscopy procedure offers minimal risks. There is a limited risk of bleeding and mild pain is a biopsy is performed.

Normal results

Normal values to look for during an anoscopy include an anal canal that appears healthy in size, color, and shape. The test also looks for no evidence of bleeding, polyps, hemorrhoids or other abnormalities.

Abnormal results

While an anoscopy is typically performed to determine is hemorrhoids are present, other abnormal finding could include polyps, abscesses, inflammation, fissures, colorectal polyps, or **cancer**.

Resources

BOOKS

Altman, Roberta, and Michael J. Sarg. "Anoscopy." *The Cancer Dictionary*. Checkmark Books, 2000, p. 18.

PERIODICALS

Colyar, Margaret. "Anascopy Basics." *The Nurse Practitioner* (October 2000): 91.

OTHER

Discovery Health. "Medical Tests: Anoscopy." May 5, 2001. < http://health.discover.com/diseasesandcond/ encyclopedia/1038.html > .

Lycos Health with WebMD. "Anoscopy." May 5, 2001. < http://webmd.lycos.com/content/asset/ adam_test_anoscopy > .

Beth A. Kapes

Anosmia

Definition

The term anosmia means lack of the sense of smell. It may also refer to a decreased sense of smell. Ageusia, a companion word, refers to a lack of taste sensation. Patients who actually have anosmia may complain wrongly of ageusia, although they retain the ability to distinguish salt, sweet, sour, and bitter–humans' only taste sensations.

Description

Of the five senses, smell ranks fourth in importance for humans, although it is much more pronounced in other animals. Bloodhounds, for example, can smell an odor a thousand times weaker than humans. Taste, considered the fifth sense, is mostly the smell of food in the mouth. The sense of smell originates from the first cranial nerves (the olfactory nerves), which sit at the base of the brain's frontal lobes, right behind the eyes and above the nose. Inhaled airborne chemicals stimulate these nerves.

There are other aberrations of smell beside a decrease. Smells can be distorted, intensified, or hallucinated. These changes usually indicate a malfunction of the brain.

Causes and symptoms

The most common cause of anosmia is nasal occlusion caused by **rhinitis** (inflammation of the

KEY TERMS

Allergen—Any substance that irritates only those who are sensitive (allergic) to it.

Corticosteroids—Cortisone, prednisone, and related drugs that reduce inflammation.

Rhinitis—Inflammation and swelling of the nasal membranes.

Nasal polyps—Drop-shaped overgrowths of the nasal membranes.

nasal membranes). If no air gets to the olfactory nerves, smell will not happen. In turn, rhinitis and **nasal polyps** (growths on nasal membranes) are caused by irritants such as allergens, infections, cigarette smoke, and other air pollutants. Tumors such as nasal polyps can also block the nasal passages and the olfactory nerves and cause anosmia. **Head injury** or, rarely, certain viral infections can damage or destroy the olfactory nerves.

Diagnosis

It is difficult to measure a loss of smell, and no one complains of loss of smell in just one nostril. So a physician usually begins by testing each nostril separately with a common, non-irritating odor such as perfume, lemon, vanilla, or coffee. Polyps and rhinitis are obvious causal agents a physician looks for. Imaging studies of the head may be necessary in order to detect brain injury, sinus infection, or tumor.

Treatment

Cessation of **smoking** is the first step. Many smokers who quit discover new tastes so enthusiastically that they immediately gain weight. Attention to reducing exposure to other nasal irritants and treatment of respiratory **allergies** or chronic upper respiratory infections will be beneficial. **Corticosteroids** are particularly helpful.

Alternative treatment

Finding and treating the cause of the loss of smell is the first approach in **naturopathic medicine**. If rhinitis is the cause, treating acute rhinitis with herbal mast cell stabilizers and herbal **decongestants** can offer some relief as the body heals. If chronic rhinitis is present, this is often related to an environmental irritant or to **food allergies**. Removal of the causative factors is the

first step to healing. Nasal steams with essential oils offer relief of the blockage and tonification of the membranes. Blockages can sometimes be resolved through naso-specific therapy—a way of realigning the nasal cavities. Polyp blockage can be addressed through botanical medicine treatment as well as **hydrotherapy**. Olfactory nerve damage may not be regenerable. Some olfactory aberrations, like intensified sense of smell, can be resolved using **homeopathic medicine**.

Prognosis

If nasal inflammation is the cause of anosmia, the chances of recovery are excellent. However, if nerve damage is the cause of the problem, the recovery of smell is much more difficult.

Resources

BOOKS

Fauci, Anthony S., et al., editors. *Harrison's Principles of Internal Medicine*. New York: McGraw-Hill, 1997.

J. Ricker Polsdorfer, MD

Anoxemia *see* **Anoxia**

Anoxia

Definition

Anoxia is a condition characterized by an absence of oxygen supply to an organ or a tissue.

Description

Anoxia results when oxygen is not being delivered to a part of the body. If the condition does not involve total oxygen deprivation, it is often called hypoxia, although the two terms have been used interchangeably. A related condition, anoxemia, occurs when the blood circulates but contains a below normal amount of oxygen.

The five types of anoxia or hypoxia include hypoxemic, anemic, affinity, stagnant, and histotoxic. Hypoxemic anoxia happens when the oxygen pressure outside the body is so low that the hemoglobin, the chemical which carries oxygen in the red blood cells (RBCs), is unable to become fully loaded with the gas. This results in too little oxygen reaching the tissues and can occur in suffocation when a person is at high

KEY TERMS

Amnesia—Loss of memory often traceable to brain tissue damage.

Anoxemia—An extreme lack of oxygen in the blood.

Hemoglobin—A chemical found in red blood cells that transports oxygen.

Myoclonus—Involuntary contractions of a muscle or group of muscles.

altitude, where the pressure of oxygen in the air is much less than at sea level.

Anemic anoxia results from a decrease in the amount of hemoglobin or RBCs in the blood, which reduces the ability to get oxygen to the tissues. Anemia may result from lack of production of red blood cells (iron deficiency), blood loss (hemorrhage), or shortened lifespan of red blood cells (autoimmune disease).

Affinity anoxia involves a defect in the chemistry of the blood such that the hemoglobin can no longer pick up as much oxygen from the air, even though the quantities are normal, reducing how much is delivered to the tissues.

Stagnant anoxia occurs when there is interference with the blood flow, although the blood and its oxygen-carrying abilities are normal. A common cause of general stagnant anoxia is heart disease or interference with the return of blood flow through the veins. Examples of local stagnant anoxia include exposure to cold, diseases that restrict circulation to the extremities, and ergot **poisoning**. When the tissue or organ itself has a reduced ability to accept and use the oxygen, it is called histotoxic anoxia. The classic example is cyanide poisoning, where the chemical inactivates a cellular enzyme necessary for the cell to use oxygen. Thus, tissue exposed to cyanide cannot use the oxygen even though it is in normal amounts in the bloodstream. Histotoxic anoxia can also be caused by exposure to **narcotics**, alcohol, formaldehyde, acetone, toluene, and certain anesthetic agents.

Causes and symptoms

Anoxia and hypoxia can be caused by any number of disease states of the blood, lungs, heart and circulation including **heart attack**, severe **asthma**, or **emphysema**. It can also result from smoke or carbon monoxide inhalation, improper exposure to anesthesia, poisoning, strangulation, **near-drowning**, or high altitude exposure

through mountain climbing or travel in an insufficiently pressurized airplane. Anoxia, and the resultant brain damage, is a particular problem with newborns during difficult births.

No matter what the cause of anoxia, the symptoms are similar. In severe cases, the patient is often confused and commonly stuporous or comatose (in a state of unconsciousness). Depending on the severity of the injury to the brain, the organ most sensitive to reduced oxygen intake, this condition can persist for hours, days, weeks, or even months or years. Seizures, myoclonic jerks (involuntary **muscle spasms** or twitches), and neck stiffness are some other symptoms of the anoxic condition.

Symptoms of more localized or less complete oxygen deprivation (hypoxia) include increased breathing rate, lightheadedness, **dizziness**, **tingling** or warm sensation, sweating, reduced field of vision, sleepiness, a bluish tint to skin, particularly the fingertips and lips, and behavior changes, often an inappropriate sense of euphoria.

Diagnosis

Diagnosis of anoxia and hypoxia is commonly made through the appearance of clinical symptoms. However, suspected reduction in oxygen reaching the tissues can be confirmed using laboratory tests. The exact test that is performed is dependent on the suspected cause of the anoxia. One systemic measure of tissue anoxia is the serum lactate (lactic acid) test. When cells are forced to produce energy without oxygen, as would happen during anoxia, lactic acid is one of the byproducts. Thus, an increase in lactic acid in the blood would indicate that tissues were starved for oxygen and are using non-oxygen pathways to produce energy. Normally, the blood contains less than 2mmol/L of lactic acid. However, some forms of anoxia do not increase lactic acid concentrations in the blood and some increases in lactic acid levels are not associated with anoxia, so an elevated value for this test is only suggestive of an anoxic or hypoxic condition.

Treatment

The exact treatment for anoxia is dependent on the cause of the reduced oxygen reaching the tissues. However, immediate restoration of tissue oxygen levels through supplementing the patient's air supply with 100% oxygen is a common first step. Secondary steps often include support of the cardiovascular system through drugs or other treatment, treatment of lung disease, transfusions, or administration of anecdotes for poisoning, as appropriate.

Prognosis

A good prognosis is dependent on the ability to treat the underlying cause of the low oxygen levels. If cardiovascular and respiratory systems can be supported adequately, recovery from the injury to the tissue is possible, although extent of injury to the brain can be difficult to assess. The exact amount of recovery varies with the amount of injury sustained, where significant injury brings a poorer prognosis. As recovery occurs, both psychological and neurological abnormalities may appear, persist, and can improve. Some problems seen after anoxia include mental confusion, personality changes, **amnesia** or other types of memory loss, **hallucinations**, and persistent myoclonus (involuntary contractions of the muscles).

Prevention

Hypoxemic anoxia can be avoided by utilizing supplemental oxygen when in high altitudes and being aware of the early symptoms of **altitude sickness** and reducing altitude once recognized. Iron supplements can avoid anemic hypoxia, although more severe anemic states are usually caused by disease or bleeding. Maintaining good cardiovascular health through proper diet and **exercise** is a good first step to avoiding the most common cause of stagnant anoxia. Avoiding exposure to the toxic chemicals that cause the condition can prevent histotoxic anoxia.

Resources

PERIODICALS

Gutierrez, Guillermo. "Metabolic Assessement of Tissue Oxygenation" *Seminars in Respiratory and Critical Care Medicine* 20 (January 1999): 11–15.

ORGANIZATIONS

Brain Injury Association. 105 N. Alfred St. Alexandria, VA 22314. (800) 444-6443. < http://www.biausa.org > .

Phoenix Project/Head Injury Hotline. Box 84151, Seattle, WA 98124. (206) 621-8558. < http://www.headinjury.com > .

OTHER

Borron, Stephen W. "Lactic Acidosis." *eMedicine.* February 7, 2001. [cited May 13, 2001]. < http://www.emedicine.com/emerg/topic291.htm > .

NINDS Anoxia/Hypoxia Information Page. The National Institute of Neurological Disorders and Stroke (NINDS). January 22, 2001. [cited May 13, 2001].

< http://www.ninds.nih.gov/health_and_medical/disorders/anoxia_doc.htm > .

Michelle Johnson, MS, JD

Antacids

Definition

Antacids are medicines that neutralize stomach acid.

Purpose

Antacids are used to relieve acid **indigestion**, upset stomach, sour stomach, and **heartburn**. Additional components of some formulations include dimethicone, to reduce gas pains (flatulence) and alginic acid, which, in combination with antacids, may help manage GERD (gastro-esophageal reflux disease). Antacids should not be confused with gastric acid inhibitors, such as the H-2 receptor blockers (cimetidine, ranitide and others) or the **proton pump inhibitors** (lansoprazole, omeprazole and others). Although all three classes of drugs act to reduce the levels of gastric acid, their mechanisms are different, and this affects the appropriate use of the drug. Antacids have a rapid onset and short duration of action, and are most appropriate for rapid relief of gastric discomfort for a short period of time.

Antacids may be divided into two classes, those that work by chemical neutralization of gastric acid, most notably sodium bicarbonate; and those that act by adsorption of the acid (non-absorbable antacids), such as calcium and magnesium salts.

The chemical antacids show the most rapid onset of action, but may cause "acid rebound," a condition in which the gastric acid returns in greater concentration after the drug effect has stopped. Also, since these antacids may contain high concentrations of sodium, they may be inappropriate in patients with **hypertension**.

Calcium and magnesium salts act by adsorption of the acid, and are less prone to the rebound effect, but may have other significant disadvantages. These antacids are particularly prone to **drug interactions**, and patients taking other medications must often avoid simultaneous administration of the medications. These antacids are more effective in liquid formulations than in tablet or capsule form, and so may be inconvenient for routine dosing.

KEY TERMS

Acid indigestion—Indigestion that results from too much acid in the stomach.

Chronic—A word used to describe a long-lasting condition. Chronic conditions often develop gradually and involve slow changes.

Heartburn—A burning sensation, usually in the center of the chest, near the breastbone.

Indigestion—A feeling of discomfort or illness that results from the inability to properly digest food.

Inflamed bowel—Irritation of the intestinal tract.

Inflammation—Pain, redness, swelling, and heat that usually develop in response to injury or illness.

Pregnancy safety categories—A system for reporting the known safety issues of drugs for use during pregnancy, The ratings range from A, proven safe by well controlled studies, to X, proven harmful.

The non-absorbable antacids may have additional uses beyond control of hyperacidity. Calcium salts may be used as diet supplements in prevention of **osteoporosis**. Aluminum carbonate is useful for binding phosphate, and has been effective in treatment and control of hyperphosphatemia or for use with a low phosphate diet to prevent formation of phosphate urinary stones. This application is particularly valuable in patients with chronic renal failure. Antacids with aluminum and magnesium hydroxides or aluminum hydroxide alone effectively prevent significant **stress** ulcer bleeding in post-operative patients or those with severe **burns**.

Recommended dosage

The dose depends on the type of antacid. Consult specific references.

When using antacids in chewable tablet form, chew the tablet well before swallowing. Drink a glass of water after taking chewable aluminum hydroxide. Lozenges should be allowed to dissolve completely in the mouth. Liquid antacids should be shaken well before using.

Precautions

Antacids should be avoided if any signs of **appendicitis** or inflamed bowel are present. These include cramping, **pain**, and soreness in the lower abdomen, bloating, and **nausea and vomiting**.

Antacids may affect the results of some medical tests, such as those that measure how much acid the stomach produces. Health care providers and patients should keep this in mind when scheduling a medical test.

Antacids that contain magnesium may cause **diarrhea**. Other types of antacids may cause **constipation**.

Avoid taking antacids containing sodium bicarbonate when the stomach is uncomfortably full from eating or drinking.

Antacids should not be given to children under six years of age.

Antacids that contain calcium or sodium bicarbonate may cause side effects, such as **dizziness**, **nausea**, and **vomiting**, in people who consume large amounts of calcium (from dairy products or calcium supplements). In some cases, this can lead to permanent kidney damage. Before combining antacids with extra calcium, check with a physician.

Some antacids contain large amounts of sodium, particularly sodium bicarbonate (baking soda). Anyone who is on a low-sodium diet should check the list of ingredients or check with a physician or pharmacist before taking an antacid product.

Excessive use of antacids may cause or increase the severity or kidney problems. Calcium based antacids may lead to renal stone formation.

PREGNANCY. Antacids are not classified under the **pregnancy** safety categories A, B, C, D and X. Occasional use of antacids in small amounts during pregnancy is considered safe. However, pregnant women should check with their physicians before using antacids or any other medicines. Pregnant women who are consuming extra calcium should be aware that using antacids that contain sodium bicarbonate or calcium can lead to serious side effects.

BREASTFEEDING. Some antacids may pass into breast milk. However, no evidence exists that the ingestion of antacids through breast milk causes problems for nursing babies whose mothers use antacids occasionally.

Side effects

Side effects are very rare when antacids are taken as directed. They are more likely when the medicine is taken in large doses or over a long time. Minor side effects include a chalky taste, mild constipation or diarrhea, thirst, stomach cramps, and whitish or speckled stools. These symptoms do not need medical attention unless they do not go away or they interfere with normal activities.

Other uncommon side effects may occur. Anyone who has unusual symptoms after taking antacids should get in touch with his or her health care provider.

Interactions

Antacids have multiple drug interactions, usually due to inhibition of absorption of other medications. In rare cases, the absorbable antacids may alter the pH of the stomach contents or urine sufficiently to alter drug absoprtion or excretion. Consult specific references.

Samuel D. Uretsky, PharmD

Antegrade pyelography *see* **Intravenous urography**

Antenatal testing

Definition

Antenatal testing includes any diagnostic procedures performed before the birth of a baby.

Purpose

These tests and exams are essential for protecting the health of a pregnant woman and her developing child.

Precautions

Some tests, such as amniocentisis, carry a small risk of a **miscarriage** or other complications that could harm the mother or baby.

Description

Women who become pregnant undergo a wide variety of tests throughout the nine months before delivery. In the early stages, physicians order blood tests to screen for possible disorders or infections, such as human **immunodeficiency** virus (HIV), which can pass from the mother to the fetus. Later, the focus shifts to checking on fetal well-being with a variety of technological tools such as ultrasound scans. Descriptions of the most common tests and procedures used during **pregnancy** are listed below.

KEY TERMS

Ultrasound — A device that records sound waves as they bounce off a developing fetus to create an image, which is projected onto a large computer screen

Breech position—When a child is oriented feet first in the mother's uterus just before delivery.

Alpha fetoprotein screen — A test that measures the level of alpha fetoprotein, a substance produced by a fetus with birth defects, in the mother's blood.

Amniocentesis— An invasive procedure that allows physicians to check for birth defects by collecting a sample of fetal cells from inside the amniotic sac.

GBS— Group B streptococci are a type of bacteria that, if passed to a can cause inflammation of the brain, spinal cord, blood or lungs. In some cases, it can result in infant death

When a woman first learns she is pregnant, her physician will run a series of routine urine and blood tests to determine her blood type, check for anemia and **gestational diabetes**, make sure she is immune to **rubella** (German **measles**) and check for infectious diseases like HIV, hepatitis, chlamydia or **syphilis**. Physicians also usually do **pelvic exam** to screen for **cervical cancer** and check the patient's blood pressure. As the pregnancy progresses, more tests will follow.

Ultrasound

Ultrasound is a device that records sound waves as they bounce off the developing fetus to create an image, which is projected onto a large computer screen. Physicians order an ultrasound scan to listen for a fetal heartbeat, determine a woman's precise due date and check for twins, among other uses. An ultrasound scan also is known as a sonogram. The procedure takes a few minutes, is painless and usually is covered by health insurance.

The ultrasound technician will ask the pregnant woman to remove her clothes and change into a gown. The technician may rub some gel on the woman's stomach, which helps the hand-held device pick up sound waves better. In certain cases, the technician may insert a plastic probe into the woman's vaginal canal to get a clearer picture of the fetus. Early in pregnancy, the test may need to be done with a full bladder.

Unlike x rays, ultrasound is safe to use during pregnancy. It does not cause any known side-effects that would harm the mother or baby.

Pregnant women usually will have their first ultrasound anytime between 8 and 12 weeks of gestation. In normal cases, the technician is able to identify a fetal heartbeat, which appears as a flashing light on the screen. Closer to the due date, physicians use ultrasound to make sure the fetus is in the correct position to exit the birth canal head first.

Sometimes an ultrasound will show that a fetus has stopped growing, or a gestational sac has formed without a fetus, and a miscarriage has occurred. Later in pregnancy, it also may show that the child is in a breech position, oriented feet first, which can cause a difficult labor.

Tests for birth defects

Most obstetricians offer parents a variety of ways to find out if their developing child might have **birth defects** such as **spina bifida** and **Down Syndrome**. An alpha fetoprotein screen can be done through a simple blood test in the doctor's office between the 16th and 18th week of gestation. It tells the odds that their child will have a severe congenital anomaly. The test works by measuring the level of alpha fetoprotein, a substance produced by a fetus with birth defects. Low levels of alpha fetoprotein in the mother's blood may indicate Down's Syndrome. In that case, the next step for most couples is **amniocentesis** because the alpha fetoprotein test can give false-positive results. Amniocentesis is a more accurate test, but it also has higher risks of complications.

This procedure typically is used to diagnose Down syndrome while a developing child is still in the womb, at 15-28 weeks.

During amniocentesis, a doctor inserts a needle through a woman's vaginal canal and inside her cervix. Using ultrasound as a guide, the doctor pierces the uterus to withdraw a sample of fluid from the amniotic sac. Afterwards, tiny cells shed by the fetus can be studied in the laboratory. Scientists can analyze DNA samples to determine if the fetus has Down syndrome or other genetic conditions. Amniocentesis also can determine the sex of the fetus.

Women who have a history of recurring miscarriages may not want to have this procedure.

Amniocentesis is usually performed in a doctor's office on an outpatient basis.

Common side effects include cramping and bleeding.

In about one out of every 1,000 cases, amniocentesis causes a needle to puncture the uterine wall, which could result in miscarriage.

In most cases, couples find out their baby does not have a birth defect.

If the results come back positive for Down's Syndrome or other serious conditions, the couple must decide if they want to end the pregnancy. Others use the knowledge to plan and prepare any special care needed for their future child.

Group B Strep

This test is for Group B streptococci (GBS) infection.

By testing for GBS, physicians can determine if a woman is at risk of passing this infection along to her child.

Women who have had a prior child with GBS, or who have a **fever** or prolonged or premature rupture of the amniotic sac may be at higher risk for this type of infection.

GBS is a type of bacteria commonly found in the vagina and rectum. Unlike regular **strep throat**, GBS can be present in a person's body without causing any symptoms, so many women do not realize they are infected with it.

To test for the presence of GBS, doctors may take a urine sample. They also may collect samples from the vagina or rectum, which are then analyzed in a lab. This test is usually performed late in pregnancy, at 35-37 weeks of gestation.

This is a routine urine test or pelvic exam with no side effects.

In many cases, doctors do not find any evidence of this type of infection.

If a woman is found to be infected with Group B strep, physicians usually wait to treat it until just before labor begins. At that time, they may give the mother **antibiotics** so the baby is not born with the infection. Newborns who are exposed to Group B strep can have inflammation of the brain, spinal cord, blood or lungs. In some cases, this serious complication can result in infant **death**.

Resources

BOOKS

Planning your Pregnancy and Birth. Washington, DC: The American College of Obstetricians and Gynecologists, 2000.

PERIODICALS

Parkey, Paula. "Birth Defects: Is Prenatal Screening Advisable?" *CBS HealthWatch* April, 2000. <http://www.cbshealthwatch.com/cx/viewarticle/214798>.

ORGANIZATIONS

American College of Obstetricians and Gynecologists. 409 12th St., S.W., P.O. Box 96920, Washington, DC 20090-6920. <http://www.acog.org>.

March of Dimes Birth Defects Foundation. 275 Mamaroneck Avenue, White Plains, NY 10605. (888) 663-4637. <http://www.modimes.org>.

Melissa Knopper

Antepartum testing

Definition

Antepartum testing consists of a variety of tests performed late in **pregnancy** to verify fetal well-being, as judged by the baby's heart rate and other characteristics. Antepartum tests include the nonstress test (NST), biophysical profile, and contraction **stress test** (CST).

Purpose

Antepartum testing is performed after 32 weeks of pregnancy so that the couple and the doctor can be warned of any problems that may necessitate further testing or immediate delivery. The results reflect the adequacy of blood flow (and oxygen delivery) to the fetus from the placenta.

Antepartum tests are usually done in pregnancies at high risk for fetal complications. Various reasons include:

- any chronic illness in the mother, such as high blood pressure or diabetes

- problems with previous pregnancies, such as **stillbirth**

- fetal complications, such as **intrauterine growth retardation** (a slowing of growth of the fetus) or **birth defects**

- problems in the current pregnancy, including **preeclampsia** (serious pregnancy-induced high blood pressure), gestational (pregnancy-related) diabetes, premature rupture of the membranes, excessive amniotic fluid (the liquid that surrounds the fetus), vaginal bleeding, or **placenta previa** (a condition in

which the placenta is positioned over the cervix instead of near the top of the uterus)

- twins or other multiple fetuses

One of the most common indications for antepartum testing is post-term pregnancy. A pregnancy should not be allowed to continue past 42 weeks. (The usual pregnancy is 40 weeks in duration). Babies should be monitored with antepartum testing starting at 41 weeks. After 41 weeks, there is an increasing risk that the placenta cannot meet the growing baby's needs for oxygen and **nutrition**. This may be reflected in decreased movements of the baby, decreased amniotic fluid, and changes in the heart rate pattern of the baby.

Description

Technology

The NST and CST use a technique called **electronic fetal monitoring** to evaluate the heartbeat of the fetus. The biophysical profile is an ultrasound examination.

NST

The NST is usually the first antepartum test used to verify fetal well-being. It is based on the principle that when the fetus moves, its heartbeat normally speeds up. The NST assesses fetal health through monitoring accelerations of the heart rate in response to the baby's own movements, i.e., in the absence of **stress**.

KEY TERMS

Amniotic fluid—The liquid that surrounds the baby within the amniotic sac. Because it is composed mostly of fetal urine, a low amount of fluid can indicate inadequate placental blood flow to the fetus.

Deceleration—A decrease in the fetal heart rate that can indicate inadequate blood flow through the placenta.

Oxytocin—A natural hormone that produces uterine contractions.

Ultrasound—A procedure in which high-frequency sound waves are used to create a picture of the baby, used alone or with antepartum tests.

Vibroacoustic stimulation—In the biophysical profile, use of an artificial larynx to produce a loud noise to "awaken" the fetus.

The mother lays down or sits, and an electronic fetal monitor is placed on her abdomen to monitor the fetal heart rate. The doctor records the baby's heartbeat on a graph or "tracing" to determine whether it demonstrates correct reactivity, or acceleration of the heart rate. To record fetal movements on the tracing, the mother presses a button every time she feels the baby move. If the baby is inactive, the mother may be asked to rub her abdomen to "awaken" it. Sometimes an instrument is used to produce a loud noise to arouse the fetus (vibroacoustic stimulation). The test usually takes between 20–45 minutes.

A baby who is receiving enough oxygen should move at least twice in a 20 minute period. The baby's heart rate should increase at least 20 beats per minute for at least 20 seconds during these movements. The NST is the simplest and cheapest antepartum test.

Biophysical profile

The biophysical profile is an ultrasound exam that can add additional information to the NST. During the biophysical profile, the examiner checks for various characteristics of the baby to evaluate its overall health. These include: fetal movement, fetal tone, breathing movements, and the amniotic fluid volume. Amniotic fluid volume is important because a decreased amount raises the possibility that the baby may be under stress. The five components of the test (NST is also included) are each given a score of 2 for normal (or present), 1 if decreased, and 0 for abnormal. The highest possible score is 10. The "modified" biophysical profile is another option; this includes only the NST and amniotic fluid volume.

CST

The CST is like the NST, except that the fetus is evaluated in response to contractions of the mother's uterus. Because it is a more complicated test, it is often used after an abnormal NST to confirm the results. Uterine contractions produce "stress" in the fetus because they temporarily stop the flow of blood and oxygen. The CST is used to confirm that the fetus does not respond to this stress by a decrease in the heart rate.

The CST is performed with the same equipment as the NST. Maternal blood pressure and fetal heart rate are recorded along with the onset, relative intensity, and duration of any spontaneous contractions. For an accurate test, the contractions should be of sufficient duration and frequency. If uterine activity does not occur naturally, a drug called oxytocin may be given to the mother intravenously (hence the test's alternate name, the oxytocin challenge test) to provoke contractions. Another option is self-stimulation of the mother's nipples, because this releases natural oxytocin. The fetal heart rate is observed until, ideally, three moderate contractions occur within 10 minutes.

Preparation

The mother should eat just before the antepartum tests to help stimulate fetal activity.

Risks

There are no appreciable risks from the NST or the biophysical profile. Ultrasound used for the biophysical profile is painless and safe because it uses no harmful radiation, and no evidence has been found that sound waves cause any adverse effects on the mother or fetus.

The frequency of antepartum testing depends on the reason for its use. All of the tests occasionally give incorrect results, which may prompt an unnecessary early delivery or cesarean. Repeat testing is important to double-check any abnormal findings.

Normal results

In general, "negative" or normal results on antepartum testing provide reassurance that the baby is healthy and should remain so for perhaps a week, with no need for immediate delivery. Unfortunately, the tests cannot guarantee that there are no problems, because falsely normal results can occur, though this is unusual. Even if all test results are normal, it is important to realize that this does not guarantee a "perfect" baby.

The NST is normal ("reactive") if two or more distinct fetal movements occur in association with appropriate accelerations of the fetal heart rate within 20 minutes. A biophysical profile score of 8-10 is considered reassuring. The CST is normal if the fetus shows no decelerations in heart rate in response to three uterine contractions within 10 minutes.

Abnormal results

A "positive" result suggests that the baby is not receiving enough oxygen for some reason. However, it is quite possible that the test result was falsely abnormal. To confirm or monitor a suspected disorder, follow-up testing with the same or an alternate test will probably be performed at least weekly.

The NST is abnormal ("nonreactive") if the fetal heart rate fails to speed up by at least 20 beats per minute at least two times during a 20-minute period. Abnormal decreases in the heart rate (decelerations) are also a cause for concern.

A biophysical profile score of 6 is considered a cause for concern and should be followed by further testing. Scores of 4 or less may require immediate delivery of the fetus.

Abnormal results on the CST include late decelerations, or abnormal slowing of the fetal heart rate after the uterine contractions. This can suggest that the baby is not receiving enough oxygen and may have difficulty withstanding the stress of labor and vaginal delivery. **Cesarean section** might be necessary so the baby can be spared the stress of labor. With either NST or CST, a severe deceleration (a period of very slow heartbeat) can also suggest fetal distress.

The ultimate outcome will depend on the woman's individual situation. In some cases, delivery can be postponed while medication is given to the mother (e.g., for high blood pressure) or the fetus (e.g., to speed up lung maturity before delivery). Depending upon the readiness of the mother's cervix, the doctor may decide to induce labor. The extra-large fetus of a diabetic woman may require cesarean delivery; severe preeclampsia also may necessitate **induction of labor** or cesarean section. The doctor will determine the most prudent course of action.

Resources

PERIODICALS

Smith-Levitin, Michelle, Boris Petrikovsky, and Elizabeth P. Schneider. "Practical Guidelines for Antepartum Fetal Surveillance." *American Family Physician* 56 (November 15, 1997): 1981-1988.

ORGANIZATIONS

American College of Obstetricians and Gynecologists. 409 12th St., S.W., P.O. Box 96920, Washington, DC 20090-6920. < http://www.acog.org >.

National Institute of Child Health and Human Development. Bldg 31, Room 2A32, MSC 2425, 31 Center Drive, Bethesda, MD 20892-2425. (800) 505-2742. < http://www.nichd.nih.gov/sids/sids.htm >.

Laura J. Ninger

▌Anthrax

Definition

Anthrax is an infection caused by the bacterium *Bacillus anthracis* that primarily affects livestock but

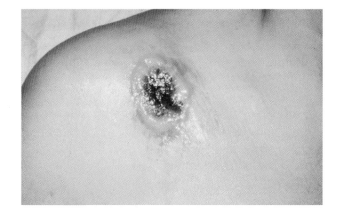

Humans suffering from anthrax often develop ulcerating nodules on the body. *Custom Medical Stock Photo. Reproduced by permission.)*

that can occasionally spread to humans, affecting either the skin, intestines, or lungs. In humans, the infection can often be treated, but it is almost always fatal in animals.

Description

Anthrax is most often found in the agricultural areas of South and Central America, southern and eastern Europe, Asia, Africa, the Caribbean, and the Middle East. In the United States, anthrax is rarely reported; however, cases of animal infection with anthrax are most often reported in Texas, Louisiana, Mississippi, Oklahoma, and South Dakota. The bacterium and its associated disease get their name from the Greek word meaning "coal" because of the characteristic coal-black sore that is the hallmark of the most common form of the disease.

During the 1800s, in England and Germany, anthrax was known either as "wool-sorter's" or "rag-picker's" disease because workers contracted the disease from bacterial spores present on hides and in wool or fabric fibers. Spores are the small, thick-walled dormant stage of some bacteria that enable them to survive for long periods of time under adverse conditions. The first anthrax vaccine was perfected in 1881 by Louis Pasteur.

The largest outbreak ever recorded in the United States occurred in 1957 when nine employees of a goat hair processing plant became ill after handling a contaminated shipment from Pakistan. Four of the five patients with the pulmonary form of the disease died. Other cases appeared in the 1970s when contaminated goatskin drumheads from Haiti were brought into the U.S. as souvenirs.

Today, anthrax is rare, even among cattle, largely because of widespread animal **vaccination**. However, some serious epidemics continue to occur among animal herds and in human settlements in developing countries due to ineffective control programs. In humans, the disease is almost always an occupational hazard, contracted by those who handle animal hides (farmers, butchers, and veterinarians) or sort wool. There are no reports of the disease spreading from one person to another.

Anthrax as a weapon

There has been a great deal of recent concern that the bacteria that cause anthrax may be used as a type of biological warfare, since it is possible to become infected simply by inhaling the spores, and inhaled anthrax is the most serious form of the disease. The bacteria can be grown in laboratories, and with a great deal of expertise and special equipment, the bacteria can be altered to be usable as a weapon.

The largest-ever documented outbreak of human anthrax contracted through spore inhalation occurred in Russia in 1979, when anthrax spores were accidentally released from a military laboratory, causing a regional epidemic that killed 69 of its 77 victims. In the United States in 2001, terrorists converted anthrax spores into a powder that could be inhaled and mailed it to intended targets, including news agencies and prominent individuals in the federal government. Because the United States government considers anthrax to be of potential risk to soldiers, the Department of Defense has begun systematic vaccination of all military personnel against anthrax. For civilians in the United States, the government has instituted a program called the National Pharmaceutical Stockpile program in which **antibiotics** and other medical materials to treat two million people are located so that they could be received anywhere in the country within twelve hours following a disaster or terrorist attack.

Causes and symptoms

The naturally occurring bacterium *Bacillus anthracis* produces spores that can remain dormant for years in soil and on animal products, such as hides, wool, hair, or bones. The disease is often fatal to cattle, sheep, and goats, and their hides, wool, and bones are often heavily contaminated.

The bacteria are found in many types of soil, all over the world, and usually do not pose a problem for humans because the spores stay in the ground. In order to infect a human, the spores have to be released from the soil and must enter the body. They can enter the body through a cut in the skin, through consuming contaminated meat, or through inhaling the spores. Once the spores are in the body, and if antibiotics are not administered, the spores become bacteria that multiply and release a toxin that affects the immune system. In the inhaled form of the infection, the immune system can become overwhelmed and the body can go into **shock**.

Symptoms vary depending on how the disease was contracted, but the symptoms usually appear within one week of exposure.

Cutaneous anthrax

In humans, anthrax usually occurs when the spores enter a cut or abrasion, causing a skin (cutaneous) infection at the site. Cutaneous anthrax, as this infection is called, is the mildest and most common form of the disease. At first, the bacteria cause an itchy, raised area like an insect bite. Within one to two days, inflammation occurs around the raised area, and a blister forms around an area of dying tissue that becomes black in the center. Other symptoms may include shivering and chills. In most cases, the bacteria remain within the sore. If, however, they spread to the nearest lymph node (or, in rare cases, escape into the bloodstream), the bacteria can cause a form of blood **poisoning** that rapidly proves fatal.

Inhalation anthrax

Inhaling the bacterial spores can lead to a rare, often-fatal form of anthrax known as pulmonary or inhalation anthrax that attacks the lungs and sometimes spreads to the brain. Inhalation anthrax begins with flu-like symptoms, namely **fever**, **fatigue**, **headache**, muscle aches, and **shortness of breath**. As early as one day after these initial symptoms appear, and as long as two weeks later, the symptoms suddenly worsen and progress to **bronchitis**. The patient experiences difficulty breathing, and finally, the patient enters a state of shock. This rare form of anthrax is often fatal, even if treated within one or two days after the symptoms appear.

Intestinal anthrax

Intestinal anthrax is a rare, often-fatal form of the disease, caused by eating meat from an animal that died of anthrax. Intestinal anthrax causes stomach and intestinal inflammation and sores or lesions (ulcers), much like the sores that appear on the skin in the cutaneous form of anthrax. The first signs of the disease are **nausea and vomiting**, loss of appetite, and fever, followed by abdominal **pain**, **vomiting** of blood, and severe bloody **diarrhea**.

Diagnosis

Anthrax is diagnosed by detecting *B. anthracis* in samples taken from blood, spinal fluid, **skin lesions**, or respiratory secretions. The bacteria may be positively identified using biochemical methods or using a technique whereby, if present in the sample, the anthrax bacterium is made to fluoresce. Blood samples will also indicate elevated antibody levels or increased amounts of a protein produced directly in response to infection with the anthrax bacterium. Polymerase chain reaction (PCR) tests amplify trace amounts of DNA to show that the anthrax bacteria are present. Additional DNA-based tests are also currently being perfected.

Treatment

In the early stages, anthrax is curable by administering high doses of antibiotics, but in the advanced stages, it can be fatal. If anthrax is suspected, health care professionals may begin to treat the patient with antibiotics even before the diagnosis is confirmed because early intervention is essential. The antibiotics used include penicillin, doxycycline, and ciprofloxacin. Because inhaled spores can remain in the body for a long time, antibiotic treatment for inhalation anthrax should continue for 60 days. In the case of cutaneous anthrax, the infection may be cured following a single dose of antibiotic, but it is important to continue treatment so as to avoid potential serious complications, such as inflammation of the membranes covering the brain and spinal cord (**meningitis**). In the setting of potential bioterrorism, cutaneous anthrax should be treated with a 60-day dose of antibiotics.

Research is ongoing to develop new antibiotics and antitoxins that would work against the anthrax bacteria and the toxins they produce. One Harvard professor, Dr. R. John Collier, and his team have been testing two possible antitoxins on rats. A Stanford microbiologist and a Penn State chemist have also been testing their new antibiotic against the bacteria that cause **brucellosis** and **tularemia**, as well as the bacteria that cause anthrax. All of these drugs are still in early investigational stages, however, and it is still unknown how these drugs would affect humans.

Prognosis

Untreated anthrax is often fatal, but **death** is far less likely with appropriate care. Ten to twenty percent of patients will die from anthrax of the skin (cutaneous anthrax) if it is not properly treated. All patients with inhalation (pulmonary) anthrax will die if untreated. Intestinal anthrax is fatal 25-75% of the time.

Prevention

Anthrax is relatively rare in the United States because of widespread animal vaccination and practices used to disinfect hides or other animal products. Anyone visiting a country where anthrax is common or where herd animals are not often vaccinated should avoid contact with livestock or animal products and avoid eating meat that has not been properly prepared and cooked.

Other means of preventing the spread of infection include carefully handling dead animals suspected of having the disease, burning (instead of burying) contaminated carcasses, and providing good ventilation when processing hides, fur, wool, or hair.

In the event that exposure to anthrax spores is known, such as in the aftermath of a terrorist attack, a course of antibiotics can prevent the disease from occurring.

In the case of contaminated mail, as was the case in the 2001 attacks, the U.S. postal service recommends certain precautions. These precautions include inspecting mail from an unknown sender for excessive tape, powder, uneven weight or lumpy spots, restrictive endorsements such as "Personal," or "Confidential," a postmark different from the sender's address, or a sender's address that seems false or that cannot be verified. Handwashing is also recommended after handling mail. In order to decontaminate batches of mail before being opened, machines that use bacteria-killing radiation could be used to sterilize the mail. These machines are similar to systems already in place on assembly lines for sterile products, such as bandages and medical devices, but this technique would not be practical for large quantities of mail. In addition, the radiation could damage some of the mail's contents, such as undeveloped photographic film. Microwave radiation or the heat from a clothes iron is not powerful enough to kill the anthrax bacteria.

For those in high-risk professions, an anthrax vaccine is available that is 93% effective in protecting against infection. To provide this immunity, an individual should be given an initial course of three injections, given two weeks apart, followed by booster injections at six, 12, and 18 months and an annual immunization thereafter.

Approximately 30% of those who have been vaccinated against anthrax may notice mild local reactions, such as tenderness at the injection site. Infrequently, there may be a severe local reaction with extensive swelling of the forearm, and a few vaccine recipients may have a more general flu-like reaction to the shot, including muscle and joint aches, headache, and fatigue. Reactions requiring hospitalization are very rare. However, this vaccine is only available to people who are at high risk, including veterinary and laboratory workers, livestock handlers, and military personnel. The vaccine is not recommended for people who have previously recovered from an anthrax infection or for pregnant women. Whether this vaccine would protect against anthrax used as a biological weapon is, as yet, unclear.

Resources

ORGANIZATIONS

Centers for Disease Control and Prevention. 1600 Clifton Rd., NE, Atlanta, GA 30333. (800) 311-3435, (404) 639-3311. < http://www.cdc.gov > .

National Institute of Allergies and Infectious Diseases, Division of Microbiology and Infectious Diseases.

Building 31, Room. 7A-50, 31 Center Drive MSC 2520, Bethesda, MD 20892. < http://www.niaid.nih.gov > .

World Health Organization, Division of Emerging and Other Communicable Diseases Surveillance and Control. Avenue Appia 20, 1211 Geneva 27, Switzerland. (+ 00 41 22) 791 21 11. < http:// www.who.int > .

OTHER

"Anthrax." *New York State Department of Health Communicable Disease Fact Sheet.* < http:// www.health.state.ny.us/nysdoh/consumer/ anthrax.htm > .

"Bacillus anthracis (Anthrax)." < http://web.bu.edu/ COHIS/infxns/bacteria/anthrax.htm > .

Begley, Sharon and Karen Springen. "Anthrax: What You Need to Know: Exposure doesn't guarantee disease, and the illness is treatable." *Newsweek* October 29, 2001: 40.

Centers for Disease Control. < http://www.cdc.gov > .

Kolata, Gina. "Antibiotics and Antitoxins." *New York Times* October 23, 2001: Section D, page 4, second column.

Park, Alice. "Anthrax: A Medical Guide." *Time* 158, no. 19 (October 29, 2001): 44.

Shapiro, Bruce. "Anthrax Anxiety." *The Nation* 273, no. 4 (November 5, 2001): 4.

Wade, Nicholas. "How a Patient Assassin Does Its Deadly Work." *New York Times* October 23, 2001: Section D, page 1.

Carol A. Turkington

Antiacne drugs

Definition

Antiacne drugs are medicines that help clear up pimples, blackheads, whiteheads, and more severe forms of **acne**.

Purpose

Different types of antiacne drugs are used for different purposes. For example, lotions, soaps, gels, and creams containing benzoyl peroxide or tretinoin may be used to clear up mild to moderately severe acne. Isotretinoin (Accutane) is prescribed only for very severe, disfiguring acne.

Acne is a skin condition that occurs when pores or hair follicles become blocked. This blockage allows a waxy material called sebum to collect inside the pores or follicles. Normally, sebum flows out onto the skin

Anti-Acne Drugs	
Brand Name (Generic Name)	Possible Common Side Effects Include:
Accutane (isotretinoin)	Dry skin, dry mouth, conjunctivitis
Benzamycin	Dry and itchy skin
Cleocin T(clindamycin phosphate)	Dry skin
Desquam-E(benzoyl peroxide)	Itching, red and peeling skin
Erythromycin topical (A/T/S, erycette, t-stat)	Burning, dry skin, **hives**, red and peeling skin
Minocin (minocycline hydrochloride)	Headache, hives, diarrhea, peeling skin, vomiting
Retin-A (tretinoin)	Darkening of the skin, blistering, crusted, or puffy skin

and hair to form a protective coating, but when it cannot get out, small swellings develop on the skin surface. Bacteria and dead skin cells can also collect that can cause inflammation. Swellings that are small and not inflamed are whiteheads or blackheads. When they become inflamed, they turn into pimples. Pimples that fill with pus are called pustules.

The severity of acne is often influenced by seasonal changes; it is typically less severe in summer than in winter. In addition, acne in girls is often affected by the menstrual cycle.

Acne cannot be cured, but acne drugs can help clear the skin. Benzoyl peroxide and tretinoin work by mildly irritating the skin. This encourages skin cells to slough off, which helps open blocked pores. Benzoyl peroxide also kills bacteria, which helps prevent whiteheads and blackheads from turning into pimples. Isotretinoin shrinks the glands that produce sebum.

Description

Benzoyl peroxide is found in many over-the-counter acne products that are applied to the skin, such as Benoxyl, Clear By Design, Neutrogena Acne, PanOxyl, and some formulations of Clean & Clear, Clearasil, and Oxy. Some benzoyl peroxide products are available without a physician's prescription; others require a prescription. Tretinoin (Retin-A) is available only with a physician's prescription and comes in liquid, cream, and gel forms, which are applied to the skin. Isotretinoin (Accutane), which is taken by mouth in capsule form, is available only with a physician's prescription. Only physicians who have experience in diagnosing and treating severe acne, such as dermatologists, should prescribe isotretinoin.

Some newer antiacne preparations combine benzoyl peroxide with **antibiotics**. One combination of benzoyl peroxide with clindamycin is sold under the trade name BenzaClin.

Many antiacne preparations contain compounds derived from plants that have anti-inflammatory properties. One group of researchers listed thirty-eight different plants that are beneficial in treating acne and other inflammatory skin conditions.

Recommended dosage

The recommended dosage depends on the type of antiacne drug. These drugs usually come with written directions for patients and should be used only as directed. Patients who have questions about how to use the medicine should check with a physician or pharmacist.

Patients who use isotretinoin usually take the medicine for a few months, then stop for at least two months. Their acne may continue to improve even after they stop taking the medicine. If the condition is still severe after several months of treatment and a two-month break, the physician may prescribe a second course of treatment.

Precautions

Isotretinoin

Isotretinoin can cause serious **birth defects**, including **mental retardation** and physical deformities. This medicine should not be used during **pregnancy**. Women who are able to bear children should not use isotretinoin unless they have very severe acne that has not cleared up with the use of other antiacne drugs. In that case, a woman who uses this drug must have a pregnancy test two weeks before beginning treatment and each month they are taking the drug. Another pregnancy test must be done one month after treatment ends. The woman must use an effective birth control method for one month before treatment begins and must continue using it throughout treatment and for one month after treatment ends. Women who are able to bear children and who want to use this medicine should discuss this information with their health care providers. Before using the medicine, they will be asked to sign a consent form stating that they understand the danger of taking isotretinoin during pregnancy and that they agree to use effective birth control.

Do not donate blood to a blood bank while taking isotretinoin or for 30 days after treatment with the drug ends. This will help reduce the chance of a pregnant woman receiving blood containing isotretinoin, which could cause birth defects.

Isotretinoin may cause a sudden decrease in night vision. If this happens, do not drive or do anything else that could be dangerous until vision returns to normal. Let the physician know about the problem.

This medicine may also make the eyes, nose, and mouth dry. Ask the physician about using special eye drops to relieve eye dryness. To temporarily relieve the **dry mouth**, chew sugarless gum, suck on sugarless candy or ice chips, or use saliva substitutes, which come in liquid and tablet forms and are available without a prescription. If the problem continues for more than two weeks, check with a physician or dentist. Mouth dryness that continues over a long time may contribute to **tooth decay** and other dental problems.

Isotretinoin may increase sensitivity to sunlight. Patients being treated with this medicine should avoid exposure to the sun and should not use tanning beds, tanning booths, or sunlamps until they know how the drug affects them.

In the early stages of treatment with isotretinoin, some people's acne seems to get worse before it starts getting better. If the condition becomes much worse or if the skin is very irritated, check with the physician who prescribed the medicine.

Benzoyl peroxide and tretinoin

When applying antiacne drugs to the skin, be careful not to get the medicine in the eyes, mouth, or inside of the nose. Do not put the medicine on skin that is wind burned, sunburned, or irritated, and do not apply it to open **wounds**.

Because such antiacne drugs as benzoyl peroxide and tretinoin irritate the skin slightly, avoid doing anything that might cause further irritation. Wash the face with mild soap and water only two or three times a day, unless the physician says to wash it more often. Avoid using abrasive soaps or cleansers and products that might dry the skin or make it peel, such as medicated cosmetics, cleansers that contain alcohol, or other acne products that contain resorcinol, sulfur or salicylic acid.

If benzoyl peroxide or tretinoin make the skin too red or too dry or cause too much peeling, check with a physician. Using the medicine less often or using a weaker strength may be necessary.

Tretinoin may increase sensitivity to sunlight. While being treated with this medicine, avoid exposure to the sun and do not use tanning beds, tanning booths, or sunlamps. If it is not possible to avoid being in the sun, use a sunscreen with a skin protection factor (SPF) of at least 15 or wear protective clothing over the treated areas. The skin may also become more sensitive to cold and wind. People who use this medicine should protect their skin from cold and wind until they know how the medicine affects them.

Benzoyl peroxide may discolor hair or colored fabrics.

Special conditions

People who have certain medical conditions or who are taking certain other medicines may have problems if they use antiacne drugs. Before using these products, be sure to let the physician know about any of these conditions:

ALLERGIES. Anyone who has had unusual reactions to etretinate, isotretinoin, tretinoin, vitamin A preparations, or benzoyl peroxide in the past should let his or her physician know before using an antiacne drug. The physician should also be told about any **allergies** to foods, dyes, preservatives, or other substances.

PREGNANCY. Women who are pregnant or who may become pregnant should check with a physician before using tretinoin or benzoyl peroxide. *Isotretinoin causes birth defects in humans and must not be used during pregnancy.*

BREASTFEEDING. No problems have been reported in nursing babies whose mothers used tretinoin or benzoyl peroxide. Women who are breastfeeding babies should not take isotretinoin, however, as it may cause problems in nursing babies.

OTHER MEDICAL CONDITIONS. Before using antiacne drugs applied to the skin, people with any of these medical problems should make sure their physicians are aware of their conditions:

• eczema. Antiacne drugs that are applied to the skin may make this condition worse.

• sunburn or raw skin. Antiacne drugs that are applied to the skin may increase the **pain** and irritation of these conditions.

In people with certain medical conditions, isotretinoin may increase the amount of triglyceride (a fatty-substance) in the blood. This may lead to heart or blood vessel problems. Before using isotretinoin, people with any of these medical problems should make sure their physicians are aware of their conditions:

• alcoholism or heavy drinking, now or in the past

• diabetes (or family history of diabetes). Isotretinoin may also change blood sugar levels.

• family history of high triglyceride levels in the blood

• severe weight problems.

USE OF CERTAIN MEDICINES. Using antiacne drugs with certain other drugs may affect the way the drugs work or may increase the chance of side effects.

Side effects

Isotretinoin

Minor discomforts such as dry mouth or nose, dry eyes, dry skin, or **itching** usually go away as the body adjusts to the drug and do not require medical attention unless they continue or are bothersome.

Other side effects should be brought to a physicians attention. These include:

• burning, redness, or itching of the eyes

• nosebleeds

• signs of inflammation of the lips, such as peeling, burning, redness or pain

Bowel inflammation is not a common side effect, but it may occur. If any of the following signs of bowel inflammation occur, stop taking isotretinoin immediately and check with a physician:

• pain in the abdomen

• bleeding from the rectum

• severe **diarrhea**

Benzoyl peroxide and tretinoin

The most common side effects of antiacne drugs applied to the skin are slight redness, dryness, peeling, and stinging, and a warm feeling to the skin. These problems usually go away as the body adjusts to the drug and do not require medical treatment.

Other side effects should be brought to a physician's attention. Check with a physician as soon as possible if any of the following side effects occur:

• blistering, crusting or swelling of the skin

• severe burning or redness of the skin

• darkening or lightening of the skin. (This effect will eventually go away after treatment with an antiacne drug ends.)

• skin rash

Other side effects are possible with any type of antiacne drug. Anyone who has unusual symptoms while using antiacne drugs should get in touch with his or her physician.

Interactions

Patients using antiacne drugs on their skin should tell their physicians if they are using any other prescription or nonprescription (over-the-counter) medicine that they apply to the skin in the same area.

Isotretinoin may interact with other medicines. When this happens, the effects of one or both drugs may change or the risk of side effects may be greater. Anyone who takes isotretinoin should let the physician know about all other medicines he or she is taking and should ask whether the possible interactions can interfere with drug therapy. Among the drugs that may interact with isotretinoin are:

• etretinate (Tegison), used to treat severe **psoriasis**. Using this medicine with isotretinoin increases side effects.

• tretinoin (Retin-A, Renova). Using this medicine with isotretinoin increases side effects.

- vitamin A or any medicine containing vitamin A. Using any vitamin A preparations with isotretinoin increases side effects. Do not take vitamin supplements containing vitamin A while taking isotretinoin.

- tetracyclines (used to treat infections). Using these medicines with isotretinoin increases the chance of swelling of the brain. Make sure the physician knows if tetracycline is being used to treat acne or another infection.

Resources

BOOKS

Beers, Mark H., MD, and Robert Berkow, MD., editors. "Acne." Section 10, Chapter 116 In *The Merck Manual of Diagnosis and Therapy*. Whitehouse Station, NJ: Merck Research Laboratories, 2002.

Beers, Mark H., MD, and Robert Berkow, MD., editors. "Warts (Verrucae)." Section 10, Chapter 115 In *The Merck Manual of Diagnosis and Therapy*. Whitehouse Station, NJ: Merck Research Laboratories, 2002.

Wilson, Billie Ann, Margaret T. Shannon, and Carolyn L. Stang. *Nurse's Drug Guide 2003*. Upper Saddle River, NJ: Prentice Hall, 2003.

PERIODICALS

Breneman, D., R. Savin, C. Van dePol, et al. "Double-Blind, Randomized, Vehicle-Controlled Clinical Trial of Once-Daily Benzoyl Peroxide/Clindamycin Topical Gel in the Treatment of Patients with Moderate to Severe Rosacea." *International Journal of Dermatology* 43 (May 2004): 381–387.

Darshan, S., and R. Doreswamy. "Patented Antiinflammatory Plant Drug Development from Traditional Medicine." *Phytotherapy Research* 18 (May 2004): 343–357.

Halder, R. M., and G. M. Richards. "Topical Agents Used in the Management of Hyperpigmentation." *Skin Therapy Letter* 9 (June-July 2004): 1–3.

Kligman, D. E., and Z. D. Draelos. "High-Strength Tretinoin for Rapid Retinization of Photoaged Facial Skin." *Dermatologic Surgery* 30 (June 2004): 864–866.

Leyden, J. J., D. Thiboutot, and A. Shalita. "Photographic Review of Results from a Clinical Study Comparing Benzoyl Peroxide 5%/Clindamycin 1% Topical Gel with Vehicle in the Treatment of Rosacea." *Cutis* 73, Supplement 6 (June 2004): 11–17.

ORGANIZATIONS

American Academy of Dermatology (AAD). P. O. Box 4014, Schaumburg, IL 60168-4014. (847) 330-0230. < http://www.aad.org. >.

American Society of Health-System Pharmacists (ASHP). 7272 Wisconsin Avenue, Bethesda, MD 20814. (301) 657-3000. < http://www.ashp.org >.

United States Food and Drug Administration (FDA). 5600 Fishers Lane, Rockville, MD 20857-0001. (888) INFO-FDA. < http://www.fda.gov >.

Nancy Ross-Flanigan
Rebecca J. Frey, PhD

Antiandrogen drugs

Definition

Antiandrogen drugs are a diverse group of medications given to counteract the effects of androgens (male sex hormones) on various body organs and tissues. Some medications in this category work by lowering the body's production of androgens while others work by blocking the body's ability to make use of the androgens that are produced. The first group of antiandrogens includes such medications as leuprolide (Lupron, Viadur, or Eligard), goserelin (Zoladex), triptorelin (Trelstar Depot), and abarelix (Plenaxis). The second group includes flutamide (Eulexin), nilutamide (Nilandron), cyproterone acetate (Cyprostat, Androcur, Cyproterone), and bicalutamide (Casodex). Flutamide, nilutamide, and bicalutamide are nonsteroidal antiandrogen drugs while cyproterone acetate is a steroidal medication.

Some drugs that were originally developed to treat other conditions are sometimes categorized as antiandrogens because their off-label uses include some of the disorders listed below. These drugs include medroxyprogesterone (**Depo-Provera**), a derivative of the female sex hormone progesterone that is used as a contraceptive and treatment for abnormal uterine bleeding; ketoconazole (Nizoral), an antifungal drug; and spironolactone (Aldactone), a diuretic.

Purpose

Antiandrogen drugs may be given for any of several conditions or disorders, ranging from skin problems to mental disorders:

- **Prostate cancer**. Antiandrogen medications may be used to treat both early-stage and advanced prostate **cancer** by lowering or blocking the supply of male sex hormones that encourage the growth and spread of the cancer.

- Androgenetic **alopecia**. Androgenetic alopecia is a type of hair loss that is genetically determined and affects both men and women. It is sometimes called pattern baldness.

- **Acne.** Acne is the end result of several factors, one of which is excessive production of sebum, a whitish semiliquid greasy substance produced by certain glands in the skin. Antiandrogens may help to clear acne by slowing down the secretion of sebum, which depends on androgen production.

- **Amenorrhea.** Amenorrhea, or the absence of menstrual periods in females of childbearing age, is sometimes caused by excessively high levels of androgens in the blood. Antiandrogen medications may help to restore normal menstrual periods.

- **Hirsutism.** Hirsutism is a condition in which women develop excessive facial and body hair in a distribution pattern usually associated with adult males. It results from abnormally high levels of androgens in the bloodstream or from increased sensitivity of the hair follicles to normal levels of androgens. Hirsutism may be a sign of **polycystic ovary syndrome** (PCOS), a condition in which the ovaries develop multiple large cysts and produce too much androgen.

- Gender reassignment. Antiandrogen drugs are often prescribed for male-to-female (MTF) transsexuals as part of the hormonal treatment that precedes gender reassignment surgery.

- Paraphilias. Paraphilias are a group of mental disorders characterized by intense and recurrent sexual urges or behaviors involving nonhuman objects, children or nonconsenting adults, or **pain** and humiliation. Antiandrogen drugs have been prescribed for men diagnosed with paraphilias in order to lower blood serum levels of testosterone and help them control their sexual urges.

- Virilization. Virilization is an extreme form of hyperandrogenism in females, marked by such changes as development of male pattern baldness, voice changes, and overdevelopment of the skeletal muscles. Antiandrogens may be given to correct this condition.

Description

- Leuprolide. Leuprolide is classified as a luteinizing hormone-releasing hormone (LHRH) agonist, which means that it resembles a chemical produced by the hypothalamus (a gland located in the brain) that lowers the level of testosterone in the bloodstream. It also reduces levels of estrogen in girls and women, and may be used to treat **endometriosis** or tumors in the uterus. It is presently

under investigation as a possible treatment for the paraphilias.

- Goserelin. Goserelin is also an LHRH agonist, and works in the same way as leuprolide.

- Triptorelin. Triptorelin is an LHRH agonist, and works in the same way as leuprolide. It is not usually given to women, however.

- Abarelix. Abarelix is a newer drug that works by blocking hormone receptors in the pituitary gland. It is recommended for the treatment of prostate cancer in men with advanced disease who refuse surgery, cannot take other hormonal treatments, or are poor candidates for surgery.

- Ketoconazole. Ketoconazole is an antifungal drug available in tablets to be taken by mouth. Its use in treating hirsutism is off-label.

- Flutamide. Flutamide is a nonsteroidal antiandrogen medication that blocks the use of androgen by the body.

- Nilutamide. Nilutamide is another nonsteroidal antiandrogen drug that works by blocking the body's use of androgens.

- Bicalutamide. Bicalutamide is a nonsteroidal antiandrogen medication that works in the same way as flutamide.

- Cyproterone acetate. Cyproterone acetate is a steroidal antiandrogen drug that works by lowering testosterone production as well as blocking the body's use of androgens.

- Medroxyprogesterone. Medroxyprogesterone is a synthetic derivative of progesterone that prevents ovulation and keeps the lining of the uterus from breaking down, thus preventing uterine bleeding.

- Spironolactone. Spironolactone is a potassium-sparing diuretic that may be given to treat androgen excess in women.

Recommended dosage

- Leuprolide. Leuprolide is available in an injectable form and as an implant. The implant form, used to treat prostate cancer, contains 22.5 mg of leuprolide and is inserted under the skin every three months. This type of slow-release medication is called depot form. A longer-acting implant that lasts 12 months is also available. Injectable leuprolide is injected once a day in a 1-mg dose to treat prostate cancer. The dosage for endometriosis or uterine tumors is 3.75 mg injected into a muscle once a month for three to six months.

- Goserelin. Goserelin is implanted under the skin of the upper abdomen. The dosage for treating cancer of the prostate is one 3.6-mg implant every 28 days or one 10.8-mg implant every 12 weeks. For treating endometriosis, the dosage is one 3.6-mg implant every 28 days for six months.

- Triptorelin. Triptorelin is given as a long-lasting injection for treatment of prostate cancer or paraphilias. The usual dose for either condition is 3.75 mg, injected into a muscle once a month.

- Abarelix. Abarelix is given in 100-mg doses by deep injection into the muscles of the buttocks. It is given on days 1, 15, and 29 of treatment, then every four weeks for a total treatment duration of 12 weeks.

- Ketoconazole. For treatment of hirsutism, 400 mg by mouth once per day.

- Flutamide. Flutamide is available in capsule as well as tablet form. For treatment of prostate cancer, 250 mg by mouth three times a day. For virilization or hyperandrogenism in women, 250 mg by mouth three times a day. It should be used in women, however, only when other treatments have proved ineffective.

- Nilutamide. To treat prostate cancer, nilutamide is taken in a single 300-mg daily dose by mouth for the first 30 days of therapy, then a single daily dose of 150 mg..

- Bicalutamide. Bicalutamide is taken by mouth in a single daily dose of 50 mg to treat prostate cancer.

- Cyproterone acetate. Cyproterone is taken by mouth three times a day in 100-mg doses to treat prostate cancer. The dose for treating hyperandrogenism or virilization in women is one 50-mg tablet by mouth each day for the first ten days of the menstrual cycle. Cyproterone acetate given to treat acne is usually given in the form of an oral contraceptive (Diane-35) that combines the drug (2 mg) with ethinyl estradiol (35 mg). Diane-35 is also taken as hormonal therapy by MTF transsexuals. The dose for treating paraphilias is 200–400 mg by injection in depot form every 1–2 weeks, or 50–200 mg by mouth daily.

- Medroxyprogesterone. For the treatment of paraphilias, given as an intramuscular 150-mg injection daily, weekly, or monthly, depending on the patient's serum testosterone levels, or as an oral dose of 100–400 mg daily. As hormonal therapy for MTF transsexuals, 10–40 mg per day. For polycystic ovary syndrome, 10 mg daily for 10 days.

- Spironolactone. For hyperandrogenism in women, 100–200 mg per day by mouth; for polycystic ovary syndrome, 50–200 mg per day. For the treatment of

acne, 200 mg per day. For hormonal therapy for MTF transsexuals, 200–400 mg per day. A topical form of spironolactone is available for the treatment of androgenetic alopecia.

Precautions

- Leuprolide. Leuprolide should not be used by pregnant or nursing women, by patients diagnosed with spinal compression, or by patients allergic to the drug. Women taking leuprolide should not try to become pregnant, and should use methods of birth control that do not contain hormones.

- Goserelin. Goserelin should not be used during **pregnancy** or **lactation**, or by patients known to be allergic to it. As with leuprolide, women taking goserelin should use methods of **contraception** that do not contain hormones.

- Triptorelin. Patients using triptorelin should see their doctor at regular intervals for monitoring of side effects.

- Abarelix. Abarelix should not be given to children or women. Because of the severity of this drug's possible side effects, doctors who prescribe it for men must be certified following successful completion of a safety program for its proper use.

- Ketoconazole. Ketoconazole should not be given to alcoholic patients or those allergic to the drug. In addition, patients using ketoconazole should have their liver function monitored by their doctor.

- Flutamide. Flutamide should not be used by pregnant women. Patients taking flutamide should have their liver function monitored carefully. They should notify their doctor at once if they have pain in the upper right side of the abdomen or a yellowish discoloration of the eyes and skin, as these are signs of liver damage. In addition, patients using this drug should not discontinue taking it without telling their doctor.

- Nilutamide. This drug should not be given to patients who are allergic to it, have severe respiratory problems, or have been diagnosed with a liver disorder. Patients taking this drug should discontinue using alcoholic beverages while they are being treated with it.

- Bicalutamide. The precautions while using this drug are the same as those for flutamide.

- Cyproterone acetate. This drug has not been approved by the Food and Drug Administration (FDA) for use in the United States, but is approved for use in Canada and the United Kingdom. It should not be used during pregnancy or lactation, or by patients with **liver disease**. Men who are taking this drug for treatment of paraphilias should not use alcohol.

- Medroxyprogesterone. This drug should not be given to patients with a history of blood clot formation in their blood vessels. It should be used with caution in patients with **asthma**, seizure disorders, migraine headaches, liver or kidney disorders, or heart disease.

- Spironolactone. This drug should not be given to patients with overly high levels of potassium in the blood or to patients with liver disease or kidney failure. It should also not be given to pregnant or lactating women.

Side effects

- Leuprolide. Side effects of leuprolide in men may include pains in the chest, groin, or legs; hot flashes, loss of interest in sex, or **impotence**; bone pain; sleep disturbances; and mood changes. Side effects in women may include amenorrhea or light and irregular menstrual periods; loss of bone density; mood changes; burning or **itching** sensations in the vagina; or pelvic pain.

- Goserelin. The side effects of goserelin may include **nausea and vomiting**; they are otherwise the same as for leuprolide.

- Triptorelin. Side effects of triptorelin include pain in the bladder, difficulty urinating, or bloody or cloudy urine; pain in the side or lower back; hot flashes or **headache**; loss of interest in sex or impotence; **vomiting** or **diarrhea**; unusual bleeding or bruising; pain at the injection site; unusual tiredness or sleep disturbances; depression or rapid mood changes. It may also cause a temporary enlargement of the tumor; this side effect is known as tumor flare.

- Abarelix. This drug may cause immediate life-threatening allergic reactions following any dose. May also cause a loss of bone mineral density, irregular heartbeat, hot flashes, sleep disturbances, **gynecomastia**, or pain in the breasts and nipples.

- Ketoconazole. The side effects of ketoconazole include **nausea** and vomiting, loss of appetite, abdominal pain, skin rash or itching, uterine bleeding, breast pain, gynecomastia, hair loss, loss of interest in sex, and decline in sperm production.

- Flutamide. Flutamide has been reported to cause breast tenderness and gynecomastia in men as well as **fatigue**, nausea, flu-like symptoms, and runny nose; darkened urine; **indigestion**, **constipation**,

diarrhea, or gas; bluish-colored or dry skin; **dizziness**; and liver damage. These side effects may be intensified in patients who smoke.

- Nilutamide. The side effects of nilutamide are the same as those for flutamide. In addition, this drug may affect the ability of the eyes to adjust to sudden changes in light intensity or may make the eyes unusually sensitive to light. Another potential side effect is difficulty breathing; this is more likely to occur in Asian patients taking this drug than in Caucasians.

- Bicalutamide. The side effects of this drug are the same as those for flutamide.

- Cyproterone acetate. Cyproterone has been reported to cause gynecomastia, impotence, loss of interest in sex, deep venous thrombosis, and possible damage to the cardiovascular system.

- Medroxyprogesterone. The side effects of this drug include high blood pressure, headache, nausea and vomiting, changes in menstrual flow, breakthrough bleeding, puffy skin (**edema**), weight gain, and sore or swollen breasts.

- Spironolactone. Spironolactone may cause fatigue, headache, and drowsiness; gynecomastia and impotence in men; abdominal cramps, nausea, vomiting, diarrhea, or loss of appetite; and skin **rashes** or itching.

Interactions

- Leuprolide. No interactions with other medications have been reported.

- Goserelin. No interactions have been reported.

- Triptorelin. No interactions have been reported.

- Abarelix. Abarelix may interact with other medications that affect heart rhythm, including procainamide, amiodarone, sotalol, and dofetilde.

- Ketoconazole. Ketoconazole interacts with a number of drugs, including rifampin, warfarin, phenytoin, **antacids**, cyclosporine, terfenadine, and astemizole. It may cause a sunburn-like skin reaction if used together with alcohol.

- Flutamide. This drug has been reported to intensify the effects of warfarin (Coumadin) and other blood-thinning medications. It has also been reported to intensify the effects of phenytoin (Dilantin), a drug given to control seizures.

- Nilutamide. Reported interactions are the same as for flutamide; in addition, nilutamide has been reported to intensify the effects of theophylline (Theo-Dur), a drug given to treat asthma.

- Bicalutamide. Reported interactions are the same as for flutamide.

- Cyproterone acetate. Patients taking oral medications to control diabetes may require dosage adjustments while taking this drug.

- Medroxyprogesterone. Patients taking phenobarbital, phenothiazine tranquilizers (chlorpromazine, perphenazine, fluphenazine, etc.), or oral medications to control diabetes should consult their doctor about dosage adjustments.

- Spironolactone. Spironolactone is reported to decrease the effectiveness of **aspirin** and anticoagulants (blood thinners). It may also interact with potassium supplements to increase the patient's blood potassium level.

Resources

BOOKS

"Amenorrhea." Section 18, Chapter 235 in *The Merck Manual of Diagnosis and Therapy*, edited by Mark H. Beers, MD, and Robert Berkow, MD. Whitehouse Station, NJ: Merck Research Laboratories, 2005.

American Psychiatric Association. *Diagnostic and Statistical Manual of Mental Disorders*, 4th edition, text revision. Washington, DC: American Psychiatric Association, 2000.

"Paraphilias." Section 15, Chapter 192 in *The Merck Manual of Diagnosis and Therapy*, edited by Mark H. Beers, MD, and Robert Berkow, MD. Whitehouse Station, NJ: Merck Research Laboratories, 2005.

"Prostate Cancer." Section 17, Chapter 233 in *The Merck Manual of Diagnosis and Therapy*, edited by Mark H. Beers, MD, and Robert Berkow, MD. Whitehouse Station, NJ: Merck Research Laboratories, 2005.

PERIODICALS

Bradford, J. M. "The Neurobiology, Neuropharmacology, and Pharmacological Treatment of the Paraphilias and Compulsive Sexual Behavior." *Canadian Journal of Psychiatry* 46 (February 2001): 26–34.

Brannon, Guy E., MD. "Paraphilias." *eMedicine*, 17 October 2002. < http://www.emedicine.com/med/topic3127.htm >.

Feinstein, Robert, MD. "Androgenetic Alopecia." *eMedicine*, 2 October 2003. < http://www.emedicine.-com/DERM/topic21.htm >.

Harper, Julie C., MD, and James Fulton, Jr., MD. "Acne Vulgaris." *eMedicine*, 29 July 2004. < http://www.-emedicine.com/derm/topic3540.htm >.

Hunter, Melissa H., MD, and Peter J. Carek, MD. "Evaluation and Treatment of Women with Hirsutism." *American Family Physician* 67 (June 15, 2003): 2565–2572.

Hyperandrogenic Disorders Task Force. "American Association of Clinical Endocrinologists Medical Guidelines for Clinical Practice for the Diagnosis and Treatment of Hyperandrogenic Disorders." *Endocrine Practice* 7 (March-April 2001): 120–135.

Krueger, R. B., and M. S. Kaplan. "Depot-Leuprolide Acetate for Treatment of Paraphilias: A Report of Twelve Cases." *Archives of Sexual Behavior* 30 (August 2001): 409–422.

Oriel, Kathleen A., MD, MS. "Medical Care of Transsexual Patients." *Journal of the Gay and Lesbian Medical Association* 4 (April 2000): 185–194.

Patel, Vipul, MD, and Raymond J. Leveille, MD. "Prostate Cancer: Neoadjuvant Androgen Deprivation." *eMedicine*, 10 March 2005. < http://www.emedicine.com/med/topic3396htm >.

Richardson, Marilyn R., MD. "Current Perspectives in Polycystic Ovary Syndrome." *American Family Physician* 68 (August 15, 2003): 697–704.

Thorneycroft, Ian, MD, PhD. "Androgen Excess." *eMedicine*, 28 February 2004. < http://www.emedicine.com/med/topic3489htm >.

ORGANIZATIONS

American Academy of Dermatology (AAD). P. O. Box 4014, Schaumburg, IL 60168-4014. (847) 330-0230. Fax: (847) 330-0050. < http://www.aad.org >.

American Association of Clinical Endocrinologists (AACE). 1000 Riverside Avenue, Suite 205, Jacksonville, FL 32204. (904) 353-7878. Fax: (904) 353-8185. < http://www.aace.com >.

American Psychiatric Association (APA). 1000 Wilson Boulevard, Suite 1825, Arlington, VA 22209-3901. (800) 368-5777 or (703) 907-7322. Fax: (703) 907-1091. < http://www.psych.org >.

Harry Benjamin International Gender Dysphoria Association, Inc. (HBIGDA). 1300 South Second Street, Suite 180, Minneapolis, MN 55454. (612) 624-9397. Fax: (612) 624-9541. < www.hbigda.org >.

National Cancer Institute (NCI). NCI Public Inquiries Office, Suite 3036A, 6116 Executive Boulevard, MSC8332, Bethesda, MD 20892-8322. (800) 4-CANCER or (800) 332-8615 (TTY). < www.nci.nih.gov >.

National Institute of Mental Health (NIMH). 6001 Executive Boulevard, Room 8184, MSC 9663, Bethesda, MD 20892-9663. (301) 443-4513 or (886) 615-NIMH. < www.nimh.nih.gov. >

United States Food and Drug Administration (FDA). 5600 Fishers Lane, Rockville, MD 20857-0001. (888) INFO-FDA. < www.fda.gov >.

OTHER

National Cancer Institute (NCI). *Prostate Cancer (PDQ®)*: Treatment, Health Professional version. < http://www.cancer.gov/cancertopics/pdq/treatment/prostate/HealthProfessional/ >.

Rebecca J. Frey, PhD

Antianemia drugs

Definition

Antianemia drugs are therapeutic agents which increase either the number of red cells or the amount of hemoglobin in the blood.

Purpose

Anemia is a general term for a large number of conditions marked by a reduction in the oxygen-carrying capacity of blood. Red blood cells carry oxygen in hemoglobin, so that anemia may be caused by a deficiency of blood or red blood cells or of hemoglobin. These conditions may be caused by a variety of other conditions. Injury can cause blood loss, which in turn can cause anemia. Nutritional deficiency, inadequate amounts of some of the **vitamins** and **minerals** that are needed for hemoglobin production, may also cause anemia. Because hemoglobin is the pigment that makes blood cells red, a lack of hemoglobin will cause the cells to be a paler color, leading to the term hypochromic, lacking in color.

Other conditions can also cause anemia. For example, certain diseases cause the condition. These can include infections and **kidney disease**, in which there is a deficiency of crythropoietin, a material produced in the kidneys which is essential for the production of red blood cells. Certain genetic conditions affect the absorption of nutrients and may lead to anemia. In sickle cell anemia, a genetic condition in which the red cells are curved rather than flat, the red cells have reduced ability to carry oxygen.

The *Merck Manual* reduces all types of anemia to three classes:

- blood loss
- inadequate production of blood
- excessive breakdown of blood cells

Anemia may be caused by one or a combination of these three factors. Drug therapy is available for many types of anemia; however, the selection of the drug depends on proper diagnosis of the cause of the anemia.

Description

Anemia caused by blood loss is normally treated with either blood volume expanders such as plasma or with related blood products. More severe blood loss may require transfusions of red blood cells.

In some cases, blood loss may be due to ulcers of the stomach or intestines. In these cases, treatment of the underlying cause will normally correct the anemia.

Iron deficiency

The most common cause of anemia in adults is iron deficiency. Although the typical American diet contains enough iron to meet normal needs, individuals who are less able to absorb and store iron may experience inadequate hemoglobin production. Although the best way to meet daily iron requirements is through improved diet, iron supplements are widely used.

Iron is normally taken in the form of ferrous sulfate. Although other iron salts are commercially available and make claims of fewer or less severe side effects, these benefits may be related to the fact that other preparations contain less iron by weight. Ferrous sulfate contains about 37% iron, while ferrous gluconate contains only about 13% iron. People who have trouble with the side effects of ferrous sulfate may benefit from some of the specialty preparations available, but ferrous sulfate normally offers the greatest amount of iron of all commercial products.

Recommended dosage

Dosage should be calculated by iron needs, based on laboratory tests. Manufacturers recommend one tablet a day, containing 65 mg of iron, as a supplement for patients over the age of 12 years.

Precautions

Iron can lead to lethal **poisoning** in children. All iron supplements should be kept carefully out of reach of children.

Some types of anemia do not respond to iron therapy, and the use of iron should be avoided in these cases. People with acquired **hemolytic anemia**, autoimmune hemolytic anemia, **hemochromatosis**, hemolytic anemia and hemosiderosis should not take iron supplements. Hemolytic anemia is caused by the increased breakdown of red blood cells. Hemochromatosis and hemosiderosis and are conditions in which there is too much, rather than too little, absorption of iron.

Iron supplements should also be avoided by people who have gastric or intestinal ulcers, **ulcerative colitis**, or **Crohn's disease**. These conditions marked by inflammation of the digestive tract, which would be made worse by use of iron.

Side effects

The most common side effects of iron consumption are stomach and intestinal problems, including stomach upset with cramps, **constipation**, **diarrhea**, **nausea**, and **vomiting**. At least 25% of patients have one or more of these side effects. The frequency and severity of the side effects increases with the dose of iron. Less frequent side effects include **heartburn** and urine discoloration.

Interactions

Iron supplements should not be taken at the same time as **antibiotics** of either the tetracycline or quinolone types. The iron will reduce the effectiveness of the antibiotic. Also, iron supplements reduces the effectiveness of levodopa, which is used in treatment of Parkinson's disease.

Iron supplements should not be used with magnesium trisilicate, an antacid, or with penicillamine, which is used for some types of arthritis.

Taking iron with vitamin C increases the absorption of iron, with no increase in side effects.

Folic acid

Folic acid is found in many common foods, including liver, dried peas, lentils, oranges, whole-wheat products, asparagus, beets, broccoli, brussel sprouts, and spinach. However, in some cases, patients have difficulty absorbing folic acid or in converting it from the form found in foods to the form that is active in blood formation. In these cases, folic acid tablets are appropriate for use.

RECOMMENDED DOSAGE. For treatment of anemia, a daily dose of 1 mg is generally used. Patients who have trouble absorbing folic acid may require higher doses.

Maintenance doses are:

- infants: 0.1 mg/day
- children (under 4 years of age): up to 0.3 mg/day
- children (over 4 years of age) and adults: 0.4 mg/day
- pregnant and lactating women: 0.8 mg/day

PRECAUTIONS. Before treating an anemia with folic acid, diagnostic tests must be performed to verify the cause of the anemia. **Pernicious anemia** caused by lack of vitamin B_{12} shows symptoms that are very similar to those of folic acid deficiency but also causes nerve damage which shows up as a **tingling** sensation and feelings of **numbness**. Giving folic acid to patients with B_{12} deficiency anemia improves the blood cell count, but the nerve damage continues to progress.

SIDE EFFECTS. Folic acid is considered extremely safe, and there are no predictable side effects. Where side effects have been reported, they have been among patients taking many times more than the normal therapeutic dose of the drug.

On rare occasions allergic reactions to folic acid have been reported.

INTERACTIONS. Phenytoins, used to treat seizure disorders, interact with folic acid with a reduction in phenytoin effectiveness and an increased risk of seizures. If the two drugs must be used together, phenytoin blood levels should be monitored, and the dose may have to be increased.

Trimethoprim (an antibacterial) and methotrexate (originally an anti-cancer drug, which is also used for arthritis and **psoriasis**) act by reducing the metabolism of folic acid. Regular blood monitoring is required, and dose adjustments may be needed.

Vitamin B_{12}

Vitamin B_{12} is also known as cyanocobalamine and hydroxocobalamine. Cyanocobalamine may be given by mouth, while hydroxocobalamine must be injected. The vitamin has many functions in the body, including maintaining the nervous system, but in treatment of anemia B_{12} is needed for the metabolism of folic acid. Lack of B_{12} causes pernicious anemia, a type of anemia which is marked by a low red cell count and lack of hemoglobin. There are many other symptoms of pernicious anemia, including a feeling of tingling or numbness, **shortness of breath**, muscle weakness, faintness, and a smooth tongue. If pernicious anemia is left untreated for more than three months, permanent damage to the nerves of the spinal cord may result.

RECOMMENDED DOSAGE. While vitamin B_{12} can be given by mouth for mild vitamin deficiency states, pernicious anemia should always be treated with injections, either under the skin (subcutaneous) or into muscle (intramuscular). Hydroxocobalamine should only be injected into muscle. Intravenous injections are not used because the vitamin is eliminated from the body too quickly when given this way. Elderly patients, whose ability to absorb vitamin B_{12} through the stomach may be impaired, should also be treated with injections only.

The normal dose of cyanocobalamine is 100 mcg (micrograms) daily for six to seven days. If improvement is seen, the dose may be reduced to 100 mcg every other day for seven doses and then 100 mcg every three to four days for two to three weeks. After that, monthly injections may be required for life.

PRECAUTIONS. Although vitamin B_{12} has a very high level of safety, commercial preparations may contain preservatives which may cause allergic responses.

In patients with pernicious anemia, treatment with vitamin B_{12} may lead to loss of potassium. Patients should be monitored for their potassium levels.

SIDE EFFECTS. Diarrhea and **itching** of the skin have been reported on rare occasions. Moreover, there have been reports of severe allergic reactions to cyanocobalamine.

INTERACTIONS. Aminosalicylic acid may reduce the effectiveness of vitamin B_{12}. Also, colchicine, a drug used for **gout**, may reduce the effectiveness of vitamin B_{12}. Other, infrequently used drugs and excessive use of alcohol may also affect the efficacy of vitamin B_{12}. Patients being treated for anemia should discuss all medications, both prescription and nonprescription, with their physician or pharmacist.

Anabolic steroids

The anabolic steroids (nandrolone, oxymetholone, oxandrolone, and stanzolol) are the same drugs that are used improperly by body builders to increase muscle mass. Two of these drugs, nandrolone and oxymetholone, are approved for use in treatment of anemia. Nandrolone is indicated for treatment of anemia caused by kidney failure, while oxymetholone may be used to treat anemia caused by insufficient red cell production, such as **aplastic anemia**.

All anabolic steroids are considered to be drugs of **abuse** under United States federal law.

RECOMMENDED DOSAGE. The information that follows is specific only to oxymetholone; however, the warnings and precautions apply to all drugs in the class of anabolic steroids.

The dosage of oxymetholone must be individualized. The most common dose is 1 to 2 mg per kilogram of body weight per day, although doses as high as 5 mg per kilogram per day have been used. The response to these drugs is slow, and it may take several months to see if there is any benefit.

PRECAUTIONS. All anabolic steroids are dangerous. The following warnings represent the most significant hazards of these drugs. For a complete list, patients should consult the manufacturer's package insert.

- Peliosis hepatitis, a condition in which liver and sometimes spleen tissue is replaced with blood-filled cysts, has occurred in patients receiving androgenic anabolic steroids. Although this condition is usually reversible by discontinuing the drug, if it is left undetected and untreated, it may lead to life-threatening liver failure or bleeding.

- Liver tumors may develop. Although most of these tumors are benign and will go away when the drug is discontinued, liver cancers may also result.

- Anabolic steroids may cause changes in blood lipids, leading to **atherosclerosis** with greatly increased risk of heart attack.

- Because anabolic steroids are derived from male sex hormones, masculinization may occur when they are used by women.

- Elderly men who use these drugs may be at increased risk of prostate enlargement and prostate **cancer**.

- Increased water retention due to anabolic steroids may lead to heart failure.

- Anabolic steroids should not be used during **pregnancy**, since this may cause masculinization of the fetus.

- Anabolic steroids should be used in children only if there is no possible alternative. These drugs may cause the long bones of the legs to stop growing prematurely, leading to reduction in adult height. Regular monitoring is essential.

- In patients with epilepsy, the frequency of seizures may be increased.

- In patients with diabetes, glucose tolerance may be altered. Careful monitoring is essential.

SIDE EFFECTS. The list of side effects associated with anabolic steroids is extremely long. The following list covers only the most commonly observed effects:

- acne

- increased urinary frequency

- breast growth in males

- breast pain

- persistent, painful erections

- masculinization in women

INTERACTIONS. Anabolic steroids should not be used in combination with anticoagulants such as warfarin. Anabolic steroids increase the effects of the anticoagulant, possibly leading to bleeding. If the combination cannot be avoided, careful monitoring is essential.

Epoetin alfa

Epoetin alfa is a synthetic form of a protein produced by the kidneys that stimulates the production and release of red blood cells. A similar drug, darepoetin alpha, is available with the same properties, but it remains active longer and so requires fewer injections each week. Because epoetin alfa is approved for more types of anemia than darepoetin, this discussion deals only with the older drug.

Epoetin alpha is approved by the Food and Drug Administration for the following uses:

- anemia associated with chronic renal failure

- anemia related to zidovudine therapy in HIV-infected patients

- anemia in cancer patients on chemotherapy

- reduction in blood transfusions in surgical patients

In addition, epoetin alpha may be useful in anemia from many other causes. These include but are not limited to anemia of **prematurity**, sickle cell anemia, and the anemia associated with **rheumatoid arthritis**.

The drug has been abused by athletes due to the theory that increasing the red blood cell count improves athletic performance. The potential benefits of misuse of the drug are limited, and the risks are significant. The United States and International Olympic Committees and the National Collegiate Athletic Association consider the use of epoetin alfa to enhance athletic ergogenic potential inappropriate and unacceptable because its use by athletes is contrary to the rules and ethical principles of athletic competition. As of the early 200s, tests to detect the misuse of epoetin alfa by athletes are increasingly reliable.

RECOMMENDED DOSAGE. Dosing schedules may vary with the cause of the anemia. All doses should be individualized. In general, epoetin alpha dosing in adults is started at 50 to 100 units per kilogram given three times a week, either by vein or subcutaneously.

The dose should be reduced if the hemoglobin level reaches 12 grams per decaliter or if the hemoglobin level increases by more than 1 gram per decaliter in any two-week period. The drug should be interrupted if hemoglobin levels reach 13 grams or more per decaliter.

The dose should be increased if the hemoglobin level does not increase by at least 2 grams per decaliter after eight weeks of treatment.

Maintenance doses, if required, should be individualized to keep the hemoglobin levels within the range of 10 to 12 grams per decaliter.

PRECAUTIONS. Epoetin alpha should not be given to patients with severe, uncontrolled **hypertension**.

Other conditions in which epoetin alpha should be used only when the benefits clearly outweigh the risks are as follows:

- constitutional aplastic anemia

- hypertension

- thromboembolism

Side effects

The most common adverse effects of erythopoetin alpha are:

- joint pain

- chest pain

- diarrhea

- swelling

- fatigue

- fever

- weakness

- headache
- high blood pressure
- irritation at injection site
- nausea
- vomiting
- rapid heart beat

A large number of additional adverse effects have been reported. Patients should consult the manufacturer's package insert for the full list.

Interactions

According to the manufacturer, as of 2004 no evidence of interaction of epoetin alfa with other drugs was observed.

Resources

BOOKS

Beers, Mark H., ed. *Merck Manual of Medical Information: Home Edition*. Riverside, NJ: Simon & Schuster, 2004.

Greer John P., et al., eds. *Wintrobe's Clinical Hematology*. Baltimore, MD: Lippincott Williams & Wilkins, 2003.

Physicians' Desk Reference 2005. Montvale, NJ: Thomson Healthcare, 2004.

PERIODICALS

Sharma, N., et al. "Vitamin supplementation: what the gastroenterologist needs to know." *Journal of Clinical Gastroenterology* 38, no. 10 (November/December 2004): 844–54.

Samuel D. Uretsky, PharmD

Antiangina drugs

Definition

Antiangina drugs are medicines that relieve the symptoms of **angina** pectoris (severe chest **pain**).

Purpose

The dull, tight chest pain of angina occurs when the heart's muscular wall is not getting enough oxygen. By relaxing the blood vessels, antiangina drugs reduce the heart's work load and increase the amount of oxygen-rich blood that reaches the heart. These drugs come in different forms, and are used in three main ways:

- taken regularly over a long period, they reduce the number of angina attacks.

Antiangina Drugs

Brand Name (Generic Name)	Possible Common Side Effects Include:
Calan (calan SR, isoptin, isoptin SR, verelan)	Constipation, dizziness, **fatigue**, headache, fluid retention, low blood pressure, nausea
Cardene (nicardipine hydrochloride)	Dizziness, headache, **indigestion**, nausea, rapid heartbeat, sleepiness, swelling of feet, flushing
Cardizem (diltiazem hydrochloride)	Dizziness, fluid retention, headache, nausea, rash
Corgard (nadolol)	Behaviorial changes, dizziness, drowsiness, tiredness
Imdur, Ismo, Monoket (isosorbide mononitrate)	Headache
Isordil (isosorbide dinitrate)	Headache, dizziness, low blood pressure
Lopressor (metroprolol tartrate)	Depression, **diarrhea**, **itching**, rash, tiredness
Nitro-Bid, Nitro-Dur, Nitrolingual Spray, Nitrostat Tables, Transderm-Nitro (nitroglycerin)	Dizziness, flushing, headache
Norvasc (amlodipine besylate)	Dizziness, fatigue, fluid retention, headache, palpitations
Procardia, Procardia XL, Adalat (nifedipine)	Constipation, dizziness, hearburn, low blood pressure, moodiness, nausea, swelling
Tenormin (atenolol)	Dizziness, fatigue, nausea, slowed heartbeat

- taken just before some activity that usually brings on an attack, such as climbing stairs, they prevent attacks.
- taken when an attack begins, they relieve the pain and pressure.

Not every form of antiangina drug can be used in every way. Some work too slowly to prevent attacks that are about to begin or to relieve attacks that have already started. These forms can be used only to reduce the number of attacks. Be sure to understand how and when to use the type of antiangina drug that has been prescribed.

Description

Antiangina drugs, also known as nitrates, come in many different forms: tablets and capsules that are swallowed; tablets that are held under the tongue, inside the lip, or in the cheek until they dissolve; stick-on patches; ointment; and in-the-mouth sprays. Commonly used antiangina drugs include isosorbide dinitrate (Isordil, Sorbitrate, and other brands) and nitroglycerin (Nitro-Bid, Nitro-Dur, Nitrolingual Spray, Nitrostat Tablets, Transderm-Nitro, and other brands). These medicines are available only with a physician's prescription.

Recommended dosage

The recommended dosage depends on the type and form of antiangina drug and may be different for different patients. Check with the physician who prescribed the drug or the pharmacist who filled the prescription for the correct dosage.

Always take antiangina drugs exactly as directed. The medicine will not work if it is not taken correctly.

Do not stop taking this medicine suddenly after taking it for several weeks or more, as this could cause angina attacks to return. If it is necessary to stop taking the drug, check with the physician who prescribed it for instructions on how to taper down gradually.

Precautions

Remember that some forms of antiangina drugs work too slowly to relieve attacks that have already started. Check with the physician who prescribed the medicine for instructions on how to use the type that has been prescribed. Patients who are using slower-acting forms to make attacks less frequent may want to ask their physicians to prescribe a fast-acting type to relieve attacks. Another method of treating the frequency of attacks is to increase the dosage of the long-acting antiangina drug. Do this only with the approval of a physician.

These medicines make some people feel light-headed, dizzy, or faint when they get up after sitting or lying down. To lessen the problem, get up gradually and hold onto something for support if possible. Antiangina drugs may also cause **dizziness**, lightheadedness, or **fainting** in hot weather or when people stand for a long time or **exercise**. Use caution in all these situations. Drinking alcohol while taking antiangina drugs may cause the same problems. Anyone who takes this medicine should limit the amount of alcohol consumed.

Because these drugs may cause dizziness, be careful when driving, using machines, or doing anything else that could be dangerous.

If the person is taking the form of nitroglycerin that is placed under the tongue and symptoms are not relieved within three doses taken about 5 minutes apart, the person should go to the hospital emergency room as soon as possible. A **heart attack** may be in progress.

Some people develop tolerance to antiangina drugs over time. That is, the drug no longer produces the desired effects. Anyone who seems to be developing a tolerance to this medicine should check with his or her physician.

Anyone who has had unusual reactions to antiangina drugs in the past should let his or her physician know before taking the drugs again. The physician should also be told about any **allergies** to foods, dyes, preservatives, or other substances.

Women who are pregnant or breastfeeding or who may become pregnant should check with their physicians before using antiangina drugs.

Older people may be especially sensitive to the effects of antiangina drugs and thus more likely to have side effects such as dizziness and lightheadedness.

Before using antiangina drugs, people with any of these medical problems should make sure their physicians are aware of their conditions:

- recent heart attack or **stroke**
- kidney disease
- liver disease
- severe anemia
- overactive thyroid
- glaucoma
- recent head injury

Side effects

A common side effect is a **headache** just after taking a dose of the medicine. These headaches usually become less noticeable as the body adjusts to the drug. Check with a physician if they are severe or they continue even after taking the medicine for a few weeks. Unless a physician says to do so, do not change the dose to avoid headaches. Other common side effects include dizziness, lightheadedness, fast pulse, flushed face and neck, **nausea** or **vomiting**, and restlessness. These problems do not need medical attention unless they do not go away or they interfere with normal activities.

Other side effects may occur. Anyone who has unusual symptoms after taking an antiangina drug should get in touch with his or her physician.

Interactions

Antiangina drugs may interact with other medicines. This may increase the risk of side effects or change the effects of one or both drugs. Anyone who takes antiangina drugs should let the physician know all other medicines he or she is taking. Among the drugs that may interact with antiangina drugs are:

- other heart medicines

- blood pressure medicines

- aspirin

- alcohol

- ergot alkaloids used in migraine headaches

Nancy Ross-Flanigan

Antiangiogenic therapy

Definition

Antiangiogenesis therapy is one of two types of drugs in a new class of medicines that restores health by controlling blood vessel growth. The other medication is called pro-angiogenic therapy.

Purpose

Antiangiogenic therapy inhibits the growth of new blood vessels. Because new blood vessel growth plays a critical role in many disease conditions, including disorders that cause blindness, arthritis, and **cancer**, angiogenesis inhibition is a "common denominator" approach to treating these diseases. Antiangiogenic drugs exert their beneficial effects in a number of ways: by disabling the agents that activate and promote cell growth, or by directly blocking the growing blood vessel cells. Angiogenesis inhibitory properties have been discovered in more than 300 substances, ranging from molecules produced naturally in animals and plants, such as green tea extract, to new chemicals synthesized in the laboratory. A number of medicines already approved by the U.S. Food and Drug Administration (FDA) have also been found to possess antiangiogenic properties, including *celecoxib* (Celebrex), *bortezomib* (Velcade), and interferon. Many inhibitors are currently being tested in clinical trials for a variety of diseases in human patients, and some in veterinary settings.

These diseases include:

- Eye disease—Excessive new blood vessels growing in the eye can cause vision loss and lead to blindness. Antiangiogenic treatments may prevent progressive loss of vision or even improve eyesight in patients.

- Arthritis—Blood vessels that invade the joint release enzymes that destroy cartilage and other tissues in arthritis. Antiangiogenic drugs may relieve the arthritic **pain** and prevent bone joint destruction caused by these pathological and destructive blood vessels.

- Cancer—Tumors recruit their own private blood supply to obtain oxygen and nourishment for cancer cells. By cutting off tumor vasculature (the arrangement of blood vessels in the body or in a particular organ or tissue), antiangiogenesis therapies may literally starve tumors, and prevent their growth and spread. Antiangiogenesis may also prove to be useful when combined with conventional **chemotherapy** or **radiation therapy**, as part of a "multiple warhead" approach to attack cancer via different strategies simultaneously.

Currently, more than 80 antiangiogenic drugs are being tested worldwide in human clinical trials sponsored by biotechnology and pharmaceutical companies, top medical centers, and the U.S. National Cancer Institute. The Angiogenesis Foundation is leading the application of antiangiogenic therapy in veterinary medicine, for treatment of certain conditions in dogs, cats, and exotic animal species.

Pro-angiogenic therapy works the opposite way as antiangiogenic therapy by using angiogenic growth factors or **gene therapy** to stimulate blood vessel growth in tissues that require an improved blood supply. A number of angiogenic growth factors and gene therapies are currently undergoing clinical trials in human patients suffering from the following conditions: ischemic heart disease, **stroke**, **peripheral vascular disease**, and chronic **wounds**.

Precautions

Since antiangiogenic therapy is still experimental, only people enrolled in a clinical trial of a particular drug therapy can use it. The only FDA-approved drug, *bevacizumab* (Avastin), is prescribed to treat colon-rectal cancer. Avastin can result in intestinal perforation and can cause wounds that have been stitched to break open, sometimes causing **death**. Intestinal perforation, sometimes associated with abscesses inside the abdomen, occurred throughout treatment with Avastin. Symptoms included abdominal pain associated with **constipation** and **vomiting**. Avastin therapy should be permanently discontinued in patients with intestinal perforation or wound breaks requiring medical intervention. Serious, and in some cases fatal, **hemoptysis** (coughing up of blood or mucus containing blood) has occurred in patients with **non-small cell lung cancer** treated with chemotherapy and Avastin.

Description

In the late 1990s, many medical researchers believed that the Holy Grail of cancer treatment had been found. Antiangiogenesis therapy was safe, elegant, and at first apparently effective. But the clinical results soon fell short of expectations. The tumors, it seemed, had found a way to circumvent even this most ingenious of treatment approaches. Despite the setbacks, however, angiogenesis remains a very tempting target, and researchers are exploring new agents and approaches to maximize the effects of antiangiogenic therapies.

Newer studies have demonstrated that in addition to differences in the regulation of new blood vessel formation in cancer compared with normal tissues, the actual blood vessels that are "created" in cancers are different from those created in normal tissues. These differences have allowed a number of antiangiogenic

drugs to be developed that specifically damage tumor-associated blood vessels and not normal vessels. The goal of these drugs is to attack cancers by damaging their blood supply. Many antiangiogenic agents also appear to hasten the death of tumor-associated blood vessels.

With the success of targeted agents such as the biotechnology company Genentech's Avastin, the only antiangiogenic drug approved by the FDA to treat cancer, new efforts are underway to widen and optimize the field of antiangiogenic agents. As oncology (the study of cancer) drug development accelerates, new indications are beginning to emerge for diseases such as ocular neovascularization and even **obesity**.

Antiangiogenic therapy represents a novel, potentially effective, and non-toxic treatment for cancer. It is likely that these drugs will provide the next major breakthrough in the management of people and pets with cancer. Antiangiogenic therapy will likely become part of the conventional treatment of cancer and will be used in combination with surgery, radiation therapy and chemotherapy. These agents are currently in clinical trials and may become available to both people and pets in the near future.

Antiangiogenic therapy offers a number of advantages over traditional therapies for cancer:

- Tumor cells often mutate and become resistant to chemotherapy. Because antiangiogenic drugs only target normal endothelial cells (a layer of cells that lines the inside of certain body cavities, such as blood vessels), these cells are less likely to develop acquired drug resistance.

- All tumors rely upon host vessels. Antiangiogenic agents are therefore effective against a broad range of cancers.

- Conventional chemotherapy and radiotherapy indiscriminately attacks all dividing cells in the body, leading to side effects such as **diarrhea**, mouth ulcers, hair loss, and weakened immunity. Antiangiogenic drugs selectively target dividing blood vessels and cause fewer side effects.

- Antiangiogenic drugs are relatively nontoxic and work at levels well below the maximum tolerated dose, so may be given in lower doses over longer periods of time.

- Antiangiogenic treatment may take weeks or even months to exhibit its full beneficial effect, but this allows for continuous, chronic control of disease.

- Antiangiogenic drugs may also serve as a powerful supplement to traditional chemotherapy or radiation therapy.

Preparation

Since antiangiogenic drugs are either injected or administered orally, little or no preparation is needed. For injections, the site should be first swabbed with alcohol.

Aftercare

Little or no aftercare is needed following the administering of antiangiogenic therapy, except for a small bandage on the injection site.

Although many of these agents are currently being tested in clinical trials, no reliable way to monitor the effects of many, if not most, of these therapeutic agents on the inhibition of the complicated process of angiogenesis exists. However, in late 2004, scientists uncovered critical information that may lead to an urgently needed method for effectively monitoring antiangiogenic cancer therapies. The research is likely to facilitate development of new antiangiogenic drugs or treatment strategies and allow for accurate determination of the optimal drug doses to use for such therapies. The researchers found that measuring peripheral blood cells can be used as a reliable way to monitor antiangiogenic drug activity, which can be used to help establish the optimal biologic dose of such drugs.

Risks

In general, early research has found the side effects of antiangiogenesis agents to be mostly minimal. Because these drugs use proteins that are produced in the human body, there is less likelihood that they will produce the bad side effects common in radiation treatments and chemotherapy. Still, one cancer study found that 6 of the 99 patients taking an antiangiogenesis drug experienced severe bleeding in the tumors being treated. Four of those patients died from this complication.

Since antiangiogenesis drugs could affect a developing fetus, they will probably not be used for pregnant women or women who might become pregnant. They may also need to be stopped before surgery, since blood vessels that are cut at such times need to repair themselves. Also, people who have damaged blood vessels (such as those with heart disease or stroke) may not be able to take these drugs. Other side effects in people are being determined. Doctors, scientists and specialists at the FDA will be monitoring these other side effects to better understand the toxicity and risks of these drugs.

Normal results

Since all antiangiogenic therapies are still experimental and in clinical trials, it is difficult to determine what normal results should be. The goal of antiangiogenic drugs is to stop the development and spread of certain diseases, especially some cancers. At least four major proteins and their receptors and signaling pathways commonly govern angiogenesis in solid tumors: platelet-derived growth factor, epidermal growth factor, vascular endothelial growth factor (VEGF), and fibroblast growth factor (basic and acidic). Therapies that either target these molecules or block their signaling pathways should be effective in preventing solid tumor growth and spread of the cancer by preventing the formation of new blood vessels.

Resources

BOOKS

Cooke, Robert. *Dr. Folkman's War: Angiogenesis and the Struggle to Defeat Cancer* Collingdale, PA: Diane Publishing Co., 2003.

Teicher, Beverly A. *Antiangiogenic Agents in Cancer Therapy* Totowa, NJ: Humana Press, 1999.

PERIODICALS

Frankish, Helen. "Researchers Target Tumour Blood Vessels With Antiangiogenic Gene Therapy." *The Lancet* (June 29, 2002): 2256.

Guttman, Cheryl. "Anti-Angiogenic Therapy Explored for Retinoblastoma." *Ophthalmology Times* (September 1, 2004): 11.

March, Keith. "New Approach for Easing Angina." *Medical Update* (December 2003): 6.

Sullivan. Michele G. "Experimental Antiangiogenic (Therapy) May Battle Drug-Resistant Tumors." *Family Practice News* (February 15, 2003): 42.

ORGANIZATION

The Angiogenesis Foundation. P.O. Box 382111, Cambridge, MA 02139. (617) 576-5708. patienthelp@angio.org. or (for veterinary information) vetmed@angio.org. http://www.angio.org.

Ken R. Wells

Antianxiety drugs

Definition

Antianxiety drugs are medicines that calm and relax people with excessive **anxiety**, nervousness, or tension, or for short-term control of social phobia disorder or specific phobia disorder.

Antianxiety Drugs

Brand Name (Generic Name)	Possible Common Side Effects Include:
Atarax (hydroxyzine hydrochloride)	Drowsiness, dry mouth
Ativan (lorazepam)	Dizziness, excessive calm, weakness
BuSpar, Buspirone (buspirone hydrochloride)	Dry mouth, dizziness, headache, fatigue, **nausea**
Centrax (pazepam)	Decreased coordination, dizziness, drowsiness, fatigue, weakness
Librium, Libritabs (chlordiazepoxide)	**Constipation**, drowsiness, nausea, swelling
Miltown, Equanil (meprobamate)	Diarrhea, bruising, **fever**, headache, nausea, rash, slurred speech
Serax (oxazepam)	Dizziness, **fainting**, headache, liver problems, decreased coordination, nausea, swelling, vertigo
Stelazine (trifluoperazine hydrochloride)	Abnormal glucose in urine, allergic reactions, blurred vision, constipation, eye spasms, fluid retention and swelling
Tranxene, Tranxene-SD (clorazepate dipotassium)	Drowsiness
Valium (diazepam)	Decreased coordination, drowsiness, light-headedness

Purpose

Antianxiety agents, or anxiolytics, may be used to treat mild transient bouts of anxiety as well as more pronounced episodes of social phobia and specific phobia. Clinically significant anxiety is marked by several symptoms. The patient experiences marked or persistent fear of one or more social or performance situations in which he or she is exposed to unfamiliar people or possible scrutiny by others, and may react in a humiliating or embarrassing way. The exposure to the feared situation produces an anxiety attack. Fear of these episodes of anxiety leads to avoidance behavior, which impairs normal social functioning, including working or attending classes. The patient is aware that these fears are unjustified.

Description

In psychiatric practice, treatment of anxiety has largely turned from traditional antianxiety agents, anxiolytics, to antidepressant therapies. In current use, the **benzodiazepines**, the best known class of anxiolytics, have been largely supplanted by **selective serotonin reuptake inhibitors** (SSRIs). Among the preferred SSRIs for **generalized anxiety disorder** are paroxetine (Paxil), escitalopram (Lexapro), and venlafaxine (Effexor), which also has norepinephrine. Other SSRIs are fluoxetine (Prozac) and sertraline (Zoloft).

Venlafaxine and Paroxetine have been shown particularly effective in relieving symptoms of social anxiety.

However, traditional anxiolytics remain useful for patients who need a rapid onset of action, or whose frequency of exposure to anxiety provoking stimuli is low enough to eliminate the need for continued treatment. While SSRIs may require three to five weeks to show any effects, and must be taken continuously, benzodiazepines may produce a response within 30 minutes, and may be dosed on an as-needed basis.

The intermediate action benzodiazepines, alprazolam (Xanax), and lorazepam (Ativan) are the appropriate choice for treatment of mild anxiety and social phobia. Diazepam (Valium) is still widely used for anxiety, but its active metabolite, desmethyldiazepam, which has a long half-life, may make this a poorer choice than other drugs in its class. There is considerable variation between individuals in metabolism of benzodiazepines, so patient response may not be predictable. As a class, benzodiazepines are used not only as anxiolytics, but also as sedatives, **muscle relaxants**, and in treatment of epilepsy and **alcoholism**. The distinctions between these uses are largely determined by onset and duration of action, and route of administration.

Buspirone (BuSpar), which is not chemically related to other classes of central nervous system drugs, is also a traditional anxiolytic, although it is now considered either a third line or adjunctive agent for use after trials of SSRIs and benzodiazepines. It is appropriate for use in patients who have either failed trials of other treatments, or who should not receive benzodiazepines because of a history of **substance abuse** problems. Buspirone, in common with antidepressants, requires a two to three week period before there is clinical evidence of improvement, and must be continuously dosed to maintain its effects.

Benzodiazepines are controlled drugs under federal law. The number of U.S. drug-abuse related trips to emergency departments involving benzodiazepine medications exceeded 100,000 in 2002. Buspirone is not a controlled substance and has no established **abuse** potential.

Recommended dosage

Benzodiazepines should be administered 30 to 60 minutes before exposure to the anticipated **stress**. Dosage should be individualized to minimize **sedation**. The normal dose of alprazolam is 0.25–0.5 mg. The usual dose of lorazepam is 2–3 mg. Doses may be repeated if necessary.

Buspirone is initially dosed at 5 mg three times a day. Patients should increase the dosage 5 mg/day, at intervals of two to three days, as needed and should not exceed 60 mg/day. Two to three weeks may be required before a satisfactory response is seen.

Precautions

Benzodiazepines should not be used in patients with **psychosis**, acute narrow angle **glaucoma**, or **liver disease**. The drugs can act as respiratory depressants and should be avoided in patients with respiratory conditions. Benzodiazepines are potentially addictive and should not be administered to patients with substance abuse disorders. Because benzodiazepines are sedative, they should be avoided in patients who must remain alert. Their use for periods over four months has not been documented. These drugs should not be used during the second and third trimester of **pregnancy**, although use during the first trimester appears to be safe. They should not be taken while breastfeeding. Physicians and pharmacists should be consulted about use in children.

Buspirone is metabolized by the liver and excreted by the kidney, and should be used with care in patients with hepatic or renal disease. The drug is classified as schedule B during pregnancy, but should not be taken during breastfeeding. Its use in children under the age of 18 years has not been studied.

In 2004, the FDA cautioned revealed that certain SSRIs could lead to increased risk of **suicide** in children and adolescents who took them for depression. Parents should check with physicians to receive more information on SSRIs when they are prescribed for teens and children with anxiety.

Side effects

The most common side effects of benzodiazepines are secondary to their CNS effects and include sedation and sleepiness; depression; lethargy; apathy; **fatigue**; hypoactivity; lightheadedness; memory impairment; disorientation; anterograde **amnesia**; restlessness; confusion; crying or sobbing; **delirium**; **headache**; slurred speech; aphonia; dysarthria; stupor; seizures; **coma**; syncope; rigidity; tremor; dystonia; vertigo; **dizziness**; euphoria; nervousness; irritability; difficulty in concentration; agitation; inability to perform complex mental functions; akathisia; hemiparesis; hypotonia; unsteadiness; ataxia; incoordination; weakness; vivid dreams; psychomotor retardation; "glassy-eyed" appearance; extrapyramidal symptoms; paradoxical reactions. Other reactions include changes in heart rate and blood pressure, changes in bowel function, severe skin rash and changes in genitourinary function. Other adverse effects have been reported.

Buspirone has a low incidence of side effects. Dizziness and drowsiness are the most commonly reported adverse effects. Other CNS effects include dream disturbances; depersonalization, dysphoria, noise intolerance, euphoria, akathisia, fearfulness, loss of interest, disassociative reaction, **hallucinations**, suicidal ideation, seizures; feelings of claustrophobia, cold intolerance, stupor and slurred speech, psychosis. Rarely, heart problems, including congestive **heart failure** and myocardial infarction, have been reported. Other adverse effects have been reported.

Interactions

The metabolism of alprazolam may be increased by: cimetidine, **oral contraceptives**, disulfiram, fluoxetine, isoniazid, ketoconazole, metoprolol, propoxyphene, propranolol and valproic acid. The absorption of all benzodiazepines is inhibited by concomitant use of **antacids**. Benzodiazepines may increase blood levels of digoxin, and reduce the efficacy of levodopa. Other **drug interactions** have been reported.

Buspirone levels will be increased by concomitant use of erythromycin, itraconazole, and nefazadone. Doses should be adjusted based on clinical response. Use of buspirone at the same time as mono-amine oxidase inhibitors (MAOIs, phenelzine, tranycypromine) may cause severe blood pressure elevations. Use of buspirone with MAOIs should be avoided.

Resources

PERIODICALS

"Abuse of Anti-anxiety Drugs Up, Study of ER Visits Shows." *Drug Week* (September 17, 2004): 225.

Finn, Robert. "Venlafaxine and Paroxetine Both Relieve Social Anxiety." *Clinical Psychiatry News* (September 2004): 41.

Sherman, Carl. "GAD Patients Often Require Combined Therapy." *Clinical Psychiatry News* (August 2004): 12–14.

Samuel D. Uretsky, PharmD
Teresa G. Odle

Antiarrhythmic drugs

Definition

Antiarrhythmic drugs are medicines that correct irregular heartbeats and slow down hearts that beat too fast.

Purpose

Normally, the heart beats at a steady, even pace. The pace is controlled by electrical signals that begin in one part of the heart and quickly spread through the whole heart. If something goes wrong with this control system, the result may be an irregular heartbeat, or an arrhythmia. Antiarrhythmic drugs correct irregular heartbeats, restoring the normal rhythm. If the heart is beating too fast, these drugs will slow it down. By correcting these problems, antiarrhythmic drugs help the heart work more efficiently.

Description

Antiarrhythmic drugs are available only with a physician's prescription and are sold in capsule (regular and extended release), tablet (regular and extended-release), and injectable forms. Commonly used antiarrhythmic drugs are disopyramide (Norpace, Norpace CR), procainamide (Procan SR, Pronestyl, Pronestyl-SR), and quinidine (Cardioquin, Duraquin, Quinidex, and other brands). *Do not confuse quinidine with quinine, which is a related medicine with different uses, such as relieving leg cramps.*

Recommended dosage

The recommended dosage depends on the type of antiarrhythmic drug and other factors. Doses may be different for different patients. Check with the physician who prescribed the drug or the pharmacist who filled the prescription for the correct dosage.

Always take antiarrhythmic drugs exactly as directed. Never take larger or more frequent doses.

Do not stop taking this medicine without checking with the physician who prescribed it. Stopping it suddenly could lead to a serious change in heart function.

Antiarrhythmic drugs work best when they are at constant levels in the blood. To help keep levels constant, take the medicine in doses spaced evenly through the day and night. Do not miss any doses. If taking medicine at night interferes with sleep, or if it is difficult to remember to take the medicine during the day, check with a health care professional for suggestions.

Precautions

Persons who take these drugs should see their physician regularly. The physician will check to make sure the medicine is working as it should and will note any unwanted side effects.

Some people feel dizzy, lightheaded, or faint when using these drugs. This medicine may cause blurred vision or other vision problems. Because of these possible problems, anyone who takes these drugs should not drive, use machines or do anything else that might be dangerous until they have found out how the drugs affect them. If the medicine does cause vision problems, wait until vision is clear before driving or engaging in other activities that require normal vision.

Antiarrhythmic drugs make some people feel lightheaded, dizzy, or faint when they get up after sitting or lying down. To lessen the problem, get up gradually and hold onto something for support if possible.

Anyone taking this medicine should not drink alcohol without his or her physician's approval.

Some antiarrhythmic drugs may change the results of certain medical tests. Before having medical tests, anyone taking this medicine should alert the health care professional in charge.

Anyone who is taking antiarrhythmic drugs should be sure to tell the health care professional in charge before having any surgical or dental procedures or receiving emergency treatment.

Antiarrhythmic drugs may cause low blood sugar in some people. Anyone who experiences symptoms of low blood sugar should eat or drink a food that

KEY TERMS

Anxiety—Worry or tension in response to real or imagined stress, danger, or dreaded situations. Physical reactions, such as fast pulse, sweating, trembling, fatigue, and weakness may accompany anxiety.

Arrhythmia—Abnormal heart rhythm.

Asthma—A disease in which the air passages of the lungs become inflamed and narrowed.

Emphysema—A lung disease in which breathing becomes difficult.

Glaucoma—A condition in which pressure in the eye is abnormally high. If not treated, glaucoma may lead to blindness.

Hallucination—A false or distorted perception of objects, sounds, or events that seems real. Hallucinations usually result from drugs or mental disorders.

Heat stroke—A severe condition caused by prolonged exposure to high heat. Heat stroke interferes with the body's temperature regulating abilities and can lead to collapse and coma.

Inflammation—Pain, redness, swelling, and heat that usually develop in response to injury or illness.

Myasthenia gravis—A chronic disease with symptoms that include muscle weakness and sometimes paralysis.

Palpitation—Rapid, forceful, throbbing, or fluttering heartbeat.

Prostate—A donut-shaped gland below the bladder in men that contributes to the production of semen.

Psoriasis—A skin disease in which people have itchy, scaly, red patches on the skin.

Systemic lupus erythematosus (SLE)—A chronic disease that affects the skin, joints, and certain internal organs.

Tourette syndrome—A condition in which a person has tics and other involuntary behavior, such as barking, sniffing, swearing, grunting, and making uncontrollable movements.

Tremor—Shakiness or trembling.

contains sugar and call a physician immediately. Signs of low blood sugar are:

- anxiety
- confusion
- nervousness

- shakiness
- unsteady walk
- extreme hunger
- headache
- nausea
- drowsiness
- unusual tiredness or weakness
- fast heartbeat
- pale, cool skin
- chills
- cold sweats

Antiarrhythmic drugs may cause **dry mouth**. To temporarily relieve the discomfort, chew sugarless gum, suck on sugarless candy or ice chips, or use saliva substitutes, which come in liquid and tablet forms and are available without a prescription. If the problem continues for more than 2 weeks, check with a physician or dentist. Mouth dryness that continues over a long time may contribute to **tooth decay** and other dental problems.

People taking antiarrhythmic drugs may sweat less, which can cause the body temperature to rise. Anyone who takes this medicine should be careful not to become overheated during **exercise** or hot weather and should avoid hot baths, hot tubs, and saunas. Overheating could lead to heat **stroke**.

Older people may be especially sensitive to the effects of antiarrhythmic drugs. This may increase the risk of certain side effects, such as dry mouth, difficult urination, and **dizziness** or lightheadedness.

The antiarrhythmic drug procainamide can cause serious blood disorders. Anyone taking this medicine should have regular blood counts and should check with a physician if any of the following symptoms occur:

- joint or muscle **pain**
- muscle weakness
- pain in the chest or abdomen
- tremors
- wheezing
- cough
- palpitations
- rash, sores, or pain in the mouth
- sore throat
- fever and chills
- loss of appetite
- **diarrhea**

- dark urine
- yellow skin or eyes
- unusual bleeding or bruising
- dizziness
- **hallucinations**
- depression

Special conditions

People with certain medical conditions or who are taking certain other medicines may have problems if they take antiarrhythmic drugs. Before taking these drugs, be sure to let the physician know about any of these conditions:

ALLERGIES. Anyone who has had unusual reactions to an antiarrhythmic drug in the past should let his or her physician know before taking this type of medicine again. Patients taking procainamide should let their physicians know if they have ever had an unusual or allergic reaction to procaine or any other "caine-type" medicine, such as xylocaine or lidocaine. Patients taking quinidine should mention any previous reactions to quinine. The physician should also be told about any **allergies** to foods, dyes, preservatives, or other substances.

CONGESTIVE HEART DISEASE. Antiarrhythmic drugs may cause low blood sugar, which can be a particular problem for people with congestive heart disease. Anyone with congestive heart disease should be familiar with the signs of low blood sugar (listed above) and should check with his or her physician about what to do if such symptoms occur.

DIABETES. Antiarrhythmic drugs may cause low blood sugar, which can be a particular problem for people with diabetes. Anyone with diabetes should be familiar with the signs of low blood sugar (listed above) and should check with his or her physician about what to do if such symptoms occur.

PREGNANCY. The effects of taking antiarrhythmic drugs in **pregnancy** have not been studied in humans. In studies of laboratory animals, this medicine increased the risk of **miscarriage**. In addition, some women who have taken these drugs while pregnant have had contractions of the uterus (womb). Women who are pregnant or who may become pregnant should check with their physicians before taking this medicine. Women who become pregnant while taking this medicine should let their physicians know right away.

BREASTFEEDING. Antiarrhythmic drugs pass into breast milk. Women who are breastfeeding should check with their physicians before taking this medicine.

OTHER MEDICAL CONDITIONS. Before using antiarrhythmic drugs, people with any of these medical problems should make sure their physicians are aware of their conditions:

- heart disorders such as structural heart disease or inflammation of the heart muscle
- congestive **heart failure**
- kidney disease
- liver disease
- diseases of the blood
- asthma or **emphysema**
- enlarged prostate or difficulty urinating
- overactive thyroid
- low blood sugar
- psoriasis
- **glaucoma**
- myasthenia gravis
- systemic lupus erythematosus

USE OF CERTAIN MEDICINES. Taking antiarrhythmic drugs with certain other drugs may affect the way the drugs work or may increase the chance of side effects.

Side effects

The most common side effects are dry mouth and throat, diarrhea, and loss of appetite. These problems usually go away as the body adjusts to the drug and do not require medical treatment. Less common side effects, such as dizziness, lightheadedness, blurred vision, dry eyes and nose, frequent urge to urinate, bloating, **constipation**, stomach pain, and decreased sexual ability, also may occur and do not need medical attention unless they do not go away or they interfere with normal activities.

More serious side effects are not common, but may occur. If any of the following side effects occur, check with the physician who prescribed the medicine as soon as possible:

- fever and chills
- difficult urination
- swollen or painful joints
- pain when breathing
- skin rash or itching

People who are especially sensitive to quinidine may have a reaction to the first dose or doses. If any of these side effects occur after taking quinidine, check with a physician immediately:

- dizziness
- ringing in the ears
- breathing problems
- vision changes
- fever
- headache
- skin rash

Other rare side effects may occur with any anti-arrhythmic drug. Anyone who has unusual symptoms after taking antiarrhythmic drugs should get in touch with his or her physician.

Interactions

Antiarrhythmic drugs may interact with other medicines. When this happens, the effects of one or both of the drugs may change or the risk of side effects may be greater. Anyone who takes antiarrhythmic drugs should let the physician know all other medicines he or she is taking. Among the drugs that may interact with antiarrhythmic drugs are:

- other heart medicines, including other antiarrhythmic drugs
- blood pressure medicine
- blood thinners
- pimozide (Orap), used to treat Tourette's syndrome

The list above does not include every drug that may interact with antiarrhythmic drugs. Be sure to check with a physician or pharmacist before combining antiarrhythmic drugs with any other prescription or nonprescription (over-the-counter) medicine.

Nancy Ross-Flanigan

Antiasthmatic drugs

Definition

Antiasthmatic drugs are medicines that treat or prevent **asthma** attacks.

Purpose

For people with asthma, the simple act of breathing can be a struggle. Their airways become inflamed and blocked with mucus during asthma attacks, narrowing the opening through which air passes. This is not such a problem when the person breathes in,

---

KEY TERMS

Asthma—A disease in which the air passages of the lungs become inflamed and narrowed.

Inflammation—Pain, redness, swelling, and heat that usually develop in response to injury or illness.

Inhalant—Medicine that is breathed into the lungs.

Mucus—Thick fluid produced by the moist membranes that line many body cavities and structures.

Nebulizer—A device that turns liquid forms of medicine into a fine spray that can be inhaled.

---

because the airways naturally expand when a person takes a breath. The real problem arises when the person with asthma tries to breathe out. The air cannot get out through the blocked airways, so it stays trapped in the lungs. With each new breath, the person can take in only a little more air, so breathing becomes shallow and takes more and more effort.

Asthma attacks can be caused by **allergies** to pollen, dust, pets or other things, but people without known allergies may also have asthma. **Exercise**, **stress**, intense emotions, exposure to cold, certain medicines and some medical conditions also can bring on attacks.

The two main approaches to dealing with asthma are avoiding substances and situations that trigger attacks and using medicines that treat or prevent the symptoms. With a combination of the two, most people with asthma can find relief and live normal lives.

Description

Three types of drugs are used in treating and preventing asthma attacks:

- **Bronchodilators** relax the smooth muscles that line the airway. This makes the airways open wider, letting more air pass through them. These drugs are used mainly to relieve sudden asthma attacks or to prevent attacks that might come on after exercise. They may be taken by mouth, injected or inhaled. Bronchodilators may be taken in pill or liquid form, but normally are used as inhalers, which go directly to the lungs and result in fewer side effects.

- **Corticosteroids** block the inflammation that narrows the airways. Used regularly, these drugs will help prevent asthma attacks. Those attacks that do occur will be less severe. However, corticosteroids cannot stop an attack that is already underway. These drugs may be taken by mouth, injected or inhaled.

- Leukotriene modifiers (montelukast and zafirlukast) are a new type of drug that can be used in place of steroids, for older children or adults who have a mild degree of asthma that persists. They work by counteracting leukotrienes, which are substances released by white blood cells in the lung that cause the air passages to constrict and promote mucus secretion. Leukotriene modifiers also fight off some forms of **rhinitis**, an added bonus for people with asthma. However, they are not proven effective in fighting seasonal allergies.

- Cromolyn also is taken regularly to prevent asthma attacks and may be used alone or with other asthma medicines. It cannot stop an attack that already has started. The drug works by preventing certain cells in the body from releasing substances that cause allergic reactions or asthma symptoms. One brand of this drug, Nasalcrom, comes in capsule and nasal spray forms and is used to treat hay **fever** and other allergies. The inhalation form of the drug, Intal, is used for asthma. It comes in aerosol canisters, in capsules that are inserted into an inhaler, and in liquid form that is used in a nebulizer.

Precautions

Using antiasthmatic drugs properly is important. Because bronchodilators provide quick relief, some people may be tempted to overuse them. However, with some kinds of bronchodilators, this can lead to serious and possibly life-threatening complications. In the long run, patients are better off using bronchodilators only as directed and also using corticosteroids, which eventually will reduce their need for bronchodilators. However, a 2004 Canadian study has questioned a standard practice of increasing steroids after asthma attacks or worsened symptoms. Also, research in 2004 showed that people with asthma who worked closely with their physicians to self-manage their asthma had fewer attacks, which reduces the need for bronchodilators. Carefully managing asthma also reduces visits to the emergency department and hospitalizations.

Corticosteroids are powerful drugs that may cause serious side effects when used over a long time. However, these problems are much less likely with the inhalant forms than with the oral and injected forms. While the oral and injected forms generally should be used only for one to two weeks, the inhalant forms may be used for long periods.

It is important to remember that leukotriene modifiers are used to prevent and manage asthma, not to stop an attack. A physician or pharmacist can advise patients on possible interactions with other drugs.

Patients who are using their antiasthmatic drugs correctly but feel their asthma is not under control should see their physicians. The physician can either increase the dose, switch to another medicine or add another medicine to the regimen. A 2004 survey showed that 70% of people with mild to moderate asthma were not taking the correct dose of asthma medication.

When used to prevent asthma attacks, cromolyn must be taken as directed every day. The drug may take as long as four weeks to start working. Unless told to do so by a physician, patients should not stop taking the drug just because it does not seem to be working. When symptoms do begin to improve, patients should continue taking all medicines that have been prescribed, unless a physician directs otherwise.

Side effects

Inhalant forms of antiasthmatic drugs may cause dryness or irritation in the throat, **dry mouth**, or an unpleasant taste in the mouth. To help prevent these problems, gargling and rinsing the mouth or taking a sip of water after each dose is recommended.

More serious side effects are not common when these medicines are used properly. However, anyone who has unusual or bothersome symptoms after taking an antiasthmatic drug should get in touch with a physician.

Interactions

A physician or pharmacist should be consulted before combining antiasthmatic drugs with any other prescription or nonprescription (over-the-counter) medicine.

Resources

PERIODICALS

"Many People With Asthma Arenót Taking the Right Amount of Medication." *Obesity, Fitness & Wellness Week* (September 25, 2004): 87.

"Study Calls Standard Asthma Management Into Doubt." *Doctor* (July 15, 2004): 4.

"What's New in: Asthma and Allergic Rhinitis." *Pulse* (September 20, 2004): 50.

Nancy Ross-Flanigan
Teresa G. Odle

Antibacterial bath *see* **Therapeutic baths**

Antibiotic-associated colitis

Definition

Antibiotic-associated colitis is an inflammation of the intestines that sometimes occurs following antibiotic treatment and is caused by toxins produced by the bacterium *Clostridium difficile*.

Description

Antibiotic-associated colitis, also called antibiotic-associated enterocolitis, can occur following antibiotic treatment. The bacteria *Clostridia difficile* are normally found in the intestines of 5% of healthy adults, but people can also pick up the bacteria while they are in a hospital or nursing home. In a healthy person, harmless resident intestinal bacteria compete with each other for food and places to "sit" along the inner intestinal wall. When **antibiotics** are given, most of the resident bacteria are killed. With fewer bacteria to compete with, the normally harmless *Clostridia difficile* grow rapidly and produce toxins. These toxins damage the inner wall of the intestines and cause inflammation and **diarrhea**.

Although all antibiotics can cause this disease, it is most commonly caused by clindamycin (Cleocin), ampicillin (Omnipen), amoxicillin (Amoxil, Augmentin, or Wymox), and any in the cephalosporin class (such as cefazolin or cephalexin). Symptoms of the condition can occur during antibiotic treatment or within four weeks after the treatment has stopped.

In approximately half of cases of antibiotic-associated colitis, the condition progresses to a more severe form of colitis called pseudomembranous enterocolitis in which pseudomembranes are excreted in the stools. Pseudomembranes are membrane-like collections of white blood cells, mucus, and the protein that causes blood to clot (fibrin) that are released by the damaged intestinal wall.

Causes and symptoms

Antibiotic-associated colitis is caused by toxins produced by the bacterium *Clostridium difficile* after treatment with antibiotics. When most of the other intestinal bacteria have been killed, *Clostridium difficile* grows rapidly and releases toxins that damage the intestinal wall. The disease and symptoms are caused by these toxins, not by the bacterium itself.

Symptoms of antibiotic-associated colitis usually begin four to ten days after antibiotic treatment has begun. The early signs and symptoms of this disease include lower abdominal cramps, an increased need to

pass stool, and watery diarrhea. As the disease progresses, the patient may experience a general ill feeling, **fatigue**, abdominal **pain**, and **fever**. If the disease proceeds to pseudomembranous enterocolitis, the patient may also experience **nausea**, **vomiting**, large amounts of watery diarrhea, and a very high fever (104-105 °F/ 40-40.5 °C). Complications of antibiotic-associated colitis include severe **dehydration**, imbalances in blood **minerals**, low blood pressure, fluid accumulation in deep skin (**edema**), enlargement of the large intestine (toxic megacolon), and the formation of a tear (perforation) in the wall of the large intestine.

The *Clostridium difficile* toxin is found in the stools of persons older than 60 years of age 20-100 times more frequently than in the stools of persons who are 10-20 years old. As a result, the elderly are much more prone to developing antibiotic-associated colitis than younger individuals.

Diagnosis

Antibiotic-associated colitis can be diagnosed by the symptoms and recent medical history of the patient, by a laboratory test for the bacterial toxin, and/or by using a procedure called endoscopy.

If the diarrhea and related symptoms occurred after the patient received antibiotics, antibiotic-associated colitis may be suspected. A stool sample may be analyzed for the presence of the *Clostridium difficile* toxin. This toxin test is the preferred diagnostic test for antibiotic-associated colitis. One frequently used test for the toxin involves adding the processed stool sample to a human cell culture. If the toxin is present in the stool sample, the cells die. It may take up to two days to get the results from this test. A simpler test, which provides results in two to three hours, is also available. Symptoms and toxin test results are usually enough to diagnose the disease.

Another tool that may be useful in the diagnosis of antibiotic-associated colitis, however, is a procedure called an endoscopy that involves inserting a thin, lighted tube into the rectum to visually inspect the intestinal lining. Two different types of endoscopy procedures, the **sigmoidoscopy** and the **colonoscopy**, are used to view different parts of the large intestine. These procedures are performed in a hospital or doctor's office. Patients are sedated during the procedure to make them more comfortable and are allowed to go home after recovering from the **sedation**.

Treatment

Diarrhea, regardless of the cause, is always treated by encouraging the individual to replace lost fluids and prevent dehydration. One method to treat antibiotic-associated colitis is to simply stop taking the antibiotic that caused the disease. This allows the normal intestinal bacteria to repopulate the intestines and inhibits the overgrowth of *Clostridium difficile*. Many patients with mild disease respond well to this and are free from diarrhea within two weeks. It is important, however, to make sure that the original disease for which the antibiotics were prescribed is treated.

Because of the potential seriousness of this disease, most patients are given another antibiotic to control the growth of the *Clostridium difficile*, usually vancomycin (Vancocin) or metronidazole (Flagyl or Protostat). Both are designed to be taken orally four times a day for 10-14 days. Upon finishing antibiotic treatment, approximately 15-20% of patients will experience a relapse of diarrhea within one to five weeks. Mild relapses can go untreated with great success, however, severe relapses of diarrhea require another round of antibiotic treatment. Instead of further antibiotic treatment, a cholestyramine resin (Questran or Prevalite) may be given. The bacterial toxins produced in the intestine stick to the resin and are passed out with the resin in the stool. Unfortunately, however, vancomycin also sticks to the resin, so these two drugs cannot be taken at the same time. Serious disease may require hospitalization so that the patient can be monitored, treated, and rehydrated.

Alternative treatment

The goal of alternative treatment for antibiotic-associated enterocolitis is to repopulate the intestinal environment with microorganisms that are normal and healthy for the intestinal tract. These microorganisms then compete for space and keep the *Clostridium difficile* from over-populating.

Several types of supplements can be used. Supplements containing *Lactobacillus acidophilus*, the bacteria commonly found in yogurt and some types of milk, *Lactobacillus bifidus*, and *Streptococcus faecium*, are available in many stores in powder, capsule, tablet, and liquid form. *Acidophilus* also acts as a mild antibiotic, which helps it to reestablish itself in the intestine, and all may aid in the production of some B **vitamins** and vitamin K. These supplements can be taken individually and alternated weekly or together following one or more courses of antibiotics.

Prognosis

With appropriate treatment and replenishment of fluids, the prognosis is generally excellent. One or more relapses can occur. Very severe colitis can cause a tear (perforation) in the wall of the large intestine that would require major surgery. Perforation of the intestine can cause a serious abdominal infection. Antibiotic-associated colitis can be fatal in people who are elderly and/or have a serious underlying illness, such as **cancer**.

Prevention

There are no specific preventative measures for this disease. Good general health can reduce the chance of developing a bacterial infection that would require antibiotic treatment and the chance of picking up the *Clostridia* bacteria. Maintaining good general health can also reduce the seriousness and length of the condition, should it develop following antibiotic therapy.

Resources

OTHER

Mayo Clinic Online. March 5, 1998. < http:// www.mayohealth.org > .

Belinda Rowland, PhD

Antibiotic prophylaxis *see* **Prophylaxis**

Antibiotics

Definition

Antibiotics may be informally defined as the subgroup of anti-infectives that are derived from bacterial sources and are used to treat bacterial infections. Other classes of drugs, most notably the **sulfonamides**,

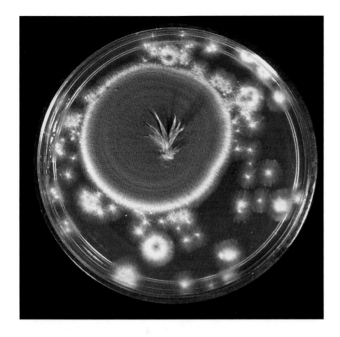

A penicillin culture. *(Photograph by P. Barber, Custom Medical Stock Photo. Reproduced by permission.)*

may be effective antibacterials. Similarly, some antibiotics may have secondary uses, such as the use of demeclocycline (Declomycin, a tetracycline derivative) to treat the syndrome of inappropriate antidiuretic hormone (SIADH) secretion. Other antibiotics may be useful in treating protozoal infections.

Purpose

Antibiotics are used for treatment or prevention of bacterial infection.

Description

Classifications

Although there are several classification schemes for antibiotics, based on bacterial spectrum (broad versus narrow) or route of administration (injectable versus oral versus topical), or type of activity (bactericidal vs. bacteriostatic), the most useful is based on chemical structure. Antibiotics within a structural class will generally show similar patterns of effectiveness, toxicity, and allergic potential.

PENICILLINS. The **penicillins** are the oldest class of antibiotics, and have a common chemical structure which they share with the cephalopsorins. The two groups are classed as the beta-lactam antibiotics, and are generally bacteriocidal—that is, they kill bacteria rather than inhibiting growth. The penicillins can be

further subdivided. The natural pencillins are based on the original penicillin G structure; penicillinase-resistant penicillins, notably methicillin and oxacillin, are active even in the presence of the bacterial enzyme that inactivates most natural penicillins. Aminopenicillins such as ampicillin and amoxicillin have an extended spectrum of action compared with the natural penicillins; extended spectrum penicillins are effective against a wider range of bacteria. These generally include coverage for *Pseudomonas aeruginaosa* and may provide the penicillin in combination with a penicillinase inhibitor.

CEPHALOSPORINS. Cephalosporins and the closely related cephamycins and carbapenems, like the pencillins, contain a beta-lactam chemical structure. Consequently, there are patterns of cross-resistance and cross-allergenicity among the drugs in these classes. The "cepha" drugs are among the most diverse classes of antibiotics, and are themselves subgrouped into 1st, 2nd and 3rd generations. Each generation has a broader spectrum of activity than the one before. In addition, cefoxitin, a cephamycin, is highly active against anaerobic bacteria, which offers utility in treatment of abdominal infections. The 3rd generation drugs, cefotaxime, ceftizoxime, ceftriaxone and others, cross the blood-brain barrier and may be used to treat **meningitis** and **encephalitis**. Cephalopsorins are the usually preferred agents for surgical **prophylaxis**.

FLUROQUINOLONES. The fluroquinolones are synthetic antibacterial agents, and not derived from bacteria. They are included here because they can be readily interchanged with traditional antibiotics. An earlier, related class of antibacterial agents, the quinolones, were not well absorbed, and could be used only to treat urinary tract infections. The fluroquinolones, which are based on the older group, are broad-spectrum bacteriocidal drugs that are chemically unrelated to the penicillins or the cephaloprosins. They are well distributed into bone tissue, and so well absorbed that in general they are as effective by the oral route as by intravenous infusion.

TETRACYCLINES. Tetracyclines got their name because they share a chemical structure that has four rings. They are derived from a species of *Streptomyces* bacteria. Broad-spectrum bacteriostatic agents, the tetracyclines may be effective against a wide variety of microorganisms, including rickettsia and amoebic parasites.

MACROLIDES. The macrolide antibiotics are derived from *Streptomyces* bacteria, and got their name because they all have a macrocyclic lactone chemical structure. Erythromycin, the prototype of this class, has a spectrum and use similar to penicillin. Newer members of the group, azithromycin and clarithyromycin, are particularly useful for their high

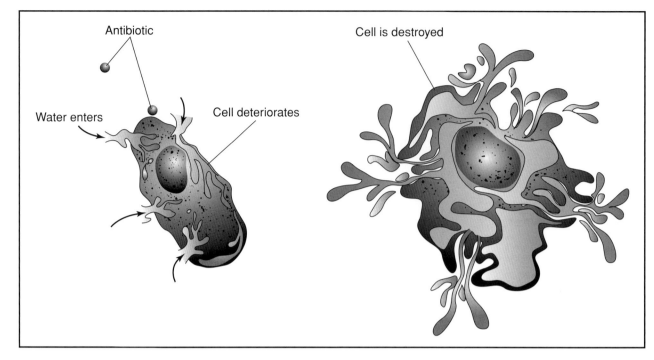

Different antibiotics destroy bacteria in different ways. Some short-circuit the processes by which bacteria receive energy. Others disturb the structure of the bacterial cell wall, as shown in the illustration above. Still others interfere with the production of essential proteins. *(Illustration by Electronic Illustrators Group.)*

KEY TERMS

Bacteria—Tiny, one-celled forms of life that cause many diseases and infections.

Inflammation—Pain, redness, swelling, and heat that usually develop in response to injury or illness.

Meningitis—Inflammation of tissues that surround the brain and spinal cord.

Microorganism—An organism that is too small to be seen with the naked eye.

Organism—A single, independent unit of life, such as a bacterium, a plant or an animal.

Pregnancy category—A system of classifying drugs according to their established risks for use during pregnancy. Category A: Controlled human studies have demonstrated no fetal risk. Category B: Animal studies indicate no fetal risk, but no human studies; or adverse effects in animals, but not in well-controlled human studies. Category C: No adequate human or animal studies; or adverse fetal effects in animal studies, but no available human data. Category D: Evidence of fetal risk, but benefits outweigh risks. Category X: Evidence of fetal risk. Risks outweigh any benefits.

---

level of lung penetration. Clarithromycin has been widely used to treat *Helicobacter pylori* infections, the cause of stomach ulcers.

OTHERS. Other classes of antibiotics include the **aminoglycosides**, which are particularly useful for their effectiveness in treating *Pseudomonas aeruginosa* infections; the lincosamindes, clindamycin and lincomycin, which are highly active against anaerobic pathogens. There are other, individual drugs which may have utility in specific infections.

Recommended dosage

Dosage varies with drug, route of administration, pathogen, site of infection, and severity. Additional considerations include renal function, age of patient, and other factors. Consult manufacturers' recommendations for dose and route.

Side effects

All antibiotics cause risk of overgrowth by non-susceptible bacteria. Manufacturers list other major hazards by class; however, the health care provider should review each drug individually to assess the degree of risk. Generally, breastfeeding is not recommended while taking antibiotics because of risk of alteration to infant's intestinal flora, and risk of masking infection in the infant. Excessive or inappropriate use may promote growth of resistant pathogens.

Penicillins: Hypersensitivity may be common, and cross allergenicity with cephalosporins has been reported. Penicillins are classed as category B during **pregnancy**.

Cephalopsorins: Several cephalopsorins and related compounds have been associated with seizures. Cefmetazole, cefoperazone, cefotetan and ceftriaxone may be associated with a fall in prothrombin activity and coagulation abnormalities. Pseudomembranous colitis has been reported with cephalosporins and other broad spectrum antibiotics. Some drugs in this class may cause renal toxicity. Pregnancy category B.

Fluroquinolones: Lomefloxacin has been associated with increased **photosensitivity**. All drugs in this class have been associated with convulsions. Pregnancy category C.

Tetracyclines: Demeclocycline may cause increased photosensitivity. Minocycline may cause **dizziness**. Do not use tetracyclines in children under the age of eight, and specifically avoid during periods of tooth development. Oral tetracyclines bind to anions such as calcium and iron. Although doxycycline and minocycline may be taken with meals, patients must be advised to take other tetracycline antibiotics on an empty stomach, and not to take the drugs with milk or other calcium-rich foods. Expired tetracycline should never be administered. Pregnancy category D. Use during pregnancy may cause alterations in bone development.

Macrolides: Erythromycin may aggravate the weakness of patients with **myasthenia gravis**. Azithromycin has, rarely, been associated with allergic reactions, including angioedema, **anaphylaxis**, and dermatologic reactions, including Stevens-Johnson syndrome and **toxic epidermal necrolysis**. Oral erythromycin may be highly irritating to the stomach and when given by injection may cause severe phlebitis. These drugs should be used with caution in patients with liver dysfunction. Pregnancy category B: Azithromycin, erythromycin. Pregnancy category C: Clarithromycin, dirithromycin, troleandomycin.

Aminoglycosides: This class of drugs causes kidney and **ototoxicity**. These problems can occur even with normal doses. Dosing should be based on renal function, with periodic testing of both kidney function and hearing. Pregnancy category D.

Recommended usage

To minimize risk of adverse reactions and development of resistant strains of bacteria, antibiotics should be restricted to use in cases where there is either known or a reasonable presumption of bacterial infection. The use of antibiotics in viral infections is to be avoided. Avoid use of fluroquinolones for trivial infections.

In severe infections, presumptive therapy with a broad-spectrum antibiotic such as a 3rd generation cephalosporin may be appropriate. Treatment should be changed to a narrow spectrum agent as soon as the pathogen has been identified. After 48 hours of treatment, if there is clinical improvement, an oral antibiotic should be considered.

Resources

PERIODICALS

"Consumer Alert: Antibiotic Resistance Is Growing!" *People's Medical Society Newsletter* 16 (August 1997): 1.

Samuel D. Uretsky, PharmD

Antibiotics, ophthalmic

Definition

Ophthalmic **antibiotics** are medicines that kill bacteria that cause eye infections.

Purpose

Ophthalmic antibiotics are applied to the eye, or under the eyelid, to treat eye infections caused by bacteria.

Description

The medicine described here, tobramycin (Tobrex), comes in the form of eye drops or ointment. It is available only with a physician's prescription.

Recommended dosage

The dosages given here are typical doses. Physicians may adjust the number of doses per day, the time between doses, and the length of treatment with the medicine, depending on the patient's particular medical problem. If the physician's directions are different from those given here, follow the physician's directions.

Adults

EYE DROPS. For mild to moderate infections, use one to two drops in the affected eye or eyes every four hours.

For severe infections, use two drops in the affected eye or eyes every two hours until the condition improves.

At that time, the physician will determine how much to use until the infection is completely cleared up.

OINTMENT. For mild to moderate infections, squeeze a half-inch ribbon of ointment into the affected eye or eyes two or three times a day. Do not let the tip of the ointment tube touch the eye.

For severe infections, squeeze a half-inch ribbon of ointment into the affected eye or eyes every three to four hours until the condition improves. At that time, the physician will determine how much to use until the infection is completely cleared up.

Children

The child's physician should determine the proper dose.

Precautions

Use this drug as often as directed, for as long as directed. Although the symptoms may have disappeared, the infection may not clear up completely if the drug is stopped too soon. Therefore, the medication may be prescribed for several days after the infection appears to have cleared. However, it is just as important to use the drug for *only* as long as directed. Using it for too long may lead to the growth of bacteria that do not respond to the drug. These bacteria may then cause infections that can be very difficult to treat. Make sure the physician or pharmacist specifies how long the medication is to be used.

Anyone who has had an allergic reaction to tobramycin or any other ingredients of Tobrex should not use this medicine. Be sure to tell the physician about any past reactions to the drug or its ingredients.

Anyone who has an allergic reaction to tobramycin should stop using it immediately and call a physician.

Women who are pregnant or breastfeeding or who plan to become pregnant should check with their physicians before using tobramycin.

Side effects

The main side effects of this medicine are **itching**, redness, and swelling of the eye or eyelid. Allergic reactions also are possible. If any of these symptoms occur, call the physician who prescribed the medicine.

Interactions

Patients who are using any other prescription or nonprescription (over-the-counter) medicines in their eyes should check with their physicians before using tobramycin.

Nancy Ross-Flanigan

Antibiotics, topical

Definition

Topical **antibiotics** are medicines applied to the skin to kill bacteria.

Purpose

Topical antibiotics help prevent infections caused by bacteria that get into minor cuts, scrapes, and **burns**. Treating minor **wounds** with antibiotics allows quicker healing. If the wounds are left untreated, the bacteria will multiply, causing **pain**, redness, swelling, **itching**, and oozing. Untreated infections can eventually spread and become much more serious.

Different kinds of topical antibiotics kill different kinds of bacteria. Many antibiotic first-aid products contain combinations of antibiotics to make them effective against a broad range of bacteria.

When treating a wound, it is not enough to simply apply a topical antibiotic. The wound must first be cleaned with soap and water and patted dry. After the antibiotic is applied, the wound should be covered with a dressing, such as a bandage or a protective gel or spray. For many years, it was thought that wounds heal best when exposed to the air. But now most experts say it is best to keep wounds clean and moist while they heal. The covering should still allow some air to reach the wound, however.

Description

Some topical antibiotics are available without a prescription and are sold in many forms, including

KEY TERMS

Bacteria—Tiny, one-celled forms of life that cause many diseases and infections.

Conception—The union of egg and sperm to form a fetus.

Fungal—Caused by a fungus.

Fungus—A member of a group of simple organisms that are related to yeast and molds.

Incontinence—The inability to control the bladder or bowel.

Inflammation—Pain, redness, swelling, and heat that usually develop in response to injury or illness.

creams, ointments, powders, and sprays. Some widely used topical antibiotics are bacitracin, neomycin, mupirocin, and polymyxin B. Among the products that contain one or more of these ingredients are Bactroban (a prescription item), Neosporin, Polysporin, and Triple Antibiotic Ointment or Cream.

Recommended dosage

The recommended dosage depends on the type of topical antibiotic. Follow the directions on the package label or ask a pharmacist for directions.

In general, topical antibiotics should be applied within four hours after injury. Do not use more than the recommended amount and do not apply it more often than three times a day. Do not apply the medicine over large areas of skin or on open wounds.

Precautions

Many public health experts are concerned about antibiotic resistance, a problem that can develop when antibiotics are overused. Over time, bacteria develop new defenses against antibiotics that once were effective against them. Because bacteria reproduce so quickly, these defenses can be rapidly passed on through generations of bacteria until almost all are immune to the effects of a particular antibiotic. The process happens faster than new antibiotics can be developed. To help control the problem, many experts advise people to use topical antibiotics only for short periods, that is, until the wound heals, and only as directed. For the topical antibiotic to work best, it should be used only to prevent infection in a fresh wound, not to treat an infection that has already started. Wounds that are not fresh may

need the attention of a physician to prevent complications such as blood **poisoning**.

Topical antibiotics are meant to be used only on the skin and only for only a few days at a time. If the wound has not healed in five days, stop using the antibiotic and call a doctor.

Do not use topical antibiotics on large areas of skin or on open wounds. These products should not be used to treat **diaper rash** in infants or incontinence rash in adults.

Only minor cuts, scrapes, and burns should be treated with topical antibiotics. Certain kinds of injuries may need medical care and should not be self-treated with topical antibiotics. These include:

- large wounds
- deep cuts
- cuts that continue bleeding
- cuts that may need stitches
- burns any larger than a few inches in diameter
- scrapes imbedded with particles that won't wash away
- animal bites
- deep puncture wounds
- eye injuries

Never use regular topical antibiotics in the eyes. Special antibiotic products are available for treating eye infections.

Although topical antibiotics control infections caused by bacteria, they may allow fungal infections to develop. The use of other medicines to treat the fungal infections may be necessary. Check with the physician or pharmacist.

Some people may be allergic to one or more ingredients in a topical antibiotic product. If an allergic reaction develops, stop using the product immediately and call a physician.

No harmful or abnormal effects have been reported in babies whose mothers used topical antibiotics while pregnant or nursing. However, pregnant women generally are advised not to use any drugs during the first 3 months after conception. A woman who is pregnant or breastfeeding or who plans to become pregnant should check with her physician before using a topical antibiotic.

Unless a physician says to do so, do not use topical antibiotics on children under two years of age.

Side effects

The most common minor side effects are itching or burning. These problems usually do not require medical treatment unless they do not go away or they interfere with normal activities.

If any of the following side effects occur, check with a doctor as soon as possible:

- rash
- swelling of the lips and face
- sweating
- tightness or discomfort in the chest
- breathing problems
- fainting or **dizziness**
- low blood pressure
- nausea
- diarrhea
- hearing loss or ringing in the ears

Other rare side effects may occur. Anyone who has unusual symptoms after using a topical antibiotic should get in touch with the physician who prescribed or the pharmacist who recommedned the medication.

Interactions

Using certain topical antibiotics at the same time as hydrocortisone (a topical corticosteroid used to treat inflammation) may hide signs of infection or allergic reaction. Do not use these two medicines at the same time unless told to do so by a health care provider.

Anyone who is using any other type of prescription or nonprescription (over-the-counter) medicine on the skin should check with a doctor before using a topical antibiotic.

Resources

PERIODICALS

Farley, Dixie. "Help for Cuts, Scrapes and Burns." *FDA Consumer* May 1996:12.

Nancy Ross-Flanigan

Antibody screening *see* **Blood typing and crossmatching**

Anticancer drugs

Definition

Anticancer, or antineoplastic, drugs are used to treat malignancies, or cancerous growths. Drug therapy may be used alone, or in combination with other treatments such as surgery or **radiation therapy**.

Purpose

Anticancer drugs are used to control the growth of cancerous cells. **Cancer** is commonly defined as the uncontrolled growth of cells, with loss of differentiation and commonly, with metastasis, spread of the cancer to other tissues and organs. Cancers are malignant growths. In contrast, benign growths remain encapsulated and grow within a well-defined area. Although benign tumors may be fatal if untreated, due to pressure on essential organs, as in the case of a benign **brain tumor**, surgery or radiation are the preferred methods of treating growths which have a well defined location. Drug therapy is used when the tumor has spread, or may spread, to all areas of the body.

Description

Several classes of drugs may be used in cancer treatment, depending on the nature of the organ involved. For example, breast cancers are commonly stimulated by estrogens, and may be treated with drugs that inactivate the sex hormones. Similarly, **prostate cancer** may be treated with drugs that inactivate androgens, the male sex hormone. However, the majority of antineoplastic drugs act by interfering with cell growth. Since cancerous cells grow more rapidly than other cells, the drugs target those cells that are in the process of reproducing themselves. As a result, antineoplastic drugs will commonly affect not only the cancerous cells, but others cells that commonly reproduce quickly, including hair follicles, ovaries and testes, and the blood-forming organs.

Newer methods of antineoplastic drug therapy have taken different approaches, including angiogenesis—the inhibition of formation of blood vessels feeding the tumor and contributing to tumor growth. Although these approaches hold promise, they are not yet in common use. Developing new anticancer drugs is the work of ongoing research. In 2003, a new technique was developed to streamline the search for effective drugs. Researchers pumped more than 23,000 chemical compounds through a screening technique to identify those that help fight cancer while leaving

Anti Cancer Drugs

Generic (Brand Name)	Clinical Uses	Common Side Effects To Drug
Altretamine(Hexalen)	Treatment of advanced ovarian cancer	Bone marrow depression, nausea and vomiting
Asparaginase(Elspar)	Commonly used in combination with other drugs; refractory acute lymphocytic leukemia	Liver, kidney, pancreas, CNS abnormalities,
Bleomycin(Blenoxane)	Lymphomas, **Hodgkin's disease**, testicular cancer	Hair loss, **stomatitis**, pulmonary toxicity, **hyperpigmentation** of skin
Busulfan(Myleran)	Chronic granulocytic leukemia	Bone marrow depression, pulmonary toxicity
Carboplatin(Paraplatin)	Pallilation of ovarian cancer	Bone marrow depression, nausea and vomiting
Carmustine	Hodgkin's disease, brain tumors, **multiple myeloma**, malignant melonoma	Bone marrow depression, nausea and vomiting, toxic damage to liver
Chlorambucil(Leukeran)	Chronic lymphocytic leukemia, non-Hodgkin's lymphomas, breast and ovarian cancer	Bone marrow depression, excess uric acid in blood
Cisplatin(Platinol)	Treatment of bladder, ovarian, uterine, testicular, head and neck cancers	Renal toxicity and ototoxicity
Cladribine(Leustatin)	Hairy cell leukemia	Bone marrow depression, nausea and vomiting, fever
Cyclophosphamide (Cytoxan)	Hodgkin's disease, non-Hodgkin's lymphomas, **neuroblastoma**. Often used with other drugs for breast, ovarian, and lung cancers; acute lymphoblastic leukemia in children; multiple myeloma	Bone marrow depression, hair loss, nausea and vomiting, inflammation of the bladder
Cytarabine(Cytosar-U)	Leukemias occurring in adults and children	Bone marrow depression, nausea and vomiting, diarrhea, stomatitis
Dacarbazine(DTIC-Dome)	Hodgkin's disease, malignant melanoma	Bone marrow depression, nausea and vomiting
Diethylstilbestrol (DES) (Stilbestrol)	**Breast cancer** in post-menopausal women, prostate cancer	Hair loss, nausea and vomiting, **edema**, excess calcium in blood; feminizing effects in men
Ethinyl estradiol(Estinyl)	Advanced breast cancer in post-menopausal women, prostate cancer	Excess calcium in blood, anorexia, edema, nausea and vomiting; feminizing effects in men
Etoposide(VePesid)	Acute leukemias, lymphomas, testicular cancer	Bone marrow depression, nausea and vomiting, hair loss

Anti Cancer Drugs (continued)

Generic (Brand Name)	Clinical Uses	Common Side Effects To Drug
Mitomycin (Mutamycin)	Bladder, breast, colon, lung, pancreas, rectum cancers, **head and neck cancer**, malignant melanoma	Bone marrow depression, nausea and vomiting, diarrhea, stomatitis, possible tissue damage
Mitotane (Lysodren)	Cancer of the adrenal cortex (inoperable)	Damage to adrenal cortex, nausea, anorexia
Mitoxantrone (Novantrone)	Acute nonlymphocytic leukemia	Cardiac **arrhythmias**, labored breating, nausea and vomiting, diarrhea, fever, congestive heart failure
Paclitaxel (Taxol)	Advanced ovarian cancer	Bone marrow depression, hair loss, nausea and vomiting, **hypotension**, allergic reactions, slow heart action, muscle and joint pain
Pentastatin (Nipent)	Hairy cell leukemia unresponsive to alpha-interferon	Bone marrow depression, fever, skin rash, liver damage, nausea and vomiting
Pipobroman (Vercyte)	Chronic granulocytic leukemia	Bone marrow depression
Plicamycin (Mithracin)	Testucular tumors	Toxicity/damage to bone marrow, kidneys, and liver
Prednisone (Meticorten)	Used in adjunct therapy for palliation of symptoms in lymphomas, acute leukemia Hodgkin's disease	May be toxic to all body systems
Procarbazine (Matulane)	Hodgkin's disease	Bone marrow depression, nausea and vomiting
Streptozocin (Zanosar)	Islet cell carcinoma of pancreas	Nausea and vomiting, toxicity to kidneys
Tamoxifen (Nolvadex)	Advanced breast cancer in post menopausal	Nausea and vomiting, ocular toxicity, hot flashes
Teniposide (Vumon)	Acute lymphocytic leukemia in children	See Etoposide
Vinblastine (Velban)	Breast cancer, Hodgkin's disease, metastatic testicular cancer	Bone marrow depression, neurotoxicity
Vincristine (Oncovin)	Acute leukemia, Hodgkin's disease, lymphomas	Constipation, neurotoxicity, possible tissue necrosis

healthy cells unharmed. The system identified nine compounds matching the profile, including one previously unidentified drug for fighting cancer. They have expanded their research to determine how the drug might be developed. This was an important step

KEY TERMS

Cataract—Clouding of the lens of the eye, leading to poor vision or blindness.

Impotent—Unable to achieve or maintain an erection of the penis.

in identifying anticancer dugs that are not completely toxic to healthy cells.

Antineoplastic drugs may be divided into two classes: cycle specific and non-cycle specific. Cycle specific drugs act only at specific points of the cell's duplication cycle, such as anaphase or metaphase, while non-cycle specific drugs may act at any point in the cell cycle. In order to gain maximum effect, antineoplastic drugs are commonly used in combinations.

Precautions

Because antineoplastic agents do not target specific cell types, they have a number of common adverse side effects. Hair loss is common due to the effects on hair follicles, and anemia, immune system impairment, and clotting problems are caused by destruction of the blood-forming organs, leading to a reduction in the number of red cells, white cells, and platelets. Because of the frequency and severity of these side effects, it is common to administer **chemotherapy** in cycles, allowing time for recovery from the drug effects before administering the next dose. Doses are often calculated, not on the basis of weight, but rather based on blood counts, in order to avoid dangerous levels of anemia (red cell depletion), **neutropenia** (white cell deficiency), or **thrombocytopenia** (platelet deficiency.)

The health professional has many responsibilities in dealing with patients undergoing chemotherapy. The patient must be well informed of the risks and benefits of chemotherapy, and must be emotionally prepared for the side effects. These may be permanent, and younger patients should be aware of the high risk of sterility after chemotherapy.

The patient must also know which side effects should be reported to the practitioner, since many adverse effects do not appear until several days after a dose of chemotherapy. When chemotherapy is self-administered, the patient must be familiar with proper use of the drugs, including dose scheduling and avoidance of drug-drug and food-drug interactions.

Appropriate steps should be taken to minimize side effects. These may include administration of anti-nauseant medications to reduce **nausea** and **vomiting**, maintaining fluid levels to reduce drug toxicity, particularly to the kidneys, or application of a scalp tourniquet to reduce blood flow to the scalp and minimize hair loss due to drug therapy.

Patients receiving chemotherapy also are at risk of infections due to reduced white blood counts. While prophylactic **antibiotics** may be useful, the health care professional should also be sure to use standard precautions, including gowns and gloves when appropriate. Patients should be alerted to avoid risks of viral contamination, and live virus immunizations are contraindicated until the patient has fully recovered from the effects of chemotherapy. Similarly, the patient should avoid contact with other people who have recently had live virus immunizations.

Other precautions which should be emphasized are the risks to pregnant or nursing women. Because antineoplastic drugs are commonly harmful to the fetus, women of childbearing potential should be cautioned to use two effective methods of birth control while receiving cancer chemotherapy. This also applies if the woman's male partner is receiving chemotherapy. Breastfeeding should be avoided while the mother is being treated.

Before prescribing or administering anticancer drugs, health care providers should inquire whether the patient has any of the following conditions:

- **chickenpox** or recent exposure to someone with chickenpox
- shingles (Herpes zoster)
- mouth sores
- current or past seizures
- head injury
- nerve or muscle disease
- hearing problems
- infection of any kind
- gout
- colitis
- intestine blockage
- stomach ulcer
- kidney stones
- kidney disease
- liver disease
- current or past alcohol **abuse**

- immune system disease
- **cataracts** or other eye problems
- high cholesterol

Other precautions

The anticancer drug methotrexate has additional precautions. Patients should be given advice on the effects of sun exposure and the use of alcohol and **pain** relievers.

Side effects

Tamoxifen

The anticancer drug tamoxifen (Nolvadex) increases the risk of cancer of the uterus in some women. It also causes cataracts and other eye problems. Women taking this drug may have hot flashes, menstrual changes, genital **itching**, vaginal discharge, and weight gain. Men who take tamoxifen may lose interest in sex or become impotent. Health care providers should keep in close contact with patients to assess the individual risks associated with taking this powerful drug.

Other anticancer drugs

These side effects are not common, but could be a sign of a serious problem. Health care providers should immediately be consulted if any of the following occur:

- black, tarry, or bloody stools
- blood in the urine
- **diarrhea**
- **fever** or chills
- cough or hoarseness
- wheezing or **shortness of breath**
- sores in the mouth or on the lips
- unusual bleeding or bruising
- swelling of the face
- red "pinpoint" spots on the skin
- redness, pain, or swelling at the point where an injectable anticancer drug is given
- pain in the side or lower back
- problems urinating or painful urination
- dizziness or faintness
- fast or irregular heartbeat

Other side effects do not need immediate care, but should have medical attention. They are:

- joint pain
- skin rash
- hearing problems or ringing in the ears
- numbness or **tingling** in the fingers or toes
- trouble walking or balance problems
- swelling of the feet or lower legs
- unusual tiredness or weakness
- loss of taste
- seizures
- dizziness
- confusion
- agitation
- headache
- dark urine
- yellow eyes or skin
- flushing of the face

In addition, there are other possible side effects that do not need medical attention unless they persist or interfere with normal activities. These include changes in menstrual period, itchy skin, nausea and vomiting, and loss of appetite.

Other rare side effects may occur. Anyone who has unusual symptoms after taking anticancer drugs should contact the physician who prescribed the medication.

Interactions

Anticancer drugs may interact with a number of other medicines. When this happens, the effects of one or both of the drugs may change or the risk of side effects may be greater. The health care provider should be aware of all other prescription or non-prescription (over-the-counter) medicines a patient is taking. The primary care provider should also be told if the patient has been treated with radiation or has taken other anticancer drugs.

Resources

PERIODICALS

"Technique Streamlines Search for Anticancer Drugs." *Cancer Weekly* April 15, 2003: 62.

Samuel D. Uretsky, PharmD
Teresa G. Odle

Anticholinergic drugs *see* **Antiparkinson drugs**

Anticlotting drugs *see* **Anticoagulant and antiplatelet drugs**

Anticoagulant and antiplatelet drugs

Definition

Anticoagulants are drugs used to prevent clot formation or to prevent a clot that has formed from enlarging. They inhibit clot formation by blocking the action of clotting factors or platelets. Anticoagulant drugs fall into three categories: inhibitors of clotting factor synthesis, inhibitors of thrombin and antiplatelet drugs.

Purpose

Anticoagulant drugs reduce the ability of the blood to form clots. Although blood clotting is essential to prevent serious bleeding in the case of skin cuts, clots inside the blood vessels block the flow of blood to major organs and cause heart attacks and strokes. Although these drugs are sometimes called blood thinners, they do not actually thin the blood. Furthermore, this type of medication will not dissolve clots that already have formed, although the drug stops an existing clot from worsening. However, another type of drug, used in **thrombolytic therapy**, will dissolve existing clots.

Anticoagulant drugs are used for a number of conditions. For example, they may be given to prevent **blood clots** from forming after the replacement of a heart valve or to reduce the risk of a **stroke** or another **heart attack** after a first heart attack. They are also used to reduce the chance of blood clots forming during open heart surgery or bypass surgery. Low doses of these drugs may be given to prevent blood clots in patients who must stay in bed for a long time after certain types of surgery.

Because anticoagulants affect the blood's ability to clot, they can increase the risk of severe bleeding and heavy blood loss. It is thus essential to take these drugs exactly as directed and to see a physician regularly as long as they are prescribed.

Description

Anticoagulant drugs, also called anticlotting drugs or blood thinners, are available only with a physician's prescription. They come in tablet and injectable forms. They fall into three groups:

- Inhibitors of clotting factor synthesis. These anticoagulants inhibit the production of certain clotting factors in the liver. One example is warfarin (brand name: coumadin).
- Inhibitors of thrombin. Thrombin inhibitors interfere with blood clotting by blocking the activity of thrombin. They include heparin, lepirudin (Refludan).

KEY TERMS

Anticoagulant—Drug used to prevent clot formation or to prevent a clot that has formed from enlarging. Anticoagulant drugs inhibit clot formation by blocking the action of clotting factors or platelets. Anticoagulant drugs fall into three groups: inhibitors of clotting factor synthesis, inhibitors of thrombin and antiplatelet drugs.

Antiplatelet drug—Drug that inhibits platelets from aggregating to form a plug. They are used to prevent clotting and alter the natural course of atherosclerosis.

Atherosclerosis—Condition characterized by deposits of fatty plaque in the arteries.

Clot—A soft, semi-solid mass that forms when blood gels.

Platelet—A small, disk-shaped body in the blood that has an important role in blood clotting: they form the initial plug at the rupture site of a blood vessel.

Thrombin—Thrombin is a protein produced by the body. It is a specific clotting factor that plays an important role in the blood clotting process.

Thrombin inhibitor—Thrombin inhibitors are one type of anticoagulant medication, used to help prevent formation of harmful blood clots in the body by blocking the activity of thrombin.

- Antiplatelet drugs. Antiplatelet drugs interact with platelets, which is a type of blood cell, to block platelets from aggregating into harmful clots. They include: **aspirin**, ticlopidine (Ticlid), clopidogrel (Plavix), tirofiban (Aggrastat), and eptifibatide (Integrilin).

Recommended dosage

The recommended dosage depends on the type of anticoagulant drug and the medical condition for which it is prescribed. The prescribing physician or the pharmacist who filled the prescription can provide information concerning the correct dosage. Usually, the physician will adjust the dose after checking the patient's clotting time.

Anticoagulant drugs must be taken exactly as directed by the physician. Larger or more frequent doses should not be taken, and the drug should also not be taken for longer than prescribed. *Taking too much of this medication can cause severe bleeding.* Anticoagulants should also be taken on schedule. A record of each dose should be kept as it is taken. If a dose is missed, it should be taken as soon as possible followed by the regular dose schedule. However, a patient who forgets to take a missed dose until the next day should not take the missed dose at all and should not double the next dose, as this could lead to bleeding. A record of all missed doses should be kept for the prescribing physician who should be informed at the scheduled visits.

Precautions

Persons who take anticoagulants should see a physician regularly while taking these drugs, particularly at the beginning of therapy. The physician will order periodic blood tests to check the blood's clotting ability. The results of these tests will help the physician determine the proper amount of medication to be taken each day.

Time is required for normal clotting ability to return after anticoagulant treatment. During this period, patients must observe the same precautions they observed while taking the drug. The length of time needed for the blood to return to normal depends on the type of anticoagulant drug that was taken. The prescribing physician will advise as to how long the precautions should be observed.

People who are taking anticoagulant drugs should tell all physicians, dentists, pharmacists, and other medical professionals who provide medical treatments or services to them that they are taking such a medication. They should also carry identification stating that they are using an anticoagulant drug.

Other prescription drugs or over-the-counter medicine–especially aspirin–should be not be taken without the prescribing physician being informed.

Because of the risk of heavy bleeding, anyone who takes an anticoagulant drug must take care to avoid injuries. Sports and other potentially hazardous activities should be avoided. Any falls, blows to the body or head, or other injuries should be reported to a physician, as internal bleeding may occur without any obvious symptoms. Special care should be taken in shaving and in brushing and flossing the teeth. Soft toothbrushes should be used and the flossing should be very gentle. Electric razors should be used instead of a blade.

Alcohol can change the way anticoagulant drugs affect the body. Anyone who takes this medicine should not have more than one to two drinks at any time and should not drink alcohol every day.

Special conditions

People with specific medical conditions or who are taking certain other medicines can have problems if they take anticoagulant drugs. Before taking these drugs, the prescribing physician should be informed about any of these conditions:

ALLERGIES. Anyone who has had unusual reactions to anticoagulants in the past should let his or her physician know before taking the drugs again. The physician should also be told about any **allergies** to beef, pork, or other foods; dyes; preservatives; or other substances.

PREGNANCY. Anticoagulants may cause many serious problems if taken during **pregnancy**. **Birth defects**, severe bleeding in the fetus, and other problems that affect the physical or mental development of the fetus or newborn are possible. The mother may also experience severe bleeding if she takes anticoagulants during pregnancy, during delivery, or even shortly after delivery. *Women should not take start taking anticoagulants during pregnancy and should not become pregnant while taking it. Any woman who becomes pregnant or suspects that she has become pregnant while taking an anticoagulant should check with her physician immediately.*

BREASTFEEDING. Some anticoagulant drugs may pass into breast milk. Blood tests can be done on nursing babies to see whether the drug is causing any problems. If it is, other medication may be prescribed to counteract the effects of the anticoagulant drug.

OTHER MEDICAL CONDITIONS. Before using anticoagulant drugs, people should inform their physician about *any* medical problems they have. They should also let the physician who prescribed the medicine know if they are being treated by any other medical physician or dentist. In addition, people who will be taking anticoagulant drugs should let their physician know if they have recently had any of the following:

- **fever** lasting more than one to two days

- severe or continuing **diarrhea**

- childbirth

- heavy or unusual menstrual bleeding

- insertion of an intrauterine contraceptive device (**IUD**)

- falls, injuries, or blows to the body or head

- any type of surgery, including dental surgery

- spinal anesthesia

- radiation treatment

USE OF CERTAIN FOODS AND MEDICINES. Many foods and drugs may affect the way the anticoagulant drugs work or may increase the risk of side effects.

Side effects

The most common minor side effects are bloating or gas. These problems usually go away as the body adjusts to the drug and do not require medical treatment.

More serious side effects may occur, especially if excessive anticoagulant is taken. If any of the following side effects occur, a physician should be notified immediately:

- bleeding gums
- sores or white spots in the mouth or throat
- unusual **bruises** or purplish areas on the skin
- unexplained nosebleeds
- unusually heavy bleeding or oozing from **wounds**
- unexpected or unusually menstrual bleeding
- blood in the urine
- cloudy or dark urine
- painful or difficult urination or sudden decrease in amount of urine
- black, tarry, or bloody stools
- coughing up blood
- **vomiting** blood or something that looks like coffee grounds
- constipation
- **pain** or swelling in the stomach or abdomen
- back pain
- stiff, swollen, or painful joints
- painful, bluish or purplish fingers or toes
- puffy or swollen eyelids, face, feet, or lower legs
- changes in the color of the face
- skin rash, **itching**, or **hives**
- yellow eyes or skin
- severe or continuing **headache**
- sore throat and fever, with or without chills
- breathing problems or **wheezing**
- tightness in the chest
- dizziness
- unusual tiredness or weakness
- weight gain.

In addition, patients taking anticoagulant drugs should check with their physicians as soon as possible if any of these side effects occur:

- nausea or vomiting
- diarrhea
- stomach pain or cramps.

Other side effects may occur. Anyone who has unusual symptoms while taking anticoagulant drugs should get in touch with his or her physician.

Interactions

Anticoagulants may interact with many other medications. When this happens, the effects of one or both of the drugs may change or the risk of side effects may be increased. *Anyone who takes anticoagulants should inform the prescribing physician about other prescription or nonprescription (over-the-counter medicines) he or she is taking–even aspirin, laxatives, vitamins, and antacids.*

Diet also affects the way anticoagulant drugs work in the body. A normal, balanced diet should be followed every day while taking such medication. No dietary changes should be made without informing first the prescribing physician, who should also be told of any illness or other condition interfering with the ability to eat normally. Diet is a very important consideration because the amount of vitamin K in the body affects how anticoagulant drugs work. Dicoumarol and warfarin act by reducing the effects of vitamin K. Vitamin K is found in meats, dairy products, leafy, green vegetables, and some multiple **vitamins** and **nutritional supplements**. For the drugs to work properly, it is best to have the same amount of vitamin K in the body all the time. Foods containing vitamin K in the diet should not be increased or decreased without consulting with the prescribing physician. If the patient takes vitamin supplements, he should check the label to see if it contains vitamin K. Because vitamin K is also produced by intestinal bacteria, a severe case of diarrhea or the use of **laxatives** may also alter a person's vitamin K levels.

Nancy Ross-Flanigan

Anticonvulsant drugs

Definition

Anticonvulsant drugs are medicines used to prevent or treat convulsions (seizures).

Purpose

Anticonvulsant drugs are used to control seizures in people with epilepsy. Epilepsy is not a single disease—it is a set of symptoms that may have different

KEY TERMS

Chronic—A word used to describe a long-lasting condition. Chronic conditions often develop gradually and involve slow changes.

Epilepsy—A brain disorder with symptoms that include seizures.

Glaucoma—A condition in which pressure in the eye is abnormally high. If not treated, glaucoma may lead to blindness.

Porphyria—A disorder in which porphyrins build up in the blood and urine.

Porphyrin—A type of pigment found in living things, such as chlorophyll which makes plants green or hemoglobin which makes blood red.

Seizure—A sudden attack, spasm, or convulsion.

Systemic lupus erythematosus (SLE)—A chronic disease with many symptoms, including weakness, fatigue, joint pain, sores on the skin, and problems with the kidneys, spleen, and other organs.

Withdrawal symptoms—A group of physical or mental symptoms that may occur when a person suddenly stops using a drug to which he or she has become dependent.

causes in different people. The common thread is an imbalance in the brain's electrical activity. This imbalance causes seizures that may affect part or all of the body and may or may not cause a loss of consciousness. Anticonvulsant drugs act on the brain to reduce the frequency and severity of seizures.

Some cases of epilepsy are brought on by head injuries, brain tumors or infections, or metabolic problems such as low blood sugar. But in some people with epilepsy, the cause is not clear.

Anticonvulsant drugs are an important part of the treatment program for epilepsy. Different kinds of drugs may be prescribed for different types of seizures. In addition to taking medicine, patients with epilepsy should get enough rest, avoid **stress**, and practice good health habits.

Some physicians believe that giving the drugs to children with epilepsy may prevent the condition from getting worse in later life. However, others say the effects are the same, whether treatment is started early or later in life. Determining when treatment begins depends on the physician and his assessment of the patient's symptoms.

Physicians also prescribe certain anticonvulsant drugs for other conditions, including **bipolar disorder** and migraine headaches.

Description

Anticonvulsant drugs may be divided into several classes. The hydantoins include pheytoin (Dilantin) and mephenytoin (Mesantoin.) Ther succimides include ethosuximide (Zarontin) and methsuccimide (Celontin.) The **benzodiazepines**, which are better known for their use as tranquilizers and sedatives, include clonazepam (Klonopin), clorazepate (Tranxene) and diazepam (Valium.) There are also a large number of other drugs which are not related to larger groups. These include carbamazepine (Tegretol), valproic acid (Depakote, Depakene) gabapentin (Neurontin), topiramate (Topamax), felbamate (Felbatol) and several others. Phenobarbital has been used as an anticonvulsant, and is still useful for some patients. The drugs are available only with a physician's prescription and come in tablet, capsule, liquid, and "sprinkle" forms.

Recommended dosage

The recommended dosage depends on the type of anticonvulsant, its strength, and the type of seizures for which it is being taken. Check with the physician who prescribed the drug or the pharmacist who filled the prescription for the correct dosage.

Do not stop taking this medicine suddenly after taking it for several weeks or more. Gradually tapering the dose may reduce the chance of withdrawal effects.

Do not change brands or dosage forms of this medicine without checking with a pharmacist or physician. If a prescription refill does not look like the original medicine, check with the pharmacist who filled the prescription.

Precautions

Patients on anticonvulsant drugs should see a physician regularly while on therapy, especially during the first few months. The physician will check to make sure the medicine is working as it should and will note unwanted side effects. The physician may also need to adjust the dosage during this period.

Valproic acid can cause serious liver damage, especially in the first 6 months of treatment. Children are particularly at risk, but anyone taking this medicine should see their physician regularly for tests of liver function and should be alert to symptoms of liver damage, such as yellow skin and eyes, facial swelling, loss of appetite, general feeling of illness, loss of appetite, and **vomiting**. If liver problems are suspected, call a physician immediately.

Felbatol has caused serious liver damage and **aplastic anemia**, a condition in which the bone marrow stops producing blood cells. Patients taking this drug should have regular blood counts, and should stop taking the drug if there are too few red blood cells.

While taking anticonvulsant drugs, do not start or stop taking any other medicines without checking with a physician. The other medicines may affect the way the anticonvulsant medicine works.

Because anticonvulsant drugs work on the central nervous system, they may add to the effects of alcohol and other drugs that slow down the central nervous system, such as **antihistamines**, cold medicine, allergy medicine, sleep aids, other medicine for seizures, tranquilizers, some **pain** relievers, and **muscle relaxants**. Anyone taking anticonvulsant drugs should check with his or her physician before drinking alcohol or taking any medicines that slow the central nervous system.

Anticonvulsant drugs may interact with medicines used during surgery, dental procedures, or emergency treatment. These interactions could increase the chance of side effects. Anyone who is taking anticonvulsant drugs should be sure to tell the health care professional in charge before having any surgical or dental procedures or receiving emergency treatment.

Some people feel drowsy, dizzy, lightheaded, or less alert when using these drugs, especially when they first begin taking them or when their dosage is increased. Anyone who takes anticonvulsant drugs should not drive, use machines or do anything else that might be dangerous until they have found out how the drugs affect them.

Anticonvulsant drugs may affect the results of certain medical tests. Before having medical tests, people who take anticonvulsant drugs should make sure that the medical professional in charge knows what they are taking.

Children may be more likely to have certain side effects from anticonvulsant drugs, such as behavior changes; tender, bleeding, or swollen gums; enlarged facial features; and excessive hair growth. Problems with the gums may be prevented by regularly brushing and flossing, massaging the gums, and having the teeth cleaned every 3 months whether the patient is a child or an adult.

Children who take high doses of this medicine for a long time may have problems in school.

Older people may be more sensitive to the effects of anticonvulsant drugs. This may increase the chance of side effects and overdoses.

Special conditions

People with certain medical conditions or who are taking certain other medicines can have problems if they take anticonvulsant drugs. Before taking these drugs, be sure to let the physician know about any of these conditions:

ALLERGIES. Anyone who has had unusual reactions to anticonvulsant drugs or to **tricyclic antidepressants** such as imipramine (Tofranil) or desipramine (Norpramin) in the past should let his or her physician know before taking the drugs again. The physician should also be told about any **allergies** to foods, dyes, preservatives, or other substances.

PREGNANCY. Some anticonvulsant drugs taken during pregnancy may cause bleeding problems in the mother during delivery and in the baby after delivery. This problem can be avoided by giving vitamin K to the mother during delivery and to the baby after birth.

Pregnancy may affect the way the body absorbs anticonvulsant drugs. Women who are prone to seizures may have more seizures during pregnancy, even though they are taking their medicine regularly. If this happens, they should check with their physicians about whether the dose needs to be increased.

BREASTFEEDING. Some anticonvulsant drugs pass into breast milk and may cause unwanted effects in babies whose mothers take the medicine. Women who are breastfeeding should check with their physicians about the benefits and risks of using anticonvulsant drugs.

DIABETES. Anticonvulsant drugs may affect blood sugar levels. Patients with diabetes who notice changes in the results of their urine or blood tests should check with their physicians.

OTHER MEDICAL CONDITIONS. Before using anticonvulsant drugs, people with any of these medical problems should make sure their physicians are aware of their conditions:

• liver disease
• kidney disease
• thyroid disease
• heart or blood vessel disease
• blood disease
• brain disease
• problems with urination
• current or past alcohol **abuse**

- behavior problems

- diabetes mellitus

- **glaucoma**

- porphyria

- systemic lupus erythematosus

- **fever** higher than 101 °F (38.3 °C) for more than 24 hours

USE OF CERTAIN MEDICINES. Taking anticonvulsant drugs with certain other drugs may affect the way the drugs work or may increase the chance of side effects.

Side effects

The most common side effects are **constipation**, mild **nausea** or vomiting, and mild **dizziness**, drowsiness, or lightheadedness. These problems usually go away as the body adjusts to the drug and do not require medical treatment. Less common side effects, such as **diarrhea**, sleep problems, aching joints or muscles, increased sensitivity to sunlight, increased sweating, hair loss, enlargement of facial features, excessive hair growth, muscle twitching, and breast enlargement in males also may occur and do not need medical attention unless they persist or are troublesome.

Other side effects may need medical attention. If any of these side effects occur, check with a physician as soon as possible:

- clumsiness or unsteadiness

- slurred speech or stuttering

- trembling

- unusual excitement, irritability, or nervousness

- uncontrolled eye movements

- blurred or double vision

- mood or mental changes

- confusion

- increase in seizures

- bleeding, tender, or swollen gums

- skin rash or itching

- enlarged glands in neck or armpits

- muscle weakness or pain

- fever

Other side effects are possible. Anyone who has unusual symptoms after taking anticonvulsant drugs should get in touch with his or her physician.

Interactions

Some anticonvulsant drugs should not be taken within two to three hours of taking **antacids** or medicine for diarrhea. These medicines may make the anticonvulsant drugs less effective. Ask the pharmacist or physician for more information.

Birth control pills may not work properly when anticonvulsant drugs are being taken. To prevent pregnancy, ask the physician or pharmacist if additional methods of birth control should be used while taking anticonvulsant drugs.

Anticonvulsant drugs may interact with many other medicines. When this happens, the effects of one or both of the drugs may change or the risk of side effects may be greater. Anyone who takes anticonvulsant drugs should let the physician know all other medicines he or she is taking. Among the drugs that may interact with certain anticonvulsant drugs are:

- airway opening drugs (**bronchodilators**) such as aminophylline, theophylline (Theo-Dur and other brands), and oxtriphylline (Choledyl and other brands)

- medicines that contain calcium, such as antacids and calcium supplements

- blood thinning drugs

- caffeine

- antibiotics such as clarithromycin (Biaxin), **erythromycins**, and **sulfonamides** (sulfa drugs)

- disulfiram (Antabuse), used to treat alcohol abuse

- fluoxetine (Prozac)

- monoamine oxidase inhibitors (MAO inhibitors) such as phenelzine (Nardil) or tranylcypromine (Parnate), used to treat conditions including depression and Parkinson's disease

- tricyclic antidepressants such as imipramine (Tofranil) or desipramine (Norpramin)

- corticosteroids

- acetaminophen (Tylenol)

- aspirin

- female hormones (estrogens)

- male hormones (androgens)

- cimetidine (Tagamet)

- central nervous system (CNS) depressants such as medicine for allergies, colds, hay fever, and **asthma**; sedatives; tranquilizers; prescription pain medicine; muscle relaxants; medicine for seizures; sleep aids; **barbiturates**; and anesthetics

- alcohol

- other anticonvulsant drugs

The list above does not include every drug that may interact with anticonvulsant drugs. Be sure to check with a physician or pharmacist before combining anticonvulsant drugs with any other prescription or nonprescription (over-the-counter) medicine.

Resources

PERIODICALS

Reynolds, E.H. "Do Anticonvulsant Drugs Alter the Natural Course of Epilepsy? Treatment Should Be Started as Early as Possible." *British Medical Journal* 310 (January 21, 1995): 176.

ORGANIZATIONS

American Epilepsy Society. 638 Prospect Avenue, Hartford, CT 06105. (203) 232-4825.

Epilepsy Foundation of America. 4351 Garden City Drive, #406, Landover, MD 20785. (800) 332-1000.

National Institute of Neurological Disorders and Stroke. P.O. Box 5801, Bethesda, MD 20824. (301) 496-5751.

Nancy Ross-Flanigan

Antidepressant drugs

Definition

Antidepressant drugs are medicines that relieve symptoms of **depressive disorders**.

Purpose

Depressive disorders may either be unipolar (depression alone) or bipolar (depression alternating with periods of extreme excitation). The formal diagnosis requires a cluster of symptoms, lasting at least two weeks. These symptoms include, but are not limited to, mood changes, insomnia or hypersomnia, and diminished interest in daily activities. The symptoms are not caused by any medical condition, drug side effect, or adverse life event. The condition is severe enough to cause clinically significant distress or impairment in social, occupational, or other important areas of functioning.

Secondary depression, or depression caused by unfavorable life events, is normally self limiting, and may best be treated with cognitive/behavioral therapy rather than drugs.

Description

Antidepressant agents act by increasing the levels of excitatory neurostransmitters, or nerve cell chemicals that act as messengers in the brain's nervous system. In 2003, a report showed that in addition to treating depression, use of antidepressant drugs may protect the brain from damage depressive episodes cause to the hippocampus, the area of the brain involved in learning and memory. Antidepressant drugs may be prescribed as a first-line treatment for depression, or in conjunction with other methods of controlling depression, such as behavioral therapy and **exercise**.

The main types of antidepressant drugs in use today are listed below, though the drugs available change frequently. For example, in mid-2003, the manufacturer of Wellbutrin released Wellbutrin XL, the only once-daily norepinephrine and dopamine reuptake inhibitor for treating depression in adults.

- **tricyclic antidepressants**, such as amitriptyline (Elavil), imipramine (Tofranil), nortriptyline (Pamelor)

- **selective serotonin reuptake inhibitors** (SSRIs or serotonin boosters), such as fluoxetine (Prozac), paroxetine (Paxil), and sertraline (Zoloft)

- **monoamine oxidase inhibitors** (MAO inhibitors), such as phenelzine (Nardil), and tranylcypromine (Parnate)

- tetracyclic compounds and atypical antidepressants which do not fall into any of the above categories

Selective serotonin reuptake inhibitors maintain levels of the excitatory neurohormone serotonin in the brain. They do not alter levels of norepinephrine. These have become the drugs of choice for a variety of psychiatric disorders, primarily because of their low incidence of severe side effects as compared with other drugs in this therapeutic class. SSRIs show similar actions and side effect profiles, but may vary in duration of action.

Tricyclic compounds, identified by their chemical structure containing three carbon rings, are an older class of antidepressants. Although generally effective, they have a high incidence of anticholinergic effects, notably dry mouth and dry eyes, which can cause discomfort. They also cause cardiac arrythmias. Because tricyclics act on both serotonin and norepinephrine, they may have some value in treatment of patients who fail to respond to SSRIs. Drugs in this class often are available at low prices, which may be significant when cost is a major factor in treatment. They also have been found useful in control of some neurologic **pain** syndromes.

Tricyclic antidepressants are similar, but may vary in severity of side effects, most notably the degree of **sedation** and the extent of the anticholinergic effects.

Tetracyclic compounds and atypical antidepressants are chemically distinct from both the major groups and each other. Although maprotilene (no brand name, marketed in generic form only) and mirtazepine (Remeron) are similar in chemical structures, they differ in their balance of activity on serotonine and norepinephrine levels.

Monoamine oxidase inhibitors (phenelzine [Nardil], tranylcypromine [Parnate]) have largely been supplanted in therapy because of their high risk of severe adverse effects, most notably severe **hypertension**. They act by inhibiting the enzyme monoamine oxidase, which is responsible for the metabolism of the stimulatory neurohormones norepinephrine, epinephrine, dopamine, and serotonin. The MAOIs are normally reserved for patients who are resistant to safer drugs. Two drugs, eldepryl (Carbex, used in treatment of Parkinson's disease) and the herb, **St. John's wort**, have some action against monoamine oxidase B, and have shown some value as antidepressants. They do not share the same risks as the non-selective MAO inhibitors.

All antidepressant agents, regardless of their structure, have a slow onset of action, typically three to five weeks. Although adverse effects may be seen as early as the first dose, significant therapeutic improvement is always delayed. Similarly, the effects of antidepressants will continue for a similar length of time after the drugs have been discontinued.

Recommended dosage

Dose varies with the specific drug and patient. Specialized references or a physician should be consulted.

Precautions

Antidepressants have many significant cautions and adverse effects. Although a few are listed here, specific references should be consulted for more complete information.

SSRIs. The most common side effect of SSRIs is excitation and insomnia. Excitation has been reported in over 20% of patients, and insomnia in 33%. Significant weight loss has been frequently reported, but most commonly in patients who are already underweight. A 2003 report showed that SSRIs also increase the risk of upper gastrointestinal tract bleeding. SSRIs may cause some sedation, and patients should be cautioned not to perform tasks requiring alertness until they have evaluated the effects of these drugs. SSRIs are **pregnancy** category C drugs. In 2003, a new report demonstrated that late-term (third trimester) use of these drugs could cause neurological symptoms in newborns, including tremor, restlessness and rigidity. Most SSRIs are excreted in breast milk, and there have been anecdotal reports of drowsiness in infants whose mothers were taking SSRIs while breastfeeding.

Most notably, a joint panel of the U.S. Food and Drug Administration (FDA) issued strong warnings to parents and physicians in 2004 about the risk of suicidal behavior in children and adolescents taking SSRIs.

Tricyclic antidepressants. Amoxepine (not marketed by brand, generic available), although a tricyclic antidepressant rather than a neuroleptic (major tranquilizer), displays some of the more serious effects of the neuroleptics, including tardive dyskinesias (drug induced involuntary movements) and neuroleptic malignant syndrome, a potentially fatal syndrome with symptoms including high fever, altered mental status, irregular pulse or blood pressure, and changes in heart rate. These adverse effects have not been reported with other tricyclic antidepressants.

The most common adverse effects of tricyclic antidepressants are sedation and the anticholinergic effects, such as dry mouth, dry eyes, and difficult urination. Alterations in heartbeat also are common, and may progress to congestive **heart failure**, **stroke**, and sudden **death**.

Tricyclic antidepressants are in pregnancy categories C or D, although there have been no formal studies of the drugs on fetal development. There are no studies of effects on newborns, but some anecdotal reports of malformations have resulted from animal studies. The drugs are excreted in breast milk.

Monoamine oxidase inhibitors. The greatest risk associated with these drugs is a hypertensive crisis which may be fatal and most often occurs when the drugs are taken with interacting foods or drugs. More common adverse reactions may include low blood pressure and slowing of heartbeat. Sedation and gastrointestinal disturbances also are common. MAOIs are in pregnancy category C. Safety in breast feeding has not been established.

Tetracyclics and atypicals. Because these drugs are individual, there are no group patterns of adverse reactions. Specific references should be consulted.

Interactions

The antidepressants have many **drug interactions**, some severe. Although a few are listed here, specific references should be consulted for more complete information.

SSRIs should not be administered with MAOIs. A wash-out period of about four weeks should be allowed before switching from one class of drugs to the other, five weeks if switching from fluoxetine (Prozac) to an MAOI.

MAOIs have many interactions, however the best known are those with foods containing the amino acid tyramine. These include aged cheese, chianti wine, and many others. Patients and providers should review the MAOI diet restrictions before using or prescribing these drugs. Because of the severity of MAOI interactions, all additions to the patient's drug regimen should be reviewed with care.

Tricyclic compounds have many interactions, and specialized references should be consulted. Specifically, it is best to avoid other drugs with anticholinergic effects. Tricyclics should not be taken with the **antibiotics** grepafloxacin and sprafloxacin, since the combination may cause serious heart arrythmias.

Tricyclic compounds should not be taken with the gastric acid inhibitor cimetidine (Tagamet), since this increases the blood levels of the tricyclic compound. Other acid inhibiting drugs do not share this interaction.

SSRIs interact with a number of other drugs that act on the central nervous system. Care should be used in combining these drugs with major or minor tranquilizers, or with anti-epileptic agents such as phenytoin (Dilantin) or carbamazepine (Tegretol). In 2003, one of the biggest concerns regarding new prescriptions for tricyclic antidepressants was data concerning overdoses from these drugs. Information in Great Britain showed that this class of antidepressants was responsible for more than 90% of all deaths from antidepressant overdose. Physicians were being advised to prescribe SSRIs in new patients, but not to change the course of those who had taken tricyclics for years with success.

Resources

PERIODICALS

"Antidepressant Drugs May Protect Brain from Damage." *Mental Health Weekly Digest* (August 18, 2003): 2.
"FDA Approves Once-daily Supplement." *Biotech Week* (September 24, 2003): 6.
"FDA Panel Urges Stronger Warnings of Child Suicide." *SCRIP World Pharmaceutical News* (February 6, 2004): 24.
"GPs Told Not to Prescribe Tricyclics." *Pulse* (October 13, 2003): 1.
"Late-term Exposure to SSRIs May Cause Neurological Symptoms in Babies." *Drug Week* (August 8, 2003): 255.
"SSRIs Increase the Risk of Upper GI Bleeding." *Psychiatric Times* (July 1, 2003): 75.

Samuel D. Uretsky, PharmD
Teresa G. Odle

Antidepressant drugs, SSRI

Definition

Purpose

SSRIs are prescribed primarily to treat mental depression. Because they are as effective as other types of antidepressants and have less serious side effects, SSRIs have become the most commonly prescribed antidepressants for all age groups, including children and adolescents.

In addition to treating depression, some SSRIs have been approved by the U.S. Food and Drug Administration (FDA) for the treatment of other disorders including:

- obsessive-compulsive disorder (OCD)
- generalized anxiety disorder
- panic disorder
- social **anxiety** disorder or social phobia
- premenstrual dysphoric disorder (PMDD) or **premenstrual syndrome** (PMS)
- post-traumatic **stress** disorder (PTSD)
- **bulimia nervosa**, an eating disorder.

SSRIs often are prescribed for other "off-label" uses including:

- various mental disorders including schizophrenia
- mania
- menopause-related symptoms such as hot flashes
- geriatric depression
- loss of mental abilities in the elderly
- nicotine withdrawal
- **alcoholism**
- premature ejaculation

The advantages of SSRIs over other types of anti-depressants include:

- Most SSRIs can be taken in one daily dose as compared with three to six daily pills.
- Because they lessen cravings for carbohydrates, SSRIs usually do not cause weight gain.
- Since SSRIs do not appear to affect the cardiovascular system, they can be prescribed for people with high blood pressure or heart conditions.
- Since SSRIs are not particularly dangerous even in high doses and are unlikely to cause permanent damage if misused, they may be prescribed for suicidal adults.

SSRIs are mood enhancers only in depressed individuals. They have little effect on people who are not clinically depressed. However some experts believe that SSRIs are over-prescribed and should be reserved for those with major disabling depression.

Description

Types of SSRIs

As of 2005, six brand-name SSRIs and generic equivalents were available in the United States:

- Celexa (citalopram hydrobromide) for treating depression
- Lexapro (escitalopram oxalate) for treating depression and generalized anxiety disorder

- Luvox (fluvoxamine) for treating OCD
- Paxil (paroxetine hydrochloride) for treating depression, generalized anxiety disorder, OCD,

panic disorder, social anxiety disorder, PMDD, and PTSD

- Prozac and Prozac Weekly (fluoxetine) for treating depression, OCD, and bulimia nervosa; marketed as Sarafem for treating PMDD

- Zoloft (sertraline) for treating depression, OCD, panic disorder, social anxiety disorder, PMDD, and PTSD.

When Prozac first became available in 1988, it was hailed as a new wonder drug and quickly became the most popular antidepressant ever prescribed. Many millions of Americans have taken Prozac and more than 70% of them claim to have benefited from it. Within a few years other SSRIs became available and, by 2000, Zoloft prescriptions outnumbered those for Prozac.

Lexapro is the newest SSRI. Celexa and Lexapro are very similar, with chemical structures unrelated to other SSRIs. Celexa is a mixture of two isomers—forms of the same chemical—whereas Lexapro is the active isomer alone. They appear to be highly selective for serotonin, only minimally inhibiting the reuptake of the neurotransmitters norepinephrine and dopamine. Paxil is structurally unrelated to other SSRIs and is more selective for serotonin than Luvox, Prozac, or Zoloft, but less selective than Celexa and Lexapro. Paxil becomes distributed widely throughout body tissues and the CNS, with only 1% remaining in the circulatory system.

Mode of action

Mental depression is believed to be related to the low activity of one or more neurotransmitters in the brain—the chemical messengers that cross the gap or synapse between nerve cells. Although it is not understood exactly how most SSRIs work, they are designed to increase the level of serotonin in the brain. This can reduce the symptoms of depression and other psychological disorders.

Serotonin is released by nerve cells and then—in a process called reuptake—is reabsorbed by the cells to be used again. SSRIs interfere with reuptake by blocking the serotonin reuptake sites on the surfaces of nerve cells, thereby making more serotonin available for brain activity. Paxil inhibits the transporter molecule that moves serotonin back into the cell. SSRIs are said to selectively interfere with the reuptake of serotonin, without affecting the uptake or activities of other neurotransmitters. In contrast, older antidepressants such as **tricyclic antidepressants** and **monoamine oxidase inhibitors** (MAOIs) affect numerous neurotransmitters, brain cell receptors, and brain processes, increasing the likelihood of serious side effects.

However it is becoming clear that the serotonin neurotransmitter system is far more complex and widespread throughout the body than was thought initially. Although serotonin receptors are particularly common in areas of the brain that control emotion, it is known now that there are at least six different types of serotonin receptors that send different signals to different parts of the brain. Serotonin also appears to affect other neurotransmitter systems—including dopamine—to at least some extent. Thus increasing the levels of serotonin may not be the only reason why SSRIs relieve depression.

Effectiveness

SSRIs are not effective for treating anxiety or depression in 20–40% of patients. However some research suggests that the use of SSRIs in the early stages of depression can prevent major **depressive disorders**.

Although different SSRIs appear to be equally effective, individuals respond differently to different SSRIs and side effects may vary. Thus finding the best SSRI for an individual may be a matter of trial-and-error. It usually takes two to four weeks after starting an SSRI before symptoms begin to improve. Luvox may take one to two months for noticeable improvement. Paxil may take as long as several months, although sleeping often improves within one or two weeks of beginning the medication. If there is no response after a few weeks or if side effects occur, the patient may be switched to another SSRI. Prozac is the most commonly prescribed SSRI for children, in part because it is available in liquid form that is easier to swallow.

Although Luvox is the only SSRI that is FDA-approved for use in children—and only for obsessive-compulsive behavior—thousands of young people have been treated with SSRIs for:

- depression

- anxiety

- OCD

- panic

- attention deficit/hyperactivity disorder (ADHD)

A 2004 study found that among depressed adolescents, 60% improved with Prozac alone, whereas 75% reported improvement with Prozac combined with cognitive behavioral therapy.

SSRIs sometimes are prescribed to relieve depression accompanying alcoholism. A recent study found that, although type A alcoholics responded to Zoloft in conjunction with a 12-step individual therapy program, type B alcoholics—those with the most severe drinking problems—did not benefit from Zoloft and, in some cases, increased their alcohol intake.

Recommended dosage

Usually SSRIs are started with a low dosage that may be gradually increased. In older adults SSRIs remain in the body longer than in younger adults. The blood levels of Paxil can be 70–80% higher in the elderly as compared with younger patients. Therefore lower doses usually are prescribed for older people. Older patients with other medical conditions or who are taking many different drugs also may need smaller or less frequent doses. The dosage of an SSRI also varies according to the individual and the condition that is being treated. SSRIs may be taken with or without food, on a full or empty stomach. However taking SSRIs with food or drink may lessen side effects such as stomach upset or **nausea**.

Celexa is supplied as tablets or as an oral solution equivalent to 2 mg per ml (0.03 oz.), taken once per day in the morning or evening:

- adults: 20 mg per day, increasing to 40 mg if necessary, to a maximum of 60 mg per day
- older adults: 20 mg per day to a maximum of 40 mg

Lexapro is supplied as 5-, 10-, or 20-mg tablets or as a 1 mg per ml (0.03 oz.) liquid. The recommended dose is 10 mg per day, with a possible increase to 20 mg per day after at least one week.

Average dosages of Luvox for treating OCD and depression are:

- adults: one 50-mg tablet at bedtime; may be increased up to a maximum of 300 mg daily; dosages of more than 100 mg per day should be divided into two doses, one taken in the evening and one in the morning
- children aged 8–17: initially one 25-mg tablet at bedtime; may be gradually increased by 25 mg per day every four to seven days, up to a maximum of 200 mg per day; daily dosages of more than 50 mg should be divided into two daily doses.

Average doses of Paxil for treating depression are:

- adults: 20 mg (10 ml, 0.3 oz.) of oral suspension, one 20-mg tablet, or one 25-mg extended-release tablet, once a day in the morning, increased by 10 mg per week to a maximum of 50 mg—25 ml (0.75 oz.) of oral suspension—or a 62.5-mg extended-release tablet

- older adults: 10 mg (5 ml, 0.15 oz.) of oral suspension or a 10-mg tablet daily, increased to a maximum of 40 mg (20 ml, 0.6 oz.); one 12.5-mg extended-release tablet daily, increased to a maximum of 50 mg

Because of its sedating effect, Paxil may be taken in the evening rather than in the morning as usually recommended. Oral suspensions need to be shaken well before measuring with a small measuring cup or measuring spoon. Extended-release tablets should be swallowed whole, not broken or chewed. Dosages may be different for treating disorders other than depression.

Typical dosages of Prozac are:

- one 10–20-mg daily capsule or solution taken in the morning; increased up to as much as 40 mg daily if there is no improvement in one month, up to an 80-mg maximum
- one 90-mg capsule per week of Prozac Weekly once the depression is under control
- one 20-mg capsule of Sarafem per day, taken in the morning, every day or for only 14 days of a menstrual cycle; maximum of 80 mg per day; Sarafem is supplied in seven-day blister packs to help keep track of the days
- children: initially one 5–10-mg capsule or solution per day.

Zoloft is available as capsules, oral solutions, or tablets:

- adults: 50 mg daily, taken in the morning or evening, up to a maximum of 200 mg daily for severely depressed individuals
- older adults: 12.5–25 mg per day, taken in the morning or evening; may be increased gradually
- for treating OCD in children aged 6–12: 25 mg per day, taken in the morning or evening; may be increased gradually to a maximum of 200 mg per day
- children aged 13–17: initially 50 mg per day, in the morning or evening, may be increased gradually to a maximum of 200 mg per day.

Zoloft oral concentrate should be mixed with 4 oz (133 ml) of water, ginger ale, lemon-lime soda, lemonade, or orange juice and taken immediately.

Missed doses of SSRIs are handled differently depending on the SSRI and the number of doses per day. An effective SSRI may be prescribed for six months or more. Some experts recommend continuing on the SSRI indefinitely to prevent the recurrence of depression.

Precautions

Medical conditions

Medical conditions that may affect the use or dosage of at least some SSRIs include:

- drug **allergies** or allergies to other substances in medications
- mania
- manic-depressive (bipolar) disorder
- brain disease or mental retardation
- seizures or epilepsy
- Parkinson s disease
- liver or severe kidney disease
- abnormal bleeding problems
- diabetes mellitus
- heart disease
- a recent heart attack
- glaucoma

SSRI use during **pregnancy** may not be safe, particularly during the third trimester. Exposure of fetuses to Celexa and other SSRIs during the late third trimester have led to very serious complications, including serotonin syndrome—a condition in which high serotonin levels cause severe problems. Symptoms in a newborn may be the result of a direct toxic effect of the SSRI or withdrawal from the drug. SSRIs pass into breast milk and may negatively affect a baby.

Suicidal tendencies

A possible link between SSRIs and **suicide** attempts in depressed adults remains controversial. Three studies in early 2005 drew conflicting conclusions concerning an association between suicidal behavior and the use of SSRIs. However a February 2005 study found a close correlation between the dramatic decrease in suicides in the United States and Europe and the introduction of SSRIs.

In October 2004, the FDA concluded that antidepressants, including SSRIs, increased the risk of suicidal thoughts and behaviors in children and adolescents who suffered from depression and other psychiatric disorders. They recommended extreme caution in prescribing SSRIs for children. In the last three months of 2004, SSRI prescriptions for children and adolescents fell by 10%.

Symptoms that may lead to suicidal tendencies can develop very suddenly in children and adolescents taking SSRIs; they may include:

- new or worsening depression
- severe worrying
- irritability
- agitation
- extreme restlessness
- frenzied excitement
- panic attacks
- insomnia
- impulsive behavior
- aggressive behavior
- thinking about, planning, or attempting to harm one's self

Withdrawal

SSRIs remain in the body for some time after the medication is stopped:

- Celexa for at least three days
- Luvox for at least 32 hours
- Paxil for at least 42 hours
- Prozac for up to five weeks
- Zoloft for at least three to five days

SSRIs can cause what the manufacturers refer to as "discontinuation syndrome" when the medication is stopped. Since this occurs most often when the drug is stopped abruptly, usually the dose is gradually reduced before stopping the drug completely. The occurrence of discontinuation syndrome depends on the SSRI, the dosage, and the length of time that the drug was used. Paxil appears to induce more serious withdrawal symptoms than other SSRIs. Symptoms of Paxil withdrawal appear within 1 to 10 days of stopping the drug. Because of its long half-life in the body, Prozac rarely causes withdrawal symptoms, although symptoms have been known to appear within 5 to 42 days of stopping Prozac.

Withdrawal symptoms may include:

- generally feeling sick
- **dry mouth**
- runny nose
- dizziness or lightheadedness
- nausea and vomiting
- diarrhea
- **headache**
- sweating
- muscle **pain**

- weakness or fatigue
- nervousness or anxiety
- restlessness or agitation
- trembling or shaking
- insomnia
- fast heart rate
- breathing difficulties
- chest pain
- confusion

Although withdrawal symptoms usually wear off, in some patients some symptoms appear to continue indefinitely.

Other precautions

Other precautions concerning SSRIs include:

- a 50% chance that an episode of depression will recur at some point after stopping the drug
- a 90% risk of recurrence following two episodes of depression
- reports of patients developing tolerance to an SSRI, requiring increased dosages for effectiveness
- the long-term effects of SSRIs are unknown
- SSRIs are expensive: at least $2–$3 per pill; over $150 for 4 oz. (133 ml) of liquid Prozac
- some insurance plans to not cover mental health medications.

Side effects

Common side effects

The most common side effects of SSRIs include:

- dry mouth
- dizziness
- sour or acid stomach or gas
- heartburn
- decreased appetite
- stomach upset
- nausea
- diarrhea
- sweating
- headache
- weakness or fatigue
- drowsiness

- insomnia
- nervousness or anxiety
- tremors
- sexual problems

Most common side effects disappear as the body adjusts to the drug. Nausea may be relieved by taking the medication with meals or temporarily dividing the dose in half.

Certain side effects occur more frequently depending on the SSRI:

- Side effects of Celexa usually are mild and disappear as the body adjusts.
- Luvox and Zoloft are more likely to cause gastrointestinal upset, including stomach irritation, nausea, and diarrhea.
- Paxil is more likely to cause dry mouth, **constipation**, and drowsiness. Paxil is significantly more sedating than other SSRIs, which may benefit patients with insomnia.
- The most common side effect of Prozac is nausea during the first two weeks on the drug; nervousness and anxiety also are common with Prozac.
- Paxil, Prozac, and Zoloft often reduce appetite.
- Up to 30% of those on Zoloft suffer headaches and 20% suffer from insomnia.

Studies with Luvox have found that children may experience different side effects than adults, the most common being:

- dry mouth
- a stuffy or bloody nose
- sweating
- drowsiness
- restlessness
- muscle twitching or tics
- tremors
- thinning hair
- abnormal thinking

Sexual side effects

Any SSRI can affect sexual interest or performance. Side effects include increased or, more often, decreased sexual interest, difficulty reaching orgasm or ejaculation, and **impotence**.

Although manufacturers initially reported that sexual problems were very rare side effects of SSRIs, most patients in clinical trials were never asked specifically about sex and were reluctant to raise the issue. After a few years it became apparent that sexual problems were commonplace among SSRI users, affecting as many as 70%. Among men taking Paxil, 23% report problems with ejaculation. Between 40% and 70% of those taking Prozac report negative sexual side effects, especially loss of interest.

Less common or rare side effects

Less common—but potentially serious—side effects of at least some SSRIs may include:

- flu-like symptoms
- sneezing
- nasal congestion or a runny nose
- sore throat
- skin rash
- itching or **tingling**, burning, or prickling of the skin
- fever
- chills
- body aches or pain
- muscle or joint pain
- abdominal cramps or pain
- vomiting
- decreased or increased appetite
- weight loss
- weight gain, especially after a year on an SSRI
- mouth watering
- increased frequency or amount of urination
- constipation
- menstrual changes or pain
- chest congestion or pain
- difficulty breathing
- taste changes, including a metallic taste in the mouth
- blurred vision or other visual changes
- loss of voice
- teeth grinding
- trembling or shaking
- hair loss
- sensitivity to sunlight
- anxiety or agitation
- abnormal dreams
- confusion

- lack of emotion, apathy
- memory loss

Rare side effects that may occur with some SSRIs include:

- symptoms of low blood sugar or sodium
- bleeding gums or nosebleeds
- unusual bruising
- irregular or slow heartbeat (less than 50 beats per minute)
- fainting
- painful urination or other difficulties with urination
- purple or red spots on the skin
- skin conditions
- red or irritated eyes
- inability to move the eyes
- swelling of the face, ankles, or hands
- increased or decreased body movements
- clumsiness
- tics or other sudden or unusual body or facial movements or postures
- changes in the breasts, including leakage of milk
- seizures
- irritability
- increased depression
- mood or mental changes
- abnormal behaviors
- difficulty concentrating
- lethargy or stupor
- hallucinations
- suicidal thoughts or tendencies

Various other SSRI side effects have been observed in clinical practice although their incidence is not known.

Symptoms of overdose

Although overdose rarely occurs with SSRIs, symptoms include two or more severe side effects occurring together. More common symptoms of SSRI overdose include:

- flushing of the face
- enlarged pupils
- fast heart rate
- upset stomach

- nausea and vomiting
- sweating
- dizziness
- irritability
- drowsiness
- insomnia
- trembling or shaking

Rare symptoms of SSRI overdose include:

- deep or fast breathing with dizziness
- fainting
- muscle pain
- weakness
- difficulty urinating
- bluish skin or lips
- fast, slow, or irregular heartbeat
- low blood pressure
- confusion
- memory loss
- seizures
- coma

Interactions

SSRIs interact with many other drugs, often in similar ways. Alcohol may increase SSRI-induced drowsiness and should not be used when taking some SSRIs. Luvox appears to cause the most serious **drug interactions**, whereas Celexa has relatively few interactions. A combination of Luvox and Clozaril can cause low blood pressure and seizures.

The interaction of SSRIs with MAOIs can be fatal. In addition to antidepressant MAOIs, the antibiotic linezolid (Zyvox) is an MAOI. There must be at least a two-week interval between stopping one drug and starting the other. There should be at least a three-week interval between an MAOI and either Paxil or Zoloft, if either type of antidepressant was taken for more than three months. Because of its long half-life in the body, it is necessary to wait five to six weeks after stopping Prozac before starting on an MAOI.

Some of the drugs that can interact negatively with SSRIs include:

- other antidepressants
- antihistamines

- various medications for anxiety, mental illness, or seizures
- sedatives and tranquilizers
- sleeping pills
- St. John's wort

Drugs that may cause severe heart problems if taken in conjunction with some SSRIs include:

- astemizole (Hismanal)
- cisapride (Propulsid)
- terfenadine (Seldane)
- thioridazine (Mellaril), which should not be taken for at least five weeks after stopping Prozac

Drugs that may affect the blood levels of an SSRI or the length of time that an SSRI remains in the body include:

- antifungal drugs
- cimetidine (Tagamet)
- erythromycin
- tricyclic antidepressants
- Dilantin and phenobarbitol, which may decrease the blood levels of Paxil

Some SSRIs may cause higher blood levels of other medications including:

- alprazolam (Xanax and others)
- anticoagulants or blood-thinners such as warfarin (Coumadin)—SSRIs can increase warfarin blood levels dramatically
- aspirin and other **nonsteroidal anti-inflammatory drugs** (NSAIDs) including ibuprofen and naproxen
- caffeine
- carbamazepine (Tegretol)
- diazepam (Valium)
- digitalis glycosides (heart medicines)
- lithium
- methadone
- phenytoin (Dilantin and others)
- propanolol (Ineral and others)
- theophylline or theophylline-containing drugs
- triazolam (Halcion and others)
- tricyclic antidepressants

Serotonin syndrome

Rarely, some drugs may interact with an SSRI to cause serotonin syndrome including:

- buspirone (BuSpar)
- bromocriptine (Parlodel)
- dextromethorphan (**cough** medicine such as Robitussin DM)
- levodopa (Sinemet)
- lithium (Eskalith)
- meperidine (Demerol)
- moclobemide (Manerex)
- nefazodone (Serzone)
- pentazocine (Talwin)
- other SSRIs
- street drugs
- sumatriptan (Imitrex)
- tramadol (Ultram)
- trazodone (Desyrel)
- tryptophan
- venlafaxine (Effexor)

Serotonin syndrome may occur shortly after the dose of a drug is increased.

Serotonin syndrome may be suspected when at least three of the following symptoms occur together:

- diarrhea
- fever
- shivering
- sweating
- restlessness
- agitation
- uncontrollable excitement
- poor coordination
- twitching
- trembling or shaking
- rigidity
- confusion
- mental changes
- fluctuating vital signs

Combined treatments

Increasingly physicians are combining an SSRI with other medications, either to increase effectiveness or to counteract side effects. Prozac sometimes is prescribed along with:

- an anti-anxiety drug such as Valium (diazepam)
- Desyrel (trazodone), a different type of antidepressant, for patients with insomnia
- lithium

Resources

BOOKS

Glenmullen, Joseph. *Prozac Backlash: Overcoming the Dangers of Prozac, Zoloft, Paxil, and Other Antidepressants with Safe, Effective Alternatives.* New York: Simon & Schuster, 2000.

Preskorn, Sheldon H., and Renato D. Alarcón, editors. *Antidepressants: Past, Present, and Future.* New York: Springer, 2004.

Trigoboff, Eileen. *Psychiatric Drug Guide.* Upper Saddle River, NJ: Pearson/Prentice Hall, 2005.

PERIODICALS

Jonsson, Patrik. "Zoloft Defense Tests Whether Pills Are Guilty; A Murder Trial Highlights Evolving Legal Debate Over Whether Antidepressants Limit Personal Accountability." *Christian Science Monitor* February 11, 2005: 3.

Sanz, Emilio J., et al. "Selective Serotonin Reuptake Inhibitors in Pregnant Women and Neonatal Withdrawal Syndrome: A Database Analysis." *Lancet* 365, no. 9458 (February 5, 2005): 482–7.

Treatment for Adolescents With Depression Study (TADS) Team. "Fluoxetine, Cognitive-Behavioral Therapy, and Their Combination for Adolescents with Depression." *Journal of the American Medical Association* 292, no. 7 (August 18, 2004): 807–20.

Whittington, Craig, J., et al. "Selective Serotonin Reuptake Inhibitors in Childhood Depression: Systematic Review of Published Versus Unpublished Data." *Lancet* 363, no. 9418 (April 24, 2004): 1341–5.

ORGANIZATIONS

National Institute of Mental Health. Office of Communications, 6001 Executive Boulevard, Room 8184, MSC 9663, Bethesda, MD 20892-9663. 866-615-6464. 301-443-4513. <http://www.nimh.nih.gov>.

U.S. Food and Drug Administration. 5600 Fishers Lane, Rockville, MD 20857-0001. 1-888-INFO-FDA (1-888-463-6332). <http://www.fda.gov>.

OTHER

CelexaTM. Forest Pharmaceuticals, Inc. January 2004 [cited March 6, 2005]. <http://www.fda.gov/medwatch/SAFETY/2004/apr_PI/Celexa_annotated_PI.pdf>.

Edelson, Ed. "Suicide Risk from Antidepressants Remains Unclear." *HealthDayNews*. National Health Information Center, U.S. Department of Health and Human Services. February 17, 2005 [cited March 6, 2005]. < http://www.healthfinder.gov/news/newsstory.asp?docid = 524064 > .

LexaproTM. Forest Pharmaceuticals, Inc. December 2003 [cited March 6, 2005]. < http://www.fda.gov/cder/foi/label/2003/21323se1-003,se8-007,21365se8-001,sc1-004_lexapro_lbl.pdf > .

Medications. National Institute of Mental Health. April 9, 2004 [cited March 13, 2005]. < http://www.nimh.nih.gov/publicat/medicate.cfm > .

Mundell, E. J. "Study: Benefits of Antidepressants Outweigh Risks." *HealthDayNews*. National Health Information Center, U.S. Department of Health and Human Services. February 2, 2005 [cited March 25, 2005]. < http://www.healthfinder.gov/news/newsstory.asp?docid = 523762 > .

Turkington, Carol, and Eliot F. Kaplan. *Selective Serotonin Reuptake Inhibitors (SSRIs)*. WebMD Medical Reference. 2001 [cited March 23, 2005]. < http://my.webmd.com/content/Article/87/99352.htm > .

Margaret Alic, Ph.D.

Antidepressants, tricyclic

Definition

Tricyclic antidepressants are medicines that relieve mental depression.

Purpose

Since their discovery in the 1950s, tricyclic antidepressants have been used to treat mental depression. Like other **antidepressant drugs**, they reduce symptoms such as extreme sadness, hopelessness, and lack of energy. Some tricyclic antidepressants are also used to treat bulimia, **cocaine** withdrawal, **panic disorder**, obsessive-compulsive disorders, certain types of chronic **pain**, and **bed-wetting** in children.

Description

Named for their three-ring chemical structure, tricyclic antidepressants work by correcting chemical imbalances in the brain. But because they also affect other chemicals throughout the body, these drugs may produce many unwanted side effects.

Tricyclic antidepressants are available only with a physician's prescription and are sold in tablet, capsule, liquid, and injectable forms. Some commonly used tricyclic antidepressants are amitriptyline (Elavil), desipramine (Norpramin), imipramine (Tofranil), nortriptyline (Pamelor), and protriptyline (Vivactil). Different drugs in this family have different effects, and physicians can choose the drug that best fits the patient's symptoms. For example, a physician might prescribe Elavil for a person with depression who has trouble sleeping, because this drug is more likely to make people feel calm and sleepy. Other tricyclic antidepressants might be more appropriate for depressed people with low energy.

Recommended dosage

The recommended dosage depends on many factors, including the patient's age, weight, general health and symptoms. The type of tricyclic antidepressant and its strength also must be considered. Check with the physician who prescribed the drug or the pharmacist who filled the prescription for the correct dosage.

Always take tricyclic antidepressants exactly as directed. Never take larger or more frequent doses, and do not take the drug for longer than directed. Do not stop taking the medicine just because it does not seem to be working. Several weeks may be needed for its effects to be felt. Visit the physician as often as recommended so that the physician can check to see if the drug is working and to note for side effects.

Do not stop taking this medicine suddenly after taking it for several weeks or more. Gradually tapering the dose may be necessary to reduce the chance of withdrawal symptoms.

Taking this medicine with food may prevent upset stomach.

Precautions

The effects of this medicine may continue for three to seven days after patients stop taking it. All precautions should be observed during this period, as well as throughout treatment with tricyclic antidepressants.

Some people feel drowsy, dizzy, or lightheaded, when taking these drugs. The drugs may also cause blurred vision. Anyone who takes these drugs should not drive, use machines or do anything else that might be dangerous until they have found out how the drugs affect them.

Because tricyclic antidepressants work on the central nervous system, they may add to the effects of alcohol and other drugs that cause drowsiness, such as **antihistamines**, cold medicine, allergy medicine,

KEY TERMS

Asthma—A disease in which the air passages of the lungs become inflamed and narrowed.

Bulimia—An eating disorder in which a person binges on food and then induces vomiting, uses laxatives, or goes without food for some time.

Chronic—A word used to describe a long-lasting condition. Chronic conditions often develop gradually and involve slow changes.

Delusion—An abnormal mental state characterized by the acceptance of something as true that is actually false or unreal, such as the belief that one is Jesus Christ.

Depression—A mental condition in which a person feels extremely sad and loses interest in life. A person with depression may also have sleep problems and loss of appetite and may have trouble concentrating and carrying out everyday activities.

Glaucoma—A condition in which pressure in the eye is abnormally high. If not treated, glaucoma may lead to blindness.

Hallucination—A false or distorted perception of objects, sounds, or events that seems real. Hallucinations usually result from drugs or mental disorders.

Obsessive-compulsive disorder—An anxiety disorder in which a person cannot prevent himself from dwelling on unwanted thoughts, acting on urges, or performing repetitious rituals, such as washing his hands or checking to make sure he turned off the lights.

Panic disorder—An disorder in which a person has sudden and intense attacks of anxiety in certain situations. Symptoms such as shortness of breath, sweating, dizziness, chest pain, and extreme fear often accompany the attacks.

Prostate—A donut-shaped gland in males below the bladder that contributes to the production of semen.

Schizophrenia—A severe mental disorder in which a person loses touch with reality and may have illogical thoughts, delusions, hallucinations, behavioral problems and other disturbances.

Seizure—A sudden attack, spasm, or convulsion.

Serotonin—A natural chemical found in the brain and other parts of the body, that carries signals between nerve cells.

Withdrawal symptoms—A group of physical or mental symptoms that may occur when a person suddenly stops using a drug to which he or she has become dependent.

sleep aids, medicine for seizures, tranquilizers, some pain relievers, and **muscle relaxants**. Anyone taking tricyclic antidepressants should check with his or her physician before drinking alcohol or taking any drugs that cause drowsiness.

These medicines make some people feel lightheaded, dizzy, or faint when they get up after sitting or lying down. To lessen the problem, get up gradually and hold onto something for support if possible.

Tricyclic antidepressants may interact with medicines used during surgery, dental procedures, or emergency treatment. These interactions could increase the chance of side effects. Anyone who is taking tricyclic antidepressants should be sure to tell the health care professional in charge before having any surgical or dental procedures or receiving emergency treatment.

These drugs may also change the results of medical tests. Before having medical tests, anyone taking this medicine should alert the health care professional in charge.

This medicine may increase sensitivity to sunlight. Even brief exposure to sun can cause a severe **sunburn** or a rash. While being treated with this tricyclic antidepressants, avoid being in direct sunlight, especially between 10 A.M. and 3 P.M.; wear a hat and tightly woven clothing that covers the arms and legs; use a sunscreen with a skin protection factor (SPF) of at least 15; protect the lips with a sun block lipstick; and do not use tanning beds, tanning booths, or sunlamps.

Tricyclic antidepressants may cause **dry mouth**. To temporarily relieve the discomfort, chew sugarless gum, suck on sugarless candy or ice chips, or use saliva substitutes, which come in liquid and tablet forms and are available without a prescription.

Children and older people are especially sensitive to the effects of tricyclic antidepressants. This increased sensitivity may increase the chance of side effects.

Special conditions

People with certain medical conditions or who are taking certain other medicines can have problems if they take tricyclic antidepressants. Before taking these drugs, be sure to let the physician know about any of these conditions:

ALLERGIES. Anyone who has had unusual reactions to tricyclic antidepressants or to carbamazepine (Tegretol), maprotiline (Ludiomil), or trazodone (Desyrel) in the past should let his or her physician know before taking tricyclic antidepressants. The physician should also be told about any **allergies** to foods, dyes, preservatives, or other substances.

PREGNANCY. Problems have been reported in babies whose mothers took tricyclic antidepressants just before delivery. Women who are pregnant or who may become pregnant should check with their physicians about the safety of using tricyclic antidepressants.

BREASTFEEDING. Tricyclic antidepressants pass into breast milk and may cause drowsiness in nursing babies whose mothers take the drugs. Women who are breastfeeding should check with their physicians before using tricyclic antidepressants.

DIABETES. Tricyclic antidepressants may affect blood sugar levels. Diabetic patients who notice changes in blood or urine test results while taking this medicine should check with their physicians.

OTHER MEDICAL CONDITIONS. Before using tricyclic antidepressants, people with any of these medical problems should make sure their physicians are aware of their conditions:

- current or past alcohol or drug **abuse**
- bipolar disorder (manic-depressive illness)
- schizophrenia
- seizures (convulsions)
- heart disease
- high blood pressure
- kidney disease
- liver disease
- overactive thyroid
- stomach or intestinal problems
- enlarged prostate
- problems urinating
- **glaucoma**
- **asthma**

USE OF CERTAIN MEDICINES. Taking tricyclic antidepressants with certain other drugs may affect the way the drugs work or may increase the chance of side effects.

Side effects

The most common side effects are **dizziness**, drowsiness, dry mouth, unpleasant taste, **headache**, **nausea**, mild tiredness or weakness, increased appetite or craving for sweets, and weight gain. These problems usually go away as the body adjusts to the drug and do not require medical treatment. Less common side effects, such as **diarrhea**, **vomiting**, sleep problems, sweating, and **heartburn** also may occur and do not need medical attention unless they do not go away or they interfere with normal activities.

More serious side effects are not common, but may occur. If any of the following side effects occur, check with the physician who prescribed the medicine as soon as possible:

- blurred vision
- eye pain
- confusion
- **hallucinations**
- fainting
- loss of balance
- swallowing problems
- difficulty speaking
- mask-like face
- shakiness or trembling
- nervousness or restlessness
- movement problems, such as shuffling walk, stiff arms and legs, or slow movement
- decreased sexual ability
- fast or irregular heartbeat
- constipation
- problems urinating

Some side effects may continue after treatment with tricyclic antidepressants has ended. Check with a physician if these symptoms occur:

- headache
- nausea, vomiting, or diarrhea
- sleep problems, including vivid dreams
- unusual excitement, restlessness, or irritability

Interactions

Life-threatening reactions, such as extrememly high blood pressure, may occur when tricyclic antidepressants are taken with other antidepressants called monoamine oxidase (MAO) inhibitors (such as Nardil and Parnate). *Do not take tricyclic antidepressants within 2 weeks of taking a MAO inhibitor. However, a patient can take an MAO inhibitor immediately after tricyclic antidepressant therapy is stopped by the physician.*

Tricyclic antidepressants may interact with many other medicines. When this happens, the effects of one or both of the drugs may change or the risk of side effects may be greater. Anyone who takes tricyclic antidepressants should let the physician know all other medicines he or she is taking. Among the drugs that may interact with tricyclic antidepressants are:

- Central nervous system (CNS) depressants such as medicine for allergies, colds, hay **fever**, and asthma; sedatives; tranquilizers; prescription pain medicine; muscle relaxants; medicine for seizures; sleep aids; **barbiturates**; and anesthetics.

- diet pills

- amphetamines

- blood thinning drugs

- medicine for overactive thyroid

- cimetidine (Tagamet)

- other antidepressant drugs, including MAO inhibitors (such as Nardil and Parnate) and antidepressants that raise serotonin levels (such as Prozac and Zoloft)

- blood pressure medicines such as clonidine (Catapres) and guanethidine monosulfate (Ismelin)

- disulfiram (Antabuse), used to treat alcohol abuse

- major tranquilizers such as thioridazine (Mellaril) and chlorpromazine (Thorazine)

- antianxiety drugs such as chlordiazepoxide (Librium) and alprazolam (Xanax)

- antiseizure medicines such as carbamazaepine (Tegretol) and phenytoin (Dilantin)

The list above does not include every drug that may interact with tricyclic antidepressants. Be sure to check with a physician or pharmacist before combining tricyclic antidepressants with any other prescription or nonprescription (over-the-counter) medicine.

Nancy Ross-Flanigan

Antidiabetic drugs

Definition

Antidiabetic drugs are medicines that help control blood sugar levels in people with **diabetes mellitus** (sugar diabetes).

Purpose

Diabetes may be divided into type I and type II, formerly termed juvenile onset or insulin-dependent, and maturity onset or non insulin-dependent. Type I is caused by a deficiency of insulin production, while type II is characterized by **insulin resistance**.

Treatment of type I diabetes is limited to insulin replacement, while type II diabetes is treatable by a number of therapeutic approaches. Many cases of insulin resistance are asymptomatic due to normal increases in insulin secretion, and others may be controlled by diet and **exercise**. Drug therapy may be directed toward increasing insulin secretion, increasing insulin sensitivity, or increasing insulin penetration of the cells.

Description

Antidiabetic drugs may be subdivided into six groups: insulin, sufonylureas, alpha-glucosidase inhibitors, biguanides, meglitinides, and thiazolidinediones.

Insulin (Humulin, Novolin) is the hormone responsible for glucose utilization. It is effective in both types of diabetes, since, even in insulin resistance, some sensitivity remains and the condition can be treated with larger doses of insulin. Most insulins are now produced by recombinant DNA techniques, and are chemically identical to natural human insulin. Isophane insulin suspension, insulin zinc suspension, and other formulations are intended to extend the duration of insulin action, and permit glucose control over longer periods of time. In 2003, research suggested that inhaled forms of insulin offered advantages to injected types, but further study was needed on its long-term effects on the lungs and cost-effectiveness.

Sulfonylureas (chlorpropamide [Diabinese], tolazamide [Tolinase], glipizide [Glucotrol] and others) act by increasing insulin release from the beta cells of the pancrease. Glimepiride (Amaryl), a member of this class, appears to have a useful secondary action in increasing insulin sensitivity in peripheral cells.

Alpha-glucosidase inhibitors (acarbose [Precose], miglitol [Glyset]) do not enhance insulin secretion. Rather, they inhibit the conversion of disaccharides and complex carbohydrates to glucose. This mechanism does not prevent conversion, but only delays it, reducing the peak blood glucose levels. Alpha-glucosidase inhibitors are useful for either monotherapy or in combination therapy with sulfonylureas or other hypoglycemic agents.

Metformin (Glucophage) is the only available member of the biguanide class. Metformin decreases hepatic (liver) glucose production, decreases intestinal absorption of glucose and increases peripheral glucose uptake and use. Metformin may be used as monotherapy (alone), or in combination therapy with a sulfonylurea.

There are two members of the meglitinide class: repaglinide (Prandin) and nateglitinide (Starlix). The mechanism of action of the meglitinides is to stimulate insulin production. This activity is both dose dependent and dependent on the presence of glucose, so that the drugs have reduced effectiveness in the presence of low blood glucose levels. The meglitinides may be used alone, or in combination with metformin. The manufacturer warns that nateglitinide should not be used in combination with other drugs that enhance insulin secretion.

Rosiglitazone (Avandia) and pioglitazone (Actos) are members of the thiazolidinedione class. They act by both reducing glucose production in the liver, and increasing insulin dependent glucose uptake in muscle cells. They do not increase insulin production. These drugs may be used in combination with metformin or a sulfonylurea.

Recommended dosage

Dosage must be highly individualized for all antidiabetic agents and is based on blood glucose levels which must be taken regularly. Patients should review specific literature that comes with antidiabetic medications for complete dosage information.

Precautions

Insulin. The greatest short term risk of insulin is **hypoglycemia**, which may be the result of either a direct overdose or an imbalance between insulin injection and level of exercise and diet. This also may occur in the presence of other conditions which reduce the glucose load, such as illness with **vomiting** and diarrhea. Treatment is with glucose in the form of glucose tablets or liquid, although severe cases may require intravenous therapy. Allergic reactions and skin reactions also may occur. Insulin is classified as category B in **pregnancy**, and is considered the drug of choice for glucose control during pregnancy. Insulin glargine (Lantus), an insulin analog which is suitable for once-daily dosing, is classified as category C, because there have been reported changes in the hearts of newborns in animal studies of this drug. The reports are essentially anecdotal, and no cause and effect relationship has been determined. Insulin is not recommended during breast feeding because either low or high doses of insulin may inhibit milk production. Insulin administered orally is destroyed in the GI tract, and represents no risk to the newborn.

Sulonylureas. All sulfonylurea drugs may cause hypoglycemia. Most patients become resistant to these drugs over time, and may require either dose adjustments or a switch to insulin. The list of adverse reactions is extensive, and includes central nervous system problems and skin reactions, among others. Hematologic reactions, although rare, may be severe and include **aplastic anemia** and **hemolytic anemia**. The administration of oral hypoglycemic drugs has been associated with increased cardiovascular mortality as compared with treatment with diet alone or diet plus insulin. The sulfonylureas are classified as category C during pregnancy, based on animal studies, although glyburide has not shown any harm to the fetus and is classified as category B. Because there may be significant alterations in blood glucose levels during pregnancy, it is recommended that patients be switched to insulin. These drugs have not been fully studied during breast feeding, but it is recommended that because their presence in breast milk might cause hypoglycemia in the newborn, breast feeding be avoided while taking sulfonylureas.

Alpha-glucosidase inhibitors are generally well tolerated, and do not cause hypoglycemia. The most common adverse effects are gastrointestinal problems, including flatulence, diarrhea, and abdominal **pain**.

These drugs are classified as category B in pregnancy. Although there is no evidence that the drugs are harmful to the fetus, it is important that rigid blood glucose control be maintained during pregnancy, and pregnant women should be switched to insulin. Alpha-glucosidase inhibitors may be excreted in small amounts in breast milk, and it is recommended that the drugs not be administered to nursing mothers.

Metformin causes gastrointestinal (stomach and digestive) reactions in about a third of patients. A rare, but very serious, reaction to metformin is lactic acidosis, which is fatal in about 50% of cases. Lactic acidosis occurs in patients with multiple medical problems, including renal (kidney-related) insufficiency. The risk may be reduced with careful renal monitoring, and careful dose adjustments to metformin. Metformin is category B during pregnancy. There have been no carefully controlled studies of the drug during pregnancy, but there is no evidence of fetal harm from animal studies. It is important that rigid blood glucose control be maintained during pregnancy, and pregnant women should be switched to insulin. Animal studies show that metformin is excreted in milk. It is recommended that metformin not be administered to nursing mothers.

Meglitinides. These drugs are generally well tolerated, with an adverse event profile similar to placebo. The drugs are classified as category C during pregnancy, based on fetal abnormalities in rabbits given about 40 times the normal human dose. It is important that rigid blood glucose control be maintained during pregnancy, and pregnant women should be switched to insulin. It is not known whether the meglitinides are excreted in human milk, but it is recommended that these drugs not be given to nursing mothers.

Thiazolidinediones. These drugs were generally well tolerated in early trials, but they are structurally related to an earlier drug, troglitazone, which was associated with liver function problems. However, in 2003, researchers reported that these drugs, which are used by more than 6 million Americans, may lead to serious side effects. Research showed that after one to 16 months of therapy with pioglitazone or rosiglitazone, some patients developed serious **edema** and signs of congestive **heart failure**. Additional studies were underway in late 2003 to determine how these drugs caused fluid build-up and if the symptoms occurred more frequently in certain age groups. The mean age of patients in the 2003 study was 69 years.

It is strongly recommended that all patients treated with pioglitazone or rosiglitazone have regular liver function monitoring. The drugs are classified as pregnancy category C, based on evidence of inhibition of fetal growth in rats given more than four times the normal human dose. It is important that rigid blood glucose control be maintained during pregnancy, and pregnant women should be switched to insulin. It is not known whether the thiazolidinediones are excreted in human milk, however they have been identified in the milk of lactating rats. It is recommended that these drugs not be administered to nursing mothers.

Interactions

The sulfonylureas have a particularly long list of **drug interactions**, several of which may be severe. Patients should review specific literature for these drugs.

The actions of oral hypoglycemic agents may be strengthened by highly protein bound drugs, including NSAIDs, salicylates, **sulfonamides**, chloramphenicol, coumarins, probenecid, MAOIs, and **beta blockers**.

The literature that accompanies each medication should list possible drug-drug or food-drug interactions.

Resources

PERIODICALS

"Inhaled Insulin Means Better Quality of Life." *Health & Medicine Week* (September 16, 2003): 189.

"Two Common Diabetes Drugs May Cause Heart Failure and Fluid Buildup." *Cardiovascular Week* (September 29, 2003): 26.

ORGANIZATIONS

American Diabetes Association. ADA National Service Center, 1660 Duke Street, Alexandria, VA 22314. (800)232-3472. < http://www.diabetes.org >.

National Diabetes Information Clearinghouse. 1 Information Way, Bethesda, MD 20892-3560. (301)654-3327. ndic@info.niddk.nih.gov.

OTHER

National Institute of Diabetes and Digestive and Kidney Diseases. < http://www.niddk.nih.gov >.

Samuel D. Uretsky, PharmD
Teresa G. Odle

Antidiarrheal drugs

Definition

Antidiarrheal drugs are medicines that relieve **diarrhea**.

KEY TERMS

Colitis—Inflammation of the colon (large bowel).

Dehydration—Excessive loss of water from the body.

Enzyme—A type of protein, produced in the body, that brings about or speeds up chemical reactions.

Nutrient—A food substance that provides energy or is necessary for growth and repair. Examples of nutrients are vitamins, minerals, carbohydrates, fats, and proteins.

Purpose

Antidiarrheal drugs help control diarrhea and some of the symptoms that go along with it. An average, healthy person has anywhere from three bowel movements a day to three a week, depending on that person's diet. Normally the stool (the material that is passed in a bowel movement) has a texture something like clay. With diarrhea, bowel movements may be more frequent, and the texture of the stool is thin and sometimes watery.

Diarrhea is not a disease, but a symptom of some other problem. The symptom may be caused by eating or drinking food or water that is contaminated with bacteria, viruses, or parasites, or by eating something that is difficult to digest. People who have trouble digesting lactose (milk sugar), for example, may get diarrhea if they eat dairy products. Some cases of diarrhea are caused by **stress**, while others are brought on by taking certain medicines.

Description

Antidiarrheal drugs work in several ways. The drug loperamide, found in Imodium A-D, for example, slows the passage of stools through the intestines. This allows more time for water and salts in the stools to be absorbed back into the body. Adsorbents, such as attapulgite (found in Kaopectate) pull diarrhea-causing substances from the digestive tract. However, they may also pull out substances that the body needs, such as enzymes and nutrients. Bismuth subsalicylate, the ingredient in Pepto-Bismol, decreases the secretion of fluid into the intestine and inhibits the activity of bacteria. It not only controls diarrhea, but relieves the cramps that often accompany diarrhea.

These medicines come in liquid, tablet, caplet, and chewable tablet forms and can be bought without a physician's prescription.

Recommended dosage

The dose depends on the type of antidiarrheal drug. Read and follow the directions on the product label. For questions about dosage, check with a physician or pharmacist. Never take larger or more frequent doses, and do not take the drug for longer than directed.

Precautions

Diarrhea usually improves within 24-48 hours. If the problem lasts longer or if it keeps coming back, diarrhea could be a sign of a more serious problem. Anyone who has any of the symptoms listed below should get medical attention as soon as possible:

- diarrhea that lasts more than two days or gets worse

- fever

- blood in the stool

- **vomiting**

- cramps or tenderness in the abdomen

- signs of **dehydration**, such as decreased urination, **dizziness** or lightheadedness, **dry mouth**, increased thirst, or wrinkled skin

Do not use antidiarrheal drugs for more than two days unless told to do so by a physician.

Severe, long-lasting diarrhea can lead to dehydration. In such cases, lost fluids and salts, such as calcium, sodium, and potassium, must be replaced.

People older than 60 should not use attapulgite (Kaopectate, Donnagel, Parepectolin), but may use other kinds of antidiarrheal drugs. However, people in this age group may be more likely to have side effects, such as severe **constipation**, from bismuth subsalicylate. Ask the pharmacist for more information.

Bismuth subsalicylate may cause the tongue or the stool to temporarily darken. This is harmless. However, do not confuse this harmless darkening of the stool with the black, tarry stools that are a sign of bleeding in the intestinal tract.

Children with flu or chicken pox should not be given bismuth subsalicylate. It can lead to **Reye's syndrome**, a life-threatening condition that affects the liver and central nervous system. To be safe, never give bismuth subsalicylate to a child under 16 years without consulting a physician. Children may have unpredictable reactions to other antidiarrheal drugs. Loperamide should not be given to children under six years and attapulgite should not be given to children under three years unless directed by a physician.

Anyone who has a history of **liver disease** or who has been taking **antibiotics** should check with his or her physician before taking the antidiarrheal drug loperamide. A physician should also be consulted before anyone with acute **ulcerative colitis** or anyone who has been advised to avoid constipation uses the drug.

Loperamide should not be used by people whose diarrhea is caused by certain infections, such as salmonella or shigella. To be safe, check with a physician before using this drug.

Anyone who has a medical condition that causes weakness should check with a physician about the best way to treat diarrhea.

Special conditions

Before taking antidiarrheal drugs, be sure to let the physician know about any of these conditions:

ALLERGIES. Anyone who has had unusual reactions to **aspirin** or other drugs containing salicylates should check with a physician before taking bismuth subsalicylate. Anyone who has developed a rash or other unusual reactions after taking loperamide should not take that drug again without checking with a physician. The physician should also be told about any **allergies** to foods, dyes, preservatives, or other substances.

PREGNANCY AND BREASTFEEDING. Women who are pregnant or breastfeeding should check with their physicians before using antidiarrheal drugs. They should also ask advice on how to replace lost fluids and salts.

OTHER MEDICAL CONDITIONS. Before using antidiarrheal drugs, people with any of these medical problems should make sure their physicians are aware of their conditions:

• dysentery
• gout
• hemophilia or other bleeding problems
• kidney disease
• stomach ulcer
• severe colitis
• liver disease

USE OF CERTAIN MEDICINES. Taking antidiarrheal drugs with certain other drugs may affect the way the drugs work or may increase the chance of side effects.

Side effects

The most common side effects of attapulgite are constipation, bloating, and fullness. Bismuth subsalicylate may cause ringing in the ears, but that side effect is rare. Possible side effects from loperamide include skin rash, constipation, drowsiness, dizziness, tiredness, dry mouth, **nausea**, vomiting, and swelling, **pain**, and discomfort in the abdomen. Some of these symptoms are the same as those that occur with diarrhea, so it may be difficult to tell if the medicine is causing the problems. Children may be more sensitive than adults to certain side effects of loperamide, such as drowsiness and dizziness.

Other rare side effects may occur with any antidiarrheal medicine. Anyone who has unusual symptoms after taking an antidiarrhea drug should get in touch with his or her physician.

Interactions

Attapulgite can decrease the effectiveness of other medicines taken at the same time. Changing the times at which the other medicines are taken may be necessary. Check with a physician or pharmacist to work out the proper dose schedule.

Bismuth subsalicylate should not be taken with aspirin or any other medicine that contains salicylate. This drug may also interact with other drugs, such as blood thinners (warfarin, for example), methotrexate, the antigout medicine probenecid, and the antidiabetes drug tolbutamide. In addition, bismuth subsalicylate may interact with any drug that interacts with aspirin. Anyone taking these drugs should check with a physician or pharmacist before taking bismuth subsalicylate.

Nancy Ross-Flanigan

Antidiuretic hormone (ADH) test

Definition

Antidiuretic hormone (ADH) test, also called the Vasopressin test, is a test for the antidiuretic hormone, which is released from the pituitary gland and acts on the kidneys to increase their reabsorption of water into the blood.

Purpose

An ADH test is used to aid in the diagnosis of **diabetes insipidus** or the syndrome of inappropriate ADH called SIADH.

KEY TERMS

Diabetes insipidus—A metabolic disorder in which the pituitary gland produces inadequate amounts of antidiuretic hormone (ADH) or the kidneys are unable to respond to release of the hormone. Primary symptoms are excessive urination and constant thirst.

Pituitary gland—The pituitary gland is sometimes referred to as the "master gland." As the most important of the endocrine glands (glands which release hormones directly into the bloodstream), it regulates and controls not only the activities of other endocrine glands but also many body processes.

Precautions

Certain drugs can either increase or decrease ADH levels. Drugs that increase ADH levels include **acetaminophen**, **barbiturates**, cholinergic agents, estrogen, nicotine, oral **hypoglycemia** agents, some **diuretics** (e.g., thiazides), cyclophosphamide, **narcotics**, and **tricyclic antidepressants**. Drugs that decrease ADH levels include alcohol, beta-adrenergic agents, morphine antagonists, and phenytoin (Dilantin).

Description

The purpose of ADH is to control the amount of water reabsorbed by the kidneys. Water is continually being taken into the body in food and drink, as well as being produced by chemical reactions in cells. Water is also continually lost in urine, sweat, feces, and in the breath as water vapor. ADH release helps maintain the optimum amount of water in the body when there is an increase in the concentration of the blood serum or a decrease in blood volume. Physical **stress**, surgery, and high levels of **anxiety** can also stimulate ADH.

Various factors can affect ADH production, thereby disturbing the body's water balance. For example, alcohol consumption reduces ADH production by direct action on the brain, resulting in a temporarily increased production of urine. This may also occur in diabetes insipidus, when the pituitary gland produces insufficient ADH, or rarely, when the kidneys fail to respond to ADH. The reverse effect of water retention can result from temporarily increased ADH production after a major operation or accident. Water retention may also be caused by the secretion of ADH by some tumors, especially of the lung.

Preparation

The test requires collection of a blood sample. The patient must be **fasting** (nothing to eat or drink) for 12 hours, be adequately hydrated, and limit physical activity for 10-12 hours before the test.

Risks

Risks for this test are minimal, but may include slight bleeding from the blood-drawing site, **fainting** or feeling lightheaded after venipuncture, or hematoma (blood accumulating under the puncture site).

Normal results

ADH normal ranges are laboratory-specific but can range from 1-5 pg/ml or 1.5 ng/L (SI units).

Abnormal results

Patients who are dehydrated, who have a decreased amount of blood in the body (hypovolemia), or who are undergoing severe physical stress (e.g., trauma, **pain** or prolonged mechanical ventilation) may exhibit increased ADH levels. Patients who are overly hydrated or who have an increased amount of blood in the body (hypervolemia) may have decreased ADH levels.

Other conditions that cause increased levels include SIADH, central nervous system tumors or infection, or **pneumonia**.

Resources

BOOKS

Pagana, Kathleen Deska. *Mosby's Manual of Diagnostic and Laboratory Tests.* St. Louis: Mosby, Inc., 1998.

Janis O. Flores

Antiemetic drugs *see* **Antinausea drugs**

Antiepileptic drugs *see* **Anticonvulsant drugs**

Antifungal drugs, systemic

Definition

Systemic antifungal drugs are medicines taken by mouth or by injection to treat deep infections caused by a fungus.

KEY TERMS

Elixir—A sweetened liquid that contains alcohol, water, and medicine.

Fetus—A developing baby inside the womb.

Fungus—A unicellular to filamentous organism that causes parasitic infections.

Ointment—A thick substance that contains medicine and is meant to be spread on the skin, or if an ophthalmic ointment, in the eye.

Systemic—A term used to describe a medicine that has effects throughout the body, as opposed to topical drugs that work on the skin. Most medicines that are taken by mouth or by injection are systemic drugs.

Purpose

Systemic antifungal drugs are used to treat infections in various parts of the body that are caused by a fungus. A fungus is an organism that can be either one-celled or filamentous. Unlike a plant, which makes its own food, or an animal, which eats plants or other animals, a fungus survives by invading and living off other living things. Fungi thrive in moist, dark places, including some parts of the body.

Fungal infections can either be systemic, meaning that the infection is deep, or topical (dermatophytic), meaning that the infection is superficial and occurs on the skin. Additionally, yeast infections can affect the mucous membranes of the body. Fungal infections on the skin are usually treated with creams or ointments (**topical antifungal drugs**). However, systemic infections, yeast infections or topical infections that do not clear up after treatment with creams or ointments may need to be treated with systemic antifungal drugs. These drugs are used, for example, to treat common fungal infections such as tinea (**ringworm**), which occurs on the skin or **candidiasis** (a yeast infection, also known as trush), which can occur in the throat, in the vagina, or in other parts of the body. They are also used to treat other deep fungal infections such as **histoplasmosis**, **blastomycosis**, and **aspergillosis**, which can affect the lungs and other organs. They are sometimes used to prevent or treat fungal infections in people whose immune systems are weakened, such as bone marrow or organ transplant patients and people with **AIDS**.

Description

Antifungal drugs are categorized depending on their route or site of action, their mechanism of action and their chemical nature.

Systemic antifungal drugs, such as capsofungin (Cancidas), flucytosine, fluconazole (Diflucan), itraconazole (Sporanox), ketoconazole (Nizoral), and miconazole (Monistat I.V.) are available only by prescription. They are available in tablet, capsule, liquid, and injectable forms.

Recommended dosage

The recommended dosage depends on the type of antifungal drug and the nature and extent of fungal infection being treated. Doses may also be different for different patients. The prescribing physician or the pharmacist can provide dosage information. Systemic antifungal drugs must be taken exactly as directed. Itraconazole and ketoconazole should be taken with food.

Fungal infections can take a long time to clear up, so it may be necessary to take the medication for several months, or even for a year or longer. It is very important to keep taking the medicine for as long as the physician says to take it, even if symptoms seem to improve. If the drug is stopped too soon, the symptoms may return.

Systemic antifungal drugs work best when their amount is kept constant in the body, meaning that they have to be taken regularly, at the same time every day, and without missing any doses.

Patients taking the liquid form of ketoconazole should use a specially marked medicine spoon or other medicine measuring device to make sure they take the correct amount. A regular household teaspoon may not hold the right amount of medicine. Ask the pharmacists about ways to accurately measure the dose of these drugs.

Precautions

If symptoms do not improve within a few weeks, the prescribing physician should be informed.

While taking this medicine, regular medical visits should be scheduled. The physician needs to keep checking for side effects throughout the antifungal therapy.

Some people feel drowsy or dizzy while taking systemic antifungal drugs. Anyone who takes these drugs should not drive, use machines or do anything else that might be dangerous until they have found out how the drugs affect them.

Liver problems, stomach problems and other problems may occur in people who drink alcohol while taking systemic antifungal drugs. Alcohol and prescription or nonprescription (over-the-counter) drugs that contain alcohol should be avoided while taking antifungal drugs. (Medicines that may contain alcohol include some **cough** syrups, tonics, and elixirs.) Alcohol should be avoided for at least a day after taking an antifungal drug.

The antifungal drug ketoconazole may make the eyes unusually sensitive to light. Wearing sunglasses and avoiding exposure to bright light may help.

Special conditions

People with certain medical conditions or who are taking certain other medicines can have problems if they take systemic antifungal drugs. Before taking these drugs, the prescribing physician should be informed about any of the following conditions:

ALLERGIES. Anyone who has had unusual reactions to systemic antifungal drugs in the past should let his or her physician know about the problem before taking the drugs again. The physician should also be told about any **allergies** to foods, dyes, preservatives, or other substances.

PREGNANCY. In laboratory studies of animals, systemic antifungal drugs have caused **birth defects** and other problems in the mother and fetus. Studies have not been done on pregnant women, so it is not known whether these drugs cause similar effects in people. Women who are pregnant or who plan to become pregnant should check with their physicians before taking systemic antifungal drugs. Any woman who becomes pregnant while taking these drugs should let her physician know immediately.

BREASTFEEDING. Systemic antifungal drugs pass into breast milk. Women who are breastfeeding should check with their physicians before using systemic antifungal drugs.

OTHER MEDICAL CONDITIONS. People who have medical conditions that deplete stomach acid (achlorhydria) or decrease stomach acid (hypochlorhydria) should be sure to inform their physicians about their condition before they use a systemic antifungal drug. These drugs are not active in their natural form, but must be converted to the active form by an acid. If these is not enough stomach acid, the drugs will be

ineffective. For people with insufficient stomach acid, it may help to take the medicine with an acidic drink, such as a cola. The patient's health care provider can suggest the best way to take the medicine.

Before using systemic antifungal drugs, people with any of these medical problems should also make sure their physicians are aware of their conditions:

- current or past alcohol **abuse**
- liver disease
- kidney disease

USE OF CERTAIN MEDICINES. Taking systemic antifungal drugs with certain other drugs may affect the way the drugs work or may increase the chance of side effects.

Side effects

Fluconazole

Although rare, severe allergic reactions to this medicine have been reported. Call a physician immediately if any of these symptoms develop after taking fluconazole (Diflucan):

- hives, itching, or swelling
- breathing or swallowing problems
- sudden drop in blood pressure
- diarrhea
- abdominal pain

Ketoconazole

Ketoconazole has caused **anaphylaxis** (a life-threatening allergic reaction) in some people after their first dose. This is a rare reaction.

Systemic antifungal drugs in general

Systemic antifungal drugs may cause serious and possibly life-threatening liver damage. Patients who take these drugs should have **liver function tests** before they start taking the medicine and as often as their physician recommends while they are taking it. The physician should be notified immediately if any of these symptoms develop:

- loss of appetite
- nausea or vomiting
- yellow skin or eyes
- unusual fatigue
- dark urine
- pale stools

The most common minor side effects of systemic antifungal drugs are **constipation**, diarrhea, nausea, vomiting, headache, drowsiness, **dizziness**, and flushing of the face or skin. These problems usually go away as the body adjusts to the drug and do not require medical treatment. Less common side effects, such as menstrual problems in women, breast enlargement in men, and decreased sexual ability in men also may occur and do not need medical attention unless they do not improve in a reasonable amount of time.

More serious side effects are not common, but may occur. If any of the following side effects occur, check with the physician who prescribed the medicine immediately:

- fever and chills
- skin rash or itching
- high blood pressure
- pain, redness, or swelling at site of injection (for injectable miconazole)

Other rare side effects are possible. Anyone who has unusual symptoms after taking systemic antifungal drugs should get in touch with his or her physician.

Interactions

Serious and possibly life-threatening side effects can result if the oral forms of itraconazole or ketoconazole or the injectable form of miconazole are taken with certain drugs. Do not take those types of systemic antifungal drugs with any of the following drugs unless the physician approves of the therapy:

- astemizole (Hismanal)
- cisapride (Propulsid)
- antacids
- theophylline-containing anti-wheezing medications

Taking an acid blocker such as cimetidine (Tagamet), famotidine (Pepcid), nizatidine (Axid), omeprazole (Prilosec), or ranitidine (Zantac) at the same time as a systemic antifungal drug may prevent the antifungal drug from working properly. For best results, take the acid blocker at least 2 hours after taking the antifungal drug.

In addition, systemic antifungal drugs may interact with many other medicines. When this happens, the effects of one or both of the drugs may change or the risk of side effects may be greater. *Anyone who takes systemic antifungal drugs should inform the prescribing physician about all other prescription and nonprescription (over-the-counter) medicines he or she is taking.* Among the drugs that may interact with systemic antifungal drugs are:

- acetaminophen (Tylenol)
- birth control pills
- male hormones (androgens)
- female hormones (estrogens)
- medicine for other types of infections
- antidepressants
- antihistamines
- muscle relaxants
- medicine for diabetes, such as tolbutamide (Orinase), glyburide (DiaBeta), and glipizide (Glucotrol)
- blood-thinning medicine, such as warfarin (Coumadin)

The list above does not include every drug that may interact with systemic antifungal drugs. Be sure to check with a physician or pharmacist before combining systemic antifungal drugs with any other medicine.

Nancy Ross-Flanigan

Antifungal drugs, topical

Definition

Topical antifungal drugs are medicines applied to the skin to treat skin infections caused by a fungus.

Purpose

Dermatologic fungal infections are usually described by their location on the body: tinea pedis (infection of the foot), tinea unguium (infection of the nails), tinia capitis (infection of the scalp.) Three types of fungus are involved in most skin infections: *Trichophyton, Epidermophyton,* and *Microsporum.* Mild infections are usually susceptible to topical therapy, however severe or resistant infections may require systemic treatment.

Description

There are a large number of drugs currently available in topical form for fungal infections. Other than the imidazoles, (miconazole [Micatin, Miconazole], clotrimazole [Lotrimin], econazole [Spectazole], ketoconazole [Nizoral], oxiconazole [Oxistat], sulconazole [Exelderm]) and the

Cream—A spreadable substance, similar to an ointment, but not as thick. Creams may be more appropriate than ointments for application to exposed skin areas such as the face and hands.

Ointment—A thick, spreadable substance that contains medicine and is meant to be used on the skin, or if a vaginal preparation, in the vagina.

Ophthalmic—Pertaining to the eye.

Otic—Pertaining to the ear.

Topical—A term used to describe medicine that has effects only in a specific area, not throughout the body, particularly medicine that is put directly on the skin.

allylamine derivatives (butenafine [Mentax], naftifine [Naftin], terbinafine [Lamisil]), the drugs in this therapeutic class are chemically distinct from each other. All drugs when applied topically have a good margin of safety, and most show a high degree of effectiveness. There are no studies comparing drugs on which to base a recommendation for drugs of choice. Although some of the topical antifungals are available over-the-counter, they may be as effective as prescription drugs for this purpose.

Traditional antifungal drugs such as undecylinic acid (Cruex, Desenex) and gentian violet (also known as crystal violet) remain available, but have a lower cure rate (complete eradication of fungus) than the newer agents and are not recommended. Tolnaftate (Tinactin) has a lower cure rate than the newer drugs, but may be used prophylactically to prevent infection.

Recommended dosage

All drugs are applied topically. Consult individual product information for specific application recommendations.

As with all topical products, selection of the dosage form may be as important as proper drug selection. Consider factors such as presence or absence of hair on the affected area, and type of skin to which the medication is to be applied. Thin liquids may preferable for application to hairy areas, creams for the hands and face, and ointments may be preferable for the trunk and legs. Other dosage forms

available include shampoos and sprays. Ciclopirox and triacetin are available in formulations for topical treatment of nail fungus as well as skin infections (ciclopirox as Penlac Nail Lacquer and triacetin as Ony-Clear Nail).

Most topical antifungal drugs require four weeks of treatment. Infections in some areas, particularly the spaces between toes, may take up to six weeks for cure.

Precautions

Most topical antifungal agents are well tolerated. The most common adverse effects are localized irritation caused by the vehicle or its components. This may include redness, itch, and a burning sensation. Some direct allergic reactions are possible.

Topical antifungal drugs should only be applied in accordance with labeled uses. They are not intended or ophthalmic (eye) or otic (ear) use. Application to mucous membranes should be limited to appropriate formulations.

The antifungal drugs have not been evaluated for safety in **pregnancy** and **lactation** on topical application under the pregnancy risk category system. Although systemic absorption is probably low, review specific references. Gentian violet is labeled with a warning against use in pregnancy.

Interactions

Topical antifungal drugs have no recognized drug-drug or food-drug interactions.

Samuel D. Uretsky, PharmD

Antigas agents

Definition

Antigas agents are medicines that relieve the uncomfortable symptoms of too much gas in the stomach and intestines.

Purpose

Excess gas can build up in the stomach and intestines for a number of reasons. Eating high-fiber foods, such as beans, grains, and vegetables is one cause. Some people unconsciously swallow air when they

KEY TERMS

Digestive tract—The stomach, intestines, and other parts of the body through which food passes.

Diverticulosis—A condition in which the colon (large intestine) develops a number of outpouchings or sacs.

Flatulence—Excess gas in the digestive tract.

Irritable colon—An intestinal disorder often accompanied by abdominal pain and diarrhea.

eat, drink, chew gum, or smoke cigarettes, which can lead to uncomfortable amounts of gas in the digestive system. Surgery and certain medical conditions, such as irritable colon, peptic ulcer, and **diverticulosis**, can also lead to gas build-up. Certain intestinal parasites can contribute to the production of severe gas - these parasites need to be treated separately with special drugs. Abdominal **pain**, pressure, bloating, and flatulence are signs of too much gas. Antigas agents help relieve the symptoms by preventing the formation of gas pockets and breaking up gas that already is trapped in the stomach and intestines.

Description

Antigas agents are sold as capsules, liquids, and tablets (regular and chewable) and can be bought without a physician's prescription. Some commonly used brands are Gas-X, Flatulex, Mylanta Gas Relief, Di-Gel, and Phazyme. The ingredient that helps relieve excess gas is simethicone. Simethicone does not relieve acid **indigestion**, but some products also contain **antacids** for that purpose. Check the label of the product or ask the pharmacist for more information.

Recommended dosage

Check the product container for dosing information. Typically, the doses should be taken after meals and at bedtime. Chewable forms should be chewed thoroughly.

Check with a physician before giving this medicine to children under age 12 years.

Precautions

Some anti-gas medicines may contain sugar, sodium, or other ingredients. Anyone who is on a special diet or is allergic to any foods, dyes, preservatives, or other substances should check with his or her physician or pharmacist before using any of these products.

Anyone who has had unusual reactions to simethicone – the active ingredient in antigas medicines – should check with his or her physician before taking these drugs.

Side effects

No common or serious side effects have been reported in people who use this medicine. However, anyone who has unusual symptoms after taking an antigas agent should get in touch with his or her physician.

Interactions

Antigas agents are not known to interact with any other drugs.

Samuel D. Uretsky, PharmD

Antigastroesophageal reflux drugs

Definition

These drugs are used to treat gastroesophageal reflux, the backward flow of stomach contents into the esophagus.

Purpose

The drug discussed here, cisapride (Propulsid), is used to treat nighttime **heartburn** resulting from gastroesophageal reflux disease (GERD). In this condition, food and stomach juices flow backward from the stomach into the esophagus, the part of the digestive tract through which food passes on its way from the mouth to the stomach. Normally, a muscular ring called the lower esophageal sphincter (LES) opens to allow food into the stomach and then closes to prevent the stomach's contents from flowing back into the esophagus. In people with GERD, this muscular ring is either weak or it relaxes at the wrong times. The main symptom is heartburn – a burning sensation centered behind the breastbone and spreading upward toward the neck and throat.

Cisapride works by strengthening the lower esophageal sphincter and making the stomach empty more quickly. This shortens the amount of time that the esophagus comes in contact with the stomach contents. Other drugs, such as H2-blockers are sometimes prescribed to reduce the amount of acid in the stomach.

Description

Cisapride is available only with a physician's prescription. Cisapride is sold in tablet and liquid forms.

Recommended dosage

The dose depends on the patient. The average dose for adults and children age 12 and over is 5-20 mg taken two to four times a day. The medicine should be taken 15 minutes before meals and at bedtime. For children under 12, the dose is based on body weight and should be determined by the child's physician.

Precautions

This medicine is effective in treating only nighttime heartburn, not daytime heartburn.

Cisapride may increase the effects of alcohol and tranquilizers.

Cisapride has caused dangerous irregular heartbeats in a few people who took it with other medicines. Anyone who takes this drug should let the physician know all other medicines he or she is taking. Patients with heart problems should check with their physicians before taking cisapride.

Anyone who has bleeding, blockage, or leakage in the stomach or intestines should not take cisapride. Cisapride should not be used by anyone who has had an unusual reaction to the drug in the past. In addition, people with any of the following medical problems should make sure their physicians are aware of their conditions:

- Epilepsy or history of seizures
- Kidney disease
- Liver disease.

The effects of taking cisapride during **pregnancy** have not been fully studied. Women who are pregnant or plan to become pregnant should check with their physicians before taking Cisapride. The drug passes into breast milk and may affect nursing babies. Women who are breastfeeding and need to take this medicine should check with their physicians. Avoiding breastfeeding while taking the drug may be necessary.

Side effects

The most common side effects are abdominal **pain**, bloating, gas, **diarrhea**, **constipation**, **nausea**, upper respiratory infections, inflammation of the nasal passages and sinuses, **headache**, and viral infections. Other side effects may occur. Anyone who has unusual or troublesome symptoms after taking this drug should get in touch with his or her physician.

Interactions

Cisapride may interact with a variety of other medicines. When this happens, the effects of one or both of the drugs may change or the risk of side effects may be greater. Anyone who takes Cisapride should let the physician know all other medicines he or she is taking. Among the drugs that may interact with cisapride are:

- Antifungal drugs such as ketoconazole (Nizoral), miconazole (Monistat), and fluconazole (Diflucan)

- Antibiotics such as clarithromycin (Biaxin) and erythromycin (E-Mycin, ERYC)

- Blood-thinners such as warfarin (Coumadin)

- H2-blockers such as cimetidine (Tagamet) and ranitidine (Zantac)

- Tranquilizers such as chlordiazepoxide (Librium), diazepam (Valium), and alprazolam (Xanax).

The list above does not include every drug that may interact with cisapride. Be sure to check with a physician or pharmacist before combining cisapride with any other prescription or nonprescription (over-the-counter) medicine.

Resources

ORGANIZATIONS

National Digestive Diseases Information Clearinghouse. 2 Information Way, Bethesda, MD 20892-3570. (800) 891-5389. < http://www.niddk.nih.gov/health/digest/nddic.htm > .

Pediatric/Adolescent Gastroesophageal Reflux Association, Inc. P.O. Box 1153, Germantown, MD 20875-1153. (301) 601-9541. < http://www.reflux.org > .

OTHER

"GERD Information Center." *Pharmaceutical Information Network*. < http://pharminfo.com/disease/gerd/gerd_info.html > .
GERD Information Resource Center. < http://www.gerd.com > .

Nancy Ross-Flanigan

Antihelminthic drugs

Definition

Antihelminthic drugs are used to treat parasitic infestations.

Purpose

Parasitic infestations are caused by protozoa or worms gaining entry into the body. Most of these organisms cause infections by being ingested in the form of eggs or larvae, usually present on contaminated food or clothing, while others gain entry through skin abrasions. Common parasitic infestations include **amebiasis**, **malaria**, **giardiasis**, hookworm, pinworm, threadworm, whipworm and tapeworm infestations. Once in the body, parasitic worms may go unnoticed if they cause no severe symptoms. However, if they multiply rapidly and spread to a major organ, they can cause very serious and even life-threatening conditions. Antihelminthic drugs are prescribed to treat these infestations. They function either by destroying the worms on contact or by paralyzing them, or by altering the permeability of their plasma membranes. The dead worms then pass out of the body in the feces.

Description

Antihelminthic drugs are available only with a prescription and are available as liquids, tablets or capsules. Some commonly used antihelminthics include: albendazole (Albenza), mebendazole (Vermox), niclosamide (Niclocide), oxamniquine (Vansil), praziquantel (Biltricide), pyrantel (Antiminth), pyantel pamoate (Antiminth) and thiabendazole (Mintezol). Some types of parasitic infestations are rarely seen in the United States, thus, the corresponding antihelminthic drugs are not widely distributed and need to be obtained from the United States Center for Disease Control (CDC) when required. These include for example bitional and ivermectin, used to treat onchocerciasis infestations. Other antihelminthic drugs, such as diethylcarbamazepine citrate (Hetrezan), used for treatment of roundworms and other parasites, is supplied directly by its manufacturer when needed.

Most antihelminthic drugs are only active against specific parasites, some are also toxic. Before treatment, the parasites must therefore be identified using tests that look for parasites, eggs or larvae in feces, urine, blood, sputum, or tissues. Thus, niclosamide is used against tapeworms, but will not be effective for the treatment of pinworm or roundworm infestations, because it acts by inhibiting ATP production in tapeworm cells. Thiabendazole (Mintezole) is the drug usually prescribed for treatment of threadworm, but a similar drug, mebendazole (Vermox) works better on whipworm by disrupting the microtubules of this worm. Praziquantel is another drug that acts by altering the membrane permeability of the worms.

Preparation

Dosage is established depending on the patient's general health status and age, the type of antihelminthic drug used, and the type of parasitic infestation being treated. The number of doses per day, the time between doses, and the length of treatment will also depend on these factors.

Antihelminthic drugs must be taken exactly as directed to completely rid the body of the parasitic infestation, and for as long as directed. A second round of treatment may be required to ensure that the infection has completely cleared.

Precautions

Some antihelminthic drugs work best when ingested along with fatty foods, such as milk or ice cream. Oral drugs should be taken with water during or after meals. The prescribing physician should be informed if the patient has a low-fat or other special diet.

Some antihelminthic drugs, such as praziquantel, come in chewable form. These tablets should not be chewed or kept in the mouth, but should swallowed whole because their bitter taste may cause gagging or **vomiting**.

Antihelminthic drugs sometimes need to be taken with other medications. For example, steroids such as prednisone are also prescribed together with the antihelminthic drug for tapeworm to reduce the inflammation that the worm may cause.

KEY TERMS

Amebiasis—Parasitic infestation caused by amebas, especially by Entamoeba histolytica.

Colitis—Inflammation of the colon (large intestine).

Feces—The solid waste that is left after digestion. Feces form in the intestines and leave the body through the anus.

Flukes—Parasite worms that look like leeches. They usually have one or more suckers for attaching to the digestive mucosa of the host. Liver flukes infest the liver, destroying liver tissue and impairing bile production and drainage.

Giardiasis—Parasitic infestation caused by a flagellate protozoan of the genus Giardia, especially by G. lamblia.

Hallucination—A false or distorted perception of objective reality. Imaginary objects, sounds, and events are perceived as real.

Hookworm—Parasitic intestinal infestation caused by any of several parasitic nematode worms of the family Ancylostomatidae. These worms have strong buccal hooks that attach to the host's intestinal lining.

Larva—The immature, early form of an organism that at birth or hatching is not like its parent and has to undergo metamorphosis before assuming adult features.

Malaria—Disease caused by the presence of sporozoan parasites of the genus Plasmodium in the red blood cells, transmitted by the bite of anopheline mosquitoes, and characterized by severe and recurring attacks of chills and fever).

Microtubules—Slender, elongated anatomical channels in worms.

Nematode—Roundworm.

Organism—A single, independent life form, such as a bacterium, a plant or an animal.

Parasite—An organism that lives in or with another organism, called the host, in parasitism, a type of association characterized by the parasite obtaining benefits from the host, such as food, and the host being injured as a result.

Parasitic—Of, or relating to a parasite.

Pinworm—Enterobius vermicularis, a nematode worm of the family Oxyuridae that causes parasitic infestation of the intestines and cecum. Pinworm is endemic in both temperate and tropical regions and common especially in school age children.

Onchocerciasis—Parasitic infestation caused by filamentous worms of the genus Onchocerca, especially O. volvulus, that is found in tropical America and is transmitted by several types of blackflies.

Protozoan—Any unicellular or multicellular organism containing nuclei and organelles (eukaryotic) of the subkingdom Protozoa.

Roundworm—Any round-bodied unsegmented worm as distinguished from a flatworm. Also called a nematode, they look similar to the common earthworm.

Tapeworm—Flat and very long (up to 30 meters) intestinal parasitic worms, similar to a long piece of tape. Common tapeworms include: T. saginata (beef tapeworm), T. solium (pork tapeworm) D. latum (fish tapeworm), H. Nana (dwarf tapeworm) and E. granulosus (dog tapeworm). General symptoms are vague abdominal discomfort, nausea, vomiting, diarrhea and weight loss.

Threadworm—Any long, thin nematode worm.

Trematode—Any parasitic flatworm of the class Trematoda, as the liver fluke.

Whipworm—A nematode worm of the family Trichuridae with a body that is thick at one end and very long and slender at the other end.

When required, pre- or post-treatment purges are also performed with magnesium or sodium sulfate.

Regular medical visits are recommended for people affected by parasitic infestations. The physician monitors whether the infection is clearing or not and also keeps track of unwanted side effects. The prescribing physician should be informed if symptoms do not disappear or if they get worse.

Hookworm or whipworm infections are also treated with iron supplements along with the antihelminthic prescription.

Some types of parasitic infestations (e.g. pinworms) can be passed from one person to another. It is then often recommended that everyone in the household of an infected person be asked to also take the prescribed antihelminthic drug.

Risks

People with the following medical conditions may have adverse reactions to antihelminthic drugs. The prescribing physician should accordingly be informed if any of these conditions are present:

- **Allergies**. Anyone who has had adverse reactions to antihelminthic drugs should inform the prescribing physician before taking the drugs again. The physician should also be informed about any other pre-existing allergies.

- Ulcers. Antihelminthic drugs are also contraindicated for persons diagnosed with ulcers of the digestive tract, especially **ulcerative colitis**.

- **Pregnancy**. There is research evidence reporting that some antihelminthic drugs cause **birth defects** or **miscarriage** in animal studies. No human birth defects have been reported, but antihelminthic drugs are usually not recommended for use during pregnancy. Pregnant women should accordingly inform the prescribing physician.

- Breastfeeding. Some antihelminthic drugs can pass into breast milk. Breastfeeding may have to be discontinued until the antihelminthic treatment has ended and breastfeeding mothers must also inform the prescribing physician.

- Other risk conditions. Any of the following medical conditions should also be reported to the prescribing physician: **Crohn's disease**, **liver disease**, **kidney disease** and worm cysts in the eyes.

Common side effects of antihelminthic drugs include **dizziness**, drowsiness, **headache**, sweating, dryness of the mouth and eyes, and ringing in the ears. Anyone taking these drugs should accordingly avoid driving, operating machines or other activities that may be dangerous until they know how they are affected by the drugs. Side effects usually wear off as the body adjusts to the drug and do not usually require medical treatment. Thiabendazole may cause the urine to have an unusual odor that can last for a day after the last dose. Other side effects of antihelminthic drugs, such as loss of appetite, **diarrhea**, **nausea**, vomiting, or abdominal cramps are less common. If they occur, they are usually mild and do not require medical attention.

More serious side effects, such as **fever**, chills, confusion, extreme weakness, **hallucinations**, severe diarrhea, nausea or vomiting, skin **rashes**, **low back pain**, dark urine, blurred vision, seizures, and **jaundice** have been reported in some cases. The patient's physician should be informed immediately if any should develop. As a rule, anyone who has unusual symptoms after starting treatment with antihelminthic drugs should notify the prescribing physician.

Antihelminthic drugs may interact with each other or with other drugs, whether prescribed or not. For example, it has been reported that use of the antihelminthic drugs pyrantel and piperazine together lowers the efficiency of pyrantel. Similarly, combining a given antihelminthic drug with another medication may increase the risk of side effects from either drug.

Nancy Ross-Flanigan

Antihemorrhoid drugs

Definition

Antihemorrhoid drugs are medicines that reduce the swelling and relieve the discomfort of **hemorrhoids** (swellings in the area around the anus).

Purpose

Hemorrhoids are bulges in the veins that supply blood to the skin and membranes of the area around the anus. They may form for various reasons. Frequent heavy lifting, sitting for long periods, or straining to have bowel movements may put **stress** on anal tissues, which can lead to hemorrhoids. Some women develop hemorrhoids during **pregnancy** as the expanding uterus puts pressure on the anal tissues. The strain of labor and delivery can also cause hemorrhoids or make existing hemorrhoids worse. Hemorrhoids sometimes result from certain medical problems, such as tumors pressing on the lower bowel.

The main symptoms of hemorrhoids are bleeding from the rectum, especially after a bowel movement, and **itching**, burning, **pain**, and general discomfort in the anal area. Over-the-counter antihemorrhoid products can relieve many of these symptoms. The products contain combinations of four main types of ingredients:

- Local anesthetics, such as benzocaine, lidocaine and tetracaine, to temporarily relieve the pain

- Vasoconstrictors, such as epinephrine base, epinephrine hydrochloride, ephedrine sulfate and phenylephrine hydrochloride that reduce swelling and relieve itching and discomfort by tightening blood vessels

- Astringents (drying agents), such as witch hazel, calamine, and zinc oxide. These help shrink hemorrhoids

KEY TERMS

Anus—The opening at the end of the intestine through which solid waste (stool) passes as it leaves the body.

Rectum—The end of the intestine closest to the anus.

Uterus—A hollow organ in a female in which a fetus develops until birth.

by pulling water out of the swollen tissue. This, in turn, helps relieve itching, burning, and irritation.

- Protectants, such as cocoa butter, lanolin, glycerin, mineral oil, and shark liver oil which soothe irritated tissues and form a protective barrier to prevent further irritation.

Description

Antihemorrhoid drugs are available as creams, ointments and suppositories. Most can be bought without a physician's prescription.

Recommended dosage

Follow package instructions for using these products. Do not use more than the recommended amount of this medicine every day. For explanations or further information about how to use antihemorrhoid drugs, check with a physician or pharmacist.

Precautions

Do not use antihemorrhoid drugs for more than seven days in a row. If the problem gets worse or does not improve, check with a physician.

If rectal bleeding continues, check with a physician. This could be a sign of a condition that needs medical attention.

Side effects

Side effects are rare, however, if a rash or any other sign of an allergic reaction occurs, stop using the medicine.

Interactions

Some antihemorrhoid drugs should not be used by people who are taking or have recently taken **monoamine oxidase inhibitors** (MAO inhibitors), such as phenelzine (Nardil) or tranylcypromine (Parnate), used to treat conditions including depression and Parkinson's disease. Anyone who is not sure if he or she has taken this type of drug should check with a physician or pharmacist before using an antihemorrhoid drug. People who are taking antidepressants or medicine for high blood pressure also should not use certain antihemorrhoid drugs. Check with a pharmacist for a list of drugs that may interact with specific antihemorrhoid drugs.

Nancy Ross-Flanigan

Antihistamines

Definition

Antihistamines are drugs that block the action of histamine (a compound released in allergic inflammatory reactions) at the H_1 receptor sites, responsible for immediate hypersensitivity reactions such as sneezing and **itching**. Members of this class of drugs may also be used for their side effects, including **sedation** and anti-emesis (prevention of **nausea and vomiting**).

Purpose

Antihistamines provide their primary action by blocking histamine H_1 at the receptor site. They have no effect on rate of histamine release, nor do they inactivate histamine. By inhibiting the activity of histamine, they can reduce capillary fragility, which produces the erythema, or redness, associated with allergic reactions. They will also reduce histamine-induced secretions, including excessive tears and salivation. Additional effects vary with the individual drug used. Several of the older drugs, called first-generation antihistamines, bind non-selectively to H_1 receptors in the central nervous system as well as to peripheral receptors, and can produce sedation, inhibition of nausea and **vomiting**, and reduction of **motion sickness**. The second-generation antihistamines bind only to peripheral H_1 receptors, and reduce allergic response with little or no sedation.

The first-generation antihistamines may be divided into several chemical classes. The side effect profile, which also determines the uses of the drugs, will vary by chemical class. The alkylamines include brompheniramine (Dimetapp) and chlorpheniramine

DANIELE BOVET (1907–1992)

A gifted researcher in therapeutic chemistry, Daniele Bovet was born in Neuchatel, Switzerland, one of four children of a professor of experimental education. Bovet studied zoology and comparative anatomy at the University of Geneva, receiving his doctor of science degree in 1929. He then joined the Pasteur Institute in Paris, becoming director of the Laboratory of Therapeutic Chemistry in 1936.

Bovet investigated histamine, thought to cause allergy symptoms. No antagonist of histamine was known, so Bovet—with his research student Anne-Marie Staub—began studying substances that blocked hormones similar to histamine. By 1937 he had produced the first antihistamine, thymoxydiethylamine. Since this substance was too toxic for human use, Bovet and Staub performed thousands more experiments seeking less toxic antihistamines. This work formed the basis for the development of subsequent clinically useful antihistamines.

ANTIHISTAMINES

Brand Name (Generic Name)	Possible Common Side Effects Include:
*Atarax (hydroxyzine hydrochloride)	Drowsiness, **dry mouth**
Benadryl (diphenhydramine hydrochloride)	**Dizziness**, sleepiness, upset stomach, decreased coordination
Hismanal (astemiozole)	Drowsiness, dry mouth, **fatigue**, weight gain
PBZ-SR (tripelennamine hydrochloride)	Dizziness, drowsiness, dry mouth and throat, chest congestion, decreased coordination, upset stomach
Periactin (cyproheptadine hydrochloride)	Chest congestion, dizziness, fluttery heartbeat, loss of appetite, **hives**, sleepiness, vision problems
Phenergan (promethazine hydrochloride)	Changes in blood pressure, dizziness, blurred vision, nausea, rash
Polaramine (dexchlorpheniramine maleate)	Drowsiness
Seldane, Seldane-D (terfenadine)	Upset stomach, **nausea**, drowsiness, **headache**, fatigue
Tavist (clemastine fumarate)	Decreased coordination, dizziness, upset stomach
Trinalin Repetabs (azatadine maleate, pseudoephedrine sulfate)	Abdominal cramps, chest **pain**, dry mouth, headache

*Also used in the treatment of **anxiety**

(Chlor-Trimeton.) These agents cause relatively little sedation, and are used primarily for treatment of allergic reactions. Promethazine (Phenergan), in contrast, is a phenothiazine, chemically related to the major tranquilizers, and while it is used for treatment of **allergies**, may also be used as a sedative, the relieve anxiety prior to surgery, as an anti-nauseant, and for control of motion sickness. Diphenhydramine (Benadryl) is chemically an ethanolamine, and in addition to its role in reducing allergic reactions, may be used as a nighttime sedative, for control of drug-induced Parkinsonism, and, in liquid form, for control of coughs. Consult more detailed references for further information.

The second generation antihistamines have no central action, and are used only for treatment of allergic reactions. These are divided into two chemical classes. Cetirizine (Zyrtec) is a piperazine derivative, and has a slight sedative effect. Loratidine (Claritin) and fexofenadine (Allegra) are members of the piperadine class and are essentially non-sedating.

Recommended dosage

Dosage varies with drug, patient and intended use. Consult more detailed references for further information.

When used for control of allergic reactions, antihistamines should be taken on a regular schedule, rather than on an as-needed basis, since they have no effect on histamine itself, nor on histamine already bound to the receptor site.

Efficacy is highly variable from patient to patient. If an antihistamine fails to provide adequate relief, switch to a drug from a different chemical class. Individual drugs may be effective in no more than 40% of patients, and provide 50% relief of allergic symptoms.

Side effects

The frequency and severity of adverse effects will vary between drugs. Not all adverse reactions will apply to every member of this class.

Central nervous system reactions include drowsiness, sedation, dizziness, faintness, disturbed coordination, lassitude, confusion, restlessness, excitation, tremor, seizures, headache, **insomnia**, euphoria, blurred vision, **hallucinations**, disorientation, disturbing dreams/nightmares, schizophrenic-like reactions, weakness, vertigo, **hysteria**, nerve pain, and convulsions. Overdoses may cause involuntary movements. Other problems have been reported.

Gastrointestinal problems include increased appetite, decreased appetite, nausea, vomiting, **diarrhea**, and **constipation**.

Hematologic reactions are rare, but may be severe. These include anemia, or breakdown of red

KEY TERMS

Allergen—A substance that causes an allergy.

Anaphylaxis—A sudden, life-threatening allergic reaction.

Hallucination—A false or distorted perception of objects, sounds, or events that seems real. Hallucinations usually result from drugs or mental disorders.

Histamine—A chemical released from cells in the immune system as part of an allergic reaction.

Pregnancy category— A system of classifying drugs according to their established risks for use during pregnancy. Category A: Controlled human studies have demonstrated no fetal risk. Category B: Animal studies indicate no fetal risk, but no human studies; or adverse effects in animals, but not in well-controlled human studies. Category C: No adequate human or animal studies; or adverse fetal effects in animal studies, but no available human data. Category D: Evidence of fetal risk, but benefits outweigh risks. Category X: Evidence of fetal risk. Risks outweigh any benefits.

blood cells; reduced platelets; reduced white cells; and bone marrow failure.

A large number of additional reactions have been reported. Not all apply to every drug, and some reactions may not be drug related. Some of the other adverse effects are chest tightness; **wheezing**; nasal stuffiness; dry mouth, nose and throat; **sore throat**; respiratory depression; sneezing; and a burning sensation in the nose.

When taking antihistamines during **pregnancy**, Chlorpheniramine (Chlor-Trimeton), dexchlorpheniramine (Polaramine), diphenhydramine (Benadryl), brompheniramine (Dimetapp), cetirizine (Zyrtec), cyproheptadine (Periactin), clemastine (Tavist), azatadine (Optimine), loratadine (Claritin) are all listed as category B. Azelastine (Astelin), hydroxyzine (Atarax), promethazine (Phenergan) are category C.

Regardless of chemical class of the drug, it is recommended that mothers not breast feed while taking antihistamines.

Contraindications

The following are absolute or relative contraindications to use of antihistamines. The significance of the contraindication will vary with the drug and dose.

- glaucoma
- hyperthyroidism (overactive thyroid)
- high blood pressure
- enlarged prostate
- heart disease
- ulcers or other stomach problems
- stomach or intestinal blockage
- liver disease
- kidney disease
- bladder obstruction
- diabetes

Interactions

Monoamine oxidase inhibitor antidepressants (phenelzine [Nardil], tranylcypromine [Parnate]) may prolong and increase the effects of some antihistamines. When used with promethazine (Phenergan) this may cause reduced blood pressure and involuntary movements.

Resources

ORGANIZATIONS

Allergy and Asthma Network. 3554 Chain Bridge Road, Suite 200. (800) 878-4403.

American Academy of Allergy, Asthma, and Immunology. 611 East Wells St, Milwaukee, WI 53202. (800) 822-2762. < http://www.aaaai.org > .

Asthma and Allergy Foundation of America. 1125 15th Street NW, Suite 502, Washington, DC 20005. (800)727-8462.

Samuel D. Uretsky, PharmD

Antihyperlipidemic drugs *see* **Cholesterol-reducing drugs**

Antihypertensive drugs

Definition

Antihypertensive drugs are medicines that help lower blood pressure.

Purpose

The overall class of antihypertensive agents lowers blood pressure, although the mechanisms of action vary greatly. In 2003, a Joint National Committee on

Antihypertensive Drugs

Brand Name (Generic Name)	Possible Common Side Effects Include:
Accupril (quinapril hydrochloride)	**Headache**, dizziness
Aldatazide	**Diarrhea**, **fever**, headache, decreased coordination
Aldactone (spironolactone)	Cramps, drowsiness, stomach disorders
Aldomet (methyldopa)	Fluid retention, headache, weak feeling
Altace (ramipril)	Headache, cough
Calan, Calan SR (verapamil hydrochloride)	**Constipation**, **fatigue**, decreased blood pressure
Capoten (captopril)	Decreased sense of taste, decreased blood pressure tiching, rash
Cardene (nicardipine Hydrochloride)	Dizziness, headache, **indigestion** and **nausea**, increased heartbeat
Cardizem (diltiazem hydrochloride)	Dizziness, fluid retention, headache, nausea, skin rash
Cardura (doxazosin mesylate)	Dizziness, fatigue, drowsiness, headache
Catapres	**Dry mouth**, drowsiness, dizziness, constipation
Corgard (nadolol)	Behaviorial changes, dizziness, decreased heartbeat, tiredness
Corzide	Dizziness, decreased heartbeat, fatigue, cold hands and feet
Diuril (chlorothiazide)	Cramps, constipation or diarrhea, dizziness, fever, increased glocose level in urine
Dyazide	Blurred vision, muscle and abdominal **pain**, fatigue
DynaCirc (isradipine)	Chest pain, fluid retention, headache, fatigue
HydroDIURIL (hydrochlorothiazide)	Upset stomach, headache, cramps, loss of appetite
Hygroton (chlorthalidone)	Anemia, constipation or diarrhea, cramps, **itching**
Hytrin (terazosin hydrochloride)	Dizziness, labored breathing, nausea, swelling
Inderal (propranolol hydrochloride)	Constipation or diarrhea, **tingling** sensation, nausea and **vomiting**
Inderide	Blurred vision, cramps, fatigue, loss of appetite
Lasix (furosemide)	Back and muscle pain, indigestion, nausea
Lopressor (metoprolol tartrate)	Diarrhea, itching/rash, tiredness
Lotensin (benazepril hydrochloride)	Nausea, dizziness, fatigue, headache
Alozol (indapamide)	Anxiety, headache, loss of energy, **muscle cramps**
Maxzide	Cramps, labored breathing, drowsiness, irritated stomach
Minipress (prazosin hdrochloride)	Headache, nausea, weakness, dizziness
Moduretic	Diarrhea, fatigue, itching, loss of appetite
Monopril (fosinopril sodium)	Nausea and vomiting, headache, cough
Normodyne (labetalol hydrochloride)	Fatigue, nausea, stuffy nose
Plendil (felodipine)	Pain in back, chest, muscles, joints, and abdomen, itching, dry mouth, respiratory problems
Procardia, Procardia X (nifedipine)	Swelling, constipation, decreased blood pressure, nausea, fatigue
Sectral (acebutolol hydrochloride)	Constipation or diarrhea, gas, chest and joint pain
Ser-Ap-Es	Blurred vision, cramps, muscle pain, dizziness
Tenex (guanfacine hydrochloride)	Headache, constipation, dry mouth, weakness
Tenoretic	Decreased heartbeat, fatigue, nausea
Tenormin (atenolol)	Nausea, fatigue, dizziness
Veseretic	Diarrhea, muscle cramps, rash

Antihypertensive Drugs (continued)

Brand Name (Generic Name)	Possible Common Side Effects Include:
Vasotec (enalapril maleate)	Chest pain, blurred vision, constipation or diarrhea, **hives**, nausea
Visken (pindolol)	Muscle cramps, labored breathing, nausea, fluid retention
Wytensin (guanabenz acetate)	Headache, drowsiness, dizziness
Zaroxolyn (metolazone)	Constipation or diarrhea, chest pain, spasms, nausea
Zestoretic (lisinopril hydrochlorothiazide)	Fatigue, headache, dizziness
Zestril (lisinopril)	Labored breathing, abdominal and chest pain, nausea, decreased blood pressure

Prevention, Detection, Evaluation, and Treatment of High Blood Pressure report said that recent clinical trials show that antihypertensive treatment can reduce incidence of **stroke** by 35-40%, **heart attack** by 20-25%, and onset of new **heart failure** by 50%. Within this therapeutic class, there are several subgroups of drugs. There are a large number of drugs used to control **hypertension**, and the drugs listed below are representative, but not the only members of their classes.

The calcium channel blocking agents, also called slow channel blockers or calcium antagonists, inhibit the movement of ionic calcium across the cell membrane. This reduces the force of contraction of muscles of the heart and arteries. Although the **calcium channel blockers** are treated as a group, there are four different chemical classes, leading to significant variations in the activity of individual drugs. Nifedipine (Adalat, Procardia) has the greatest effect on the blood vessels, while verapamil (Calan, Isoptin) and diltiazem (Cardizem) have a greater effect on the heart muscle itself.

Peripheral **vasodilators** such as hydralazine (Apresoline), isoxuprine (Vasodilan), and **minoxidil** (Loniten) act by relaxing blood vessels.

There are several groups of drugs that act by reducing adrenergic nerve stimulation, the excitatory nerve stimulation that causes contraction of the muscles in the arteries, veins, and heart. These drugs include the beta-adrenergic blockers and alpha/beta adrenergic blockers. There are also non-specific adrenergic blocking agents.

Beta-adrenergic blocking agents include propranolol (Inderal), atenolol (Tenormin), and pindolol (Visken). Propranolol acts on the beta-adrenergic receptors anywhere in the body, and has been used as a treatment for emotional **anxiety** and rapid heart

KEY TERMS

Adrenergic—Activated by adrenalin (norepinephrine), loosely applied to the sympathetic nervous system responses.

Angioedema—An allergic skin disease characterized by patches of confined swelling involving the skin the layers beneath the skin, the mucous membranes, and sometimes the viscera—called also angioneurotic edema, giant urticaria, Quincke's disease, or Quincke's edema.

Arteries—Blood vessels that carry blood away from the heart to the cells, tissues, and organs of the body.

Laryngospasm—Spasmodic closure of the larynx.

Pregnancy category—A system of classifying drugs according to their established risks for use during pregnancy. Category A: Controlled human studies have demonstrated no fetal risk. Category B: Animal studies indicate no fetal risk, but no human studies; or adverse effects in animals, but not in well--controlled human studies. Category C: No adequate human or animal studies; or adverse fetal effects in animal studies, but no available human data. Category D: Evidence of fetal risk, but benefits outweigh risks. Category X: Evidence of fetal risk. Risks outweigh any benefits.

Sympathetic nervous system—The part of the autonomic nervous system that is concerned especially with preparing the body to react to situations of stress or emergency; it contains chiefly adrenergic fibers and tends to depress secretion, decrease the tone and contractility of smooth muscle, and increase heart rate.

beat. Atenolol and acebutolol (Sectral) act specifically on the nerves of the heart and circulation.

There are two alpha/beta adrenergic blockers, labetolol (Normodyne, Trandate) and carvedilol (Coreg). These work similarly to the **beta blockers**.

The ACE II inhibitors, losartan (Cozaar), candesartan (Atacand), irbesartan (Avapro), telmisartan (Micardis), valsartan (Diovan) and eprosartan (Teveten) directly inhibit the effects of ACE II rather than blocking its production. Their actions are similar to the ACE inhibitors, but they appear to have a more favorable side effect and safety profile.

In addition to these drugs, other classes of drugs have been used to lower blood pressure, most notably the thiazide **diuretics**. There are 12 thiazide diuretics marketed in the United States, including hydrochlorothiazide (Hydrodiuril, Esidrex), indapamide (Lozol), polythiazide (Renese), and hydroflumethiazide (Diucardin). The drugs in this class appear to lower blood pressure through several mechanisms. By promoting sodium loss they lower blood volume. At the same time, the pressure of the walls of blood vessels, the peripheral vascular resistance, is lowered. Thiazide diuretics are commonly used as the first choice for reduction of mild hypertension, and may be used in combination with other antihypertensive drugs.

Debate continued in 2003 as to the best drugs to lower blood pressure. One study seemed to prove that diuretics were the best initial choice, but a study from Australia said that ACE inhibitors were a superior choice. However, many physicians agreed that the best treatment for a particular patient depends on his or her particular age, economic situation, genetic factors and other existing illnesses and conditions.

While designed to lower cholesterol rather than blood pressure, a large clinical trial reported in 2003 that people with high blood pressure may one day benefit from taking them. In the trial, participants with increased risk for heart disease, even if it was not from **high cholesterol**, benefited from taking statins.

Recommended dosage

Recommended dosage varies with patient, drug, severity of hypertension, and whether the drug is being used alone or in combination with other drugs. Specialized references can be consulted for further information.

Precautions

Because of the large number of classes and individual drugs in this group, specialized references offer more complete information.

Peripheral vasodilators may cause **dizziness** and orthostatic hypotension—a rapid lowering of blood pressure when the patient stands up in the morning. Patients taking these drugs must be instructed to rise from bed slowly. **Pregnancy** risk factors for this group are generally category C. Hydralazine has been shown to cause **cleft palate** in animal studies, but there is no human data available. Breastfeeding is not recommended.

ACE inhibitors generally are well tolerated, but rarely may cause dangerous reactions including laryngospasm and angioedema. Persistent **cough** is a common side effect. ACE inhibitors should not be used in pregnancy. When used in pregnancy during the second and third trimesters, angiotension-converting inhibitors (ACEIs) can cause injury to and even **death** in the developing fetus. When pregnancy is detected, discontinue the ACE inhibitor as soon as possible. Breastfeeding is not recommended.

ACE II inhibitors are generally well tolerated and do not cause cough. Pregnancy risk factor is category C during the first trimester and category D during the second and third trimesters. Drugs that act directly on the renin-angiotensin system can cause fetal and neonatal morbidity and death when administered to pregnant women. Several dozen cases have been reported in patients who were taking ACE inhibitors. When pregnancy is detected, AIIRAs should be discontinued as soon as possible. Breastfeeding is not recommended.

Thiazide diuretics commonly cause potassium depletion. Patients should have potassium supplementation either through diet or potassium supplements. Pregnancy risk factor is category B (chlorothiazide, chlorthalidone, hydrochlorothiazide, indapamide, metolazone) or category C (bendroflumethiazide, benzthiazide, hydroflumethiazide, methyclothiazide, trichlormethiazide). Routine use during normal pregnancy is inappropriate. Thiazides are found in breast milk. Breastfeeding is not recommended.

Beta blockers may cause a large number of adverse reactions including dangerous heart rate abnormalities. Pregnancy risk factor is category B (acebutolol, pindolol, sotalol) or category C (atenolol, labetalol, esmolol, metoprolol, nadolol, timolol, propranolol, penbutolol, carteolol, bisoprolol). Breastfeeding is not recommended. In 2003, a report announced that adavances in **pharmacogenetics** mean that in the future, physicians may be able to use a patients genetic information to make certain prescribing decisions for antihypertensives.

Interactions

Specific drug references should be consulted, since interactions vary for antihypertensive drugs.

Resources

PERIODICALS

Belden, Heidi. "Debate Continues Over Best Drug for Hypertension." *Drug Topics* (April 21, 2003): 32.

Mechcatie, Elizabeth. "Genetics Will Guide Prescribing for Hypertension: Genotype Predicts Response to Drug." *Internal Medicine News* (July 1, 2003): 48-51.

"New Hypertension Guidelines: JNC-7." *Clinical Cardiology Alert* (July 2003): 54-63.

"Studies Show Thatá Statins Benefits People With High Blood Pressure." *Harvard Health Letter* (June 2003).

Samuel D. Uretsky, PharmD
Teresa G. Odle

Anti-hyperuricemic drugs

Definition

Anti-hyperuricemic drugs are used to treat hyperuricemia, the state of having too much uric acid in the blood.

Purpose

Anti-hyperuricemic drugs decrease the levels of uric acid in the blood, either by increasing the rate at which uric acid is excreted in the urine, or by preventing the formation of excess uric acid.

Precautions

Before taking any medication, patients should notify their physician of all other medications that they are currently taking. Patients should also notify their physician of any health problems they are currently experiencing. Patients must notify physicians if they have kidney problems, since this might affect the type of drug administered. Patients must also notify their physician if they are allergic to any of the medications used to treat acute or long-term **gout**. Since all of these factors contribute to the disease, patients suffering from gout should attempt to lose weight, avoid excess alcohol consumption, and avoid foods high in purines, such as asparagus, sardines, lobster, avocado, and peas.

Description

Gout and hyperuricemia

Persons with high levels of uric acid (hyperuricemia) may experience gout. Commonly gout occurs in males in their 40s and 50s. Gout is defined by the attacks of (arthritic) painful, reddened joints, and is often accompanied by hard lumps in the painful joints. The most common joint affected is the big toe. **Kidney stones**, and/or poor kidney function may also be associated with hyperuricemia, but may not be considered gout if the patient does not have painful joints. In persons with gout (and associated symptoms), uric acid forms crystals, which then cause the aforementioned symptoms. Although uric acid levels must be high in order for patients to have crystals form, and therefore have gout, most persons with high uric acid levels don't ever have symptoms. Thus, recent criteria for use of anti-hyperuricemic agents suggest that patients who have never experienced symptoms of gout should not receive drug therapy, unless their hyperuricemia is associated with **cancer** (may lead to kidney damage) or certain rare genetic disorders (McGill, Rheumatologist, University of Sydney, Australia, 2000).

Acute gout attacks

When patients experience acute attacks of gout, drugs that lower the levels of uric acid can cause an acute gout attack or cause an attack to become more severe. Thus, drugs that lower uric acid levels and are used to treat gout in the long term are not used in the short term. Medications used in acute gout attacks include non-steroidal anti-inflammatory drugs (such as indomethacin), colchicine, and **corticosteroids**. Colchicine causes side effects in a large number of individuals (usually diarhhea). The most important factor in the effective treatment of gout may not be the drug used, but how quickly it is administered after an acute attack has begun.

Long-term treatment

Long-term treatment of gout or hyperuricemia usually involves one of four drugs: allopurinol, probenicid, sulphinpyrazone, or benzbromarone (as of 2001, benzbromarone was not available for use in the United States). While allopurinol decreases the amount of uric acid that is produced (and may help prevent acute attacks of gout), the other drugs all increase the rate at which uric acid is excreted in the urine. As previously mentioned, lowering the concentration of uric acid can cause gout attacks. Thus, patients taking these medications should have the dose slowly increased (and uric acid levels slowly lowered) to prevent acute attacks of gout. Patients may also be treated with colchicine or non-steroidal anti-inflammatory drugs to prevent acute attacks of gout (corticosteroids are not used in this scenario because over the long term corticosteroids have deleterious side effects). In 2004, the FDA was seeking trial data on a new drug called oxypurinol (Oxyprim) for treating chronic gout. These medications may have to be taken for life to prevent further gout attacks.

Resources

PERIODICALS

Coghill, Kim. "FDA Panel Discusses Endpoints for Approval of Gout Products." *Bioworld Today* June 3, 2004.

Michael V Zuck, PhD
Teresa G. Odle

Anti-insomnia drugs

Definition

Anti-insomnia drugs are medicines that help people fall asleep or stay asleep.

Purpose

Physicians prescribe anti-insomnia drugs for short-term treatment of insomnia—a sleep problem in which people have trouble falling asleep or staying asleep or wake up too early and can't go back to sleep. These drugs should be used only for occasional treatment of temporary sleep problems and should not be taken for more than a week or two at a time. People whose sleep problems last longer than this should see a physician. Their sleep problems could be a sign of another medical problem.

Description

The anti-insomnia drug described here, zolpidem (Ambien), is a classified as a central nervous system (CNS) depressant. CNS depressants are medicines that slow the nervous system. Physicians also prescribe medicines in the benzodiazepine family, such as flurazepam (Dalmane), quazepam (Doral), triazolam (Halcion), estazolam (ProSom), and temazepam (Restoril), for **insomnia**. Benzodiazepine drugs are described in the essay on **antianxiety drugs**. Zaleplon (Sonata) is another anti-insomnia drug that is not related to other drugs with the same effect. The **barbiturates**, such as pentobarbital (Nembutal) and secobarbital (Seconal) are no longer commonly used to treat insomnia because they are too dangerous if they are taken in overdoses. For patients with mild insomnia, some **antihistamines**, such as diphenhydramine (Benadryl) or hydroxyzine (Atarax) may be used, since these also cause sleepiness.

Zolpidem is available only with a physician's prescription and comes in tablet form.

Anti-Insomnia Drugs	
Brand Name (Generic Name)	**Possible Common Side Effects Include:**
Ambien (zolpidem tartrate)	Daytime drowsiness, **dizziness**, headache
Dalmane (flurazepam hydrochloride)	Decreased coordination, lightheadedness, dizziness
Doral (quazepam)	Daytime drowsiness, headache, dry mouth, **fatigue**
Halcion (triazolam)	Decreased coordination, chest pain, memory impairment
ProSom (estazolam)	Dizziness, headache, nausea, weakness
Restoril (temazepam)	Dizziness, fatigue, nausea, headache, sluggishness

KEY TERMS

Asthma—A disease in which the air passages of the lungs become inflamed and narrowed.

Bronchitis—Inflammation of the air passages of the lungs.

Emphysema—A lung disease in which breathing becomes difficult.

Hallucination—A false or distorted perception of objects, sounds, or events that seems real. Hallucinations usually result from drugs or mental disorders.

Sleep apnea—A condition in which a person temporarily stops breathing during sleep.

Withdrawal symptoms—A group of physical or mental symptoms that may occur when a person suddenly stops using a drug to which he or she has become dependent.

Recommended dosage

The recommended dose for adults is 5-10 mg just before bedtime. The medicine works quickly, often within 20 minutes, so it should be taken right before going to bed.

For older people and others who may be more sensitive to the drug's effects, the recommended starting dosage is 5 mg just before bedtime.

Zolpidem may be taken with food or on an empty stomach, but it may work faster when taken on an empty stomach. Check with a physician or pharmacists for instructions on how to take the medicine.

Precautions

Zolpidem is meant only for short-term treatment of insomnia. If sleep problems last more than seven to 10 days, check with a physician. Longer-lasting sleep problems could be a sign of another medical problem. Also, this drug may lose its effectiveness when taken every night for more than a few weeks.

Some people feel drowsy, dizzy, confused, lightheaded, or less alert the morning after they have taken zolpidem. The medicine may also cause clumsiness, unsteadiness, double vision, or other vision problems the next day. For these reasons, anyone who takes these drugs should not drive, use machines or do anything else that might be dangerous until they have found out how zolpidem affects them.

This medicine has caused cause behavior changes in some people, similar to those seen in people whose behavior changes when they drink alcohol. Examples include giddiness and rage. More extreme changes, such as confusion, agitation, and **hallucinations**, also are possible. Anyone who starts having strange or unusual thoughts or behavior while taking this medicine should get in touch with his or her physician.

Zolpidem and other sleep medicines may cause a special type of temporary memory loss, in which the person does not remember what happens between the time they take the medicine and the time its effects wear off. This is usually not a problem, because people go to sleep right after taking the medicine and stay asleep until its effects wear off. But it could be a problem for anyone who has to wake up before getting a full night's sleep (seven to eight hours). In particular, travelers should not take this medicine on airplane flights of less than seven to eight hours.

Because zolpidem works work on the central nervous system, it may add to the effects of alcohol and other drugs that slow down the central nervous system, such as antihistamines, cold medicine, allergy medicine, medicine for seizures, tranquilizers, some **pain** relievers, and **muscle relaxants**. Zolpidem may also add to the effects of anesthetics, including those used for dental procedures. The combined effects of zolpidem and alcohol or other CNS depressants (drugs that slow the central nervous system) can be very dangerous, leading to unconsciousness or even **death**. People who take zolpidem should not drink alcohol and should check with their physicians before taking any other CNS depressant. Anyone who shows signs of an overdose or of the effects of combining zolpidem drugs with alcohol or other drugs should have immediate emergency help. Warning signs include severe drowsiness, severe **nausea** or **vomiting**, breathing problems, and staggering.

Anyone who takes zolpidem for more than 1–2 weeks should not stop taking it without first checking with a physician. Stopping the drug abruptly may cause rebound insomnia; increased difficulty falling asleep for the first one of two nights after the drug has been discontinued. In rare cases, withdrawal symptoms, such as vomiting, cramps, and unpleasant feelings may occur. Gradual tapering may be necessary.

Older people may be more sensitive to the effects of zolpidem. This may increase the chance of side effects, such as confusion, and may also increase the risk of falling.

In people with breathing problems, zolpidem may worsen the symptoms.

Special conditions

People with certain other medical conditions or who are taking certain other medicines can have problems if they take zolpidem. Before taking this medicine, be sure to let the physician know about any of these conditions:

ALLERGIES. Anyone who has had unusual reactions to zolpidem in the past should let his or her physician know before taking the drugs again. The physician should also be told about any **allergies** to foods, dyes, preservatives, or other substances.

PREGNANCY. Women who are pregnant or who may become pregnant should check with their physicians about the safety of using zolpidem during **pregnancy**.

BREASTFEEDING. Women who are breastfeeding should check with their physicians before using zolpidem.

OTHER MEDICAL CONDITIONS. Before using zolpidem, people with any of these medical problems should make sure their physicians are aware of their conditions:

- Chronic lung diseases (**emphysema**, **asthma**, or chronic bronchitis)
- Liver disease
- Kidney disease
- Current or past alcohol or drug abuse
- Depression
- Sleep apnea

USE OF CERTAIN MEDICINES. Taking zolpidem with certain other drugs may affect the way the drugs work or may increase the chance of side effects.

Side effects

The most common minor side effects are daytime drowsiness or a "drugged" feeling, vision problems, memory problems, nightmares or unusual dreams, vomiting, nausea, abdominal or stomach pain, **diarrhea**, **dry mouth**, **headache**, and general feeling of discomfort or illness. These problems usually go away as the body adjusts to the drug and do not require medical treatment.

More serious side effects are not common, but may occur. If any of the following side effects occur, check with the physician who prescribed the medicine as soon as possible:

- Confusion
- Depression
- Clumsiness or unsteadiness

Patients who take zolpidem may notice side effects for several weeks after they stop taking the drug. They should check with their physicians if these or other troublesome symptoms occur:

- Agitation, nervousness, feelings of panic
- Uncontrolled crying
- Worsening of mental or emotional problems
- Seizures
- Tremors
- Lightheadedness
- Sweating
- Flushing
- Nausea or abdominal or stomach cramps
- Muscle cramps
- Unusual tiredness or weakness

Other rare side effects may occur. Anyone who has unusual symptoms after taking zolpidem should get in touch with his or her physician.

Interactions

Zolpidem may interact with other medicines. When this happens, the effects of one or both of the drugs may change or the risk of side effects may be greater. Anyone who takes zolpidem should let the physician know all other medicines he or she is taking. Among the drugs that may interact with zolpidem are:

- Other central nervous system (CNS) depressants such as medicine for allergies, colds, hay **fever**, and asthma; sedatives; tranquilizers; prescription pain medicine; muscle relaxants; medicine for seizures; barbiturates; and anesthetics.

- The major tranquilizer chlorpromazine (Thorazine).

- Tricyclic antidepressants such as imipramine (Tofranil) and amitriptyline (Elavil).

Nancy Ross-Flanigan

Anti-itch drugs

Definition

Anti-itch drugs are medicines taken by mouth or by injection to relieve **itching**.

Purpose

The medicine described here, hydroxyzine, is a type of antihistamine used to relieve itching caused by allergic reactions. An allergic reaction occurs when the body is unusually sensitive to some substance, such as pollen, dust, mold, or certain foods or medicine. The body reacts by releasing a chemical called histamine that causes itching and other symptoms, such as sneezing and watery eyes. **Antihistamines** reduce the symptoms by blocking the effects of histamine.

Hydroxyzine is also prescribed for **anxiety** and to help people relax before or after having **general anesthesia**.

Description

Anti-itch drugs, also called antipruritic drugs, are available only with a physician's prescription and come in tablet and injectable forms. Some commonly used brands of the anti-itch drug hydroxyzine are Atarax and Vistaril.

Recommended dosage

When prescribed for itching, the usual dosage for adults is 25 mg, three to four times a day. For children over six years of age, the usual dosage 50-100 mg per

day, divided into several small doses. The usual dosage for children under six years of age is 50 mg per day, divided into several small doses.

The dosage may be different for different people. Check with the physician who prescribed the drug or the pharmacist who filled the prescription for the correct dosage, and take the medicine exactly as directed.

Precautions

This medicine should not be used for more than four months at a time because its effects can wear off. See a physician regularly while taking the medicine to determine whether it is still needed.

Hydroxyzine may add to the effects of alcohol and other drugs that slow down the central nervous system, such as other antihistamines, cold medicine, allergy medicine, sleep aids, medicine for seizures, tranquilizers, some **pain** relievers, and **muscle relaxants**. Anyone taking hydroxyzine should not drink alcohol and should check with his or her physician before taking any of the above.

Some people feel drowsy or less alert when using this medicine. Anyone who takes it should not drive, use machines, or do anything else that might be dangerous until they have found out how the drugs affect them.

Anyone who has had unusual reactions to hydroxyzine in the past should let his or her physician know before taking the medicine again. The physician should also be told about any **allergies** to foods, dyes, preservatives, or other substances.

A woman who is pregnant or who may become pregnant should check with her physician before taking this medicine. In studies of laboratory animals, hydroxyzine has caused **birth defects** when taken during **pregnancy**. Although the drug's effects on pregnant women have not been fully studied, physicians advise against taking it in early pregnancy.

BREASTFEEDING. Women who are breastfeeding should also check with their physicians before using hydroxyzine. The medicine may pass into breast milk and may cause problems in nursing babies whose mothers take it.

Side effects

The most common side effect, drowsiness, usually goes away as the body adjusts to the drug. If it does not, reducing the dosage may be necessary. Other side effects, such as **dry mouth**, also may occur and do not need medical attention unless they continue.

More serious side effects are not common, but may occur. If any of the following side effects occur, check with the physician who prescribed the medicine as soon as possible:

- Twitches or **tremors**
- Convulsions (seizures).

Interactions

Hydroxyzine may interact with other medicines. When this happens, the effects of one or both of the drugs may change or the risk of side effects may be greater. Anyone who takes hydroxyzine should let the physician know all other medicines he or she is taking. Among the drugs that may interact with hydroxyzine are:

- Barbiturates such as phenobarbital and secobarbital (Seconal)
- Opioid (narcotic) pain medicines such as meperidine (Demerol) and oxycodone (Percocet)
- Non-narcotic pain medicines such as **acetaminophen** (Tylenol) and ibuprofen (Motrin, Advil).

The list above may not include every drug that interacts with hydroxyzine. Be sure to check with a physician or pharmacist before combining hydroxyzine with any other prescription or nonprescription (over-the-counter) medicine.

Nancy Ross-Flanigan

Antimalarial drugs

Definition

Antimalarial drugs are medicines that prevent or treat **malaria**.

KEY TERMS

Glucose—A simple sugar that serves as the body's main source of energy.

Hypoglycemia—Abnormally low levels of glucose in the blood.

Organism—An individual of some type of life form, such as a plant or an animal.

Parasite—An organism that lives and feeds in or on another organism (the host) and does nothing to benefit the host.

Protozoa—Animal-like, one-celled organisms, some of which cause diseases in people.

Psoriasis—A skin disease in which people have itchy, scaly, red patches on the skin.

Purpura—A spotty or patchy purplish rash caused by bleeding under the surface of the skin.

Purpose

Antimalarial drugs treat or prevent malaria, a disease that occurs in tropical, subtropical, and some temperate regions of the world. The disease is caused by a parasite, *Plasmodium*, which belongs to a group of one-celled organisms known as protozoa. The only way to get malaria is to be bitten by a certain type of mosquito that has bitten someone who has the disease. Thanks to mosquito control programs, malaria has been eliminated in the United States, almost all of Europe, and large parts of Central and South America. However, mosquito control has not worked well in other parts of the world, and malaria continues to be a major health problem in parts of Africa, Southeast Asia, Latin America, Haiti, the Dominican Republic, and some Pacific Islands. Every year, some 30,000 Americans and Europeans who travel to these areas get malaria. People planning to travel to the tropics are often advised to take antimalarial drugs before, during, and after their trips, to help them avoid getting the disease and bringing it home with them. These drugs kill *Plasmodium* or prevent its growth.

In recent years, some strains of *Plasmodium* have become resistant to antimalarial drugs, and medical researchers have stepped up efforts to develop a malaria vaccine. In early 1997, researchers reported encouraging results from a small study of one vaccine and planned to test the vaccine in Africa.

Description

Antimalarial drugs are available only with a physician's prescription. They come in tablet, capsule, and injectable forms. Among the commonly used antimalarial drugs are chloroquine (Aralen), mefloquine (Lariam), primaquine, pyrimethamine (Daraprim), and quinine. Other drugs are constantly in development. In early 2004, scientists were researching promising new agents called beat-amino hydroxamates and amino acid-conjugated quinolinamines.

Recommended dosage

Recommended dosage depends on the type of antimalarial drug, its strength, and the form in which it is being used (such as tablet or injection). The dosage may also be different for different people. The physician who prescribed the drug or the pharmacist who filled the prescription can recommend the correct dosage. This medicine should be taken exactly as directed and for the full time of treatment. If the drug is being taken to treat malaria, it should not be stopped just because symptoms begin to improve. Symptoms may return if the drug is stopped too soon. Larger or more frequent doses than the physician has ordered should never be taken, nor should the drug be taken for longer than directed.

Travelers taking this medicine to prevent malaria may be told to take it for one to two weeks before their trip and for four weeks afterward, as well as for the whole time they are away. It is important to follow these directions.

Antimalarial drugs work best when they are taken on a regular schedule. When taken once a week to prevent malaria, they should be taken on the same day every week. When taken daily or several times a day to treat malaria, they should be taken at the same time every day. Doses should not be missed or skipped.

Some antimalarial drugs should be taken with meals or with milk to prevent upset stomach. Others must be taken with a full glass of water. It is important to follow directions along with the prescription.

Precautions

Antimalarial drugs may cause lightheadedness, **dizziness**, blurred vision and other vision changes. Anyone who takes these drugs should not drive, use machines or do anything else that might be dangerous until they have found out how the drugs affect them.

The antimalarial drug mefloquine (Lariam) has received attention because of reports that it causes panic attacks, **hallucinations**, **anxiety**, depression,

paranoia, and other mental and mood changes, sometimes lasting for months after the last dose. In fact, the U.S. Food and Drug Administration (FDA) began requiring warnings with Lariam beginning in July 2003 because of serious psychiatric effects caused by the drug. Pharmacists are required to include a 2,000-word medication guide detailing the warnings. Anyone who has unexplained anxiety, depression, restlessness, confusion, or other troubling mental or mood changes after taking mefloquine should call a physician right away. Switching to a different antimalarial drug may be an alternative and can allow the side effects to stop.

Anyone taking antimalarial drugs to prevent malaria who develops a **fever** or flu-like symptoms while taking the medicine or within 2-3 months after traveling to an area where malaria is common should call a physician immediately.

If the medicine is being taken to treat malaria, and symptoms stay the same or get worse, The patient should check with the physician who prescribed the medicine.

Patients who take this medicine over a long period of time need to have a physician check them periodically for unwanted side effects.

Babies and children are especially sensitive to the antimalarial drug chloroquine. Not only are they more likely to have side effects from the medicine, but they are also at greater risk of being harmed by an overdose. A single 300-mg tablet could kill a small child. *This medicine should be kept out of the reach of children and safety vials should be used.*

Special conditions

People with certain medical conditions or who are taking certain other medicines can have problems if they take antimalarial drugs. Before taking these drugs, the physician should know about any of these conditions:

ALLERGIES. Anyone who has had unusual reactions to antimalarial drugs or related medicines in the past should let his or her physician know before taking the drugs again. The physician should also be told about any **allergies** to foods, dyes, preservatives, or other substances.

PREGNANCY. In laboratory animal studies, some antimalarial drugs cause **birth defects**. But it is also risky for a pregnant woman to get malaria. Untreated malaria can cause premature birth, **stillbirth**, and **miscarriage**. When given in low doses to prevent malaria, antimalarial drugs have not been reported to cause birth defects in humans. If possible, pregnant women should avoid traveling to areas where they could get malaria. If travel is necessary, women who are pregnant or who may become pregnant should check with their physicians about the use of antimalarial drugs.

BREASTFEEDING. Some antimalarial drugs pass into breast milk. Although no problems have been reported in nursing babies whose mothers took antimalarial drugs, babies and young children are particularly sensitive to some of these drugs. Women who are breastfeeding should check with their physicians before using antimalarial drugs.

OTHER MEDICAL CONDITIONS. Before using antimalarial drugs, people who have any of these medical problems (or have had them in the past) should make sure their physicians are aware of their conditions:

- Blood disease
- Liver disease
- Nerve or brain disease or disorder, including seizures (convulsions)
- Past or current mental disorder
- Stomach or intestinal disease
- Deficiency of the enzyme glucose-6-phosphate dehydrogenase (G6PD), which is important in the breakdown of sugar in the body
- Deficiency of the enzyme nicotinamide adenine dinucleotide (NADH) methemoglobin reductase
- Psoriasis
- Heart disease
- Family or personal history of the genetic condition favism (a hereditary allergic condition)
- Family or personal history of **hemolytic anemia**, a condition in which red blood cells are destroyed
- Purpura
- Hypoglycemia (low blood sugar)
- Blackwater fever (a serious complication of one type of malaria)
- Myasthenia gravis (a disease of the nerves and muscles).

USE OF CERTAIN MEDICINES. Taking antimalarial drugs with certain other drugs may affect the way the drugs work or may increase the chance of side effects.

Side effects

High doses of the antimalarial drug pyrimethamine may cause blood problems that can interfere with healing and increase the risk of infection. People taking this drug should be careful not to injure their gums when brushing or flossing their teeth or using toothpicks. If possible, dental work should be postponed until treatment is complete and the blood has returned to normal.

The most common side effects of antimalarial drugs are **diarrhea**, **nausea** or **vomiting**, stomach cramps or **pain**, loss of appetite, **headache**, **itching**, difficulty concentrating, dizziness, lightheadedness, and sleep problems. These problems usually go away as the body adjusts to the drug and do not require medical treatment. Less common side effects, such as hair loss or loss of color in the hair; skin rash; or blue-black discoloration of the skin, fingernails, or inside of the mouth also may occur and do not need medical attention unless they are long-lasting.

More serious side effects are not common, but may occur. If any of the following side effects occur, the physician who prescribed the medicine should be contacted immediately:

- Blurred vision or any other vision changes
- Convulsions (seizures)
- Mood or mental changes
- Hallucinations
- Anxiety
- Confusion
- Weakness or unusual tiredness
- Unusual bruising or bleeding
- Hearing loss or ringing or buzzing in the ears
- Fever, with or without sore throat
- Slow heartbeat
- Pain in the back or legs
- Dark urine
- Pale skin
- Taste changes
- Soreness, swelling, or burning sensation in the tongue.

Other rare side effects may occur. Anyone who has unusual symptoms after taking an antimalarial drug should get in touch with his or her physician.

GALE ENCYCLOPEDIA OF MEDICINE 323

Interactions

Some antimalarial drugs may interact with other medicines. When this happens, the effects of one or both of the drugs may change or the risk of side effects may be greater. Anyone who takes antimalarial drugs should let the physician know all other medicines he or she is taking. Among the drugs that interact with some antimalarial drugs are:

- Beta blockers such as atenolol (Tenormin), propranolol (Inderal), and metoprolol (Lopressor)
- Calcium channel blockers such as diltiazem (Cardizem), nicardipene (Cardene), and nifedipine (Procardia)
- Other antimalarial drugs
- Quinidine, used to treat abnormal heart rhythms
- Antiseizure medicines such as vaproic acid derivatives (Depakote or Depakene)
- Oral typhoid vaccine
- Diabetes medicines taken by mouth
- Sulfonamides (sulfa drugs)
- Vitamin K
- Anticancer drugs
- Medicine for overactive thyroid
- Antiviral drugs such as zidovudine (Retrovir).

The list above does not include every medicine that may interact with every antimalarial drug. It is advised to check with a physician or pharmacist before combining an antimalarial drug with any other prescription or nonprescription (over-the-counter) medicine.

Resources

PERIODICALS

"Amino Acid-conjugated Quinolinamines Are Potent Antimalarials." *Drug Week* (March 12, 2004): 142.

"FDA Requires Warnings on Anti-malaria Drug Lariam." *Consumer Reports* (January 2004): 45.

"Glycosylated Beta-amino Hydroxamates Show Promise as Antimalarials." *Malaria Weekly* (February 2, 2004): 2.

OTHER

"Should You Take Lariam?" *Travel Health Information Page.* < http://travelhealth.com/lariam.htm >.

Nancy Ross-Flanigan
Teresa G. Odle

Antimicrobial agents *see* **Antibiotics**

Antimigraine drugs

Definition

Antimigraine drugs are medicines used to prevent or reduce the severity of migraine headaches.

Purpose

Migraine headaches usually cause a throbbing **pain** on one side of the head. **Nausea, vomiting, dizziness**, increased sensitivity to light and sound, and other symptoms may accompany the pain. The attacks may last for several hours or for a day or more and may come as often as several times a week. Some people who get migraine headaches have warning signals before the headaches begin, such as restlessness, **tingling** in an arm or leg, or seeing patterns of flashing lights. This set of signals is called an aura. The antimigraine drugs discussed in this section are meant to be taken as soon as the pain begins, to relieve the pain and other symptoms. Other types of drugs, such as antiseizure medicines, antidepressants, **calcium channel blockers** and **beta blockers**, are sometimes prescribed to prevent attacks in people with very severe or frequent migraines.

Description

Migraine is thought to be caused by electrical and chemical imbalances in certain parts of the brain. These imbalances affect the blood vessels in the brain – first tightening them up, then widening them. As the blood vessels widen, they stimulate the release of chemicals that increase sensitivity to pain and cause inflammation and swelling. Antimigraine drugs are believed to work by correcting the imbalances and by tightening the blood vessels.

Examples of drugs in this group are ergotamine (Cafergot), naratriptan (Amerge), sumatriptan (Imitrex), rizatriptan (Maxalt), almotriptan (Axert), and zolmitriptan (Zomig). Methysergide maleate (Sansert) may be used by patients whose headaches are not controlled by other drugs, while some patients do well on other drugs. For example, combinations or ergotamine and **caffeine** may be very effective. The caffeine acts by constricting blood vessels to relieve the **headache**. Sometimes, an analgesic such as **acetaminophen**, caffeine, and a barbiturate which acts as a sedative, are combined, as in Fioricet and similar compounds. These medicines are available only with a physician's prescription and come in several forms. Ergotamine is available as tablets

Antimigraine Drugs	
Brand Name (Generic Name)	**Possible Common Side Effects Include:**
Cafergot	Nausea, increased blood pressure, fluid retention, numbness, increased heart rate, tingling sensation
Imitrex (sumatriptan succinate)	Burning, flushing, neck pain, inflammation at injection site, sore throat, tingling sensation
Inderal (propranolol hydrochloride)	Constipation or **diarrhea**, headache, nausea, rash
Midrin	Dizziness, rash

KEY TERMS

Anticonvulsant—A type of drug given to prevent seizures. Some patients with migraines can be treated effectively with an anticonvulsant.

Aura—A set of warning symptoms, such as seeing flashing lights, that some people have 10–30 minutes before a migraine attack.

Inflammation—Pain, redness, swelling, and heat that usually develop in response to injury or illness.

Status migrainosus—The medical term for an acute migraine headache that lasts 72 hours or longer.

and rectal suppositories; sumatriptan as tablets, injections, and nasal spray; and zolmitriptan as tablets.

Antimigraine drugs are used to treat headaches once they have started. These drugs should not be taken to prevent headaches.

Some patients are given anti-epileptic drugs, which are also known as anticonvulsants, to treat migraine headaches. As of 2003, sodium valproate (Epilim) is the only anticonvulsant approved by the Food and Drug Administration (FDA) for prevention of migraine. Such newer anticonvulsants as gabapentin (Neurontin) and topiramate (Topamax) are being evaluated as migraine preventives as of early 2004.

Recommended dosage

Recommended dosage depends on the type of drug. Typical recommended dosages for adults are given below for each type of drug.

Ergotamine

Take at the first sign of a migraine attack. Patients who get warning signals (aura) may take the drug as soon as they know a headache is coming.

TABLETS. No more than 6 tablets for any single attack.

No more than 10 tablets per week.

SUPPOSITORIES. No more than 2 suppositories for any single attack.

No more than 5 suppositories per week.

Naratriptan

Take as soon as pain or other migraine symptoms begin. Also effective if taken any time during an attack. Do not take the drug until the pain actually starts as not all auras result in a migraine.

TABLETS. Usual dose is one 1-mg tablet taken with water or other liquid.

Doses of 2.5-mg may be used, but they may cause more side effects.

If the headache returns or if there is only partial response, the dose may be repeated once after 4 hours, for a maximum dose of 5 mg in a 24-hour period. Larger doses do not seem to offer any benefit.

Sumatriptan

Take as soon as pain or other migraine symptoms begin. Also effective if taken any time during an attack. Do not take the drug until the pain actually starts as not all auras result in a migraine.

TABLETS. Usual dose is one 25-mg tablet, taken with water or other liquid.

Doses should be spaced at least 2 hours apart.

Anyone with **liver disease** should consult with a physician for proper dosing.

INJECTIONS. No more than 6 mg per dose, injected under the skin.

No more than two 6-mg injections per day. These doses should be taken at least 1 hour apart.

Zolmitriptan

Take as soon as symptoms begin.

TABLETS. Usual dose is 1–5 mg. Additional doses may be taken at 2-hour intervals.

No more than 10 mg per 24 hour period.

General dosage advice

Always take antimigraine drugs exactly as directed. Never take larger or more frequent doses, and do not take the drug for longer than directed.

If possible, lie down and relax in a dark, quiet room for a few hours after taking the medicine.

Precautions

These drugs should be used only to treat the type of headache for which they were prescribed. Patients should not use them for other headaches, such as those caused by **stress** or too much alcohol, unless directed to do so by a physician.

Anyone whose headache is unlike any previous headache should check with a physician before taking these drugs. If the headache is far worse than any other, emergency medical treatment should be sought immediately.

Taking too much of the antimigraine drug ergotamine (Cafergot), can lead to ergot **poisoning**. Symptoms include headache, muscle pain, **numbness**, coldness, and unusually pale fingers and toes. If not treated, the condition can lead to **gangrene** (tissue death).

Sumatriptan (Imitrex), naratriptan (Amerge), rizatriptan (Maxalt) and zolmitriptan (Zomig) may interact with ergotamine. These drugs should not be taken within 24 hours of taking any drug containing ergotamine.

Some antimigraine drugs work by tightening blood vessels in the brain. Because these drugs also affect blood vessels in other parts of the body, people with coronary heart disease, circulatory problems, or high blood pressure should not take these medicines unless directed to do so by their physicians.

About 40% of all migraine attacks do not respond to treatment with triptans or any other medication. If the headache lasts longer than 72 hours—a condition known as status migrainosus—the patient may be given narcotic medications to bring on sleep and stop the attack. Patients with status migrainosus are often hospitalized because they are likely to be dehydrated from severe **nausea and vomiting**.

Special conditions

People with certain other medical conditions or who are taking certain other medicines can have problems if they take antimigraine drugs. Before taking these drugs, be sure to let the physician know about any of these conditions:

ALLERGIES. Anyone who has had unusual reactions to ergotamine, caffeine, sumatriptan, zolmitriptan, or other antimigraine drugs in the past should let his or her physician know before taking the drugs again. The physician should also be told about any **allergies** to foods, dyes, preservatives, or other substances.

PREGNANCY. Women who are pregnant should not take ergotamine (Cafergot). The effects of other antimigraine drugs during **pregnancy** have not been well studied. Any woman who is pregnant or plans to become pregnant should let her physician know before an antimigraine drug is prescribed.

BREASTFEEDING. Some antimigraine drugs can pass into breast milk and may cause serious problems in nursing babies. Women who are breastfeeding should check with their physicians about whether to stop breastfeeding while taking the medicine.

OTHER MEDICAL CONDITIONS. Before using antimigraine drugs, people with any of these medical problems should make sure their physicians know about their conditions:

- Coronary heart disease
- Angina (crushing chest pain)
- Circulatory problems or blood vessel disease
- High blood pressure
- Liver problems
- Kidney problems
- Any infection
- Eye problems.

USE OF CERTAIN MEDICINES. Taking antimigraine drugs certain other drugs may affect the way the drugs work or may increase the chance of side effects.

Side effects

The most common side effects are fluid retention, flushing; high blood pressure; unusually fast or slow heart rate; numbness; tingling; **itching**; nausea; vomiting; weakness; neck or jaw pain and stiffness; feelings of tightness, heaviness, warmth, or coldness; **sore throat**; and discomfort of the mouth and tongue.

More serious side effects are not common, but they may occur. If any of the following side effects occur, call a physician immediately:

- Tightness in the chest
- Bluish tinge to the skin
- Cold arms and legs

- Signs of gangrene, such as coldness, dryness, and a shriveled or black appearance of a body part

- Dizziness

- Drowsiness

- Shortness of breath or **wheezing**

- Skin rash

- Swelling of the eyelids or face.

Possible side effects with anticonvulsants include dizziness, drowsiness, emotional upset, skin rash, temporary hair loss, nausea, and irregular menstrual periods.

Other side effects may occur with any antimigraine drug. Anyone who has unusual symptoms after taking this medicine should get in touch with his or her physician.

Alternative treatments

There are two herbal remedies that are reported to be effective as alternative treatments for migraine. One is feverfew (*Tanacetum parthenium*), an herb related to the daisy that is traditionally used in England to prevent migraines. Published studies indicate that feverfew can reduce the frequency and intensity of migraines. It does not, however, relieve pain once the headache has begun. The other herbal remedy is butterbur root (*Petasites hybridus*). Petadolex is a natural preparation made from butterbur root that has been sold in Germany since the 1970s as a migraine preventive. Petadolex has been available in the United States since December 1998.

Interactions

Antimigraine drugs may interact with other medicines. When this happens, the effects of one or both of the drugs may change, or the risk of side effects may be greater. Anyone who takes these drugs should let the physician know all other medicines he or she is taking. Among the drugs that may interact with antimigraine drugs are:

- Beta blockers such as atenolol (Tenormin) and propranolol (Inderal)

- Drugs that tighten blood vessels such as epinephrine (EpiPen) and pseudoephedrine (Sudafed)

- Nicotine such as cigarettes or Nicoderm, Habitrol, and other **smoking-cessation drugs**

- Certain **antibiotics**, such as erythromycin and clarithromycin (Biaxin)

- Monoamine oxidase inhibitors such as phenelzine (Nardil) and tranylcypromine (Parnate)

- Certain antidepressants, such as sertraline (Zoloft), fluoxetine (Prozac), and paroxetine (Paxil)

- Fluvoxamine (Luvox), prescribed for obsessive compulsive disorder or chronic pain.

Anticonvulsants should not be taken together with **aspirin**, alcohol, or tranquilizers.

Remember naratriptan, sumatriptan, rizatriptan and zolmitriptan may interact with ergotamine. These drugs should not be taken within 24 hours of taking any drug containing ergotamine.

Resources

BOOKS

American Psychiatric Association.*Diagnostic and Statistical Manual of Mental Disorders*. 4th ed., revised. Washington, DC: American Psychiatric Association, 2000.

Beers, Mark H., MD, and Robert Berkow, MD., editors. "Headache." Section 14, Chapter 168 In *The Merck Manual of Diagnosis and Therapy*. Whitehouse Station, NJ: Merck Research Laboratories, 2002.

Beers, Mark H., MD, and Robert Berkow, MD., editors. "Psychogenic Pain Syndromes." Section 14, Chapter 167 In *The Merck Manual of Diagnosis and Therapy*. Whitehouse Station, NJ: Merck Research Laboratories, 2002.

Pelletier, Kenneth R., MD. *The Best Alternative Medicine*, Part II. "CAM Therapies for Specific Conditions: Headache." New York: Simon & Schuster, 2002.

PERIODICALS

Ceballos Hernansanz, M. A., R. Sanchez Roy, A. Cano Orgaz, et al. "Migraine Treatment Patterns and Patient Satisfaction with Prior Therapy: A Substudy of a Multicenter Trial of Rizatriptan Effectiveness." *Clinical Therapeutics* 25 (July 2003): 2053–2069.

Corbo, J. "The Role of Anticonvulsants in Preventive Migraine Therapy." *Current Pain and Headache Reports* 7 (February 2003): 63–66.

Dodick, D. W. "A Review of the Clinical Efficacy and Tolerability of Almotriptan in Acute Migraine." *Expert Opinion in Pharmacotherapy* 4 (July 2003): 1157–1163.

Dowson, A. J., and B. R. Charlesworth. "Patients with Migraine Prefer Zolmitriptan Orally Disintegrating Tablet to Sumatriptan Conventional Oral Tablet." *International Journal of Clinical Practice* 57 (September 2003): 573–576.

Johannessen, C. U., and S. I. Johannessen. "Valproate: Past, Present, and Future." *CNS Drug Review* 9 (Summer 2003): 199–216.

Sahai, Soma, MD, Robert Cowan, MD, and David Y. Ko, MD. "Pathophysiology and Treatment of Migraine and Related Headache." *eMedicine* April 30, 2002.

Tepper, S. J., and D. Millson. "Safety Profile of the Triptans." *Expert Opinion on Drug Safety* 2 (March 2003): 123–132.

Nancy Ross-Flanigan
Rebecca J. Frey, PhD

Antimyocardial antibody test

Definition

Testing for antimyocardial antibodies is done when evaluating a person for heart damage or heart disease.

Purpose

Antimyocardial antibodies are autoantibodies. Normal antibodies are special proteins built by the body as a defense against foreign material entering the body. Autoantibodies are also proteins built by the body, but instead of attacking foreign material, they inappropriately attack the body's own cells. Antimyocardial antibodies attack a person's heart muscle, or myocardium.

This test may be done on a person who recently had trauma to the heart, such as heart surgery or a myocardial infarction (**heart attack**). It also may be done on someone with heart disease, such as **cardiomyopathy** or **rheumatic fever**.

Although the presence of antimyocardial antibodies does not diagnose heart damage or disease, there is a connection between the presence of these antibodies and damage to the heart. The amount of damage, however, cannot be predicted by the amount of antibodies.

These antibodies usually appear after heart surgery or the beginning of disease, but they may be present before surgery or the onset of disease. In 30% of people with myocardial infarction and 70% of people having heart surgery, antimyocardial antibodies will appear within two to three weeks and stay for three to eight weeks.

Description

A 5-10 mL sample of venous blood is drawn from the patient's arm in the region of the inner elbow. Antimyocardial antibodies are detected by combining a patient's serum (clear, thin, sticky fluid in blood) with cells from animal heart tissue, usually that of a monkey. Antimyocardial antibodies in the serum bind to the heart tissue cells. A fluorescent dye is then added

---

KEY TERMS

Antibody—A special protein built by the body as a defense against foreign material entering the body.

Antimyocardial antibody—An autoantibody that attacks a person's own heart muscle, or myocardium.

Autoantibody— An antibody that attacks the body's own cells or tissues.

Myocardial infarction—A block in the blood supply to the heart, resulting in what is commonly called a heart attack.

Myocardium—The muscular middle layer of the heart.

Titer—A dilution of a substance with an exact known amount of fluid. For example, one part of serum diluted with four parts of saline is a titer of 1:4.

---

to the mixture. This dye will attach to any antibodies and heart tissue cells bound together. The final mixture is studied under a microscope that is designed to show fluorescence. If fluorescent cells are seen under the microscope, the test is positive.

When the test is positive, the next step is to find out how much antibody is present. The patient's serum is diluted, or titered, and the test is done again. The serum is then further diluted and the test repeated until the serum is so dilute that fluorescence is no longer seen. The last dilution that showed fluorescence is the titer reported.

Preparation

No **fasting** or special prepartion is needed. Before the test is done it should be explained to the patient.

Aftercare

Discomfort or bruising may occur at the puncture site after the blood is drawn or the person may feel dizzy or faint. Pressure to the puncture site until the bleeding stops reduces bruising. Warm packs on the puncture site relieve discomfort.

Normal results

Antimyocardial antibodies are not normally seen in healthy individuals.

Abnormal results

A positive result means that antimyocardial antibodies are present and that heart disease or damage is likely. Further testing may be needed as other autoantibodies could also be present, causing a false abnormal test.

Resources

BOOKS

Pagana, Kathleen Deska. *Mosby's Manual of Diagnostic and Laboratory Tests.* St. Louis: Mosby, Inc., 1998.

Nancy J. Nordenson

Antinausea Drugs

Brand Name (Generic Name)	Possible Common Side Effects Include:
Compazine (phochlorperazine)	Involuntary muscle spasms, dizziness, jitteriness, puckering of the mouth
Phenergan (promethazine hydrochloride)	Dizziness, dry mouth, nausea and vomiting, rash
Reglan (metoclopramide hydrochloride)	Fatigue, drowsiness, restlessness
Tigan (trimethobenzamide hydrochloride)	Blurred vision, **diarrhea**, cramps, **headache**
Zofan (ondansetron hydrochloride)	Constipation, headache, fatigue, abdominal pain

Antinausea drugs

Definition

Antinausea drugs are medicines that control nausea—a feeling of sickness or queasiness in the stomach with an urge to vomit. These drugs also prevent or stop **vomiting**. Drugs that control vomiting are called antiemetic drugs.

Purpose

Antinausea drugs such as prochlorperazine (Compazine), usually control both **nausea and vomiting**. Prochlorperazine is also sometimes prescribed for symptoms of mental disorders, such as **schizophrenia**.

Another commonly prescribed antinausea drug is promethazine (Phenergan). Promethazine also may be prescribed to relieve allergy symptoms and apprehension, as well as **motion sickness**.

Description

Prochlorperazine is available only with a physician's prescription. It is sold in syrup, capsule, tablet, injection, and suppository forms.

Recommended dosage

To control **nausea** and vomiting in adults, the usual dose is:

- Tablets—one 5-mg or 10-mg tablet three to four times a day
- Extended-release capsules—one 15-mg capsule first thing in the morning or one 10-mg capsule every 12 hours
- Suppository—25 mg, twice a day

KEY TERMS

Anesthetic—Medicine that causes a loss of feeling, especially pain. Some anesthetics also cause a loss of consciousness.

Antihistamine—Medicine that prevents or relieves allergy symptoms.

Central nervous system—The brain and spinal cord.

Spasm—Sudden, involuntary tensing of a muscle or a group of muscles.

Tranquilizer—Medicine that has a calming effect and is used to treat anxiety and mental tension.

- Syrup—5-10 mg three to four times a day
- Injection—5-10 mg injected into a muscle three to four times a day.

Doses for children must be determined by a physician.

Promethazine may be administered in pill, syrup, chewable tablet, or extended release capsule form by prescription only. For severe nausea, it may be administered by injection or via a suppository. The physician recommends dose depending on the patient's condition.

Precautions

Prochlorperazine may cause a movement disorder called **tardive dyskinesia**. Signs of this disorder are involuntary twitches and **muscle spasms** in the face and body and jutting or rolling movements of the tongue. The condition may be permanent. Older people, especially women, are particularly at risk of developing this problem when they take prochlorperazine.

Some people feel drowsy, dizzy, lightheaded, or less alert when using this medicine. The drug may also cause blurred vision, and movement problems. For these reasons, anyone who takes this drug should not drive, use machines or do anything else that might be dangerous until they have found out how the drug affects them.

Prochlorperazine makes some people sweat less, which can allow the body to overheat. The drug may also make the skin and eyes more sensitive to the sun. People who are taking prochlorperazine should try to avoid extreme heat and exposure to the sun. When going outdoors, they should wear protective clothing, a hat, a sunscreen with a skin protection factor (SPF) of at least 15, and sunglasses that block ultraviolet (UV) light. Saunas, sunlamps, tanning booths, tanning beds, hot baths, and hot tubs should be avoided while taking this medicine. Anyone who must be exposed to extreme heat while taking the drug should check with his or her physician.

This medicine adds to the effects of alcohol and other drugs that slow down the central nervous system, such as **antihistamines**, cold and flu medicines, tranquilizers, sleep aids, anesthetics, some **pain** medicines, and **muscle relaxants**. Drinking alcohol while taking prochlorperazine is not advised and patients should check with the physician who prescribed the drug before combining it with any other medicines.

Do not stop taking this medicine without checking with the physician who prescribed it. Stopping the drug suddenly can cause **dizziness**, nausea, vomiting, **tremors**, and other side effects. When stopping the medicine, it may be necessary to taper down the dose gradually.

Prochlorperazine may cause false **pregnancy** tests.

Women who are pregnant (or planning to become pregnant) or breast feeding should check with their physicians before using antinausea medicines.

Before using prochlorperazine, people with any of the medical problems should make sure their physicians are aware of their conditions:

- Previous sensitivity or allergic reaction to prochlorperazine
- Heart disease
- Glaucoma
- Brain tumor
- Intestinal blockage
- Abnormal blood conditions, such as leukemia
- Exposure to pesticides.

Some people may experience side effects from promethazine including:

- **dry mouth**
- drowsiness
- confusion
- **fatigue**
- difficulty coordinating movements
- stuffy nose.

A physician should be contacted immediately if a patient experiences the following effects while taking promethazine:

- vision problems
- ringing in the ears
- tremors
- insomnia
- excitement
- restlessness
- yellowing of the skin or eyes
- skin rash.

Side effects

Many side effects are possible with prochlorperazine, including, but not limited to, **constipation**, dizziness, drowsiness, decreased sweating, dry mouth, stuffy nose, movement problems, changes in menstrual period, increased sensitivity to sun, and swelling or pain in breasts. Anyone who has unusual or troublesome symptoms after taking prochlorperazine should get in touch with his or her physician.

Side effects associated with promethazine include those listed above and interactions with various medications that may cause complications or lessen the effects of the drug. A physician should be notified of other medications the patient is on when taking promethazine.

Interactions

Prochlorperazine may interact with other medicines. When this happens, the effects of one or both of the drugs may change or the risk of side effects may be greater. Among the drugs that may interact with prochlorperazine are antiseizure drugs such as phenytoin (Dilantin) and carbamazepine (Tegretol), anticoagulants such as warfarin (Coumadin), and drugs that slow the central nervous system such as alprazolam (Xanax), diazepam (Valium), and secobarbital (Seconal). Not every drug that interacts with prochlorperazine is listed here. A physician or pharmacist can advise patients about prescription or nonprescription (over-the-counter) drugs that might interact with Prochlorperazine.

Resources

PERIODICALS

Flake, Zachary A., Robert D. Scalley, and Austin G. Bailey. "Practical Selection of Antiemetics." *American Family Physician* March 1, 2004: 1169.

OTHER

"Promethazine" *Medline Plus Drug Information.* < http://www.nlm.nih.gov/medlineplus/druginfo/medmaster/a682284.html#precautions >.

Nancy Ross-Flanigan
Teresa G. Odle

Antinuclear antibody test

Definition

The antinuclear antibody (ANA) test is a test done early in the evaluation of a person for autoimmune or rheumatic disease, particularly **systemic lupus erythematosus** (SLE).

Purpose

In autoimmune diseases, the body makes antibodies that work against its own cells or tissues. Rheumatic diseases (diseases that affect connective tissue, including the joints, bone, and muscle) are also associated with these antibodies. Autoantibodies are proteins built by the body, but instead of guarding against foreign material (including bacteria, viruses, and fungi) as normal antibodies do, they attack the body's own cells.

Autoimmune and rheumatic diseases can be difficult to diagnose. People with the same disease can have very different symptoms. A helpful strategy in the diagnosis of these diseases is to find and identify an autoantibody in the person's blood.

The antinuclear antibody test looks for a group of autoantibodies that attack substances found in the center (nucleus) of all cells. It is useful as a screen for many autoantibodies associated with diseases that affect the entire body (systemic diseases).

This test is particularly useful when diagnosing a person with symptoms of SLE, an illness that affects many body organs and tissues. If the test is negative, it is unlikely that the person has SLE; if the test is positive, more tests are done to confirm whether the person has SLE or another related disease. Other diseases, such as **scleroderma**, **Sjögren's syndrome**, **Raynaud's disease**, **rheumatoid arthritis**, and **autoimmune hepatitis**, often have a positive test for antinuclear antibodies.

Description

Five to 10 mL of blood is needed for this test. The antinuclear antibody test is done by adding a person's serum to commercial cells mounted on a microscope slide. If antinuclear antibodies are in the serum, they bind to the nuclei of cells on the slide. Next, a second antibody is added to the mixture. This antibody is "tagged" with a fluorescent dye so that it can be seen. The second antibody attaches to any antibodies and cells bound together and, because of the fluorescent "tag," the areas with antinuclear antibodies seem to glow, or fluoresce, when the slide is viewed under an ultraviolet microscope.

If fluorescent cells are seen, the test is positive. When positive, the serum is diluted, or titered, and the test done again. These steps are repeated until the serum is so dilute it no longer gives a positive result. The last dilution that shows fluorescence is the titer reported.

The pattern of fluorescence within the cells gives the physician clues as to what the disease might be. The test result includes the titer and the pattern.

This test is also called the fluorescent antinuclear antibody test or FANA. Results are available within one to three days.

Preparation

No special preparations or diet changes are required before a person undergoes an antinuclear antibody test.

Aftercare

Discomfort or bruising may occur at the puncture site or the person may feel dizzy or faint. Pressure to the puncture site until the bleeding stops reduces bruising. Warm packs relieve discomfort.

Normal results

Normal results will be negative, showing no antinuclear antibodies.

Abnormal results

A positive test in a person with symptoms of an autoimmune or rheumatic disease helps the physician make a diagnosis. More than 95% of people with SLE have a positive ANA test. Scleroderma has a 60-71% positive rate; Sjögren's disease, 50-60%, and rheumatoid arthritis, 25-30%.

Several factors must be considered when interpreting a positive test. Diseases other than autoimmune diseases can cause autoantibodies. Some healthy people have a positive test. More testing is done after a positive test to identify individual autoantibodies associated with the various diseases.

Resources

BOOKS

Lehman, Craig A. *Saunders Manual of Clinical Laboratory Science.* Philadelphia: W. B. Saunders Co., 1998.

Nancy J. Nordenson

▌Antiparkinson drugs

Definition

Antiparkinson drugs are medicines that relieve the symptoms of Parkinson's disease and other forms of parkinsonism.

Purpose

Antiparkinson drugs are used to treat symptoms of parkinsonism, a group of disorders that share four main symptoms: tremor or trembling in the hands,

Antiparkinson Drugs

Brand Name (Generic Name)	Possible Common Side Effects Include:
Artane (trihexyphenidyl hydrochloride)	Dry mouth, nervousness, blurred vision, nausea
Benadryl (diphenhydramine hydrochloride)	Dizziness, sleepiness, upset stomach, decreased coordination
Cogentin (benztropine mesylate)	Constipation, dry mouth, nausea and vomiting, rash
Eldepryl (selegiline hydrochloride)	Abdominal and back **pain**, drowsiness, decreased coordination
Parlodel (bromocriptine mesylate)	Constipation, decreased blood pressure, abdominal cramps
Sinemet CR	Involuntary body movements, confusion, nausea, hallucinations

arms, legs, jaw, and face; stiffness or rigidity of the arms, legs, and trunk; slowness of movement (bradykinesia); and poor balance and coordination. Parkinson's disease is the most common form of parkinsonism and is seen more frequently with advancing age. Other forms of the disorder may result from viral infections, environmental toxins, **carbon monoxide poisoning**, and the effects of treatment with **antipsychotic drugs**.

The immediate cause of Parkinson's disease or Parkinsonian-like syndrome is the lack of the neurotransmitter dopamine in the brain. Drug therapy may take several forms, including replacement of dopamine, inhibition of dopamine metabolism to increase the effects of the dopamine already present, or sensitization of dopamine receptors. Drugs may be used singly or in combination.

Description

Levodopa (Larodopa) is the mainstay of Parkinson's treatment. The drug crosses the blood-brain barrier, and is converted to dopamine. The drug may be administered alone, or in combination with carbidopa (Lodosyn) which inhibits the enzyme responsible for the destruction of levodopa. The limitation of levodopa or levodopa-carbidopa therapy is that after approximately two years of treatment, the drugs cease to work reliably. This has been termed the "on-off phenomenon." Additional treatment strategies have been developed to retard the progression of Parkinsonism, or to find alternative approaches to treatment.

Anticholinergic drugs reduce some of the symptoms of Parkinsonism, and reduce the reuptake of dopamine, thereby sustaining the activity of the natural neurohormone. They may be effective in all stages of the disease. All drugs with anticholinergic

KEY TERMS

Anorexia—Lack or loss of appetite.

Anticholiginginc—An agent that blocks the parasympathetic nerves and their actions.

Bradykinesia—Extremely slow movement.

Bruxism—Compulsive grinding or clenching of the teeth, especially at night.

Carbon monoxide—A colorless, odorless, highly poisonous gas.

Central nervous system—The brain and spinal cord.

Chronic—A word used to describe a long-lasting condition. Chronic conditions often develop gradually and involve slow changes.

Hallucination—A false or distorted perception of objects, sounds, or events that seems real. Hallucinations usually result from drugs or mental disorders.

Heat stroke—A severe condition caused by prolonged exposure to high heat. Heat stroke interferes with the body's temperature regulating abilities and can lead to collapse and coma.

Parkinsonism—A group of conditions that all have these typical symptoms in common: tremor, rigidity, slow movement, and poor balance and coordination.

Pregnancy category— A system of classifying drugs according to their established risks for use during pregnancy. Category A: Controlled human studies have demonstrated no fetal risk. Category B: Animal studies indicate no fetal risk, but no human studies; or adverse effects in animals, but not in well-controlled human studies. Category C: No adequate human or animal studies; or adverse fetal effects in animal studies, but no available human data. Category D: Evidence of fetal risk, but benefits outweigh risks. Category X: Evidence of fetal risk. Risks outweigh any benefits.

Seizure—A sudden attack, spasm, or convulsion.

Spasm—Sudden, involuntary tensing of a muscle or a group of muscles.

Tremor—Shakiness or trembling.

properties, the naturally occurring belladonna alkaloids (atropine, scopolamine, hyoscyamine), some **antihistamines** with anticholinergic properties, and synthetics such as benztropin (Cogentin), procyclidine (Kemadrin) and biperiden (Akineton) are members of this group. Although the anticholinergic drugs have only limited activity against Parkinson's disease, they are useful in the early stages, and may be adjuncts to levodopa as the disease progresses.

Amantadine (Symmetrel), was developed for prevention of **influenza** virus infection, but has anti-Parkinsonian properties. Its mechanism of action is not known.

Bromocriptine (Parlodel) is a prolactin inhibitor, which is used for a variety of indications including amenorrhea/galactorrhea, female **infertility**, and acromegaly. It appears to work by direct stimulation of the dopamine receptors. Bromocriptine is used as a late adjunct to levodopa therapy, and may permit reduction in levodopa dosage. Pergolide (Permax) is similar to bromocriptine, but has not been studied as extensively in Parkinson's disease.

Entacapone (Comtan) appears to act by maintaining levels of dopamine through enzyme inhibition. It is used as an adjunct to levodopa was the patient is beginning to experience the on-off effect. Tolcapone (Tasmar) is a similar agent, but has demonstrated the potential for inducing severe liver failure. As such, tolcapone is reserved for cases where all other adjunctive therapies have failed or are contraindicated.

Selegeline (Carbex, Eldepryl) is a selective monoamine oxidase B (MAO-B) inhibitor, however its mechanism of action in Parkinsonism is unclear, since other drugs with MAO-B inhibition have failed to show similar anti-Parkinsonian effects. Selegeline is used primarily as an adjunct to levodopa, although some studies have indicated that the drug may be useful in the early stages of Parkinsonism, and may delay the progression of the disease.

Pramipexole (Mirapex) and ropinirole (Requip) are believed to act by direct stimulation of the dopamine receptors in the brain. They may be used alone in early Parkison's disease, or as adjuncts to levodopa in advanced stages.

Recommended dosage

Dosages of anti-Parkinsonian medications must be highly individualized. All doses must be carefully titrated. Consult specific references.

Precautions

There are a large number of drugs and drug classes used to treat Parkinson's disease, and individual references should be consulted.

The anticholinergics have a large number of adverse effects, all related to their primary mode of activity. Their cardiovascular effects include tachycardia, **palpitations**, **hypotension**, postural hypotension, and mild bradycardia. They may also cause a wide range of central nervous system effects, including disorientation, confusion, memory loss, **hallucinations**, psychoses, agitation, nervousness, **delusions**, **delirium**, **paranoia**, euphoria, excitement, lightheadedness, **dizziness**, **headache**, listlessness, depression, drowsiness, weakness, and giddiness. **Dry mouth**, dry eyes and gastrointestinal distress are common problems. **Sedation** has been reported with some drugs in this group, but this may be beneficial in patients who suffer from **insomnia**. **Pregnancy** risk factor is C. Because anticholinergic drugs may inhibit milk production, their use during breastfeeding is not recommended. Patients should be warned that anticholinergic medications will inhibit perspiration, and so **exercise** during periods of high temperature should be avoided.

Levodopa has a large number of adverse effects. Anorexia, loss of appetite, occurs in roughly half the patients using this drug. Symptoms of gastrointestinal upset, such as **nausea and vomiting**, have been reported in 80% of cases. Other reported effects include increased hand tremor; headache; dizziness; **numbness**; weakness and faintness; **bruxism**; confusion; insomnia; nightmares; hallucinations and delusions; agitation and **anxiety**; malaise; **fatigue** and euphoria. Levodopa has not been listed under the pregnancy risk factor schedules, but should be used with caution. Breastfeeding is not recommended.

Amantadine is generally well tolerated, but may cause dizziness and **nausea**. It is classified as pregnancy schedule C. Since amantadine is excreted in breast milk, breastfeeding while taking amantidine is not recommended.

Pergolide and bromocriptine have been generally well tolerated. **Orthostatic hypotension** are common problems, and patients must be instructed to risk slowly from bed. This problem can be minimized by low initial doses with small dose increments. Hallucinations may be a problem. Bromocriptine has not been evaluated for pregnancy risk, while pergolide is category B. Since both drugs may inhibit **lactation**, breastfeeding while taking these drugs is not recommended.

Pramipexole and ropinirole cause orthostatic hypotension, hallucinations and dizziness. The two drugs are in pregnancy category C. In animals, ropinirole has been shown to have adverse effects on embryo-fetal development, including teratogenic effects, decreased fetal body weight, increased fetal **death** and digital malformation. Because these drugs inhibit prolactin secretion, they should not be taken while breastfeeding.

Side effects

The most common side effects are associated with the central nervous system, and include dizziness, lightheadedness, mood changes and hallucinations. Gastrointestinal problems, including nausea and **vomiting**, are also common.

Interactions

All anti-Parkinsonian regimens should be carefully reviewed for possible **drug interactions**. Note that combination therapy with anti-Parkinsonian drugs is, in itself, use of additive and potentiating interactions between drugs, and so careful dose adjustment is needed whenever a drug is added or withdrawn.

Samuel D. Uretsky, PharmD

Antiplatelet drugs *see* **Anticoagulant and antiplatelet drugs**

Antiprotozoal drugs

Definition

Antiprotozoal drugs are medicines that treat infections caused by protozoa.

Purpose

Antiprotozoal drugs are used to treat a variety of diseases caused by protozoa. Protozoa are animal-like, one-celled animals, such as amoebas. Some are parasites that cause infections in the body. African **sleeping sickness**, **giardiasis**, **amebiasis**, *Pneumocystis carinii* **pneumonia** (PCP), and **malaria** are examples of diseases caused by protozoa.

Description

Antiprotozoal drugs come in liquid, tablet, and injectable forms and are available only with a doctor's prescription. Some commonly used antiprotozoal drugs are metronidazole (Flagyl), eflornithine

KEY TERMS

Amebiasis—An infection caused by an ameba, which is a type of protozoan.

Fetus—A developing baby inside the womb.

Giardiasis—A condition in which the intestines are infected with *Giardia lamblia*, a type of protozoan.

Inflammation—Pain, redness, swelling, and heat that usually develop in response to injury or illness.

Parasite—An organism that lives and feeds in or on another organism (the host) and does nothing to benefit the host.

Pneumocystis carinii pneumonia—A severe lung infection caused by a parasitic protozoan. The disease mainly affects people with weakened immune systems, such as people with AIDS.

(Ornidyl), furazolidone (Furoxone), hydroxychloroquine (Plaquenil), iodoquinol (Diquinol, Yodoquinol, Yodoxin), and pentamidine (Pentam 300).

Recommended dosage

The recommended dosage depends on the type of antiprotozoal drug, its strength, and the medical problem for which it is being used. Check with the physician who prescribed the drug or the pharmacist who filled the prescription for the correct dosage. Always take antiprotozoal drugs exactly as directed.

Precautions

Some people feel dizzy, confused, lightheaded, or less alert when using these drugs. The drugs may also cause blurred vision and other vision problems. For these reasons, anyone who takes these drugs should not drive, use machines or do anything else that might be dangerous until they have found out how the drugs affect them.

The antiprotozoal drug furazolidone may cause very dangerous side effects when taken with certain foods or beverages. Likewise, metronidazole (Flagyl) can cause serious liver damage if taken with alcohol. Check with the physician who prescribed the drug or the pharmacist who filled the prescription for a list of products to avoid while taking these medicines.

Anyone who has ever had unusual reactions to antiprotozoal drugs or related medicines should let his or her physician know before taking the drugs again.

The physician should also be told about any **allergies** to foods, dyes, preservatives, or other substances.

Some antiprotozoal drugs may cause problems with the blood. This can increase the risk of infection or excessive bleeding. Patients taking these drugs shouldbe careful not to injure their gums when brushing or flossing their teeth or using a toothpick. They shouldcheck with the physician before having any dentalwork done. Care should also be taken to avoidcuts from razors, nail clippers, or kitchen knives, orhousehold tools. Anyone who has any of these symptoms while taking antiprotozoal drugs should call the physician immediately:

- Fever or chills
- Signs of cold or flu
- Signs of infection, such as redness, swelling, or inflammation
- Unusual bruising or bleeding
- Black, tarry stools
- Blood in urine or stools
- Pinpoint red spots on the skin
- Unusual tiredness or weakness.

Anyone taking this medicine should also check with a physician immediately if any of these symptoms occur:

- Blurred vision or other vision changes
- Skin rash, **hives**, or **itching**
- Swelling of the neck
- Clumsiness or unsteadiness
- Numbness, **tingling**, **pain**, or weakness in the hands or feet
- Decrease in urination.

Children are especially sensitive to the effects of some antiprotozoal drugs. *Never give this medicine to a child unless directed to do so by a physician, and always keep this medicine out of the reach of children. Use safety vials.*

The effects of antiprotozoal drugs on pregnant women have not been studied. However, in experiments with pregnant laboratory animals, some antiprotozoal drugs cause **birth defects** or **death** of the fetus. Women who are pregnant or who plan to become pregnant should check with their physicians before taking antiprotozoal drugs. Mothers who are breastfeeding should also check with their physicians about the safety of taking these drugs.

Before using antiprotozoal drugs, people with any of these medical problems should make sure their physicians are aware of their conditions:

- Anemia or other blood problems
- Kidney disease
- Heart disease
- Low blood pressure
- Diabetes
- Hypoglycemia (low blood sugar)
- Liver disease
- Stomach or intestinal disease
- Nerve or brain disease or disorder, including convulsions (seizures)
- Psoriasis (a skin condition)
- Hearing loss
- Deficiency of the enzyme glucose-6-phosphate dehydrogenase (G6PD)
- Eye or vision problems
- Thyroid disease.

Side effects

The most common side effects are **diarrhea, nausea, vomiting,** and stomach pain. These problems usually go away as the body adjusts to the drug and do not require medical treatment.

Other rare side effects may occur. Anyone who has unusual symptoms after taking an antiprotozoal drug should get in touch with his or her physician.

Interactions

Antiprotozoal drugs may interact with other medicines. When this happens, the effects of one or both of the drugs may change or the risk of side effects may be greater. Anyone who takes antiprotozoal drugs should let the physician know all other medicines he or she is taking. Among the drugs that may interact with antiprotozoal drugs are:

- Alcohol
- Anticancer drugs
- Medicine for overactive thyroid
- Antiviral drugs such as zidovudine (Retrovir)
- Antibiotics
- Medicine used to relieve pain or inflammation
- Amphetamine
- Diet pills (appetite suppressants)

- Monoamine oxidase inhibitors (MAO inhibitors) such as phenelzine (Nardil) and tranylcypromine (Parnate), used to treat conditions including depression and Parkinson's disease.
- Tricyclic antidepressants such as amitriptyline (Elavil) and imipramine (Tofranil)
- Decongestants such as phenylephrine (Neo-Synephrine) and pseudoephedrine (Sudafed)
- Other antiprotozoal drugs.

The list above does not include every medicine that may interact with an antifungal drug. Be sure to check with a physician or pharmacist before combining antifungal drugs with any other prescription or nonprescription (over-the-counter) medicine.

Nancy Ross-Flanigan

Antipruritic drugs *see* **Anti-itch drugs**

Antipsychotic drugs

Definition

Antipsychotic drugs are a class of medicines used to treat **psychosis** and other mental and emotional conditions.

Purpose

Psychosis is defined as "a serious mental disorder (as **schizophrenia**) characterized by defective or lost contact with reality often with **hallucinations** or delusions." Psychosis is an end-stage condition arising from a variety of possible causes. Anti-psychotic drugs control the symptoms of psychosis, and in many cases are effective in controlling the symptoms of other disorders that may lead to psychosis, including bipolar mood disorder (formerly termed manic-depressive), in which the patient cycles from severe depression to feelings of extreme excitation. This class of drugs is primarily composed of the major tranquilizers; however, lithium carbonate, a drug that is largely specific to bipolar mood disorder, is commonly classified among the antipsychotic agents.

Description

The antipsychotic agents may be divided by chemical class. The phenothiazines are the oldest group, and include chlorpromazine (Thorazine), mesoridazine

Antipsychotic Drugs

Brand Name (Generic Name)	Possible Common Side Effects Include:
Clozaril (clozapine)	Seizures, agranulocytosis, **dizziness**, increased blood pressure
Compazine (prochlorperazine)	Involuntary **muscle spasms**, dizziness, jitteriness, puckering of the mouth
Haldol (haloperidol)	Involuntary muscle spasms, blurred vision, **dehydration**, **headache**, puckering of the mouth
Mellaril (thioridazine)	Involuntary muscle spasms, **constipation** and **diarrhea**, sensitivity to light
Navane (thiothixene)	Involuntary muscle spasms, dry mouth, rash, hives
Risperdal (risperidone)	Involuntary muscle spasms, abdominal and chest **pain**, **fever**, headache
Stelazine (trifluoperazine hydrochloride)	Involuntary muscle spasms, drowsiness, fatigue
Thorazine (chlorpromazine)	Involuntary muscle spasms, labored breathing, fever, puckering of the mouth
Triavil	Involuntary muscle spasms, disorientation, excitability, lightheadedness

(Serentil), prochlorperazine (Compazine), and thioridazine (Mellaril). These drugs are essentially similar in action and adverse effects. They may also be used as anti-emetics, although prochlorperazine is the drug most often used for this indication.

The phenylbutylpiperadines are haloperidol (Haldol) and pimozide (Orap). They find primary use in control of Tourette's syndrome. Haloperidol has been extremely useful in controlling aggressive behavior.

The debenzapine derivatives, clozapine (Clozaril), loxapine (Loxitane), olanzapine (Zyprexa) and quetiapine (Seroquel), have been effective in controlling psychotic symptoms that have not been responsive to other classes of drugs.

The benzisoxidil group is composed of resperidone (Resperidal) and ziprasidone (Geodon). Resperidone has been found useful for controlling bipolar mood disorder, while ziprasidone is used primarily as second-line treatment for schizophrenia.

In addition to these drugs, the class of antipsychotic agents includes lithium carbonate (Eskalith, Lithonate), which is used for control of bipolar mood disorder, and thiothixene (Navane), which is used in the treatment of psychosis.

Newer agents

Some newer antipsychotic drugs have been approved by the Food and Drug administration

(FDA) in the early 2000s. These drugs are sometimes called second-generation antipsychotics or SGAs. Aripiprazole (Abilify), which is classified as a partial dopaminergic agonist, received FDA approval in August 2003. Two drugs that are still under investigation, a neurokinin antagonist and a serotonin 2A/2C antagonist respectively, show promise in the treatment of schizophrenia and **schizoaffective disorder**.

Recommended dosage

Dose varies with the drug, condition being treated, and patient response. See specific references.

Precautions

Neuroleptic malignant syndrome (NMS). NMS is a rare, idiosyncratic combination of extra-pyramidal symptoms (EPS), hyperthermia, and autonomic disturbance. Onset may be hours to months after drug initiation, but once started, proceeds rapidly over 24 to 72 hours. It is most commonly associated with haloperidol, long-acting fluphenazine, but has occurred with thiothixene, thioridazine, and clozapine, and may occur with other agents. NMS is potentially fatal, and requires intensive symptomatic treatment and immediate discontinuation of neuroleptic treatment. There is no established treatment. Most patients who develop NMS will have the same problem if the drug is restarted.

Agranulocytosis has been associated with clozapine. This is a potentially fatal reaction, but can be prevented with careful monitoring of the white **blood count**. There are no well-established risk factors for developing agranulocytosis, and so all patients treated with this drug must follow the clozapine Patient Management System. For more information, the reader should call 1-800-448-5938.

Anticholinergic effects, particularly **dry mouth**, have been reported with all of the phenothiazines, and can be severe enough to cause patients to discontinue their medication.

Photosensitization is a common reaction to chlorpromazine. Patients must be instructed to use precautions when exposed to sunlight.

Lithium carbonate commonly causes increased frequency of urination.

The so-called atypical antipsychotics are associated with a substantial increase in the risk of developing **diabetes mellitus**. A study done at the University of Rochester (New York) reported in 2004 that 15.2% of patients receiving atypical antipsychotics developed diabetes, compared with 6.3% of patients taking other antipsychotic medications.

Antipsychotic drugs are **pregnancy** category C. (Clozapine is category B.) The drugs in this class appear to be generally safe for occasional use at low doses during pregnancy, but should be avoided near time of delivery. Although the drugs do not appear to be teratogenic, when used near term, they may cross the placenta and have adverse effects on the newborn infant, including causing involuntary movements. There is no information about safety in breast feeding.

As a class, the antipsychotic drugs have a large number of potential side effects, many of them serious. Because of the potential severity of side effects, these drugs must be used with special caution in children. Specific references should be consulted.

Interactions

Because the phenothiazines have anticholinergic effects, they should not be used in combination with other drugs that may have similar effects.

Because the drugs in this group may cause **hypotension**, or low blood pressure, they should be used with extreme care in combination with blood pressure-lowering drugs.

The antipsychotic drugs have a large number of **drug interactions**. Consult specific references.

Resources

BOOKS

Beers, Mark H., MD, and Robert Berkow, MD., editors. "Childhood Psychosis." Section 19, Chapter 274 In *The Merck Manual of Diagnosis and Therapy*. Whitehouse Station, NJ: Merck Research Laboratories, 2002.

Beers, Mark H., MD, and Robert Berkow, MD., editors. "Psychiatric Emergencies." Section 15, Chapter 194 In *The Merck Manual of Diagnosis and Therapy*. Whitehouse Station, NJ: Merck Research Laboratories, 2002.

Wilson, Billie Ann, Margaret T. Shannon, and Carolyn L. Stang. *Nurse's Drug Guide 2003*. Upper Saddle River, NJ: Prentice Hall, 2003.

PERIODICALS

DeLeon, A., N. C. Patel, and M. L. Crismon. "Aripiprazole: A Comprehensive Review of Its Pharmacology, Clinical Efficacy, and Tolerability." *Clinical Therapeutics* 26 (May 2004): 649–666.

Emsley, R., H. J. Turner, J. Schronen, et al. "A Single-Blind, Randomized Trial Comparing Quetiapine and Haloperidol in the Treatment of Tardive Dyskinesia." *Journal of Clinical Psychiatry* 65 (May 2004): 696–701.

Lamberti, J. S., J. F. Crilly, K. Maharaj, et al. "Prevalence of Diabetes Mellitus among Outpatients with Severe Mental Disorders Receiving Atypical Antipsychotic Drugs." *Journal of Clinical Psychiatry* 65 (May 2004): 702–706.

Meltzer, H. Y., L. Arvanitis, D. Bauer, et al. "Placebo-Controlled Evaluation of Four Novel Compounds for the Treatment of Schizophrenia and Schizoaffective Disorder." *American Journal of Psychiatry* 161 (June 2004): 975–984.

Stahl, S. M. "Anticonvulsants as Mood Stabilizers and Adjuncts to Antipsychotics: Valproate, Lamotrigine, Carbamazepine, and Oxcarbazepine and Actions at Voltage-Gated Sodium Channels." *Journal of Clinical Psychiatry* 65 (June 2004): 738–739.

ORGANIZATIONS

American Society of Health-System Pharmacists (ASHP). 7272 Wisconsin Avenue, Bethesda, MD 20814. (301) 657-3000. < http://www.ashp.org >.

United States Food and Drug Administration (FDA). 5600 Fishers Lane, Rockville, MD 20857-0001. (888) INFO-FDA. < http://www.fda.gov >.

Samuel D. Uretsky, PharmD
Rebecca J. Frey, PhD

Antipsychotic drugs, atypical

Definition

The atypical antipsychotic agents, sometimes called the "novel" antipsychotic agents are a group of drugs which are different chemically from the older drugs used to treat **psychosis**. The "conventional" **antipsychotic drugs** are classified by their chemical structures as the phenothiazines, thioxanthines (which are chemically very similar to the phenothiazines), butyrophenones, diphenylbutylpiperadines and the indolones. All of the atypical antipsychotic agents are chemically classified as dibenzepines. They are considered *atypical* or *novel* because they have different side effects from the conventional antipsychotic agents. The atypical drugs are far less likely to cause extra-pyramidal side-effects(EPS), drug induced involuntary movements, than are the older drugs. The atypical antipsychotic drugs may also be effective in some cases that are resistant to older drugs.

The drugs in this group are clozapine (Clozaril), loxapine (Loxitane), olanzapine (Zyprexa), and quetiapine (Seroquel).

Purpose

The antipsychotic drugs are used to treat severe emotional disorders. Although there may be different names for these disorders, depending on severity and how long the symptoms last, psychotic disorders all cause at least one of the following symptoms:

Loxapine has also been used to treat **anxiety** with mental depression.

Recommended dosage

The recommended dose depends on the drug, the patient, and the condition being treated. The normal practice is to start each patient at a low dose, and gradually increase the dose until a satisfactory response is achieved. The odse should be held at the lowest level that gives satisfactory results.

Clozapine usually requires doses between 300 and 600 milligrams a day, but some people require as much as 900 milligrams/day. Doses higher than 900 milligrams/day are not recommended.

Loxapine is usually effective at doses of 60-100 milligrams/day, but may be used in doses as high as 250 mg/day if needed.

Olanzapine doses vary with the condition being treated. The usual maximum dose is 20 milligrams/day.

Quetiapine may be dosed anywhere from 150-750 milligrams/day, depending on how well the patient responds.

Precautions

Although the atypical antipsychotics are generally safe, clozapine has been associated with severe agranulocytosis, a shortage of white blood cells. For this reason, people who may be treated with clozapine should have blood counts before starting the drug, blood counts every week for as long as they are using clozapine, and blood counts every week for the first 4 weeks after they stop taking clozapine. If there is any evidence of a drop in the white **blood count** while using clozapine, the drug should be stopped.

Atypical antipsychotics should not be used in patients with liver damage, brain or circulatory problems, or some types of blood problems.

Allergies

People who have had an allergic reaction to one of the atypical antipsychotics should not use that medication again. However, sometimes it is possible to use a different drug from the same group safely.

Pregnancy

The atypical antipsychotics have not been proved safe in **pregnancy**. They should be used only when clearly needed and when potential benefits outweigh potential hazards to the fetus. These drugs have not been reported in human milk.

Side effects

Although the atypical antipsychotics are less likely to cause involuntary movements than the older antipsychotic drugs, they still have a large number of adverse effects. The following list is not complete. Review each drug individually for a full list of possible adverse effects.

Interactions

Taking atypical antipsychotic medications with certain other drugs may affect the way the drugs work or may increase the chance of side effects. While taking antipsychotic drugs, do not take any other prescription or nonprescription (over-the-counter) drugs without first checking with a physician.

Because the atypical antipsychotics may cause lowering of blood pressure, care should be used when these drugs are taken at the same time as other drugs which lower blood pressure.

Quetiapine has many interactions. Doses should be carefully adjusted when quetiapine is used with ketoconazole, itraconazole, fluconazole, erythromycin, carbamazepine, **barbiturates**, rifampin or glucocorticoids including prednisone, dexamethasone and methylprednisolone.

These drugs will also require dose adjustments when used with anti-Parkinson medications.

Resources

BOOKS

Brain Basics: An Integrated Biological Approach to Understanding and Assessing Human Behavior. Phoenix: Biological-Psychiatry-Institute, June 1999.

PERIODICALS

McDougle, C. J. "A double-blind, placebo-controlled study of risperidone addition in serotonin reuptake inhibitor-refractory obsessive-compulsive disorder." *Archives of General Psychiatry* August 2000: 794.

Samuel D. Uretsky, PharmD

▌Anti-rejection drugs

Definition

Anti-rejection drugs are daily medications taken by organ transplant patients to prevent organ rejection.

Purpose

Anti-rejection drugs, which are also called immunosuppressants, help to suppress the immune system's response to a new organ. When a new organ is placed inside a patient s body, the patient's immune system recognizes the organ as foreign tissue and tries to reject it.

Description

When a physician prescribes anti-rejection drugs, the patient's risk of rejection and susceptibility to side effects are considered. The most common drugs prescribed to prevent organ rejection are cyclosporine, prednisone, azathioprine, tacrolimus or FK506, mycophenolate mofetil, sirolimus, and OKT3, as well as ATGAM and Thymoglobulin. As is true with all medications, each of these drugs has benefits and drawbacks. Cyclosporine, which is one of the most frequently used anti-rejection drugs, is usually combined with prednisone. An extremely powerful medicine, cyclosporine is usually taken by a patient over the course of his or her lifetime. Cortisol, which is the naturally produced form of prednisone in a person's body, helps the body manage **stress**, such as infections or organ rejection. Taking prednisone results in less cortisol production in a person's body, thus minimizing the risk of rejection. Azathioprine, which needs to be taken with food to avoid stomach upset, is frequently combined with cyclosporine, prednisone, or tacrolimus. Mycophenolate mofetil is a relatively new immunosuppressant that is similar to azathioprine; therefore, the two drugs should not be taken together. It is preferable to take mycophenolate mofetil on an empty stomach; however, like azathioprine, it can be taken with food because it, too, can cause stomach problems, such as **heartburn** and **nausea**. Like azathioprine, mycophenolate mofetil is not a stand-alone drug; instead, it must be used, in combination with other medications. This is also the case with regard to sirolimus.

Physicians prescribe either mycophenolate mofetil or azathioprine (in combination with other **immunosuppressant drugs**) to help patients cope with acute bouts of organ rejection. The medications work by interfering with the multiplication process of white blood cells, which is part of the body's natural defense system when foreign invaders, such as a new organ, are detected. However, researchers at Duke University and the University of Florida found that mycophenolate mofetil doesn't work any better than azathioprine, but costs significantly more. Aside from cost, another consideration also needs to be the type of organ transplanted, because acute rejection rates differ. For example, six months after surgery, approximately 15% of kidney recipients will have an acute rejection episode as compared to approximately 60% of lung recipients. And because study results vary depending on the organ transplanted, more research is needed with regard to the success of mycophenolate mofetil as compared to azathioprine.

OKT3 prevents is prescribed to prevent organ rejection immediately after surgery and is also used to treat acute rejection episodes; ATGAM and Thymoglobulin, which are similar to OKT3, are used for the same reasons. All three drugs are given intravenously.

Tacrolimus, which is also known as FK506, is a fairly new drug that is considered by many experts to be as effective as cyclosporine. An alternative drug choice for patients that cannot tolerate cyclosporine, tacrolimus has been the subject of much research in recent years. Used to treat rejection episodes that are acute or chronic in nature, tacrolimus is being studied to see if using it will allow patients to reduce their dosage of prednisone without organ rejection.

In a presentation at the 2003 American Transplant Congress, surgeons from the University of Pittsburgh reported that an innovative clinical protocol developed by Dr. Thomas E. Starzl was implemented, which reduced the dosage of tacrolimus needed by lung transplant patients with excellent success. Patients required lower doses of prednisone as well. In fact, in some cases, patients were taking tacrolimus only once a day (rather than twice a day) or only four times a week. Over the long-term, physicians hope that there will be less risk of lung recipients developing the kinds of complications normally associated with high levels of immunosuppressants, such as kidney dysfunction, which is a common problem faced by lung transplant patients.

Dr. Thomas E. Strazl, the renowned physician often referred to as the modern-day father of transplantation, developed the protocol based on the knowledge that some of his patients had stopped taking their daily pills with no ill effects. Starzl theorized that giving several drugs to a patient immediately after surgery, which was the normal practice, might inhibit the immune system from developing a tolerance for the new organ. Therefore, his new protocol embraced a different approach. Shortly before the transplantation, patients were given a drug that killed their T-cells and after the

operation, patients received only one anti-rejection medicine rather than the multi-pill cocktail normally prescribed. In an article published by *Lancet* in 2003, Starzl and colleagues reported the results of their pilot study involving 82 two kidney, liver, pancreas or small bowel transplant patients treated according to the new drug protocol. Out of the 72 patients with successful transplants after one year, over half the patients were taking anti-rejection medication either every other day, three times per week or twice per week. Amazingly, 11 of the patients were taking only one pill a week and they exhibited no signs of organ rejection or complications. Certainly more research needs to be conducted, but these results are very promising.

Recommended dosage

The dosages vary depending on the drug or drug combination being taken by the patient. In general, cyclosporine is taken every 12 hours in liquid or capsule form. Tacrolimus is generally taken every 12 hours as well. The level of either drug in a patient's blood is monitored carefully and doses are adjusted accordingly in order to not only prevent reject, but also unpleasant side effects. Azathioprine is taken once a day in tablet form, whereas mycophenolate mofetil is generally taken every 12 hours. High doses of prednisone are usually given at first and then tapered down slowly.

Precautions

Patients should discuss proper storage methods with regard to their medications. Sirolimus, for example, should be stored at room temperature with special care taken to keep it out of excessive heat and humidity.

Although pregnant women taking anti-rejection drugs have delivered healthy babies, women planning on becoming pregnant while taking anti-rejection drugs should talk with their physicians regarding any possible complications. For example, the safety of taking mycophenolate mofetil during **pregnancy** or while breastfeeding is questionable and not advised.

Side effects

Side effects vary depending on the individual and the drug therapy chosen. Patients should talk with their doctors regarding the various side effects they can expect and under what conditions emergency medical care needs to be sought.

Interactions

It is essential that patients talk with their pharmacist and transplant team before taking any medications, regardless of whether they are prescription or over-the-counter drugs to ensure that the combinations will not interact. For example, **antacids** can diminish the effectiveness of mycophenolate mofetil and drugs used to treat **high cholesterol** may increase the potency of sirolimus. In addition, certain food products can also alter the potency of some anti-rejection drugs. For example, grapefruit and grapefruit juice can cause cyclosporine blood levels to increase.

Resources

PERIODICALS

Mazariegos, G. V., Zahorchak, A. F., Reyes, J., et al. "Dendritic cell subset ratio in peripheral blood correlates with successful withdrawal of immunosuppression in liver transplant patients." *American Journal of Transplantation* 3 (2003): 689–696.

Starzl, T. E., Murase, N., Abu-Elmagd, K., et al. "Tolerogenic immunosuppression for organ transplantation." *Lancet* 361 (2003): 1502–1510.

OTHER

Ross, Melanie Fridl "Duke/UF Researchers compare anti-rejection medicines in lung transplant patients." *University of Florida* 9 Aug 2001 University of Florida News. 22 Feb 2005 < http://www.napa.ufl.edu/2001news/antireject.htm >.

Rossi, Lisa "Studies of liver transplant patients off anti-rejection drugs have altered cell profile." *University of Pittsburgh Medical Center* 2 June 2003 University of Pittsburgh Medical Center. 22 Feb 2005 < http://www.eurekalert.org/pub_releases/2003-06/uopm-so1060203.php >.

Srikameswaran, Anita "Protocol reduces transplant patients need for anti-rejection drugs." *Post-Gazette.com Health and Science* 2 May 2003 PG Publishing Company, Inc. 22 Feb 2005 < http://www.post-gazette.com/healthscience/20030502starzlhealth2p2.asp >.

University of Pittsburgh Medical Center "Our Experts: Thomas E. Starzl, M.D., Ph.D." *University of Pittsburgh Medical Center* 2005 University of Pittsburgh Medical Center. 22 Feb 2005 < http://newsbureau.upmc.com/Bios/BioStarzl.htm >.

Lee Ann Paradise

Antiretroviral drugs

Definition

Antiretroviral drugs inhibit the reproduction of retroviruses—viruses composed of RNA rather than DNA. The best known of this group is HIV, human **immunodeficiency** virus, the causative agent of **AIDS**.

Purpose

Antiretroviral agents are virustatic agents which block steps in the replication of the virus. The drugs are not curative; however continued use of drugs, particularly in multi-drug regimens, significantly slows disease progression.

Description

There are three main types of antiretroviral drugs, although only two steps in the viral replication process are blocked. Nucleoside analogs, or nucleoside reverse transcriptase inhibitors (NRTIs), such as didanosine (ddI, Videx), lamivudine (3TC, Epivir), stavudine (d4T, Zerit), zalcitabine (ddC, Hivid), and zidovudine (AZT, Retrovir), act by inhibiting the enzyme reverse transcriptase. Because a retrovirus is composed of RNA, the virus must make a DNA strand in order to replicate itself. Reverse transcriptase is an enzyme that is essential to making the DNA copy. The nucleoside reverse transcriptase inhibitors are incorporated into the DNA strand. This is a faulty DNA molecule that is incapable of reproducing.

The **non-nucleoside reverse transcriptase inhibitors** (NNRTIs), such as delavirdine (Rescriptor), loviride, and nevirapine (Viramune) act by binding directly to the reverse transcriptase molecule, inhibiting its activity.

A fourth class of drugs was under clinical trials in 2003. Called fusion inhibitors, they block HIV from fusing with healthy cells. The first to receive FDA approval will likely be a drug called Enfurvitide.

Because HIV mutates readily, the virus can develop resistance to single drug therapy. However, treatment with drug combinations appears to produce a durable response. Proper treatment appears to slow the progression of HIV infections and reduce the frequency of opportunistic infections. One of the most notable advances in recent years has been the success of highly active antiretroviral therapy (HAART). This multidrug approach reduced the risk of opportunistic infections in persons with HIV/AIDS and slowed the progression of the disease and **death**. Usually, patients receive triple combination therapy, however research in 2003 showed a new once-daily regimen of quadruple therapy effective. The combination included adefovir, lamivudine, didanosine, and efavirenz. In short, the scientific community continues to make rapid advancements in developing and evaluating antiretroviral drug therapy. It is best to keep well informed and frequently check with a physician.

Antiviral drugs—Medicines that cure or control virus infections.

Bioavailability—A measure of the amount of drug that is actually absorbed from a given dose.

Hypoxemia—Lower than normal oxygenation of arterial blood.

Immune system—The body's natural defenses against disease and infection.

Inflammation—Pain, redness, swelling, and heat that usually develop in response to injury or illness.

Pancreas—A gland located beneath the stomach. The pancreas produces juices that help break down food and secretes insulin that helps the body use sugar for energy.

Insomnia—A sleep disorder characterized by inability to either fall asleep or to stay asleep.

Mutates—Undergoes a spontaneous change in the make-up of genes or chromosomes.

Pregnancy category— A system of classifying drugs according to their established risks for use during pregnancy. Category A: Controlled human studies have demonstrated no fetal risk. Category B: Animal studies indicate no fetal risk, but no human studies; or adverse effects in animals, but not in well-controlled human studies. Category C: No adequate human or animal studies; or adverse fetal effects in animal studies, but no available human data. Category D: Evidence of fetal risk, but benefits outweigh risks. Category X: Evidence of fetal risk. Risks outweigh any benefits.

Retrovirus—A virus composed of ribonucleic acid (RNA) instead of deoxynucleic acid (DNA).

Virus—A tiny, disease-causing particle that can reproduce only in living cells.

Recommended dosage

Doses must be individualized based on the patient and use of interacting drugs. The optimum combinations of antiretroviral drugs have not been determined, nor is there agreement on the stage of infection at which to start treatment. In fact, starting treatment too early has led to unwanted side effects in some patients or problems with patient readiness to comply. Treatment should begin when the time and circumstances are right.

Precautions

Although the antiretroviral drugs fall into several groups, each drug has a unique pattern of adverse effects and **drug interactions**. Since the drugs are used in various combinations, the frequency and severity of adverse effects will vary with the combination. Although most drug combinations show a higher rate of adverse events than single drug therapy, some patterns are not predictable. For example, indinavir has been reported to cause **insomnia** in 3% of patients, however, when used in combination with zidovudine, only 1.5% of patients complained of sleep difficulties.

The most severe adverse effects associated with the protease inhibitors are kidney and liver toxicity. Patients also have reported a syndrome of abdominal distention (selling and expansion) and increased body odor, which may be socially limiting. Hemophilic patients have reported increased bleeding tendencies while taking protease inhibitors. The drugs are **pregnancy** category B. There have been no controlled studies of safety in pregnancy. HIV-infected mothers are advised not to breast feed in order to prevent transmission of the virus to the newborn.

The nucleoside reverse transcriptase inhibitors have significant levels of toxicity. Lactic acidosis in the absence of hypoxemia and severe liver enlargement with fatty degeneration have been reported with zidovudine and zalcitabine, and are potentially fatal. Rare cases of liver failure, considered possibly related to underlying **hepatitis B** and zalcitabine monotherapy, have been reported.

Abacavir has been associated with fatal hypersensitivity reactions. Didanosine has been associated with severe **pancreatitis**. Nucleoside reverse transcriptase inhibitors are pregnancy category C. There is limited information regarding safety during pregnancy. Zidovudine has been used during pregnancy to reduce the risk of HIV infection to the infant. HIV-infected mothers are advised not to breast feed in order to prevent transmission of the virus to the newborn.

Efavirenz has been associated with a high frequency of skin rash, 27% in adults and 40% in children. Nevirapine has been associated with severe liver damage and skin reactions. All of the non-nucleoside reverse transcriptase inhibitors are pregnancy category C, based on animal studies.

Using antiretroviral drugs in combination also helps lower risk of developing viral resistance. Fifty percent of patients who fail antiretroviral therapy are resistant to one class of drug. Recent research into multiple drugs and combinations is promising.

Interactions

Because of the high frequency of drug interactions associated with AIDS therapy, specialized references should be consulted. Use of recreational drugs while on antiretroviral therapy can trigger potentially lethal side effects or negate the positive effects of the therapy.

Saquinavir is marketed in both hard and soft gelatin capsules. Because saquinavir in the hard gelatin capsule formulation (Invirase) has poor bioavailability, it is recommended that this formulation only be used in combination with other drugs which interact to raise saquinavir blood levels. Saquinavir soft gelatin capsules (Fortovase) are the preferred dosage form of this drug.

Resources

PERIODICALS

"Grant Awarded for Evaluation of Once-Daily Antiretroviral." *Virus Weekly* (November 26, 2002): 12.

Isaac, A., and D. Pillay. "New Drugs for Treating Drug Resistant HIV–1: Clinical Management of Virological Failure Remains an Important and Difficult Issue for HIV Physicians." *Sexualy Transmitted Diseases* (June 2003): 176–183.

"New Therapy Strategies Focusing on Long Term: DrugsÆ Impact on Heart is Debated." *AIDS Alert* April 2003: 45.

"Once-Daily Quadruple Regimen Safe, Effective." *AIDS Weekly* (October 7, 2003): 4.

"Recreational Drugs can Reduce Safety, Efficacy of Antiretroviral Agents." *AIDS Weekly* (December 16, 2003): 3.

Thanker, H.K., and M.H. Snow. "HIV Viral Suppression in the Era of Antiretroviral Therapy." *Postgraduate Medical Journal* (January 2003): 36.

ORGANIZATIONS

Project Inform. 205 13th Street, #2001, San Francisco, CA 94103. (415) 558-8669. < http://www.projinf.org >.

OTHER

AIDS Clinical Trials Information Service website and telephone information line. Sponsored by Centers for Disease Control and Prevention, Food and Drug Administration, National Institute of Allergy and Infectious Diseases, and National Library of Medicine. (800) TRIALS-A or (800) 874-2572. < http://actis.org >.

HIV/AIDS Treatment Information Service website and telephone information line. Sponsored by Agency for Health Care Policy and Research, Centers for Disease Control and Prevention, Health Resources and Services Administration, Indian Health Service, National Institutes of Health, and Substance Abuse and Mental Health Services Administration. (800) HIV-0440 (800) 448-0440. < http://www.hivatis.org >.

Project Inform National HIV/AIDS Treatment Hotline. (800) 822-7422.

Samuel D. Uretsky, PharmD
Teresa G. Odle

Antirheumatic drugs

Definition

Antirheumatic drugs are drugs used to treat **rheumatoid arthritis**.

Purpose

Rheumatoid arthritis is a progressive form of arthritis that has devastating effects on joints and general health. It is classified as an auto-immune disease, because the disease is caused by the body's own immune system acting against the body itself. Symptoms include painful, stiff, swollen joints, **fever**, **fatigue**, and loss of appetite.

In recent years, there has been a change in attitude concerning the treatment of rheumatoid arthritis. Physicians now use Disease Modifying Anti-Rheumatic Drugs (DMARDs) early in the history of the disease and are less inclined to wait for crippling stages before resorting to the more potent drugs. Fuller understanding of the side-effects of non-steroidal anti-inflammatory drugs (NSAIDs) has also stimulated reliance on other types of antirheumatic drugs.

Description

The major classes of antirheumatic drugs include:

- Nonsteroidal Anti-Inflammatory Drugs (NSAIDs. Drugs belonging to this class bring symptomatic relief of both inflammation and **pain**, but have a limited effect on the progressive bone and cartilage loss associated with rheumatoid arthritis. They act by slowing the body's production of prostaglandins. Common NSAIDs include: ibuprofen (Motrin, Nuprin or Advil), naproxen (Naprosyn, Aleve) and indomethacin (Indocin).

- **Corticosteroids**. These drugs are very powerful anti-inflammatory agents. They are the synthetic analogs of cortisone, produced by the body. Corticosteroids are used to reduce inflammation and suppress

KEY TERMS

Anti-inflammatory drugs—A class of drugs that lower inflammation and that includes NSAIDs and corticosteroids.

Arthritis—A painful condition that involves inflammation of one or more joints.

Conception—The union of egg and sperm to form a fetus.

Corticosteroids—A class of drugs that are synthetic versions of the cortisone produced by the body. They rank among the most powerful anti-inflammatory agents.

Cortisone—Glucocorticoid produced by the adrenal cortex in response to stress. Cortisone is a steroid and has anti-inflammatory and immunosuppressive properties.

Cytotoxic drugs—Drugs that function by destroying cells.

Disease Modifying Anti-Rheumatic Drugs (DMARDs)—A class of antirheumatic drugs, including chloroquine, methotrexate, cyclosporine, and gold compounds, that influence the disease process itself and do not only treat its symptoms.

Inflammation—A process occurring in body tissues, characterized by increased circulation and the accumulation of white blood cells. Inflammation also occurs in disorders such as arthritis and causes harmful effects.

Inflammatory—Pertaining to inflammation.

Immune response—Physiological response of the body controlled by the immune system that involves the production of antibodies to fight off specific foreign substances or agents (antigens).

Immune system—The sum of the defence mechanisms of the body that protects it against foreign substances and organisms causing infection.

Immunosuppressive—Any agent that suppresses the immune response of an individual.

Immunosuppresive cytotoxic drugs—A class of drugs that function by destroying cells and suppressing the immune response.

Methotrexate—A drug that interferes with cell growth and is used to treat rheumatoid arthritis as well as various types of cancer. Side-effects may include mouth sores, digestive upsets, skin rashes, and hair loss.

Non steroidal—Not containing steroids or cortisone. Usually refers to a class of drugs called Non Steroidal Anti-Inflammatory Drugs (NSAID).

Nonsteroidal Anti-Inflammatory Drugs (NSAIDs)—A class of drugs that is used to relieve pain, and symptoms of inflammation, such as ibuprofen and ketoprofen.

Osteoarthritis—A form of arthritis that occurs mainly in older people and involves the gradual degeneration of the cartilage of the joints.

Prostaglandins—Prostaglandins are produced by the body and are responsible for inflammation features, such as swelling, pain, stiffness, redness and warmth.

---

activity of the immune system. The most commonly prescribed are prednisone and dexamethasone.

- Disease Modifying Anti-Rheumatic Drugs (DMARDs). DMARDs influence the disease process itself and do not only treat symptoms, hence their name. DMARDs also have anti-inflammatory effects, and most were borrowed from the treatment of other diseases, such as **cancer** and **malaria**. Antimalarials DMARDs include chloroquine (Aralen) and hydroxychloroquine (Plaquenil). Powerful DMARDs include: methotrexate (Rheumatrex), sulfasalazine, cyclosporine, azathioprine (Imuran) and cyclophosphamide (Cytoxan), azathioprine, sulfasalazine, penicillamine, and organic gold compounds such as aurothioglucose (Solganol), gold sodium thiomalate (Aurolate) and auranofin (Ridaura).

- Slow-Acting Antirheumatic Drugs (SAARDs). SAARDs are a special class of DMARDs and the effect of these drugs is slow acting and not so quickly apparent as that of the NSAIDs. Examples are hydroxychloroquine and aurothioglucose.

- Immunosuppresive cytotoxic drugs. This class of drugs is used if treatment with NSAIDs and SAARDs have no effect. Immunosuppresive drugs have a stabilizing effect on the immune system. Since the inflammation associated with chronic arthritis is due to malfunctions of the immune system, use of this class of drugs has been shown to be beneficial for the treatment of rheumatoid arthritis as well. Examples are: methotrexate, mechlorethamine, cyclophosphamide, chlorambucil, and azathioprine.

Recommended dosage

Recommended dosage depends on the type of drug. The prescribing physician or the pharmacist provide information for the correct dosage. The drugs must be taken exactly as directed.

When taking methotrexate for rheumatoid arthritis, it should be taken only *once or twice a week as prescribed,* not every day. Taking it every day can lead to a fatal overdose.

Precautions

Many antirheumatic drugs such as, for example, azathioprine (Imuran) and methotrexate (Rheumatrex), are very powerful drugs. They are usually prescribed in severe cases, when all other treatments have failed. Thus, they may have serious side effects, so it is important to be monitored closely by a physician while taking any of these drugs.

Side effects

Hydroxychloroquine (Plaquenil) may cause vision problems. Anyone taking it should see an ophthalmologist (a physician who specializes in treating eyes) for a thorough **eye examination** every six months.

Methotrexate and penicillamine may cause **birth defects**. Women taking these drugs must stop taking them during **pregnancy** and for several months before a planned pregnancy. Methotrexate may also cause lung damage or fertility problems and should not be taken by anyone with serious kidney or **liver disease** or by anyone who drinks alcohol.

Azathioprine may cause birth defects if either the man or woman is using it at the time of conception. Anyone who uses this drug and is sexually active should consult with a physician about an effective birth control method.

Other common side effects of antirheumatic drugs include abdominal cramps, **diarrhea**, **dizziness**, loss of appetite, **headache**, **nausea**, **vomiting**, fever and chills, and mouth sores. A variety of other side effects may occur. Anyone who has unusual symptoms while taking antirheumatic drugs should notify the treating physician.

The gold compounds may cause serious blood problems by reducing the ability of the blood forming organs to produce blood cells. These drugs may decrease the number of white blood cells, red blood cells, or both. Patients taking these drugs should have regular blood counts.

Entanercept (Enbrel) may also cause blood problems, and some patients who received this drug have developed eye problems and **multiple sclerosis**. It is not certain whether these reactions were caused by entanercept, but multiple sclerosis has been seen in patients taking other drugs which act against tumor necrosis factor.

Interactions

Antirheumatic drugs may interact with a variety of other medicines or other antirheumatic drugs. When this happens, the effects of one or both of the drugs may change, or the risk of side effects may be greater. Anyone who takes this type of drug should inform the prescribing physician about any other medication he or she is taking. Among the drugs that may interact with antirheumatic drugs are phenytoin (Dilantin), **aspirin**, sulfa drugs such as Bactrim and Gantrisin, tetracycline and some other **antibiotics** and cimetidine (Tagamet). NSAIDs such as ibuprofen (Motrin, Advil) are also known to interact with other classes of antirheumatic drugs.

Nancy Ross-Flanigan

▌Antiseptics

Definition

An antiseptic is a substance which inhibits the growth and development of microorganisms. For practical purposes, antiseptics are routinely thought of as topical agents, for application to skin, mucous membranes, and inanimate objects, although a formal definition includes agents which are used internally, such as the urinary tract antiseptics.

Purpose

Antiseptics are a diverse class of drugs which are applied to skin surfaces or mucous membranes for their anti-infective effects. This may be either bacteriocidal or bacteriostatic. Their uses include cleansing of skin and wound surfaces after injury, preparation of skin surfaces prior to injections or surgical procedures, and routine disinfection of the oral cavity as part of a program of **oral hygiene**. Antiseptics are also used for disinfection of inanimate objects, including instruments and furniture surfaces.

Commonly used antiseptics for skin cleaning include benzalkonium chloride, chlorhexidine, hexachlorophine, iodine compounds, mercury compounds, alcohol and hydrogen peroxide. Other agents which have been used for this purpose, but have largely been supplanted by more effective or safer agents, include

KEY TERMS

Antibiotic—A medicine used to treat infections.

Bacteria—Tiny, one-celled forms of life that cause many diseases and infections.

Mucous membrane—The moist lining of a body cavity or structure, such as the mouth or nose.

Residue—Traces that remain after most of the rest of the material is gone.

boric acid and volatile oils such as methyl salicylate (oil of wintergreen.)

Chlorhexidine shows a high margin of safety when applied to mucous membranes, and has been used in oral rinses and preoperative total body washes.

Benzalkonium chloride and hexachlorophine are used primarily as hand scrubs or face washes. Benzalkonium may also find application is a disinfecting agent for instruments, and in low concentration as a preservative for drugs including ophthalmic solutions. Benzalkonium chloride is inactivated by organic compounds, including soap, and must not be applied to areas which have not been fully rinsed.

Iodine compounds include tincture of iodine and povidone iodine compounds. Iodine compounds have the broadest spectrum of all topical anti-infectives, with action against bacteria, fungi, viruses, spores, protozoa, and yeasts. Iodine tincture is highly effective, but its alcoholic component is drying and extremely irritating when applied to abraided (scraped or rubbed) skin. Povidone iodine, an organic compound, is less irritating and less toxic, but not as effective. Povidone iodine has been used for hand scrubs and disinfection of surgical sites. Aqueous solutions of iodine have also been used as antiseptic agents, but are less effective than alcoholic solutions and less convenient to use that the povidone iodine compounds.

Hydrogen peroxide acts through the liberation of oxygen gas. Although the antibacterial activity of hydrogen peroxide is relatively weak, the liberation of oxygen bubbles produces an effervescent action, which may be useful for wound cleansing through removal of tissue debris. The activity of hydrogen peroxide may be reduced by the presence of blood and pus. The appropriate concentration of hydrogen peroxide for antiseptic use is 3%, although higher concentrations are available.

Thimerosol (Mersol) is a mercury compound with activity against bacteria and yeasts. Prolonged use may result in mercury toxicity.

Recommended dosage

Dosage varies with product and intended use. Consult individualized references.

Precautions

Precautions vary with individual product and use. Consult individualized references.

Hypersensitivity reactions should be considered with organic compounds such as chlorhexidine, benzalkonium and hexachlorophine.

Skin dryness and irritation should be considered with all products, but particularly with those containing alcohol.

Systemic toxicity may result from ingestion of iodine containing compounds or mercury compounds.

Chlorhexidine should not be instilled into the ear. There is one anecdotal report of deafness following use of chlorhexidine in a patient with a **perforated eardrum**. Safety in **pregnancy** and breastfeeding have not been reported, however there is one anecdotal report of an infant developing slowed heartbeat apparently related to maternal use of chlorhexidine.

Iodine compounds should be used sparingly during pregnancy and **lactation** due to risk of infant absorption of iodine with alterations in thyroid function.

Interactions

Antiseptics are not known to interact with any other medicines. However, they should not be used together with any other topical cream, solution, or ointment.

Resources

PERIODICALS

Farley, Dixie. "Help for Cuts, Scrapes and Burns." *FDA Consumer* May 1996: 12.

Samuel D. Uretsky, PharmD

Antispasmodic drugs

Definition

Antispasmodic drugs relieve cramps or spasms of the stomach, intestines, and bladder.

KEY TERMS

Heat stroke—A serious condition that results from exposure to extreme heat. The body loses its ability to cool itself. Severe headache, high fever, and hot, dry skin may result. In severe cases, a person with heat stroke may collapse or go into a coma.

Hiatal hernia—A condition in which part of the stomach protrudes through the diaphragm.

Hyperthyroidism—Secretion of excess thyroid hormones by the thyroid gland.

Inflammation—Pain, redness, swelling, and heat that usually develop in response to injury or illness.

Myasthenia gravis—A condition in which certain muscles weaken and may become paralyzed.

Reflux esophagitis—Inflammation of the lower esophagus caused by the backflow of stomach contents.

Spasm—Sudden, involuntary tensing of a muscle or a group of muscles

Ulcerative colitis—Long-lasting and repeated inflammation of the colon with the development of sores.

Purpose

Antispasmodic drugs have been used to treat stomach cramps. Traditionally, they were used to treat stomach ulcers, but for this purpose they have largely been replaced by the acid inhibiting compoundsa, the H-2 receptor blockers such as cimetidine and ranitidine and the proton pump inhibtors such as omeprazole, lansoprazole and rabetazole.

Most of the drugs used for this purpose as "anticholinergics", since they counteract the effects of the neurohormone acetylcholine. Some of these drugs are derived from the plant belladonna, also known as Deadly Nightshade. There is also a group of drugs with similar activity, but not taken from plant sources. The anticholingergics decrease both the movements of the stomach and intestine, and also the secretions of stomach acid and digestive enzymes. They may be used for other purposes including treatment of Parkinson's Disease, and bladder urgency. Because these drugs inhibit secretions, they cause **dry mouth** and dry eyes because of reduced salivation and tearing. Dicyclomine is an antispasmodic with very lettle effect on secretions. It is used to treat **irritable bowel syndrome**.

Description

Dicyclomine is available only with a prescription and is sold as capsules, tablets (regular and extended-release forms), and syrup.

Recommended dosage

The usual dosage for adults is 20 mg, four times a day. However, the physician may recommend starting at a lower dosage and gradually increasing the dose to reduce the chance of unwanted side effects.

The dosage for children depends on the child's age. Check with the child's physician for the correct dosage.

Precautions

Dicyclomine makes some people sweat less, which allows the body to overheat and may lead to heat prostration (**fever** and heat **stroke**). Anyone taking this drug should try to avoid extreme heat. If that is not possible, check with the physician who prescribed the drug. If heat prostration occurs, stop taking the medicine and call a physician immediately.

This medicine can cause drowsiness and blurred or double vision. People who take this drug should not drive, use machines, or do anything else that might be dangerous until they have found out how the medicine affects them.

Dicyclomine should not be given to infants or children unless the physician decides the use of this drug is necessary. Dicyclomine should not be used by women who are breast feeding. Women who are pregnant or plan to become pregnant should check with their physicians before using this drug.

Anyone with the following medical conditions should not take dicyclomine unless directed to do so by a physician:

- Previous sensitivity or allergic reaction to dicyclomine
- Glaucoma
- Myasthenia gravis
- Blockage of the urinary tract, stomach, or intestines
- Severe **ulcerative colitis**
- Reflux esophagitis.

In addition, patients with these conditions should check with their physicians before using dicyclomine:

- Liver disease
- Kidney disease
- High blood pressure
- Heart problems
- Enlarged prostate gland
- Hiatal **hernia**
- Autonomic neuropathy (a nerve disorder)
- Hyperthyroidism.

Side effects

The most common side effects are **dizziness**, drowsiness, lightheadedness, **nausea**, nervousness, blurred vision, dry mouth, and weakness. Other side effects may occur. Anyone who has unusual symptoms after taking dicyclomine should get in touch with his or her physician.

Interactions

Dicyclomine may interact with other medicines. When this happens, the effects of one or both of the drugs may change or the risk of side effects may be greater. Among the drugs that may interact with Dicyclomine are:

- Antacids such as Maalox
- Antihistamines such as clemastine fumarate (Tavist)
- Bronchodilators (airway opening drugs) such as albuterol (Proventil, Ventolin)
- Corticosteroids such as prednisone (Deltasone)
- Monoamine oxidase inhibitors (MAO inhibitors) such as phenelzine (Nardil) and tranylcypromine (Parnate)
- Tranquilizers such as diazepam (Valium) and alprazolam (Xanax).

The list above does not include every drug that may interact with dicyclomine. Be sure to check with a physician or pharmacist before combining dicyclomine with any other prescription or nonprescription (over-the-counter) medicine.

Nancy Ross-Flanigan

Antistreptolysin O titer (ASO) *see*
Streptococcal antibody tests

Antithrombin III deficiency *see*
Hypercoagulation disorders

Antituberculosis drugs

Definition

Antituberculosis drugs are medicines used to treat **tuberculosis**, an infectious disease that can affect the lungs and other organs.

Purpose

Tuberculosis is a disease caused by Mycobacterium tuberculae, a bacteria that is passed between people through the air. The disease can be cured with proper drug therapy, but because the bacteria may become resistant to any single drug, combinations of antituberculosis drugs are used to treat tuberculosis (TB) are normally required for effective treatment. At the start of the 20th Century, tuberculosis was the most common cause of **death** in the United States, but was largely eliminated with better living conditions. It is most common in areas of crowding and poor ventilation, such as crowded urban areas and prisons. In some areas, the **AIDS** epidemic has been accompanied by an increase in the prevalence of tuberculosis.

Some antituberculosis drugs also are used to treat or prevent other infections such as *Mycobacterium avium* complex (MAC), which causes disease throughout the bodies of people with AIDS or other diseases of the immune system.

Description

Antituberculosis drugs are available only with a physician's prescription and come in tablet, capsule, liquid and injectable forms. Some commonly used antituberculosis drugs are cycloserine (Seromycin), ethambutol (Myambutol), ethionamide (Trecator-SC), isoniazid (Nydrazid, Laniazid), pyrazinamide, rifabutin (Mycobutin), and rifampin (Rifadin, Rimactane).

Recommended dosage

The recommended dosage depends on the type of antituberculosis drug and may be different for different patients. Check with the physician who prescribed the medicine or the pharmacist who filled the prescription for the proper dosage. The physician may gradually increase the dosage during treatment. Be sure to follow the physician's orders. Patients who are infected with HIV must usually take larger combinations of drugs for a longer period of time than is needed for patients with an unimpaired immune system.

KEY TERMS

Bacteria—Tiny, one-celled forms of life that cause many diseases and infections.

Feces—(Also called stool.) The solid waste that is left after food is digested. Feces form in the intestines and pass out of the body through the anus.

Fetus—A developing baby inside the womb.

Gout—A disease in which uric acid, a waste product that normally passes out of the body in urine, collects in the joints and the kidneys. This causes arthritis and kidney stones.

Immune system—The body's natural defenses against disease and infection.

Microorganism—An organism (life form) that is too small to be seen with the naked eye.

Platelets—Disk-shaped bodies in the blood that are important in clotting.

Seizure—A sudden attack, spasm, or convulsion.

Some antituberculosis drugs must be taken with other drugs. If they are taken alone, they may encourage the bacteria that cause tuberculosis to become resistant to drugs used to treat the disease. When the bacteria become resistant, treating the disease becomes more difficult.

To clear up tuberculosis completely, antituberculosis drugs must be taken for as long as directed. This may mean taking the medicine every day for a year or two or even longer. Symptoms may improve very quickly after treatment with this medicine begins. However, they may come back if the medicine is stopped too quickly. Do not stop taking the medicine just because symptoms improve.

Because people may neglect to take their medication for tuberculosis, it is common to have tuberculosis centers develop a program of Directly Observed Therapy (DOT.) In these programs, patients come to the hospital or clinic, and take their medication in front of an observer. These programs may be annoying to the patients, but are justified by the risks to public health if tuberculosis germs which have become resistant to drugs were to be spread.

Cycloserine works best when it is at constant levels in the blood. To help keep levels constant, take the medicine in doses spaced evenly through the day and night. Do not miss any doses. If taking medicine at night interferes with sleep, or if it is difficult to

remember to take the medicine during the day, check with a health care professional for suggestions.

Do not take **antacids** that contain aluminum, such as Maalox, within 1 hour of taking isoniazid, as this may keep the medicine from working.

Precautions

Seeing a physician regularly while taking antituberculosis drugs is important. The physician will check to make sure the medicine is working as it should and will watch for unwanted side effects. These visits also will help the physician know if the dosage needs to be changed.

Symptoms should begin to improve within a few weeks after treatment begins with antituberculosis drugs. If they do not, or if they become worse, check with a physician.

Some people feel drowsy, dizzy, confused, or less alert when using these drugs. Some may also cause vision changes, clumsiness, or unsteadiness. Because of these possible problems, anyone who takes antituberculosis drugs should not drive, use machines, or do anything else that might be dangerous until they have found out how the medicine affects them.

Daily doses of pyridoxine (vitamin B_6) may lessen or prevent some side effects of ethionamide or isoniazid. If the physician who prescribed the medicine recommends this, be sure to take the pyridoxine every day.

Certain kinds of cheese (such as Swiss and Cheshire) and fish (such as tuna and skipjack) may cause an unusual reaction in people taking isoniazid. Symptoms of this reaction include fast or pounding heartbeat, sweating or a hot feeling, chills or a clammy feeling, **headache**, lightheadedness, and red or itchy skin. This reaction is very rare. However, if any of these symptoms occur, check with a physician as soon as possible.

Rifabutin and rifampin will make saliva, sweat, tears, urine, feces, and skin turn reddish orange to reddish brown. This is nothing to worry about. However, the discolored tears may permanently stain soft contact lenses (but not hard contact lenses). To avoid ruining contact lenses, do not wear soft contacts while taking these medicines.

Rifampin may temporarily lower the number of white blood cells. Because the white blood cells are important in fighting infection, this effect increases the chance of getting an infection. This drug also may lower the number of platelets that play an important role in clotting. To reduce the risk of bleeding and infection in the mouth while taking this medicine, be especially careful when brushing and flossing the teeth. Check with a physician or dentist for suggestions on how to keep the teeth and mouth clean without causing injuries. Put off any dental work until blood counts return to normal.

Rifampin may affect the results of some medical tests. Before having medical tests, anyone taking this medicine should alert the health care professional in charge.

People who have certain medical conditions may have problems if they take antituberculosis drugs. For example:

- cycloserine or isoniazid may increase the risk of seizures (convulsions) in people with a history of seizures.

- the dosage of cycloserine may need to be adjusted for people with **kidney disease**.

- ethambutol or pyrazinamide may cause or worsen attacks of **gout** in people who are prone to having them.

- ethambutol may cause or worsen eye damage.

- diabetes may be harder to control in patients who take ethionamide.

- isoniazid may cause false results on some urine sugar tests, and pyrazinamide may cause false results on urine ketone tests. Diabetic patients who either of these medicines should discuss the possibility of false test results with their physicians.

- people with **liver disease** or a history of alcohol **abuse** may be more likely to develop hepatitis when taking isoniazid and are more likely to have side effects that affect the liver when taking rifampin.

- in people with kidney disease, ethambutol, ethionamide, or isoniazid may be more likely to cause side effects.

- side effects are also more likely in people with liver disease who take pyrazinamide.

Before taking antituberculosis drugs, be sure to let the physician know about these or any other medical problems.

In laboratory tests of pregnant animals, high doses of some antituberculosis drugs have caused **birth defects** and other problems in the fetus or newborn. However, pregnant women with tuberculosis need to take antituberculosis drugs to clear up their disease. Knowing that many women have had healthy babies after taking these drugs during pregnancy may be reassuring. Pregnant women who need to take this medicine and are worried about birth defects or other problems should talk to their physicians.

Anyone who has had unusual reactions to antituberculosis drugs or to niacin should let his or her physician know before taking any antituberculosis drug. The physician should also be told about any **allergies** to foods, dyes, preservatives, or other substances.

Patients who are on special **diets**, such as low-sodium or low-sugar diets, should make sure their physicians know. Some antituberculosis medicines may contain sodium, sugar, or alcohol.

Side effects

Cycloserine

In some people, this medicine causes depression and thoughts of **suicide**. If this happens, check with a physician immediately. Switching to another medicine will usually stop these troubling thoughts and feelings. Also let the physician know immediately about any other mood or mental changes; such as nervousness, nightmares, anxiety, confusion, or irritability; and about symptoms such as muscle twitches, convulsions, or speech problems.

Headache is a common side effect that usually goes away as the body adjusts to this medicine. This problem does not need medical attention unless it continues or it interferes with everyday life.

Ethambutol

This medicine may cause eye **pain** or vision changes, including loss of vision or changes in color vision. Check with a physician immediately if any of these problems develop.

In addition, anyone who has any of these symptoms while taking ethambutol should check with a physician immediately:

- painful or swollen joints, especially in the knee, ankle, or big toe

- a tight, hot sensation in the skin over painful or swollen joints

- chills.

Other side effects may occur but do not need medical attention unless they are bothersome or they do not go away as the body adjusts to the medicine. These include: headache, confusion, nausea and **vomiting**, stomach pain, and loss of appetite.

Ethionamide

Check with a physician immediately if eye pain, blurred vision, or other vision changes occur while taking this medicine.

Symptoms such as unsteadiness, clumsiness and pain, **numbness**, **tingling**, or burning in the hands or feet could be the first signs of nerve problems that may become more serious. If any of these symptoms occur, check with a physician immediately. Other side effects that should be brought to a physician's attention immediately include yellow eyes or skin and mood or mental changes such as depression or confusion.

Less serious side effects such as **dizziness**, **nausea** or vomiting, appetite loss, sore mouth, or metallic taste may also occur. These problems usually go away as the body adjusts to the medicine. They do not need medical attention unless they continue or they interfere with normal activities.

Isoniazid

This medicine may cause serious liver damage, especially in people over 40 years of age. However, taking medicine for tuberculosis is very important for people with the disease. Anyone who has tuberculosis and has been advised to take this drug should thoroughly discuss treatment options with his or her physician.

Recognizing the early signs of liver and nerve damage can help prevent the problems from getting worse. If any of these symptoms occur, check with a physician immediately:

- unusual tiredness or weakness
- clumsiness or unsteadiness
- pain, numbness, tingling, or burning in the hands and feet
- loss of appetite
- vomiting

This medicine may also cause less serious side effects such as **diarrhea** and stomach pain. These usually go away as the body adjusts to the medicine and do not need medical attention unless they continue.

If eye pain, blurred vision, or other vision changes occur while taking this medicine, check with a physician immediately.

Pyrazinamide

Check with a physician immediately if pain in the joints occurs.

Rifabutin

Check with a physician immediately if a skin rash occurs.

Rifampin

Stop taking rifampin and check with a physician immediately if any of the following symptoms occur. These symptoms could be early signs of problems that may become more serious. Getting prompt medical attention could prevent them from getting worse.

- unusual tiredness or weakness
- nausea or vomiting
- loss of appetite

In addition, anyone who has any of these symptoms while taking rifampin should check with a physician immediately:

- breathing problems
- fever
- chills
- shivering
- headache
- dizziness
- itching
- skin rash or redness
- muscle and bone pain

Other side effects, such as diarrhea and stomach pain, may occur with this medicine, but should go away as the body adjusts to the drug. Medical treatment is not necessary unless these problems continue.

Other side effects may occur with any antituberculosis drug. Anyone who has unusual symptoms while taking an antituberculosis drug should get in touch with his or her physician.

Interactions

Taking cycloserine and ethionamide together may increase the risk of seizures and other nervous system problems. These and other side effects also are more likely in people who drink alcohol while taking cycloserine. To avoid these problems, *do not drink alcohol while taking cycloserine* and check with a physician before combining cycloserine and ethionamide.

Drinking alcohol regularly may prevent isoniazid from working properly and may increase the chance of liver damage. Anyone taking this medicine should strictly limit the use of alcohol. Check with a health care professional for advice on the amount of alcohol that may safely be used.

Many drugs may interact with isoniazid or rifampin, increasing the chance of liver damage or other side effects. Among these drugs are acetaminophen (Tylenol), birth control pills and other drugs that contain female hormones, and the antiseizure drugs divalproex (Depakote) and valproic acid (Depakene). For a complete list of drugs that may have this effect, check with a pharmacist.

Isoniazid may also decrease the effects of the antifungal drug ketoconazole (Nizoral) and the antituberculosis drug rifampin (Rifadin).

Rifampin may make many drugs less effective. Among the drugs that may be affected are diabetes medicines taken by mouth (oral hypoglycemics), digitalis heart drugs, many antifungal drugs, and birth control pills. Because it makes birth control pills less effective, taking rifampin may increase the chance of becoming pregnant. Women who take this medicine along with birth control pills should use an additional form of birth control. For a complete list of drugs that may be affected by rifampin, check with a pharmacist.

Using rifabutin with the antiretroviral drug zidovudine (AZT, Retrovir) may make the zidovudine less effective. Consult with a physician if both drugs are prescribed.

Not every drug that may interact with an antituberculosis drug is listed here. Be sure to check with a physician or pharmacist before combining an antituberculosis drug with any other prescription or nonprescription (over-the-counter) medicine.

Resources

PERIODICALS

Cornwall, Janet. "Tuberculosis: A Clinical Problem of International Importance." *The Lancet* (August 30, 1997): 660.

Nancy Ross-Flanigan

▌Antiulcer drugs

Definition

'Antiulcer drugs are a class of drugs, exclusive of the antibacterial agents, used to treat ulcers in the stomach and the upper part of the small intestine.

Antiulcer Drugs	
Brand Name (Generic Name)	**Possible Common Side Effects Include:**
Axid (nitzatidine)	Diarrhea, headache, **nausea and vomiting**, sore throat
Carafate (sucralfate)	**Constipation, insomnia, hives**, upset stomach, vomiting
Cytotec (misoprostol)	Cramps, diarrhea, nausea, gas, headache, **menstrual disorders** (including heavy bleeding and severe cramping)
Pepcid (famotidine)	Constipation or diarrhea, dizziness, **fatigue**, fever
Prilosec (omeprazole)	Nausea and vomiting, headache, diarrhea, abdominal pain
Tagamet (cimetidine)	Headache, breast development in men, depression and disorientation
Zantac (ranitidine hydrochloride)	Headache, constipation or diarrhea, joint pain

Purpose

Recurrent gastric and duodenal ulcers are caused by *Helicobacter pylori* infections, and are treated with combination treatments that incorporate antibiotic therapy with gastric acid suppression. Additionally, bismuth compounds have been used. The primary class of drugs used for gastric acid suppression are the proton pump inhibitors, omeprazole, lansoprazole, pantoprazole and rabeprazole. The H-2 receptor blocking agents, cimetidine, famotidine, nizatidine, and ranitidine have been used for this purpose, but are now more widely used for maintenance therapy after treatment with the proton pump inhibitors. Sucralfate, which acts by forming a protective coating over the ulcerate lesion, is also used in ulcer treatment and may be appropriate for patients in whom other classes of drugs are not indicated, or those whose gastric ulcers are caused by non-steroidal anti-inflammatory drugs (NSAIDs) rather than *H. pylori* infections.

Description

The **proton pump inhibitors** block the secretion of gastric acid by the gastric parietal cells. The extent of inhibition of acid secretion is dose related. In some cases, gastric acid secretion is completely blocked for over 24 hours on a single dose. In addition to their role in treatment of gastric ulcers, the proton pump inhibitors are used to treat syndromes of excessive acid secretion (Zollinger-Ellison Syndrome) and gastroesophageal reflux disease (GERD).

Histamine H-2 receptor blockers stop the action of histamine on the gastric parietal cells, inhibiting the secretion of gastric acid. These drugs are less effective than the proton pump inhibitors, but may achieve a 75–79% reduction in acid secretion. Higher rates of acid inhibition may be achieved when the drug is administered by the intravenous route. The H-2 receptor blockers may also be used to treat **heartburn** and hypersecretory syndromes. When given before surgery, the H-2 receptor blockers are useful in prevention of aspiration **pneumonia**.

Sucralfate (Carafate), a substituted sugar molecule with no nutritional value, does not inhibit gastric acid, but rather, reacts with existing stomach acid to form a thick coating that covers the surface of an ulcer, protecting the open area from further damage. A secondary effect is to act as an inhibitor of the digestive enzyme pepsin. Sucralfate does not bind to the normal stomach lining. The drug has been used for prevention of **stress** ulcers, the type seen in patients exposed to physical stress such as **burns** and surgery. It has no systemic effects.

Recommended dosage

The doses of the proton pump inhibitors and H-2 receptor blockers vary depending on the drug and condition being treated. Consult individual references.

The dose of sucralfate for acute ulcer therapy is 1 gram four times a day. After the ulcer has healed, maintenance treatment may continue at 1 gram two times daily.

Precautions

The proton pump inhibitors are generally well tolerated, and the most common adverse effects are **diarrhea**, **itching**, skin rash, **dizziness** and headache. Muscle aches and a higher than normal rate of respiratory infections are among the other adverse reactions reported. Omeprazole has an increased rate of fetal deaths in animal studies. It is not known if these drugs are excreted in human milk, but because of reported adverse effects to infants in animal studies, it is recommended that proton pump inhibitors not be used by nursing mothers.

The H-2 receptor blockers vary widely in their adverse effects. Although they are generally well tolerated, cimetidine may cause confusion in elderly patients, and has an antiandrogenic effect that may cause **sexual dysfunction** in males. Famotidine has been reported to cause **headache** in 4.7% of patients. It is advisable that mothers not take H-2 receptor blockers while nursing.

Sucralfate is well tolerated. It is poorly absorbed, and its most common side effect is constipation in 2% of patients. Diarrhea, **nausea**, **vomiting**, gastric discomfort, **indigestion**, flatulence, dry mouth, rash, pruritus (itching), back **pain**, headache, dizziness, sleepiness, and vertigo have been reported, as well as rare allergic responses. Because sucralfate releases small amounts of aluminum into the system, it should be used with caution in patients with renal insufficiency. There is no information available about sucralfate's safety in breastfeeding.

Interactions

Proton pump inhibitors may increase the pH of the stomach. This will inactivate some antifungal drugs that require an acid medium for effectiveness, notable itraconazole and ketoconazole.

H-2 receptor blocking agents have a large number of **drug interactions**. Consult individualized references.

Sucralfate should not be used with aluminum containing **antacids**, because of the risk of increased aluminum absorption. Sucralfate may inhibit absorption and reduce blood levels of anticoagulants, digoxin, quinidine, ketoconazole, quinolones and phenytoin.

Resources

ORGANIZATIONS

Digestive Disease National Coalition. 507 Capitol Court NE, Suite 200, Washington, DC 20003. (202) 544-7497.

National Digestive Diseases Information Clearinghouse. 2 Information Way, Bethesda, MD 20892-3570. nddic@aerie.com. < http://www.niddk.nih.gov/ Brochures/NDDIC.htm > .

OTHER

Duodenal UlcerFact sheet. Johns Hopkins Health Information Adult Health Advisor. < http:// csi.intelihealth.com > .

National Institute of Diabetes and Digestive and Kidney Diseases. < http://www.niddk.nih.gov > .

PharmInfoNet's Digestive Disease Center. < http:// pharminfo.com/disease.gastro.html > .

Stomach Ulcer (Gastric Ulcer). Fact sheet. Johns Hopkins Health Information Adult Health Advisor. < http:// csi.intelihealth.com > .

Samuel D. Uretsky, PharmD

Antiviral drugs

Definition

Antiviral drugs are medicines that cure or control virus infections.

Purpose

Antivirals are used to treat infections caused by viruses. Unlike antibacterial drugs, which may cover a wide range of pathogens, antiviral agents tend to be narrow in spectrum, and have limited efficacy.

Description

Exclusive of the antiretroviral agents used in HIV (AIDS) therapy, there are currently only 11 antiviral drugs available, covering four types of virus. Acyclovir (Zovirax), famciclovir (Famvir), and valacyclovir (Valtrex) are effective against herpesvirus, including herpes zoster and herpes genitalis. They may also be of value in either conditions caused by herpes, such as **chickenpox** and **shingles**. These drugs are not curative, but may reduce the **pain** of a herpes outbreak and shorten the period of viral shedding.

Amantadine (Symmetrel), oseltamivir (Tamiflu), rimantidine (Flumadine), and zanamivir (Relenza) are useful in treatment of **influenza** virus. Amantadine,

rimantadine, and oseltamivir may be administered throughout the flu season as preventatives for patients who cannot take influenza virus vaccine.

Cidofovir (Vistide), foscarnet (Foscavir), and ganciclovir (Cytovene) have been beneficial in treatment of cytomegalovirus in immunosupressed patients, primarily HIV-positive patients and transplant recipients. Ribavirin (Virazole) is used to treat respiratory syncytial virus. In combination with interferons, ribavirin has shown some efficacy against **hepatitis C**, and there have been anecdotal reports of utility against other types of viral infections.

As a class, the antivirals are not curative, and must be used either prophylactically or early in the development of an infection. Their mechanism of action is typically to inactivate the enzymes needed for viral replication. This will reduce the rate of viral growth, but will not inactive the virus already present. Antiviral therapy must normally be initiated within 48 hours of the onset of an infection to provide any benefit. Drugs used for influenza may be used throughout the influenza season in high risk patients, or within 48 hours of exposure to a known carrier. Antiherpetic agents should be used at the first signs of an outbreak. Anti-cytomegaloviral drugs must routinely be used as part of a program of secondary **prophylaxis** (maintenance therapy following an initial response) in order to prevent reinfection in immunocompromised patients.

Recommended dosage

Dosage varies with the drug, patient age and condition, route of administration, and other factors. See specific references.

Precautions

Ganciclovir is available in intravenous injection, oral capsules, and intraoccular inserts. The capsules should be reserved for prophylactic use in organ transplant patients, or for HIV infected patients who cannot be treated with the intravenous drug. The toxicity profile of this drug when administered systemically includes granulocytopenia, anemia and **thrombocytopenia**. The drug is in pregnancy category C, but has caused significant fetal abnormalities in animal studies including cleft palate and organ defects. Breast feeding is not recommended.

Cidofovir causes renal toxicity in 53% of patients. Patients should be well hydrated, and renal function should be checked regularly. Other common adverse effects are **nausea and vomiting** in 65% or patients, asthenia in 46% and **headache** and **diarrhea**, both reported in 27% of cases. The drug is category C in **pregnancy**, due to fetal abnormalities in animal studies. Breast feeding is not recommended.

Foscarnet is used in treatment of immunocompromised patients with cytomegalovirus infections and in acyclovir-resistant herpes simples virus. The primary hazard is renal toxicity. Alterations in electrolyte levels may cause seizures. Foscarnet is category C during pregnancy. The drug has caused skeletal abnormailities in developing fetuses. It is not known whether foscarnet is excreted in breast milk, however the drug does appear in breast milk in animal studies.

Valaciclovir is metabolized to acyclovir, so that the hazards of the two drugs are very similar. They are generally well tolerated, but **nausea** and headache are common adverse effects. They are both pregnancy category B. Although there have been no reports of fetal abnormalities attributable to either drug, the small number of reported cases makes it impossible to draw conclusions regarding safety in pregnancy. Acyclovir is found in breast milk, but no adverse effects have been reported in the newborn. Famciclovir is similar in actions and adverse effects.

Ribavirin is used by aerosol for treatment of hospitalized infants and young children with severe lower respiratory tract infections due to respiratory syncytial virus (RSV). When administered orally, the drug has been used in adultys to treat other viral diseases including acute and chronic hepatitis, herpes genitalis, **measles**, and Lassa fever, however there is relatively little information about these uses. In rare cases, initiation of ribavirin therapy has led to deterioration of respiratory function in infants. Careful monitoring is essential for safe use.

The anti-influenza drugs are generally well tolerated. Amantadine, which is also used for treatment of Parkinsonism, may show more frequent CNS effects, including **sedation** and **dizziness**. Rapid discontinuation of amantidine may cause an increase in Parkinsonian symptoms in patients using the drug for that purpose. All are schedule C for pregnancy. In animal studies, they have caused fetal malformations in doses several times higher than the normal human dose. Use caution in breast feeding.

Interactions

Consult specific references for information on **drug interactions**.

Use particular caution in HIV-positive patients, since these patients are commonly on multi-drug regimens with a high frequency of interactions. Ganciclovir should not be used with other drugs which cause hematologic toxicity, and cidofovir should not be used with other drugs that may cause kidney damage.

Resources

PERIODICALS

Gray, Mary Ann. "Antiviral Medications." *Orthopaedic Nursing* 15 (November-December 1996): 82.

Samuel D. Uretsky, PharmD

Anxiety

Definition

Anxiety is a multisystem response to a perceived threat or danger. It reflects a combination of biochemical changes in the body, the patient's personal history and memory, and the social situation. As far as we know, anxiety is a uniquely human experience. Other animals clearly know fear, but human anxiety involves an ability, to use memory and imagination to move backward and forward in time, that animals do not appear to have. The anxiety that occurs in post-traumatic syndromes indicates that human memory is a much more complicated mental function than animal memory. Moreover, a large portion of human anxiety is produced by anticipation of future events. Without a sense of personal continuity over time, people would not have the "raw materials" of anxiety.

It is important to distinguish between anxiety as a feeling or experience, and an anxiety disorder as a psychiatric diagnosis. A person may feel anxious without having an anxiety disorder. In addition, a person facing a clear and present danger or a realistic fear is not usually considered to be in a state of anxiety. In addition, anxiety frequently occurs as a symptom in other categories of psychiatric disturbance.

Description

Although anxiety is a commonplace experience that everyone has from time to time, it is difficult to describe concretely because it has so many different potential causes and degrees of intensity. Doctors sometimes categorize anxiety as an emotion or an affect depending on whether it is being described by the person having it (emotion) or by an outside observer (affect). The word *emotion* is generally used for the biochemical changes and feeling state that underlie a person's internal sense of anxiety. *Affect* is used to describe the person's emotional state from an observer's perspective. If a doctor says that a patient has an anxious affect, he or she means that the patient

> **KEY TERMS**
>
> **Affect**—An observed emotional expression or response. In some situations, anxiety would be considered an inappropriate affect.
>
> **Anxiolytic**—A type of medication that helps to relieve anxiety.
>
> **Autonomic nervous system (ANS)**—The part of the nervous system that supplies nerve endings in the blood vessels, heart, intestines, glands, and smooth muscles, and governs their involuntary functioning. The autonomic nervous system is responsible for the biochemical changes involved in experiences of anxiety.
>
> **Endocrine gland**—A ductless gland, such as the pituitary, thyroid, or adrenal gland, that secretes its products directly into the blood or lymph.
>
> **Free-floating anxiety**—Anxiety that lacks a definite focus or content. .
>
> **Hyperarousal**—A state or condition of muscular and emotional tension produced by hormones released during the fight-or-flight reaction.
>
> **Hypothalamus**—A portion of the brain that regulates the autonomic nervous system, the release of hormones from the pituitary gland, sleep cycles, and body temperature.
>
> **Limbic system**—A group of structures in the brain that includes the hypothalamus, amygdala, and hippocampus. The limbic system plays an important part in regulation of human moods and emotions. Many psychiatric disorders are related to malfunctioning of the limbic system.
>
> **Phobia**—In psychoanalytic theory, a psychological defense against anxiety in which the patient displaces anxious feelings onto an external object, activity, or situation.

appears nervous or anxious, or responds to others in an anxious way (for example, the individual is shaky, tremulous, etc.).

Although anxiety is related to fear, it is not the same thing. Fear is a direct, focused response to a specific event or object, and the person is consciously aware of it. Most people will feel fear if someone points a loaded gun at them or if they see a tornado forming on the horizon. They also will recognize that they are afraid. Anxiety, on the other hand, is often unfocused, vague, and hard to pin down to a specific cause. In this form it is called free-floating anxiety.

Sometimes anxiety being experienced in the present may stem from an event or person that produced pain and fear in the past, but the anxious individual is not consciously aware of the original source of the feeling. It is anxiety's aspect of remoteness that makes it hard for people to compare their experiences of it. Whereas most people will be fearful in physically dangerous situations, and can agree that fear is an appropriate response in the presence of danger, anxiety is often triggered by objects or events that are unique and specific to an individual. An individual might be anxious because of a unique meaning or memory being stimulated by present circumstances, not because of some immediate danger. Another individual looking at the anxious person from the outside may be truly puzzled as to the reason for the person's anxiety.

Causes and symptoms

Anxiety can have a number of different causes. It is a multidimensional response to stimuli in the person's environment, or a response to an internal stimulus (for example, a hypochondriac's reaction to a stomach rumbling) resulting from a combination of general biological and individual psychological processes.

Physical

In some cases, anxiety is produced by physical responses to **stress**, or by certain disease processes or medications.

THE AUTONOMIC NERVOUS SYSTEM (ANS). The nervous system of human beings is "hard-wired" to respond to dangers or threats. These responses are not subject to conscious control, and are the same in humans as in lower animals. They represent an evolutionary adaptation to the animal predators and other dangers with which all animals, including primitive humans, had to cope. The most familiar reaction of this type is the so-called "fight-or-flight" response. This response is the human organism's automatic "red alert" in a life-threatening situation. It is a state of physiological and emotional hyperarousal marked by high muscle tension and strong feelings of fear or anger. When a person has a fight-or-flight reaction, the level of stress hormones in their blood rises. They become more alert and attentive, their eyes dilate, their heartbeat increases, their breathing rate increases, and their digestion slows down, allowing more energy to be available to the muscles.

This emergency reaction is regulated by a part of the nervous system called the autonomic nervous system, or ANS. The ANS is controlled by the hypothalamus, a specialized part of the brainstem that is among a group of structures called the limbic system. The limbic system controls human emotions through its connections to glands and muscles; it also connects to the ANS and "higher" brain centers, such as parts of the cerebral cortex. One problem with this arrangement is that the limbic system cannot tell the difference between a realistic physical threat and an anxiety-producing thought or idea. The hypothalamus may trigger the release of stress hormones by the pituitary gland, even when there is no external and objective danger. A second problem is caused by the biochemical side effects of too many "false alarms" in the ANS. When a person responds to a real danger, his or her body gets rid of the stress hormones by running away or by fighting. In modern life, however, people often have fight-or-flight reactions in situations in which they can neither run away nor lash out physically. As a result, their bodies have to absorb all the biochemical changes of hyperarousal, rather than release them. These biochemical changes can produce anxious feelings, as well as muscle tension and other physical symptoms associated with anxiety. They may even produce permanent changes in the brain, if the process occurs repeatedly. Moreover, chronic physical disorders, such as coronary artery disease, may be worsened by anxiety, as chronic hyperarousal puts undue stress on the heart, stomach, and other organs.

DISEASES AND DISORDERS. Anxiety can be a symptom of certain medical conditions. Some of these diseases are disorders of the endocrine system, such as Cushing's syndrome (overproduction of cortisol by the adrenal cortex), and include over- or underactivity of the thyroid gland. Other medical conditions that can produce anxiety include **respiratory distress syndrome**, mitral valve prolapse, porphyria, and chest **pain** caused by inadequate blood supply to the heart (angina pectoris).

A study released in 2004 showed that people who had experienced traumatic bone injuries may have unrecognized anxiety in the form of **post-traumatic stress disorder**. This disorder can result from witnessing or experiencing an event involving serious injury, or threatened **death** (or experiencing the death or threatened death of another.)

MEDICATIONS AND SUBSTANCE USE. Numerous medications may cause anxiety-like symptoms as a side effect. They include birth control pills; some thyroid or **asthma** drugs; some psychotropic agents; occasionally, local anesthetics; **corticosteroids; antihypertensive drugs**; and nonsteroidal anti-inflammatory drugs (like flurbiprofen and ibuprofen).

Although people do not usually think of **caffeine** as a drug, it can cause anxiety-like symptoms when consumed in sufficient quantity. Patients who consume caffeine rich foods and beverages, such as chocolate, cocoa, coffee, tea, or carbonated soft drinks (especially cola beverages), can sometimes lower their anxiety symptoms simply by reducing their intake of these substances.

Withdrawal from certain prescription drugs, primarily beta blockers and corticosteroids, can cause anxiety. Withdrawal from drugs of abuse, including **LSD**, **cocaine**, alcohol, and opiates, can also cause anxiety.

Learned associations

Some aspects of anxiety appear to be unavoidable byproducts of the human developmental process. Humans are unique among animals in that they spend an unusually long period of early life in a relatively helpless condition, and a sense of helplessness can lead to anxiety. The extended period of human dependency on adults means that people may remember, and learn to anticipate, frightening or upsetting experiences long before they are capable enough to feel a sense of mastery over their environment. In addition, the fact that anxiety disorders often run in families indicates that children can learn unhealthy attitudes and behaviors from parents, as well as healthy ones. Also, recurrent disorders in families may indicate that there is a genetic or inherited component in some **anxiety disorders**. For example, there has been found to be a higher rate of anxiety disorders (panic) in identical twins than in fraternal twins.

CHILDHOOD DEVELOPMENT AND ANXIETY. Researchers in early childhood development regard anxiety in adult life as a residue of childhood memories of dependency. Humans learn during the first year of life that they are not self-sufficient and that their basic survival depends on the care of others. It is thought that this early experience of helplessness underlies the most common anxieties of adult life, including fear of powerlessness and fear of being unloved. Thus, adults can be made anxious by symbolic threats to their sense of competence and/or significant relationships, even though they are no longer helpless children.

SYMBOLIZATION. The psychoanalytic model gives considerable weight to the symbolic aspect of human anxiety; examples include phobic disorders, obsessions, compulsions, and other forms of anxiety that are highly individualized. The length of the human maturation process allows many opportunities for children and adolescents to connect their experiences with certain objects or events that can bring back feelings in later life. For example, a person who was frightened as a child by a tall man wearing glasses may feel panicky years later by something that reminds him of that person or experience without consciously knowing why.

Freud thought that anxiety results from a person's internal conflicts. According to his theory, people feel anxious when they feel torn between desires or urges toward certain actions, on the one hand, and moral restrictions, on the other. In some cases, the person's anxiety may attach itself to an object that represents the inner conflict. For example, someone who feels anxious around money may be pulled between a desire to steal and the belief that stealing is wrong. Money becomes a symbol for the inner conflict between doing what is considered right and doing what one wants.

PHOBIAS. Phobias are a special type of anxiety reaction in which the person's anxiety is concentrated on a specific object or situation that the person then tries to avoid. In most cases, the person's fear is out of all proportion to its "cause." Prior to the *Diagnostic and Statistical Manual of Mental Disorders,* 4th edition *(DSM-IV)*, these specific phobias were called simple phobias. It is estimated that 10-11% of the population will develop a phobia in the course of their lives. Some phobias, such as **agoraphobia** (fear of open spaces), claustrophobia (fear of small or confined spaces), and social phobia, are shared by large numbers of people. Others are less common or unique to the patient.

Social and environmental stressors

Anxiety often has a social dimension because humans are social creatures. People frequently report feelings of high anxiety when they anticipate and, therefore, fear the loss of social approval or love. Social phobia is a specific anxiety disorder that is marked by high levels of anxiety or fear of embarrassment in social situations.

Another social stressor is prejudice. People who belong to groups that are targets of bias are at higher risk for developing anxiety disorders. Some experts think, for example, that the higher rates of phobias and **panic disorder** among women reflects their greater social and economic vulnerability.

Some controversial studies indicate that the increase in violent or upsetting pictures and stories in news reports and entertainment may raise the anxiety level of many people. Stress and anxiety management programs often suggest that patients cut down their exposure to upsetting stimuli.

Anxiety may also be caused by environmental or occupational factors. People who must live or work around sudden or loud noises, bright or flashing lights, chemical vapors, or similar nuisances, which they cannot avoid or control, may develop heightened anxiety levels.

Existential anxiety

Another factor that shapes human experiences of anxiety is knowledge of personal mortality. Humans are the only animals that appear to be aware of their limited life span. Some researchers think that awareness of death influences experiences of anxiety from the time that a person is old enough to understand death.

Symptoms of anxiety

In order to understand the diagnosis and treatment of anxiety, it is helpful to have a basic understanding of its symptoms.

SOMATIC. The somatic or physical symptoms of anxiety include headaches, **dizziness** or lightheadedness, **nausea** and/or **vomiting**, **diarrhea**, **tingling**, pale complexion, sweating, **numbness**, difficulty in breathing, and sensations of tightness in the chest, neck, shoulders, or hands. These symptoms are produced by the hormonal, muscular, and cardiovascular reactions involved in the fight-or-flight reaction. Children and adolescents with **generalized anxiety disorder** show a high percentage of physical complaints.

BEHAVIORAL. Behavioral symptoms of anxiety include pacing, trembling, general restlessness, hyperventilation, pressured speech, hand wringing, or finger tapping.

COGNITIVE. Cognitive symptoms of anxiety include recurrent or obsessive thoughts, feelings of doom, morbid or fear-inducing thoughts or ideas, and confusion, or inability to concentrate.

EMOTIONAL. Feeling states associated with anxiety include tension or nervousness, feeling "hyper" or "keyed up," and feelings of unreality, panic, or terror.

DEFENSE MECHANISMS. In psychoanalytic theory, the symptoms of anxiety in humans may arise from or activate a number of unconscious defense mechanisms. Because of these defenses, it is possible for a person to be anxious without being consciously aware of it or appearing anxious to others. These psychological defenses include:

- Repression. The person pushes anxious thoughts or ideas out of conscious awareness.

- Displacement. Anxiety from one source is attached to a different object or event. Phobias are an example

of the mechanism of displacement in psychoanalytic theory.

- Rationalization. The person justifies the anxious feelings by saying that any normal person would feel anxious in their situation.

- Somatization. The anxiety emerges in the form of physical complaints and illnesses, such as recurrent headaches, stomach upsets, or muscle and joint pain.

- Delusion formation. The person converts anxious feelings into conspiracy theories or similar ideas without reality testing. Delusion formation can involve groups as well as individuals.

Other theorists attribute some drug **addiction** to the desire to relieve symptoms of anxiety. Most addictions, they argue, originate in the use of mood-altering substances or behaviors to "medicate" anxious feelings.

Diagnosis

The diagnosis of anxiety is difficult and complex because of the variety of its causes and the highly personalized and individualized nature of its symptom formation. There are no medical tests that can be used to diagnose anxiety by itself. When a doctor examines an anxious patient, he or she will first rule out physical conditions and diseases that have anxiety as a symptom. Apart from these exclusions, the **physical examination** is usually inconclusive. Some anxious patients may have their blood pressure or pulse rate affected by anxiety, or may look pale or perspire heavily, but others may appear physically completely normal. The doctor will then take the patient's medication, dietary, and occupational history to see if they are taking prescription drugs that might cause anxiety, if they are abusing alcohol or mood-altering drugs, if they are consuming large amounts of caffeine, or if their workplace is noisy or dangerous. In most cases, the most important source of diagnostic information is the patient's psychological and social history. The doctor may administer a brief psychological test to help evaluate the intensity of the patient's anxiety and some of its features. Some tests that are often given include the Hamilton Anxiety Scale and the Anxiety Disorders Interview Schedule (ADIS). Many doctors will check a number of chemical factors in the blood, such as the level of thyroid hormone and blood sugar.

Treatment

Not all patients with anxiety require treatment, but for more severe cases, treatment is recommended. Because anxiety often has more than one cause and is experienced in highly individual ways, its treatment usually requires more than one type of therapy. In addition, there is no way to tell in advance how patients will respond to a specific drug or therapy. Sometimes the doctor will need to try different medications or methods of treatment before finding the best combination for the particular patient. It usually takes about six to eight weeks for the doctor to evaluate the effectiveness of a treatment regimen.

Medications

Medications are often prescribed to relieve the physical and psychological symptoms of anxiety. Most agents work by counteracting the biochemical and muscular changes involved in the fight-or-flight reaction. Some work directly on the chemicals in the brain that are thought to underlie the anxiety.

ANXIOLYTICS. Anxiolytics are sometimes called tranquilizers. Most anxiolytic drugs are either **benzodiazepines** or **barbiturates**. Barbiturates, once commonly used, are now rarely used in clinical practice. Barbiturates work by slowing down the transmission of nerve impulses from the brain to other parts of the body. They include such drugs as phenobarbital (Luminal) and pentobarbital (Nembutal). Benzodiazepines work by relaxing the skeletal muscles and calming the limbic system. They include such drugs as chlordiazepoxide (Librium) and diazepam (Valium). Both barbiturates and benzodiazepines are potentially habit-forming and may cause withdrawal symptoms, but benzodiazepines are far less likely than barbiturates to cause physical dependency. Both drugs also increase the effects of alcohol and should never be taken in combination with it.

Two other types of anxiolytic medications include meprobamate (Equanil), which is now rarely used, and buspirone (BuSpar), a new type of anxiolytic that appears to work by increasing the efficiency of the body's own emotion-regulating brain chemicals. Buspirone has several advantages over other anxiolytics. It does not cause dependence problems, does not interact with alcohol, and does not affect the patient's ability to drive or operate machinery. However, buspirone is not effective against certain types of anxiety, such as panic disorder.

ANTIDEPRESSANTS AND BETA-BLOCKERS. For some anxiety disorders, such as obsessive-compulsive disorder and panic type anxiety, a type of drugs used to treat depression, **selective serotonin reuptake inhibitors** (SSRIs; such as Prozac and Paxil), are the treatment of choice. A newer drug that has been shown as effective as Paxil is called escitalopram oxalate (Lexapro). Because anxiety often coexists with symptoms of depression, many doctors prescribe antidepressant medications for anxious/depressed patients. While SSRIs are more common, antidepressants are sometimes prescribed, including **tricyclic antidepressants** such as imipramine (Tofranil) or **monoamine oxidase inhibitors** (MAO inhibitors) such as phenelzine (Nardil).

Beta-blockers are medications that work by blocking the body's reaction to the stress hormones that are released during the fight-or-flight reaction. They include drugs like propranolol (Inderal) or atenolol (Tenormin). Beta-blockers are sometimes given to patients with post-traumatic anxiety symptoms. More commonly, the beta-blockers are given to patients with a mild form of social phobic anxiety, such as fear of public speaking.

Psychotherapy

Most patients with anxiety will be given some form of psychotherapy along with medications. Many patients benefit from insight-oriented therapies, which are designed to help them uncover unconscious conflicts and defense mechanisms in order to understand how their symptoms developed. Patients who are extremely anxious may benefit from supportive psychotherapy, which aims at symptom reduction rather than personality restructuring.

Two newer approaches that work well with anxious patients are **cognitive-behavioral therapy** (CBT), and relaxation training. In CBT, the patient is taught to identify the thoughts and situations that stimulate his or her anxiety, and to view them more realistically. In the behavioral part of the program, the patient is exposed to the anxiety-provoking object, situation, or internal stimulus (like a rapid heart beat) in gradual stages until he or she is desensitized to it. Relaxation training, which is sometimes called anxiety management training, includes breathing exercises and similar techniques intended to help the patient prevent hyperventilation and relieve the muscle tension associated with the fight-or-flight reaction. Both CBT and relaxation training can be used in group therapy as well as individual treatment. In addition to CBT, support groups are often helpful to anxious patients, because they provide a social network and lessen the embarrassment that often accompanies anxiety symptoms.

Psychosurgery

Surgery on the brain is very rarely recommended for patients with anxiety; however, some patients with severe cases of **obsessive-compulsive disorder** (OCD) have been helped by an operation on a part of the brain that is involved in OCD. Normally, this operation is attempted after all other treatments have failed.

Alternative treatment

Alternative treatments for anxiety cover a variety of approaches. **Meditation** and mindfulness training are thought beneficial to patients with phobias and panic disorder. **Hydrotherapy** is useful to some anxious patients because it promotes general relaxation of the nervous system. **Yoga**, aikido, t'ai chi, and dance therapy help patients work with the physical, as well as the emotional, tensions that either promote anxiety or are created by the anxiety.

Homeopathy and traditional Chinese medicine approach anxiety as a symptom of a systemic disorder. Homeopathic practitioners select a remedy based on other associated symptoms and the patient's general constitution. Chinese medicine regards anxiety as a blockage of *qi*, or vital force, inside the patient's body that is most likely to affect the lung and large intestine meridian flow. The practitioner of Chinese medicine chooses **acupuncture** point locations and/or herbal therapy to move the qi and rebalance the entire system in relation to the lung and large intestine.

Prognosis

The prognosis for resolution of anxiety depends on the specific disorder and a wide variety of factors, including the patient's age, sex, general health, living situation, belief system, social support network, and responses to different anxiolytic medications and forms of therapy.

Prevention

Humans have significant control over thoughts, and, therefore, may learn ways of preventing anxiety by changing irrational ideas and beliefs. Humans also have some power over anxiety arising from social and environmental conditions. Other forms of anxiety, however, are built into the human organism and its life cycle, and cannot be prevented or eliminated.

Resources

PERIODICALS

"Lexapro Found to be as Effective as Paxil." *Mental Health Weekly Digest* (April 12, 2004): 16.

Masi, Gabriele, et al. "Generalized Anxiety Disorder in Referred Children and Adolescents." *Journal of the American Academy of Child and Adolescent Psychiatry* (June 2004): 752–761.

"Patients With Traumatic Bone Injuries Have Unrecognized Anxiety." *Health & Medicine Week* (June 28, 2004): 824.

Rebecca J. Frey, PhD
Teresa G. Odle

Anxiety disorders

Definition

The **anxiety** disorders are a group of mental disturbances characterized by anxiety as a central or core symptom. Although anxiety is a commonplace experience, not everyone who experiences it has an anxiety disorder. Anxiety is associated with a wide range of physical illnesses, medication side effects, and other psychiatric disorders.

The revisions of the *Diagnostic and Statistical Manual of Mental Disorders (DSM)* that took place after 1980 brought major changes in the classification of the anxiety disorders. Prior to 1980, psychiatrists classified patients on the basis of a theory that defined anxiety as the outcome of unconscious conflicts in the patient's mind. *DSM-III* (1980), *DSM-III-R* (1987), and *DSM-IV* (1994) introduced and refined a new classification that considered recent discoveries about the biochemical and post-traumatic origins of some types of anxiety. The present definitions are based on the external and reported symptom patterns of the disorders rather than on theories about their origins.

Description

Anxiety disorders are the most common form of mental disturbance in the United States population. It is estimated that 28 million people suffer from an anxiety disorder every year. These disorders are a serious problem for the entire society because of their interference with patients' work, schooling, and family life. They also contribute to the high rates of alcohol and substance **abuse** in the United States. Anxiety disorders are an additional problem for health professionals because the physical symptoms of anxiety frequently bring people to primary care doctors or emergency rooms.

DSM-IV defines 12 types of anxiety disorders in the adult population. They can be grouped under seven headings:

- Panic disorders with or without **agoraphobia**. The chief characteristic of **panic disorder** is the occurrence of panic attacks coupled with fear of their recurrence. In clinical settings, agoraphobia is usually not a disorder byitself, but is typically associated with some form of panic disorder. Patients with agoraphobia are afraid of places or situations in which they might have a panic attack and be unable to leave or to find help. About 25% of patients with panic disorder develop **obsessive-compulsive disorder** (OCD).

- **Phobias**. These include specific phobias and social phobia. A phobia is an intense irrational fear of a specific object or situation that compels the patient to avoid it. Some phobias concern activities or objects that involve some risk (for example, flying or driving) but many are focused on harmless animals or other objects. Social phobia involves a fear of being humiliated, judged, or scrutinized. It manifests itself as a fear of performing certain functions in the presence of others, such as public speaking or using public lavatories.

- Obsessive-compulsive disorder (OCD). This disorder is marked by unwanted, intrusive, persistent thoughts or repetitive behaviors that reflect the patient's anxiety or attempts to control it. It affects between 2-3% of the population and is much more common than was previously thought.

- **Stress** disorders. These include **post-traumatic stress disorder** (PTSD) and acute stress disorder. Stress disorders are symptomatic reactions to traumatic events in the patient's life.

- **Generalized anxiety disorder** (GAD). GAD is the most commonly diagnosed anxiety disorder and occurs most frequently in young adults.

- Anxiety disorders due to known physical causes. These include general medical conditions or **substance abuse**.

- Anxiety disorder not otherwise specified. This last category is not a separate type of disorder, but is included to cover symptoms that do not meet the specific *DSM-IV* criteria for other anxiety disorders.

All *DSM-IV* anxiety disorder diagnoses include a criterion of severity. The anxiety must be severe enough to interfere significantly with the patient's occupational or educational functioning, social activities or close relationships, and other customary activities.

The anxiety disorders vary widely in their frequency of occurrence in the general population, age of onset, family patterns, and gender distribution. The stress disorders and anxiety disorders caused by

---

KEY TERMS

Agoraphobia—Abnormal anxiety regarding public places or situations from which the patient may wish to flee or in which he or she would be helpless in the event of a panic attack.

Compulsion—A repetitive or ritualistic behavior that a person performs to reduce anxiety. Compulsions often develop as a way of controlling or "undoing" obsessive thoughts.

Obsession—A repetitive or persistent thought, idea, or impulse that is perceived as inappropriate and distressing.

Panic attack—A time-limited period of intense fear accompanied by physical and cognitive symptoms. Panic attacks may be unexpected or triggered by specific cues.

---

medical conditions or substance abuse are less age- and gender-specific. Whereas OCD affects males and females equally, GAD, panic disorder, and specific phobias all affect women more frequently than men. GAD and panic disorders are more likely to develop in young adults, while phobias and OCD can begin in childhood.

Anxiety disorders in children and adolescents

DSM-IV defines one anxiety disorder as specific to children, namely, separation anxiety disorder. This disorder is defined as anxiety regarding separation from home or family that is excessive or inappropriate for the child's age. In some children, separation anxiety takes the form of school avoidance.

Children and adolescents can also be diagnosed with panic disorder, phobias, generalized anxiety disorder, and the post-traumatic stress syndromes.

Causes and symptoms

The causes of anxiety include a variety of individual and general social factors, and may produce physical, cognitive, emotional, or behavioral symptoms. The patient's ethnic or cultural background may also influence his or her vulnerability to certain forms of anxiety. Genetic factors that lead to biochemical abnormalities may also play a role.

Anxiety in children may be caused by suffering from abuse, as well as by the factors that cause anxiety in adults.

Diagnosis

The diagnosis of anxiety disorders is complicated by the variety of causes of anxiety and the range of disorders that may include anxiety as a symptom. Many patients who suffer from anxiety disorders have features or symptoms of more than one disorder. Patients whose anxiety is accounted for by another psychic disorder, such as schizophrenia or major depression, are not diagnosed with an anxiety disorder. A doctor examining an anxious patient will usually begin by ruling out diseases that are known to cause anxiety and then proceed to take the patient's medication history, in order to exclude side effects of prescription drugs. Most doctors will ask about **caffeine** consumption to see if the patient's dietary habits are a factor. The patient's work and family situation will also be discussed. Often, primary care physicians will exhaust resources looking for medical causes for general patient complaints which may indicate a physical illness. In 2004, the Anxiety Disorders Association of American published guidelines to better aid physicians in diagnosing and managing generalized anxiety disorder. Laboratory tests for blood sugar and thyroid function are also common.

Diagnostic testing for anxiety

There are no laboratory tests that can diagnose anxiety, although the doctor may order some specific tests to rule out disease conditions. Although there is no psychiatric test that can provide definite diagnoses of anxiety disorders, there are several short-answer interviews or symptom inventories that doctors can use to evaluate the intensity of a patient's anxiety and some of its associated features. These measures include the Hamilton Anxiety Scale and the Anxiety Disorders Interview Schedule (ADIS).

Treatment

For relatively mild anxiety disorders, psychotherapy alone may suffice. In general, doctors prefer to use a combination of medications and psychotherapy with more severely anxious patients. Most patients respond better to a combination of treatment methods than to either medications or psychotherapy in isolation. Because of the variety of medications and treatment approaches that are used to treat anxiety disorders, the doctor cannot predict in advance which combination will be most helpful to a specific patient. In many cases the doctor will need to try a new medication or treatment over a six- to eight-week period in order to assess its effectiveness. Treatment trials do not necessarily mean that the patient cannot be helped or that the doctor is incompetent.

Although anxiety disorders are not always easy to diagnose, there are several reasons why it is important for patients with severe anxiety symptoms to get help. Anxiety doesn't always go away by itself; it often progresses to panic attacks, phobias, and episodes of depression. Untreated anxiety disorders may eventually lead to a diagnosis of major depression, or interfere with the patient's education or ability to keep a job. In addition, many anxious patients develop addictions to drugs or alcohol when they try to "medicate" their symptoms. Moreover, since children learn ways of coping with anxiety from their parents, adults who get help for anxiety disorders are in a better position to help their families cope with factors that lead to anxiety than those who remain untreated.

Alternative treatment

Alternative treatments for anxiety cover a variety of approaches. **Meditation** and mindfulness training are thought beneficial to patients with phobias and panic disorder. **Hydrotherapy** is useful to some anxious patients because it promotes general relaxation of the nervous system. **Yoga**, aikido, t'ai chi, and dance therapy help patients work with the physical, as well as the emotional, tensions that either promote anxiety or are created by the anxiety.

Homeopathy and traditional Chinese medicine approach anxiety as a symptom of a systemic disorder. Homeopathic practitioners select a remedy based on other associated symptoms and the patient's general constitution. Chinese medicine regards anxiety as a blockage of *qi*, or vital force, inside the patient's body that is most likely to affect the lung and large intestine meridian flow. The practitioner of Chinese medicine chooses **acupuncture** point locations and/or herbal therapy to move the qi and rebalance the entire system in relation to the lung and large intestine.

Prognosis

The prognosis for recovery depends on the specific disorder, the severity of the patient's symptoms, the specific causes of the anxiety, and the patient's degree of control over these causes.

Prevention

Anxiety is an unavoidable feature of human existence. However, humans have some power over their reactions to anxiety-provoking events and situations. Cognitive therapy and meditation or mindfulness training appear to be beneficial in helping people lower their long-term anxiety levels.

Resources

PERIODICALS

"Guidelines to Assist Primary Care Physicians in Diagnosing GAD." *Psychiatric Times* (July 1, 2004): 16.

Rebecca J. Frey, PhD
Teresa G. Odle

Anxiolytics *see* **Antianxiety drugs**

Aortic aneurysm

Definition

An aneurysm is an abnormal bulging or swelling of a portion of a blood vessel. The aorta, which can develop these abnormal bulges, is the large blood vessel that carries oxygen-rich blood away from the heart to the rest of the body.

Description

The aorta carries oxygen-rich blood to the body, and is therefore called an artery. Because the aorta is an artery, its walls are made of up three layers; a thin inner layer, a muscular middle layer (that gives the vessel its flexibility under pressure from the filling blood), and a fiber-like outer layer that gives the vessel strength to not burst when the heart pumps blood to the body.

Aortic aneurysms occur when a weakness develops in part of the wall of the aorta; three basic types are usually found. If all three layers of the vessel are affected and weakness develops along an extended area of the vessel, the weakened area will appear as a large, bulging region of blood vessel; this is called a fusiform aneurysm. If weakness develops between the inner and outer layers of the aortic wall, a bulge results as blood from the interior of the vessel is pushed around the damaged region in the wall and collects between these layers. This is called a dissecting aneurysm because one layer is "dissected" or separated from another. If damage occurs to only the middle (muscular) layer of the vessel, a sack-like bulge can form; therefore, this is a saccular aneurysm.

Causes and symptoms

Aortic aneurysms occur in different portions of the aorta, which begins in the chest (at the heart) and travels downward through the abdomen. Aneurysms found in the region of the aorta within the chest are

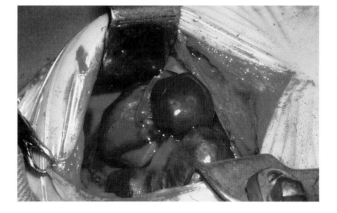

Surgery being performed to correct aortic aneurysm. *(Custom Medical Stock Photo. Reproduced by permission.)*

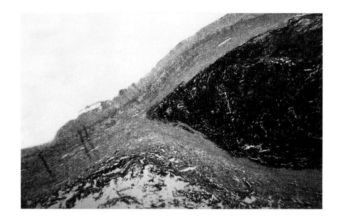

An aneurysm in progress. An aneurysm is an abnormal bulging or swelling of a portion of a blood vessel. *(Custom Medical Stock Photo. Reproduced by permission.)*

called thoracic aortic aneurysms. Aneurysms that occur in the part of the aorta within the abdomen are called abdominal aortic aneurysms.

Thoracic aortic aneurysms do not usually produce any noticeable symptoms. However, as the aneurysm becomes larger, chest, shoulder, neck, lower back, or abdominal **pain** can result. Abdominal aortic aneurysms occur more often in men, and these aneurysms can cause pain in the lower back, hips, and abdomen. A painful abdominal aortic aneurysm usually means that the aneurysm could burst very soon.

Most abdominal aortic aneurysms are caused by **atherosclerosis**, a condition caused when fat (mostly cholesterol) carried in the blood builds up in the inner wall of the aorta. As more and more fat attaches to the aortic wall, the wall itself becomes abnormally weak and often results in an aneurysm or bulge.

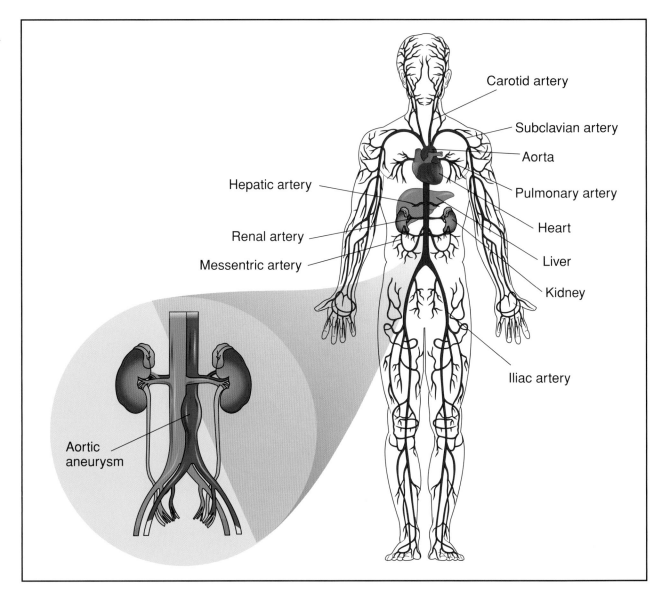

Aortic aneurysms occur when a weakness develops in a part of the wall of the aorta. The aorta is the large blood vessel that carries oxygen-rich blood away from the heart to the rest of the body. *(Illustration by Electronic Illustrators Group.)*

KEY TERMS

Atherosclerosis—The accumulation of fat on the inner wall of an artery. This fat is largely made up of cholesterol being carried in the blood.

Dacron—A synthetic polyester fiber used to surgically repair damaged sections of blood vessel walls.

Aortic aneurysms are also caused by a breakdown of the muscular middle layer of the artery wall, by high blood pressure, by direct injury to the chest, and although rare, by bacteria that can infect the aorta.

Diagnosis

Silent, stable aneurysms are often detected when a person has an x ray as part of a routine examination or for other medical reasons. Otherwise, when chest, abdominal, or back pain is severe, aortic aneurysm is suspected and x-ray (radiographic) studies can confirm or rule out that condition.

Treatment

Aortic aneurysms are potentially life-threatening conditions. Small aneurysms should be monitored for their rate of growth and large aneurysms require consideration for a surgical repair. The most common method of surgical repair is to cut out the bulging section of artery wall and sew a Dacron fiber material into its place in the vessel wall.

Prognosis

Only 1-2% of people die from having surgical repair of an aortic aneurysm. However, if the aneurysm is untreated and eventually ruptures, less than half of the people with ruptured aneurysms will survive. The challenge for the physician is to decide when or if to do the preventive surgery.

Prevention

Aneuryms can develop in people with atherosclerosis. High blood pressure can also lead to this condition. Although no definite prevention exists, lifestyle and dietary changes that help lower blood pressure and the amount of fat in the blood stream may slow the development of aneurysms.

Resources

PERIODICALS

van der Vleit, J. Adam, and Albert P. M. Boll. "Abdominal Aortic Aneurysm." *The Lancet* 349 (March 22, 1997): 863.

ORGANIZATIONS

American Heart Association. 7320 Greenville Ave. Dallas, TX 75231. (214) 373-6300. < http://www.americanheart.org > .

National Heart, Lung and Blood Institute. P.O. Box 30105, Bethesda, MD 20824-0105. (301) 251-1222. < http://www.nhlbi.nih.gov > .

Dominic De Bellis, PhD

Aortic dissection

Definition

Aortic dissection is a rare, but potentially fatal, condition in which blood passes through the inner lining and between the layers of the aorta. The dissecting aorta usually does not burst, but has an abnormal second channel within it.

Description

A defect in the inner lining of the aorta allows an opening or tear to develop. The aorta is the main artery of the body and is an area of high blood

pressure. When a defect develops, blood pressure can force the tear to open and allow blood to pass through. Since the blood is under pressure, it eventually splits (dissecting) the middle layer of the blood vessel, creating a new channel for blood. The length of the channel grows over time and can result in the closing off of connection points to other arteries. This can lead to **heart attack**, strokes, abdominal **pain**, and nerve damage. Blood may leak from the dissection and collect in the chest an around the heart.

A second mechanism leading to aortic dissection is medial hemorrhage. A medial hemorrhage occurs in the middle layer of the blood vessel and spills through the inner lining of the aorta wall. This opening then allows blood from the aorta to enter the vessel wall and begin a dissection. Approximately 2,000 cases of aortic dissection occur yearly in the United States.

Causes and symptoms

Aortic dissection is caused by a deterioration of the inner lining of the aorta. There are a number of conditions that predispose a person to develop defects of the inner lining, including high blood pressure, Marfan's disease, **Ehlers-Danlos syndrome**, connective tissue diseases, and defects of heart development which begin during fetal development. A dissection can also occur accidentally following insertion of a catheter, trauma, or surgery. The main symptom is sudden, intense pain. The pain can be so intense as to immobilize the patient and cause him to fall to the ground. The pain is frequently felt in both the chest and in the back, between the shoulder blades. The extent of the pain is proportional to the length of the dissection.

Diagnosis

The pain experienced by the patient is the first symptom of aortic dissection and is unique. The pain is usually described by the patient as "tearing, ripping, or stabbing." This is in contrast to the pain associated with heart attacks. The patient frequently has a reduced or absent pulse in the extremities. A murmur may be heard if the dissection is close to the heart. An enlarged aorta will usually appear in the chest x rays and ultrasound exams of most patients. The use of a blood dye in angiograms and/or CT scans (**computed tomography scans**) will aid in diagnosing and visualizing the dissection.

Treatment

Because of the potentially fatal nature of aortic dissection, patients are treated immediately. Drugs are administered to reduce the blood pressure and heart rate. If the dissection is small, drug therapy alone may be used. In other cases, surgery is performed. In surgery, damaged sections of the aorta are removed and a synthetic graft is often used to reconstruct the damaged vessel.

Prognosis

Depending on the nature and extent of the dissection, **death** can occur within a few hours of the start of a dissection. Approximately 75% of untreated people die within two weeks of the start of a dissection. Of those who are treated, 40% survive more than 10 years. Patients are usually given long term treatment with drugs to reduce their blood pressure, even if they have had surgery.

Resources

BOOKS

Alexander, R. W., R. C. Schlant, and V. Fuster, editors. *The Heart*. 9th ed. New York: McGraw-Hill, 1998.

John T. Lohr, PhD

Aortic incompetence *see* **Aortic valve insufficiency**

Aortic regurgitation *see* **Aortic valve insufficiency**

Aortic stenosis *see* **Aortic valve stenosis**

Aortic valve insufficiency

Definition

The aortic valve separates the left ventricle of the heart (the heart's largest pumping chamber) from the aorta, the large artery that carries oxygen-rich blood out of the left ventricle to the rest of the body. In aortic valve insufficiency, the aortic valve becomes leaky, causing blood to flow backwards into the left ventricle.

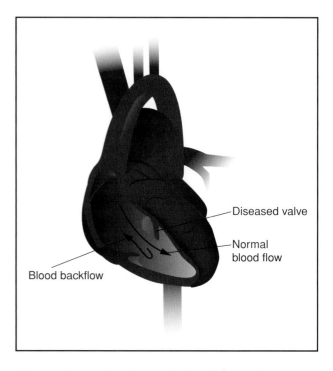

A human heart with a diseased valve that doesn't open and close properly, allowing blood to backflow to the heart. *(Illustration by Argosy, Inc.)*

Description

Aortic valve insufficiency occurs when this valve cannot properly close after blood that is leaving the heart's left ventricle enters the aorta. With each contraction of the heart more and more blood flows back into the left ventricle, causing the ventricle to become overfilled. This larger-than-normal amount of blood that collects in the left ventricle puts pressure on the walls of the heart, causing the heart muscle to increase in thickness (hypertrophy). If this thickening continues, the heart can be permanently damaged.

Aortic valve insufficiency is also know as aortic valve regurgitation because of the abnormal reversed flow of blood leaking through the poorly functioning valve.

Causes and symptoms

The faulty working of the aortic valve can be caused by a birth defect; by abnormal widening of the aorta (which can be caused by very high blood pressure and a variety of other less common conditions); by various diseases that cause large amounts of swelling (inflammation) in different areas of the body, like **rheumatic fever**; and, although rarely, by the sexually transmitted disease, **syphilis**.

About 75% of people with aortic valve insufficiency are men. Rheumatic (inflammatory) diseases have been the main cause of this condition in both men and women.

Aortic valve insufficiency can remain unnoticed for 10 to 15 years. In cases of severe insufficiency a person may notice a variety of symptoms, including an uncomfortable pounding of the heart when lying down, a very rapid or hard heart beat (**palpitations**), **shortness of breath**, chest **pain**, and if untreated for very long times, swelling of the liver, ankles, and belly.

Diagnosis

A poorly functioning or insufficient aortic valve can be identified when a doctor listens to the heart during a **physical examination**. A **chest x ray**, an electrocardiogram (ECG, an electrical printout of the heart beats), as well as an echocardiogram (a test that uses sound waves to create an image of the heart and its valves), can further evaluate or confirm the condition.

Treatment

Aortic insufficiency is usually corrected by having the defective valve surgically replaced. However, such an operation is done in severe cases. Before the condition worsens, certain drugs can be used to help manage this condition.

Drugs that remove water from the body, drugs that lower blood pressure, and drugs that help the heart beat more effectively can each be used for this condition. Reducing the amount of salt in the diet also helps lower the amount of fluid the body holds and can help the heart to work more efficiently as well.

In cases of a severely malfunctioning valve that has been untreated for a long time, surgery is the treatment of choice, especially if the heart is not functioning normally. Human heart valves can be replaced with man-made valves or with valves taken from pig hearts.

Prognosis

Although drug treatment can help put off the need for surgical valve replacement, it is important to replace the faulty valve before the heart muscle itself is damaged beyond recovery.

Resources

PERIODICALS

Condos Jr., William R. "Decade-old Heart Drug May Have a New Use." *San Diego Business Journal* 18 (21 July 1997): 24.

ORGANIZATIONS

American Heart Association. 7320 Greenville Ave. Dallas, TX 75231. (214) 373-6300. <http://www.americanheart.org>.

National Heart, Lung and Blood Institute. P.O. Box 30105, Bethesda, MD 20824-0105. (301) 251-1222. <http://www.nhlbi.nih.gov>.

Dominic De Bellis, PhD

Aortic valve stenosis

Definition

When aortic valve stenosis occurs, the aortic valve, located between the aorta and left ventricle of the heart, is narrower than normal size.

Description

A normal aortic valve, when open, allows the free flow of blood from the left ventricle to the aorta. When the valve narrows, as it does with stenosis, blood flow is impeded. Because it is more difficult for blood to flow through the valve, there is increased strain on the heart. This can cause the left ventricle to enlarge and malfunction, resulting in reduced blood supply to the heart muscle and body, as well as fluid build up in the lungs.

Cause and symptoms

Aortic valve stenosis can occur because of a birth defect in the formation of the valve. Calcium deposits may form on the valve with **aging**, causing the valve to become stiff and narrow. Stenosis can also occur as a result of **rheumatic fever**. Mild aortic stenosis may produce no symptoms at all. The most common symptoms, depending on the severity of the disease, are chest **pain**, blackouts, and difficulty breathing.

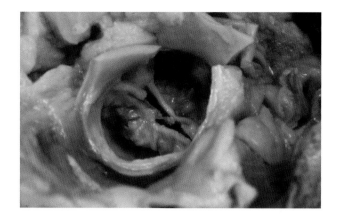

A close-up view of a calcified stenosis of the aortic valve.
(Custom Medical Stock Photo. Reproduced by permission.)

Diagnosis

Using a stethoscope, a physician may hear a murmur and other abnormal heart sounds. An ECG, also called an electrocardiogram, records the electrical activity of the heart. This technique and **chest x ray** can show evidence that the left ventricle is enlarged. An x ray can also reveal calcium deposits on the valve, as well as congestion in the lungs. **Echocardiography** can pick up thickening of the valve, heart size, and whether or not the valve is working properly. This is a procedure in which high frequency sound waves harmlessly bounce off organs in the body. Cardiac catheterization, in which a contrast dye is injected in an artery using a catheter, is the key tool to confirm stenosis and gauge its severity.

Treatment

Treatment depends on the symptoms and how the heart's function is affected. The valve can be opened without surgery by using a balloon catheter, but this is often a temporary solution. The procedure involves inserting a deflated balloon at the end of a catheter through the arteries to the valve. Inflating the balloon should widen the valve. In severe stenosis, heart valve replacement is recommended, most often involving open-heart surgery. The valve can be replaced with a mechanical valve, a valve from a pig, or by moving the patient's other heart valve (pulmonary) into the position of the aortic valve and then replacing the pulmonary valve with an mechanical one. Anyone with aortic stenosis needs to take **antibiotics** (amoxicillin, erythromycin, or clindamycin) before dental and some other surgical procedures, to prevent a heart valve infection.

Prognosis

The prognosis for aortic valve stenosis depends on the severity of the disease. With surgical repair, the disease is curable. Patients suffering mild stenosis can usually lead a normal life; a minority of the patients progress to severe disease. Anyone with moderate stenosis should avoid vigorous physical activity. Most of these patients end up suffering some kind of coronary heart disease over a 10 year period. Because it is a progressive disease, moderate and severe stenosis will be treated ultimately with surgery. Severe disease, if left untreated, leads to death within 2 to 4 years once the symptoms start.

Prevention

There is no way to prevent aortic stenosis.

Resources

BOOKS

Bender, Jeffrey R. "Heart Valve Disease." In *Yale University School of Medicine Heart Book*, edited by Barry L. Zaret, et al. New York: HearstBooks, 1992.

OTHER

"Aortic Stenosis." *Ochsner Heart and VascularInstitute.*
< http://www.ochsner.org/pedcard/as.htm > .
Rahimtoola, Aly. "Aortic Stenosis." *Loyola University
Health System Page.* < http://www.luhs.org > .

Jeanine Barone, Physiologist

Apgar testing

Definition

Apgar testing is the assessment of the newborn rating color, heart rate, stimulus response, muscle tone, and respirations on a scale of zero to two, for a maximum possible score of 10. It is performed twice, first at one minute and then again at five minutes after birth.

Purpose

Apgar scoring was originally developed in the 1950s by the anesthesiologist Virginia Apgar to assist practitioners attending a birth in deciding whether or not a newborn was in need of resuscitation. Using a scoring method fosters consistency and standardization among different practitioners. A February 2001 study published in the *New England Journal of Medicine* investigated whether Apgar scoring continues to be relevant. Researchers concluded that "The Apgar scoring system remains as relevant for the prediction of neonatal survival today as it was almost 50 years ago."

Description

The five areas are scored as follows:

- Appearance, or color: 2 if the skin is pink all over; 1 for **acrocyanosis**, where the trunk and head are pink, but the arms and legs are blue; and 0 if the whole body is blue. Newborns with naturally darker skin color will not be pink. However, pallor is still noticeable, especially in the soles and palms. Color is related to the neonate's ability to oxygenate its body and extremities, and is dependent on heart rate and respirations. A perfectly healthy newborn will often receive a score of 9 because of some blueness in the hands and feet.

- Pulse (heart rate): 2 for a pulse of 100+ beats per minute (bpm); 1 for a pulse below 100 bpm; 0 for no pulse. Heart rate is assessed by listening with a stethoscope to the newborn's heart and counting the number of beats.

- Grimace, or reflex irritability: 2 if the neonate coughs, sneezes, or vigorously cries in response to a stimulus (such as the use of nasal suctioning, stroking the back to assess for spinal abnormalities, or having the foot tapped); 1 for a slight cry or grimace in response to the stimulus; 0 for no response.

- Activity, or muscle tone: 2 for vigorous movements of arms and legs; 1 for some movement; 0 for no movement, limpness.

- Respirations: 2 for visible breathing and crying; 1 for slow, weak, irregular breathing; 0 for apnea, or no breathing. A crying newborn can adequately oxygenate its lungs. Respirations are best assessed by watching the rise and fall of the neonate's abdomen, as infants are diaphragmatic breathers.

The combined first letters in these five areas spell Apgar.

Preparation

No preparation is needed to perform the test. However, while being born the neonate may receive nasal and oral suctioning to remove mucus and amniotic fluid. This may be done when the head of the newborn is safely out, while the mother rests before she continues to push.

Aftercare

Since the test is primarily observational in nature, no aftercare is needed. However, the test may flag the need for immediate intervention or prolonged observation.

Normal results

The maximum possible score is 10, the minimum is zero. It is rare to receive a true 10, as some acrocyanosis in the newborn is considered normal, and therefore not a cause for concern. Most infants score between 7 and 10. These infants are expected to have an excellent outcome. A score of 4, 5, or 6 requires immediate intervention, usually in the form of oxygen and respiratory assistance, or perhaps just suctioning if breathing has been obstructed by mucus. While suctioning is being done, a source of oxygen may be placed near, but not over the newborn's nose and mouth. This form of oxygen is referred to as *blow-by.* A score in the 4-6 range indicates that the neonate is having some difficulty adapting to extrauterine life.

DR. VIRGINIA APGAR (1909–1974)

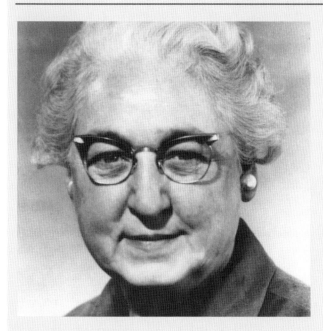

(AP/Wide World Photos. Reproduced by permission.)

As one of very few female medical students at Columbia University College of Physicians and Surgeons in New York during the early 1930s and one of the first women to graduate from its medical school, Apgar knew that her goal of becoming a surgeon would not be achieved easily in a male-dominated profession. Reluctantly, she switched her medical specialty to anesthesiology, she embraced her new field with typical intelligence and energy. At this time, anesthesiology was a relatively new field, having been left by the doctors mostly to the attention of nurses. Apgar realized immediately how much in need of scientifically trained personnel was this significant part of surgery, and she set out to make anesthesiology a separate medical discipline. By 1937, she had become the fiftieth physician to be certified as an anesthesiologist in the United States. The following year she was appointed director of anesthesiology at the Columbia-Presbyterian Medical Center, becoming the first woman to head a department at that institution.

As the attending anesthesiologist who assisted in the delivery of thousands of babies during these years, Apgar realized that infants had died from respiratory or circulatory complications that early treatment could have prevented. Apgar decided to bring her considerable research skills to this childbirth dilemma, and her careful study resulted in her publication of the Apgar Score System in 1952.

KEY TERMS

Acrocyanosis—A slight cyanosis, or blueness of the hands and feet of the neonate is considered normal. This impaired ability to fully oxygenate the extremities is due to an immature circulatory system which is still in flux.

Amniotic fluid—The protective bag of fluid that surrounds the fetus while growing in the uterus.

Neonate—A term referring to the newborn infant, from birth until one month of age.

Neonatologist—A physician who specializes in problems of newborn infants.

Pallor—Extreme paleness in the color of the skin.

This may be due to medications given to the mother during a difficult labor, or at the very end of labor, when these medications have an exaggerated effect on the neonate.

Abnormal results

With a score of 0-3, the newborn is unresponsive, apneic, pale, limp and may not have a pulse. Interventions to resuscitate will begin immediately. The test is repeated at five minutes after birth and both scores are documented. Should the resuscitation effort continue into the five-minute time period, interventions will not stop in order to perform the test. The one-minute score indicates the need for intervention at birth. It addresses survival and prevention of birth-related complications resulting from inadequate oxygen supply. Poor oxygenation may be due to inadequate neurological and/or chemical control of respiration. The five-minute score appears to have a more predictive value for morbidity and normal development, although research studies on this are inconsistent in their conclusions.

Resources

BOOKS

Feinbloom, Richard I. *Pregnancy, Birth and the EarlyMonths.* Cambridge, MA: Perseus Publishing, 2000.

Pillitteri, Adele. *Maternal & Child Nursing; Care of the Childbearing and Childrearing Family*. 3rd ed. Philadelphia: Lippincott, 1999.

PERIODICALS

Casey, B. M., D. D. McIntire, and K. J. Leveno. "The Continuing Value of Apgar Score for the Assessment of Newborn Infants". *New England Journal of Medicine* 344 (February 15, 2000): 467-71.

OTHER

Apgar, Virginia. *A Proposal for a New Method of Evaluation of the Newborn Infant*. < http://www.apgarfamily.com/ Apgar_Paper.html >.
The National Childbirth Trust. < http:// www.nctpregnancyandbabycare.com >.
Pregnancy Weekly.com < http:// www.pregnancyweekly.com >.

Esther Csapo Rastegari, RN, BSN, EdM

Aphasia

Definition

Aphasia is condition characterized by either partial or total loss of the ability to communicate verbally or using written words. A person with aphasia may have difficulty speaking, reading, writing, recognizing the names of objects, or understanding what other people have said. Aphasia is caused by a brain injury, as may occur during a traumatic accident or when the brain is deprived of oxygen during a **stroke**. It may also be caused by a **brain tumor**, a disease such as Alzheimer's, or an infection, like **encephalitis**. Aphasia may be temporary or permanent. Aphasia does not include speech impediments caused by loss of muscle control.

Description

To understand and use language effectively, an individual draws upon word memory–stored information on what certain words mean, how to put them together, and how and when to use them properly. For a majority of people, these and other language functions are located in the left side (hemisphere) of the brain. Damage to this side of the brain is most commonly linked to the development of aphasia. Interestingly, however, left-handed people appear to have language areas in both the left and right hemispheres of the brain and, as a result, may develop aphasia from damage to either side of the brain.

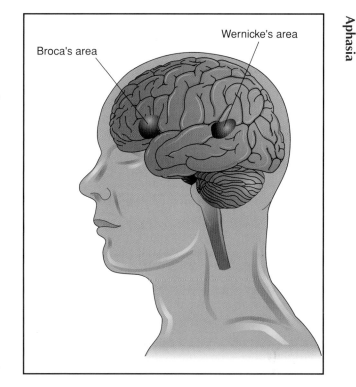

Broca's area

Wernicke's area

Broca's aphasia results from damage to the frontal lobe of the language-dominant area of the brain. Individuals with Broca's aphasia may become mute or may be able to use single-word statements or full sentences, although it may require great effort. Wernicke's aphasia is caused by damage to the temporal lobe of the language-dominant area of the brain. People with this condition speak in long, uninterrupted sentences, but the words used are often unnecessary and unintelligible. *(Illustration by Electronic Illustrators Group.)*

Stroke is the most common cause of aphasia in the United States. Approximately 500,000 individuals suffer strokes each year, and 20% of these individuals develop some type of aphasia. Other causes of brain damage include head injuries, brain tumors, and infection. About half of the people who show signs of aphasia have what is called temporary or transient aphasia and recover completely within a few days. An estimated one million Americans suffer from some form of permanent aphasia. As yet, no connection between aphasia and age, gender, or race has been found.

Aphasia is sometimes confused with other conditions that affect speech, such as dysarthria and **apraxia**. These condition affect the muscles used in speaking rather than language function itself. Dysarthria is a speech disturbance caused by lack of control over the muscles used in speaking, perhaps due to nerve damage. Speech apraxia is a speech disturbance in which language comprehension and muscle control are retained, but the memory of how to use the muscles to form words is not.

KEY TERMS

Anomic aphasia—A condition characterized by either partial or total loss of the ability to recall the names of persons or things as a result of a stroke, head injury, brain tumor, or infection.

Broca's aphasia—A condition characterized by either partial or total loss of the ability to express oneself, either through speech or writing. Hearing comprehension is not affected. This condition may result from a stroke, head injury, brain tumor, or infection.

Computed tomography (CT)—An imaging technique that uses cross-sectional x rays of the body to create a three-dimensional image of the body's internal structures.

Conduction aphasia—A condition characterized by the inability to repeat words, sentences, or phrases as a result of a stroke, head injury, brain tumor, or infection.

Frontal lobe—The largest, most forward-facing part of each side or hemisphere of the brain.

Global aphasia—A condition characterized by either partial or total loss of the ability to communicate verbally or using written words as a result of widespread injury to the language areas of the brain. This condition may be caused by a stroke, head injury, brain tumor, or infection. The exact language abilities affected vary depending on the location and extent of injury.

Hemisphere—One of the two halves or sides-the left and the right-of the brain.

Magnetic resonance imaging (MRI)—An imaging technique that uses a large circular magnet and radio waves to generate signals from atoms in the body. These signals are used to construct images of internal structures.

Subcortical aphasia—A condition characterized by either partial or total loss of the ability to communicate verbally or using written words as a result of damage to non language-dominated areas of the brain. This condition may be caused by a stroke, head injury, brain tumor, or infection.

Temporal lobe—The part of each side or hemisphere of the brain that is on the side of the head, nearest the ears.

Transcortical aphasia—A condition characterized by either partial or total loss of the ability to communicate verbally or using written words that does not affect an individual's ability to repeat words, phrases, and sentences.

Wernicke's aphasia—A condition characterized by either partial or total loss of the ability to understand what is being said or read. The individual maintains the ability to speak, but speech may contain unnecessary or made-up words.

Causes and symptoms

Aphasia can develop after an individual sustains a brain injury from a stroke, head trauma, tumor, or infection, such as herpes encephalitis. As a result of this injury, the pathways for language comprehension or production are disrupted or destroyed. For most people, this means damage to the left hemisphere of the brain. (In 95 to 99% of right-handed people, language centers are in the left hemisphere, and up to 70% of left-handed people also have left-hemisphere language dominance.) According to the traditional classification scheme, each form of aphasia is caused by damage to a different part of the left hemisphere of the brain. This damage affects one or more of the basic language functions: speech, naming (the ability to identify an object, color, or other item with an appropriate word or term), repetition (the ability to repeat words, phrases, and sentences), hearing comprehension (the ability to

understand spoken language), reading (the ability to understand written words and their meaning), and writing (the ability to communicate and record events with text).

The traditional classification scheme includes eight types of aphasia:

- Broca's aphasia, also called motor aphasia, results from damage to the front portion or frontal lobe of the language-dominant area of the brain. Individuals with Broca's aphasia may be completely unable to use speech (**mutism**) or may be able to use single-word statements or even full sentences, though these sentences may require a great deal of effort to construct. Small words, such as conjunctions (and, or, but) and articles (the, an, a), may be omitted, leading to a "telegraph" quality in their speech. Hearing comprehension is usually not affected, so they are able to understand other people's speech and conversation and can follow commands. Often, they may experience weakness on the right side of their bodies, which can make it difficult to write. Reading ability is impaired, and they may have difficulty finding the right word when speaking. Individuals with Broca's aphasia may become frustrated and depressed because they are aware of their language difficulties.

• Wernicke's aphasia is caused by damage to the side portion or temporal lobe of the language-dominant area of the brain. Individuals with Wernicke's aphasia speak in long, uninterrupted sentences; however, the words used are frequently unnecessary or even made-up. They have a great deal of difficulty understanding other people's speech, sometimes to the point of being unable to understand spoken language at all. Reading ability is diminished, and although writing ability is retained, what is written may be abnormal. No physical symptoms, such as the right-sided weakness seen with Broca's aphasia, are typically observed. Also, in contrast to Broca's aphasia, individuals with Wernicke's aphasia are not aware of their language errors.

• Global aphasia is caused by widespread damage to the language areas of the left hemisphere. As a result, all basic language functions are affected, but some areas may be more affected than others. For example, an individual may have difficulty speaking but may be able to write well. The individual may experience weakness and loss of feeling on the right side of their body.

• Conduction aphasia, also called associative aphasia, is rather uncommon. Individuals with conduction aphasia are unable to repeat words, sentences, and phrases. Speech is fairly unbroken, although individuals may frequently correct themselves and words may be skipped or repeated. Although able to understand spoken language, it may also be difficult for the individual with conduction aphasia to find the right word to describe a person or object. The impact of this condition on reading and writing ability varies. As with other types of aphasia, right-sided weakness or sensory loss may be present.

• Anomic or nominal aphasia primarily influences an individual's ability to find the right name for a person or object. As a result, an object may be described rather than named. Hearing comprehension, repetition, reading, and writing are not affected, other than by this inability to find the right name. Speech is fluent, except for pauses as the individual tries to recall the right name. Physical symptoms are variable, and some individuals have no symptoms of one-sided weakness or sensory loss.

• Transcortical aphasia is caused by damage to the language areas of the left hemisphere outside the primary language areas. There are three types of aphasia: transcortical motor aphasia, transcortical sensory aphasia, and mixed transcortical aphasia. All of the transcortical aphasias are distinguished from other types by the individual's ability to repeat words, phrases, or sentences. Other language functions may also be impaired to varying degrees, depending on the extent and particular location of brain damage.

As researchers continue to learn more about the brain's structure and function, new types of aphasia are being recognized. One newly recognized type of aphasia, subcortical aphasia, mimics the symptoms of other traditional types of aphasia but involves language disorders that are not typical. This type of aphasia is associated with injuries to areas of the brain typically not identified with language and language processing.

Diagnosis

Following brain injury, an initial bedside assessment is made to determine whether language function has been affected. If the individual experiences difficulty communicating, attempts are made to determine whether this difficulty arises from impaired language comprehension or an impaired ability to speak. A typical examination involves listening to spontaneous speech and evaluating the individual's ability to recognize and name objects, comprehend what is heard, and repeat sample words and phrases. The individual may also be asked to read text aloud and explain what the passage means. In addition, writing ability is evaluated by having the individual copy text, transcribe dictated text, and write something without prompting.

A speech pathologist or neuropsychologist may be asked to conduct more extensive examinations using in-depth, standardized tests. Commonly used tests include the Boston Diagnostic Aphasia Examination, the Western Aphasia Battery, and possibly, the Porch Index of Speech Ability.

The results of these tests indicate the severity of the aphasia and may also provide information regarding the exact location of the brain damage. This more extensive testing is also designed to provide the information necessary to design an individualized speech therapy program. Further information about the location of the damage is gained through the use of imaging technology, such as **magnetic resonance imaging** (MRI) and **computed tomography scans** (CT).

Treatment

Initially, the underlying cause of aphasia must be treated or stabilized. To regain language function, therapy must begin as soon as possible following the injury. Although there are no medical or surgical procedures currently available to treat this condition, aphasia resulting from stroke or **head injury** may improve through the use of speech therapy. For most individuals, however, the primary emphasis is placed on making the most of retained language abilities and learning to use other means of communication to compensate for lost language abilities.

Speech therapy is tailored to meet individual needs, but activities and tools that are frequently used include the following:

- **Exercise** and practice. Weakened muscles are exercised by repetitively speaking certain words or making facial expressions, such as smiling.

- Picture cards. Pictures of everyday objects are used to improve word recall and increase vocabulary. The names of the objects may also be repetitively spoken aloud as part of an exercise and practice routine.

- Picture boards. Pictures of everyday objects and activities are placed together, and the individual points to certain pictures to convey ideas and communicate with others.

- Workbooks. Reading and writing exercises are used to sharpen word recall and regain reading and writing abilities. Hearing comprehension is also redeveloped using these exercises.

- Computers. Computer software can be used to improve speech, reading, recall, and hearing comprehension by, for example, displaying pictures and having the individual find the right word.

Prognosis

The degree to which an individual can recover language abilities is highly dependent on how much brain damage occurred and the location and cause of the original brain injury. Other factors include the individual's age, general health, motivation and willingness to participate in speech therapy, and whether the individual is left or right handed. Language areas may be located in both the left and right hemispheres in left-handed individuals. Left-handed individuals are, therefore, more likely to develop aphasia following brain injury, but because they have two language centers, may recover more fully because language abilities can be recovered from either side of the brain. The intensity of therapy and the time between diagnosis and the start of therapy may also affect the eventual outcome.

Prevention

Because there is no way of knowing when a stroke, traumatic head injury, or disease will occur, very little can be done to prevent aphasia. The extent of recovery, however, in some cases, can be affected by an individual's willingness to cooperate and participate in speech therapy directly following the injury.

Resources

BOOKS

Lyon, Jon G., and Marianne B. Simpson. *Coping with Aphasia.* San Diego: Singular Publishing Group, 1998.

ORGANIZATIONS

National Aphasia Association. 156 5th Ave., Suite 707, New York, NY 10010. (800) 922-4622. < http:// www.aphasia.org > .

Julia Barrett

Apheres *see* **Transfusion**

Aplastic anemia

Definition

Aplastic anemia is a disorder in which the bone marrow greatly decreases or stops production of blood cells.

Description

The bone marrow (soft tissue that is located within the hard outer shell of the bones) is responsible for the production of all types of blood cells. The mature forms of these cells include red blood cells, which carry oxygen throughout the body; white blood cells, which fight infection; and platelets, which are involved in clotting. In aplastic anemia, the basic structure of the marrow becomes abnormal, and those cells responsible for generating blood cells (hematopoietic cells) are greatly decreased in number or absent. These hematopoietic cells are replaced by large quantities of fat.

Yearly, aplastic anemia strikes about 5-10 people in every one million. Although aplastic anemia strikes both males and females of all ages, there are two age groups that have an increased risk. Both young adults

KEY TERMS

Bone marrow—A substance found in the cavities of bones, especially the long bones and the sternum (breast bone). The bone marrow contains those cells that are responsible for the production of the blood cells (red blood cells, white blood cells, and platelets).

Bone marrow transplant—A procedure in which a quantity of bone marrow is extracted through a needle from a donor, and then passed into a patient to replace the patient's diseased or absent bone marrow.

Hematopoietic cells—Those cells that are lodged within the bone marrow, and which are responsible for producing the cells which circulate in the blood (red blood cells, white blood cells, and platelets).

(between 15-30 years of age) and the elderly (over the age of 60) have higher rates of aplastic anemia than the general population. While the disorder occurs worldwide, young adults in Asia have a higher disease rate than do populations in North America and Europe.

Causes and symptoms

Aplastic anemia falls into three basic categories, based on the origin of its cause: idiopathic, acquired, and hereditary.

In about 60% of cases, aplastic anemia is considered to be idiopathic, meaning that the cause of the disorder is unknown.

Acquired aplastic anemia refers to those cases where certain environmental factors and physical conditions seem to be associated with development of the disease. Acquired aplastic anemia can be associated with:

- exposure to drugs, especially anti-cancer agents, **antibiotics**, anti-inflammatory agents, seizure medications, and antithyroid drugs (drugs given to stop the functioning of an overactive thyroid)

- exposure to radiation

- chemical exposure (especially to the organic solvent benzene and certain insecticides)

- infection with certain viruses (especially those causing viral hepatitis, as well as Epstein-Barr virus, parvovirus, and HIV, the virus that can cause **AIDS**)

- pregnancy

- certain other disorders, including a disease called paroxysmal nocturnal hemoglobinuria, an autoimmune

reaction called graft-vs-host disease (which occurs when the body's immune system attacks and destroys the body's own cells), and certain connective tissue diseases

Hereditary aplastic anemia is relatively rare, but occurs in Fanconi's anemia, Shwachman-Diamond syndrome, and dyskeratosis congenita.

Symptoms of aplastic anemia tend to be those of other **anemias**, including **fatigue**, weakness, tiny reddish-purple marks (petechiae) on the skin (evidence of pinpoint hemorrhages into the skin), evidence of abnormal bruising, and bleeding from the gums, nose, intestine, or vagina. The patient is likely to appear pale. If the anemia progresses, decreased oxygen circulating in the blood may lead to an increase in heart rate and the sudden appearance of a new heart murmur.

Diagnosis

The **blood count** in aplastic anemia will reveal low numbers of all formed blood cells. Red blood cells will appear normal in size and coloration, but greatly decreased in number. Cells called reticulocytes (very young red blood cells, which are usually produced in great numbers by the bone marrow in order to compensate for a severe anemia) will be very low in number. Platelets and white blood cells will also be decreased in number, though normal in structure.

A sample of the patient's bone marrow will need to be removed by needle (usually from the hip bone) and examined under a microscope. If aplastic anemia is present, this examination will reveal very few or no hematopoietic cells, and replacement with fat.

Treatment

The first step in the treatment of aplastic anemia involves discontinuing exposure to any substance that may be causing the disorder. Although it would seem that blood transfusions would be helpful in this disease, in fact, they only serve as a temporary help, and may complicate future attempts at **bone marrow transplantation**.

The most successful treatment for aplastic anemia is bone marrow transplantation. To do this, a marrow donor (often a sibling) must be identified. There are a number of tissue markers that must be examined to determine whether a bone marrow donation is likely to be compatible with the patient's immune system. Compatibility is necessary to avoid complications, including the destruction of the donor marrow by the patient's own immune system.

Patients who cannot undergo bone marrow transplant can be treated with a number of agents, including antithymocyte globulin (ATG), cyclophosphamide, steroids, and cyclosporine. These agents all have the potential to cause a number of troublesome side-effects and may have a success rate of only 60% to 80%. Still, even among those patients who have a good response, many later suffer a relapse (return) of aplastic anemia. Researchers are trying to identify the molecules in certain stem cells that the immune system targets in aplastic anemia.

Prognosis

Aplastic anemia is a life-threatening illness. Without treatment, it will almost surely progress to **death**. Survival depends on how severe the disease is at diagnosis, which type of treatment a patient is eligible for, and what kind of response their body has to that treatment. The worst-prognosis type of aplastic anemia is one associated with very low numbers of a particular type of white blood cell. These patients have a high chance of dying from overwhelming bacterial infections. In fact, 80% of all patients treated with blood transfusions alone die within 18 months to two years. Patients who undergo bone marrow transplantation have a 60-90% chance of being cured of the disease.

Resources

PERIODICALS

Marsh, Judith C.W., Edward C. Gordon-Smith. "Insights Into the Autoimmune Nature of Aplastic Anemia." *The Lancet* (July 24, 2004): 308.

ORGANIZATIONS

Aplastic Anemia Foundation of America. P.O. Box 613, Annapolis, MD 21404. (800) 747-2820. < http:// www.aplastic.org > .

Rosalyn Carson-DeWitt, MD
Teresa G. Odle

Aplastic crisis *see* **Fifth disease**

Appendectomy

Definition

Appendectomy is the surgical removal of the appendix. The appendix is a worm-shaped hollow pouch attached to the cecum, the beginning of the large intestine.

Purpose

Appendectomies are performed to treat **appendicitis**, an inflamed and infected appendix.

Precautions

Since appendicitis occurs most commonly in males between the ages of 10-14 and in females between the ages of 15-19, appendectomy is most often performed during this time. The diagnosis of appendicitis is most difficult in the very young (less than two years of age) and in the elderly.

Description

Appendectomy is considered a major surgical operation. Therefore, a general surgeon must perform this operation in the operating room of a hospital. An anesthesiologist is also present during the operation to administer an anesthetic. Most often the anesthesiologist uses a general anesthetic technique whereby patients are put to sleep and made **pain** free by administering drugs in the vein or by agents inhaled through a tube placed in the windpipe. Occasionally a spinal anesthetic may be used.

After the patient is anesthetized, the general surgeon can remove the appendix either by using the traditional open procedure (in which a 2-3 in [5-7.6 cm] incision is made in the abdomen) or via **laparoscopy** (in which four 1 in [2.5cm] incisions are made in the abdomen).

Traditional open appendectomy

When the surgeon uses the open approach, he makes an incision in the lower right section of the abdomen. Most incisions are less than 3 in (7.6 cm) in length. The surgeon then identifies all of the organs in the abdomen and examines them for other disease or abnormalities. The appendix is located and brought up into the **wounds**. The surgeon separates the appendix from all the surrounding tissue and its attachment to the cecum and then removes it. The site where the appendix was previously attached, the cecum, is closed and returned to the abdomen. The muscle layers and then the skin are sewn together.

Laproscopic appendectomy

When the surgeon conducts a laproscopic appendectomy, four incisions, each about 1 in (2.5 cm) in length, are made. One incision is near the umbilicus, or navel, and one is between the umbilicus and the pubis. Two other incisions are smaller and are in the right

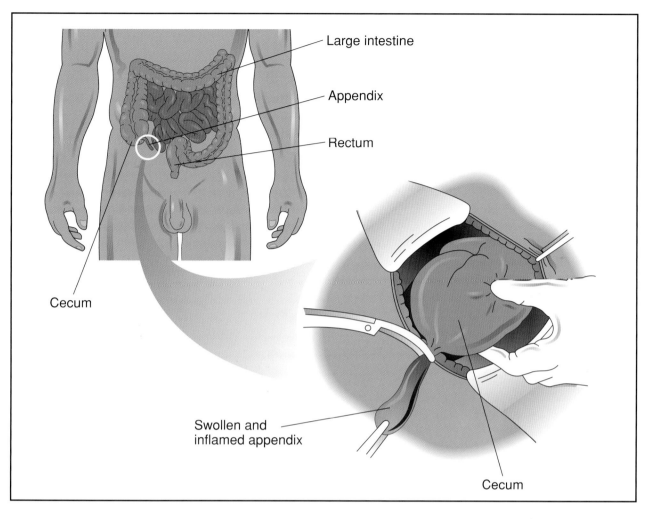

A traditional open appendectomy. After the surgeon makes an incision in the lower right section of the abdomen, he/she pulls the appendix up, separates it from the surrounding tissue and its attachment to the cecum, and then removes it. *(Illustration by Electronic Illustrators Group.)*

side of the lower abdomen. The surgeon then passes a camera and special instruments through these incisions. With the aid of this equipment, the surgeon visually examines the abdominal organs and identifies the appendix. Similarly, the appendix is freed from all of its attachments and removed. The place where the appendix was formerly attached, the cecum, is stitched. The appendix is removed through one of the incisions. The instruments are removed and then all of the incisions are closed.

Studies and opinions about the relative advantages and disadvantages of each method are divided. A skilled surgeon can perform either one of these procedures in less than one hour. However, laproscopic appendectomy (LA) always takes longer than traditional appendectomy (TA). The increased time required to do a LA increases the patient's exposure to anesthetics, which increases the risk of complications. The increased time requirement also escalates fees charged by the hospital for operating room time and by the anesthesiologist. Since LA also requires specialized equipment, the fees for its use also increases the hospital charges. Patients with either operation have similar pain medication needs, begin eating **diets** at comparable times, and stay in the hospital equivalent amounts of time. LA is of special benefit in women in whom the diagnosis is difficult and gynecological disease (such as **endometriosis**, pelvic inflammatory disease, ruptured ovarian follicles, ruptured ovarian cysts, and tubal pregnancies) may be the source of pain and not appendicitis. If LA is done in these patients, the pelvic organs can be more thoroughly examined and a definitive diagnosis made prior to removal of the appendix. Most surgeons select

KEY TERMS

Abscess—A collection of pus buried deep in the tissues or in a body cavity.

Anesthesiologist—A physician who has special training and expertise in the delivery of anesthetics.

Anesthetics—Drugs or methodologies used to make a body area free of sensation or pain.

Cecum—The beginning of the large intestine and the place where the appendix attaches to the intestinal tract.

General surgeon—A physician who has special training and expertise in performing a variety of operations.

Pelvic organs— The organs inside of the body that are located within the confines of the pelvis. This includes the bladder and rectum in both sexes and the uterus, ovaries, and fallopian tubes in females.

Pubis—The anterior portion of the pelvis located in the anterior abdomen.

Thrombophlebitis—Inflammation of the veins, usually in the legs, which causes swelling and tenderness in the affected area.

Umbilicus—The navel.

either TA or LA based on the individual needs and circumstances of the patient.

Insurance plans do cover the costs of appendectomy. Fees are charged independently by the hospital and the physicians. Hospital charges include fees for operating and recovery room use, diagnostic and laboratory testing, as well as the normal hospital room charges. Surgical fees vary from region to region and range between $250-$750. The anesthesiologist's fee depends upon the health of the patient and the length of the operation.

Preparation

Once the diagnosis of appendicitis is made and the decision has been made to perform an appendectomy, the patient undergoes the standard preparation for an operation. This usually takes only one to two hours and includes signing the operative consents, patient identification procedures, evaluation by the anesthesiologist, and moving the patient to the operating suites of the hospital. Occasionally, if the patient has been ill for a prolonged period of time or has had protracted

vomiting, a delay of few to several hours may be necessary to give the patient fluids and antibiotics.

Aftercare

Recovery from an appendectomy is similar to other operations. Patients are allowed to eat when the stomach and intestines begin to function again. Usually the first meal is a clear liquid diet–broth, juice, soda pop, and gelatin. If patients tolerate this meal, the next meal usually is a regular diet. Patients are asked to walk and resume their normal physical activities as soon as possible. If TA was done, work and physical education classes may be restricted for a full three weeks after the operation. If a LA was done, most patients are able to return to work and strenuous activity within one to three weeks after the operation.

Risks

Certain risks are present when any operation requires a general anesthetic and the abdominal cavity is opened. **Pneumonia** and collapse of the small airways (**atelectasis**) often occurs. Patients who smoke are at a greater risk for developing these complications. Thrombophlebitis, or inflammation of the veins, is rare but can occur if the patient requires prolonged bed rest. Bleeding can occur but rarely is a blood **transfusion** required. Adhesions (abnormal connections to abdominal organs by thin fibrous tissue) is a known complication of any abdominal procedure such as appendectomy. These **adhesions** can lead to intestinal obstruction which prevents the normal flow of intestinal contents. **Hernia** is a complication of any incision, However, they are rarely seen after appendectomy because the abdominal wall is very strong in the area of the standard appendectomy incision.

The overall complication rate of appendectomy depends upon the status of the appendix at the time it is removed. If the appendix has not ruptured the complication rate is only about 3%. However, if the appendix has ruptured the complication rate rises to almost 59%. Wound infections do occur and are more common if the appendicitis was severe, far advanced, or ruptured. An **abscess** may form in the abdomen as a complication of appendicitis.

Occasionally, an appendix will rupture prior to its removal, spilling its contents into the abdominal cavity. **Peritonitis** or a generalized infection in the abdomen will occur. Treatment of peritonitis as a result of a ruptured appendix includes removal of what remains of the appendix, insertion of drains (rubber tubes that promote the flow of infection inside the abdomen to outside of the body), and **antibiotics**. **Fistula** formation (an abnormal connection between the cecum and the skin) rarely occurs. It is only seen if the appendix has a broad attachment to the cecum and the appendicitis is far advanced causing destruction of the cecum itself.

Normal results

Most patients feel better immediately after an operation for appendicitis. Many patients are discharged from the hospital within 24 hours after the appendectomy. Others may require a longer stay–three to five days. Almost all patients are back to their normal activities within three weeks.

The mortality rate of appendicitis has dramatically decreased over time. Currently, the mortality rate is estimated at one to two per 1,000,000 cases of appendicitis. **Death** is usually due to peritonitis, intra abdominal abscess or severe infection following rupture.

The complications associated with undiagnosed, misdiagnosised, or delayed diagnosis of appendectomy are very significant. The diagnosis is of appendicitis is difficult and never certain. This has led surgeons to perform an appendectomy any time that they feel appendicitis is the diagnosis. Most surgeons feel that in approximately 20% of their patients, a normal appendix will be removed. Rates much lower than this would seem to indicate that the diagnosis of appendicitis was being frequently missed.

Resources

PERIODICALS

McCall, J. L., K. Sharples, and F. Jafallah. "Systematic Review of Randomized Controlled Trial Comparing Laproscopic with Open Appendectomy." *British Journal of Surgery* 84, no. 8 (August 1997): 1045-1950.

OTHER

"Appendectomy." ThriveOnline. < http://thriveonline.oxygen.com > .

"The Appendix." Mayo Clinic Online. < http://www.mayohealth.org > .

Mary Jeanne Krob, MD, FACS

▌Appendicitis

Definition

Appendicitis is an inflammation of the appendix, which is the worm-shaped pouch attached to the

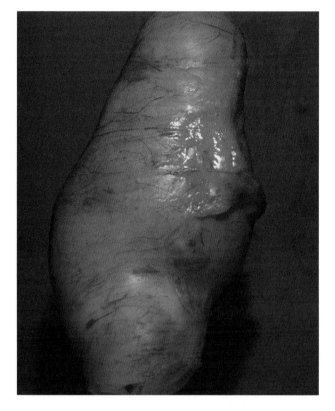

An extracted appendix. *(Photograph by Lester V. Bergman, Corbis Images. Reproduced by permission.)*

cecum, the beginning of the large intestine. The appendix has no known function in the body, but it can become diseased. Appendicitis is a medical emergency, and if it is left untreated the appendix may rupture and cause a potentially fatal infection.

Description

Appendicitis is the most common abdominal emergency found in children and young adults. One person in 15 develops appendicitis in his or her lifetime. The incidence is highest among males aged 10-14, and among females aged 15-19. More males than females develop appendicitis between **puberty** and age 25. It is rare in the elderly and in children under the age of two.

The hallmark symptom of appendicitis is increasingly severe abdominal **pain**. Since many different conditions can cause abdominal pain, an accurate diagnosis of appendicitis can be difficult. A timely diagnosis is important, however, because a delay can result in perforation, or rupture, of the appendix. When this happens, the infected contents of the appendix spill into the abdomen, potentially causing a serious infection of the abdomen called **peritonitis**.

KEY TERMS

Appendectomy (or appendicectomy)—Surgical removal of the appendix.

Appendix—The worm-shaped pouch attached to the cecum, the beginning of the large intestine.

Laparotomy—Surgical incision into the loin, between the ribs and the pelvis, which offers surgeons a view inside the abdominal cavity.

Peritonitis—Inflammation of the peritoneum, membranes lining the abdominal pelvic wall.

Other conditions can have similar symptoms, especially in women. These include pelvic inflammatory disease, ruptured ovarian follicles, ruptured ovarian cysts, tubal pregnancies, and **endometriosis**. Various forms of stomach upset and bowel inflammation may also mimic appendicitis.

The treatment for acute (sudden, severe) appendicitis is an **appendectomy**, surgery to remove the appendix. Because of the potential for a life-threatening ruptured appendix, persons suspected of having appendicitis are often taken to surgery before the diagnosis is certain.

Causes and symptoms

The causes of appendicitis are not well understood, but it is believed to occur as a result of one or more of these factors: an obstruction within the appendix, the development of an ulceration (an abnormal change in tissue accompanied by the death of cells) within the appendix, and the invasion of bacteria.

Under these conditions, bacteria may multiply within the appendix. The appendix may become swollen and filled with pus (a fluid formed in infected tissue, consisting of while blood cells and cellular debris), and may eventually rupture. Signs of rupture include the presence of symptoms for more than 24 hours, a **fever**, a high white blood cell count, and a fast heart rate. Very rarely, the inflammation and symptoms of appendicitis may disappear but recur again later.

The distinguishing symptom of appendicitis is pain beginning around or above the navel. The pain, which may be severe or only achy and uncomfortable, eventually moves into the right lower corner of the abdomen. There, it becomes more steady and more severe, and often increases with movement, coughing,

and so forth. The abdomen often becomes rigid and tender to the touch. Increasing rigidity and tenderness indicates an increased likelihood of perforation and peritonitis.

Loss of appetite is very common. **Nausea and vomiting** may occur in about half of the cases and occasionally there may be **constipation** or **diarrhea**. The temperature may be normal or slightly elevated. The presence of a fever may indicate that the appendix has ruptured.

Diagnosis

A careful examination is the best way to diagnose appendicitis. It is often difficult even for experienced physicians to distinguish the symptoms of appendicitis from those of other abdominal disorders. Therefore, very specific questioning and a thorough physical examination are crucial. The physician should ask questions, such as where the pain is centered, whether the pain has shifted, and where the pain began. The physician should press on the abdomen to judge the location of the pain and the degree of tenderness.

The typical sequence of symptoms is present in about 50% of cases. In the other half of cases, less typical patterns may be seen, especially in pregnant women, older patients, and infants. In pregnant women, appendicitis is easily masked by the frequent occurrence of mild abdominal pain and **nausea** from other causes. Elderly patients may feel less pain and tenderness than most patients, thereby delaying diagnosis and treatment, and leading to rupture in 30% of cases. Infants and young children often have diarrhea, **vomiting**, and fever in addition to pain.

While laboratory tests cannot establish the diagnosis, an increased white cell count may point to appendicitis. **Urinalysis** may help to rule out a urinary tract infection that can mimic appendicitis.

Patients whose symptoms and **physical examination** are compatible with a diagnosis of appendicitis are usually taken immediately to surgery, where a laparotomy (surgical exploration of the abdomen) is done to confirm the diagnosis. In cases with a questionable diagnosis, other tests, such as a computed tomography scan (CT) may be performed to avoid unnecessary surgery. An ultrasound examination of the abdomen may help to identify an inflamed appendix or other condition that would explain the symptoms. Abdominal x-rays are not of much value except when the appendix has ruptured.

Often, the diagnosis is not certain until an operation is done. To avoid a ruptured appendix, surgery may be recommended without delay if the symptoms point clearly to appendicitis. If the symptoms are not clear, surgery may be postponed until they progress enough to confirm a diagnosis.

When appendicitis is strongly suspected in a woman of child-bearing age, a diagnostic laparoscopy (an examination of the interior of the abdomen) is sometimes recommended before the appendectomy in order to be sure that a gynecological problem, such as a ruptured ovarian cyst, is not causing the pain. In this procedure, a lighted viewing tube is inserted into the abdomen through a small incision around the navel.

A normal appendix is discovered in about 10-20% of patients who undergo laparotomy, because of suspected appendicitis. Sometimes the surgeon will remove a normal appendix as a safeguard against appendicitis in the future. During the surgery, another specific cause for the pain and symptoms of appendicitis is found for about 30% of these patients.

Treatment

The treatment of appendicitis is an immediate appendectomy. This may be done by opening the abdomen in the standard open appendectomy technique, or through **laparoscopy**. In laparoscopy, a smaller incision is made through the navel. Both methods can successfully accomplish the removal of the appendix. It is not certain that laparoscopy holds any advantage over open appendectomy. When the appendix has ruptured, patients undergoing a laparoscopic appendectomy may have to be switched to the open appendectomy procedure for the successful management of the rupture. If a ruptured appendix is left untreated, the condition is fatal.

Prognosis

Appendicitis is usually treated successfully by appendectomy. Unless there are complications, the patient should recover without further problems. The mortality rate in cases without complications is less than 0.1%. When an appendix has ruptured, or a severe infection has developed, the likelihood is higher for complications, with slower recovery, or death from disease. There are higher rates of perforation and mortality among children and the elderly.

Prevention

Appendicitis is probably not preventable, although there is some indication that a diet high in green vegetables and tomatoes may help prevent appendicitis.

Resources

PERIODICALS

Van Der Meer, Antonia. "Do You Know the Warning Signs of Appendicitis?" *Parents Magazine* (April 1997): 49.

Caroline A. Helwick

Appendix removal *see* **Appendectomy**

Appetite-enhancing drugs

Definition

Appetite-enhancing drugs are a diverse group of medications given to prevent undesired weight loss in the elderly and in patients suffering from such diseases as **AIDS** and **cancer**, which often result in wasting of the body's muscle tissue as well as overall weight loss. The medical term for these drugs is orexigenic, which is derived from the Greek word for "appetite" or "desire." None of the orexigenic drugs in common use as of 2005, however, were originally formulated or prescribed as appetite stimulants; they range from **antihistamines** and antiemetics (drugs given to treat or prevent **nausea and vomiting**) to antidepressants and synthetic hormones. The medications most often used in the early 2000s include mirtazapine (Remeron), a tetracyclic antidepressant; cyproheptadine (Periactin), an antihistamine; dronabinol (Marinol, THC), an antiemetic; nandrolone, oxymetholone, and oxandrolone (Anadrol-50, Durabolin, Hybolin, Oxandrin, and other brand nam! es), which are anabolic steroids related to the male sex hormone testosterone; and megestrol acetate (Megace), a synthetic derivative of the female sex hormone progesterone. In addition to these prescription drugs, fish oil (eicosapentaenoic acid or EPA) has been recommended as an alternative or complementary treatment for undesired weight loss.

Purpose

The reader should note the distinction between appetite and hunger in order to understand why a group of such different medications could be used to stimulate the desire for food. Hunger is defined as the body's basic physical need for food, whether in terms of calorie content or specific nutrients. Appetite, on the other hand, refers to the complex desires in humans for food and drink that are often conditioned or influenced by previous experiences or cultural factors as well as by a person's present health status.

People may have an appetite for food in the absence of hunger; conversely, they may be hungry in the physical sense but have little or no appetite. Loss of appetite may lead to a type of **malnutrition** known as undernutrition, which is characterized by food intake that falls below a recommended daily allowance of calories or by the body's inability to make use of the nutrients in the food that is consumed.

People may become anorexic (lose their appetite for food) for a variety of physical, emotional, and social reasons:

- Sensory changes related to **aging**. Elderly persons often experience a partial loss of the senses of taste and smell, which means that they may not enjoy their meals as much as they did when they were younger. In addition, many elderly persons feel full after eating relatively small amounts of food. It is thought that this early feeling of fullness is caused by increased secretion of gastric hormones known as cholecystokinins.

- Gastrointestinal disorders. Patients with such disorders as Crohn's disease or gastric atonia (abnormally slow emptying of the stomach) may lose their appetite for food.

- Severe diseases that affect the entire body, particularly cancer and AIDS. Patients with these diseases may develop cachexia, a potentially life-threatening condition characterized by unintended weight loss and wasting of lean muscle tissue. Cachexia is often accompanied by loss of appetite.

- Medication side effects. In addition to the drugs used in cancer **chemotherapy**, such drugs as fluoxetine (Prozac), digoxin (Lanoxin), quinidine (Duraquin, Cardioquin), hydralazine (Alazine, Apresoline), certain **antibiotics**, and vitamin A may cause loss of appetite.

- Emotional **stress**. Many people do not feel like eating before examinations, job interviews, public speaking, artistic performances, athletic competitions, or similar stressful situations.

- Depression and other **mood disorders**. Loss of appetite is a common feature of depressive episodes as well as of major depressive disorder.

- Cultural factors. The types of food that people find appetizing are influenced by their respective cultures; for example, Westerners usually find the use of cats and dogs for food in China and Korea upsetting or disgusting because they regard these animals as domestic pets rather than dietary items. In addition, many people lose their appetite when they discover insects, hair, or other evidence of unsanitary conditions in their food, or when they find that a dish's ingredients violate the dietary laws of their religion.

- Social isolation. Research indicates that human appetite for food is stimulated by eating in the company of others. Loss of appetite in many elderly people is associated with living alone.

- Previous experience. People who have developed **food poisoning** after eating contaminated or improperly refrigerated salads, raw clams or oysters, or similar foods may develop a long-term distaste for the food that made them sick.

Given the complexity and variety of factors that influence the desire for food in humans, doctors often use such questionnaires as the Mini Nutritional Assessment or the **Nutrition** Screening Index before prescribing any appetite-enhancing drug. Many patients can be successfully treated by changes in the type or dosage of medications they are taking for other conditions, or by therapy directed at an underlying mood disorder or gastrointestinal disease. Others can be helped by changes in their living situations that allow them to share mealtimes with others or by assistance in preparing foods that they particularly enjoy. The American Academy of Home Care Physicians (AAHCP) noted in a report published in May 2004 that the use of orexigenic drugs in the elderly is "controversial and not generally FDA-approved."

Description

Orexigenic drugs used in the United States as of 2005 are classified as follows:

- Mirtazapine. Mirtazapine is a tetracyclic antidepressant that was approved by the Food and Drug Administration (FDA) in 1996 for the treatment of major depression. Although researchers do not fully understand why mirtazapine relieves mood disorders, they think that it increases the levels of noradrenaline and serotonin (chemicals that transmit nerve impulses across the gaps between cells) in the brain. Mirtazapine is most often prescribed as an appetite stimulant for patients who have been previously diagnosed with depression.

- Cyproheptadine. Cyproheptadine is an antihistamine given to relieve the symptoms of colds, nasal **allergies**, and hay **fever**. It is also prescribed to relieve the **itching** associated with insect **bites and stings**, poison ivy, and poison oak. It appears to be most effective in treating loss of appetite in children and adults diagnosed with cystic fibrosis.

KEY TERMS

Anabolic steroids—A group of drugs derived from the male sex hormone testosterone, most commonly prescribed to promote growth or to help the body repair tissues weakened by severe illness or aging. Some anabolic steroids are given as appetite stimulants.

Anorexia—Loss of appetite for food.

Antiemetic—A type of medication given to relieve or prevent nausea and vomiting. Some appetite-enhancing drugs are also used as antiemetics.

Appetite—The natural instinctive desire for food. It should be distinguished from hunger, which is the body's craving or need for food (either calories or specific nutrients).

Cachexia—A condition of general ill health, malnutrition, undesired weight loss, and physical weakness, often associated with cancer.

Off-label—Referring to the use of a drug for a condition or disorder not listed in the official FDA labeling.

Orexigenic—The medical term for drugs that increase or stimulate the appetite.

Palliative—Referring to drugs or other therapies intended to relieve the symptoms of a disease rather than to cure it.

Undernutrition—A type of malnutrition caused by inadequate food intake or the body's inability to make use of needed nutrients.

• Dronabinol. Dronabinol is a synthetic version of tetrahydrocannabinol (THC), the mood-altering compound found in **marijuana** (*Cannabis sativa*). Marijuana has been known as an appetite stimulant for centuries, having been recommended for that purpose by Ayurvedic practitioners and by the Arabic physician Al Badri, who first described its orexigenic properties in 1251. Dronabinol is most commonly used to treat the **nausea** and **vomiting** associated with AIDS and with cancer chemotherapy.

• Anabolic steroids. These drugs are given to older persons to increase muscle mass and strength, or to help patients recovering from severe illness or injury to regain lost weight.

• Megestrol acetate. Megestrol acetate was first approved by the FDA in 1976 for palliative treatment of metastatic breast or **endometrial cancer**. It received additional approval in 1993 for the

treatment of anorexia or unexplained weight loss in patients with AIDS. Researchers do not fully understand how the drug prevents the growth of cancer cells or how it stimulates appetite.

• Fish oil. Fish oil is recommended by some practitioners as a nutritional supplement for weight loss caused by cancer or AIDS. It is thought that the **omega-3 fatty acids** in fish oil help to reduce the inflammation associated with some forms of cancer therapy as well as helping patients regain lost weight. Although some studies question the effectiveness of fish oil as a complementary treatment for undesired weight loss, the National Center for Complementary and Alternative Medicine (NCCAM) is recruiting patients as of April 2005 for a clinical trial of fish oil as a dietary supplement to maintain weight in patients with pancreatic cancer. The study will be completed in September 2007.

Recommended dosage

Recommended dosages for orexigenic drugs are as follows:

• Mirtazapine. Mirtazapine is available in 15- and 30-mg tablets or disintegrating tablets. The usual starting dose is 15 mg once daily, usually at bedtime. The drug can be taken with or without food, as the patient prefers.

• Cyproheptadine. Cyproheptadine is taken by mouth, either as tablets or in liquid form. Adults are usually given 4 mg three or four times per day. Children between 2 and 6 years of age are usually given 12 mg per day in 3–4 divided doses while older children are given 16 mg per day in divided doses.

• Dronabinol. As an appetite stimulant, dronabinol is given as a 2.5-mg capsule twice a day, before lunch and dinner. Some AIDS patients may be given as much as 10 mg per day.

• Anabolic steroids. Oxandrolone and oxymetholone are available in the United States and Canada as tablets, while nandrolone is given by injection. To build up body tissues after injury or serious illness, the adult dosage of oxandrolone is a 2.5-mg tablet taken by mouth two to four times daily for a period of four weeks, although the total daily dosage may be raised as high as 20 mg. To treat anemia, oxymetholone is prescribed according to the patient's body weight, usually 0.45–2.3 mg per pound of body weight per day in adults and children. Nandrolone is given by injection every three to four weeks for a period of 12 weeks. The usual dosage for women and girls over 14 is 50–100 mg; for men and boys over 14,

50–200 mg; for children between the ages of 2 and 13, 15–50 mg.

- Megestrol acetate. Megestrol acetate is given as a liquid suspension in 200-mg doses every 6 hours.

- Fish oil. A recommended dose for cancer-induced weight loss is 12 g daily, taken by mouth. Fish oil is available in capsules as well as liquid forms.

Precautions

Precautions for orexigenic drugs are as follows:

- Mirtazapine. In January 2005 the FDA required labeling changes for mirtazapine to warn of the increased risk of **suicide** or self-harm in children or adolescents taking this drug. Mirtazapine should not be given to children below 18 years of age, and should be used with caution in pregnant or lactating women. Patients taking mirtazapine should not stop taking it without telling their doctor; it should not be discontinued abruptly but taken in progressively smaller doses over a period of time. This precaution is particularly important in patients who have been taking the drug for a long time.

- Cyproheptadine. This drug should not be given to patients who suffer acute **asthma** attacks or are hypersensitive to antihistamines. It should not be given to patients who have taken phenelzine (Nardil), tranylcypromine (Parnate), or other MAO inhibitors within the last two weeks. Cyproheptadine should be used cautiously in the elderly and in patients with **glaucoma**, high blood pressure, or cardiovascular disease.

- Dronabinol. Patients taking dronabinol should be closely supervised by their doctor, as the drug may cause unpredictable changes in blood pressure and heart rate. In addition, it may make certain mental disorders worse. It also has a high potential for **abuse**; for this reason, it should be used cautiously in patients with a history of alcohol or drug abuse. Dronabinol should not be used by nursing mothers because it passes into breast milk. It should be used with great caution in children or patients diagnosed with severe mental illness because of its effects on the mind. Patients taking dronabinol should notify their dentist or surgeon before any procedure requiring local or **general anesthesia**, as the drug may intensify the effects of the anesthetic. In addition, these patients should not drive a car or operate dangerous machinery until they know whether dronabinol makes them dizzy, drowsy, or uncoordinated.

- Anabolic steroids. Patients taking these drugs must follow a diet high in protein and calories in order to benefit from the medications, and should be carefully supervised by their doctor because of possible side effects. Children or teenagers taking these drugs should have x-rays every six months to make sure they are growing normally, as anabolic steroids can interfere with growth. Patients with diabetes should check their blood sugar levels with extra care, as these drugs may cause rapid changes in blood sugar levels.

- Megestrol acetate. This drug should not be used by pregnant or lactating women, or by women planning to become pregnant. Women of childbearing age who are taking megestrol should use a reliable form of contraception.

- Fish oil. Fish oil is not a prescription drug; however, patients who choose to take cod liver oil as their fish oil supplement should make sure that they are not getting more than the safe maximum daily allowances of **vitamins** A and D. These vitamins tend to build up in the body and may reach toxic levels. The maximum safe daily level of vitamin A for adults is 3000 micrograms (mcg).

Side effects

Side effects reported for orexigenic drugs are as follows:

- Mirtazapine. Mirtazapine may cause mood changes, including worsening depression or thoughts of suicide. It may also cause panic attacks, irritability, difficulty with impulse control, abnormal levels of excitement, or difficulty sleeping. Physical side effects may include sleepiness, **dry mouth**, **constipation**, nausea and vomiting, flu-like symptoms, chest **pain**, and rapid heartbeat. Patients who have any of these side effects should consult their doctor at once.

- Cyproheptadine. Side effects include drowsiness, **fatigue**, dry mouth, skin rash, chest congestion, **headache**, **diarrhea**, nausea and vomiting, difficulty urinating, and blurred vision. Patients who experience urinary or vision problems should consult their doctor at once.

- Dronabinol. Dronabinol may cause a variety of changes in mental status, including **delirium**, confusion, **hallucinations**, memory loss, **delusions**, euphoria (false sense of well-being), nervousness or **anxiety**. Because of the possibility of severe mental side effects, *anyone who has taken an overdose of dronabinol needs immediate emergency medical help.* The drug may also cause clumsiness or lightheadedness, dry mouth, fatigue, headache, sweating, facial flushing, diarrhea or constipation, muscle pains, high blood pressure, seizures, problems in urinating, red eyes, or vomiting.

- Anabolic steroids. These drugs have been reported to cause a rare form of **liver disease**; patients who notice yellowing of the eyes or skin, or black, tarry stools, **sore throat** and fever, vomiting of blood, or purplish or reddish spots on the body should contact their doctor at once. Other side effects include feeling chilly, diarrhea, **muscle cramps**, unusual increase or decrease in sexual desire, **acne** or oily skin, bone pain, nausea, or vomiting. Women may notice deepening of the voice, hair loss, unnatural hair growth (**hirsutism**), or irregular menstrual periods. Adult males may notice enlargement of the breasts (**gynecomastia**), frequent need to urinate, or frequent erections. Elderly males may have difficulty urinating.

- Megestrol acetate. Side effects of megestrol acetate include swelling of the hands, feet, or lower legs; headaches; sore breasts; or decreased sexual desire. Men taking this drug may become impotent. Women may notice vaginal bleeding or abdominal pain.

- Fish oil. Some people taking fish oil as a dietary supplement experience an increased tendency to burp followed by a fishy taste in the mouth.

Interactions

Most orexigenic drugs interact with a number of other medications:

- Mirtazapine. Mirtazapine may cause high blood pressure or abnormally high body temperature if taken together with MAO inhibitors (furazolidone, phenelzine, procarbazine, selegiline, or tranylcypromine). It intensifies the sedating (sleep-inducing) effects of alcohol, benzodiazepine tranquilizers, antihistamines, **tricyclic antidepressants**, narcotic pain relievers, and some medications given for high blood pressure.

- Cyproheptadine. Cyproheptadine intensifies and prolongs the effects of other antihistamines, alcohol, **barbiturates**, narcotic pain relievers, benzodiazepine tranquilizers, and antidepressant medications.

- Dronabinol. Dronabinol intensifies the effects of alcohol and other medications that act as **central nervous system depressants**. These groups of drugs include barbiturates, benzodiazepine tranquilizers, tetracyclic and tricyclic antidepressants, narcotic pain relievers, antiseizure medications, antihistamines, **muscle relaxants**, and anesthetics, including dental anesthetics.

- Anabolic steroids. Anabolic steroids may intensify the effects of blood thinners (**aspirin**, coumadin, warfarin). They may increase the risk of liver damage in patients who are taking phenothiazines, valproic acid, **oral contraceptives** containing estrogen, gold salts, methotrexate, carbamazepine, amiodarone, mercaptopurine, phenytoin, plicamycin, disulfiram, daunorubicin, chloroquine, methyldopa, or naltrexone.

- Megestrol acetate. No significant interactions with other drugs have been reported. Patients taking megestrol acetate should, however, notify their physician of all other drugs and dietary supplements (including herbal preparations) that they use on a regular basis, as dosage adjustments are sometimes needed.

- Fish oil. Fish oil has been reported to intensify the effects of such blood-thinning medications as coumadin and warfarin. Persons who take these drugs and wish to use fish oil as a dietary supplement should consult their doctor first.

Resources

BOOKS

"Malnutrition." Section 1, Chapter 2 in *The Merck Manual of Diagnosis and Therapy*, edited by Mark H. Beers, MD, and Robert Berkow, MD. Whitehouse Station, NJ: Merck Research Laboratories, 2004.

"Protein-Energy Undernutrition." Section 8, Chapter 61 in *The Merck Manual of Geriatrics*, edited by Mark H. Beers, MD, and Robert Berkow, MD. Whitehouse Station, NJ: Merck Research Laboratories, 2004.

Wilson, Billie A., Margaret T. Shannon, and Carolyn L. Stang. *Nurses Drug Guide 2000*, Stamford, CT: Appleton & Lange, 2000.

PERIODICALS

Anttila, S. A., and E. V. Leinonen. "A Review of the Pharmacological and Clinical Profile of Mirtazapine." *CNS Drug Reviews* 7 (Fall 2001): 249–264.

Grinspoon, S., and K. Mulligan. "Weight Loss and Wasting in Patients Infected with Human Immunodeficiency Virus." *Clinical Infectious Diseases* 36 (April 1, 2003) (Supplement 2): S69–S78.

Holder, H. "Nursing Management of Nutrition in Cancer and Palliative Care." *British Journal of Nursing* 12 (June 12–25, 2003): 667–674.

Homnick, D. N., B. D. Homnick, A. J. Reeves, et al. "Cyproheptadine Is an Effective Appetite Stimulant in Cystic Fibrosis." *Pediatric Pulmonology* 38 (August 2004): 129–134.

Jatoi, A., K. Rowland, C. L. Loprinzi, et al. "An Eicosapentaenoic Acid Supplement Versus Megestrol Acetate Versus Both for Patients with Cancer-Associated Wasting: A North Central Cancer Treatment Group and National Cancer Institute of

Canada Collaborative Project." *Journal of Clinical Oncology* 22 (June 15, 2004): 2469–2476.

Jatoi, A., H. E. Windschitl, C. L. Loprinzi, et al. "Dronabinol Versus Megestrol Acetate Versus Combination Therapy for Cancer-Associated Anorexia: A North Central Cancer Treatment Group Study." *Journal of Clinical Oncology* 20 (January 15, 2002): 567–573.

Morley, J. E. "Orexigenic and Anabolic Agents." *Clinics in Geriatric Medicine* 18 (November 2002): 853–866.

Vickers, S. P., and G. A. Kennett. "Cannabinoids and the Regulation of Ingestive Behaviour." *Current Drug Targets* 6 (March 2005): 215–223.

ORGANIZATIONS

American Academy of Home Care Physicians (AAHCP). P. O. Box 1037, Edgewood, MD 21040-0337. (410) 676-7966. Fax: (410) 676-7980. < http://www.aahcp.org > .

American Psychiatric Association (APA). 1000 Wilson Boulevard, Suite 1825, Arlington, VA 22209-3901. (800) 368-5777 or (703) 907-7322. Fax: (703) 907-1091. < http://www.psych.org > .

American Society of Health-System Pharmacists (ASHP). 7272 Wisconsin Avenue, Bethesda, MD 20814. (301) 657-3000. < www.ashp.org > .

National Cancer Institute (NCI). NCI Public Inquiries Office, Suite 3036A, 6116 Executive Boulevard, MSC8332, Bethesda, MD 20892-8322. (800) 4-CANCER or (800) 332-8615 (TTY). < www.nci.nih.gov > .

United States Food and Drug Administration (FDA). 5600 Fishers Lane, Rockville, MD 20857-0001. (888) INFO-FDA. < www.fda.gov > .

OTHER

Food and Drug Administration (FDA) MedWatch, January 2005. "Summary View: Safety Labeling Changes Approved by FDA Center for Drug Evaluation and Research (CDER)—January 2005." < http://www.fda.gov/medwatch/SAFETY/2005/jan05_quickview.htm > .

Morley, John E., David R. Thomas, and Margaret-Mary G. Wilson. "Appetite and Orexigenic Drugs." St. Louis, MO: Council for Nutrition, Clinical Strategies in Long-Term Care, 2001.

National Center for Complementary and Alternative Medicine (NCCAM). "Clinical Trial: A Fish Oil Supplement to Maintain Body Weight in Pancreatic Cancer Patients." < http://clinicaltrials.gov/show/NCT00094562 > .

Taler, George, MD, and Christine Ritchie, MD. "Unintended Weight Loss Guidelines.". Edgewood, MD: American Academy of Home Care Physicians, 2004.

Rebecca J. Frey, PhD

Applied kinesiology *see* **Kinesiology, applied**

Apraxia

Definition

Apraxia is neurological condition characterized by loss of the ability to perform activities that a person is physically able and willing to do.

Description

Apraxia is caused by brain damage related to conditions such as **head injury**, **stroke**, **brain tumor**, and Alzheimer's disease. The damage affects the brain's ability to correctly signal instructions to the body. Forms of apraxia include the inability to say some words or make gestures.

Various conditions cause apraxia, and it can affect people of all ages. A baby might be born with the condition. A car accident or fall that resulted in head trauma could lead to apraxia.

From 500,000 to 750,000 people need to be hospitalized each year for head injuries according to the American Medical Association (AMA). Men between the ages of 18 and 24 form the largest group of people with head injuries. While not all severe injuries result in apraxia, men in that age group are at risk.

Risk factors for strokes include high blood pressure, diabetes, and heart disease. Cigarette **smoking** also puts a person at risk for a stroke. Brain tumors are abnormal tissue growths in the skull. They may be secondary tumors caused by the spread of **cancer** through the body.

There is more than one type of apraxia, and a person may have one or more form of this condition. Furthermore, a milder form of apraxia is called dyspraxia.

Causes and symptoms

Apraxia is caused by conditions that affect parts of the brain that control movements. Apraxia is a result of damage to the brain's cerebral hemispheres. These are the two halves of the cerebrum and are the location of brain activities such as voluntary movements.

Apraxia causes a lapse in carrying out movements that a person knows how to do, is physically able to perform, and wants to do. A person may be willing and able to do something like bathe. However, the brain does not send the signals that allow the person to perform the necessary sequence of activities to do this correctly.

KEY TERMS

CT scanning—Computer tomography scanning is a diagnostic imaging tool that uses x rays sent through the body at different angles.

MRI—Magnetic resonance imaging is a diagnostic imaging tool that utilizes an electromagnetic field and radio waves.

Types of apraxia

There are several types of apraxia, and a patient could be diagnosed with one or more forms of this condition. The types of apraxia include:

- Buccofacial or orofacial apraxia is the inability of a person to follow through on commands involving face and lip motions. These activities include coughing, licking the lips, whistling, and winking. Also known as facial-oral apraxia, it is the most common form of apraxia, according to the National Institute of Neurological Disorders and Stroke (NINDS).

- Limb-kinetic apraxia is the inability to make precise movements with an arm or leg.

- Ideomotor apraxia is the inability to make the proper movement in response to a command to pantomime an activity like waving.

- Constructional apraxia is the inability to copy, draw, or build simple figures.

- Ideational apraxia is the inability to do an activity that involves performing a series of movements in a sequence. A person with this condition could have trouble dressing, eating, or bathing. It is also known as conceptual apraxia.

- Oculomotor apraxia is characterized by difficulty moving the eyes.

- Verbal apraxia is a condition involving difficulty coordinating mouth and speech movements. It is referred to as apraxia of speech by organizations including the American Speech Language Hearing Association (ASHA).

A baby who does not coo or babble may display a symptom of apraxia of speech, according to ASHA. A young child may only say a few consonant sounds, and an older child may have difficulty imitating speech. An adult also has this difficulty. Other symptoms include saying the wrong words. A person wants to say "kitchen," but says "bipem" instead, according to an ASHA report.

A person diagnosed with apraxia may also have **aphasia**, a condition caused by damage to the brain's speech centers. This results in difficulty reading, witting, speaking, and understanding when others speak.

Post-apraxia changes

A person with apraxia could experience frustration about difficulty communicating or trouble performing tasks. In some cases, the condition could affect the person's ability to live independently.

Diagnosis

Diagnosis of apraxia could begin with testing of its underlying cause. Testing for conditions like a stroke or cancer includes the MRI (**magnetic resonance imaging**) and CT scanning (computer tomography scanning). A **brain biopsy** is used to measure changes caused by Alzheimer's disease. In all cases, the physician takes a family history. Head trauma that could cause apraxia is first treated in the emergency room.

Other diagnostic treatment is related to identifying the type of apraxia. For example, the physician may ask the patient to demonstrate how to blow out a candle, wave, use a fork, or use a toothbrush.

Assessment for speech apraxia in children includes a hearing evaluation to determine if difficulty in speaking is related to a **hearing loss**. If the condition appears related to apraxia, a speech-language pathologist examines muscle development in the jaw, lips, and tongue. The examination of adults and children includes an evaluation of how words are pronounced individually and in conversation. The pathologist observes how the patient breathes when speaking and the ability to perform actions like smiling.

The costs of diagnosis vary because the process could include examinations and diagnostic screening related to the underlying cost of the apraxia. Insurance generally covers part of these costs.

Treatment

The treatment for apraxia usually involves **rehabilitation** through speech-language therapy, physical therapy, or occupational therapy. In addition, treatment such as **chemotherapy** is administered for the condition that caused the apraxia.

Family education is an important component of apraxia treatment. The rehabilitation process takes time, and relatives can offer encouragement and support to the patient. They may be asked to help the patient with in-home exercises. Furthermore, family members sometimes need to take on the role of caregivers.

Speech-language therapy

Speech-language therapy focuses on helping the patients learn or regain communication skills. Therapists teach exercises to strengthen facial muscles used in speech. Other exercises concentrate on patients learning to correctly pronounce sounds and then turn those sounds into words.

In cases where apraxia limits the ability to speak, therapists help patients develop alternate means of communication. These alternatives range from gesturing to using a portable computer that writes and produces speech, according to ASHA.

Occupational and physical therapies

Occupational and physical therapies focus on helping patients regain the skills impaired by apraxia. Physical therapy exercises concentrate on areas such as mobility and balance. Occupational therapy helps patients relearn daily living skills.

Treatment costs

The costs of therapy vary by the type of treatment, regional location, and where the therapy is offered. Fees can range for $40 per hour for in-office speech therapy for a child to $85 per hour for in-home physical or occupational therapy for a senior citizen. Part of therapy costs may be covered by insurance.

Alternative treatment

Most alternative treatments target Alzheimer's disease and other conditions that cause apraxia. Herbal remedies thought to help people with Alzheimer's include **ginkgo biloba**, a plant extract. However, organizations including the Alzheimer's Association caution that the effectiveness and safety of this herbal remedy has not been evaluated by the U.S. Food and Drug Administration. The government does not require a review of supplements like ginkgo. Furthermore, there is a risk of internal bleeding if ginkgo is taken in combination with **aspirin** and blood-thinning medications.

Prognosis

The prognosis for apraxia depends on factors such as what caused the condition. While Alzheimer's is a degenerative condition, a child with verbal apraxia or a stroke patient could make progress.

In some cases, treatment helps a person to relearn or acquire skills needed to function. A caregiver may be required, and some people with **dementia** require supervised, longterm care.

Prevention

The methods of preventing apraxia focus on preventing the underlying causes of this condition. This may not be entirely possible when there is a family history of conditions such as stroke, dementia, and cancer. However, a person at risk by not smoking, exercising, and eating a diet based on the American Heart Association guidelines.

Head injury can be prevented by wearing a helmet when participating in activities like sports and bicycling. Wearing a seatbelt when in a vehicle also helps reduce the risk of head injury.

Resources

BOOKS

PERIODICALS

ORGANIZATIONS

American Speech Language Hearing Association. 10801 Rockville Pike, Rockville, MD 20852-3279. 800-638-8255. < http://www.asha.org > .

Alzheimer's Association. 225 North Michigan Avenue, Floor 17, Chicago, IL 60601. 800-272-3900. < http://www.alz.org > .

National Institute of Neurological Disorders and Stroke, NIH Neurological Institute. P.O. Box 5801, Bethesda, MD 20824. 800-352-9424. < http://www.ninds.nih.gov > .

National Rehabilitation Information Center. 4200 Forbes Boulevard Suite 202, Lanham, MD 20706-4829. 800-346-2742. < http://www.naric.com > .

National Stroke Association. 9707 East Easter Lane, Englewood, CO 80112. 1-800-787-6537. < http://www.stroke.org > .

OTHER

"Apraxia in Adults." American Speech Language Hearing Association. 2005. [cited March 29, 2005]. < http://www.asha.org/public/speech/disorders/apraxia_adults.htm > .

"Childhood Apraxia of Speech." American Speech Language Hearing Association. 2005. [cited March 29, 2005]. < http://www.asha.org/public/speech/disorders/Developmental-Apraxia-of-Speech.htm > .

Jacobs, Daniel H., M.D."Apraxia and Related Syndromes." e-medicine. October 27, 2004 [cited March 29, 2005]. < http://www.emedicine.com/neuro/topic438.htm > .

"NINDS Apraxia Information Page." National Institute of Neurological Disorders and Stroke February 09, 2005 [cited March 29, 2005]. < http://www.ninds.nih.gov/disorders/apraxia/apraxia.htm > .

Liz Swain,

APSGN *see* **Acute poststreptococcal glomerulonephritis**

APTT *see* **Partial thromboplastin time**

Arachnodactyly *see* **Marfan syndrome**

Arbovirus encephalitis

Definition

Encephalitis is a serious inflammation of the brain, Arbovirus encephalitis is caused by a virus from the Arbovirus group. The term *arbovirus* stands for *Arthro-pod-borne virus* because these viruses are passed to humans by members of the phylum Arthropoda (which includes insects and spiders).

Description

Of the huge number of arboviruses known to exist, about 80 types are responsible for human disease. In addition to the virus, there are usually two other types of living creatures involved in the cycle leading to human disease. When large quantities of virus are present in an arthropod (often a tick or mosquito), the viruses are passed to a bird or small mammal when the arthropod attempts to feed on the blood of that creature. The virus thrives within the new host, sometimes causing illness, sometimes not. More ticks or mosquitoes are infected with the virus when they feed on the host's blood. Eventually, a tick or mosquito bites a human, and the virus is passed along. Just a few types of arboviruses cycle only between arthropods and humans, with no intermediate stop in a bird or small mammal.

Because the arboviruses require an arthropod to pass them along to humans, the most common times of year for these illnesses include summer and fall, when mosquitoes and ticks are most prevalent. Damp environments favor large populations of mosquitoes, and thus also increase the risk of arbovirus infections.

The major causes of arbovirus encephalitis include the members of the viral families alphavirus (causing Eastern equine encephalitis, Western equine encephalitis, and Venezuelan equine encephalitis), flavivirus (responsible for St. Louis encephalitis, **Japanese encephalitis**, Tick-borne encephalitis, Murray Valley encephalitis, Russian spring-summer encephalitis, and Powassan), and bunyavirus (causing California encephalitis).

In the United States, the most important types of arbovirus encephalitis include Western equine encephalitis (WEE), Eastern equine encephalitis (EEE), St. Louis encephalitis, and California encephalitis. WEE strikes young infants in particular, with a 5% chance of **death** from the illness. Of those who survive, about 60% suffer permanent brain damage. EEE strikes infants and children, with a 20% chance of death, and a high rate of permanent brain damage among survivors. St. Louis encephalitis tends to strike adults older than 40 years of age, and older patients tend to have higher rates of death and long-term disability from the infection. California virus primarily strikes 5-18 year olds, with a lower degree of permanent brain damage.

Causes and symptoms

Encephalitis occurs because specific arboviruses have biochemical characteristics which cause them to be particularly attracted to the cells of the brain and the nerves. The virus causes cell death and inflammation, with **fever** and swelling within the brain and nerves. The membranous coverings of the brain and spinal cord (the meninges) may also become inflamed, a condition called **meningitis**. The brain is swollen, and patches of bleeding occur throughout the brain and spinal cord.

Patients with encephalitis suffer from headaches, fever, **nausea and vomiting**, stiff neck, and sleepiness. As the disease progresses, more severe symptoms develop, including **tremors**, confusion, seizures, **coma**, and **paralysis**. Loss of function occurs when specific nerve areas are damaged and/or killed.

Diagnosis

Early in the disease, laboratory testing of blood may reveal the presence of the arbovirus. The usual technique used to verify the presence of arbovirus involves injecting the patient's blood into the brain of a newborn mouse, then waiting to see if the mouse develops encephalitis. Diagnosis is usually based on the patient's symptoms, history of tick or mosquito bites, and knowledge that the patient has been in an area known to harbor the arbovirus.

Treatment

Treatment is mostly supportive, meaning it is directed at improving the symptoms, but does not shorten the course of the illness. The main concerns of treatment involve lowering fever, treating **pain**, avoiding **dehydration** or other chemical imbalances, and decreasing swelling in the brain with steroids.

Prognosis

Prognosis depends on the particular type of arbovirus causing disease, and on the age and prior health status of the patient. Death rates range all the way up to 20% for arbovirus encephalitis, and the rates of lifelong effects due to brain damage reach 60% for some types of arboviruses.

Prevention

Prevention involves avoiding contact with arthropods which carry these viruses. This means wearing appropriate insect repellents, and dressing properly in areas known to be infested. Insecticides and the avoidance of collections of standing water (which are good breeding ground for arthropods) is also effective at decreasing arthropod populations.

There are immunizations available against EEE and WEE. These have primarily been used to safeguard laboratory workers who have regular exposure to these viruses.

Resources

BOOKS

Stoffman, Phyllis. *The Family Guide to Preventing and Treating 100 Infectious Diseases.* New York: John Wiley & Sons, 1995.

Rosalyn Carson-DeWitt, MD

ARDS *see* **Adult respiratory distress syndrome**

▌Aromatherapy

Definition

Aromatherapy is the therapeutic use of plant-derived, aromatic essential oils to promote physical and psychological well-being. It is sometimes used in combination with massage and other therapeutic techniques as part of a holistic treatment approach.

Aromatherapy Oils

Name	Description	Conditions treated
Bay laurel	Antiseptic, diuretic, sedative, etc.	Digestive problems, bronchitis, **common cold**, **influenza**, and **scabies** and lice. CAUTION: Don't use if pregnant.
Clary sage	Relaxant, anticonvulsive, antiinflammatory, and antiseptic	Menstrual and menopausal symptoms, burns, eczema, and **anxiety**. CAUTION: Don't use if pregnant.
Eucalyptus	Antiseptic, antibacterial, astringent, expectorant, and analgesic	Boils, breakouts, **cough**, common cold, influenza, and **sinusitis**. CAUTION: Not to be taken orally.
Chamomile	Sedative, antiinflammatory, antiseptic, and pain reliever	Hay **fever**, burns, **acne**, arthritis, digestive problems, **sunburn**, and menstrual an menopausal symptoms.
Lavender	Analgesic, antiseptic, calming/soothing	**Headache**, depression, insomnia, stress, **sprains**, and nausea.
Peppermint	Pain reliever	**Indigestion**, nausea, headache, **motion sickness**, and muscle pain.
Rosemary	Antiseptic, stimulant, and diuretic	Indigestion, gas, bronchitis, fluid retention, and influenza. CAUTION: Don't use if pregnant or have epilepsy or hypertension.
Tarragon	Diuretic, laxative, antispasmodic, and stimulant	Menstrual and menopausal symptoms, gas, and indigestion. CAUTION: Don't use if pregnant.
Tea tree	Antiseptic and soothing	Common cold, bronchitis, abscesses, acne, vaginitis, and burns.
Thyme	Stimulant, antiseptic, antibacterial, and antispasmodic	Cough, **laryngitis**, **diarrhea**, gas, and intestinal worms. CAUTION: Don't use if pregnant or have hypertension.

Purpose

Aromatherapy offers diverse physical and psychological benefits, depending on the essential oil or oil combination and method of application used. Some common medicinal properties of essential oils used in aromatherapy include: analgesic, antimicrobial, antiseptic, anti-inflammatory, astringent, sedative, antispasmodic, expectorant, diuretic, and sedative. Essential oils are used to treat a wide range of symptoms and conditions, including, but not limited to, gastrointestinal discomfort, skin conditions, menstrual **pain** and irregularities, stress-related conditions, **mood disorders**, circulatory problems, respiratory infections, and **wounds**.

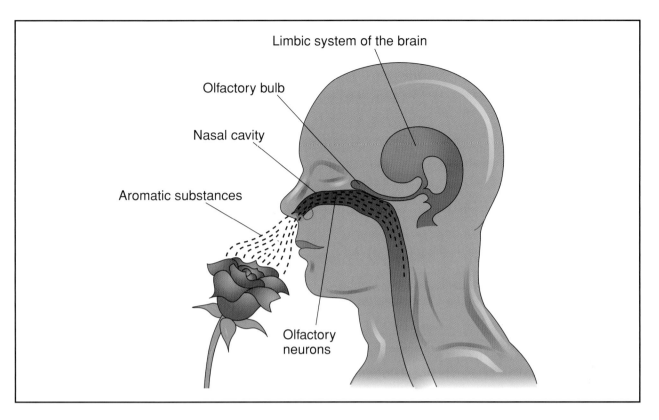

Limbic system of the brain

Olfactory bulb

Nasal cavity

Aromatic substances

Olfactory neurons

As a holistic therapy, aromatherapy is believed to benefit both the mind and body. Here, the aromatic substances from a flower stimulates the olfactory bulb and neurons. The desired emotional response (such as relaxation) is activated from the limbic system of the brain. *(Illustration by Electronic Illustrators Group.)*

Description

Origins

Aromatic plants have been employed for their healing, preservative, and pleasurable qualities throughout recorded history in both the East and West. As early as 1500 B.C. the ancient Egyptians used waters, oils, incense, resins, and ointments scented with botanicals for their religious ceremonies.

There is evidence that the Chinese may have recognized the benefits of herbal and aromatic remedies much earlier than this. The oldest known herbal text, Shen Nung's *Pen Ts'ao* (c. 2700-3000 B.C.) catalogs over 200 botanicals. Ayurveda, a practice of traditional Indian medicine that dates back over 2,500 years, also used aromatic herbs for treatment.

The Romans were well-known for their use of fragrances. They bathed with botanicals and integrated them into their state and religious rituals. So did the Greeks, with a growing awareness of the medicinal properties of herbs, as well. Greek physician and surgeon Pedanios Dioscorides, whose renown herbal text

De Materia Medica (60 A.D.) was the standard textbook for Western medicine for 1,500 years, wrote extensively on the medicinal value of botanical aromatics. The *Medica* contained detailed information on over 500 plants and 4,740 separate medicinal uses for them, including an entire section on aromatics.

Written records of herbal distillation are found as early as the first century A.D., and around 1000 A.D., the noted Arab physician and naturalist Avicenna described the distillation of rose oil from rose petals, and the medicinal properties of essential oils in his writings. However, it wasn't until 1937, when French chemist René-Maurice Gattefossé published *Aromatherapie: Les Huiles essentielles, hormones végétales*, that aromatherapie, or aromatherapy, was introduced in Europe as a medical discipline. Gattefossé, who was employed by a French perfumeur, discovered the healing properties of lavender oil quite by accident when he suffered a severe burn while working and used the closest available liquid, lavender oil, to soak it in.

In the late 20th century, French physician Jean Valnet used botanical aromatics as a front line

KEY TERMS

Antiseptic—Inhibits the growth of microorganisms.

Bactericidal—An agent that destroys bacteria (e.g., *Staphylococci aureus, Streptococci pneumoniae, Escherichia coli, Salmonella enteritidis*).

Carrier oil—An oil used to dilute essential oils for use in massage and other skin care applications.

Contact dermatitis—Skin irritation as a result of contact with a foreign substance.

Essential oil—A volatile oil extracted from the leaves, fruit, flowers, roots, or other components of a plant and used in aromatherapy, perfumes, and foods and beverages.

Holistic—A practice of medicine that focuses on the whole patient, and addresses the social, emotional, and spiritual needs of a patient as well as their physical treatment.

Phototoxic—Causes a harmful skin reaction when exposed to sunlight.

Remedy antidote—Certain foods, beverages, prescription medications, aromatic compounds, and other environmental elements that counteract the efficacy of homeopathic remedies.

Steam distillation—A process of extracting essential oils from plant products through a heating and evaporation process.

Volatile—Something that vaporizes or evaporates quickly when exposed to air.

---

treatment for wounded soldiers in World War II. He wrote about his use of essential oils and their healing and antiseptic properties, in his 1964 book *Aromatherapie, traitement des maladies par les essences des plantes*, which popularized the use of essential oils for medical and psychiatric treatment throughout France. Later, French biochemist Mauguerite Maury popularized the cosmetic benefits of essential oils, and in 1977 Robert Tisserand wrote the first English language book on the subject, *The Art of Aromatherapy*, which introduced massage as an adjunct treatment to aromatherapy and sparked its popularity in the United Kingdom.

In aromatherapy, essential oils are carefully selected for their medicinal properties. As essential oils are absorbed into the bloodstream through application to the skin or inhalation, their active components trigger certain pharmalogical effects (e.g., pain relief).

In addition to physical benefits, aromatherapy has strong psychological benefits. The volatility of an oil, or the speed at which it evaporates in open air, is thought to be linked to the specific psychological effect of an oil. As a rule of thumb, oils that evaporate quickly are considered emotionally uplifting, while slowly-evaporating oils are thought to have a calming effect.

Essential oils commonly used in aromatherapy treatment include:

- Roman chamomile (*Chamaemelum nobilis*). An anti-inflammatory and analgesic. Useful in treating **otitis media** (earache), skin conditions, menstrual pains, and depression.

- Clary sage (*Salvia sclarea*). This natural astringent is not only used to treat oily hair and skin, but is also said to be useful in regulating the menstrual cycle, improving mood, and controlling high blood pressure. Clary sage should not be used by pregnant women.

- Lavender (*Lavandula officinalis*). A popular aromatherapy oil which mixes well with most essential oils, lavender has a wide range of medicinal and cosmetic applications, including treatment of insect bites, **burns**, respiratory infections, intestinal discomfort, **nausea**, migraine, **insomnia**, depression, and **stress**.

- Myrtle (*Myrtus communis*). Myrtle is a fungicide, disinfectant, and antibacterial. It is often used in steam aromatherapy treatments to alleviate the symptoms of **whooping cough**, **bronchitis**, and other respiratory infections.

- Neroli (bitter orange), (*Citrus aurantium*). Citrus oil extracted from bitter orange flower and peel and used to treat **sore throat**, insomnia, and stress and anxiety-related conditions.

- Sweet orange (*Citrus sinensis*). An essential oil used to treat stomach complaints and known for its reported ability to lift the mood while relieving stress.

- Peppermint (*Mentha piperita*). Relaxes and soothes the stomach muscles and gastrointestinal tract. Peppermint's actions as an anti-inflammatory, antiseptic, and antimicrobial also make it an effective skin treatment, and useful in fighting cold and flu symptoms.

- Rosemary (*Rosmarinus officinalis*). Stimulating essential oil used to treat muscular and rheumatic complaints, as well as low blood pressure, gastrointestinal problems, and headaches.

- Tea tree (*Melaleuca alternifolia*). Has bactericidal, virucidal, fungicidal, and anti-inflammatory properties that make it a good choice for fighting infection. Recommended for treating sore throat and respiratory infections, vaginal and bladder infections, wounds, and a variety of skin conditions.

- Ylang ylang (*Cananga odorata*). A sedative essential oil sometimes used to treat **hypertension** and tachycardia.

Essential oils contain active agents that can have potent physical effects. While some basic aromatherapy home treatments can be self-administered, medical aromatherapy should always be performed under the guidance of an aromatherapist, herbalist, massage therapist, nurse, or physician.

Inhalation

The most basic method of administering aromatherapy is direct or indirect inhalation of essential oils. Several drops of an essential oil can be applied to a tissue or handkerchief and gently inhaled. A small amount of essential oil can also be added to a bowl of hot water and used as a steam treatment. This technique is recommended when aromatherapy is used to treat respiratory and/or skin conditions. Aromatherapy steam devices are also available commercially. A warm bath containing essential oils can have the same effect as steam aromatherapy, with the added benefit of promoting relaxation. When used in a bath, water should be lukewarm rather than hot to slow the evaporation of the oil.

Essential oil diffusers, vaporizers, and light bulb rings can be used to disperse essential oils over a large area. These devices can be particularly effective in aromatherapy that uses essential oils to promote a healthier home environment. For example, eucalyptus and tea tree oil are known for their antiseptic qualities and are frequently used to disinfect sickrooms, and citronella and geranium can be useful in repelling insects.

Direct application

Because of their potency, essential oils are diluted in a carrier oil or lotion before being applied to the skin to prevent an allergic skin reaction. The carrier oil can be a vegetable or olive based one, such as wheat germ or avocado. Light oils, such as safflower, sweet almond, grapeseed, hazelnut, apricot seed, or peach kernel, may be absorbed more easily by the skin. Standard dilutions of essential oils in carrier oils range from 2–10%. However, some oils can be used at higher concentrations, and others should be diluted further for safe and effective use. The type of carrier oil used and the therapeutic use of the application may also influence how the essential oil is mixed. Individuals should seek guidance from a healthcare professional and/or aromatherapist when diluting essential oils.

Massage is a common therapeutic technique used in conjunction with aromatherapy to both relax the body and thoroughly administer the essential oil treatment. Essential oils can also be used in hot or cold compresses and soaks to treat muscle aches and pains (e.g., lavender and ginger). As a sore throat remedy, antiseptic and soothing essential oils (e.g., tea tree and sage) can be thoroughly mixed with water and used as a gargle or mouthwash.

Internal use

Some essential oils can be administered internally in tincture, infusion, or suppository form to treat certain symptoms or conditions; however, this treatment should never be self-administered. Essential oils should only be taken internally under the supervision of a qualified healthcare professional.

As non-prescription botanical preparations, the essential oils used in aromatherapy are typically not paid for by health insurance. The self-administered nature of the therapy controls costs to some degree. Aromatherapy treatment sessions from a professional aromatherapist are not covered by health insurance in most cases, although aromatherapy performed in conjunction with physical therapy, nursing, therapeutic massage, or other covered medical services may be. Individuals should check with their insurance provider to find out about their specific coverage.

The adage "You get what you pay for" usually applies when purchasing essential oils, as bargain oils are often adulterated, diluted, or synthetic. Pure essential oils can be expensive; and the cost of an oil will vary depending on its quality and availability.

Preparations

The method of extracting an essential oil varies by plant type. Common methods include water or steam distillation and cold pressing. Quality essential oils should be unadulterated and extracted from pure botanicals. Many aromatherapy oils on the market are synthetic and/or diluted, contain solvents, or are extracted from botanicals grown with pesticides or herbicides. To ensure best results, essential oils should be made from pure organic botanicals and labeled by their full botanical name. Oils should always be stored dark bottles out of direct light.

Before using essential oils on the skin, individuals should perform a skin patch test by applying a small amount of the diluted oil behind the wrist and covering it with a bandage or cloth for up to 12 hours. If redness or irritation occurs, the oil should be diluted further and a second skin test performed, or it should be avoided altogether. Individuals should never apply undiluted essential oils to the skin unless advised to do so by a trained healthcare professional.

Precautions

Individuals should only take essential oils internally under the guidance and close supervision of a health-care professional. Some oils, such as eucalyptus, wormwood, and sage, should never be taken internally. Many essential oils are highly toxic and should never be used at all in aromatherapy. These include (but are not limited to) bitter almond, pennyroyal, mustard, sassafras, rue, and mugwort.

Citrus-based essential oils, including bitter and sweet orange, lime, lemon, grapefruit, and tangerine, are phototoxic, and exposure to direct sunlight should be avoided for at least four hours after their application.

Other essential oils, such as cinnamon leaf, black pepper, juniper, lemon, white camphor, eucalyptus blue gum, ginger, peppermint, pine needle, and thyme can be extremely irritating to the skin if applied in high enough concentration or without a carrier oil or lotion. Caution should always be exercised when applying essential oils topically. Individuals should never apply undiluted essential oils to the skin unless directed to do so by a trained healthcare professional and/or aromatherapist.

Individuals taking homeopathic remedies should avoid black pepper, camphor, eucalyptus, and peppermint essential oils. These oils may act as a remedy antidote to the homeopathic treatment.

Children should only receive aromatherapy treatment under the guidance of a trained aromatherapist or healthcare professional. Some essential oils may not be appropriate for treating children, or may require additional dilution before use on children.

Certain essential oils should not be used by pregnant or nursing women or by people with specific illnesses or physical conditions. Individuals suffering from any chronic or acute health condition should inform their healthcare provider before starting treatment with any essential oil.

Asthmatic individuals should not use steam inhalation for aromatherapy, as it can aggravate their condition.

Essential oils are flammable, and should be kept away from heat sources.

Side effects

Side effects vary by the type of essential oil used. Citrus-based essential oils can cause heightened sensitivity to sunlight. Essential oils may also cause **contact dermatitis**, an allergic reaction characterized by redness and irritation. Anyone experiencing an allergic reaction to an essential oil should discontinue its use and contact their healthcare professional for further guidance. Individuals should do a small skin patch test with new essential oils before using them extensively (see "Preparations" above).

Research and general acceptance

The antiseptic and bactericidal qualities of some essential oils (such as tea tree and peppermint) and their value in fighting infection has been detailed extensively in both ancient and modern medical literature.

Recent research in mainstream medical literature has also shown that aromatherapy has a positive psychological impact on patients, as well. Several clinical studies involving both post-operative and chronically ill subjects showed that massage with essential oils can be helpful in improving emotional well-being, and consequently, promoting the healing process.

Today, the use of holistic aromatherapy is widely accepted in Europe, particularly in Great Britain, where it is commonly used in conjunction with massage as both a psychological and physiological healing tool. In the United States, where aromatherapy is often misunderstood as solely a cosmetic treatment, the mainstream medical community has been slower to accept it.

Resources

BOOKS

Schnaubelt, Kurt. *Medical Aromatherapy: Healing With Essential Oils.* Berkeley, CA: Frog Ltd, 1999.

ORGANIZATIONS

National Association of Holistic Aromatherapy. 836 Hanley Industrial Court, St. Louis, MO 63144. (888) ASK-NAHA. < http://www.naha.org > .

Paula Anne Ford-Martin

Arrhythmias

Definition

An arrhythmia is an abnormality in the heart's rhythm, or heartbeat pattern. The heartbeat can be too slow, too fast, have extra beats, skip a beat, or otherwise beat irregularly.

Description

Arrhythmias are deviations from the normal cadence of the heartbeat, which cause the heart to pump improperly. The normal heartbeat starts in the right atrium, where the heart's natural pacemaker (the sinus node) sends an electrical signal to the center of the heart to the atrioventricular node. The atrioventricular node then sends signals into the main pumping chamber to make the ventricle contract. Arrhythmias occur when the heartbeat starts in a part of the heart other than the sinus node, an abnormal rate or rhythm develops in the sinus node, or a heart conduction "block" prevents the electrical signal from traveling down the normal pathway.

More than four million Americans have arrhythmias, most of which are harmless. Middle-aged adults commonly experience arrhythmias. As people age, the probability of experiencing an arrhythmia increases. Arrhythmias often occur in people who do not have heart disease. In people with heart disease, it is usually the heart disease which is dangerous, not the arrhythmia. Arrhythmias often occur during and after heart attacks. Some types of arrhythmias, such as **ventricular tachycardia**, are serious and even life threatening. In the United States, arrhythmias are the primary cause of **sudden cardiac death**, accounting for more than 350,000 deaths each year.

Slow heart rates (less than 60 beats per minute) are called bradycardias, while fast heart rates (more than 100 beats per minute) are called tachycardias. Bradycardia can result in poor circulation of blood, and, hence, a lack of oxygen throughout the body, especially the brain. Tachycardias also can compromise the heart's ability to pump effectively because the ventricles do not have enough time to completely fill.

Arrhythmias are characterized by their site of origin: the atria or the ventricles. Supraventricular arrhythmias occur in the upper areas of the heart and are less serious than ventricular arrhythmias. **Ventricular fibrillation** is the most serious arrhythmia and is fatal unless medical help is immediate.

Causes and symptoms

In many cases, the cause of an arrhythmia is unknown. Known causes of arrhythmias include heart disease, **stress**, **caffeine**, tobacco, alcohol, diet pills, and **decongestants** in **cough** and cold medicines.

Symptoms of an arrhythmia include a fast heartbeat, pounding or fluttering chest sensations, skipping a heartbeat, "flip-flops," **dizziness**, faintness, **shortness of breath**, and chest pains.

Diagnosis

Examination with a stethoscope, electrocardiograms, and electrophysiologic studies is used to diagnose arrhythmias. Sometimes arrhythmias can be identified by listening to the patient's heart through a stethoscope, but, since arrhythmias are not always present, they may not occur during the physical exam.

An electrocardiogram (ECG) shows the heart's activity and may reveal a lack of oxygen from poor circulation (**ischemia**). Electrodes covered with conducting jelly are placed on the patient's chest, arms, and legs. They send impulses of the heart's activity through an electrical activity monitor (oscilloscope) to a recorder that traces them on paper. The test takes about 10 minutes and is performed in a physician's office. Another type of ECG, commonly known as the **exercise stress test**, measures how the heart and blood vessels respond to exertion while the patient is exercising on a treadmill or a stationary bike. This test is performed in a physician's office or an exercise laboratory and takes 15-30 minutes. Other types of ECGs include 24-hour ECG monitoring and transtelephonic monitoring. In 24-hour ECG (Holter) monitoring, the patient wears a small, portable tape recorder connected to disks on his/her chest that record the heart's rhythm during daily activities. Transtelephonic monitoring can identify arrhythmias that occur infrequently. Similar to **Holter monitoring**, transtelephonic monitoring can continue for days or weeks, and it enables patients to send the ECG via telephone to a monitoring station when an arrhythmia is felt, or the patient can store the information in the recorder and transmit it later.

Electrophysiologic studies are invasive procedures performed in a hospital to identify the origin of serious arrhythmias and responses to various treatments. They involve **cardiac catheterization**, in which catheters tipped with electrodes are passed from a vein in the arm or leg through the blood vessels into the heart. The electrodes record impulses in the heart, highlighting where the arrhythmia starts. During the procedure, physicians can test the effects of various drugs by provoking an arrhythmia through the electrodes and trying different drugs. The procedure takes one to three hours, during which the patient is awake but mildly sedated. Local anesthetic is injected at the catheter insertion sites.

Treatment

Many arrhythmias do not require any treatment. For serious arrhythmias, treating the underlying heart disease sometimes controls the arrhythmia. In some cases, the arrhythmia itself is treated with drugs, electrical shock (**cardioversion**), automatic implantable defibrillators, artificial **pacemakers**, **catheter ablation**, or surgery. Supraventricular arrhythmias often can be treated with drug therapy. Ventricular arrhythmias are more complex to treat.

Drug therapy can manage many arrhythmias, but finding the right drug and dose requires care and can take some time. Common drugs for suppressing arrhythmias include beta-blockers, **calcium channel blockers**, quinidine, digitalis preparations, and procainamide. Because of their potential serious side effects, stronger, desensitizing drugs are used only to treat life-threatening arrhythmias. All of the drugs used to treat arrhythmias have possible side effects, ranging from mild complications with beta-blockers and calcium channel blockers to more serious effects of desensitizing drugs that can, paradoxically, cause arrhythmias or make them worse. Response to drugs is usually measured by ECG, Holter monitor, or electrophysiologic study.

In emergency situations, cardioversion or **defibrillation** (the application of an electrical shock to the chest wall) is used. Cardioversion restores the heart to its normal rhythm. It is followed by drug therapy to prevent recurrence of the arrhythmia.

Artificial pacemakers that send electrical signals to make the heart beat properly can be implanted under the skin during a simple operation. Leads from the pacemaker are anchored to the right side of the heart. Pacemakers are used to correct bradycardia and are sometimes used after surgical or catheter ablation.

Automatic implantable defibrillators correct life-threatening ventricular arrhythmias by recognizing them and then restoring a normal heart rhythm by pacing the heart or giving it an electric shock. They are implanted within the chest wall without major surgery and store information for future evaluation by physicians. Automatic implantable defibrillators have proven to be more effective in saving lives than drugs alone. They often are used in conjunction with drug therapy.

Ablation, a procedure to alter or remove the heart tissue causing the arrhythmia in order to prevent a recurrence, can be performed through a catheter or surgery. Supraventricular tachycardia can be treated successfully with ablation. Catheter ablation is performed in a catheterization laboratory with the patient under **sedation**. A catheter equipped with a device that maps the heart's electrical pathways is inserted into a vein and is threaded into the heart. High-frequency radio waves are then used to remove the pathway(s) causing the arrhythmia. Surgical ablation is similar in principle but it is performed in a hospital, using a cold probe instead of radio waves to destroy tissue. Ablation treatments are used when medications fail.

Maze surgery treats atrial fibrillation by making multiple incisions through the atrium to allow electrical impulses to move effectively. This is often recommended for patients who have not responded to drugs or cardioversion.

Alternative treatment

Since some arrhythmias can be life threatening, a conventional medical doctor should always be consulted first. **Acupuncture** can correct an insignificant number (1.5%) of atrial fibrillation cases. For new, minor arrhythmias, acupuncture may be effective in up to 70% of cases, but this figure may not differ much from placebo therapy. Both western and Chinese herbal remedies are also used in the treatment of arrhythmias. Since hawthorn (*Crataegus laevigata*) dilates the blood vessels and stimulates the heart muscle, it may help to stabilize arrhythmias. It is gentle and appropriate for home use, unlike foxglove (*Digitalis purpurea*), an herb whose action on the heart is too potent for use without supervision by a qualified practitioner. Homeopathic practitioners may prescribe remedies such as *Lachesis* and aconite or monkshood (*Aconitum napellus*) to treat mild arrhythmias.

Prognosis

Advances in diagnostic techniques, new drugs, and medical technology have extended the lives of many patients with serious arrhythmias. Diagnostic techniques enable physicians to accurately identify arrhythmias, while new drugs, advances in pacemaker technology, the development of implantable defibrillators, and progress in ablative techniques offer effective treatments for many types of arrhythmia.

Prevention

Some arrhythmias can be prevented by managing stress, controlling **anxiety**, and avoiding caffeine, alcohol, decongestants, **cocaine**, and cigarettes.

Resources

ORGANIZATIONS

American Heart Association. 7320 Greenville Ave. Dallas, TX 75231. (214) 373-6300. <http://www.americanheart.org>.

National Heart, Lung and Blood Institute. PO Box 30105, Bethesda, MD 20824-0105. (301) 251-1222. <http://www.nhlbi.nih.gov>.

Texas Heart Institute. Heart Information Service. PO Box 20345, Houston, TX 77225-0345. <http://www.tmc.edu/thi>.

Lori De Milto

▌ Art therapy

Definition

Art therapy, sometimes called creative arts therapy or expressive arts therapy, encourages people to express and understand emotions through artistic expression and through the creative process.

Purpose

Art therapy provides the client-artist with critical insight into emotions, thoughts, and feelings. Key benefits of the art therapy process include:

- Self-discovery. At its most successful, art therapy triggers an emotional catharsis.

- Personal fulfillment. The creation of a tangible reward can build confidence and nurture feelings of self-worth. Personal fulfillment comes from both the creative and the analytical components of the artistic process.

- Empowerment. Art therapy can help people visually express emotions and fears that they cannot express through conventional means, and can give them some sense of control over these feelings.

- Relaxation and **stress** relief. Chronic stress can be harmful to both mind and body. Stress can weaken and damage the immune system, can cause **insomnia** and depression, and can trigger circulatory problems (like high blood pressure and irregular heartbeats). When used alone or in combination with other relaxation techniques such as **guided imagery**, art therapy can effectively relieve stress.

- Symptom relief and physical **rehabilitation**. Art therapy can also help patients cope with **pain**. This therapy can promote physiological healing when patients identify and work through anger, resentment, and other emotional stressors. It is often prescribed to accompany pain control therapy for chronically and terminally ill patients.

Description

Origins

Humans have expressed themselves with symbols throughout history. Masks, ritual pottery, costumes, other objects used in rituals, cave drawings, Egyptian hieroglyphics, and Celtic art and symbols are all visual records of self-expression and communication through art. Art has also been associated spiritual power, and artistic forms such as the Hindu and

KEY TERMS

Catharsis—Therapeutic discharge of emotional tension by recalling past events.

Mandala—A design, usually circular, that appears in religion and art. In Buddhism and Hinduism, the mandala has religious ritual purposes and serves as a yantra (a geometric emblem or instrument of contemplation).

Organic illness—A physically, biologically based illness.

Buddhist mandala and Native American sand painting are considered powerful healing tools.

In the late nineteenth century, French psychiatrists Ambrose Tardieu and Paul-Max Simon both published studies on the similar characteristics of and symbolism in the artwork of the mentally ill. Tardieu and Simon viewed art therapy as an effective diagnostic tool to identify specific types of mental illness or traumatic events. Later, psychologists would use this diagnostic aspect to develop psychological drawing tests (the Draw-A-Man test, the Draw-A-Person Questionnaire [DAP.Q]) and projective personality tests involving visual symbol recognition (e.g., the Rorschach Inkblot Test, the Thematic Apperception Test [TAT], and the Holtzman Inkblot Test [HIT]).

The growing popularity of milieu therapies at psychiatric institutions in the twentieth century was an important factor in the development of art therapy in the United States. Milieu therapies (or environmental therapy) focus on putting the patient in a controlled therapeutic social setting that provides the patient with opportunities to gain self-confidence and interact with peers in a positive way. Activities that encourage self-discovery and empowerment such as art, music, dance, and writing are important components of this approach.

Educator and therapist Margaret Naumburg was a follower of both Freud and Jung, and incorporated art into psychotherapy as a means for her patients to visualize and recognize the unconscious. She founded the Walden School in 1915, where she used students' artworks in psychological counseling. She published extensively on the subject and taught seminars on the technique at New York University in the 1950s. Today, she is considered the founder of art therapy in the United States.

In the 1930s, Karl, William, and Charles Menninger introduced an art therapy program at their Kansas-based psychiatric hospital, the Menninger Clinic. The Menninger Clinic employed a number of artists in residence in the following years, and the facility was also considered a leader in the art therapy movement through the 1950s and 60s. Other noted art therapy pioneers who emerged in the 50s and 60s include Edith Kramer, Hanna Yaxa Kwiatkowska (National Institute of Mental Health), and Janie Rhyne.

Art therapy, sometimes called expressive art or art psychology, encourages self-discovery and emotional growth. It is a two part process, involving both the creation of art and the discovery of its meaning. Rooted in Freud and Jung's theories of the subconscious and unconscious, art therapy is based on the assumption that visual symbols and images are the most accessible and natural form of communication to the human experience. Patients are encouraged to visualize, and then create, the thoughts and emotions that they cannot talk about. The resulting artwork is then reviewed and its meaning interpreted by the patient.

The "analysis" of the artwork produced in art therapy typically allows patients to gain some level of insight into their feelings and lets them to work through these issues in a constructive manner. Art therapy is typically practiced with individual, group, or family psychotherapy (talk therapy). While a therapist may provide critical guidance for these activities, a key feature of effective art therapy is that the patient/artist, not the therapist, directs the interpretation of the artwork.

Art therapy can be a particularly useful treatment tool for children, who frequently have limited language skills. By drawing or using other visual means to express troublesome feelings, younger patients can begin to address these issues, even if they cannot identify or label these emotions with words. Art therapy is also valuable for adolescents and adults who are unable or unwilling to talk about thoughts and feelings.

Beyond its use in mental health treatment, art therapy is also used with traditional medicine to treat organic diseases and conditions. The connection between mental and physical health is well documented, and art therapy can promote healing by relieving stress and allowing the patient to develop coping skills.

Art therapy has traditionally centered on visual mediums, like paintings, sculptures, and drawings. Some mental healthcare providers have now broadened the definition to include music, film, dance, writing, and other types of artistic expression.

Art therapy is often one part of a psychiatric inpatient or outpatient treatment program, and can take place in individual or **group therapy** sessions. Group art therapy sessions often take place in hospital, clinic, shelter, and community program settings. These group therapy sessions can have the added benefits of positive social interaction, empathy, and support from peers. The client-artist can learn that others have similar concerns and issues.

Preparations

Before starting art therapy, the therapist may have an introductory session with the client-artist to discuss art therapy techniques and give the client the opportunity to ask questions about the process. The client-artist's comfort with the artistic process is critical to successful art therapy.

The therapist ensures that appropriate materials and space are available for the client-artist, as well as an adequate amount of time for the session. If the individual artist is exploring art as therapy without the guidance of a trained therapist, adequate materials, space, and time are still important factors in a successful creative experience.

The supplies used in art therapy are limited only by the artist's (and/or therapist's) imagination. Some of the materials often used include paper, canvas, poster board, assorted paints, inks, markers, pencils, charcoals, chalks, fabrics, string, adhesives, clay, wood, glazes, wire, bendable metals, and natural items (like shells, leaves, etc.). Providing artists with a variety of materials in assorted colors and textures can enhance their interest in the process and may result in a richer, more diverse exploration of their emotions in the resulting artwork. Appropriate tools such as scissors, brushes, erasers, easels, supply trays, glue guns, smocks or aprons, and cleaning materials are also essential.

An appropriate workspace should be available for the creation of art. Ideally, this should be a bright, quiet, comfortable place, with large tables, counters, or other suitable surfaces. The space can be as simple as a kitchen or office table, or as fancy as a specialized artist's studio.

The artist should have adequate time to become comfortable with and explore the creative process. This is especially true for people who do not consider themselves "artists" and may be uncomfortable with the concept. If performed in a therapy group or one-on-one session, the art therapist should be available to answer general questions about materials and/or the creative process. However, the therapist should be careful not to influence the creation or interpretation of the work.

Precautions

Art materials and techniques should match the age and ability of the client. People with impairments, such as traumatic brain injury or an organic neurological condition, may have difficulties with the self-discovery portion of the art therapy process depending on their level of functioning. However, they may still benefit from art therapy through the sensory stimulation it provides and the pleasure they get from artistic creation.

While art is accessible to all (with or without a therapist to guide the process), it may be difficult to tap the full potential of the interpretive part of art therapy without a therapist to guide the process. When art therapy is chosen as a therapeutic tool to cope with a physical condition, it should be treated as a supplemental therapy and not as a substitute for conventional medical treatments.

Research and general acceptance

A wide body of literature supports the use of art therapy in a mental health capacity. And as the mind-body connection between psychological well-being and physical health is further documented by studies in the field, art therapy gains greater acceptance by mainstream medicine as a therapeutic technique for organic illness.

Resources

BOOKS

Ganim, Barbara. *Art and Healing: Using expressive art toheal your body, mind, and spirit.* New York: Three Rivers Press, 1999.

ORGANIZATIONS

American Art Therapy Association.1202 Allanson Rd., Mundelein, IL 60060-3808. 888-290-0878 or 847-949-6064. Fax: 847-566-4580. E-mail: arttherapy@ntr.net <http://www.arttherapy.org>.

Paula Anne Ford-Martin

Arterial blood gas analysis *see* **Blood gas analysis**

Arterial embolism

Definition

An embolus is a blood clot, bit of tissue or tumor, gas bubble, or other foreign body that circulates in the blood stream until it becomes stuck in a blood vessel.

Description

When a blood clot develops in an artery and remains in place, it is called a thrombosis. If all or part of the blockage breaks away and lodges in another part of the artery, it is called an **embolism**. Blockage of an artery in this manner can be the result of a blood clot, fat cells, or an air bubble.

When an embolus blocks the flow of blood in an artery, the tissues beyond the plug are deprived of normal blood flow and oxygen. This can cause severe damage and even death of the tissues involved.

Emboli can affect any part of the body. The most common sites are the legs and feet. When the brain is affected, it is called a **stroke**. When the heart is involved, it is called a **heart attack** or myocardial infarction (MI).

Causes and symptoms

A common cause of embolus is when an artery whose lining has become thickened or damaged, usually with age, allows cholesterol to build up more easily than normal on the artery wall. If some of the cholesterol breaks off, it forms an embolus. Emboli also commonly form from **blood clots** in a heart that has been damaged from heart attack or when the heart contracts abnormally from atrial fibrillation.

Other known causes are fat cells that enter the blood after a major bone fracture, infected blood cells, **cancer** cells that enter the blood stream, and small gas bubbles.

Symptoms of an embolus can begin suddenly or build slowly over time, depending on the amount of blocked blood flow.

If the embolus is in an arm or leg, there will be muscle **pain**, **numbness** or **tingling**, pale skin color, lower temperature in the limb, and weakness or loss of muscle function. If it occurs in an internal organ, there is usually pain and/or loss of the organ's function.

Diagnosis

The following tests can be used to confirm the presence of an arterial embolism:

- Electrocardiogram, also known as an EKG or ECG. For this test, patches that detect electrical impulses from the heart are attached to the chest and extremities. The information is displayed on a monitor screen or a paper tape in the form of waves. Reduced blood and oxygen supply to the heart shows as a change in the shape of the waves.

- Noninvasive vascular tests. These involve measuring blood pressure in various parts of the body and comparing the results from each location. When there is a decrease in blood pressure beyond what is normal between two points, a blockage is presumed to be present.

- **Angiography**. In this procedure, a colored liquid material (a dye, or contrast material) that can be seen with x rays is injected into the blood stream through a small tube called a catheter. As the dye fills the arteries, they are easily seen on x ray motion pictures. If there is a blockage in the artery, it shows up as a sudden cut off in the movement of contrast material. Angiography is an expensive procedure and does carry some risk. The catheter may cause a blood clot to form, blocking blood flow. There is also the risk of poking the catheter through the artery or heart muscle. Some people may be allergic to the dye. The risk of any of these injuries occurring is small.

Treatment

Arterial embolism can be treated with medication or surgery, depending on the extent and location of the blockage.

Medication to dissolve the clot is usually given through a catheter directly into the affected artery. If the embolus was caused by a blood clot, medications that thin the blood will help reduce the risk of another embolism.

A surgeon can remove an embolus by making an incision in the artery above the blockage and, using a catheter inserted past the embolus, drag it out through the incision.

If the condition is severe, a surgeon may elect to bypass the blocked vessel by grafting a new vessel in its place.

Prognosis

An arterial embolism is serious and should be treated promptly to avoid permanent damage to the affected area. The outcome of any treatment depends on the location and seriousness of the embolism. New arterial emboli can form even after successful treatment of the first event.

Prevention

Prevention may include diet changes to reduce cholesterol levels, medications to thin the blood, and practicing an active, healthy lifestyle.

Resources

ORGANIZATIONS

American Heart Association. 7320 Greenville Ave. Dallas, TX 75231. (214) 373-6300. < http://www.americanheart.org > .

OTHER

"Arterial Embolism." HealthAnswers.com. < http://www.healthanswers.com > .

Dorothy Elinor Stonely

Arteriogram *see* **Angiography**

Arteriography *see* **Angiography**

Arteriosclerosis *see* **Atherosclerosis**

▌ Arteriovenous fistula

Definition

An arteriovenous **fistula** is an abnormal channel or passage between an artery and a vein.

Description

An arteriovenous fistula is a disruption of the normal blood flow pattern. Normally, oxygenated blood flows to the tissue through arteries and capillaries.

Following the release of oxygen in the tissues, the blood returns to the heart in veins. An arteriovenous fistula is an abnormal connection of an artery and a vein. The blood bypasses the capillaries and tissues, and returns to the heart. Arterial blood has a higher blood pressure than veins and causes swelling of veins involved in a fistula. Although both the artery and the vein retain their normal connections, the new opening between the two will cause some arterial blood to shunt into the vein because of the blood pressure difference.

Causes and symptoms

There are two types of arteriovenous fistulas, congenital and acquired. A congenital arteriovenous fistula is one that formed during fetal development. It is a birth defect. In congenital fistulas, blood vessels of the lower extremity are more frequently involved than other areas of the body. Congenital fistulas are not common. An acquired arteriovenous fistula is one that develops after a person is born. It usually occurs when an artery and vein that are side-by-side are damaged and the healing process results in the two becoming linked. After catheterizations, arteriovenous fistulas may occur as a complication of the arterial puncture in the leg or arm. Fistulas also form without apparent cause. In the case of patients on hemodialysis, physicians perform surgery to create a fistula. These patients receive many needle sticks to flush their blood through dialysis machines and for routine blood analysis testing. The veins used may scar and become difficult to use. Surgery is used to connect an artery and vein so that arterial blood pressure and flow rate widens the vein and decreases the chance of **blood clots** forming inside the vein.

The main symptoms of arteriovenous fistulas near the surface of the skin are bulging and discolored veins. In some cases, the bulging veins can be mistaken for **varicose veins**. Other fistulas can cause more serious problems depending on their location and the blood vessels involved.

Diagnosis

Using a stethoscope, a physician can detect the sound of a pulse in the affected vein (bruit). The sound is a distinctive to-and-fro sound. Dye into the blood can be tracked by x ray to confirm the presence of a fistula.

Treatment

Small arteriovenous fistulas can be corrected by surgery. Fistulas in the brain or eye are very difficult to treat. If surgery is not possible or very difficult, injection therapy may be used. Injection therapy is the injection of substances that cause the blood to clot at the site of the injection. In the case of an arteriovenous fistula, the blood clot should stop the passage of blood from the artery to the vein. Surgery is usually used to correct acquired fistulas once they are diagnosed.

Resources

BOOKS

Alexander, R. W., R. C. Schlant, and V. Fuster, eds. *The Heart.* 9th ed. New York: McGraw-Hill, 1998.

Berkow, Robert, ed. *Merck Manual of Medical Information.* Whitehouse Station, NJ: Merck Research Laboratories, 2004.

Braunwald, E. *Heart Disease.* Philadelphia: W. B. Saunders Co., 1997.

John T. Lohr, PhD

Arteriovenous malformations

Definition

Arteriovenous malformations are blood vessel defects that occur before birth when the fetus is growing in the uterus (prenatal development). The blood vessels appear as a tangled mass of arteries and veins. They do not possess the capillary (very fine blood vessels) bed which normally exists in the common area where the arteries and veins lie in close proximity (artery-vein interface). An arteriovenous malformation (AVM) may hemorrhage, or bleed, leading to serious complications that can be life-threatening.

Description

AVMs represent an abnormal interface between arteries and veins. Normally, arteries carry oxygenated blood to the body's tissues through progressively smaller blood vessels. The smallest are capillaries, which form a web of blood vessels (the capillary bed) through the body's tissues. The arterial blood moves through tissues by these tiny pathways, exchanging its load of oxygen and nutrients for carbon dioxide and other waste products produced by the body cells (cellular wastes). The blood is carried

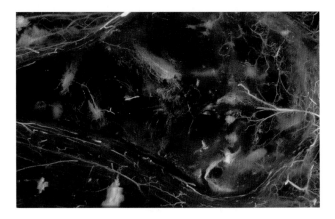

Arteriovenous malformations. *(Custom Medical Stock Photo. Reproduced by permission.)*

away by progressively larger blood vessels, the veins. AVMs lack a capillary bed and arterial blood is moved (shunted) directly from the arteries into the veins.

AVMs can occur anywhere in the body and have been found in the arms, hands, legs, feet, lungs, heart, liver, and kidneys. However, 50% of these malformations are located in the brain, brainstem, and spinal cord. Owing to the possibility of hemorrhaging, such AVMs carry the risk of stroke, **paralysis**, and the loss of speech, memory, or vision. An AVM that hemorrhages can be fatal.

Approximately three of every 100,000 people have a cerebral AVM and roughly 40-80% of them will experience some bleeding from the abnormal blood vessels at some point. The annual risk of an AVM bleeding is estimated at about 1-4%. After age 55, the risk of bleeding decreases. Pre-existing high blood pressure or intense physical activity do not seem to be associated with AVM hemorrhage, but **pregnancy** and labor could cause a rupture or breaking open of a blood vessel. An AVM hemorrhage is not as dangerous as an aneurysmal rupture. (An aneurysm is a swollen, blood filled vessel where the pressure of the blood causes the wall to bulge outward.) There is an approximate 10% fatality rate associated with AVM hemorrhage, compared to a 50% fatality rate for ruptured aneurysms.

Although AVMs are congenital defects, meaning a person is born with them, they are rarely discovered before age 20. A genetic link has been proposed for some AVMs, but studies are only suggestive, not positive. The majority of AVMs are discovered in people age 20-40. Medical researchers estimate that the malformations are created during days 45-60 of fetal development. A second theory suggests that AVMs are primitive structures that are left over from the

KEY TERMS

Aneurysm—A weak point in a blood vessel where the pressure of the blood causes the vessel wall to bulge outwards.

Angiography—A mapping of the brain's blood vessels, using x-ray imaging.

Capillary bed—A dense network of tiny blood vessels that enables blood to fill a tissue or organ.

Hydrocephalus—Swelling of the brain caused by an accumulation of fluid.

Lumbar puncture—A diagnostic procedure in which a needle is inserted into the lower spine to withdraw a small amount of cerebrospinal fluid. This fluid is examined to assess trauma to the brain.

Saccular aneurysm—A type of aneurysm that resembles a small sack of blood attached to the outer surface of a blood vessel by a thin neck.

period when fetal blood circulating systems began to develop.

However they form, AVMs have blood vessels that are abnormally fragile. The arteries that feed into the malformation are unusually swollen and thin walled. They lack the usual amount of smooth muscle tissue and elastin, a fibrous connective tissue. These blood vessels commonly accumulate deposits of calcium salts and hyalin. The venous part of the malformation receives blood directly from the artery. Without the intervening capillary bed, the veins receive blood at a higher pressure than they were designed to handle. This part of the malformation is also swollen (dilated) and thin walled. There is a measurable risk of an aneurysm forming near an AVM, increasing the threat of hemorrhage, brain damage, and death. Approximately 10-15% of AVMs are accompanied by saccular aneurysms, a type of aneurysm that looks like a small sac attached to the outer wall of the blood vessel.

Although the malformation itself lacks capillaries, there is often an abnormal proliferation of capillaries next to the defect. These blood vessels feed into the malformation, causing it to grow larger in some cases. As the AVM receives more blood through this "steal," adjacent brain tissue does not receive enough. These areas show abnormal nerve cell growth, cell death, and deposits of calcium in that area (calcification). Nerve cells within the malformation may demonstrate abnormal growth and are believed to be nonfunctional.

Causes and symptoms

Most people do not realize that they have an AVM unless it hemorrhages enough to produce symptoms. Small AVMs are more likely to hemorrhage. If a hemorrhage occurs, it produces a sudden, severe **headache**. The headache may be focused in one specific area or it may be more general. It can be mistaken for a migraine in some cases. The headache is accompanied by other symptoms, such as **vomiting**, a stiff neck, sleepiness, lethargy, confusion, irritability, or weakness anywhere in the body. Seizures occur in about a quarter of AVM cases. A person may experience decreased, double, or blurred vision. Hemorrhaging from an AVM is generally less dangerous than hemorrhaging from an aneurysm, with a survival rate of 80-90%.

Other symptoms occur less frequently, but sometimes appear alongside major symptoms such as the sudden severe headache. Additional warning signs of a bleeding AVM are impaired speech or smell, **fainting**, facial paralysis, a drooping eyelid, dizziness, and ringing or buzzing in the ears.

Although large AVMs are less likely to hemorrhage, they can induce symptoms based on their mass alone. Large AVMs exert pressure against brain tissue, cause abnormal development in the surrounding brain tissue, and slow down or block blood flow. **Hydrocephalus**, a swelling of brain tissue caused by accumulated fluids, may develop. The warning signs associated with a large non-bleeding AVM are similar to the symptoms of a small malformation that is bleeding. Unexplained headaches, seizures, dizziness, and neurological symptoms, such as sensory changes, are signals that demand medical attention.

Diagnosis

Based on the clinical symptoms such as severe headache and neurological problems, and after a complete **neurologic exam**, a computed tomography scan (CT) of the head will be done. In some cases, a whooshing sound from arteries in the neck or over the eye or jaw (called a bruit), can be heard with a stethoscope. The CT scan will reveal whether there has been bleeding in the brain and can identify AVMs larger than 1 inch (2.5 cm). **Magnetic resonance imaging** (MRI) is also used to identify an AVM. A lumbar puncture, or spinal tap, may follow the MRI or CT scan. A lumbar puncture involves removing a small amount of cerebrospinal fluid from the lower part of the spine. Blood cells or blood breakdown products in the cerebrospinal fluid indicate bleeding.

To pinpoint where the blood is coming from, a cerebral **angiography** is done. This procedure uses x rays to map out the blood vessels in the brain, including the vessels that feed into the malformation. The information gained from angiography complements the MRI and helps distinguish the precise location of the AVM.

Treatment

Neurosurgeons consider several factors before deciding on a treatment option. There is some debate over whether or not to treat AVMs that have not ruptured and are not causing any symptoms. The risks and benefits of proceeding with treatment need to be measured on an individual basis, taking into account factors such as the person's age and general health, as well as the AVM's size and location. Several treatment options are available, both for symptomatic or asymptomatic AVMs. These treatment options may be used alone or in combination.

Surgery

Removing the AVM is the surest way of preventing it from causing future problems. Both small and large AVMs can be handled in surgery. Surgery is recommended for superficial AVMs, but may be too dangerous for deep or very large AVMs. Unless it is an emergency situation, an AVM that has hemorrhaged is treated conservatively for several weeks. Conservative treatment consists of managing the immediate symptoms and allowing the patient's condition to stabilize. Surgery requires **general anesthesia** and a longer period of recuperation than any other treatment option.

Radiation

Radiation is particularly useful to treat small (under 1 in) malformations that are deep within the brain. Ionizing radiation is directed at the malformation, destroying the AVM without damaging the surrounding tissue. Radiation treatment is accomplished in a single session and it is not necessary to open the skull. However, success can only be measured over the course of the following two years. A year after the procedure, 50-75% of treated AVMs are completely blocked; two years after radiation treatment, the percentage increases to 85-95%.

Embolization

Embolization involves plugging up access to the malformation. This technique does not require opening the skull to expose the brain and can be used to treat deep AVMs. Using x-ray images as a guide, a catheter is threaded through the artery in the thigh (femoral artery) to the affected area. The patient remains awake during the procedure and medications can be administered to prevent discomfort. The blood vessel leading into the AVM is assessed for its importance to the rest of the brain before a balloon or other blocking agent is inserted via the catheter. The block chokes off the blood supply to the malformation. There may be a mild headache or **nausea** associated with the procedure, but patients may resume normal activities after leaving the hospital. At least two to three embolization procedures are usually necessary at intervals of two to six weeks. At least a three-day hospital stay is associated with each embolization.

Prognosis

Approximately 10% of AVM cases are fatal. Seizures and neurological changes may be permanent in another 10-30% cases of AVM rupture. If an AVM bleeds once, it is about 20% likely to bleed again in the next year. As time passes from the initial hemorrhage, the risk for further bleeding drops to about 3-4%. If the AVM has not bled, it is possible, but not guaranteed, that it never will. Untreated AVMs can grow larger over time and rarely go away by themselves. Once an AVM is removed and a person has recovered from the procedure, there should be no further symptoms associated with that malformation.

Resources

PERIODICALS

Henning, Mast. "Risk of Spontaneous Hemorrhage after Diagnosis of Cerebral Arteriovenous Malformation." *The Lancet* 350 (October 11, 1997): 1065.

ORGANIZATIONS

American Chronic Pain Association. PO Box 850, Rocklin, CA 95677-0850. (916) 632-0922. < http://members. tripod.com/~widdy/ACPA.html > .

Arteriovenous Malformation Support Group. 168 Six Mile Canyon Road, Dayton, NV 89403. (702) 246-0682.

National Chronic Pain Outreach Association, Inc. P.O. Box 274, Millboro, VA 24460. (540) 997-5004.

Julia Barrett

Arthritis *see* **Juvenile arthritis; Osteoarthritis; Psoriatic arthritis; Rheumatoid arthritis**

Arthrocentesis *see* **Joint fluid analysis**

Arthrogram *see* **Arthrography**

Arthrography

Definition

Arthrograpy is a procedure involving multiple x rays of a joint using a fluoroscope, or a special piece of x-ray equipment which shows an immediate x-ray image. A contrast medium (in this case, a contrast iodine solution) injected into the joint area helps highlight structures of the joint.

Purpose

Frequently, arthrography is ordered to determine the cause of unexplained joint **pain**. This fluoroscopic procedure can show the internal workings of specific joints and outline soft tissue structures. The procedure may also be conducted to identify problems with the ligaments, cartilage, tendons, or the joint capsule of the hip, shoulder, knee, ankle or wrist. An arthrography procedure may locate cysts in the joint area, evaluate problems with the joint's arrangement and function, or indicate the need for **joint replacement** (prostheses). The most commonly studied joints are the knee and shoulder.

Precautions

Patients who are pregnant or may be pregnant should not have this procedure unless the benefits of the findings outweigh the risk of radiation exposure. Patients who are known to be allergic to iodine need to discuss this complication with their physician. Patients who have a known allergy to shellfish are more likely to be allergic to iodine contrast.

Description

Arthrograpy may be referred to as "joint radiography" or "x rays of the joint." The term arthrogram may be used interchangeably with arthrography. The joint area will be cleaned and a local anesthetic will be injected into the tissues around the joint to reduce pain. Next, if fluids are present in the joint, the physician may suction them out (aspirate) with a needle. These fluids may be sent to a laboratory for further study. Contrast agents are then injected into the joint through the same location by attaching the aspirating needle to a syringe containing the contrast medium. The purpose of contrast agents in x-ray procedures is to help highlight details of areas under study by making them opaque. Agents for arthrography are generally air and water-soluble dyes, the most common

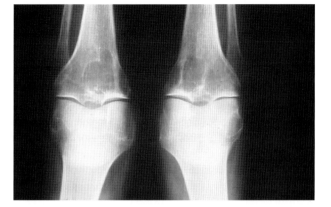

An x-ray image of the knees of a patient with cysts caused by rheumatoid arthritis. The cysts appear as dark areas just below the knee joints. *(Custom Medical Stock Photo. Reproduced by permission.)*

KEY TERMS

Aspirate—Remove fluids by suction, often through a needle.

Contrast (agent, medium)—A substance injected into the body that illuminates certain structures that would otherwise be hard to see on the radiograph (film).

Fluoroscope—A device used in some radiology procedures that provides immediate images and motion on a screen much like those seen at airport baggage security stations.

Radiologist—A medical doctor specially trained in radiology (x ray) interpretation and its use in the diagnosis of diseases and injuries.

X ray—A form of electromagnetic radiation with shorter wavelengths than normal light. X rays can penetrate most structures.

containing iodine. Air and iodine may be used together or independently. After the contrast agent is administered, the site of injection will be sealed and the patient may be asked to move the joint around to distribute the contrast.

Before the contrast medium can be absorbed by the joint itself, several films will be quickly taken under the guidance of the fluoroscope. The patient will be asked to move the joint into a series of positions, keeping still between positioning. Sometimes, the patient will experience some **tingling** or discomfort during the procedure, which is normal and due to the contrast. Following fluoroscopic tracking of the contrast, standard x rays of the area may also be taken. The entire procedure will last about one hour.

Preparation

It is important to discuss any known sensitivity to local anesthetics or iodine prior to this procedure. A physician should explain the procedure and the risks associated with contrast agents and ask the patient to sign an informed consent. If iodine contrast will be administered, the patient may be instructed not to eat before the exam. The timeframe of **fasting** may extend from only 90 minutes prior to the exam up to the night before. There is no other preparation necessary.

Aftercare

The affected joint should be rested for approximately 12 hours following the procedure. The joint may be wrapped in an elastic bandage and the patient should receive instructions on the care and changing of the bandage. Noises in the joint such as cracking or clicking are normal for a few days following arthrography. These noises are the result of liquid in the joints. Swelling may also occur and can be treated with application of ice or cold packs. A mild pain reliever can be used to lessen pain in the first few days. However, if any of these symptoms persist for more than a few days, patients are advised to contact their physician.

Risks

In some patients iodine can cause allergic reactions, ranging from mild **nausea** to severe cardiovascular or nervous system complications. Since the contrast dye is put into a joint, rather than into a vein, allergic reactions are rare. Facilities licensed to perform contrast exams should meet requirements for equipment, supplies and staff training to handle a possible severe reaction. Infection or joint damage are possible, although not frequent, complications of arthrography.

Normal results

A normal arthrography exam will show proper placement of the dye or contrast medium throughout the joint structures, joint space, cartilage and ligaments.

Abnormal results

The abnormal placement of dye may indicate **rheumatoid arthritis**, cysts, joint dislocation, rupture

of the rotator cuff, tears in the ligament and other conditions. The entire lining of the joint becomes opaque from the technique, which allows the radiologist to see abnormalities in the intricate workings of the joint. In the case of recurrent shoulder **dislocations**, arthrography results can be used to evaluate damage. Patients with hip prostheses may receive arthrography to evaluate proper placement or function of their prostheses.

Resources

ORGANIZATIONS

American College of Radiology. 1891 Preston White Drive, Reston, VA 22091. (800) 227-5463. < http:// www.acr.org > .

Arthritis Foundation. 1300 W. Peachtree St., Atlanta, GA 30309. (800) 283-7800. < http://www.arthritis.org > .

Teresa Odle

Arthroplasty

Definition

Arthroplasty is surgery to relieve **pain** and restore range of motion by realigning or reconstructing a joint.

Purpose

The goal of arthroplasty is to restore the function of a stiffened joint and relieve pain. Two types of arthroplastic surgery exist. Joint resection involves removing a portion of the bone from a stiffened joint, creating a gap between the bone and the socket, to improve the range of motion. Scar tissue eventually fills the gap. Pain is relieved and motion is restored, but the joint is less stable.

Interpositional reconstruction is surgery to reshape the joint and add a prosthetic disk between the two bones forming the joint. The prosthesis can be made of plastic and metal or from body tissue such as fascia and skin. When interpositional reconstruction fails, total **joint replacement** may be necessary. Joint replacement is also called total joint arthroplasty.

In recent years, joint replacement has become the operation of choice for most knee and hip problems. Elbow, shoulder, ankle, and finger joints are more likely to be treated with joint resection or interpositional reconstruction.

KEY TERMS

Fascia—Thin connective tissue covering or separating the muscles and internal organs of the body.

Rheumatoid arthritis—A joint disease of unknown origins that may begin at an early age, causing deformity and loss of function in the joints.

Arthroplasty is performed on people suffering from severe pain and disabling joint stiffness that result from **osteoarthritis** or **rheumatoid arthritis**. Joint resection, rather than joint replacement, is more likely to be performed on people with rheumatoid arthritis, especially when the elbow joint is involved. Total joint replacement is usually reserved for people over the age of 60.

Precautions

If both the bone and socket of a joint are damaged, joint replacement is usually the preferred treatment.

Description

Arthroplasty is performed under general or regional anesthesia in a hospital, by an orthopedic surgeon. Certain medical centers specialize in joint surgery and tend to have higher success rates than less specialized centers.

In joint resection, the surgeon makes an incision at the joint, then carefully removes minimum amount of bone necessary to allow free motion. The more bone that remains, the more stable the joint. Ligament attachments are preserved as much as possible. In interpositional reconstruction, both bones of the joint are reshaped, and a disk of material is placed between the bones to prevent their rubbing together. Length of hospital stay depends on which joint is treated, but is normally only a few days.

Preparation

Prior to arthroplasty, all the standard preoperative blood and urine tests are performed. The patient meets with the anesthesiologist to discuss any special conditions that affect the administration of anesthesia.

Aftercare

Patients who have undergone arthroplasty must be careful not to over **stress** or destabilize the joint. Physical therapy is begun immediately. **Antibiotics** are given to prevent infection.

Risks

Joint resection and interpositional reconstruction do not always produce successful results, especially in patients with rheumatoid arthritis. Repeat surgery or total joint replacement may be necessary. As with any major surgery, there is always a risk of an allergic reaction to anesthesia or that **blood clots** will break loose and obstruct the arteries.

Normal results

Most patients recover with improved range of motion in the joint and relief from pain.

Resources

BOOKS

"Joint Replacement." In *Everything You Need to Know About Medical Treatments.* Springhouse, PA: Springhouse Corp., 1996.

OTHER

"Darrach's Procedure." *Wheeless' Textbook of Orthopaedics Page.* < http://www.medmedia.com/ooa1/119.htm >.

Tish Davidson, A.M.

Arthroscopic surgery

Definition

Arthroscopic surgery is a procedure to visualize, diagnose, and treat joint problems. The name is derived from the Greek words *arthron,* which means *joint,* and *skopein,* which means *to look at.*

Purpose

Arthroscopic surgery is used to identify, monitor, and diagnose joint injuries and disease; or to remove bone or cartilage or repair tendons or ligaments. Diagnostic arthroscopic surgery is performed when medical history, physical exam, x rays, and other tests such as MRIs or CTs don't provide a definitive diagnosis.

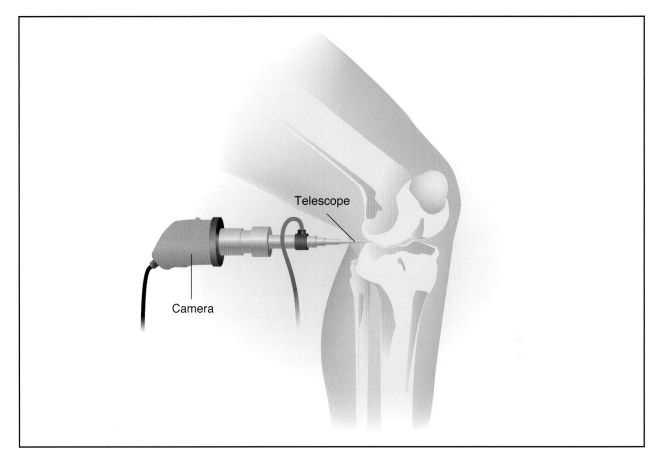

An arthroscope uses optical fibers to form an image of the damged cartilage, which it sends to a television monitor that helps the surgeon perform surgery. *(Illustration by Argosy Inc.)*

Precautions

Diagnostic arthroscopic surgery should not be performed unless conservative treatment does not fix the problem.

Description

In arthroscopic surgery, an orthopedic surgeon uses an arthroscope, a fiber-optic instrument, to see the inside of a joint. After making an incision about the size of a buttonhole in the patient's skin, a sterile sodium chloride solution is injected to distend the joint. The arthroscope, an instrument the size of a pencil, is then inserted into the joint. The arthroscope has a lens and a lighting system through which the structures inside the joint are transmitted to a miniature television camera attached to the end of the arthroscope. The surgeon uses irrigation and suction to remove blood and debris from the joint before examining it. Other incisions may be made in order to see other parts of the joint or to insert additional instruments. Looking at the interior of the joint on the television screen, the surgeon can then determine the amount or type of injury and, if necessary, take a biopsy specimen or repair or correct the problem. Arthroscopic surgery can be used to remove floating bits of cartilage and treat minor tears and other disorders. When the procedure is finished, the arthroscope is removed and the joint is irrigated. The site of the incision is bandaged.

Arthroscopic surgery is used to diagnose and treat joint problems, most commonly in the knee, but also in the shoulder, elbow, ankle, wrist, and hip. Some of the most common joint problems seen with an arthroscope are:

- inflammation in the knee, shoulder, elbow, wrist, or ankle

- injuries to the shoulder (rotator cuff tendon tears, impingement syndrome, and recurrent dislocations), knee (cartilage tears, wearing down of or injury to the cartilage cushion, and anterior cruciate ligament tears with instability), and wrist (carpal tunnel syndrome)

• loose bodies of bone and/or cartilage in the knee, shoulder, elbow, ankle, or wrist

Corrective arthroscopic surgery is performed with instruments that are inserted through additional incisions. Arthritis can sometimes be treated with arthroscopic surgery. Some problems are treated with a combination of arthroscopic and standard surgery.

Also called **arthroscopy**, the procedure is performed in a hospital or outpatient surgical facility. The type of anesthesia (local, spinal, or general) and the length of the procedure depends on the joint operated on and the complexity of the suspected problem. Arthroscopic surgery rarely takes more than an hour. Most patients who have arthroscopic surgery are released that same day; some patients stay in the hospital overnight.

Considered the most important orthopedic development in the 20th century, arthroscopic surgery is widely used. The use of arthroscopic surgery on famous athletes has been well publicized. It is estimated that 80% of orthopedic surgeons practice arthroscopic surgery. Arthroscopic surgery was initially a diagnostic tool used prior to open surgery, but as better instruments and techniques were developed, it began to be used to actually treat a variety of joint problems. New techniques currently under development are likely to lead to other joints being treated with arthroscopic surgery in the future. Recently, lasers were introduced in arthroscopic surgery and other new energy sources are being explored. Lasers and electromagnetic radiation can repair rather than resect injuries and may be more cost effective than instruments.

Preparation

Before the procedure, blood and urine studies and x rays of the joint will be conducted.

Aftercare

Immediately after the procedure, the patient will spend several hours in the recovery room. An ice pack will be put on the joint that was operated on for up to 48 hours after the procedure. Pain medicine, prescription or non-prescription, will be given. The morning after the surgery, the dressing can be removed and replaced by adhesive strips. The patient should call his/her doctor upon experiencing an increase in **pain**, swelling, redness, drainage or bleeding at the site of the surgery, signs of infection (**headache**, muscle aches, **dizziness**, **fever**), or **nausea** or **vomiting**.

It takes several days for the puncture **wounds** to heal, and several weeks for the joint to fully recover. Many patients can resume their daily activities, including going back to work, within a few days of the procedure. A **rehabilitation** program, including physical therapy, may be suggested to speed recovery and improve the future functioning of the joint.

Risks

Complications are rare in arthroscopic surgery, occurring in less than 1% of patients. These include infection and inflammation, blood vessel clots, damage to blood vessels or nerves, and instrument breakage.

Resources

PERIODICALS

Wilkinson, Todd. "Pop, Crackle, Snap." *Women's Sports & Fitness* (April 1998): 68.

Lori De Milto

Arthroscopy

Definition

Arthroscopy is the examination of a joint, specifically, the inside structures. The procedure is performed by inserting a specifically designed illuminated device into the joint through a small incision. This instrument is called an arthroscope. The procedure of arthroscopy is primarily associated with the process of diagnosis. However, when actual repair is performed, the procedure is called **arthroscopic surgery**.

Purpose

Arthroscopy is used primarily by doctors who specialize in treating disorders of the bones and

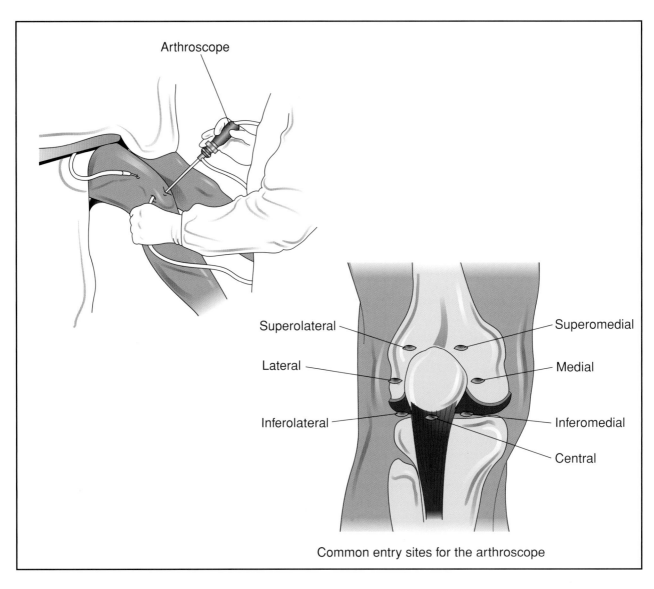

Arthroscope

Superolateral

Superomedial

Lateral

Medial

Inferolateral

Inferomedial

Central

Common entry sites for the arthroscope

Arthroscopy is primarily used to help diagnose joint problems. This procedure, most commonly associated with knee and shoulder problems, allows accurate examination and diagnosis of damaged joint ligaments, surfaces, and other related joint structures. The illustration above indicates the most common entry sites, or portals, in knee arthroscopy. *(Illustration by Electronic Illustrators Group.)*

related structures (orthopedics) to help diagnose joint problems. Once described as essential for those who primarily care for athletic injuries, arthroscopy is now a technique commonly used by orthopedic surgeons for the treatment of patients of all ages. This procedure is most commonly used to diagnose knee and shoulder problems, although the elbow, hip, wrist, and ankle may also be examined with an arthroscope.

A joint is a complex system. Within a joint, ligaments attach bones to other bones, tendons attach muscles to bones, cartilage lines and helps protect the ends of bones, and a special fluid (synovial fluid) cushions and lubricates the structures. Looking inside the joint allows the doctors to see exactly which structures are damaged. Arthroscopy also permits earlier diagnosis of many types of joint problems which had been difficult to detect in previous years.

Precautions

Most arthroscopic procedures today are performed in same-day surgery centers where the patient is admitted just before surgery. A few hours following the procedure, the patient is allowed to return home,

KEY TERMS

Hemarthrosis—A condition of blood within a joint.

Pulmonary embolus—Blockage of an artery of the lung by foreign matter such as fat, tumor, tissue, or a clot originating from a vein.

Thrombophlebitis—Inflamation of a vein with the formation of a thrombus or clot.

although usually someone else must drive. Depending on the type of anesthesia used, the patient may be told not to eat for several hours before arriving. Before the procedure, the anesthesiologist will ask if the patient has any known **allergies** to local or general anesthetics. Airway obstruction is always possible in any patient who receives a **general anesthesia**. Because of this, oxygen, suction, and monitoring equipment must be available. The patient's cardiac status should always be monitored in the event that any cardiac abnormalities arise during the arthroscopy.

Description

The arthroscope is an instrument used to look directly into the joint. It contains magnifying lenses and glass-coated fibers that send concentrated light into the joint. A camera attached to the arthroscope allows the surgeon to see a clear image of the joint. This image is then transferred to a monitor located in the operating room at the time of the arthroscopy. This video technology is also important for documentation of the arthroscopic procedure. For example, if the surgeon decides after the arthroscopic examination that a conventional approach to surgically expose or "open" the joint (arthrotomy) must be used, a good photographic record will be useful when the surgeon returns to execute the final surgical plan.

The procedure requires the surgeon to make several small incisions (portals) through the skin's surface into the joint. Through one or two of the portals, a large-bore needle, called a cannula, is attached to tubing and inserted into the joint. The joint is inflated with a sterile saline solution to expand the joint and ensure clear arthroscopic viewing. Often, following a recent traumatic injury to a joint, the joint's natural fluid may be cloudy, making interior viewing of the joint difficult. In this condition, a constant flow of the saline solution is necessary. This inflow of saline solution may be through the cannula with the outflow

through the arthroscope, or the positions may be reversed. The arthroscope is placed through one of the portals to view and evaluate the condition of the joint.

Preparation

Before an arthroscopy can take place, the surgeon completes a thorough medical history and evaluation. Important for the accuracy of this diagnostic procedure, a medical history and evaluation may discover other disorders of the joint or body parts, proving the procedure unnecessary. This is always an important preliminary step, because **pain** can often be referred to a joint from another area of the body. Anatomical models and pictures are useful aids to explain to the patient the proposed arthroscopy and what the surgeon may be looking at specifically.

Proper draping of the body part is important to prevent contamination from instruments used in arthroscopy, such as the camera, light cords, and inflow and outflow drains placed in the portals. Draping packs used in arthroscopy include disposable paper gowns and drapes with adhesive backing. The surgeon may also place a tourniquet above the joint to temporarily block blood flow to the area during the arthroscopic exam.

General or **local anesthesia** may be used during arthroscopy. Local anesthesia is usually used because it reduces the risk of lung and heart complications and allows the patient to go home sooner. The local anesthetic may be injected in small amounts in multiple locations in skin and joint tissues in a process called infiltration. In other cases, the anesthetic is injected into the spinal cord or a main nerve supplying the area. This process is called a "block," and it blocks all sensation below the main trunk of the nerve. For example, a femoral block anesthetizes the leg from the thigh down (its name comes from femur, the thighbone). Most patients are comfortable once the skin, muscles, and other tissues around the joint are numbed by the anesthetic; however, some patients are also given a sedative if they express **anxiety** about the procedure. (It's important for the patient to remain still during the arthroscopic examination.)

General anesthesia, in which the patient becomes unconcious, may be used if the procedure may be unusually complicated or painful. For example, people who have relatively "tight" joints may be candidates for general anesthesia because the procedure may take longer and cause more discomfort.

Aftercare

The portals are closed by small tape strips or stitches and covered with dressings and a bandage. The patient spends a short amount of time in the recovery room after arthroscopy. Most patients can go home after about an hour in the recovery room. Pain medication may be prescribed for a short period; however, many patients find various over-the-counter pain relievers sufficient.

Following the surgical procedure, the patient needs to be aware of the signs of infection, which include redness, warmth, excessive pain, and swelling. The risk of infection increases if the incisions become wet too early following surgery. Because of this, it is good practice to cover the joint with plastic (for example, a plastic bag) while showering after arthroscopy.

The use of crutches is commonplace after arthroscopy, with progression to independent walking on an "as tolerated" basis by the patient. Generally, a **rehabilitation** program, supervised by a physical therapist, follows shortly after the arthroscopy to help the patient regain mobility and strength of the affected joint and limb.

Risks

The incidence of complications is low compared to the high number of arthroscopic procedures performed every year. Possible complications include infection, swelling, damage to the tissues in the joint, **blood clots** in the leg veins (**thrombophlebitis**), leakage of blood into the joint (hemarthrosis), blood clots that move to the lung (pulmonary embolus), and injury to the nerves around the joint.

Normal results

The goal of arthroscopy is to diagnose a joint problem causing pain and/or restrictions in normal joint function. For example, arthroscopy can be a useful tool in locating a tear in the joint surface of the knee or locating a torn ligament of the shoulder. Arthroscopic examination is often followed by arthroscopic surgery performed to repair the problem with appropriate arthroscopic tools. The final result is to decrease pain, increase joint mobility, and thereby improve the overall quality of the patient's activities of daily living.

Abnormal results

Less optimal results that may require further treatment include adhesive capsulitis. In this condition, the joint capsule that naturally forms around the joint becomes thickened, forming **adhesions**. This results in a stiff and less mobile joint. This problem is frequently corrected by manipulation and mobilization of the joint with the patient placed under general anesthesia.

Resources

PERIODICALS

Glassman, Scott. "Advances in Treating Shoulder Injuries." *Advanced Magazine for Physical Therapists* (December 1997): 10-12.

Jeffrey P. Larson, RPT

Artificial insemination *see* **Infertility therapies**

Asbestosis

Definition

Asbestosis is chronic, progressive inflammation of the lung. It is not contagious.

Description

Asbestosis is a consequence of prolonged exposure to large quantities of asbestos, a material once widely used in construction, insulation, and manufacturing. When asbestos is inhaled, fibers penetrate the breathing passages and irritate, fill, inflame, and scar lung tissue. In advanced asbestosis,, the lungs shrink, stiffen, and become honeycombed (riddled with tiny holes).

Legislation has reduced use of asbestos in the United States, but workers who handle automobile brake shoe linings, boiler insulation, ceiling acoustic tiles, electrical equipment, and fire-resistant materials are still exposed to the substance. Asbestos is used in the production of paints and plastics. Significant amounts can be released into the atmosphere when old buildings or boats are razed or remodeled.

Asbestosis is most common in men over 40 who have worked in asbestos-related occupations. Smokers or heavy drinkers have the greatest risk of developing this disease. Between 1968 and 1992, more than 10,000 Americans over the age of 15 died as a result of asbestosis. Nearly 25% of those who died lived in California or New Jersey, and most of them had worked in the construction or shipbuilding trades.

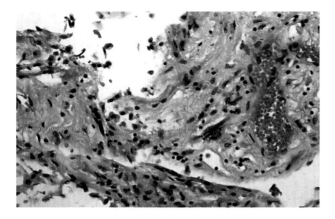

Micrograph of asbestos fibers embedded in lung tissue.
(Photograph by Dr. E. Walker, Custom Medical Stock Photo. Reproduced by permission.)

Causes and symptoms

Occupational exposure is the most common cause of asbestosis, but the condition also strikes people who inhale asbestos fiber or who are exposed to waste products from plants near their homes. Family members can develop the disease as a result of inhaling particles of asbestos dust that cling to workers' clothes.

It is rare for asbestosis to develop in anyone who hasn't been exposed to large amounts of asbestos on a regular basis for at least 10 years. Symptoms of the disease do not usually appear until 15–20 years after initial exposure to asbestos.

The first symptom of asbestosis is usually shortness of breath following **exercise** or other physical activity. The early stages of the disease are also characterized by a dry **cough** and a generalized feeling of illness.

As the disease progresses and lung damage increases, **shortness of breath** occurs even when the patient is at rest. Recurrent respiratory infections and coughing up blood are common. So is swelling of the feet, ankles, or hands. Other symptoms of advanced asbestosis include chest pain, hoarseness, and restless sleep. Patients who have asbestosis often have clubbed (widened and thickened) fingers. Other potential complications include heart failure, collapsed (deflated) lung, and **pleurisy** (inflammation of the membrane that protects the lung).

Diagnosis

Screening of at-risk workers can reveal lung inflammation and lesions characteristic of asbestosis. Patients' medical histories can identify occupations, hobbies, or other situations likely to involve exposure to asbestos fibers.

X rays can show shadows or spots on the lungs or an indistinct or shaggy outline of the heart that suggests the presence of asbestosis. Blood tests are used to measure concentrations of oxygen and carbon dioxide. Pulmonary function tests can be used to assess a patient's ability to inhale and exhale, and a computed tomography scan (CT) of the lungs can show flat, raised patches associated with advanced asbestosis.

Treatment

The goal of treatment is to help patients breathe more easily, prevent colds and other respiratory infections, and control complications associated with advanced disease. Ultrasonic, cool-mist humidifiers or controlled coughing can loosen bronchial secretions.

Regular exercise helps maintain and improve lung capacity. Although temporary bed rest may be recommended, patients are encouraged to resume their regular activities as soon as they can.

Anyone who develops symptoms of asbestosis should see a family physician or lung disease specialist. A doctor should be notified if someone who has been diagnosed with asbestosis:

- coughs up blood
- continues to lose weight
- is short of breath
- has chest **pain**
- develops a sudden **fever** of 101°F (38.3°C) or higher
- develops unfamiliar, unexplained symptoms

Prognosis

Asbestosis can't be cured, but its symptoms can be controlled. Doctors don't know why the health of some patients deteriorates and the condition of others remain the same, but believe the difference may be due to varying exposures of asbestos. People with asbestosis who smoke, particularly those who smoke more than one pack of cigarettes each day, are at increased risk for developing lung **cancer** and should be strongly advised to quit smoking.

Prevention

Workers in asbestosis-related industries should have regular x rays to determine whether their lungs are healthy. A person whose lung x ray shows a shadow should eliminate asbestos exposure even if no symptoms of the condition have appeared.

Anyone who works with asbestos should wear a protective mask or a hood with a clean-air supply and obey recommended procedures to control asbestos dust. Anyone who is at risk of developing asbestosis should:

- not smoke
- be vaccinated against **influenza** and **pneumonia**
- exercise regularly to maintain cardiopulmonary fitness
- avoid crowds and people who have respiratory infections

A person who has asbestosis should exercise regularly, relax, and conserve energy whenever necessary.

Resources

BOOKS

Burton, George G., John E. Hodgkin, and Jeffrey J. Ward, editors. *Respiratory Care: A Guide to Clinical Practice.* 4th ed. Philadelphia: Lippincott, 1997.

ORGANIZATIONS

American Lung Association. 1740 Broadway, New York, NY 10019. (800) 586-4872. < http://www.lungusa.org > .

Maureen Haggerty

Ascariasis *see* **Roundworm infections**

Ascending cholangitis *see* **Cholangitis**

Ascending contrast phlebography *see* **Venography**

Ascites

Definition

Ascites is an abnormal accumulation of fluid in the abdomen.

Description

Rapidly developing (acute) ascites can occur as a complication of trauma, perforated ulcer, appendicitis, or inflammation of the colon or other tube-shaped organ (**diverticulitis**). This condition can also develop when intestinal fluids, bile, pancreatic juices, or bacteria invade or inflame the smooth, transparent membrane that lines the inside of the abdomen (peritoneum). However, ascites is more often associated with **liver disease** and other long-lasting (chronic) conditions.

Types of ascites

Cirrhosis, which is responsible for 80% of all instances of ascites in the United States, triggers a series of disease-producing changes that weaken the kidney's ability to excrete sodium in the urine.

Pancreatic ascites develops when a cyst that has thick, fibrous walls (pseudocyst) bursts and permits pancreatic juices to enter the abdominal cavity.

Chylous ascites has a milky appearance caused by lymph that has leaked into the abdominal cavity. Although chylous ascites is sometimes caused by trauma, abdominal surgery, **tuberculosis**, or another peritoneal infection, it is usually a symptom of lymphoma or some other **cancer**.

Cancer causes 10% of all instances of ascites in the United States. It is most commonly a consequence of disease that originates in the peritoneum (peritoneal carcinomatosis) or of cancer that spreads (metastasizes) from another part of the body.

Endocrine and renal ascites are rare disorders. Endocrine ascites, sometimes a symptom of an endocrine system disorder, also affects women who are taking fertility drugs. Renal ascites develops when blood levels of albumin dip below normal. Albumin is the major protein in blood plasma. It functions to keep fluid inside the blood vessels.

Causes and symptoms

Causes

The two most important factors in the production of ascites due to chronic liver disease are:

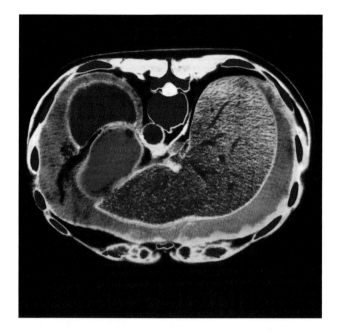

A computed tomography (CT) scan of an axial section through the abdomen, showing ascites. At right is the liver occupying much of the abdomen; the stomach and spleen are also seen. Around these organs is fluid giving rise to this condition. *(Custom Medical Stock Photo. Reproduced by permission.)*

KEY TERMS

Computed tomography scan (CT)—An imaging technique in which cross-sectional x rays of the body are compiled to create a three-dimensional image of the body's internal structures.

Interferon—A protein formed when cells are exposed to a virus. Interferon causes other noninfected cells to develop translation inhibitory protein (TIP). TIP blocks viruses from infecting new cells.

Paracentesis—A procedure in which fluid is drained from a body cavity by means of a catheter placed through an incision in the skin.

Systemic lupus erythematosus—An inflammatory disease that affects many body systems, including the skin, blood vessels, kidneys, and nervous system. It is characterized, in part, by arthritis, skin rash, weakness, and fatigue.

Ultrasonography—A test using sound waves to measure blood flow. Gel is applied to a hand-held transducer that is pressed against the patient's body. Images are displayed on a monitor.

- Low levels of albumin in the blood that cause a change in the pressure necessary to prevent fluid exchange (osmotic pressure). This change in pressure allows fluid to seep out of the blood vessels.

- An increase in the pressure within the branches of the portal vein that run through liver (portal **hypertension**). Portal hypertension is caused by the scarring that occurs in cirrhosis. Blood that cannot flow through the liver because of the increased pressure leaks into the abdomen and causes ascites.

Other conditions that contribute to ascites development include:

- hepatitis

- heart or kidney failure

- inflammation and fibrous hardening of the sac that contains the heart (constrictive pericarditis)

Persons who have **systemic lupus erythematosus** but do not have liver disease or portal hypertension occasionally develop ascites. Depressed thyroid activity sometimes causes pronounced ascites, but inflammation of the pancreas (**pancreatitis**) rarely causes significant accumulations of fluid.

Symptoms

Small amounts of fluid in the abdomen do not usually produce symptoms. Massive accumulations may cause:

- rapid weight gain

- abdominal discomfort and distention

- shortness of breath

- swollen ankles

Diagnosis

Skin stretches tightly across an abdomen that contains large amounts of fluid. The navel bulges or lies flat, and the fluid makes a dull sound when the doctor taps the abdomen. Ascitic fluid may cause the flanks to bulge.

Physical examination generally enables doctors to distinguish ascites from pregnancy, intestinal gas, obesity, or ovarian tumors. Ultrasound or **computed tomography scans (CT)** can detect even small amounts of fluid. Laboratory analysis of fluid extracted by inserting a needle through the abdominal wall (diagnostic paracentesis) can help identify the cause of the accumulation.

Treatment

Reclining minimizes the amount of salt the kidneys absorb, so treatment generally starts with bed rest and a low-salt diet. Urine-producing drugs (diuretics) may be prescribed if initial treatment is ineffective. The weight and urinary output of patients using diuretics must be carefully monitored for signs of :

- hypovolemia (massive loss of blood or fluid)

- azotemia (abnormally high blood levels of nitrogen-bearing materials)

- potassium imbalance

- high sodium concentration. If the patient consumes more salt than the kidneys excrete, increased doses of **diuretics** should be prescribed

Moderate-to-severe accumulations of fluid are treated by draining large amounts of fluid (large-volume paracentesis) from the patient's abdomen. This procedure is safer than diuretic therapy. It causes fewer complications and requires a shorter hospital stay.

Large-volume paracentesis is also the preferred treatment for massive ascites. Diuretics are sometimes used to prevent new fluid accumulations, and the procedure may be repeated periodically.

Alternative treatment

Dietary alterations, focused on reducing salt intake, should be a part of the treatment. In less severe cases, herbal diuretics like dandelion (*Taraxacum officinale*) can help eliminate excess fluid and provide potassium. Potassium-rich foods like low-fat yogurt, mackerel, cantaloupe, and baked potatoes help balance excess sodium intake.

Prognosis

The prognosis depends upon the condition that is causing the ascites. Carcinomatous ascites has a very bad prognosis. However, salt restriction and diuretics can control ascites caused by liver disease in many cases.

Therapy should also be directed towards the underlying disease that produces the ascites. Cirrhosis should be treated by abstinence from alcohol and appropriate diet. The new interferon agents maybe helpful in treating chronic hepatitis.

Prevention

Modifying or restricting use of salt can prevent most cases of recurrent ascites.

Resources

BOOKS

Berkow, Robert, editor. *The Merck Manual of Medical Information*. Whitehouse Station, NJ: Merck Research Laboratories, 1997.

ORGANIZATIONS

American Liver Foundation. 1425 Pompton Ave., Cedar Grove, NJ 07009. (800) 223-0179. <http://www.liverfoundation.org>.

OTHER

"Hepatic and Liver Disorders." *The Meck Page*. April 20, 1998. <http://www.merck.com>.

Maureen Haggerty

Ascorbic acid deficiency *see* **Scurvy**

ASD *see* **Atrial septal defect**

Asian American health *see* **Minority health**

Asian flu *see* **Influenza**

Aspartate aminotransferase test

Definition

The Aspartate aminotransferase test measures levels of AST, an enzyme released into the blood when certain organs or tissues, particularly the liver and heart, are injured. Aspartate aminotransferase (AST) is also known as serum glutamic oxaloacetic transaminase (SGOT).

Purpose

The determination of AST levels aids primarily in the diagnosis of **liver disease**. In the past, the AST test was used to diagnose **heart attack** (myocardial infarction or MI) but more accurate blood tests have largely replaced it for cardiac purposes.

Description

AST is determined by analysis of a blood sample, usually from taken from a venipuncture site at the bend of the elbow.

AST is found in the heart, liver, skeletal muscle, kidney, pancreas, spleen, lung, red blood cells, and brain tissue. When disease or injury affects these tissues, the cells are destroyed and AST is released into the bloodstream. The amount of AST is directly

KEY TERMS

Cirrhosis—Disease of the liver caused by chronic damage to its cells.

Myocardial infarction—Commonly known as a heart attack. Sudden death of part of the heart muscle, characterized, in most cases, by severe, unremitting chest pain.

related to the number of cells affected by the disease or injury, but the level of elevation depends on the length of time that the blood is tested after the injury. Serum AST levels become elevated eight hours after cell injury, peak at 24-36 hours, and return to normal in three to seven days. If the cellular injury is chronic (ongoing), AST levels will remain elevated.

One of the most important uses for AST determination has formerly been in the diagnosis of a heart attack, or MI. AST can assist in determining the timing and extent of a recent MI, although it is less specific than creatine phosphokinase (CPK), CKMB, myglobin, troponins, and lactic dehydrogenase (LDH). Assuming no further cardiac injury occurs, the AST level rises within 6-10 hours after an acute attack, peaks at 12-48 hours, and returns to normal in three to four days. Myocardial injuries such as **angina** (chest **pain**) or **pericarditis** (inflammation of the pericardium, the membrane around the heart) do not increase AST levels.

AST is also a valuable aid in the diagnosis of liver disease. Although not specific for liver disease, it can be used in combination with other enzymes to monitor the course of various liver disorders. Chronic, silent hepatitis (**hepatitis C**) is sometimes the cause of elevated AST. In **alcoholic hepatitis**, caused by excessive alcohol ingestion, AST values are usually moderately elevated; in acute viral hepatitis, AST levels can rise to over 20 times normal. Acute extrahepatic (outside the liver) obstruction (e.g. gallstone), produces AST levels that can quickly rise to 10 times normal, and then rapidly fall. In cases of **cirrhosis**, the AST level is related to the amount of active inflammation of the liver. Determination of AST also assists in early recognition of toxic hepatitis that results from exposure to drugs toxic to the liver, like **acetaminophen** and cholesterol lowering medications.

Other disorders or diseases in which the AST determination can be valuable include acute **pancreatitis**, muscle disease, trauma, severe burn, and **infectious mononucleosis**.

Preparation

The physician may require discontinuation of any drugs that might affect the test. These types include such drugs as antihypertensives (for treatment of high blood pressure), coumarin-type anticoagulants (blood-thinning drugs), digitalis, erythromycin (an antibiotic), **oral contraceptives**, and opiates, among others. The patient may also need to cut back on strenuous activities temporarily, because **exercise** can also elevate AST for a day or two.

Risks

Risks for this test are minimal, but may include slight bleeding from the blood-drawing site, **fainting** or feeling lightheaded after venipuncture, or hematoma (blood accumulating under the puncture site).

Normal results

Normal ranges for the AST are laboratory-specific, but can range from 3-45 units/L (units per liter).

Abnormal results

Striking elevations of AST (400-4000 units/L) are found in almost all forms of acute hepatic necrosis, such as viral hepatitis and carbon tetrachloride **poisoning**. In alcoholics, even moderate doses of the analgesic acetaminophen have caused extreme elevations (1, 960-29, 700 units/L). Moderate rises of AST are seen in **jaundice**, cirrhosis, and metastatic carcinoma. Approximately 80% of patients with infectious mononucleosis show elevations in the range of 100-600 units/L.

Resources

BOOKS

Pagana, Kathleen Deska. *Mosby's Manual of Diagnostic and Laboratory Tests.* St. Louis: Mosby, Inc., 1998.

Janis O. Flores

Asperger's syndrome *see* **Pervasive developmental disorders**

Aspergilloma *see* **Aspergillosis**

Aspergillosis

Definition

Aspergillosis refers to several forms of disease caused by a fungus in the genus *Aspergillus*. Aspergillosis fungal infections can occur in the ear canal, eyes, nose, sinus cavities, and lungs. In some individuals, the infection can even invade bone and the membranes that enclose the brain and spinal cord (**meningitis**).

Description

Aspergillosis is primarily an infection of the lungs caused by the inhalation of airborne spores of the fungus *Aspergillus*. Spores are the small particles that most fungi use to reproduce. Although virtually everyone is exposed to this fungus in their daily environment, it rarely causes disease. When *Aspergillus* does cause disease, however, it usually occurs in those individuals with weakened immune systems (immunocompromised) or who have a history of respiratory ailments. Because it does not present distinctive symptoms, aspergillosis is generally thought to be underdiagnosed and underreported. Furthermore, many patients with the more severe forms of aspergillosis tend to have multiple, complex health problems, such as **AIDS** or a blood disorder like leukemia, which can further complicate diagnosis and treatment.

Once considered particularly rare, the incidence of reported aspergillosis has risen somewhat with the development of more sophisticated methods of diagnosis and advances made in other areas of medicine, such as with the increased use of certain chemotherapeutic and corticosteroid drugs that are extremely useful in treating various types of **cancer** but that decrease the individual's immune response, making them more susceptible to other diseases like aspergillosis.

Our advanced ability to perform tissue and organ transplants has also increased the number of people vulnerable to fungal infections. Transplant recipients, particularly those receiving bone marrow or heart transplants, are highly susceptible to *Aspergillus*, which may be circulating in the hospital air.

Aspergillosis can be a serious, potentially deadly threat for two primary reasons:

- Aspergillosis usually occurs in those individuals who are already ill or have weakened immune systems, such as patients who have undergone **chemotherapy** for cancer.

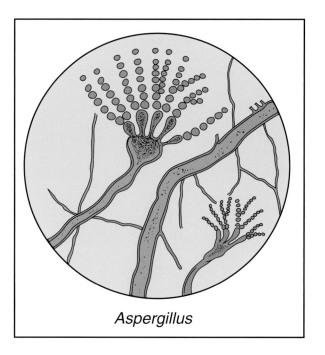

Aspergillus

Aspergillosis is an infection of the lungs caused by inhalation of airborne spores of the fungus ***Aspergillus***. *(Illustration by Electronic Illustrators Group).*

KEY TERMS

Antibody—A specific protein produced by the immune system in response to a specific foreign protein or particle called an antigen.

Aspergilloma—A ball or mass made of *Aspergillus* fungi that can form in the lungs of patients with suppressed immune systems.

Bronchial lavage—A procedure that involves repeatedly washing the inside of the bronchial tubes of the lung.

Hemoptysis—Spitting up blood from the lungs or sputum stained with blood.

Immunocompromised—A state in which the immune system is suppressed or not functioning properly.

Meningitis—Inflammation of the membranes covering the brain and spinal cord, called the meninges.

Nebulizer—A device that produces an extremely fine mist that is readily inhalable.

Spores—The small, thick-walled reproductive structures of fungi.

Sputum—Mucus and other matter coughed up from the airways.

- None of the currently available antifungal drugs are reliably effective against *Aspergillus*.

Causes and symptoms

Airborne *Aspergillus* spores enter the body primarily through inhalation but can also lodge in the ear or eye. Normally functioning immune systems are generally able to cope without consequent development of aspergillosis.

It is important to make distinctions between the various forms of aspergillosis, as the treatment and prognosis varies considerably among types. Aspergillosis as a diagnosis refers to three general forms:

- Allergic bronchopulmonary aspergillosis (ABPA) is seen in patients with long-standing asthma, particularly in patients taking oral **corticosteroids** for a long period of time. This is usually the least serious and most treatable form.

- Aspergilloma refers to the mass formed when fungal spores settle into or colonize areas of the lung that have been pitted and scarred as a result of tuberculosis or prior **pneumonia**. There are several available treatments, although the success rate varies with each treatment.

- Invasive fungal infection refers to rare cases in which the fungus spreads throughout the body via the blood stream and invades other organ systems. Once established, invasive fungal infections are extremely difficult to cure and, as a result, the associated **death** rate is extremely high.

Diagnosis

Aspergillosis can be quite difficult to diagnose because the symptoms, such as coughing and **wheezing**, if present at all, are common to many respiratory disorders. Furthermore, blood and sputum cultures are not very helpful. The presence of *Aspergillus* is so common, even in asthmatics, that a positive culture alone is insufficient for a diagnosis. Other, potentially more useful, screening tools include examining the sample obtained after repeatedly washing the bronchial tubes of the lung with water (bronchial lavage), but examining a tissue sample (biopsy) is the most reliable diagnostic tool. Researchers are currently attempting to develop a practical, specific, and rapid blood test that would confirm *Aspergillus* infection.

Signs of ABPA include a worsening of bronchial **asthma** accompanied by a low-grade fever. Brown flecks or clumps may be seen in the sputum. Pulmonary function tests may show decreased blood flow, suggesting an obstruction within the lungs. Elevated blood levels of an antibody produced in response to *Aspergillus* and of certain immune system cells may indicate a specific allergic-type immune system response.

A fungal mass (aspergilloma) in the lung usually does not produce clear symptoms and is generally diagnosed when seen on chest x rays. However, 70% or more of patients spit up blood from the lungs (**hemoptysis**) at least once, and this may become repetitive and serious. Hemoptysis, then, is another indication that the patient may be suffering from an aspergilloma.

In patients with lowered immune systems who are at risk for developing invasive aspergillosis, the physician may use a combination of blood culture with visual diagnostic techniques, such as computed tomography scans (CT) and radiography, to arrive at a likely diagnosis.

Treatment

The treatment method selected depends on the form of aspergillosis. ABPA can usually be treated with many of the same drugs used to treat asthma, such as systemic steroids. Long-term therapy may be required, however, to prevent recurrence. Antifungal agents are not recommended in the treatment of ABPA. In cases of aspergilloma, it may become necessary to surgically remove or reduce the size of a fungal mass, especially if the patient continues to spit up blood. In aspergillosis cases affecting the nose and nasal sinuses, surgery may also be required.

In non-ABPA cases, the use of antifungal drugs may be indicated. In such cases, amphotericin B (Fungizone) is the first-line therapy. The prescribed dose will depend on the patient's condition but usually begins with a small test dose and then escalates. Less than one-third of patients are likely to respond to amphotericin B, and its side effects often limit its use. For patients who do not respond to oral amphotericin B, another option is a different formulation of the same drug called liposomal amphotericin B.

For patients who fail to respond or who cannot tolerate amphotericin B, another drug called itraconazole (Sporanox), given 400-600 mg daily, has also been approved. Treatment generally lasts about 3 months. Giving itraconazole can produce adverse reactions if prescribed in combination with certain other drugs by increasing the concentrations of both drugs in the blood and creating a potentially life-threatening situation. Even antacids can significantly affect itraconazole levels. As a result, drug levels must be continually monitored to ensure that absorption is occurring at acceptable levels.

Two other methods of treatment are being studied: direct instillation of an antifungal agent into the lungs and administration of antifungals using a nebulizer. Instilling or injecting amphotericin B or itraconazole directly into the lung cavity or into the fungal ball (aspergilloma) itself has been helpful in stopping episodes of hemoptysis, but not in preventing future recurrences. Furthermore, many patients with aspergillomas are poor risks for surgery because their lung function is already compromised. As a result, instillation of a fungal agent should only be considered in those who have significant hempotysis.

A popular method of treating some respiratory disorders is to add a liquid drug to another carrier liquid and aerosolize or produce a fine mist that can be inhaled into the lungs through a device called a nebulizer. However, this has not yet been shown to improve the patient's condition in cases of aspergillosis, possibly because the drug is not reaching the aspergilloma.

At this point, preventative therapy for aspergillosis is not suggested for susceptible individuals, primarily because overuse of the drugs used to fight fungal infections may lead to the development of drug-resistant aspergillosis against which current antifungal drugs are no longer effective.

Prognosis

The likelihood of recovery from aspergillosis depends on any underlying medical conditions, the patient's general health, and the specific type of aspergillosis. If the problem is based on an allergic response, as in ABPA, the patient will likely respond well to systemic steroids.

Patients who require **lung surgery**, especially those who have problems with coughing up blood, have a mortality rate of about 7-14%, and complications or recurrence may result in a higher overall death rate. However, by treating aspergilloma with other, non-surgical methods, that risk rises to 26%, making surgery a better option in some cases.

Unfortunately, the prognosis for the most serious form, invasive aspergillosis, is quite poor, largely because these patients have little resilience due to their underlying disorders. Death rates have ranged from about 50% in some studies to as high as 95% for bone-marrow recipients and patients with AIDS. The course of the illness can be rapid, resulting in death within a few months of diagnosis.

Prevention

Fungal infection by *Aspergillus* presents a major challenge, particularly in the patient with a suppressed immune system (immunocompromised). Hospitals and government health agencies continually seek ways to minimize exposure for hospitalized patients. Practical suggestions are minimal but include moving leaf piles away from the house. Unfortunately, overall avoidance of this fungus is all but impossible because it is present in the environment virtually everywhere. Research efforts are being directed at enhancing patients' resistance to *Aspergillus* rather than trying to eliminate exposure to the fungus. Given the growing number of people with immune disorders or whose immune systems have been suppressed in the course of treating another disease, research and clinical trials for new antifungal agents will be increasingly important in the future.

Resources

ORGANIZATIONS

American College of Allergy, Asthma, and Immunology. 85 West Algonquin Road, Suite 550, Arlington Heights, IL 60005. < http://allergy.mcg.edu > .

OTHER

"Lung, Allergic and Immune Diseases: Mold Allergy: Prevention Techniques." National Jewish Medical and Research. < http://nationaljewish.org/main.html > .
Office of Rare Diseases (ORD) at National Institutes of Health, Bldg. 31,1BO3, Bethesda, MD 20892-2082. (301) 402-4336 < http://rarediseases.info.nih.gov/ord > .

Jill S. Lasker

Aspirin

Definition

Aspirin is a medicine that relieves **pain** and reduces fever.

Purpose

Aspirin is used to relieve many kinds of minor aches and pains–headaches, toothaches, muscle pain, menstrual cramps, the joint pain from arthritis, and aches associated with colds and flu. Some people take aspirin daily to reduce the risk of stroke, heart attack, or other heart problems.

Description

Aspirin–also known as acetylsalicylic acid–is sold over the counter and comes in many forms, from the familiar white tablets to chewing gum and rectal suppositories. Coated, chewable, buffered, and extended release forms are available. Many other over-the-counter medicine contain aspirin. Alka-Seltzer Original Effervescent Antacid Pain Reliever, for example, contains aspirin for pain relief and sodium bicarbonate to relieve acid indigestion, heartburn, and sour stomach.

Aspirin belongs to a group of drugs called salicylates. Other members of this group include sodium salicylate, choline salicylate, and magnesium salicylate. These drugs are more expensive and no more effective than aspirin. However, they are a little easier on the stomach. Aspirin is quickly absorbed into the bloodstream and provides quick and relatively long-lasting pain relief. Aspirin also reduces inflammation. Researchers believe these effects come about because aspirin blocks the production of pain-producing chemicals called prostaglandins.

In addition to relieving pain and reducing inflammation, aspirin also lowers **fever** by acting on the part of the brain that regulates temperature. The brain then signals the blood vessels to widen, which allows heat to leave the body more quickly.

Recommended dosage

Adults

TO RELIEVE PAIN OR REDUCE FEVER. One to two tablets every three to four hours, up to six times per day.

TO REDUCE THE RISK OF STROKE. One tablet four times a day or two tablets twice a day.

TO REDUCE THE RISK OF HEART ATTACK. Check with a physician for the proper dose and number of times per week aspirin should, if at all, be taken.

Children

Check with a physician.

Precautions

Aspirin–even children's aspirin–should never be given to children or teenagers with flu-like symptoms or **chickenpox**. Aspirin can cause **Reye's syndrome**, a life-threatening condition that affects the nervous system and liver. As many as 30% of children and teenagers who develop Reye's syndrome die. Those who survive may have permanent brain damage.

KEY TERMS

Diuretic—Medicine that increases the amount of urine produced and relieves excess fluid buildup in body tissues. Diuretics may be used in treating high blood pressure, lung disease, premenstrual syndrome, and other conditions.

Inflammation—Pain, redness, swelling, and heat that usually develop in response to injury or illness.

NSAIDs—Nonsteroidal anti-inflammatory drugs. Drugs such as ketoprofen and ibuprofen which relieve pain and reduce inflammation.

Polyp—A lump of tissue protruding from the lining of an organ, such as the nose, bladder, or intestine. Polyps can sometimes block the passages in which they are found.

Prostaglandin—A hormonelike chemical produced in the body. Prostaglandins have a wide variety of effects, and may be responsible for the production of some types of pain and inflammation.

Reye's syndrome—A life-threatening disease that affects the liver and the brain and sometimes occurs after a viral infection, such as flu or chickenpox. Children or teenagers who are given aspirin for flu or chickenpox are at increased risk of developing Reye's syndrome.

Rhinitis—Inflammation of the membranes inside the nose.

Salicylates—A group of drugs that includes aspirin and related compounds. Salicylates are used to relieve pain, reduce inflammation, and lower fever.

Check with a physician before giving aspirin to a child under 12 years for arthritis, rheumatism, or any condition that requires long-term use of the drug.

No one should take aspirin for more than 10 days in a row unless told to do so by a physician. Anyone with fever should not take aspirin for more than 3 days without a physician's consent. Do not to take more than the recommended daily dosage.

People in the following categories should not use aspirin without first checking with their physician:

- Pregnant women. Aspirin can cause bleeding problems in both the mother and the developing fetus. Aspirin can also cause the infant's weight to be too low at birth.

- Women who are breastfeeding. Aspirin can pass into breast milk and may affect the baby.

- People with a history of bleeding problems.
- People who are taking blood-thinning drugs, such as warfarin (Coumadin).
- People with a history of ulcers.
- People with a history of **asthma**, nasal polyps, or both. These people are more likely to be allergic to aspirin.
- People who are allergic to fenoprofen, ibuprofen, indomethacin, ketoprofen, meclofenamate sodium, naproxen, sulindac, tolmetin, or the orange food-coloring tartrazine. They may also be allergic to aspirin.
- People with **AIDS** or AIDS-related complex who are taking AZT (zidovudine). Aspirin can increase the risk of bleeding in these patients.
- People taking certain other drugs (discussed in Interactions).
- People with liver damage or severe kidney failure.

Aspirin should not be taken before surgery, as it can increase the risk of excessive bleeding. Anyone who is scheduled for surgery should check with his or her surgeon to find out how long before surgery to avoid taking aspirin.

Aspirin can cause stomach irritation. To reduce the likelihood of that problem, take aspirin with food or milk or drink a full 8-oz glass of water with it. Taking coated or buffered aspirin can also help. Be aware that drinking alcohol can make the stomach irritation worse.

Stop taking aspirin immediately and call a physician if any of these symptoms develop:

- ringing or buzzing in the ears
- hearing loss
- **dizziness**
- stomach pain that does not go away

Do not take aspirin that has a vinegary smell. That is a sign that the aspirin is too old and ineffective. Flush such aspirin down the toilet.

Because aspirin can increase the risk of excessive bleeding, do not take aspirin daily over long periods–to reduce the risk of **stroke** or **heart attack**, for example–unless advised to do so by a physician.

Side effects

The most common side effects include stomachache, **heartburn**, loss of appetite, and small amounts of blood in stools. Less common side effects are rashes, hives, fever, vision problems, liver damage, thirst, stomach ulcers, and bleeding. People who are allergic to aspirin or those who have asthma, **rhinitis**, or polyps in the nose may have trouble breathing after taking aspirin.

Interactions

Aspirin may increase, decrease, or change the effects of many drugs. Aspirin can make drugs such as methotrexate (Rheumatrex) and valproic acid (Depakote, Depakene) more toxic. If taken with blood-thinning drugs, such as warfarin (Coumadin) and dicumarol, aspirin can increase the risk of excessive bleeding. Aspirin counteracts the effects of other drugs, such as angiotensin-converting enzyme (ACE) inhibitors and beta blockers, which lower blood pressure, and medicines used to treat gout (probenecid and sulfinpyrazone). Blood pressure may drop unexpectedly and cause **fainting** or dizziness if aspirin is taken along with nitroglycerin tablets. Aspirin may also interact with **diuretics**, diabetes medicines, other nonsteroidal anti-inflammatory drugs (NSAIDs), seizure medications, and steroids. Anyone who is taking these drugs should ask his or her physician whether they can safely take aspirin.

Resources

PERIODICALS

"What's the Best Pain Reliever? Depends on Your Pain." *Consumer Reports* May 1996: 62.

Nancy Ross-Flanigan

AST *see* **Aspartate aminotransferase test**

Astemizole *see* **Antihistamines**

Asthma

Definition

Asthma is a chronic (long-lasting) inflammatory disease of the airways. In those susceptible to asthma, this inflammation causes the airways to narrow periodically. This, in turn, produces **wheezing** and breathlessness, sometimes to the point where the patient gasps for air. Obstruction to air flow either stops spontaneously or responds to a wide range of treatments, but continuing inflammation makes the

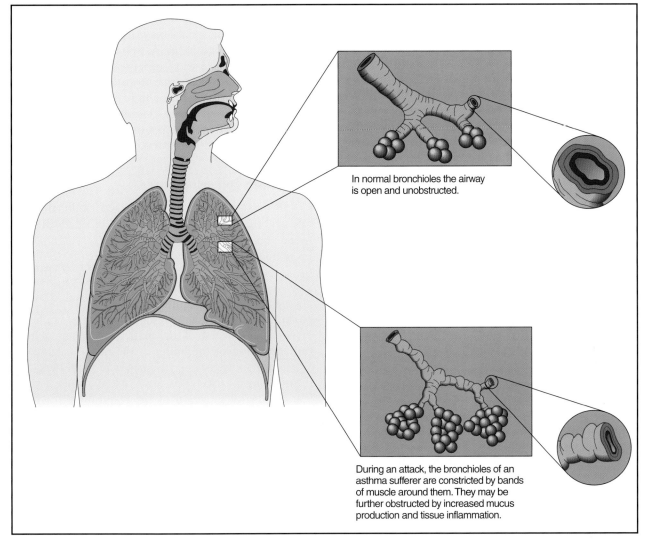

In normal bronchioles the airway is open and unobstructed.

During an attack, the bronchioles of an asthma sufferer are constricted by bands of muscle around them. They may be further obstructed by increased mucus production and tissue inflammation.

A comparison of normal bronchioles and those of an asthma sufferer. *(Illustration by Hans & Cassady.)*

airways hyper-responsive to stimuli such as cold air, **exercise**, dust mites, pollutants in the air, and even **stress** and **anxiety**.

Description

Between 17 million and 26 million Americans have asthma, and the number seems to be increasing. In about 1992, the number with asthma was about 10 million, and had risen 42% from 1982, just 10 years prior. Not only is asthma becoming more frequent, but it also is a more severe disease than before, despite modern drug treatments. Asthma accounts for almost 500,000 hospitalizations, two million emergency department visits, and 5,000 deaths in the United States each year.

The changes that take place in the lungs of asthmatic persons makes the airways (the "breathing tubes," or *bronchi* and the smaller *bronchioles*) hyper-reactive to many different types of stimuli that don't affect healthy lungs. In an asthma attack, the muscle tissue in the walls of bronchi go into spasm, and the cells lining the airways swell and secrete mucus into the air spaces. Both these actions cause the bronchi to become narrowed (bronchoconstriction). As a result, an asthmatic person has to make a much greater effort to breathe in air and to expel it.

Cells in the bronchial walls, called mast cells, release certain substances that cause the bronchial muscle to contract and stimulate mucus formation. These substances, which include histamine and a group of chemicals called leukotrienes, also bring white blood cells into the area, which is a key part of the inflammatory response. Many patients with asthma are prone to react to such "foreign" substances as pollen, house dust mites, or animal dander; these are called allergens. On the other hand, asthma affects many patients who are not allergic in this way.

Asthma usually begins in childhood or adolescence, but it also may first appear during adult years. While the symptoms may be similar, certain important aspects of asthma are different in children and adults.

Child-onset asthma

Nearly one-third on the 17 to 26 million Americans with asthma are children. When asthma begins in childhood, it often does so in a child who is likely, for genetic reasons, to become sensitized to common allergens in the environment (atopic person). When these children are exposed to house-dust mites, animal proteins, fungi, or other potential allergens, they produce a type of antibody that is intended to engulf and destroy the foreign materials. This has the effect of making the airway cells sensitive to particular materials. Further exposure can lead rapidly to an asthmatic response. This condition of atopy is present in at least one-third and as many as one-half of the general population. When an infant or young child wheezes during viral infections, the presence of allergy (in the child or a close relative) is a clue that asthma may well continue throughout childhood.

Adult-onset asthma

Allergenic materials may also play a role when adults become asthmatic. Asthma can actually start at any age and in a wide variety of situations. Many adults who are not allergic have conditions such as **sinusitis** or nasal polyps, or they may be sensitive to **aspirin** and related drugs. Another major source of adult asthma is exposure at work to animal products, certain forms of plastic, wood dust, or metals.

Causes and symptoms

In most cases, asthma is caused by inhaling an allergen that sets off the chain of biochemical and tissue changes leading to airway inflammation, bronchoconstriction, and wheezing. Because avoiding (or at least minimizing) exposure is the most effective way of treating asthma, it is vital to identify which allergen or irritant is causing symptoms in a particular patient. Once asthma is present, symptoms can be set off or made worse if the patient also has **rhinitis** (inflammation of the lining of the nose) or sinusitis. When, for some reason, stomach acid passes back up the esophagus (acid reflux), this can also make asthma worse. A viral infection of the respiratory tract can also inflame an asthmatic reaction. Aspirin and a type of drug called beta-blockers, often used to treat high blood pressure, can also worsen the symptoms of asthma.

The most important inhaled allergens giving rise to attacks of asthma are:

- animal dander
- mites in house dust
- fungi (molds) that grow indoors
- cockroach allergens
- pollen
- occupational exposure to chemicals, fumes, or particles of industrial materials in the air

Inhaling tobacco smoke, either by **smoking** or being near people who are smoking, can irritate the airways and trigger an asthmatic attack. Air pollutants can have a similar effect. In addition, there are three important factors that regularly produce attacks in certain asthmatic patients, and they may sometimes be the sole cause of symptoms. They are:

- inhaling cold air (cold-induced asthma)
- exercise-induced asthma (in certain children, asthma is caused simply by exercising)
- stress or a high level of anxiety

Wheezing is often obvious, but mild asthmatic attacks may be confirmed when the physician listens to the patient's chest with a stethoscope. Besides wheezing and being short of breath, the patient may **cough** and may report a feeling of "tightness" in the chest. Children may have **itching** on their back or neck at the start of an attack. Wheezing is often loudest when the patient breathes out, in an attempt to expel used air through the narrowed airways. Some asthmatics are free of symptoms most of the time but may occasionally be short of breath for a brief time. Others spend much of their days (and nights) coughing and wheezing, until properly treated. Crying or even laughing may bring on an attack. Severe episodes are often seen when the patient gets a viral respiratory tract infection or is exposed to a heavy load of an allergen or irritant. Asthmatic attacks may last only a few minutes or can go on for hours or even days (a condition called status asthmaticus).

Being short of breath may cause a patient to become very anxious, sit upright, lean forward, and use the muscles of the neck and chest wall to help breathe. The patient may be able to say only a few words at a time before stopping to take a breath. Confusion and a bluish tint to the skin are clues that the oxygen supply is much too low, and that emergency treatment is needed. In a severe attack that lasts for some time, some of the air sacs in the lung may rupture so that air collects within the chest. This makes it even harder to breathe in enough air.

Diagnosis

Apart from listening to the patient's chest, the examiner should look for maximum chest expansion while taking in air. Hunched shoulders and contracting neck muscles are other signs of narrowed airways. **Nasal polyps** or increased amounts of nasal secretions are often noted in asthmatic patients. Skin changes, like **atopic dermatitis** or eczema, are a tipoff that the patient has allergic problems.

Inquiring about a family history of asthma or **allergies** can be a valuable indicator of asthma. The diagnosis may be strongly suggested when typical symptoms and signs are present. A test called spirometry measures how rapidly air is exhaled and how much is retained in the lungs. Repeating the test after the patient inhales a drug that widens the air passages (a bronchodilator) will show whether the airway narrowing is reversible, which is a very typical finding in asthma. Often patients use a related instrument, called a peak flow meter, to keep track of asthma severity when at home.

Often, it is difficult to determine what is triggering asthma attacks. Allergy skin testing may be used, although an allergic skin response does not always mean that the allergen being tested is causing the asthma. Also, the body's immune system produces antibody to fight off the allergen, and the amount of antibody can be measured by a blood test. This will show how sensitive the patient is to a particular allergen. If the diagnosis is still in doubt, the patient can inhale a suspect allergen while using a spirometer to detect airway narrowing. Spirometry can also be repeated after a bout of exercise if exercise-induced asthma is a possibility. A chest x ray will help rule out other disorders.

Treatment

Patients should be periodically examined and have their lung function measured by spirometry to make sure that treatment goals are being met. These goals are to prevent troublesome symptoms, to maintain lung function as close to normal as possible, and to allow patients to pursue their normal activities including those requiring exertion. The best drug therapy is that which controls asthmatic symptoms while causing few or no side-effects.

Drugs

METHYLXANTHINES. The chief methylxanthine drug is theophylline. It may exert some anti-inflammatory effect, and is especially helpful in controlling nighttime symptoms of asthma. When, for some reason, a patient cannot use an inhaler to maintain long-term control, sustained-release theophylline is a good alternative. The blood levels of the drug must be measured periodically, as too high a dose can cause an abnormal heart rhythm or convulsions.

BETA-RECEPTOR AGONISTS. These drugs, which are **bronchodilators**, are the best choice for relieving sudden attacks of asthma and for preventing attacks from being triggered by exercise. Some agonists, such as albuterol, act mainly in lung cells and have little effect on other organs, such as the heart. These drugs generally start acting within minutes, but their effects last only four to six hours. Longer-acting brochodilators have been developed. They may last up to 12 hours. Bronchodilators may be taken in pill or liquid form, but normally are used as inhalers, which go directly to the lungs and result in fewer side effects.

STEROIDS. These drugs, which resemble natural body hormones, block inflammation and are extremely effective in relieving symptoms of asthma. When steroids are taken by inhalation for a long period, asthma attacks become less frequent as the airways become less sensitive to allergens. This is the strongest medicine for asthma, and can control even severe cases over the long term and maintain good lung function. Steroids can cause numerous side-effects, however, including bleeding from the stomach, loss of calcium from bones, **cataracts** in the eye, and a diabetes-like state. Patients using steroids for lengthy periods may also have problems with wound healing, may gain weight, and may suffer mental problems. In children, growth may be slowed. Besides being inhaled, steroids may be taken by mouth or injected, to rapidly control severe asthma.

LEUKOTRIENE MODIFIERS. Leukotriene modifiers (montelukast and zafirlukast) are a new type of drug that can be used in place of steroids, for older children or adults who have a mild degree of asthma that persists. They work by counteracting leukotrienes, which are substances released by white blood cells in the lung that cause the air passages to constrict and promote mucus secretion. Leukotriene modifiers also fight off some forms of rhinitis, an added bonus for people with asthma. However, they are not proven effective in fighting seasonal allergies.

OTHER DRUGS. Cromolyn and nedocromil are anti-inflammatory drugs that are often used as initial treatment to prevent asthmatic attacks over the long term in children. They can also prevent attacks when given before exercise or when exposure to an allergen cannot be avoided. These are safe drugs but are expensive, and must be taken regularly even if there are no symptoms. Anti-cholinergic drugs, such as atropine, are useful in controlling severe attacks when added to an inhaled beta-receptor agonist. They help widen the airways and suppress mucus production.

If a patient's asthma is caused by an allergen that cannot be avoided and it has been difficult to control symptoms by drugs, immunotherapy may be worth trying. Typically, increasing amounts of the allergen are injected over a period of three to five years, so that the body can build up an effective immune response. There is a risk that this treatment may itself cause the airways to become narrowed and bring on an asthmatic attack. Not all experts are enthusiastic about immunotherapy, although some studies have shown that it reduces asthmatic symptoms caused by

exposure to house-dust mites, ragweed pollen, and cat dander.

Managing asthmatic attacks

A severe asthma attack should be treated as quickly as possible. It is most important for a patient suffering an acute attack to be given extra oxygen. Rarely, it may be necessary to use a mechanical ventilator to help the patient breathe. A beta-receptor agonist is inhaled repeatedly or continuously. If the patient does not respond promptly and completely, a steroid is given. A course of steroid therapy, given after the attack is over, will make a recurrence less likely.

Maintaining control

Long-term asthma treatment is based on inhaling a beta-receptor agonist using a special inhaler that meters the dose. Patients must be instructed in proper use of an inhaler to be sure that it will deliver the right amount of drug. Once asthma has been controlled for several weeks or months, it is worth trying to cut down on drug treatment, but this must be done gradually. The last drug added should be the first to be reduced. Patients should be seen every one to six months, depending on the frequency of attacks.

Starting treatment at home, rather than in a hospital, makes for minimal delay and helps the patient to gain a sense of control over the disease. All patients should be taught how to monitor their symptoms so that they will know when an attack is starting, and those with moderate or severe asthma should know how to use a flow meter. They should also have a written "action plan" to follow if symptoms suddenly become worse, including how to adjust their medication and when to seek medical help. A 2004 report said that a review of medical studies revealed that patients with self-management written action plans had fewer hospitalizations, fewer emergency department visits, and improved lung function. They also had a 70% lower mortality rate. If more intense treatment is necessary, it should be continued for several days. Over-the-counter "remedies" should be avoided. When deciding whether a patient should be hospitalized, the past history of acute attacks, severity of symptoms, current medication, and whether good support is available at home all must be taken into account.

Referral to an asthma specialist should be considered if:

• there has been a life-threatening asthma attack or severe, persistent asthma

- treatment for three to six months has not met its goals
- some other condition, such as nasal polyps or chronic lung disease, is complicating asthma
- special tests, such as allergy skin testing or an allergen challenge, are needed
- intensive steroid therapy has been necessary

Special populations

INFANTS AND YOUNG CHILDREN. It is especially important to closely watch the course of asthma in young patients. Treatment is cut down when possible and if there is no clear improvement, some other treatment should be tried. If a viral infection leads to severe asthmatic symptoms, steroids may help. The health care provider should write out an asthma treatment plan for the child's school. Asthmatic children often need medication at school to control acute symptoms or to prevent exercise-induced attacks. Proper management will usually allow a child to take part in play activities. Only as a last resort should activities be limited.

THE ELDERLY. Older persons often have other types of obstructive lung disease, such as chronic bronchitis or **emphysema**. This makes it important to know to what extent the symptoms are caused by asthma. Giving steroids for two to three weeks can help determine this. Side-effects from beta-receptor agonist drugs (including a speeding heart and tremor) may be more common in older patients. These patients may benefit from receiving an anti-cholinergic drug, along with the beta-receptor agonist. If theophylline is given, the dose should be limited, as older patients are less able to clear this drug from their blood. Steroids should be avoided, as they often make elderly patients confused and agitated. Steroids may also further weaken the bones.

Prognosis

Most patients with asthma respond well when the best drug or combination of drugs is found, and they are able to lead relatively normal lives. More than one-half of affected children stop having attacks by the time they reach 21 years of age. Many others have less frequent and less severe attacks as they grow older. Urgent measures to control asthma attacks and ongoing treatment to prevent attacks are equally important. A small minority of patients will have progressively more trouble breathing and run a risk of going into respiratory failure, for which they must receive intensive treatment.

Prevention

Minimizing exposure to allergens

There are a number of ways to cut down exposure to the common allergens and irritants that provoke asthmatic attacks, or to avoid them altogether:

- If the patient is sensitive to a family pet, removing the animal or at least keeping it out of the bedroom (with the bedroom door closed), as well as keeping the pet away from carpets and upholstered furniture and Removing hair and feathers.

- To reduce exposure to house dust mites, removing wall-to-wall carpeting, keeping humidity down, and using special pillows and mattress covers. Cutting down on stuffed toys, and washing them each week in hot water.

- If cockroach allergen is causing asthma attacks, killing the roaches (using poison, traps, or boric acid rather than chemicals). Taking care not to leave food or garbage exposed.

- Keeping indoor air clean by vacuuming carpets once or twice a week (with the patient absent), avoiding using humidifiers. Using air conditioning during warm weather (so that the windows can be closed).

- Avoiding exposure to tobacco smoke.

- Not exercising outside when air pollution levels are high.

- When asthma is related to exposure at work, taking all precautions, including wearing a mask and, if necessary, arranging to work in a safer area.

More than 80% of people with asthma have rhinitis and recent research emphasizes that treating rhinitis helps benefit ashtma. Prescription nasal steroids and other methods to control rhinitis (in addition to avoiding known allergens) can help prevent asthma attacks. It is also important for patients to keep open communication with physicians to ensure that the correcnt amount of medication is being taken.

Resources

PERIODICALS

"Many People With Asthma ArenÆt Taking the Right Amount of Medication." *Obesity, Fitness & Wellness Week* (September 25, 2004): 87.

Mintz, Matthew. "Asthma Update: Part 1. Diagnosis, Monitoring, and Prevention of Disease Progression." *American Family Physician* September 1, 2004: 893.

Solomon, Gina, Elizabeth H. Humphreys, and Mark D. Miller. "Asthma and the Environment: Connecting the Dots: What Role do Environmental Exposures Play in the Rising Prevalence and Severity of Asthma?" *Contemporary Peditatrics* August 2004: 73–81.

"WhatÆs New in: Asthma and Allergic Rhinitis." *Pulse* September 20, 2004: 50.

ORGANIZATIONS

Asthma and Allergy Foundation of America. 1233 20th Street, NW, Suite 402, Washington, DC 20036. (800) 727-8462. < http://www.aafa.org > .

Mothers of Asthmatics, Inc. 3554 Chain Bridge Road, Suite 200, Fairfax, VA 22030. (800) 878-4403.

National Asthma Education Program. 4733 Bethesda Ave., Suite 350, Bethesda, MD 20814. (301) 495-4484.

National Jewish Medical and Research Center. 1400 Jackson St., Denver, CO 80206. (800) 222-LUNG.

David A. Cramer, MD
Teresa G. Odle

Astigmatism

Definition

Astigmatism is the result of an inability of the cornea to properly focus an image onto the retina. The result is a blurred image.

Description

The cornea is the outermost part of the eye. It is a transparent layer that covers the colored part of the eye (iris), pupil, and lens. The cornea bends light and helps to focus it onto the retina where specialized cells (photo receptors) detect light and transmit nerve impulses via the optic nerve to the brain where the image is formed. The cornea is dome shaped. Any incorrect shaping of the cornea results in an incorrect focusing of the light that passes through that part of the cornea. The bending of light is called refraction and focusing problems with the cornea are called diseases of refraction or refractive disorders. Astigmatism is an image distortion that results from an improperly shaped cornea. Usually the cornea is spherically shaped, like a baseball. However, in astigmatism the cornea is elliptically shaped, more like a football. There is a long meridian and a short meridian. These two meridians generally have a constant curvature and are generally perpendicular to each other

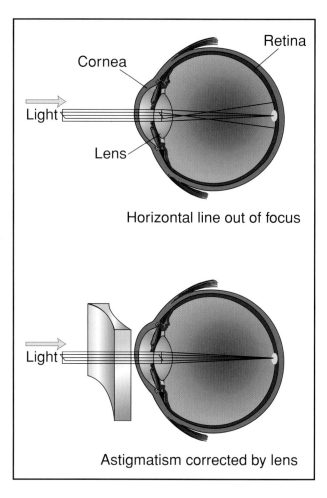

Horizontal line out of focus

Astigmatism corrected by lens

Astigmatism can be treated by the use of cylindrical lenses. The lenses are shaped to counteract the shape of the sections of the cornea that are causing the difficulty. *(Illustration by Electronic Illustrators Group.)*

(regular astigmatism). Irregular astigmatism may have more than two meridians of focus and they may not be 90° apart. A point of light, therefore, going through an astigmatic cornea will have two points of focus, instead of one nice sharp image on the retina. This will cause the person to have blurry vision. What the blur looks like will depend upon the amount and the direction of the astigmatism. A person with nearsightedness (**myopia**) or farsightedness (**hyperopia**) may see a dot as a blurred circle. A person with astigmatism may see the same dot as a blurred oval or frankfurter-shaped blur.

Some cases of astigmatism are caused by problems in the lens of the eye. Minor variations in the curvature of the lens can produce minor degrees of astigmatism (lenticular astigmatism). In these patients, the cornea is usually normal in shape. Infants, as a group, have the least amount of astigmatism. Astigmatism may increase during childhood, as the eye is developing.

Causes and symptoms

The main symptom of astigmatism is blurring. People can also experience headaches and eyestrain. Parents can notice that a child may have astigmatism when the child can see some part of a pattern or picture more clearly than others. For example, lines going across may seem clearer than lines going up and down.

Regular astigmatism can be caused by the weight of the upper eyelid resting on the eyeball creating distortion, surgical incisions in the cornea, trauma or scarring to the cornea, the presence of tumors in the eyelid, or a developmental factor. Irregular astigmatism can be caused by scarring or keratoconus. Keratoconus is a condition in which the cornea thins and becomes cone shaped. It usually occurs around **puberty** and is more common in women. Although the causes of keratoconus are unknown, it may be hereditary or a result of chronic eye rubbing, as in people with **allergies**. The center of the cone may not be in line with the center of the cornea. Diabetes can play a role in the development of astigmatism. High blood sugar levels can cause shape changes in the lens of the eye. This process usually occurs slowly and, often, is only noticed when the diabetic has started treatment to control their blood sugar. The return to a more normal blood sugar allows the lens to return to normal and this change is sometimes noticed by the patient as farsightedness. Because of this, diabetics should wait until their blood sugar is under control for at least one month to allow vision to stabilize before being measured for eyeglasses.

Diagnosis

Patients seek treatment because of blurred vision. A variety of tests can be used to detect astigmatism during the eye exam. The patient may be asked to describe the astigmatic dial, a series of lines that radiate outward from a center. People with astigmatism will see some of the lines more clearly than others. One diagnostic instrument used is the keratometer. This measures the curvature of the central cornea. It measures the amount and direction of the curvature. A corneal topographer can measure a larger area of the cornea. It can measure the central area and mid-periphery of the cornea. A keratoscope projects a series of concentric light rings onto the cornea. Misshapen areas of the cornea are revealed by noting areas of the light pattern that do not appear concentric on the cornea. Because these instruments are measuring the cornea, it is also important to have a refraction in case the lens is also contributing to the astigmatism. The refraction measures the optics or visual status of the eye and the result is the eyeglass prescription. The refraction is when the patient is looking at an eye chart and the doctor is putting different lenses in front of the patient's eyes and asks which one looks better.

Treatment

Astigmatism can be treated by the use of cylindrical lenses. They can be in eyeglasses or contact lenses. The unit of measure describing the power of the lens system or lens is called the diopter (D). The lenses are shaped to counteract the shape of the sections of cornea that are causing the difficulty. Because the correction is in one direction, it is written in terms of the axis the correction is in. On a prescription, for example, it may say $-1.00 \times 180°$. Cylinders correct astigmatism, minus spheres correct myopia, and plus spheres correct hyperopia.

There is some debate as to whether people with very small amounts of astigmatism should be treated. Generally, if visual acuity is good and the patient experiences no overt symptoms, treatment is not necessary. When treating larger amounts of astigmatism, or astigmatism for the first time, the doctor may not totally correct the astigmatism. The cylindrical correction in the eyeglasses may make the floor appear to tilt, thus making it difficult for the patient at first. Generally, the doctor will place lenses in a trial frame to allow the patient to try the prescription at the exam. It may take a week or so to get used to the glasses, however, if the patient is having a problem they should contact their doctor, who might want to recheck the prescription.

Contact lenses that are used to correct astigmatism are called toric lenses. When a person blinks, the contact lens rotates. In toric lenses, it is important for the lens to return to the same position each time. Lenses have thin zones, or cut-off areas (truncated), or have other ways to rotate and return to the correct position. Soft toric lenses are available in a variety of prescriptions, materials, and even in tints. Patients should ask their doctors about the possibility of toric lenses.

In 1997, the Food and Drug Administration (FDA) approved laser treatment of astigmatism. Patients considering this should make sure the surgeon has a lot of experience in the procedure and discuss the possible side effects or risks with the doctor. In the case of keratoconus, a corneal transplant is performed if the astigmatism can not be corrected with hard contact lenses.

Prognosis

Astigmatism is a condition that may be present at birth. It may also be acquired if something is distorting the cornea. Vision can generally be corrected with eyeglasses or contact lenses. The major risks of surgery (aside from the surgical risks) are over and under correction of the astigmatism. There is no cure for over correction. Under correction can be solved by repeating the operation.

Resources

BOOKS

Berkow, Robert, editor. *Merck Manual of Medical Information.* Whitehouse Station, NJ: Merck Research Laboratories, 2004.

John T. Lohr, PhD

Aston-Patterning

Definition

Aston-Patterning is an integrated system of movement education, bodywork, ergonomic adjustments, and fitness training that recognizes the relationship between the body and mind for well being. It helps people who seek a remedy from acute or chronic **pain** by teaching them to improve postural and movement patterns.

Purpose

Aston-Patterning assists people in finding more efficient and less stressful ways of performing the

JUDITH ASTON

Judith Aston was born in Long Beach, California. She graduated from University of California at Los Angeles with a B.A. and a M.F.A. in dance. Her interest in movement arose from working as a dancer. In 1963 Aston established her first movement education program for dancers, actors, and athletes at Long Beach City College.

Five years later, while recovering from injuries sustained during two consecutive automobile accidents, Aston met Ida Rolf, the developer of Rolfing. Aston began working for Rolf, teaching a movement education program called Rolf-Aston Structural Patterning that emphasized using the body with minimum effort and maximum precision.

In time, Rolf and Aston's views on movement diverged, and the partnership was dissolved in 1977. Aston formed her own company called the Aston Paradigm Corporation in Lake Tahoe, California. This company provides training and certification for Aston practitioners. She also began exploring how environmental conditions affect body movement, foreshadowing the ergonomic movement in the workplace that developed in the 1990s. Over time, Aston has expanded her movement work to include a fitness program for older adults. Today, Judith Aston serves as director of Aston Paradigm Corporation.

simple movements of everyday life to dissipate tension in the body. This is done through massage, alteration of the environment, and fitness training.

Description

Seeking to solve movement problems, Aston-Patterning helps make the most of their own unique body types rather than trying to force them to conform to an ideal. Unlike **Rolfing**, it doesn't strive for linear symmetry. Rather it works with asymmetry in the human body to develop patterns of alignment and movement that feel right to the individual. Aston also introduced the idea of working in a three-dimensional spinal pattern. Aston-Patterning sessions have four general components. They are:

- A personal history that helps the practitioner assess the client's needs.

- Pre-testing, in which the practitioner and the client explore patterns of movement and potential for improvement.

- Movement education and bodywork, including massage, myofacial release, and arthrokinetics, to help release tension and make new movement patterns easier.

KEY TERMS

Rolfing—Developed by Dr. Ida Rolf (1896–1979), rolfing is a systematic approach to relieving stress patterns and dysfunctions in the body's structure through the manipulation of the highly pliant myofacial (connective) tissue. It assists the body in reorganizing its major segments into vertical alignment.

• Post-testing, when pre-testing movements are repeated, allowing the client to feel the changes that have taken place and integrate them into daily life.

Aston-Patterning requires more participation from the client than many bodywork techniques. The massage aspect of Aston-Patterning is designed around a three-dimensional, non-compressive touch that releases patterns of tension in the body. It is gentler than Rolfing. Myokinetics uses touch to release tension in the face and neck. Arthrokinetics addresses tension at bones and joints. This massage is accompanied by education about how new movement patterns may be established.

In addition to Aston-Patterning sessions, clients are also helped to examine their environment for factors, such as seating or sleeping arrangements, that may limit their body function and introduce tension. Finally, they may choose to participate in the Aston fitness training program that includes loosening techniques based on self-massage, toning, stretching, and cardiovascular fitness.

Preparations

No special preparation need be taken.

Precautions

No special precautions are necessary when participating.

Side effects

No undesirable side effects are reported. Usually clients report a diminution of tension, improved body movement, and an enhanced feeling of well being.

Research and general acceptance

Aston-Patterning is an outgrowth of Rolfing, which has been shown to be of benefit in a limited number of controlled studies. Little controlled research has been done on the either benefits or limitations of Aston-Patterning. Its claims have been neither proven nor disproved, although anecdotally many clients report relief from pain and tension and also improved body movement.

Resources

ORGANIZATIONS

Aston Training Center. P. O. Box 3568, Incline Village, NV 89450. (775) 831-8228. Astonpat@aol.com < http://www.aston-patterning.com > .

Tish Davidson, A.M.

Astrocytoma *see* **Brain tumor**

Ataxia-telangiectasia

Definition

Ataxia-telangiectasia (A-T), also called Louis-Bar syndrome, is a rare, genetic neurological disorder of childhood that progressively destroys part of the motor control area of the brain, leading to a lack of balance and coordination. A-T also affects the immune system and increases the risk of leukemia and lymphoma in affected individuals.

Description

The disorder first appeared in the medical literature in the mid-1920s, but was not named specifically until 1957. The name is a combination of two recognized abnormalities: ataxia (lack of muscle control) and telangiectasia (abnormal dilatation of capillary vessels that often result in tumors and red **skin lesions**). However, A-T involves more than just the sum of these two findings. Other associated A-T problems include immune system deficiencies, extreme sensitivity to radiation, and blood cancers.

Medical researchers initially suspected that multiple genes (the units responsible for inherited features) were involved. However, in 1995, mutations in a single large gene were identified as causing A-T. Researchers named the gene ATM for A-T, mutated. Subsequent research revealed that ATM has a significant role in regulating cell division. The symptoms associated with A-T reflect the main role of the AT gene, which is to induce several cellular responses to DNA damage, such as preventing damaged DNA from being reproduced. When the AT gene is mutated into ATM, the

KEY TERMS

Angioma—A tumor (such as a hemangioma or lymphangioma) that mainly consists of blood vessels or lymphatic vessels.

Antibody—Any of a large number of proteins produced by specialized blood cells after stimulation by an antigen and that act specifically against the antigen in an immune response.

Antigen—Any substance (such as a toxin or enzyme) capable of stimulating an immune response in the body.

Ataxia—The inability to control voluntary muscle movement, most frequently resulting from disorders in the brain or spinal cord.

Autosomal—Relating to any of the chromosomes except for X and Y, the sex chromosomes.

Cerebellum—The part of the brain responsible for coordination of voluntary movements.

Gamma-globulin—An extract of human blood that contains antibodies.

Immune response—A response from the body to an antigen that occurs when the antigen is identified as foreign and that induces the production of antibodies and lymphocytes capable of destroying the antigen or making it harmless.

Immunoglobulin—A protein in the blood that is the component part of an antibody.

Leukemia—A cancer of blood cells characterized by the abnormal increase in the number of white blood cells in the tissues. There are many types of leukemias and they are classified according to the type of white blood cell involved.

Lymphoma—A blood cancer in which lymphocytes, a variety of white blood cells, grow at an unusually rapid rate.

Mutation—Any change in the hereditary material of genes.

Purkinje's cells—Large branching cells of the nervous system.

Recessive—Producing little or no phenotypic effect when occurring in heterozygous condition with a contrasting allele.

Telangiectases—Spidery red skin lesions caused by dilated blood vessels.

Telangiectasia—Abnormal dilation of capillary blood vessels leading to the formation of telangiectases or angiomas.

Thymus—A gland located in the front of the neck that coordinates the development of the immune system.

signaling networks are affected and the cell no longer responds correctly to minimize the damage.

A-T is very rare, but it occurs in every population world wide, with an estimated frequency of between 1/40,000 and 1/100,000 live births. But it is believed that many A-T cases, particularly those who die at a young age, are never properly diagnosed. Therefore, this disease may actually be much more prevalent. According to the A-T Project Foundation, an estimated 1% (2.5 million in the United States) of the general population carries defective A-T genes. Carriers of one copy of this gene do not develop A-T, but have a significantly increased risk of **cancer**. This makes the A-T gene one of the most important cancer-related genes identified to date.

Causes and symptoms

The ATM gene is autosomal recessive, meaning the disease occurs only if a defective gene is inherited from both parents. Infants with A-T initially often appear very healthy. At around age two, ataxia and nervous system abnormalities becomes apparent. The root cause of A-T-associated ataxia is cell death in the brain, specifically the large branching cells of the nervous system (Purkinje's cells) which are located in the cerebellum. A toddler becomes clumsy, loses balance easily and lacks muscle control. Speech becomes slurred and more difficult, and the symptoms progressively worsen. Between ages two and eight, telangiectases, or tiny, red "spider" veins, appear on the cheeks and ears and in the eyes.

By age 10-12, children with A-T can no longer control their muscles. Immune system deficiencies become common, and affected individuals are extremely sensitive to radiation. Immune system deficiencies vary between individuals but include lower-than-normal levels of proteins that function as antibodies (immunoglobulins) and white blood cells (blood cells not containing "iron" proteins). The thymus gland, which aids in development of the body's immune system, is either missing or has developed abnormally. Intelligence is normal, but growth may be retarded owing to immune system or hormonal deficiencies. Individuals with A-T are also sometimes afflicted with diabetes, prematurely graying hair, and difficulty swallowing. As the children grow older, the immune system becomes weaker and less capable of fighting infection. In the later stages, recurrent respiratory infections and blood cancers, such as leukemia or lymphoma, are common.

Diagnosis

Diagnosis relies on recognizing the hallmarks of A-T: progressive ataxia and telangiectasia. However, this may be difficult as ataxia symptoms do appear prior to telangiectasia symptoms by several years. Other symptoms can vary between individuals; for example, 70% of individuals with A-T have a high incidence of respiratory infection, 30% do not. The identification of the ATM gene raises hopes that screening, and perhaps treatment, may be possible.

Treatment

There is currently no cure for A-T, and treatment focuses on managing the individual's multiple symptoms. Physical therapy and speech therapy can help the patient adjust to ataxia. Injections of gamma globulin, or extracts of human blood that contain antibodies, are used to strengthen the weakened immune system. High-dose vitamin administrations may also be prescribed. Research continues in many countries to find effective treatments. Individuals and families living with this disorder may benefit from attending support groups.

Prognosis

A-T is a fatal condition. Children with A-T become physically disabled by their early teens and typically die by their early 20s, usually from the associated blood cancers and malignancies. In very rare cases, individuals with A-T may experience slower progression and a slightly longer life span, surviving into their 30s. A-T carriers have a five-fold higher risk than non-carriers of developing certain cancers, especially **breast cancer**.

Prevention

Medical researchers are investigating methods for screening individuals who may be carriers of the defective gene. Prenatal testing for A-T is possible but not done routinely, because commercial screening tests have yet to be developed.

Ataxia *see* **Movement disorders**

Atelectasis

Definition

Atelectasis is a collapse of lung tissue affecting part or all of one lung. This condition prevents normal oxygen absoption to healthy tissues.

Description

Atelectasis can result from an obstruction (blockage) of the airways that affects tiny air scas called alveoli. Alveoli are very thin-walled and contain a rich blood supply. They are important for lung function, since their purpose is the exchange of oxygen and carbon dioxide. When the airways are blocked by a mucous "plug," foreign object, or tumor, the alveoli are unable to fill with air and collapse of lung tissue can occur in the affected area. Atelectasis is a potential complication following surgery, especially in individuals who have undergone chest or abdominal operations resulting in associated abdominal or chest **pain** during breathing. Congenital atelectasis can result from a failure of the lungs to expand at birth. This congenital condition may be localized or may affect all of both lungs.

Causes and symptoms

Causes of atelectasis include insufficient attemps at respiration by the newborn, bronchial obstruction, or absence of **surfactant** (a substance secreted by alveoli that maintains the stability of lung tissue by reducing the surface tension of fluids that coat the lung). This lack of surfactant reduces the surface area available for effective gas exchange causing it to collapse if severe. Pressure on the lung from fluid or air can cause atelectasis as well as obstruction of lung air passages by thick mucus resulting from various infections and lung diseases. Tumors and inhaled objects can also cause obstruction of the airway, leading to atelectasis.

Anyone undergoing chest or abdominal surgery using **general anesthesia** is at risk to develop atelectasis, since breathing is often shallow after surgery to

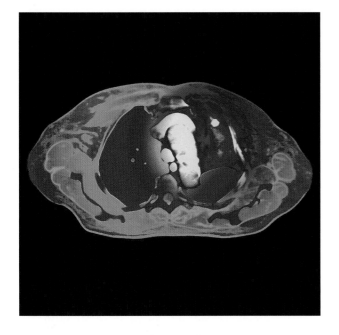

A computed tomography (CT) scan through a patient's chest. The collapsed lung appears at the right of the image. *(Photo Researchers, Inc. Reproduced by permission.)*

avoid pain from the surgical incision. Any significant decrease in airflow to the alveoli contributes to pooling of secretions, which in turn can cause infection. Chest injuries causing shallow breathing, including fractured ribs, can cause atelectasis. Common symptoms of atelectasis include **shortness of breath** and decreased chest wall expansion. If atelectasis only afects a small area of the lung, symptoms are ususally minimal. If the condition affects a large area of the lung and develops quickly, the individual may turn blue (cyanotic) or pale, have extreme shortness of breath, and feel a stabbing pain on the affected side. **Fever** and increased heart rate may be present if infection accompanies atelectasis.

Diagnosis

To diagnose atelectasis, a doctor starts by recording the patient's symptoms and performing a thorough **physical examination**. When the doctor listens to the lungs through a stethoscope (ausculation), diminished or bronchial breath sounds may be heard. By tapping on the chest (percussion) while listening through the stethoscope, the doctor can often tell if the lung is collapsed. A **chest x ray** that shows an airless area in the lung confirms the diagnosis of atelectasis. If an obstruction of the airways is suspected, a computed tomography scan (CT) or **bronchoscopy** may be performed to locate the cause of the blockage.

Treatment

If atelectasis is due to obstruction of the airway, the first step in treatment is to remove the cause of the blockage. This may be done by coughing, suctioning, or bronchoscopy. If a tumor is the cause of atelectasis, surgery may be necessary to remove it. **Antibiotics** are commonly used to fight the infection that often accompanies atelectasis. In cases where recurrent or long-lasting infection is disabling or where significant bleeding occurs, the affected section of the lung may be surgically removed.

Prognosis

If atelectasis is caused by a thick mucus "plug" or inhaled foreign object, the patient usually recovers completely when the blockage is removed. If it is caused by a tumor, the outcome depends on the nature of the tumor involved. If atelectasis is a result of surgery, other post-operative conditions and/or complications affect the prognosis.

Prevention

When recovering from surgery, frequent repositioning in bed along with coughing and deep breathing are important. Coughing and breathing deeply every one to two hours after any surgical operation with general anesthesia is recommended. Breathing exercises and the use of breathing devices, such as an incentive spirometer, may also help prevent atelectasis. Although smokers have a higher risk of developing atelectasis following surgery, stopping **smoking** six to eight weeks before surgery can help reduce the risk. Increasing fluid intake during respiratory illness or after surgery (by mouth or intravenously) helps lung secretions to remain loose. Increasing humidity may also be beneficial.

Postural drainage techniques can be learned from a respiratory therapist or physical therapist and are a useful tool for anyone affected with a respiratiory illness that could cause atelectasis. Because **foreign objects** blocking the airway can cause atelectasis, it is very important to keep small objects that might be inhaled away from young children.

Resources

ORGANIZATIONS

National Heart, Lung and Blood Institute. PO Box 30105, Bethesda, MD 20824-0105. (301) 251-1222. < http:// www.nhlbi.nih.gov > .

Jeffrey P. Larson, RPT

Atenolol *see* **Beta blockers**

Atherectomy

Definition

Atherectomy is a non-surgical procedure to open blocked coronary arteries or vein grafts by using a device on the end of a catheter to cut or shave away atherosclerotic plaque (a deposit of fat and other substances that accumulate in the lining of the artery wall).

Purpose

Atherectomy is performed to restore the flow of oxygen-rich blood to the heart, to relieve chest **pain**, and to prevent heart attacks. It may be done on patients with chest pain who have not responded to other medical therapy and on certain of those who are candidates for balloon **angioplasty** (a surgical procedure in which a balloon catheter is used to flatten plaque against an artery wall) or coronary artery bypass graft surgery. It is sometimes performed to remove plaque that has built up after a **coronary artery bypass graft surgery**.

Precautions

Atherectomy should not be performed when the plaque is located where blood vessels divide into branches, when plaque is angular or inside an angle of a blood vessel, on patients with weak vessel walls, on ulcerated or calcium-hardened lesions, or on blockages through which a guide wire won't pass.

Description

Atherectomy uses a rotating shaver or other device placed on the end of a catheter to slice away or destroy plaque. At the beginning of the procedure, medications to control blood pressure, dilate the coronary arteries, and prevent **blood clots** are administered. The patient is awake but sedated. The catheter is inserted into an artery in the groin, leg, or arm, and threaded through the blood vessels into the blocked coronary artery. The cutting head is positioned against the plaque and activated, and the plaque is ground up or suctioned out.

The types of atherectomy are rotational, directional, and transluminal extraction. Rotational atherectomy uses a high speed rotating shaver to grind up plaque. Directional atherectomy was the first type approved, but is no longer commonly used; it scrapes plaque into an opening in one side of the catheter. Transluminal extraction coronary atherectomy uses a device that cuts plaque off vessel walls and vacuums it into a bottle. It is used to clear bypass grafts.

Performed in a **cardiac catheterization** lab, atherectomy is also called removal of plaque from the coronary arteries. It can be used instead of, or along with, balloon angioplasty. Atherectomy is successful about 95% of the time. Plaque forms again in 20-30% of patients.

Preparation

The day before atherectomy, the patient takes medication to prevent blood clots and may be asked to bathe and shampoo with an antiseptic skin cleaner.

Aftercare

After the procedure, the patient spends several days in the hospital's cardiac monitoring area. For at least 20 minutes, pressure is applied to a dressing on the insertion site. For the first hour, an electrocardiogram and close monitoring are conducted; vital signs are

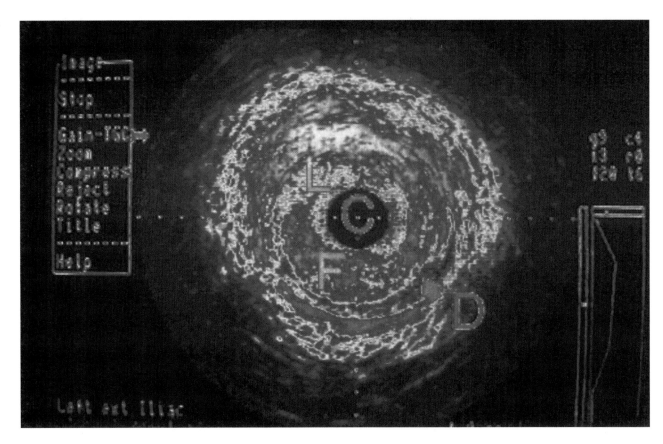

In this digitized ultrasound of a blood vessel, C is the catheter, D is the dissection, and F is the artherosclerotic flap. *(Custom Medical Stock Photo. Reproduced by permission.)*

KEY TERMS

Atherosclerotic plaque—A deposit of fat and other substances that accumulate in the lining of the artery wall.

Balloon angioplasty—A surgical procedure in which a balloon catheter is used to flatten plaque against an artery wall.

Coronary arteries—The two main arteries that provide blood to the heart. The coronary arteries surround the heart like a crown, coming out of the aorta, arching down over the top of the heart, and dividing into two branches. These are the arteries where coronary artery disease occurs.

Hematoma—A localized collection of blood, usually clotted, due to a break in the wall of blood vessel.

---

checked every 15 minutes. Pain medication is then administered. The puncture site is checked once an hour or more. For most of the first 24 hours, the patient remains in bed.

Risks

Chest pain is the most common complication of atherectomy. Other common complications are injury to the blood vessel lining, plaque that re-forms, blood clots (hematoma), and bleeding at the site of insertion. More serious but less frequent complications are blood vessel holes, blood vessel wall tears, or reduced blood flow to the heart.

Resources

BOOKS

McPhee, Stephen, et al., editors. *Current Medical Diagnosis and Treatment, 1998.* 37th ed. Stamford: Appleton & Lange, 1997.

ORGANIZATIONS

American Heart Association. 7320 Greenville Ave. Dallas, TX 75231. (214) 373-6300. < http:// www.americanheart.org > .

Texas Heart Institute. Heart Information Service. PO Box 20345, Houston, TX 77225-0345. < http:// www.tmc.edu/thi > .

Lori De Milto

Atherosclerosis

Definition

Atherosclerosis is the build up of a waxy plaque on the inside of blood vessels. In Greek, *athere* means *gruel*, and *skleros* means *hard*. Atherosclerosis is often called arteriosclerosis. Arteriosclerosis (from the Greek *arteria*, meaning *artery*) is a general term for hardening of the arteries. Arteriosclerosis can occur in several forms, including atherosclerosis.

Description

Atherosclerosis, a progressive process responsible for most heart disease, is a type of arteriosclerosis or hardening of the arteries. An artery is made up of several layers: an inner lining called the endothelium, an elastic membrane that allows the artery to expand and contract, a layer of smooth muscle, and a layer of connective tissue. Arteriosclerosis is a broad term that includes a hardening of the inner and middle layers of the artery. It can be caused by normal **aging**, by high blood pressure, and by diseases such as diabetes. Atherosclerosis is a type of arteriosclerosis that affects only the inner lining of an artery. It is characterized by plaque deposits that block the flow of blood.

Plaque is made of fatty substances, cholesterol, waste products from the cells, calcium, and fibrin, a stringy material that helps clot blood. The plaque formation process stimulates the cells of the artery wall to produce substances that accumulate in the inner layer. Fat builds up within these cells and around them, and they form connective tissue and calcium. The inner layer of the artery wall thickens, the artery's diameter is reduced, and blood flow and oxygen delivery are decreased. Plaques can rupture or crack open, causing the sudden formation of a blood clot (thrombosis). Atherosclerosis can cause a **heart attack** if it completely blocks the blood flow in the heart (coronary) arteries. It can cause a **stroke** if it completely blocks the brain (carotid) arteries. Atherosclerosis can also occur in the arteries of the neck, kidneys, thighs, and arms, causing kidney failure or **gangrene** and **amputation**.

Causes and symptoms

Atherosclerosis can begin in the late teens, but it usually takes decades to cause symptoms. Some people experience rapidly progressing atherosclerosis during their thirties, others during their fifties or sixties. Atherosclerosis is complex. Its exact cause is still unknown. It is thought that atherosclerosis is caused by a response to damage to the endothelium from high cholesterol, high blood pressure, and cigarette **smoking**. A person who has all three of these risk factors is eight times more likely to develop atherosclerosis than is a person who has none. Physical inactivity, diabetes, and obesity are also risk factors for atherosclerosis. High levels of the amino acid **homocysteine** and abnormal levels of protein-coated fats called lipoproteins also raise the risk of **coronary artery disease**. These substances are the targets of much current research. The role of triglycerides, another fat that circulates in the blood, in forming atherosclerotic plaques is unclear. High levels of triglycerides are often associated with diabetes, **obesity**, and low levels of high-density lipoproteins (HDL cholesterol). The more HDL ("good") cholesterol, in the blood, the less likely is coronary artery disease. These risk factors are all modifiable. Non-modifiable risk factors are heredity, sex, and age.

Risk factors that can be changed:

- Cigarette/tobacco smoke–Smoking increases both the chance of developing atherosclerosis and the chance of dying from coronary heart disease. Second hand smoke may also increase risk.

- High blood cholesterol–Cholesterol, a soft, waxy substance, comes from foods such as meat, eggs, and other animal products and is produced in the liver. Age, sex, heredity, and diet affect cholesterol. Total blood cholesterol is considered high at levels above 240 mg/dL and borderline at 200-239 mg/dL. High-risk levels of low-density lipoprotein (LDL cholesterol) begin at 130-159 mg/dL.

- High triglycerides–Most fat in food and in the body takes the form of triglycerides. Blood triglyceride levels above 400 mg/dL have been linked to coronary artery disease in some people. Triglycerides, however, are not nearly as harmful as LDL cholesterol.

- High blood pressure–Blood pressure of 140 over 90 or higher makes the heart work harder, and over time, both weakens the heart and harms the arteries.

- Physical inactivity–Lack of **exercise** increases the risk of atherosclerosis.

- Diabetes mellitus–The risk of developing atherosclerosis is seriously increased for diabetics and can be lowered by keeping diabetes under control. Most diabetics die from heart attacks caused by atherosclerosis.

- Obesity–Excess weight increases the strain on the heart and increases the risk of developing atherosclerosis even if no other risk factors are present.

Risk factors that cannot be changed:

- Heredity–People whose parents have coronary artery disease, atherosclerosis, or stroke at an early

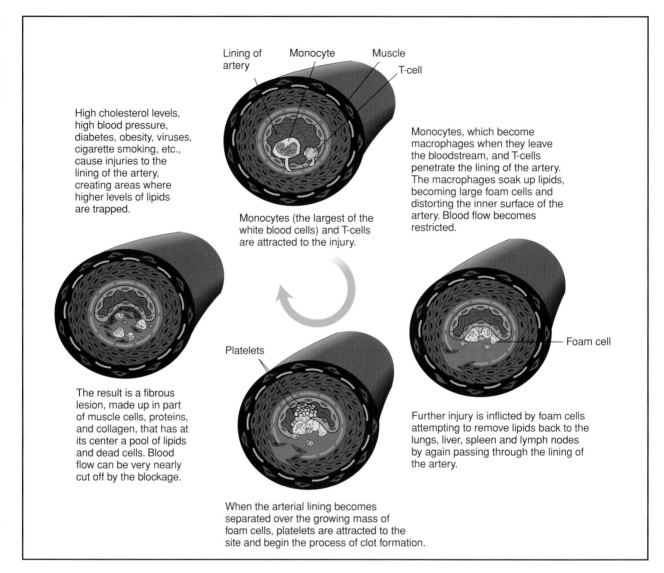

High cholesterol levels, high blood pressure, diabetes, obesity, viruses, cigarette smoking, etc., cause injuries to the lining of the artery, creating areas where higher levels of lipids are trapped.

Monocytes (the largest of the white blood cells) and T-cells are attracted to the injury.

Monocytes, which become macrophages when they leave the bloodstream, and T-cells penetrate the lining of the artery. The macrophages soak up lipids, becoming large foam cells and distorting the inner surface of the artery. Blood flow becomes restricted.

The result is a fibrous lesion, made up in part of muscle cells, proteins, and collagen, that has at its center a pool of lipids and dead cells. Blood flow can be very nearly cut off by the blockage.

When the arterial lining becomes separated over the growing mass of foam cells, platelets are attracted to the site and begin the process of clot formation.

Further injury is inflicted by foam cells attempting to remove lipids back to the lungs, liver, spleen and lymph nodes by again passing through the lining of the artery.

The progression of atherosclerosis. *(Illustration by Hans & Cassady.)*

age are at increased risk. The high rate of severe **hypertension** among African-Americans puts them at increased risk.

- Sex–Before age 60, men are more likely to have heart attacks than women are. After age 60, the risk is equal among men and women.

- Age–Risk is higher in men who are 45 years of age and older and women who are 55 years of age and older.

Symptoms differ depending upon the location of the atherosclerosis.

- In the coronary (heart) arteries: Chest **pain**, heart attack, or sudden **death**.

- In the carotid (brain) arteries: Sudden **dizziness**, weakness, loss of speech, or blindness.

- In the femoral (leg) arteries: Disease of the blood vessels in the outer parts of the body (peripheral vascular disease) causes cramping and **fatigue** in the calves when walking.

- In the renal (kidney) arteries: High blood pressure that is difficult to treat.

Diagnosis

Physicians may be able to make a diagnosis of atherosclerosis during a physical exam by means of a stethoscope and gentle probing of the arteries with the hand (palpation). More definite tests are **electrocardiography**, **echocardiography** or ultrasonography of the arteries (for example, the carotids), radionuclide scans, and **angiography**.

An electrocardiogram shows the heart's activity. Electrodes covered with conducting jelly are placed on the patient's body. They send impulses of the heart to a recorder. The test takes about 10 minutes and is performed in a physician's office. Exercise electrocardiography (**stress test**) is conducted while the patient exercises on a treadmill or a stationary bike. It is performed in a physician's office or an exercise laboratory and takes 15-30 minutes.

Echocardiography, cardiac ultrasound, uses sound waves to create an image of the heart's chambers and valves. A technician applies gel to a hand-held transducer, presses it against the patient's chest, and images are displayed on a monitor. This technique cannot evaluate the coronary arteries directly. They are too small and are in motion with the heart. Severe coronary artery disease, however, may cause abnormal heart motion that is detected by echocardiography. Performed in a cardiology outpatient diagnostic laboratory, the test takes 30-60 minutes. Ultrasonography is also used to assess arteries of the neck and thighs.

Radionuclide angiography and thallium (or sestamibi) scanning enable physicians to see the blood flow through the coronary arteries and the heart chambers. Radioactive material is injected into the bloodstream. A device that uses gamma rays to produce an image of the radioactive material (gamma camera) records pictures of the heart. Radionuclide angiography is usually performed in a hospital's nuclear medicine department and takes 30-60 minutes. Thallium scanning is usually done after an exercise **stress** test or after injection of a vasodilator, a drug to enlarge the blood vessels, like dipyridamole (Persantine). Thallium is injected, and the scan is done then and again four hours (and possibly 24 hours) later. Thallium scanning is usually performed in a hospital's nuclear medicine department. Each scan takes 30-60 minutes.

Coronary angiography is the most accurate diagnostic method and the only one that requires entering the body (invasive procedure). A cardiologist inserts a catheter equipped with a viewing device into a blood vessel in the leg or arm and guides it into the heart. The patient has been given a contrast dye that makes the heart visible to x rays. Motion pictures are taken of the contrast dye flowing though the arteries. Plaques and blockages, if present, are well defined. The patient is awake but has been given a sedative. Coronary angiography is performed in a **cardiac catheterization** laboratory and takes from 30 minutes to two hours.

Treatment

Treatment includes lifestyle changes, lipid-lowering drugs, percutaneous transluminal coronary **angioplasty**, and coronary artery bypass surgery. Atherosclerosis requires lifelong care.

Patients who have less severe atherosclerosis may achieve adequate control through lifestyle changes and drug therapy. Many of the lifestyle changes that prevent disease progression–a low-fat, low-cholesterol diet, losing weight (if necessary), exercise, controlling blood pressure, and not smoking–also help prevent the disease.

Most of the drugs prescribed for atherosclerosis seek to lower cholesterol. Many popular lipid-lowering drugs can reduce LDL-cholesterol by an average of 25-30% when combined with a low-fat, low-cholesterol diet. Lipid-lowering drugs include bile acid resins, "statins" (drugs that effect HMG-CoA reductase, an enzyme that controls the processing of cholesterol), niacin, and fibric acid derivatives such as gemfibrozil (Lobid). **Aspirin** helps prevent thrombosis and a variety of other medications can be used to treat the effects of atherosclerosis.

Percutaneous transluminal coronary angioplasty and bypass surgery are invasive procedures that improve blood flow in the coronary arteries. Percutaneous transluminal coronary angioplasty (coronary angioplasty) is a non-surgical procedure in which a catheter tipped with a balloon is threaded from a blood vessel in the thigh into the blocked artery. The balloon is inflated, compresses the plaque to enlarge the blood vessel, and opens the blocked artery. Coronary angioplasty is performed by a cardiologist in a hospital and generally requires a hospital stay of one or two days. It is successful about 90% of the time, but for one-third of patients the artery narrows again within six months. It can be repeated and a "stent" may be placed in the artery to help keep it open (see below).

In coronary artery bypass surgery (bypass surgery), a detour is built around the blockage with a healthy vein or artery, which then supplies oxygen-rich blood to the heart. It is major surgery appropriate for patients with blockages in two or three major coronary arteries or severely narrowed left main coronary arteries, and for those who have not responded to other treatments. It is performed in a hospital under **general anesthesia** and uses a heart-lung machine. About 70% of patients experience full relief; about 20% partial relief.

Three other semi-experimental surgical procedures may be used to treat atherosclerosis. In atherectomy, a cardiologist shaves off and removes strips of plaque from the blocked artery. In laser angioplasty, a catheter with a laser tip is inserted to burn or break down the plaque. A metal coil called a stent may be permanently implanted to keep a blocked artery open.

Alternative treatment

Alternative therapies that focus on diet and lifestyle can help prevent, retard, or reverse atherosclerosis. Herbal therapies that may be helpful include: hawthorn (*Crataegus laevigata*), notoginseng root (*Panax notoginseng*), garlic (*Allium sativum*), ginger (*Zingiber officinale*), hot red or chili peppers, yarrow (*Achillea millefolium*), and alfalfa (*Medicago sativum*). Relaxation techniques including yoga, meditation, guided imagery, biofeedback, and counseling and other "talking" therapies may also be useful to prevent or slow the progress of the disease. Dietary modifications focus on eating foods that are low in fats (especially saturated fats), cholesterol, sugar, and animal proteins and high in fiber and antioxidants (found in fresh fruits and vegetables). Liberal use of onions and garlic is recommended, as is eating raw and cooked fish, especially cold-water fish like salmon. Smoking, alcohol, and stimulants like coffee should be avoided. Chelation therapy, which uses **anticoagulant drugs** and nutrients to dissolve plaque and flush it through the kidneys, is controversial. Long-term remedies can be prescribed by specialists in ayurvedic medicine, which combines diet, herbal remedies, relaxation and exercise, and homeopathy, which treats a disease with small doses of a drug that causes the symptoms of the disease.

Prognosis

Atherosclerosis can be successfully treated but not cured. Recent clinical studies have shown that atherosclerosis can be delayed, stopped, and even reversed by aggressively lowering LDL cholesterol. New diagnostic techniques enable physicians to identify and treat atherosclerosis in its earliest stages. New technologies and surgical procedures have extended the lives of many patients who would otherwise have died. Research continues.

Prevention

A healthy lifestyle–eating right, regular exercise, maintaining a healthy weight, not smoking, and controlling hypertension–can reduce the risk of developing atherosclerosis, help keep the disease from progressing, and sometimes cause it to regress.

- Eat right-A healthy diet reduces excess levels of LDL cholesterol and triglycerides. It includes a variety of foods that are low in fat and cholesterol and high in fiber; plenty of fruits and vegetables; and limited sodium. Fat should comprise no more than 30%, and saturated fat no more than 8-10%, of total daily calories according to the American Heart Association. Cholesterol should be limited to about 300 milligrams per day and sodium to about 2,400 milligrams. The "Food Guide" Pyramid developed by the U.S. Departments of Agriculture and Health and Human Services provides daily guidelines: 6-11 servings of bread, cereal, rice, and pasta; 3-5 servings of vegetables; 2-4 servings of fruit; 2-3 servings of milk, yogurt, and cheese; and 2-3 servings of meat, poultry, fish, dry beans, eggs, and nuts. Fats, oils, and sweets should be used sparingly. Mono-unsaturated oils, like olive and rapeseed (Canola) are good alternatives to use for cooking.

- Exercise regularly–Aerobic exercise can lower blood pressure, help control weight, and increase HDL ("good") cholesterol. It may keep the blood vessels more flexible. Moderate to intense aerobic exercise lasting about 30 minutes (or three 10-minute exercise periods) four or more times per week is recommended, according to the Centers for Disease Control and Prevention and the American College of Sports Medicine. Aerobic exercise includes walking, jogging, and cycling, active gardening, climbing stairs, or brisk housework. A physician should be consulted before exercise if a person has atherosclerosis or is at increased risk for it.

- Maintain a desirable body weight–Losing weight can help reduce total and LDL cholesterol, reduce triglycerides, and boost HDL cholesterol. It may also reduce blood pressure. Eating right and exercising are two key components in maintaining a desirable body weight.

- Do not smoke or use tobacco–Smoking has many adverse effects on the heart but quitting can repair damage. Ex-smokers face the same risk of heart disease as non-smokers within five to 10 years of quitting. Smoking is the worst thing a person can do to their heart and lungs.

- Seek treatment for hypertension–High blood pressure can be controlled through lifestyle changes–reducing sodium and fat, exercising, managing stress, quitting smoking, and drinking alcohol in moderation–and medication. Drugs that provide effective treatment are: **diuretics**, beta-blockers, sympathetic nerve inhibitors, **vasodilators**, angiotensin converting enzyme inhibitors, and calcium antagonists. Hypertension usually has no symptoms so it must be checked to be known. Like cholesterol, hypertension is called a "silent killer."

Resources

PERIODICALS

Morgan, Peggy. "What Your Heart Wishes You Knew About Cholesterol." *Prevention* (September 1997): 96.

ORGANIZATIONS

American Heart Association. 7320 Greenville Ave. Dallas, TX 75231. (214) 373-6300. < http:// www.americanheart.org > .

National Heart, Lung and Blood Institute. PO Box 30105, Bethesda, MD 20824-0105. (301) 251-1222. < http:// www.nhlbi.nih.gov > .

Texas Heart Institute. Heart Information Service. PO Box 20345, Houston, TX 77225-0345. < http:// www.tmc.edu/thi > .

Lori De Milto

Athetosis *see* **Movement disorders**

Athlete's foot

Definition

A common fungus infection between the toes in which the skin becomes itchy and sore, cracking and peeling away. Athlete's foot (also known as tinea pedis or foot **ringworm**) can be treated, but it can be tenacious and difficult to clear up completely.

Description

Athlete's foot is a very common condition of itchy, peeling skin on the feet. In fact, it's so common that most people will have at least one episode at least once in their lives. It's less often found in women and children under age 12. (Symptoms that look like athlete's foot in young children most probably are caused by some other skin condition).

Because the fungi grow well in warm, damp areas, they flourish in and around swimming pools, showers, and locker rooms. Tinea pedis got its common name because the infection was common among athletes who often used these areas.

Causes and symptoms

Athlete's foot is caused by a fungal infection that most often affects the fourth and fifth toe webs. *Trichophyton rubrum*, *T. mentagrophytes*, and *Epidermophyton floccosum*, the fungi that cause athlete's foot, are unusual in that they live exclusively on dead body tissue (hair, the outer layer of skin, and nails). The fungus grows best in moist, damp, dark places with poor ventilation. The problem doesn't occur among people who usually go barefoot.

Many people carry the fungus on their skin. However, it will only flourish to the point of causing athlete's foot if conditions are right. Many people believe athlete's foot is highly contagious, especially in public swimming pools and shower rooms. Research has shown, however, that it is difficult to pick up the infection simply by walking barefoot over a contaminated damp floor. Exactly why some people develop the condition and others don't is not well understood.

Sweaty feet, tight shoes, synthetic socks that don't absorb moisture well, a warm climate, and not drying the feet well after swimming or bathing, all contribute to the overgrowth of the fungus.

Symptoms of athlete's foot include itchy, sore skin on the toes, with scaling, cracking, inflammation, and blisters. Blisters that break, exposing raw patches of

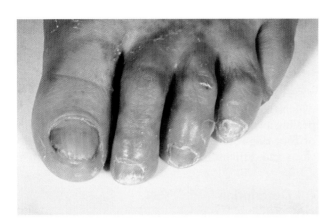

Athlete's foot fungus on toes of patient. *(Custom Medical Stock Photo. Reproduced by permission.)*

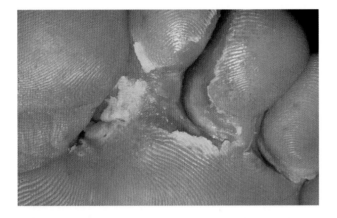

Athlete's foot fungus on bottom of patient's foot. *(Custom Medical Stock Photo. Reproduced by permission.)*

tissue, can cause pain and swelling. As the infection spreads, **itching** and burning may get worse.

If it's not treated, athlete's foot can spread to the soles of the feet and toenails. Stubborn toenail infections may appear at the same time, with crumbling, scaling and thickened nails, and nail loss. The infection can spread further if patients scratch and then touch themselves elsewhere (especially in the groin or under the arms). It's also possible to spread the infection to other parts of the body via contaminated bed sheets or clothing.

Diagnosis

Not all foot **rashes** are athlete's foot, which is why a physician should diagnose the condition before any remedies are used. Using nonprescription products on a rash that is not athlete's foot could make the rash worse.

A dermatologist can diagnose the condition by physical examination and by examining a preparation of skin scrapings under a microscope. This test, called a KOH preparation, treats a sample of tissue scraped from the infected area with heat and potassium hydroxide (KOH). This treatment dissolves certain substances in the tissue sample, making it possible to see the fungi under the microscope.

Treatment

Athlete's foot may be resistant to medication and should not be ignored. Simple cases usually respond well to antifungal creams or sprays (clotrimazole, ketoconazole, miconazole nitrate, sulconazole nitrate, or tolnaftate). If the infection is resistant to topical treatment, the doctor may prescribe an oral antifungal drug.

Untreated athlete's foot may lead to a secondary bacterial infection in the skin cracks.

Alternative treatment

A footbath containing cinnamon has been shown to slow down the growth of certain molds and fungi, and is said to be very effective in clearing up athlete's foot. To make the bath:

• heat four cups of water to a boil

• add eight to 10 broken cinnamon sticks

• reduce heat and simmer five minutes

• remove and let the mixture steep for 45 minutes until lukewarm

• soak feet

Other herbal remedies used externally to treat athlete's foot include: a foot soak or powder containing goldenseal (*Hydrastis canadensis*); tea tree oil (*Melaleuca* spp.); or calendula (*Calendula officinalis*) cream to help heal cracked skin.

Prognosis

Athlete's foot usually responds well to treatment, but it is important to take all medication as directed by a dermatologist, even if the skin appears to be free of fungus. Otherwise, the infection could return. The toenail infections that may accompany athlete's foot, however, are typically very hard to treat effectively.

Prevention

Good personal hygiene and a few simple precautions can help prevent athlete's foot. To prevent spread of athlete's foot:

• wash feet daily

• dry feet thoroughly (especially between toes)

- avoid tight shoes (especially in summer)
- wear sandals during warm weather
- wear cotton socks and change them often if they get damp
- don't wear socks made of synthetic material
- go barefoot outdoors when possible
- wear bathing shoes in public bathing or showering areas
- use a good quality foot powder
- don't wear sneakers without socks
- wash towels, contaminated floors, and shower stalls well with hot soapy water if anyone in the family has athlete's foot.

Resources

BOOKS

Thompson, June, et al. *Mosby's Clinical Nursing.* St. Louis: Mosby, 1998.

ORGANIZATIONS

American Podiatric Medical Association. 9312 Old Georgetown Road, Bethesda, MD 20814-1698. (301) 571-9200. <http://www.apma.org>.

Carol A. Turkington

Athletic heart syndrome

Definition

Athletic heart syndrome is the adaptation of an athlete's heart in response the physiologic stresses of strenuous physical training. It can be difficult to distinguish a significant medical condition from an athletic heart.

Description

The heart adapts to physical demands by enlarging, especially the left ventricle. Enlargement increases the cardiac output, the amount of blood pumped with each beat of the heart. The exact type of adaptation depends on the nature of the physical demand. There are two types of demand, static and dynamic. Static demand involves smaller groups of muscles under extreme resistance for brief period. An example is weight lifting. Dynamic training involves larger groups of muscles at lower resistance for extended periods of time. Examples are aerobic training and tennis.

Cardiac enlargement is associated with dynamic training. The heart's response to static training is hypertrophy, thickening of the muscle walls of the heart. As the wall of the heart adapts, there are changes in the electrical conducting system of the heart. Because of the larger volume of blood being pumped with each heart beat, the heart rate when at rest decreases below the normal level for nonathletes.

Sudden unexpected **death** (SUD) is the death of an athlete, usually during or shortly after physical activity. Often, there is no warning that the person will experience SUD, although in some cases, warning signs appear which cause the person to seek medical advice. Importantly, cases of death occurring during physical activity are not caused by athletic heart syndrome, but by undiagnosed heart disorders.

Causes and symptoms

Athletic heart syndrome is the consequence of a normal adaptation by the heart to increased physical activity. The changes in the electrical conduction system of the heart may be pronounced and diagnostic, but should not cause problems. In the case of SUD, other heart problems are involved. In 85-97% of the cases of SUD, an underlying structural defect of the heart has been noted.

Diagnosis

The changes in the heart beat caused by the electrical conduction system of the heart are detectable on an electrocardiogram. Many of the changes seen in athletic heart syndrome mimic those of various heart diseases. Careful examination must be made to distinguish heart disease from athletic heart syndrome.

Prognosis

The yearly rate for occurrence of SUD in people less than 35 years of age is less than 7 incidents per 100,000. Of all SUD cases, only about 8% are **exercise** related. On a national basis, this means that each year approximately 25 athletes experience SUD. In persons over age 35, the incidence of SUD is approximately 55 in 100,000, with only 3% of the cases occurring during exercise.

Resources

BOOKS

Alexander, R. W., R. C. Schlant, and V. Fuster, editors. *The Heart.* 9th ed. New York: McGraw-Hill, 1998.

John T. Lohr, PhD

Atkins diet

Definition

The Atkins diet is a high-protein, high-fat, and very low-carbohydrate regimen. It emphasizes meat, cheese, and eggs, while discouraging foods such as bread, pasta, fruit, and sugar. It is a form of ketogenic diet.

Purpose

The primary benefit of the diet is rapid and substantial weight loss. By restricting carbohydrate intake, the body will burn more fat stored in the body. Since there are no limits on the amount of calories or quantities of foods allowed on the diet, there is little hunger between meals. According to Atkins, the diet can alleviate symptoms of conditions such as **fatigue**, irritability, headaches, depression, and some types of joint and muscle **pain**.

Description

The regimen is a low-carbohydrate, or ketogenic diet, characterized by initial rapid weight loss, usually due to water loss. Drastically reducing the amount of carbohydrate intake causes liver and muscle glycogen loss, which has a strong but temporary diuretic effect. Long-term weight loss occurs because with a low amount of carbohydrate intake, the body burns stored fat for energy.

The four-step diet starts with a two-week induction program designed to rebalance an individual's metabolism. Unlimited amounts of fat and protein are allowed but carbohydrate intake is restricted to 20 grams per day. Foods allowed include butter, oil, meat, poultry, fish, eggs, cheese, and cream. The daily amount of carbohydrates allowed equals about three cups of salad vegetables, such as lettuce, cucumbers, and celery.

The second stage is for ongoing weight loss. It allows 20-40 grams of carbohydrates a day. When the individual is about 10 pounds from their desired weight, they begin the pre-maintenance phase. This gradually adds one to three servings a week of high carbohydrate foods, such as a piece of fruit or slice of whole-wheat bread. When the desired weight is reached, the maintenance stage begins. It allows 40-60 grams of carbohydrates per day.

Opinion from the general medical community remains mixed on the Atkins diet. There have been no significant long-term scientific studies on the diet.

A number of leading medical and health organizations, including the American Medical Association, American Dietetic Association (ADA), and the American Heart Association oppose it. It is drastically different than the dietary intakes recommended by the U.S. Department of Agriculture and the National Institutes of Health. Much of the opposition is because the diet is lacking in some **vitamins** and nutrients, and because it is high in fat. In a hearing before the U.S. Congress on February 24, 2000, an ADA representative called the Atkins diet "hazardous" and said it lacked scientific credibility.

Preparations

No advance preparation is needed to go on the diet. However, as with most **diets**, it is generally considered appropriate to consult with a physician and to have a physical evaluation before starting such a nutritional regimen. The evaluation should include blood tests to determine levels of cholesterol, triglycerides, glucose, insulin, and uric acid. A glucose tolerance test is also recommended.

Precautions

Adherence to the Atkins diet can result in vitamin and mineral deficiencies. In his books, Atkins recommends a wide-range of **nutritional supplements**, including a multi-vitamin. Among his recommendations, Atkins suggests the following daily dosages: 300-600 micrograms (mcg) of chromium picolinate, 100-400 milligrams (mg) of pantetheine, 200 mcg of selenium, and 450-675 mcg of biotin.

The diet is not recommended for lacto-ovo vegetarians, since it cannot be done as successfully without protein derived from animal products. Also, vegans cannot follow this diet, since a vegan diet is too high in carbohydrates, according to Atkins. Instead, he recommends vegetarians with a serious weight problem give up **vegetarianism**, or at least include fish in their diet.

Side effects

According to Atkins, the diet causes no adverse side effects. Many health care professionals disagree. In a fact sheet for the Healthcare Reality Check Web site (< http://www.hcrc.org >), Ellen Coleman, a registered dietician and author, said the diet may have serious side effects for some people. She said complications associated with the diet include ketosis, **dehydration**, electrolyte loss, calcium depletion, weakness, **nausea**, and kidney problems.

DR. ROBERT C. ATKINS (1930–2003)

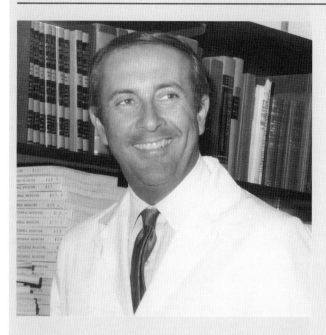

(AP/Wide World Photos. Reproduced by permission.)

Dr. Robert C. Atkins graduated from the University of Michigan in 1951 and received his medical degree from Cornell University Medical School in 1955 with a specialty in cardiology. As an internist and cardiologist he developed the Atkins Diet in the early 1970s. The diet is a ketogenic diet—a high protein, high fat, and very low carbohydrate regimen resulting in ketosis. It emphasizes meat, cheese, and eggs, while discouraging foods such as bread, pasta, fruit, and sugar. It first came to public attention in 1972 with the publication of *Dr. Atkins' Diet Revolution*. The book quickly became a bestseller but unlike most other fad diet books, this one has remained popular. At last count, it had been reprinted 28 times and sold more than 10 million copies worldwide. Since then, Atkins has authored a number of other books on his diet theme, including *Dr. Atkins' New Diet Revolution* (1992), *Dr. Atkins' Quick and Easy New Diet Cookbook* (1997), and *The Vita-Nutrient Solution: Nature's Answer to Drugs* (1998).

Atkins has seen about 60,000 patients in his more than 30 years of practice. He has also appeared on numerous radio and television talk shows, has his own syndicated radio program, *Your Health Choices*, and authors the monthly newsletter *Dr. Atkins' Health Revelations*. Atkins has received the World Organization of Alternative Medicine's Recognition of Achievement Award and been named the National Health Federation's Man of the Year. He was the director of the Atkins Center for Complementary Medicine which he founded in the early 1980s until his death. The center is located at 152 E. 55th St., New York, NY 10022.

KEY TERMS

Biotin—A B complex vitamin, found naturally in yeast, liver, and egg yolks.

Carbohydrates—Neutral compounds of carbon, hydrogen, and oxygen found in sugar, starches, and cellulose.

Hypertension—Abnormally high arterial blood pressure, which if left untreated can lead to heart disease and stroke.

Ketogenic diet—A diet that supplies an abnormally high amount of fat, and small amounts of carbohydrates and protein.

Ketosis—An abnormal increase in ketones in the body, usually found in people with uncontrolled diabetes mellitus.

Pantetheine—A growth factor substance essential in humans, and a constituent of coenzyme A.

Triglycerides—A blood fat lipid that increases the risk for heart disease.

"It is certainly riskier for overweight individuals with medical problems such as heart disease, **hypertension**, **kidney disease**, and diabetes than it is for overweight people with no health problems," she said.

People with diabetes taking insulin are at risk of becoming hypoglycemic if they do not eat appropriate carbohydrates. Also, persons who **exercise** regularly may experience low energy levels and muscle fatigue from low carbohydrate intake.

Resources

BOOKS

Atkins, Dr. Robert C. *Dr. Atkins' Age-Defying Diet Revolution.* New York: St. Martin's Press. 1999.

PERIODICALS

Cray, Dan, et al. "The Low-Carb Diet Craze." *Time* November 1, 1999: 72-79.

Gotthardt, Melissa Meyers. "The New Low-Carb Diet Craze." *Cosmopolitan* February 2000: 148.

Merrell, Woodson. "How I Became a Low-Carb Believer." *Time* November 1, 1999: 80.

Turner, Richard. "The Trendy Diet That Sizzles." *Newsweek* September 6, 1999: 60.

OTHER

Atkins Center for Complementary Medicine. 152 E. 55th St., New York, NY 10022. 212-758-2110. <http://www.atkinscenter.com>.

Ken R. Wells

Atopic dermatitis

Definition

Eczema is a general term used to describe a variety of conditions that cause an itchy, inflamed skin rash. Atopic **dermatitis**, a form of eczema, is a non-contagious disorder characterized by chronically inflamed skin and sometimes intolerable itching.

Description

Atopic dermatitis refers to a wide range of diseases that are often associated with stress and allergic disorders that involve the respiratory system, like **asthma** and hay **fever**. Although atopic dermatitis can appear at any age, it is most common in children and young adults. Symptoms usually abate before the age of 25 and do not affect the patient's general health.

About one in ten babies develop a form of atopic dermatitis called infantile eczema. Characterized by skin that oozes and becomes encrusted, infantile eczema most often occurs on the face and scalp. The condition usually improves before the child's second birthday, and medical attention can keep symptoms in check until that time.

When atopic dermatitis develops after infancy, inflammation, blistering, oozing, and crusting are less pronounced. The patient's sores become dry, turn from red to brownish-gray, and skin may thicken and become scaly. In dark-skinned individuals, this condition can cause the complexion to lighten or darken. **Itching** associated with this condition is usually worst at night. It can be so intense that patients scratch until their sores bleed, sometimes causing scarring and infection.

Atopic dermatitis affects about 3% of the population of the United States, and about 80% of the people who have the condition have one or more relatives with the same condition or a similar one. Symptoms tend to be most severe in females. Atopic dermatitis can erupt on any part of the skin, and crusted, thickened patches on the fingers, palms, or the soles of the feet can last for years. In teenagers and young adults, atopic dermatitis often appears on one or more of the following areas:

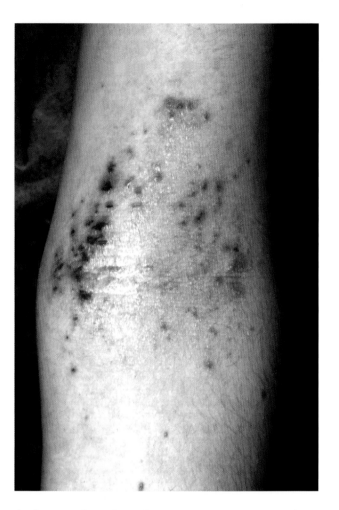

A close-up view of atopic dermatitis in the crook of the elbow of a 12-year-old patient. *(Custom Medical Stock Photo. Reproduced by permission.)*

- elbow creases
- backs of the knees
- ankles
- wrists
- face
- neck
- upper chest
- palms and between the fingers

Causes and symptoms

While allergic reactions often trigger atopic dermatitis, the condition is thought to be the result of an inherited over-active immune system or a genetic defect that causes the skin to lose abnormally large amounts of moisture. The condition can

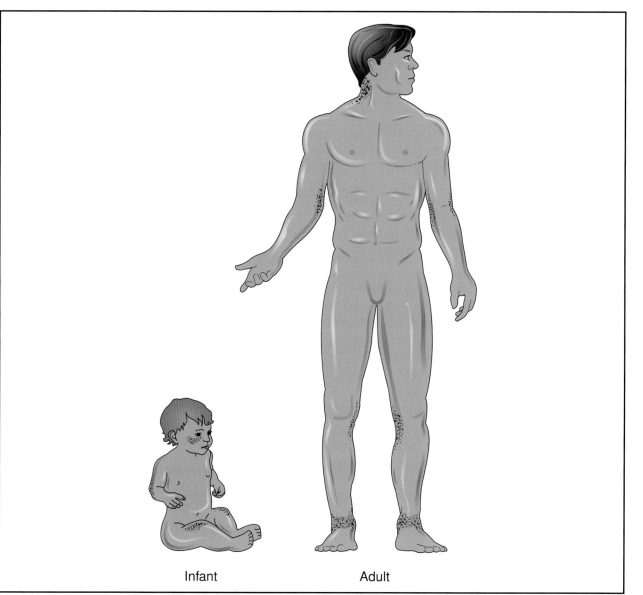

Infant   Adult

Atopic dermatitis can erupt on any part of the skin. In infants, it often appears on the face, scalp, and knees, while it develops on the elbows, neck, back of the knees, and ankles in adults. *(Illustration by Electronic Illustrators Group.)*

be aggravated by a cycle that develops in which the skin itches, the patient scratches, the condition worsens, the itching worsens, the patient scratches, etc.

This cycle must be broken by relieving the itching to allow the skin time to heal. If the skin becomes broken, there is also a risk of developing skin infections which, if not recognized and treated promptly, can become more serious.

Symptoms of atopic dermatitis include the following:

- an itchy rash and dry, thickened skin on areas of the body where moisture can be trapped

- continual scratching

- chronic **fatigue**, caused when itching disrupts sleep

An individual is more at-risk for developing the condition if there is a personal or family history of atopic dermatitis, hay fever, asthma, or other allergies. Exposure to any of the following can cause a flare-up:

- hot or cold temperatures
- wool and synthetic fabrics
- detergents, fabric softeners, and chemicals
- use of drugs that suppress immune-system activity

Certain foods, such as peanuts, cow's milk, eggs, and fish, can trigger symptoms of atopic dermatitis. A small percentage of patients with atopic dermatitis find that their symptoms worsen after having been exposed to dust, feather pillows, rough-textured fabrics, or other materials to which dust adheres.

Diagnosis

Diagnosis of atopic dermatitis is usually based on the patient's symptoms and personal and family health history. Skin tests do not generally provide reliable information about this condition.

Treatment

Atopic dermatitis cannot be cured, but the severity and duration of symptoms can be controlled. A dermatologist should be consulted when symptoms first appear, and is likely to recommend warm baths to loosen encrusted skin, followed by applications of petroleum jelly or vegetable shortening to prevent the skin's natural moisture from escaping.

Externally applied (topical) steroids or preparations containing coal tar can relieve minor itching, but coal tar has an unpleasant odor, stains clothes, and may increase skin-cancer risk. Excessive use of steroid creams in young children can alter growth. Pregnant women should not use products that contain coal tar. Topical steroids can cause itching, burning, **acne**, permanent stretch marks, and thinning and spotting of the skin. Applying topical steroids to the area around the eyes can cause **glaucoma**.

Oral **antihistamines**, such as diphenhydramine (Benadryl), can relieve symptoms of allergy-related atopic dermatitis. More concentrated topical steroids are recommended for persistent symptoms. A mild tranquilizer may be prescribed to reduce **stress** and help the patient sleep, and **antibiotics** are used to treat secondary infections.

Cortisone ointments should be used sparingly, and strong preparations should never be applied to the face, groin, armpits, or rectal area. Regular medical monitoring is recommended for patients who use cortisone salves or lotions to control widespread symptoms. Oral cortisone may be prescribed if the patient does not respond to other treatments, but patients who take the medication for more than two weeks have a greater-than-average risk of developing severe symptoms when the treatment is discontinued.

Allergy shots rarely improve atopic dermatitis and sometimes aggravate the symptoms. Since **food allergies** may trigger atopic dermatitis, the doctor may suggest eliminating certain foods from the diet if other treatments prove ineffective.

If symptoms are extremely severe, ultraviolet light therapy may be prescribed, and a wet body wrap recommended to help the skin retain moisture. This technique, used most often with children, involves sleeping in a warm room while wearing wet pajamas under dry clothing, rain gear, or a nylon sweatsuit. The patient's face may be covered with wet gauze covered by elastic bandages, and his hands encased in wet socks covered by dry ones.

A physician should be notified if the condition is widespread or resists treatment, or the skin oozes, becomes encrusted, or smells, as this may indicate an infection.

Alternative treatment

Alternative therapies can sometimes bring relief or resolution of atopic dermatitis when conventional therapies are not helping. If the condition becomes increasingly widespread or infected, a physician should be consulted.

Helpful alternative treatments for atopic dermatitis may include:

- Taking regular brisk walks, followed by bathing in warm water sprinkled with essential oil of lavender (*Lavandula officinalis*); lavender oil acts as a nerve relaxant for the whole body including the skin
- Supplementing the diet daily with zinc, fish oils, vitamin A, vitamin E, and evening primrose oil (*Oenothera biennis*)–all good sources of nutrients for the skin
- Reducing or eliminating red meat from the diet
- Eliminating or rotating potentially allergic foods such as cow's milk, peanuts, wheat, eggs, and soy
- Implementing **stress reduction** techniques in daily life.

Herbal therapies also can be helpful in treating atopic dermatitis. Western herbal remedies used in the treatment of this condition include burdock (*Arctium lappa*) and *Ruta* (*Ruta graveolens*). Long-term herbal therapy requires monitoring and should be guided by an experienced practitioner.

Other alternative techniques that may be useful in the treatment of atopic dermatitis include:

- Acupressure (**acupuncture** without needles) to relieve tension that may trigger a flare
- Aromatherapy, using essential oils like lavender, thyme (*Thymus vulgaris*), jasmine (*Jasminum officinale*) and chamomile (*Matricaria recutita*) in hot water, to add a soothing fragrance to the air
- Shiatsu massage and **reflexology**, performed by licensed practitioners, to alleviate symptoms by restoring the body's natural balance
- Homeopathy, which may temporarily worsen symptoms before relieving them, and should be supervised by a trained alternative healthcare professional
- Hydrotherapy, which uses water, ice, liquid, and steam, to stimulate the immune system
- Juice therapy to purify the liver and relieve bowel congestion
- Yoga to induce a sense of serenity.

Prognosis

Atopic dermatitis is unpredictable. Although symptoms occur less often with age and sometimes disappear altogether, they can recur without warning. Atopic dermatitis lowers resistance to infection and increases the risk of developing **cataracts**. Sixty percent of patients with atopic dermatitis will experience flares and remissions throughout their lives.

Prevention

Research has shown that babies weaned from breast milk before they are four months old are almost three times more likely than other babies to develop recurrent eczema. Feeding eggs or fish to a baby less than one year old can activate symptoms, and babies should be shielded from such irritants as mites, molds, pet hair, and smoke.

Possible ways to prevent flare-ups include the following:

- eliminate activities that cause sweating
- lubricate the skin frequently
- avoid wool, perfumes, fabric softeners, soaps that dry the skin, and other irritants
- avoid sudden temperature changes

A doctor should be notified whenever any of the following occurs:

- fever or relentless itching develop during a flare
- an unexplained rash develops in someone who has a personal or family history of eczema or asthma
- inflammation does not decrease after seven days of treatment with an over-the-counter preparation containing coal tar or steroids
- a yellow, tan, or brown crust or pus-filled blisters appear on top of an existing rash
- a person with active atopic dermatitis comes into contact with someone who has cold sores, **genital herpes**, or another viral skin disease

Resources

ORGANIZATIONS

American Academy of Dermatology. 930 N. Meacham Road, P.O. Box 4014, Schaumburg, IL 60168-4014. (847) 330-0230. Fax: (847) 330-0050. < http://www.aad.org > .

Maureen Haggerty

Atrial ectopic beats

Definition

Atrial ectopic beats (AEB) refers to a contraction of the upper heart chamber which occurs before it would be expected. Atrial ectopic beats are also known as premature atrial beats, premature atrial complex (PAC), or atrial extrasystole.

Description

An AEB is usually a harmless disturbance in the normal rhythm of the heart. It can occur only occasionally, in a regular pattern, or several may occur in sequence and then disappear. Most often, the person is unaware of the event.

Causes and symptoms

As people age, extra beats tend to happen more frequently even in perfectly healthy individuals. AEB may be triggered or increased by **stress, caffeine, smoking**, and some medicines. Cold remedies containing ephedrine or pseudoephedrine have been known to increase the incidence of atrial ectopic beats. AEB may also be the result of an enlarged atria, lung disease, or the result of reduced blood supply to that area of the heart.

If a person is aware of the event, the first symptom of AEB is usually a feeling that the heart has skipped or missed a beat. This is often accompanied by a feeling that the heart is thumping or pounding in the chest. The thumping or pounding is caused by the fact that when there is an AEB, the pause before the next beat is usually longer than normal. The next beat must be stronger than usual to pump the accumulated blood out of the chamber.

Diagnosis

Diagnosis of AEB is often suspected on the basis of the patient's description of the occurrence. An electrocardiogram (ECG) can confirm the diagnosis. An ECG shows the heart beat as three wave forms. The first wave is called P, the second is called QRS, and the last is T. An atrial ectopic beat will show up on the ECG as a P wave that occurs closer than usual to the preceding T wave.

Treatment

Atrial ectopic beats do not usually require treatment. If treatment is necessary because the beats occur frequently and cause intolerable discomfort, the doctor may prescribe medication.

Prognosis

Occasional AEB usually have no significance. If they increase in frequency, they can lead to atrial tachycardia or fibrillation and to a decrease in cardiac output.

Prevention

AEB cannot usually be prevented. Aggravating factors can be addressed, like excessive stimulants, and uncontrolled pulmonary disorders.

Resources

ORGANIZATIONS

American Heart Association. 7320 Greenville Ave. Dallas, TX 75231. (214) 373-6300. < http:// www.americanheart.org > .

Dorothy Elinor Stonely

Atrial extrasystole *see* **Atrial ectopic beats**

Atrial fibrillation and flutter

Definition

Atrial fibrillation and flutter are abnormal heart rhythms in which the atria, or upper chambers of the heart, are out of sync with the ventricles, or lower chambers of the heart. In atrial fibrillation, the atria "quiver" chaotically and the ventricles beat irregularly. In atrial flutter, the atria beat regularly and faster than the ventricles.

Description

Atrial fibrillation and flutter are two types of cardiac **arrhythmias**, irregularities in the heart's rhythm. Nearly 2 million Americans have atrial fibrillation, according to the American Heart Association. It is the most common chronic arrhythmia. Atrial flutter is less common, but both of these arrhythmias can cause a blood clot to form in the heart. This can lead to a **stroke** or a blockage carried by the blood flow (an **embolism**) anywhere in the body's arteries. Atrial fibrillation is responsible for about 15% of strokes.

The atria are the heart's two small upper chambers. In atrial fibrillation, the heart beat is completely irregular. The atrial muscles contract very quickly and irregularly; the ventricles, the heart's two large lower chambers, beat irregularly but not as fast as the atria. When the atria fibrillate, blood that is not completely pumped out can pool and form a clot. In atrial flutter, the heart beat is usually very fast but steady. The atria beat faster than the ventricles.

Atrial fibrillation often occurs in people with various types of heart disease. Atrial fibrillation may also result from an inflammation of the heart's covering (**pericarditis**), chest trauma or surgery, pulmonary disease, and certain medications. Atrial fibrillation is more common in older people; about 10% of people over the age of 75 have it. Atrial flutter and fibrillation usually occur in people with hypertensive or coronary heart disease and other types of heart disorders.

Causes and symptoms

In most cases, the cause of atrial fibrillation and flutter can be found, but often it cannot. Causes of these heart beat abnormalities include:

- many types of heart disease
- **stress** and anxiety
- **caffeine**

KEY TERMS

Arrhythmia—A variation in the normal rhythm of the heart beat. Atrial fibrillation and flutter are two types of arrhythmia.

Atria—The two small upper chambers of the heart that receive blood from the lungs and the body.

Stroke—A brain attack caused by a sudden disruption of blood flow to the brain, in this case because of a blood clot.

Ventricles—The two large lower chambers of the heart that pump blood to the lungs and to the rest of the body.

- alcohol
- tobacco
- diet pills
- some prescription and over-the-counter medications
- open heart surgery

Symptoms, when present, include:

- a fluttering feeling in the chest
- a pulse that feels like the heart is skipping, racing, jumping, or is irregular
- low energy
- a faint or dizzy feeling
- pressure or discomfort in the chest
- shortness of breath
- anxiety

Diagnosis

A doctor can sometimes hear these arrhythmias using an instrument (a stethoscope) to listen to the sounds within the chest. Atrial fibrillation and flutter are usually diagnosed through electrocardiography (EKGs), an **exercise stress test**, a 24-hour Holter EKG monitor, or a telephone cardiac monitor. An EKG shows the heart's activity and may reveal a lack of oxygen (**ischemia**). Electrodes covered with conducting jelly are placed on the patient's chest, arms, and legs. The electrodes send impulses of the heart's activity through a monitor (called an oscilloscope) to a recorder that traces the pattern of the impulses onto paper. The test takes about 10 minutes and is performed in a doctor's office. The exercise stress test measures how the heart and blood vessels respond to work when the patient is exercising on a treadmill or a stationary bike. This test is performed in a doctor's office within an exercise laboratory and takes 15-30 minutes.

In 24-hour EKG (Holter) monitoring, the patient wears a small, portable tape recorder connected to disks on his/her chest that record the heart's rhythm during normal activities. An EKG called transtelephonic monitoring identifies arrhythmias that occur infrequently. Like **Holter monitoring**, transtelephonic monitoring continues for days or weeks and enables patients to send the EKG via telephone to a monitoring station when an arrhythmia is felt, or to store the information in the recorder and transmit it later. Doctors can also use high-frequency sound waves (**echocardiography**) to determine the structure and function of the heart. This diagnostic method is often helpful to evaluate for underlying heart disease.

Treatment

Atrial fibrillation and flutter are usually treated with medications and/or electrical shock (cardioversion). In some cases, removal of a small portion of the heart (ablation), implantation of a pacemaker or a cardioverter defibrillator, or maze surgery is needed.

If the heart rate cannot be quickly controlled, electrical **cardioversion** may be used. Cardioversion, the electric shock to the chest wall, is usually performed emergencies. This device briefly suspends the heart's activity and allows it to return to a normal rhythm.

Ablation destroys the heart tissue that causes the arrhythmia. The tissue can be destroyed by catheterization or surgery. Radiofrequency catheter ablation, performed in a **cardiac catheterization** laboratory, can cure atrial flutter and control the heart rate in atrial fibrillation. The patient is awake but sedated. A thin tube called a catheter is inserted into a vein and is threaded into the heart. At the end of the catheter, a device maps the electrical pathways of the heart. A cardiologist, a doctor specializing in the heart, uses this map to identify the pathway(s) causing the arrhythmia, and then eliminates it (them) with bursts of high-frequency radio waves. Surgical ablation is performed in an operating room under general anesthesia. Computerized mapping techniques are combined with a cold probe to destroy arrhythmia-causing tissue. Ablation is generally successful. When ablation is used for atrial fibrillation, it is usually followed by implantation of a pacemaker as well as drug therapy.

A pacemaker is a battery-powered device about the size of a matchbox that is surgically implanted near the collarbone to regulate the heart beat. Lead wires threaded to the right side of the heart supply electrical energy to pace the atria and ventricles. The implantable cardioverter defibrillator is a treatment for serious arrhythmias. The battery-powered device senses an abnormal heart rhythm and automatically provides electrical shock(s). The shock(s) suspends heart activity and then allows the heart to initiate a normal rhythm. Wire electrodes on the device are attached to the heart. Some of the electrodes are attached to the outside of the heart and some are attached to the inside of the heart through veins. The newest implantable cardioverter defibrillators can be implanted in the chest wall and do not require open chest surgery. These devices weigh less than 10 oz and generally last seven or eight years. An implantable cardioverter defibrillator is usually used with drug therapy, but the amount medication is reduced. In maze surgery, often the last resort, surgeons create a maze of stitches (sutures) that help the heart's electrical impulses travel effectively.

Most of the drugs used for treatment have potential side effects and should be carefully monitored by a doctor. The goal of treatment is to control the rate and rhythm of the heart and to prevent the formation of **blood clots**. If the arrhythmia is caused by heart disease, the heart disease will also be treated. The American Heart Association recommends aggressive treatment.

A digitalis drug, most commonly digoxin, is usually prescribed to control the heart rate. Digitalis drugs slow the heart's electrical impulses, helping to restore the normal rate and rhythm. These drugs also increase the ability of the heart's muscular layer to contract and pump properly. Beta-blockers and calcium channel blockers can also be used for this purpose. Beta-blockers slow the speed of electrical impulses through the heart. Some **calcium channel blockers** dampen the heart's response to erratic electrical impulses.

To prevent blood clots, **aspirin** or warfarin (Coumadin) is administered. Warfarin, however, has potential bleeding side effects, especially in older patients. Amiodarone is fairly effective for atrial flutter. This drug is often able to maintain the heart's proper rhythm and can also help control the heart rate when the flutter occurs.

Prognosis

Patients with atrial fibrillation and flutter can live a normal life for many years as long as the arrhythmia is controlled and serious blood clots are prevented.

Prevention

Atrial fibrillation and flutter can sometimes be prevented when the cause can be identified and controlled. Depending on the cause, prevention could include:

- treating the underlying heart disease
- reducing stress and anxiety
- reducing or stopping consumption of caffeine, alcohol, or tobacco; and/or
- discontinuing diet pills or other medications (over-the-counter or prescription)

Resources

PERIODICALS

Kosinski, Daniel, et al. "Catheter Ablation for Atrial Flutter and Fibrillation: An Effective Alternative to Medical Therapy." *Postgraduate Medicine*103, no. 1 (January 1998): 103-110.

ORGANIZATIONS

American Heart Association. 7320 Greenville Ave. Dallas, TX 75231. (214) 373-6300. < http://www.americanheart.org > .

National Heart, Lung and Blood Institute. PO Box 30105, Bethesda, MD 20824-0105. (301) 251-1222. < http://www.nhlbi.nih.gov > .

Texas Heart Institute. Heart Information Service. PO Box 20345, Houston, TX 77225-0345. < http://www.tmc.edu/thi > .

Lori De Milto

Atrial flutter *see* **Atrial fibrillation and flutter**

Atrial septal defect

Definition

An atrial septal defect is an abnormal opening in the wall separating the left and right upper chambers (atria) of the heart.

Description

During the normal development of the fetal heart, there is an opening in the wall (the septum) separating the left and right upper chambers of the heart. Normally, this opening closes before birth, but if it does not, the child is born with a hole between the left and right atria. This abnormal opening is called an atrial septal defect and causes blood from the left atrium to flow into the right atrium.

Different types of atrial septal defects can occur, and they are classified according to where in the separating wall they are found. The most commonly found atrial septal defect occurs in the middle of the atrial septum and accounts for about 70% of all atrial septal defects. Abnormal openings can form in the upper and lower parts of the atrial septum as well.

Causes and symptoms

Abnormal openings in the atrial septum occur during fetal development and are twice as common in females as in males. These abnormalities can go unnoticed if the opening is small, producing no abnormal symptoms. If the defect is big, large amounts of blood flowing from the left to the right atrium will cause the right atrium to swell to hold the extra blood.

People born with an atrial septal defect can have no symptoms through their twenties, but by age 40, most people with this condition have symptoms that can include **shortness of breath**, rapid abnormal beating of the atria (atrial fibrillation), and eventually **heart failure**.

Diagnosis

Atrial septal defects can be identified by various methods. Abnormal changes in the sound of the heart beats can be heard when a doctor listens to the heart with a stethoscope. In addition, a **chest x ray**, an electrocardiogram (ECG, an electrical printout of the heartbeats), and an echocardiogram (a test that uses sound waves to form a detailed image of the heart) can also be used to identify this condition.

An atrial septal defect can also be diagnosed by using a test called **cardiac catheterization**. This test involves inserting a very thin tube (catheter) into the heart's chambers to measure the amount of oxygen present in the blood within the heart. If the heart has an opening between the atria, oxygen-rich blood from the left atrium enters the right atrium. Through cardiac catheterization, doctors can detect the higher-than-normal amount of oxygen in the heart's right atrium, right ventricle, and the large blood vessels that carry blood to the lungs, where

---

KEY TERMS

Cardiac catheterization—A test that involves having a tiny tube inserted into the heart through a blood vessel.

Dacron—A synthetic polyester fiber used to surgically repair damaged sections of heart muscle and blood vessel walls.

Echocardiogram—A test that uses sound waves to generate an image of the heart, its valves, and chambers.

---

the blood would normally subsequently get its oxygen.

Treatment

Atrial septal defects often correct themselves without medical treatments by the age of two. If this dose not happen, surgery is done by sewing the hole closed, or by sewing a patch of Dacron material or a piece of the sac that surrounds the heart (the pericardium), over the opening.

Some patients can have the defect fixed by having an clam-shaped plug placed over the opening. This plug is a man-made device that is put in place through a catheter inserted into the heart.

Prognosis

Individuals with small defects can live a normal life, but larger defects require surgical correction. Less than 1% of people younger than 45 years of age die from corrective surgery. Five to ten percent of patients can die from the surgery if they are older than 40 and have other heart-related problems. When an atrial septal defect is corrected within the first 20 years of life, there is an excellent chance for the individual to live normally.

Resources

ORGANIZATIONS

American Heart Association. 7320 Greenville Ave. Dallas, TX 75231. (214) 373-6300. < http:// www.americanheart.org > .

Dominic De Bellis, PhD

Atrioventricular block *see* **Heart block**

Attapulgite *see* **Antidiarrheal drugs**

Attention-deficit/ Hyperactivity disorder (ADHD)

Definition

Attention-deficit/hyperactivity disorder (ADHD) is a developmental disorder characterized by distractibility, hyperactivity, impulsive behaviors, and the inability to remain focused on tasks or activities.

Description

ADHD, also known as hyperkinetic disorder (HKD) outside of the United States, is estimated to affect 3-9% of children, and afflicts boys more often than girls. Although difficult to assess in infancy and toddlerhood, signs of ADHD may begin to appear as early as age two or three, but the symptom picture changes as adolescence approaches. Many symptoms, particularly hyperactivity, diminish in early adulthood, but impulsivity and inattention problems remain with up to 50% of ADHD individuals throughout their adult life.

Children with ADHD have short attention spans, becoming easily bored and/or frustrated with tasks. Although they may be quite intelligent, their lack of focus frequently results in poor grades and difficulties in school. ADHD children act impulsively, taking action first and thinking later. They are constantly moving, running, climbing, squirming, and fidgeting, but often have trouble with gross and fine motor skills and, as a result, may be physically clumsy and awkward. Their clumsiness may extend to the social arena, where they are sometimes shunned due to their impulsive and intrusive behavior.

Causes and symptoms

The causes of ADHD are not known. However, it appears that heredity plays a major role in the development of ADHD. Children with an ADHD parent or sibling are more likely to develop the disorder themselves. In 2004, scientists reported at least 20 candidate genes that might contribute to ADHD, but no single gene stood out as the gene causing the condition. Before birth, ADHD children may have been exposed to poor maternal **nutrition**, viral infections, or maternal **substance abuse**. In early childhood, exposure to lead or other toxins can cause ADHD-like symptoms. Traumatic brain injury or neurological disorders may also trigger

Drugs Used To Treat ADHD

Brand Name (Generic Name)	Possible Common Side Effects Include:
Cylert (pemoline)	Insomnia
Dexedrine (dextroamphetamine sulfate)	Excessive stimulation, restlessness
Ritalin (methylphenidate hydrochloride)	Insomnia, nervousness, loss of appetite

KEY TERMS

Conduct disorder—A behavioral and emotional disorder of childhood and adolescence. Children with a conduct disorder act inappropriately, infringe on the rights of others, and violate societal norms.

Nervous tic—A repetitive, involuntary action, such as the twitching of a muscle or repeated blinking.

Oppositional defiant disorder—A disorder characterized by hostile, deliberately argumentative, and defiant behavior toward authority figures.

ADHD symptoms. Although the exact cause of ADHD is not known, an imbalance of certain neurotransmitters, the chemicals in the brain that transmit messages between nerve cells, is believed to be the mechanism behind ADHD symptoms.

A widely publicized study conducted by Dr. Ben Feingold in the early 1970s suggested that allergies to certain foods and food additives caused the characteristic hyperactivity of ADHD children. Although some children may have adverse reactions to certain foods that can affect their behavior (for example, a rash might temporarily cause a child to be distracted from other tasks), carefully controlled follow-up studies have uncovered no link between **food allergies** and ADHD. Another popularly held misconception about food and ADHD is that the consumption of sugar causes hyperactive behavior. Again, studies have shown no link between sugar intake and ADHD. It is important to note, however, that a nutritionally balanced diet is important for normal development in *all* children.

Psychologists and other mental health professionals typically use the criteria listed in the *Diagnostic and Statistical Manual of Mental Disorders, Fourth*

Edition (DSM-IV) as a guideline for determining the presence of ADHD. For a diagnosis of ADHD, *DSM-IV* requires the presence of at least six of the following symptoms of inattention, or six or more symptoms of hyperactivity and impulsivity combined:

Inattention:

- fails to pay close attention to detail or makes careless mistakes in schoolwork or other activities
- has difficulty sustaining attention in tasks or activities
- does not appear to listen when spoken to
- does not follow through on instructions and does not finish tasks
- has difficulty organizing tasks and activities
- avoids or dislikes tasks that require sustained mental effort (e.g., homework)
- is easily distracted
- is forgetful in daily activities

Hyperactivity:

- fidgets with hands or feet or squirms in seat
- does not remain seated when expected to
- runs or climbs excessively when inappropriate (in adolescents and adults, feelings of restlessness)
- has difficulty playing quietly
- is constantly on the move
- talks excessively

Impulsivity:

- blurts out answers before the question has been completed
- has difficulty waiting for his or her turn
- interrupts and/or intrudes on others

Diagnosis

The first step in determining if a child has ADHD is to consult with a pediatrician. The pediatrician can make an initial evaluation of the child's developmental maturity compared to other children in his or her age group. The physician should also perform a comprehensive **physical examination** to rule out any organic causes of ADHD symptoms, such as an overactive thyroid or vision or hearing problems.

If no organic problem can be found, a psychologist, psychiatrist, neurologist, neuropsychologist, or learning specialist is typically consulted to perform a comprehensive ADHD assessment. A complete medical, family, social, psychiatric, and educational history

is compiled from existing medical and school records and from interviews with parents and teachers. Interviews may also be conducted with the child, depending on his or her age. Along with these interviews, several clinical inventories may also be used, such as the Conners Rating Scales (Teacher's Questionnaire and Parent's Questionnaire), Child Behavior Checklist (CBCL), and the Achenbach Child Behavior Rating Scales. These inventories provide valuable information on the child's behavior in different settings and situations. In addition, the Wender Utah Rating Scale has been adapted for use in diagnosing ADHD in adults.

It is important to note that mental disorders such as depression and **anxiety** disorder can cause symptoms similar to ADHD. A complete and comprehensive psychiatric assessment is critical to differentiate ADHD from other possible mood and behavioral disorders. **Bipolar disorder**, for example, may be misdiagnosed as ADHD.

Public schools are required by federal law to offer free ADHD testing upon request. A pediatrician can also provide a referral to a psychologist or pediatric specialist for ADHD assessment. Parents should check with their insurance plans to see if these services are covered.

Treatment

Psychosocial therapy, usually combined with medications, is the treatment approach of choice to alleviate ADHD symptoms. Psychostimulants, such as dextroamphetamine (Dexedrine), pemoline (Cylert), and methylphenidate (Ritalin) are commonly prescribed to control hyperactive and impulsive behavior and increase attention span. They work by stimulating the production of certain neurotransmitters in the brain. Possible side effects of stimulants include nervous tics, irregular heartbeat, loss of appetite, and **insomnia**. However, the medications are usually well-tolerated and safe in most cases. In 2004, longer-acting stimulants had been released to treat adult ADHD.

In 2004, the American Academy of Child and Adolescent Psychiatry listed the first nonstimulant as a first-line therapy for ADHD. Called atomoxetine HCl (Strattera), it is a norepinephrine reuptake inhibitor.

In children who do not respond well to stimulant therapy, **tricyclic antidepressants** such as desipramine (Norpramin, Pertofane) and amitriptyline (Elavil) are sometimes recommended. Reported side effects of these drugs include persistent dry mouth, sedation, disorientation, and cardiac arrhythmia (particularly with desipramine). Other medications prescribed for ADHD therapy include buproprion (Wellbutrin), an antidepressant; fluoxetine (Prozac), an **SSRI** antidepressant; and carbamazepine (Tegretol, Atretol), an anticonvulsant drug. Clonidine (Catapres), an antihypertensive medication, has also been used to control aggression and hyperactivity in some ADHD children, although it should not be used with Ritalin. A child's response to medication will change with age and maturation, so ADHD symptoms should be monitored closely and prescriptions adjusted accordingly.

Behavior modification therapy uses a reward system to reinforce good behavior and task completion and can be implemented both in the classroom and at home. A tangible reward such as a sticker may be given to the child every time he completes a task or behaves in an acceptable manner. A chart system may be used to display the stickers and visually illustrate the child's progress. When a certain number of stickers are collected, the child may trade them in for a bigger reward such as a trip to the zoo or a day at the beach. The reward system stays in place until the good behavior becomes ingrained.

A variation of this technique, **cognitive-behavioral therapy**, works to decrease impulsive behavior by getting the child to recognize the connection between thoughts and behavior, and to change behavior by changing negative thinking patterns.

Individual psychotherapy can help an ADHD child build self-esteem, give them a place to discuss their worries and anxieties, and help them gain insight into their behavior and feelings. Family therapy may also be beneficial in helping family members develop coping skills and in working through feelings of guilt or anger parents may be experiencing.

ADHD children perform better within a familiar, consistent, and structured routine with positive reinforcements for good behavior and real consequences for bad. Family, friends, and caretakers should all be educated on the special needs and behaviors of the ADHD child. Communication between parents and teachers is especially critical to ensuring an ADHD child has an appropriate learning environment.

Alternative treatment

A number of alternative treatments exist for ADHD. Although there is a lack of controlled studies to prove their efficacy, proponents report that they are successful in controlling symptoms in some ADHD patients. Some of the more popular alternative treatments include:

- EEG (electroencephalograph) **biofeedback**. By measuring brainwave activity and teaching the ADHD patient which type of brainwave is associated with attention, EEG biofeedback attempts to train patients to generate the desired brainwave activity.

- Dietary therapy. Based in part on the Feingold food allergy diet, dietary therapy focuses on a nutritional plan that is high in protein and complex carbohydrates and free of white sugar and salicylate-containing foods such as strawberries, tomatoes, and grapes.

- Herbal therapy. Herbal therapy uses a variety of natural remedies to address the symptoms of ADHD, such as ginkgo (*Gingko biloba*) for memory and mental sharpness and chamomile (*Matricaria recutita*) extract for calming. The safety of herbal remedies has not been demonstrated in controlled studies. For example, it is known that gingko may affect blood coagulation, but controlled studies have not yet evaluated the risk of the effect.

- **Homeopathic medicine**. The theory of homeopathic medicine is to treat the whole person at a core level. Constitutional homeopathic care requires consulting with a well-trained homeopath who has experience working with ADD and ADHD individuals.

Prognosis

Untreated, ADHD negatively affects a child's social and educational performance and can seriously damage his or her sense of self-esteem. ADHD children have impaired relationships with their peers, and may be looked upon as social outcasts. They may be perceived as slow learners or troublemakers in the classroom. Siblings and even parents may develop resentful feelings towards the ADHD child.

Some ADHD children also develop a conduct disorder problem. For those adolescents who have both ADHD and a **conduct disorder**, as many as 25% go on to develop antisocial personality disorder and the criminal behavior, substance **abuse**, and high rate of **suicide** attempts that are symptomatic of it. Children diagnosed with ADHD are also more likely to have a learning disorder, a mood disorder such as depression, or an anxiety disorder.

Approximately 70-80% of ADHD patients treated with stimulant medication experience significant relief from symptoms, at least in the short-term. Approximately one-half of ADHD children seem to "outgrow" the disorder in adolescence or early adulthood; the other half will retain some or all symptoms of ADHD as adults. With early identification and intervention, careful compliance with a treatment program, and a supportive and nurturing home and school environment, ADHD children can flourish socially and academically.

Resources

PERIODICALS

"AACAP Guidelines Include Strattera as a First-line ADHD Therapy Option." *Drug Week* (May 28, 2004): 54.

"More Long-acting Stimulants to Treat Adult ADHD." *SCRIP World Pharmaceutical News* (May 14, 2004): 101-23.

"Study Updates Genetics of ADHD." *Drug Week* (May 21, 2004): 55.

ORGANIZATIONS

American Academy of Child and Adolescent Psychiatry. (AACAP). 3615 Wisconsin Ave. NW, Washington, DC 20016. (202) 966-7300. < http://www.aacap.org > .

Children and Adults with Attention Deficit Disorder (CH.A.D.D.). 8181 Professional Place, Suite 201.

National Attention Deficit Disorder Association. (ADDA). 9930 Johnnycake Ridge Road, Suite 3E, Mentor, OH 44060. (800) 487-2282. < http://www.add.org > .

Paula Anne Ford-Martin
Teresa G. Odle

Attention deficit disorder *see* **Attention-deficit/Hyperactivity disorder (ADHD)**

Atypical mycobacterial infections *see* **Mycobacterial infections, atypical**

Atypical pneumonia *see* **Mycoplasma infections**

Audiometry

Definition

Audiometry is the testing of a person's ability to hear various sound frequencies. The test is performed with the use of electronic equipment called an audiometer. This testing is usually administered by a trained technician called an audiologist.

Purpose

Audiometry testing is used to identify and diagnose hearing loss. The equipment is used in health screening programs, for example in grade schools, to detect hearing problems in children. It is also used in the doctor's office or hospital audiology department to diagnose hearing problems in children, adults, and

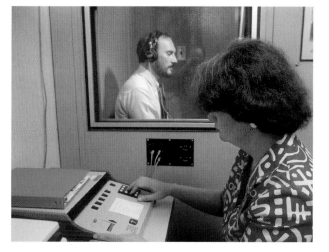

An audiologist conducting a hearing test. *(Custom Medical Stock Photo. Reproduced by permission.)*

the elderly. With correct diagnosis of a person's specific pattern of hearing impairment, the right type of therapy, which might include **hearing aids**, corrective surgery, or speech therapy, can be prescribed.

Precautions

Testing with audiometry equipment is simple and painless. No special precautions are required.

Description

A trained audiologist (a specialist in detecting **hearing loss**) uses an audiometer to conduct audiometry testing. This equipment emits sounds or tones, like musical notes, at various frequencies, or pitches, and at differing volumes or levels of loudness. Testing is usually done in a soundproof testing room.

The person being tested wears a set of headphones that blocks out other distracting sounds and delivers a test tone to one ear at a time. At the sound of a tone, the patient holds up a hand or finger to indicate that the sound is detected. The audiologist lowers the volume and repeats the sound until the patient can no longer detect it. This process is repeated over a wide range of tones or frequencies from very deep, low sounds, like the lowest note played on a tuba, to very high sounds, like the pinging of a triangle. Each ear is tested separately. It is not unusual for levels of sensitivity to sound to differ from one ear to the other.

A second type of audiometry testing uses a headband rather than headphones. The headband is worn with small plastic rectangles that fit behind the ears to conduct sound through the bones of the skull. The patient being tested senses the tones that are transmitted as vibrations through the bones to the inner ear. As with the headphones, the tones are repeated at various frequencies and volumes.

The results of the audiometry test may be recorded on a grid or graph called an audiogram. This graph is generally set up with low frequencies or tones at one end and high ones at the other end, much like a piano keyboard. Low notes are graphed on the left and high notes on the right. The graph also charts the volume of the tones used; from soft, quiet sounds at the top of the chart to loud sounds at the bottom. Hearing is measured in units called decibels. Most of the sounds associated with normal speech patterns are generally spoken in the range of 20-50 decibels. An adult with normal hearing can detect tones between 0-20 decibels.

Speech audiometry is another type of testing that uses a series of simple recorded words spoken at various volumes into headphones worn by the patient being tested. The patient repeats each word back to the audiologist as it is heard. An adult with normal hearing will be able to recognize and repeat 90-100% of the words.

Preparation

The ears may be examined with an otoscope prior to audiometry testing to determine if there are any blockages in the ear canal due to ear wax or other material.

Normal results

A person with normal hearing will be able to recognize and respond to all of the tone frequencies

administered at various volumes in both ears by the audiometry test. An adult with normal hearing can detect a range of low and high pitched sounds that are played as softly as between nearly 0-20 decibels. Normal speech is generally spoken in the range of 20-50 decibels.

Abnormal results

Audiometry test results are considered abnormal if there is a significant or unexplained difference between the levels of sound heard between the two ears, or if the person being tested is unable to hear in the normal range of frequencies and volume. The pattern of responses displayed on the audiogram can be used by the audiologist to identify if a significant hearing loss is present and if the patient might benefit from hearing aids or corrective surgery.

Resources

ORGANIZATIONS

American Academy of Audiology. 8201 Greensboro Drive, Suite 300, McLean, VA 22102. (703) 610-9022. < http:// audiology.org > .

Audiology Awareness Campaign. 3008 Millwood Ave., Columbia, SC 29205. (800) 445-8629.

OTHER

"How to Read Your Hearing Test." *Hearing Alliance of America.* < http://www.earinfo.com > .

"Understanding Your Audiogram." *The League for the Hard of Hearing.* < http://www.lhh.org > .

Altha Roberts Edgren

Auditory integration training

Definition

Auditory integration training, or AIT, is one specific type of music/auditory therapy based upon the work of French otolaryngologists Dr. **Alfred Tomatis** and Dr. Guy Berard.

Origins

The premise upon which most auditory integration programs are based is that distortion in how things are heard contributes to commonly seen behavioral or **learning disorders** in children. Some of these disorders include **attention deficit/hyperactive disorder (ADHD)**, **autism**, **dyslexia**, and central

ALFRED TOMATIS (1920–)

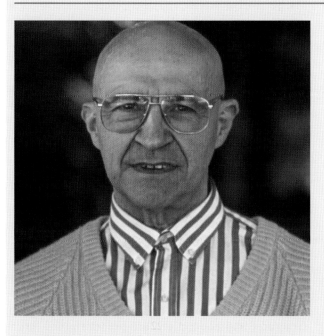

(Photograph by V. Brynner. Gamma Liaison. Reproduced by permission.)

Internationally renowned French otolaryngologist, psychologist, educator and inventor Alfred Tomatis perceived the importance of sound and hearing early in his career. He took his degree as a Doctor of Medicine from the University of Paris and specialized in ear, nose and throat medicine. The son of two opera singers, Tomatis early in his career treated some of his parents' fellow opera singers. From these experiences with the sound of music, he developed the principle that has come to be known as the Tomatis Effect, i.e. that the human voice can only sing what it hears.

Tomatis has been called the Einstein of the ear. It was his research that made the world aware that the ears of an infant in utero are already functioning at four and half months of age. Just as the umbilical cord provides nourishment to the unborn infant's body, Tomatis postulated that the sound of the mother's voice is also a nutrient heard by the fetus. This sound literally charges and stimulates the growth of the brain.

Tomatis took this further, into the realm of language. Tomatis concluded that the need to communicate and to be understood are among our most basic needs. He was a pioneer in perceiving that language problems convert into social problems for people. "Language is what characterizes man and makes him different from other creatures," Tomatis is quoted as saying. The techniques he developed to teach people how to listen effectively are internationally respected tools used in the treatment of autism, attention-deficit disorder, and other learning disabilities.

His listening program, the invention of the Electronic Ear, and his work with the therapeutic use of sound and music for the past fifty years have made Tomatis arguably the best known and most successful ear specialist in the world. There are more than two hundred Tomatis Centers worldwide, treating a vast variety of problems related to the ability to hear.

auditory processing disorders (CAPD). Training the patient to listen can stimulate central and cortical organization.

Auditory integration is one facet of what audiologists call central auditory processing. The simplest definition of central auditory processing, or CAP, is University of Buffalo Professor of Audiology Jack Katz's, which is: "What we do with what we hear." Central auditory integration is actually the perception of sound, including the ability to attend to sound, to remember it, retaining it in both the long- and short-term memory, to be able to listen to sound selectively, and to localize it.

Guy Berard developed one of the programs commonly used. Berard's auditory integration training consists of twenty half-hour sessions spent listening to musical sounds via a stereophonic system. The music is random, with filtered frequencies, and the person listens through earphones. These sound waves vibrate and **exercise** structures in the middle ear. This is normally done in sessions twice a day for 10 days.

Alfred Tomatis is also the inventor of the Electronic Ear. This device operates through a series of filters, and reestablishes the dominance of the right ear in hearing. The basis of Tomatis' work is a series of principles that follow:

- The most important purpose of the ear is to adapt sound waves into signals that charge the brain.

- Sound is conducted via both air and bone. It can be considered something that nourishes the nervous system, either stimulating or destimulating it.

- Just as seeing is not the same as looking, hearing is not the same as listening. Hearing is passive. Listening is active.

- A person's ability to listen affects all language development for that person. This process influences every aspect of self-image and social development.

- The capacity to listen can be changed or improved through auditory stimulation using musical and vocal sounds at high frequencies.
- Communication begins in the womb. As early as the beginning of the second trimester, fetuses can hear sounds. These sounds literally cause the brain and nervous system of the baby to develop.

Description

A quartet of CAP defects have been identified that can unfavorably alter how each person processes sound. Among these are:

- Phonetic decoding, a problem that occurs when the brain incorrectly decodes what is being heard. Sounds are unrecognizable, often because the person speaking talks too fast.
- Tolerance-fading memory, a condition with little or poor tolerance for background sounds.
- Auditory integration involves a person's ability to put together things heard with things seen. Characteristically there are long response delays and trouble with phonics, or recognizing the symbols for sounds.
- The fourth problem area, often called auditory organization, overlaps the previous three. It is characterized by disorganization in handling auditory and other information.

Certain audiological tests are carried out to see if the person has a CAP problem, and if so, how severe it is. Other tests give more specific information regarding the nature of the CAP problem. They include:

- Puretone air-conduction threshold testing, which measures peripheral **hearing loss**. If loss is found, then bone-conduction testing, or evaluation of the vibration of small bones in the inner ear, is also carried out.
- Word discrimination scores (WDS) determines a person's clarity in hearing ideal speech. This is done by presenting 25–50 words at 40 decibels above the person's average sound threshold in each ear. Test scores equal the percentage of words heard correctly.
- Immittance testing is made up of two parts, assessing the status of, and the protective mechanisms of the middle ear.
- Staggered sporadic word (SSW) testing delivers 40 compound words in an overlapping way at 50 decibels above threshold to each ear of the person being tested. This test provides expanded information that makes it possible to break down CAP problems into the four basic types.

- Speech in noise discrimination (SN) testing is similar to Staggered Sporadic Word testing except that other noise is also added and the percentage correct in quiet is compared with that correct when there is added noise.
- Phonemic synthesis (PS) determines serious learning problems. The types of errors made in sounding out written words or associating written letters with the sounds they represent help in determining the type and severity of CAP problems.

Purpose

Upon completion of an auditory integration training program, the person's hearing should be capable of perceiving all frequencies at, or near, the same level. Total improvement from this therapy, in both hearing and behavior, can take up to one year.

Research and general acceptance

Auditory integration training is based upon newly learned information about the brain. Though brain structures and connections are predetermined, probably by heredity, another factor called *plasticity* also comes into play. Learning, we now know, continues from birth to **death**. Plasticity is the ability of the brain to actually change its structuring and connections through the process of learning.

Problems with auditory processing are now viewed as having a wide–reaching ripple effect on our society. It is estimated that 30–40% of children starting school have language-learning skills that can be described as poor. CAP difficulties are a factor in several different learning disabilities. They affect not only academic success, but also nearly every aspect of societal difficulties. One example to illustrate this is a 1989 University of Buffalo study where CAP problems were found to be present in a surprising 97% of youth inmates in an upstate New York corrections facility.

Resources

OTHER

Cooper, Rachel. "What is Auditory Integration Training?" December 2000. < http://www.vision3d.com/adhd > .

Dejean, Valerie. *About the Tomatis Method, 1997.* Tomatis Auditory Training Spectrum Center, Bethseda, MD.

The Spectrum Center. "Auditory Integration and AlfredTomatis." December 2000. < http://listeningtraining.com > .

Joan Schonbeck

Australia antigen-associated hepatitis *see* **Hepatitis B**

Autism

Definition

Autism is a severe disorder of brain function marked by problems with social contact, intelligence and language, together with ritualistic or compulsive behavior and bizarre responses to the environment.

Description

Autism is a lifelong disorder that interferes with the ability to understand what is seen, heard, and touched. This can cause profound problems in personal behavior and in the ability to relate to others. A person with autism must learn how to communicate normally and how to relate to people, objects and events. However, not all patients suffer the same degree of impairment. There is a full spectrum of symptoms, which can range from mild to severe.

Autism occurs in as many as one or two per 1,000 children. It is found four times more often in boys (usually the first-born) and occurs around the world in all races and social backgrounds. Autism usually is evident in the first three years of life, although in some children it's hard to tell when the problem develops. Sometimes the condition isn't diagnosed until the child enters school.

While a person with autism can have symptoms ranging from mild to severe, about 10% have an extraordinary ability in one area, such as in mathematics, memory, music, or art. Such children are known as "autistic savants" (formerly known as "idiot savants.").

Causes and symptoms

Autism is a brain disorder that affects the way the brain uses or transmits information. Studies have found abnormalities in several parts of the brain that almost certainly occurred during fetal development. The problem may be centered in the parts of the brain responsible for processing language and information from the senses.

There appears to be a strong genetic basis for autism. Identical twins are more likely to both be affected than twins who are fraternal (not genetically identical). In a family with one autistic child, the chance of having another child with autism is about 1 in 20, much higher than in the normal population. Sometimes, relatives of an autistic child have mild behaviors that look very much like autism, such as repetitive behaviors and social or communication problems. Research also has found that some emotional disorders (such as manic depression) occur more often in families of a child with autism.

At least one group of researchers has found a link between an abnormal gene and autism. The gene may be just one of at least three to five genes that interact in some way to cause the condition. Scientists suspect that a faulty gene or genes might make a person vulnerable to develop autism in the presence of other factors, such as a chemical imbalance, viruses or chemicals, or a lack of oxygen at birth.

In a few cases, autistic behavior is caused by a disease such as:

- rubella in the pregnant mother
- tuberous sclerosis
- fragile X syndrome
- encephalitis
- untreated **phenylketonuria**

The severity of the condition varies between individuals, ranging from the most severe (extremely unusual, repetitive, self- injurious, and aggressive behavior) to very mild, resembling a personality disorder with some learning disability.

Profound problems with social interaction are the most common symptoms of autism. Infants with the disorder won't cuddle; they avoid eye contact and don't seem to want or need physical contact or affection. They may become rigid or flaccid when they are held, cry when picked up, and show little interest in human contact. Such a child doesn't smile or lift his arms in anticipation of being picked up. He forms no attachment to parents nor shows any normal anxiety toward strangers. He doesn't learn typical games of childhood, such as peek-a-boo.

Language problems

The child with autism may not speak at all; if he does, it is often in single words. He may endlessly repeat words or phrases that are addressed to him and may reverse pronouns ("You go sleep" instead of "I want to go to sleep").

Restricted interests and activity

Usually a child with autism has many problems playing normally. He probably won't act out adultroles during play time, and instead of enjoying fantasy play, he may simply repeatedly mimic the actions of someone else. Bizarre behavior patterns are very common among autistic children and may include complex rituals, screaming fits, rhythmic rocking, arm flapping, finger

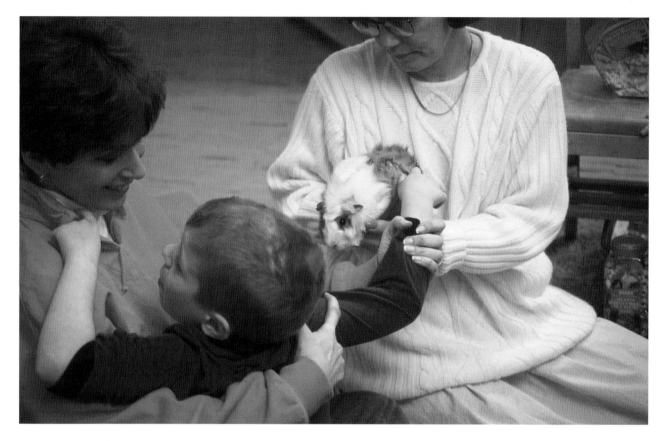

This autistic child is encouraged to interact with the guinea pig in an effort to improve his social interaction. *(Helen B. Senisi. Photo Researchers, Inc. Reproduced by permission.)*

twiddling, and crying without tears. Autistic children may play with their own saliva, feces or urine.They may be self-destructive, biting their own hands, gouging at their eyes, pulling their hair, or banging their head.

Sensory problems

The sensory world poses a real problem to many autistic children, who seem overwhelmed by their own senses. A child with autism may ignore objects or become obsessed with them, continually watching the object or the movement of his fingers over it. Many of these children may react to sounds by banging their head or flapping fingers. Some high-functioning autistic adults who have written books about their childhood experiences report that sounds were often excruciatingly painful to them, forcing them to withdraw from their environment or try to cope by withdrawing into their own world of sensation and movement.

Intellectual problems

Most autistic children appear to be moderately mentally retarded. They may giggle or cry for no

reason, have no fear of real danger, but exhibit terror of harmless objects.

Diagnosis

There is no medical test for autism. Because the symptoms of autism are so varied, the condition may go undiagnosed for some time (especially in those with mild cases or if other handicaps are also present). It may be confused with other diseases, such as fragile X syndrome, tuberous sclerosis, and untreated phenylketonuria.

Autism is diagnosed by observing the child's behavior, communication skills, and social interactions. Medical tests should rule out other possible causes of autistic symptoms. Criteria that mental health experts use to diagnose autism include:

- problems with developing friendships
- problems with make-believe or social play
- endlessly repeated words or strings of words
- difficulty in carrying on a conversation

KEY TERMS

Antidepressants—A type of medication that is used to treat depression; it is also sometimes used to treat autism.

Asperger syndrome—Children who have autistic behavior but no problems with language.

Encephalitis—A rare inflammation of the brain caused by a viral infection. It has been linked to the develoment of autism.

Fragile X syndrome—A genetic condition related to the X chromosome that affects mental, physical and sensory development.

Major tranquilizers—The family of drugs that includes the psychotropic or neuroleptic drugs, sometimes used to help autistic people. They carry significant risk of side effects, including Parkinsonism and movement disorders, and should be prescribed with caution.

Opiate blockers—A type of drug that blocks the effects of natural opiates in the system. This makes some people, including some people with autism, appear more responsive to their environment.

Phenylketonuria (PKU)—An enzyme deficiency present at birth that disrupts metabolism and causes brain damage. This rare inherited defect may be linked to the development of autism.

Rubella—Also known as German measles. When a woman contracts rubella during pregnancy, her developing infant may be damaged. One of the problems that may result is autism.

Stimulants—A class of drugs, including Ritalin, used to treat people with autism. They may make children calmer and better able to concentrate, but they also may limit growth or have other side effects.

Tuberous sclerosis—A genetic disease that causes skin problems, seizures, and mental retardation. It may be confused with autism.

• obsessions with rituals or restricted patterns

• preoccupation with parts of objects

Some children have a few of the symptoms of autism, but not enough to be diagnosed with the "classical" form of the condition. Children who have autistic behavior but no problems with language may be diagnosed with "Asperger syndrome." Children who seem normal at first but who begin to show autistic behavior as they get older might be diagnosed with "childhood disintegrative disorder" (CDD). These problems are sometimes called "autistic spectrum disorders." It is also important to rule out other problems that seem similar to autism.

Treatment

There is no cure for autism. Treatments are aimed at reducing specific symptoms. Because the symptoms vary so widely from one person to the next, there is not a single approach that works for every person. A spectrum of interventions include training in music, listening, vision, speech and language, and senses. Special **diets** and medications may also be prescribed.

Studies show that people with autism can improve significantly with proper treatment. A child with autism can learn best with special teachers in a structured program that emphasizes individual instruction. The two most-often studied types of treatment are:

Educational or behavioral treatment

Typically, behavioral techniques are used to help the child respond and decrease symptoms. This might include positive reinforcement (food and rewards) to boost language and social skills. This training includes structured, skill-oriented instruction designed to boost social and language abilities. Training needs to begin as early as possible, since early intervention appears to influence brain development.

Most experts believe that modern treatment is most effective when carried out at home, although treatment may also take place in a psychiatric hospital, specialized school, or day care program.

Medication

No single medication has yet proved highly effective for the major features of autism. However, a variety of drugs can control self-injurious, aggressive, and other of the more difficult behaviors. Drugs also can control epilepsy, which afflicts up to 20% of people with autism.

Five types of drugs are sometimes prescribed to help the behavior problems of people with autism:

• stimulants, such as methylphenidate (Ritalin)

• antidepressants, such as fluroxamine (Luvox)

• opiate blockers, such as naltrexone (ReVia)

- antipsychotics
- tranquilizers.

Today, most experts recommend a complex treatment regimen that begins early and continues through the teenage years. Behavioral therapies are used in conjunction with medications.

Alternative treatment

Many parents report success with megavitamin therapy. Some studies have shown that vitamin B_6 improves eye contact and speech and lessens tantrum behavior. Vitamin B_6 causes fewer side effects than other medications and is considered safe when used in appropriate doses. However, not many health practitioners advocate its use in the treatment of autism, citing that the studies showing its benefit were flawed.

DMG (dimethylglycine)

This compound, available in many health food stores, is legally classified as a food, not a vitamin or drug. Some researchers claim that it improves speech in children with autism. Those who respond to this treatment will usually do so within a week. Again, many doctors do not feel that the studies are adequate to promote this treatment.

Exercise

One researcher found that vigorous **exercise** (20 minutes or longer, three or four days a week) seems to decrease hyperactivity, aggression, self-injury and other autistic symptoms.

Prognosis

While there is no cure, with appropriate treatment the negative behaviors of autism may improve. Earlier generations placed autistic children in institutions; today, even severely disabled children can be helped in a less restrictive environment to develop to their highest potential. Many can eventually become more responsive to others as they learn to understand the world around them, and some can lead nearly normal lives.

People with autism have a normal life expectancy. Some people with autism can handle a job; they do best with structured jobs that involve a degree of repetition.

Prevention

Until the cause of autism is discovered, prevention is not possible.

Resources

ORGANIZATIONS

Autism Network International. PO Box 448, Syracuse, NY 13210.

Autism Research Institute. 4182 Adams Ave., San Diego, CA 92116. (619) 281-7165.

Autism Society of America. 7910 Woodmont Avenue, Suite 300, Bethesda, Maryland 20814-3067. (800) 328-8476. < http://www.autism-society.org > .

National Alliance for Autism Research. < naar@naar.org > .

National Autism Hotline. c/o Autism Services Center, PO Box 507, 605 Ninth St., Huntington, WV 25710. (304) 525-8014.

National Fragile X Foundation. PO Box 190488, San Francisco, CA 94119. (800) 688-8765. < http://www.nfxf.org > .

National Institute of Neurological Disorders and Stroke. PO Box 5801, Bethesda, MD 20824. (800) 352-9424. < http://www.ninds.nih.gov/index.htm > .

OTHER

Autism Society of America. 7910 Woodmont Avenue. < http://www.autism-society.org > .

National Alliance for Autism Research (NAAR). < http://www.naar.org > .

National Information Center for Children and Youth with Disabilities. < http://www.nichcy.org/transitn.htm > .

Carol A. Turkington

Autograft *see* **Skin grafting**

Autoimmune disorders

Definition

Autoimmune disorders are conditions in which a person's immune system attacks the body's own cells, causing tissue destruction.

Description

Autoimmunity is accepted as the cause of a wide range of disorders, and it is suspected to be responsible for many more. Autoimmune diseases are classified as either general, in which the autoimmune reaction takes place simultaneously in a number of tissues, or organ specific, in which the autoimmune reaction targets a single organ.

Autoimmune disorders include the following:

- **Systemic lupus erythematosus**. A general autoimmune disease in which antibodies attack a number of different tissues. The disease recurs periodically and is seen mainly in young and middle-aged women.

• **Rheumatoid arthritis**. Occurs when the immune system attacks and destroys the tissues that line bone joints and cartilage. The disease occurs throughout the body, although some joints may be more affected than others.

• Goodpasture's syndrome. Occurs when antibodies are deposited in the membranes of both the lung and kidneys, causing both inflammation of kidney glomerulus (**glomerulonephritis**) and lung bleeding. It is typically a disease of young males.

• Grave's disease. Caused by an antibody that binds to specific cells in the thyroid gland, causing them to make excessive amounts of thyroid hormone.

• Hashimoto's **thyroiditis**. Caused by an antibody that binds to cells in the thyroid gland. Unlike in Grave's disease, however, this antibody's action results in less thyroid hormone being made.

• Pemphigus vulgaris. A group of autoimmune disorders that affect the skin.

• Myasthenia gravis. A condition in which the immune system attacks a receptor on the surface of muscle cells, preventing the muscle from receiving nerve impulses and resulting in severe muscle weakness.

• **Scleroderma**. Also called CREST syndrome or progressive systemic sclerosis, scleroderma affects the connective tissue.

• Autoimmune **hemolytic anemia**. Occurs when the body produces antibodies that coat red blood cells.

• Autoimmune thrombocytopenic purpura. Disorder in which the immune system targets and destroys blood platelets.

• **Polymyositis** and **Dermatomyositis**. Immune disorders that affect the neuromuscular system.

• **Pernicious anemia**. Disorder in which the immune system attacks the lining of the stomach in such a way that the body cannot metabolize vitamin B_{12}.

• Sjögren's syndrome. Occurs when the exocrine glands are attacked by the immune system, resulting in excessive dryness.

• **Ankylosing spondylitis**. Immune system induced degeneration of the joints and soft tissue of the spine.

• Vasculitis. A group of autoimmune disorders in which the immune system attacks and destroys blood vessels.

• Type I **diabetes mellitus**. May be caused by an antibody that attacks and destroys the islet cells of the pancreas, which produce insulin.

• Amyotrophic lateral schlerosis. Also called Lou Gehrig's disease. An immune disorder that causes the death of neurons which leads to progressive loss of muscular control.

• Guillain-Barre syndrome. Also called infectious polyneuritis. Often occurring after an infection or an immunization (specifically Swine flu), the disease affects the myelin sheath, which coats nerve cells. It causes progressive muscle weakness and **paralysis**.

• **Multiple sclerosis**. An autoimmune disorder that may involve a virus affects the central nervous system, causing loss of coordination and muscle control.

Causes and symptoms

To further understand autoimmune disorders, it is helpful to understand the workings of the immune system. The purpose of the immune system is to defend the body against attack by infectious microbes (germs) and **foreign objects**. When the immune system attacks an invader, it is very specific—a particular immune system cell will only recognize and target one type of invader. To function properly, the immune system must not only develop this specialized knowledge of individual invaders, but it must also learn how to recognize and not destroy cells that belong to the body itself. Every cell carries protein markers on its surface that identifies it in one of two ways: what kind of cell it is (e.g. nerve cell, muscle cell, blood cell, etc.) and to whom that cell belongs. These markers are called major histocompatability complexes (MHCs). When functioning properly, cells of the immune system will not attack any other cell with markers identifying it as belonging to the body. Conversely, if the immune system cells do not recognize the cell as "self," they attach themselves to it and put out a signal that the body has been invaded, which in turn stimulates the production of substances such as antibodies that engulf and destroy the foreign particles. In case of autoimmune disorders, the immune system cannot distinguish between "self" cells and invader cells. As a result, the same destructive operation is carried out on the body's own cells that would normally be carried out on bacteria, viruses, and other such harmful entities.

The reasons why immune systems become dysfunctional in this way is not well understood. However, most researchers agree that a combination of genetic, environmental, and hormonal factors play into autoimmunity. Researchers also speculate that certain mechanisms may trigger autoimmunity. First, a substance that is normally restricted to one part of the body, and therefore not usually exposed to the immune system, is released into other areas

KEY TERMS

Autoantibody—An antibody made by a person that reacts with their own tissues.

Paresthesias— A prickly, tingling sensation.

where it is attacked. Second, the immune system may mistake a component of the body for a similar foreign component. Third, cells of the body may be altered in some way, either by drugs, infection, or some other environmental factor, so that they are no longer recognizable as "self" to the immune system. Fourth, the immune system itself may be damaged, such as by a genetic mutation, and therefore cannot function properly.

The symptoms of the above disorders include:

- Systemic lupus erythematosus. Symptoms include fever, chills, **fatigue**, weight loss, skin **rashes** (particularly the classic "butterfly" rash on the face), vasculitis, polyarthralgia, patchy hair loss, sores in the mouth or nose, lymph-node enlargement, gastric problems, and, in women, irregular periods. About half of those who suffer from lupus develop cardiopulmonary problems, and some may also develop urinary problems. Lupus can also effect the central nervous system, causing seizures, depression, and psychosis.

- Rheumatoid arthritis. Initially may be characterized by a low-grade **fever**, loss of appetite, weight loss, and a generalized **pain** in the joints. The joint pain then becomes more specific, usually beginning in the fingers, then spreading to other areas, such as the wrists, elbows, knees, and ankles. As the disease progresses, joint function diminishes sharply and deformities occur, particularly the characteristic "swan's neck" curling of the fingers.

- Goodpasture's syndrome. Symptoms are similar to that of iron deficiency anemia, including fatigue and pallor. Symptoms involving the lungs may range from a cough that produces bloody sputum to outright hemorrhaging. Symptoms involving the urinary system include blood in the urine and/or swelling.

- Grave's disease. This disease is characterized by an enlarged thyroid gland, weight loss without loss of appetite, sweating, heart **palpitations**, nervousness, and an inability to tolerate heat.

- Hashimoto's thyroiditis. This disorder generally displays no symptoms.

- Pemphigus vulgaris. This disease is characterized by blisters and deep lesions on the skin.

- Myasthenia gravis. Characterized by fatigue and muscle weakness that at first may be confined to certain muscle groups, but then may progress to the point of paralysis. Myasthenia gravis patients often have expressionless faces as well as difficulty chewing and swallowing. If the disease progresses to the respiratory system, artificial respiration may be required.

- Scleroderma. Disorder is usually preceded by Raynaud's phenomenon. Symptoms that follow include pain, swelling, and stiffness of the joints, and the skin takes on a tight, shiny appearance. The digestive system also becomes involved, resulting in weight loss, appetite loss, diarrhea, **constipation**, and distention of the abdomen. As the disease progresses, the heart, lungs, and kidneys become involved, and malignant **hypertension** causes death in approximately 30% of cases.

- Autoimmune hemolytic anemia. May be acute or chronic. Symptoms include fatigue and abdominal tenderness due to an enlarged spleen.

- Autoimmune thrombocytopenic purpura. Characterized by pinhead-size red dots on the skin, unexplained **bruises**, bleeding from the nose and gums, and blood in the stool.

- Polymyositis and Dermatomyositis. In polymyositis, symptoms include muscle weakness, particularly in the shoulders or pelvis, that prevents the patient from performing everyday activities. In dermatomyositis, the same muscle weakness is accompanied by a rash that appears on the upper body, arms, and fingertips. A rash may also appear on the eyelids, and the area around the eyes may become swollen.

- Pernicious anemia. Signs of pernicious anemia include weakness, sore tongue, bleeding gums, and **tingling** in the extremities. Because the disease causes a decrease in stomach acid, nausea, **vomiting**, loss of appetite, weight loss, **diarrhea**, and constipation are possible. Also, because Vitamin B_{12} is essential for the nervous system function, the deficiency of it brought on by the disease can result in a host of neurological problems, including weakness, lack of coordination, blurred vision, loss of fine motor skills, loss of the sense of taste, ringing in the ears, and loss of bladder control.

- Sjögren's syndrome. Characterized by excessive dryness of the mouth and eyes.

- Ankylosing spondylitis. Generally begins with lower back pain that progresses up the spine. The pain may eventually become crippling.

- Vasculitis. Symptoms depend upon the group of veins affected and can range greatly.

- Type I diabetes mellitus. Characterized by fatigue and an abnormally high level of glucose in the blood (hyperglycemia).

- Amyotrophic lateral schlerosis. First signs are stumbling and difficulty climbing stairs. Later, **muscle cramps** and twitching may be observed as well as weakness in the hands making fastening buttons or turning a key difficult. Speech may become slowed or slurred. There may also be difficulty swallowing. As respiratory muscles atrophy, there is increased danger of aspiration or lung infection.

- Guillain-Barre syndrome. Muscle weakness in the legs occurs first, then the arms and face. Paresthesias (a prickly, tingling sensation) is also felt. This disorder affects both sides of the body and may involve paralysis and the muscles that control breathing.

- Multiple sclerosis. Like Lou Gehrig's disease, the first symptom may be clumsiness. Weakness or exhaustion is often reported, as well as blurry or double vision. There may be dizziness, depression, loss of bladder control, and muscle weakness so severe that the patient is confined to a wheelchair.

Diagnosis

A number of tests are involved in the diagnosis of autoimmune diseases, depending on the particular disease; e.g. blood tests, cerebrospinal fluid analysis, electromylogram (measures muscle function), and **magnetic resonance imaging** of the brain. Usually, these tests determine the location and extent of damage or involvement. They are useful in charting progress of the disease and as baselines for treatment.

The principle tool, however, for authenticating autoimmune disease is antibody testing. Such tests involve measuring the level of antibodies found in the blood and determining if they react with specific antigens that would give rise to an autoimmune reaction. An elevated amount of antibodies indicates that a humoral immune reaction is occurring. Since elevated antibody levels are also seen in common infections, they must be ruled out as the cause for the increased antibody levels.

Antibodies can also be typed by class. There are five classes of antibodies, and they can be separated in the laboratory. The class IgG is usually associated with autoimmune diseases. Unfortunately, IgG class antibodies are also the main class of antibody seen in normal immune responses.

The most useful antibody tests involve introducing the patient's antibodies to samples of his or her own tissue, usually thyroid, stomach, liver, and kidney tissue. If antibodies bind to the "self" tissue, it is diagnostic for an autoimmune disorder. Antibodies from a person without an autoimmune disorder would not react to "self" tissue.

Treatment

Treatment of autoimmune diseases is specific to the disease, and usually concentrates on alleviating or preventing symptoms rather than correcting the underlying cause. For example, if a gland involved in an autoimmune reaction is not producing a hormone such as insulin, administration of that hormone is required. Administration of a hormone, however, will restore the function of the gland damaged by the autoimmune disease.

The other aspect of treatment is controlling the inflammatory and proliferative nature of the immune response. This is generally accomplished with two types of drugs. Steroid compounds are used to control inflammation. There are many different steroids, each having side effects. The proliferative nature of the immune response is controlled with immunosuppressive drugs. These drugs work by inhibiting the replication of cells and, therefore, also suppress non-immune cells leading to side effects such as anemia.

Systemic **enzyme therapy** is a new treatment that is showing results for rheumatoid arthritis, multiple sclerosis, ankylosing spondylitis, and other inflammatory diseases. Enzymes combinations of pancreatin, trypsin, chymotrypsin, bromelain, and papain help stimulate the body's own defenses, accelerate inflammation in order to reduce swelling and improve circulation, and break up the immune complexes within the bloodstream. Symptoms have been reduced using this treatment.

Other treatments that hold some promise are irradiation of the spleen and **gene therapy**. Splenic irradiation is touted to be a safe, alternative for patients with autoimmune blood diseases, especially autoimmune hemolytic anemia, or others with compromised immune systems, such as HIV patients and the elderly. It is reported to have few side effects and seems to be working. Cytokine and cytokine inhibitor genes injected directly into muscle tissue also appear to be effective in treating Type I diabetes mellitus, systemic lupus erythematosus, thyroditis, and arthritis.

Prognosis

Prognosis depends upon the pathology of each autoimmune disease.

Prevention

Most autoimmune diseases cannot be prevented. Though the mechanisms involved in how these diseases affect the body are known, it is still unclear why the body turns on itself. Since more women than men seem to be affected by some of these disorders (e.g. lupus), some researchers are looking into hormones as a factor. This, and gene therapy, may be the preventatives of the future.

Resources

PERIODICALS

Cichoke, Anthony J. "Natural Relief for Autoimmune Disorders." *Better Nutrition.* 62, no. 6 (June 2000): 24.

Henderson, Charles W. "Gene Therapy Uses Vectors EncodingCytokines or Cytokine Inhibitors (for treatment of autoimmune disorders)." *ImmunotherapyWeekly* September 27, 2000: pNA.

Riccio, Nina M. "Autoimmune Disorder: When the Body AttacksItself." *Current Health 2* 26, no. 5 (January 2000): 13.

"Splenic Irradiation Is an Option for Patients with AutoimmuneDisorders and Those with HIV." *AIDS Weekly* (April 9, 2001): pNA.

Janie F. Franz

Autoimmune hepatitis *see* **Hepatitis, autoimmune**

Autologous transfusion *see* **Transfusion**

Autologous transplant *see* **Bone marrow transplantation**

Automatic implantable cardioverter-defibrillator *see* **Implantable cardioverter-defibrillator**

Autopsy

Definition

An autopsy is a postmortem assessment or examination of a body to determine the cause of death. An autopsy is performed by a physician trained in pathology.

Purpose

Most autopsies advance medical knowledge and provide evidence for legal action. Medically, autopsies determine the exact cause and circumstances of **death**,

---

KEY TERMS

Acquired immunodeficiency syndrome (AIDS) — A group of diseases resulting from infection with the human immunodeficiency virus (HIV). A person infected with HIV gradually loses immune function, becoming less able to resist aliments and cancers, resulting in eventual death.

Computed tomography scan (CT scan) —The technique used in diagnostic studies of internal bodily structures in the detection of tumors or brain aneurysms. This diagnostic test consists of a computer analysis of a series of cross-sectional scans made along a single axis of a bodily structure or tissue that is used to construct a three-dimensional image of that structure

Creutzfeld-Jakob disease—A rare, often fatal disease of the brain, characterized by gradual dementia and loss of muscle control that occurs most often in middle age and is caused by a slow virus.

Hepatitis—Inflammation of the liver, caused by infectious or toxic agents and characterized by jaundice, fever, liver enlargement, and abdominal pain.

Magnetic resonance imaging (MRI)—A diagnostic tool that utilizes nuclear magnetic energy in the production of images of specific atoms and molecular structures in solids, especially human cells, tissues, and organs.

Postmortem—After death.

---

discover the pathway of a disease, and provide valuable information to be used in the care of the living. When foul play is suspected, a government coroner or medical examiner performs autopsies for legal use. This branch of medical study is called forensic medicine. Forensic specialists investigate deaths resulting from violence or occurring under suspicious circumstances.

Benefits of research from autopsies include the production of new medical information on diseases such as **toxic shock syndrome**, acquired **immunodeficiency** syndrome (**AIDS**). Organ donation, which can potentially save the lives of other patients, is also another benefit of autopsies.

Precautions

When performed for medical reasons, autopsies require formal permission from family members or the legal guardian. (Autopsies required for legal reasons when foul play is suspected do not need the consent of next of kin.) During the autopsy, very concise notes and documentation must be made for both medical and legal reasons. Some religious groups prohibit autopsies.

Description

An autopsy can be described as the examination of a deceased human body with a detailed exam of the person's remains. This procedure dates back to the Roman era when few human dissections were performed; autopsies were utilized, however, to determine the cause of death in criminal cases. At the beginning of the procedure the exterior body is examined and then the internal organs are removed and studied. Some pathologists argue that more autopsies are performed than necessary. However, recent studies show that autopsies can detect major findings about a person's condition that were not suspected when the person was alive. And the growing awareness of the influence of genetic factors in disease has also emphasized the importance of autopsies.

Despite the usefulness of autopsies, fewer autopsies have been performed in the United States during the past 10-20 years. A possible reason for this decline is concern about malpractice suits on the part of the treating physician. Other possible reasons are that hospitals are performing fewer autopsies because of the expense or because modern technology, such as CT scans and magnetic resonance imaging, can often provide sufficient diagnostic information. Nonetheless, federal regulators and pathology groups have begun to establish new guidelines designed to increase the number and quality of autopsies being performed.

Many experts are concerned that if the number of autopsies increases, hospitals may be forced to charge families a fee for the procedure as autopies are not normally covered by insurance companies or Medicare. Yet, according to several pathologists, the benefit of the procedure for families and doctors does justify the cost. In medical autopsies, physicians remain cautious to examine only as much of the body as permitted according to the wishes of the family. It is important to note that autopsies can also provide peace of mind for the bereaved family in certain situations.

Preparation

If a medical autopsy is being performed, written permission is secured from the family of the deceased

Aftercare

Once the autopsy has been completed, the body is prepared for final arrangements according to the family's wishes

Risks

There are some risks of disease transmission from the deceased. In fact, some physicans may refuse to do autopsies on specific patients because of a fear of contracting diseases such as AIDS, hepatitis, or Creutzfeld-Jakob disease.

Normal results

In most situations the cause of death is determined from the procedure of an autopsy without any transmission of disease.

Abnormal results

Abnormal results would include inconclusive results from the autopsy and transmission of infectious disease during the autopsy.

Resources

ORGANIZATIONS

American Medical Association. 515 N. State St., Chicago, IL 60612. (312) 464-5000. < http://www.ama-assn.org > .

Jeffrey P. Larson, RPT

Aviation medicine

Definition

Also known as aerospace medicine, flight medicine, or space medicine, aviation medicine is a medical specialty that focuses on the physical and psychological conditions associated with flying and space travel.

Purpose

Since flying airplanes and spacecraft involves great risk and physical demands, such as changes in gravity and oxygen, pilots and astronauts need medical experts to protect their safety and the public's safety.

Description

Pressure changes

In the United States, the Federal Aviation Administration (FAA) requires all pilots who fly above 14,500 ft (4,420 m) to be prepared for pressure changes caused by lower oxygen levels at high altitude. Pilots must either have a pressurized cabin or access to an oxygen mask. Without these protections, they could experience hypoxia, or altitude sickness. Hypoxia reduces the amount of oxygen in the brain, causing such symptoms as **dizziness**, shortness of breath, and mental confusion. These symptoms could cause the pilot to lose control of the plane. Hypoxia can be treated with **oxygen therapy**.

Rapid altitude increases and decreases can cause pain because there is an air pocket in the middle portion of the ear. To equalize pressure in the ear, physicians typically advise pilots and passengers to clear their sinuses by plugging their nose and blowing until the eardrums "pop." Other options include yawning, swallowing or chewing gum. For people with a cold or a severely blocked middle ear, the use of **decongestants**, **antihistamines**, or nasal sprays may help. Without taking steps to equalize pressure, the tympanic membrane could rupture, causing hearing loss, vertigo, dizziness, and **nausea**.

Gravity's impact

Fighter pilots who fly high-performance jets can experience health problems during rapid acceleration and when executing tight turns at high speed. During these moves, a pilot experiences extreme gravity conditions that can pull blood away from the brain and heart and into the lower body. This can cause the pilot to have tunnel vision or pass out. To prevent these potentially deadly situations, the military requires fighter pilots to wear special flight suits, or G suits, which have compartments that fill with air or fluid to keep blood from pooling in the lower body.

Some pilots, like the Blue Angels, use a technique called the Valsalva Maneuver instead of G suits to prevent black outs during high-performance flying. The Valsalva Maneuver involves grunting and tightening the abdominal muscles to stop blood from collecting in the wrong parts of the body.

PREVENTIVE CARE. Since any routine health problem that affects a pilot could mean the loss of hundreds of lives, aviation medicine specialists who work for commercial airlines and the military take special care to educate pilots about proper diet, **exercise** and preventive health tools. For example, physicians may frequently screen pilots for vision changes caused by **glaucoma** or cataracts. They also will check for **hearing loss** and encourage the pilot to wear earplugs or headphones to buffer engine noise. To monitor for heart disease, physicians will check blood pressure and may order diagnostic tests such as an ECG or **stress test**.

Motion sickness

Many people experience nausea, vertigo, and disorientation when they first arrive in space. This is caused by changes in the fluid in the inner ear, which is sensitive to gravity and affects our sense of spatial orientation. The symptoms typically ease after several days, but often recur when the astronaut returns to Earth. To treat this condition, physicians give astronauts **motion sickness** medication, such as lorazepam.

Bone and muscle loss

In zero-gravity conditions, astronauts lose bone and muscle mass. On earth, the natural resistance of gravity helps build stronger muscles and bones during normal weight-bearing activities like walking or even sitting at a desk. In space, however, astronauts must work harder to prevent bone and muscle loss. Exercise is an important treatment. Crew members may use an exercise cycle or resistive rubber bands to stay in shape. Physicians also may give them medication to prevent bone loss and prescribe **nutritional supplements**, such as a mixture of essential amino acids and carbohydrates, to limit muscle atrophy.

Radiation

Another health threat to space travelers is radiation. Harmful rays can alter the DNA in human cells and cause **cancer**. Excess radiation also can weaken the immune system. To prevent these problems, physicians may give astronauts nutritional supplements. For example, research has show that n-3 fatty acids found in fish oil reduce DNA damage.

Cardiovascular issues

When astronauts return to earth after a long mission, they tend to feel dizzy and black out. Scientists are concerned about this dilemma because it could be dangerous if the crew members need to make an emergency exit. One way to prevent this problem, which is caused by a drop in blood pressure, is to have the astronauts drink extra fluids and increase salt intake to increase blood volume. Physicians also may prescribe medication that causes blood vessels to contract. As another precaution, astronauts also put on protective flight suits, or G suits, before they re-enter the earth's atmosphere.

Resources

PERIODICALS

Aviation, Space and Environmental Medicine. Monthly peer-reviewed journal published by the Aerospace Medical Association. Contact theeditor: 3212 Swandale Dr., San Antonio, TX 78230-4404. (210) 342-5670. ASEMJournal@worldnet.att.net.

ORGANIZATIONS

Aerospace Medical Association. 320 S. Henry St., Alexandria, VA 22314-3579. (703) 739-2240. < http:// www.asma.org > .
National Space Biomedical Research Institute. One Baylor Plaza, NA-425, Houston, TX 77030. (713) 798-7412. info@www.nsbri.org. < http://www.nsbri.org > .
Wright State University Aerospace Medicine Program. P.O. Box 92, Dayton, Ohio 45401-0927. (937) 276-8338. < http://www.med.wright.edu > .

OTHER

Federal Aviation Administration Office of Aviation Medicine. < http://www.faa.gov/avr/aamhome.htm > .
National Aeronautics and Space Administration Aerospace Medicine. < http://spacelink.msfc.nasa.gov > .
Society of USAF Flight Surgeons Online Catalog. < http:// www.sam.brooks.af.mil/ram/rammain.htm > .

Melissa Knopper

AVM *see* **Arteriovenous malformations**

Avoidant personality disorder *see* **Personality disorders**

Avulsions *see* **Wounds**

▌Ayurvedic medicine

Definition

Ayurvedic medicine is a system of healing that originated in ancient India. In Sanskrit, *ayur* means life or living, and *veda* means knowledge, so Ayurveda has been defined as the "knowledge of living" or the "science of longevity." Ayurvedic medicine utilizes diet, **detoxification** and purification techniques, herbal and mineral remedies, **yoga**, breathing exercises, **meditation**, and **massage therapy** as holistic healing methods. Ayurvedic medicine is widely practiced in modern India and has been steadily gaining followers in the West.

Purpose

According to the original texts, the goal of Ayurveda is prevention as well as promotion of the body's own capacity for maintenance and balance. Ayurvedic treatment is non-invasive and non-toxic, so it can be used safely as an alternative therapy or alongside conventional therapies. Ayurvedic physicians claim that their methods can also help stress-related, metabolic, and chronic conditions. Ayurveda has been used to treat **acne**, **allergies**, **asthma**, **anxiety**, arthritis, **chronic fatigue syndrome**, colds, colitis, **constipation**, depression, diabetes, flu, heart disease, **hypertension**, immune problems, inflammation, **insomnia**, nervous disorders, **obesity**, skin problems, and ulcers.

Ayurvedic physicians seek to discover the roots of a disease before it gets so advanced that more radical treatments are necessary. Thus, Ayurveda seems to be limited in treating severely advanced conditions, traumatic injuries, acute **pain**, and conditions and injuries requiring invasive surgery. Ayurvedic techniques have also been used alongside **chemotherapy** and surgery to assist patients in recovery and healing.

Description

Origins

Ayurvedic medicine originated in the early civilizations of India some 3,000-5,000 years ago. It is mentioned in the *Vedas*, the ancient religious and philosophical texts that are the oldest surviving literature in the world, which makes Ayurvedic medicine the oldest surviving healing system. According to the texts, Ayurveda was conceived by enlightened wise men as a system of living harmoniously and maintaining the body so that mental and spiritual awareness could be possible. Medical historians believe that

DEEPAK CHOPRA (1946–)

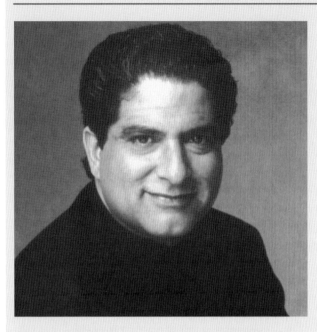

(AP/Wide World Photos. Reproduced by permission.)

Deepak Chopra was born in India and studied medicine at the All India Institute of Medical Science. He left his home for the United States in 1970 and completed residencies in internal medicine and endocrinology. He went on to teaching posts at major medical institutions—Tufts University and Boston University schools of medicine—while establishing a very successful private practice. By the time he was thirty-five, Chopra had become chief of staff at New England Memorial Hospital.

Disturbed by Western medicine's reliance on medication, he began a search for alternatives and discovered one in the teachings of the Maharishi Mahesh Yogi, an Indian spiritualist who had gained a cult following in the late sixties teaching Transcendental Meditation (TM). Chopra began practicing TM fervently and eventually met the Maharishi. In 1985 Chopra established the Ayurvedic Health Center for Stress Management and Behavioral Medicine in Lancaster, Massachusetts, where he began his practice of integrating the best aspects of Eastern and Western medicine.

In 1993, he published *Creating Affluence: Wealth Consciousness in the Field of All Possibilities,* and the enormously successful best seller, *Ageless Body, Timeless Mind.* In the latter he presents his most radical thesis: that aging is not the inevitable deterioration of organs and mind that we have been traditionally taught to think of it as. It is a process that can be influenced, slowed down, and even reversed with the correct kinds of therapies, almost all of which are self-administered or self-taught. He teaches that applying a regimen of nutritional balance, meditation, and emotional clarity characterized by such factors as learning to easily and quickly express anger, for instance, can lead to increased lifespans of up to 120 years.

Ayurvedic ideas were transported from ancient India to China and were instrumental in the development of Chinese medicine.

Today, Ayurvedic medicine is used by 80% of the population in India. Aided by the efforts of **Deepak Chopra** and the Maharishi, it has become an increasingly accepted alternative medical treatment in America during the last two decades. Chopra is an M.D. who has written several bestsellers based on Ayurvedic ideas. He also helped develop the Center for Mind/Body Medicine in La Jolla, California, a major Ayurvedic center that trains physicians in Ayurvedic principles, produces herbal remedies, and conducts research and documentation of its healing techniques.

Key ideas

To understand Ayurvedic treatment, it is necessary to have an idea how the Ayurvedic system views the body. The basic life force in the body is *prana,* which is also found in the elements and is similar to the Chinese notion of *chi.* As Swami Vishnudevananda, a yogi and expert, put it, "Prana is in the air, but is not the oxygen, nor any of its chemical constituents. It is in food, water, and in the sunlight, yet it is not vitamin, heat, or light-rays. Food, water, air, etc., are only the media through which the prana is carried."

In Ayurveda, there are five basic elements that contain prana: earth, water, fire, air, and ether. These elements interact and are further organized in the human body as three main categories or basic physiological principles in the body that govern all bodily functions known as the *doshas.* The three doshas are *vata, pitta, and kapha.* Each person has a unique blend of the three doshas, known as the person's *prakriti,* which is why Ayurvedic treatment is always individualized. In Ayurveda, disease is viewed as a state of imbalance in one or more of a person's doshas, and an Ayurvedic physician strives to adjust and balance them, using a variety of techniques.

The vata dosha is associated with air and ether, and in the body promotes movement and lightness.

Ayurvedic Body Types

	Vata	Pitta	Kapha
Physical characteristics	Thin. Prominent features. Cool, dry skin. Constipation. Cramps.	Average build. Fair, thin hair. Warm, moist skin. Ulcers, heartburn, and hemorrhoids. Acne.	Large build. Wavy, thick hair. Pale, cool, oily skin. Obesity, allergies, and sinus problems. High cholesterol.
Emotional characteristics	Moody. Vivacious. Imaginative. Enthusiastic. Intuitive.	Intense. Quick tempered. Intelligent. Loving. Articulate.	Relaxed. Not easily angered. Affectionate. Tolerant. Compassionate.
Behavioral characteristics	Unscheduled sleep and meal times. Nervous disorders. Anxiety.	Orderly. Structured sleep and meal times. Perfectionist.	Slow, graceful. Long sleeper and slow eater. Procrastination.

Vata people are generally thin and light physically, dry-skinned, and very energetic and mentally restless. When vata is out of balance, there are often nervous problems, hyperactivity, sleeplessness, lower back pains, and headaches.

Pitta is associated with fire and water. In the body, it is responsible for metabolism and digestion. Pitta characteristics are medium-built bodies, fair skin, strong digestion, and good mental concentration. Pitta imbalances show up as anger and aggression and stress-related conditions like **gastritis**, ulcers, liver problems, and hypertension.

The kapha dosha is associated with water and earth. People characterized as kapha are generally large or heavy with more oily complexions. They tend to be slow, calm, and peaceful. Kapha disorders manifest emotionally as greed and possessiveness, and physically as obesity, **fatigue**, **bronchitis**, and sinus problems.

Diagnosis

In Ayurvedic medicine, disease is always seen as an imbalance in the dosha system, so the diagnostic process strives to determine which doshas are underactive or overactive in a body. Diagnosis is often taken over a course of days in order for the Ayurvedic physician to most accurately determine what parts of the body are being affected. To diagnose problems, Ayurvedic physicians often use long questionnaires and interviews to determine a

person's dosha patterns and physical and psychological histories. Ayurvedic physicians also intricately observe the pulse, tongue, face, lips, eyes, and fingernails for abnormalities or patterns that they believe can indicate deeper problems in the internal systems. Some Ayurvedic physicians also use laboratory tests to assist in diagnosis.

Treatment

Ayurvedic treatment seeks to re-establish balance and harmony in the body's systems. Usually the first method of treatment involves some sort of detoxification and cleansing of the body, in the belief that accumulated toxins must be removed before any other methods of treatment will be effective. Methods of detoxification include therapeutic **vomiting**, **laxatives**, medicated **enemas**, **fasting**, and cleansing of the sinuses. Many Ayurvedic clinics combine all of these cleansing methods into intensive sessions known as *panchakarma*. Panchakarma can take several days or even weeks and they are more than elimination therapies. They also include herbalized oil massage and herbalized **heat treatments**. After purification, Ayurvedic physicians use herbal and mineral remedies to balance the body as well. Ayurvedic medicine contains a vast knowledge of the use of herbs for specific health problems.

Ayurvedic medicine also emphasizes how people live their lives from day to day, believing that proper lifestyles and routines accentuate balance, rest, diet, and prevention. Ayurveda recommends yoga as a form of **exercise** to build strength and health, and also advises massage therapy and self-massage as ways of increasing circulation and reducing **stress**. Yogic breathing techniques and meditation are also part of a healthy Ayurvedic regimen, to reduce stress and improve mental energy.

Of all treatments, though, diet is one of the most basic and widely used therapy in the Ayurvedic system. An Ayurvedic diet can be a very well planned and individualized regimen. According to Ayurveda, there are six basic tastes: sweet, sour, salty, pungent, bitter, and astringent. Certain tastes and foods can either calm or aggravate a particular dosha. For instance, sweet, sour, and salty decrease vata problems and increase kapha. Sour, salty, and pungent can increase pitta. After an Ayurvedic physician determines a person's dosha profile, they will recommend a specific diet to correct imbalances and increase health. The Ayurvedic diet emphasizes primarily vegetarian foods of high quality and freshness, tailored to the season and time of day. Cooling foods are eaten in the summer and heating ones in the winter, always within a person's dosha requirements. In daily routine, the heaviest meal of the day should be lunch, and dinner should eaten well before bedtime, to allow for complete digestion. Also, eating meals in a calm manner with proper chewing and state of mind is important, as is combining foods properly and avoiding overeating.

Cost

Costs of Ayurvedic treatments can vary, with initial consultations running anywhere from $40 to over $100, with follow-up visits costing less. Herbal treatments may cost from $10 to $50 per month, and are often available from health food or bulk herb stores. Some clinics offer panchakarma, the intensive Ayurvedic detoxification treatment, which can include overnight stays for up to several weeks. The prices for these programs can vary significantly, depending on the services and length of stay. Insurance reimbursement may depend on whether the primary physician is a licensed M.D.

Preparations

Ayurveda is a mind/body system of health that contains some ideas foreign to the Western scientific model. Those people considering Ayurveda should approach it with an open mind and willingness to experiment. Also, because Ayurveda is a whole-body system of healing and health, patience and discipline are helpful, as some conditions and diseases are believed to be brought on by years of bad health habits and require time and effort to correct. Finally, the Ayurvedic philosophy believes that each person has the ability to heal themselves, so those considering Ayurveda should be prepared to bring responsibility and participation into the treatment.

Precautions

An Ayurvedic practitioner should always be consulted.

Side effects

During Ayurvedic detoxification programs, some people report fatigue, muscle soreness, and general sickness. Also, as Ayurveda seeks to release mental stresses and psychological problems from the patient, some people can experience mental disturbances and depression during treatment, and psychological counseling may be part of a sound program.

Research and general acceptance

Because Ayurveda had been outside the Western scientific system for years, research in the United States is new. Another difficulty in documentation arises because Ayurvedic treatment is very individualized; two people with the same disease but different dosha patterns might be treated differently. Much more scientific research has been conducted over the past several decades in India. Much research in the United States is being supported by the Maharishi Ayur-Ved organization, which studies the Ayurvedic products it sells and its clinical practices.

Some Ayurvedic herbal mixtures have been proven to have high antioxidant properties, much stronger than **vitamins** A, C, and E, and some have also been shown in laboratory tests to reduce or eliminate tumors in mice and to inhibit **cancer** growth in human lung tumor cells. In a 1987 study at MIT, an Ayurvedic herbal remedy was shown to significantly reduce **colon cancer** in rats. Another study was performed in the Netherlands with Maharishi Ayur-Ved products. A group of patients with chronic illnesses, including asthma, chronic bronchitis, hypertension, eczema, **psoriasis**, constipation, **rheumatoid arthritis**, headaches, and non-insulin dependent **diabetes mellitus**, were given Ayurvedic treatment. Strong results were observed, with nearly 80% of the patients improving and some chronic conditions being completely cured.

Other studies have shown that Ayurvedic therapies can significantly lower cholesterol and blood pressure in stress-related problems. Diabetes, acne, and allergies have also been successfully treated with Ayurvedic remedies. Ayurvedic products have been shown to increase short-term memory and reduce headaches. Also, Ayurvedic remedies have been used successfully to support the healing process of patients undergoing chemotherapy, as these remedies have been demonstrated to increase immune system activity.

Resources

BOOKS

Lad, Dr. Vasant. *The Complete Book of Ayurvedic Home Remedies*. Minneapolis: Three Rivers Press, 1999.

ORGANIZATIONS

American Institute of Vedic Studies. P.O. Box 8357, Santa Fe, NM 87504. (505) 983-9385

Ayurveda Holistic Center. Bayville, Long Island, NY. (516)759-7731 mail@Ayurvedahc.com < http://www.Ayurvedahc.com >.

Ayurvedic and Naturopathic Medical Clinic. 10025 NE 4th Street, Bellevue, WA 98004. (206)453-8022.

Ayurvedic Institute. 11311 Menaul, NE Albuquerque, New Mexico 87112. (505) 291-9698. info@Ayurveda.com < http://www.Ayurveda.com >.

Bastyr University of Natural Health Sciences. 144 N.E. 54th Street, Seattle, WA 98105. (206) 523-9585.

Center for Mind/Body Medicine. P.O. Box 1048, La Jolla, CA 92038. (619)794-2425.

College of Maharishi Ayur-Ved, Maharishi International University. 1000 4th Street, Fairfield, IA 52557. (515) 472-7000.

National Institute of Ayurvedic Medicine. (914) 278-8700. drgerson@erols.com. < http://www.niam.com >.

Rocky Mountain Institute of Yoga and Ayurveda. P.O. Box 1091, Boulder, CO 80306. (303) 443-6923.

OTHER

"Inside Ayurveda: An Independent Journal of Ayurvedic Health Care." P.O. Box 3021, Quincy, CA 95971. < http://www.insideayurveda.com >.

Douglas Dupler, MA

Azithromycin *see* Erythromycins
AZT *see* Antiretroviral drugs

B

B-cell count *see* **Lymphocyte typing**

Babesiosis

Definition

Babesiosis is an infection of red blood cells caused by the single-celled parasite, *Babesia microti*, which is spread to humans by a tick bite.

Description

Babesiosis is a rare, tick-transmitted disease that is caused most often by the single-celled parasite *Babesia microti*. By 1995, fewer than 500 cases of babesiosis had been reported in the United States. The disease occurs primarily in New England and New York, especially on the coastal islands. However, cases have occurred in other parts of the United States. Because of tick activity, the risk for babesiosis is highest during June and July.

Ticks are small, blood-sucking arachnids. Although some ticks carry diseasecausing organisms, most do not. *Babesia microti* is spread to humans through the bite of the tick *Ixodes scapularis* (also called *Ixodes dammini*). *Ixodes scapularis*, called the "blacklegged deer tick," usually feeds on deer and mice. A tick picks up the parasites by feeding on an infected mouse and then passes them on by biting a new host, possibly a human. To pass on the parasites, the tick must be attached to the skin for 36-48 hours. Once in the bloodstream, *Babesia microti* enters a red blood cell, reproduces by cell division, and destroys the cell, causing anemia. Humans infected with *Babesia microti* produce antibodies that can be helpful in diagnosing the infection.

Causes and symptoms

Babesia microti live and divide within red blood cells, destroying the cells and causing anemia. The majority of people who are infected have no visible symptoms. In those who become ill, symptoms appear one to six weeks following the tick bite. Because the ticks are small, many patients have no recollection of a tick bite. The symptoms are flu-like and include tiredness, loss of appetite, **fever**, drenching sweats, and muscle **pain**. **Nausea**, **vomiting**, **headache**, shaking chills, blood in the urine, and depression can occur.

Persons who are over 40 years old, have had their spleen removed (splenectomized), and/or have a serious disease (**cancer**, **AIDS**, etc.) are at a greater risk for severe babesiosis. In severe cases of babesiosis, up to 85% of the blood cells can be infected. This causes a serious, possibly fatal, blood deficiency.

Diagnosis

Babesiosis can be diagnosed by examining a blood sample microscopically and detecting the presence of *Babesia microti* within the blood cells. The blood can also be checked for the presence of antibodies to the parasite.

Treatment

In serious cases, babesiosis is treated with a combination of clindamycin (Cleocin) and quinine. Clindamycin is given by injection and quinine is given orally three to four times a day for four to seven days. To reduce the number of parasites in the blood, severely ill patients have been treated with blood transfusions.

Prognosis

Otherwise healthy patients will recover completely. Babesiosis may last several months without treatment and is a severe, potentially fatal disease in splenectomized patients.

Prevention

The only prevention for babesiosis is to minimize exposure to ticks by staying on trails when walking through the woods, avoiding tall grasses, wearing long sleeves and tucking pant legs into socks, wearing insect repellent, and checking for ticks after an outing. Remove a tick as soon as possible by grasping the tick with tweezers and gently pulling. Splenectomized people should avoid northeastern coastal regions during the tick season.

Resources

OTHER

Mayo Clinic Online. March 5, 1998. < http://www.mayohealth.org > .

Belinda Rowland, PhD

Bach flower remedies *see* **Flower remedies**

Bacillary angiomatosis

Definition

A life-threatening but curable infection that causes an eruption of purple lesions on or under the skin that resemble **Kaposi's sarcoma**. The infection, which occurs almost exclusively in patients with **AIDS**, can be a complication of **cat-scratch disease**.

Description

Bacillary angiomatosis is a re-emerging bacterial infection that is identical or closely related to one which commonly afflicted thousands of soldiers during World War I. Today, the disease, caused by two versions of the same bacteria, is linked to homeless AIDS patients and to those afflicted with cat-scratch disease.

The infection is rarely seen today in patients who don't have HIV. According to the U.S. Centers for Disease Control and Prevention (CDC), an HIV patient diagnosed with bacillary angiomatosis is considered to have progressed to full-blown AIDS.

Causes and symptoms

Scientists have recently isolated two varieties of the Bartonella bacteria as the cause of bacillary angiomatosis: *Bartonella* (formerly *Rochalimaea quintana*) and *B. henselae* (cause of cat-scratch disease).

B. quintana infection is known popularly as **trench fever**, and is the infection associated with body lice that sickened European troops during World War I. Lice carry the bacteria, and can transmit the infection to humans. The incidence of trench **fever** was believed to have faded away with the end of World War I. It was not diagnosed in the United States until 1992, when 10 cases were reported among homeless Seattle men.

The related bacteria *B. henselae* was first identified several years ago as the cause of cat-scratch fever. It also can lead to bacillary angiomatosis in AIDS patients. Bacillary angiomatosis caused by this bacteria is transmitted to AIDS patients from cat fleas.

These two different types of bacteria both cause bacillary angiomatosis, a disease which is characterized by wildly proliferating blood vessels that form tumor-like masses in the skin and organs. The nodules that appear in bacillary angiomatosis are firm and don't turn white when pressed. The lesions can occur anywhere on the body, in numbers ranging from one to 100. They are rarely found on palms of the hands, soles of the feet, or in the mouth. As the number of lesions increase, the patient may develop a high fever, sweats, chills, poor appetite, **vomiting**, and weight loss. If untreated, the infection may be fatal.

In addition to the basic disease process, the two different types of bacteria cause some slightly different symptoms. Patients infected with *B. henselae* also experience blood-filled cysts within the liver and abnormal liver function, whereas *B. quintana* patients may have tumor growths in the bone.

Diagnosis

This life-threatening but curable infection is often misdiagnosed, because it may be mistaken for other conditions (such as Kaposi's sarcoma). A blood test developed in 1992 by the CDC detects antibodies to the bacteria. It can be confirmed by reviewing symptoms, history and negative tests for other diseases that cause swollen lymph glands. It isn't necessary to biopsy a small sample of the lymph node unless there is a question of cancer of the lymph node or some other disease.

Treatment

Recent research indicates that **antibiotics** used to treat other HIV opportunistic infections can both prevent and treat bacillary angiomatosis. Treatment is usually given until the lesions disappear, which typically takes three or four weeks. A severely affected lymph node or blister may have to be drained, and a heating pad may help swollen, tender lymph glands. **Acetaminophen** (Tylenol) may relieve **pain**, aches, and fever over 101 °F (38.3 °C).

Prognosis

In most cases, prompt antibiotic treatment in patients with AIDS cured the infection caused by either variety of the bacteria, and patients may resume normal life. Early diagnosis is crucial to a cure.

Prevention

Studies suggest that antibiotics may prevent the disease. Patients also should be sure to treat cats for fleas.

Resources

PERIODICALS

Koehler, J. E. "Zoonoses: Cats, Fleas and Bacteria." *Journal of the American Medical Association* 271 (1994): 531-535.

Carol A. Turkington

Bacillary dysentery *see* **Shigellosis**

Bacitracin *see* **Antibiotics, topical**

Bacteremia

Definition

Bacteremia is an invasion of the bloodstream by bacteria.

Description

Bacteremia occurs when bacteria enter the bloodstream. This may occur through a wound or infection, or through a surgical procedure or injection. Bacteremia may cause no symptoms and resolve without treatment, or it may produce **fever** and other symptoms of infection. In some cases, bacteremia leads to septic shock, a potentially life-threatening condition.

Causes and symptoms

Causes

Several types of bacteria live on the surface of the skin or colonize the moist linings of the urinary tract, lower digestive tract, and other internal surfaces. These bacteria are normally harmless as long as they are kept in check by the body's natural barriers and the immune system. People in good health with strong immune systems rarely develop bacteremia. However, when bacteria are introduced directly into the circulatory system, especially in a person who is ill or undergoing aggressive medical treatment, the immune system may not be able to cope with the invasion, and symptoms of bacteremia may develop. For this reason, bacteremia is most common in people who are already affected by or being treated for some other medical problem. In addition, medical treatment may bring a person in contact with new types of bacteria that are more invasive than those already residing in that person's body, further increasing the likelihood of bacterial infection.

Conditions which increase the chances of developing bacteremia include:

- immune suppression, either due to HIV infection or drug therapy

- antibiotic therapy which changes the balance of bacterial types in the body

- prolonged or severe illness

- alcoholism or other drug **abuse**

- malnutrition

- diseases or drug therapy that cause ulcers in the intestines, e.g. **chemotherapy** for cancer

KEY TERMS

Colostomy—Surgical creation of an artificial anus on the abdominal wall by cutting into the colon and bringing it up to the surface.

Gastrostomy—Surgical creation of an artificial opening into the stomach through the abdominal wall to allow tube feeding.

Jejunostomy—Surgical creation of an opening to the middle portion of the small intestine (jejunum), through the abdominal wall.

Septic shock—A life-threatening drop in blood pressure caused by bacterial infection.

Common immediate causes of bacteremia include:

• drainage of an **abscess**, including an abscessed tooth

• urinary tract infection, especially in the presence of a bladder catheter

• decubitus ulcers (pressure sores)

• intravenous procedures using unsterilized needles, including IV drug use

• prolonged IV needle placement

• use of **ostomy** tubes, including **gastrostomy** (surgically making a new opening into the stomach), jejunostomy (surgically making an opening from the abdominal wall into the jejunum), and **colostomy** (surgically creating an articifical opening into the colon).

The bacteria most likely to cause bacteremia include members of the *Staphylococcus, Streptococcus, Pseudomonas, Haemophilus,* and *Esherichia coli* (*E. coli*) genera.

Symptoms

Symptoms of bacteremia may include:

• fever over 101 °F (38.3 °C)

• chills

• malaise

• abdominal **pain**

• nausea

• vomiting

• diarrhea

• anxiety

• shortness of breath

• confusion

Not all of these symptoms are usually present. In the elderly, confusion may be the only prominent symptom. Bacteremia may lead to **septic shock**, whose symptoms include decreased consciousness, rapid heart and breathing rates and multiple organ failures.

Diagnosis

Bacteremia is diagnosed by culturing the blood for bacteria. Samples may need to be tested several times over several hours. Blood analysis may also reveal an elevated number of white blood cells. Blood pressure is monitored closely; a decline in blood pressure may indicate the onset of septic **shock**.

Treatment

Bacteremia may cause no symptoms, but may be discovered through a blood test for another condition. In this situation, it may not need to be treated, except in patients especially at risk for infection, such as those with heart valve defects or whose immune systems are suppressed.

Prognosis

Prompt antibiotic therapy usually succeeds in clearing bacteria from the bloodstream. Recurrence may indicate an undiscovered site of infection. Untreated bacteria in the blood may spread, causing infection of the heart (**endocarditis** or **pericarditis**) or infection of the covering of the central nervous system (meningitis).

Prevention

Bacteremia can be prevented by preventing the infections which often precede it. Good personal hygiene, especially during viral illness, may reduce the risk of developing bacterial infection. Treating bacterial infections quickly and thoroughly can minimize the risk of spreading infection. During medical procedures, the burden falls on medical professionals to minimize the number and duration of invasive procedures, to reduce patients' exposure to sources of bacteria when being treated, and to use scrupulous technique.

Resources

OTHER

The Merck Page. April 13, 1998. < http://www.merck.com >.

Richard Robinson

Bacterial meningitis *see* **Meningitis**

Bacterial vaginosis

Definition

Bacterial vaginosis (BV) is a type of vaginal infection in which the normal balance of bacteria in the vagina is disrupted, allowing the overgrowth of harmful anaerobic bacteria at the expense of protective bacteria.

Description

BV is the most, common and the most serious type of vaginal infection in women of childbearing age. As many as 10 to 26 percent of pregnant women in the United States have BV; BV has been found in 12 to 25 percent of women in routine clinic populations, and in 32 to 64 percent of women in clinics for **sexually transmitted diseases** (STDs). BV is different than vaginal yeast infections and requires different methods of treatment.

In most cases, BV does not have lasting effects on women. However, there can be risks associated with BV:

Causes and symptoms

Bacteria that dominate the vaginal flora in a BV infection include *Gardnerella vaginalis* or *Mobiluncus*, although other bacteria, such as **Escherichia coli** from the rectum have also been shown to cause the disease. The overgrowth of these harmful bacteria are at the expense of the protective bacteria lactobacilli, which secrete a natural disinfectant, hydrogen peroxide, that maintains the healthy, normal balance of vaginal microorganisms. The factors that upset the normal balance of bacteria in the vagina are not well-understood; however, the following activities or behaviors that have been associated with BV include:

- having a new sex partner or multiple sex partners

- **stress**

- douching

- using an intrauterine device (**IUD**) for contraception

BV is not transmitted through toilet seats, bedding, swimming pools, or touching of objects. Women who have not had sexual intercourse rarely have BV. However BV is not considered an STD, although it does appear to act like an STD in women who have sex with women.

The main symptom of BV is a thin, watery or foamy, white (milky) or gray vaginal discharge with an unpleasant, foul, fish-like or musty odor. The odor is sometimes stronger after a woman has sex, when the semen mixes with the vaginal secretions. Burning or

pain during urination can also be present with BV. **Itching** on the outside of the vagina and redness can also occur, but are seen less frequently. However, many women with BV do not exhibit any symptoms.

Diagnosis

BV is diagnosed through a examination of the vagina by a health care provider. A woman who suspects that she may have BV should not douche or use a feminine hygiene spray before the appointment with the health care provider. Laboratory tests are conducted on a sample of the vaginal fluid to see if the bacteria present are those associated with BV. The health care provider may also check to see if there is decreased vaginal acidity. Potassium hydroxide, when added to a vaginal discharge sample, enhances vaginal odors and allows the health care provider to determine if the odor is fishy or foul.

Treatment

In a few cases, BV might clear up without treatment. However, all women with symptoms of BV should be treated to relieve symptoms and to avoid the development of complications such as pelvic inflammatory disease (PID). In most cases, male partners are not treated, but female sexual partners should be examined to see if they have BV and require treatment.

BV is treated with prescription **antibiotics** such as metronidazole or clindamycin creams or oral metronidazole (both are antibiotics that can also be used by pregnant women, although at different doses). Metronidazole kills anaerobic bacteria but does not harm the protective lactobacilli. Drinking alcohol should be avoided when taking metronidazole, for this medicine can cause severe **nausea and vomiting** when combined with alcohol.

For postmenopausal women, in addition to the use of antibiotics, the health care provider may also prescribe estrogen suppositories or topical cream to thicken and lubricate vaginal tissues. Sexual activity should be avoided during treatment; a **condom** should be used if the woman does have sexual intercourse.

The woman should be tested after treatment to ensure that the infection has been cured.

Alternative treatment

Supplement therapies are available in addition to the use of prescription medicines to ease recovery.

Herbal therapies

Fresh garlic (*Allium sativum*) has antibacterial properties and can be added to a woman's diet. A fresh, peeled garlic wrapped in gauze can also be inserted into the vagina to help treat BV. The insert should be changed twice daily.

To soothe itching or irritation of the vaginal tissues, a woman can bathe the tissues in an infusion of fresh chickweed (*Stellaria media*). The infusion is made by pouring one cup of boiling water on one to two teaspoons of the herb, steeping for five minutes, and allowing the mixture to cool before use.

Prognosis

- Pregnant women with BV often have babies of low birth weight (less than 5.5 pounds) or who are premature

- Bacteria that cause BV may also cause **pelvic inflammatory disease** (PID), an infection of the uterus and fallopian tubes. The risk of a woman with BV developing PID is higher after the woman undergoes surgical procedures such as a **hysterectomy** or an abortion. PID can result in **infertility** and can also increase the risk of an ectopic pregnancy

- BV may increase the risk of a woman becoming infected with HIV, the virus that causes AIDS

- A woman with BV and HIV is more likely to pass HIV to her sexual partner

- BV increases the chance that a woman will contract other STDs, such as chlamydia and gonorrhea

    BV can be successfully treated with antibiotics.

- practicing abstinence

- delaying having sex for the first time, as younger people who have sex are more likely to contract BV and STDs

- limiting the number of sexual partners

- having a sexual relationship with only one partner who does not have an STD

- practicing safer sex, which means using a condom every time when having sex

Prevention

Since the development of BV often appears to be associated with sexual activities, recommended ways to avoid BV include:

Other ways to prevent BV include:

- discontinuing the use of tampons for six months

- practicing good hygiene by wiping from front to back (away from the vagina) after bowel movements to avoid spreading bacteria from the rectum to the vagina

- wearing cotton panties and panty-hose with a cotton crotch and avoiding tight or latex clothing to keep the vagina cool and dry

- avoiding the use of perfumed soaps and feminine sprays

- lowering stress levels

- avoiding douching, as douching removes some of the normal bacteria in the vagina that protects women from infection

- finishing the course of antibiotic treatment, even if the symptoms are relieved, to prevent reoccurrence of the disease

- routinely being tested for BV during regular gynecological examinations

Some physicians recommend that all women who have a hysterectomy or an abortion be treated for BV, to reduce the risk of developing PID.

Resources

BOOKS

Icon Health Publications. *Bacterial Vaginosis - a Medical Dictionary, Bibliography, and Annotated Research Guide to Internet References.* San Diego, CA: Icon Health Publications, 2003.

Parker, James N. and Parker, Philip M., editors. *The Official Patient's Sourcebook on Vaginitis.* San Diego, CA: Icon Health Publications, 2002.

Parker, James N. and Parker, Philip M., editors. *The Official Patient's Sourcebook on Bacterial Vaginosis.* San Diego, CA: Icon Health Publications, 2003.

Time-Life Books. *Vaginal Problems The Medical Advisor..* Richmond, VA: Time-Life Books, 1996.

PERIODICALS

ORGANIZATIONS

American Social Health Association, P.O. Box 13827, Research Triangle Park, NC 27709. Telephone: (919) 361-8400; Fax: (919) 361-8425; Web site: http://www.ashastd.org/.

3M National Vaginitis Association. 3M Center, 275-3W-01, P.O. Box 33275 Saint Paul, MN 55133-3275. Website: www3.3m.com/pdas-nva/

National Women's Health Information Center. U.S. Department of Health and Human Services. Telephone: (800) 994-9662: Website: www.4woman.gov

OTHER

3M National Vaginitis Association. *Women's Guide to Vaginal Infections.* Brochure available for download: www3.3m.com/pdas-nva/cons_addresources.html

Judith Sims

Bacteroides infection *see* **Anaerobic infections**

Bad breath

Definition

Bad breath, sometimes called halitosis, is an unpleasant odor of the breath.

Description

Bad breath is likely to be experienced by most adults at least occasionally. Bad breath, either real or imagined, can have a significant impact on a person's social and professional life.

Causes and symptoms

Bad breath can be caused by a number of problems. Oral diseases, fermentation of food particles in the mouth, sinus infections, and unclean dentures can all contribute to mouth odor. Many non-oral diseases, such as lung infections, kidney failure, or severe **liver disease**, can also cause bad breath, though rarely. Many people think that bad breath can originate in the stomach or intestines; this is extremely rare. The esophagus is usually collapsed and closed, and, although a belch may carry odor up from the stomach, the chance of bad breath being caused from air continually escaping from the stomach is remote. Cigarette smoke can cause bad breath, not only in the cigarette smoker, but also in one who is constantly exposed to second-hand smoke.

Diagnosis

The easiest way to determine if one has bad breath is to ask someone who is trustworthy and discrete.

This is usually not too difficult. Another, more private, method of determining if one has bad breath is to lick one's wrist, wait until it dries, then smell the area. Scraping the rear area of the tongue with a plastic spoon, then smelling the spoon, is another method one can use to assess bad breath.

Treatment

The most effective treatment of bad breath is to treat the cause. Poor oral hygiene can be improved by regular brushing and flossing, as well as regular dental checkups. Gentle brushing of the tongue should be part of daily **oral hygiene**. In addition to good oral hygiene, the judicious use of mouthwashes is helpful. Mouth dryness, experienced at night or during **fasting**, or due to certain medications and medical conditions, can contribute to bad breath. Dryness can be avoided by drinking adequate amounts of water. Chewing gum may be beneficial.

As mentioned, some medications, such as some high blood pressure medications, can cause dry mouth. If this problem is significant, a medication change, under the supervision of one's health care provider, may improve the dry-mouth condition. Oral or sinus infections, once diagnosed, can be treated medically, usually with **antibiotics**. Lung infections and kidney or liver problems will, of course, need medical treatment.

Alternative treatment

Depending on the cause, a multitude of alternative therapeutic remedies can be used. For example, **sinusitis** can be treated with steam inhalation of essential oils and/or herbs.

Prognosis

Most bad breath can be treated successfully with good oral hygiene and/or medical care. Occasionally, for patients who feel that these therapies are unsuccessful, some delusional or obsessive behavior pattern might pertain, and mental health counseling may be appropriate.

Resources

ORGANIZATIONS

American Dental Association. 211 E. Chicago Ave., Chicago, IL 60611. (312) 440-2500. < http://www.ada.org >.

American Medical Association. 515 N. State St., Chicago, IL 60612. (312) 464-5000. < http://www.ama-assn.org > .

Joseph Knight, PA

Balance and coordination tests

Definition

Balance is the ability to maintain a position. Coordination is the capacity to move through a complex set of movements. Balance and coordination depend on the interaction of multiple body organs and systems including the eyes, ears, brain and nervous system, cardiovascular system, and muscles. Tests or examination of any or all of these organs or systems may be necessary to determine the causes of loss of balance, **dizziness**, or the inability to coordinate movement or activities.

Purpose

Tests of balance and coordination, and the examination of the organs and systems that influence balance and coordination, can help to identify causes of dizziness, **fainting**, falling, or incoordination.

Precautions

Tests for balance and coordination should be conducted in a safe and controlled area where patients will not experience injury if they become dizzy or fall.

Description

Assessment of balance and coordination can include discussion of the patient's medical history and a complete **physical examination** including evaluation of the heart, head, eyes, and ears. A slow pulse or heart rate, or very low blood pressure may indicate a circulatory system problem, which can cause dizziness or fainting. During the examination, the patient may be asked to rotate the head from side to side while sitting up or while lying down with the head and neck extended over the edge of the examination table. If these tests produce dizziness or a rapid twitching of the eyeballs (**nystagmus**), the patient may have a disorder of the inner ear, which is responsible for maintaining balance.

An examination of the eyes and ears may also give clues to episodes of dizziness or incoordination. The patient may be asked to focus on a light or on a distant point or object, and to look up, down, left, and right

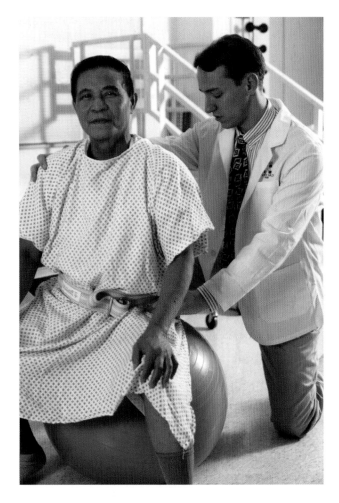

A patient sits on a ball, working on his balance. He wears a belt so that the physical therapist can catch him if he loses balance. *(Custom Medical Stock Photo. Reproduced by permission.)*

moving only the eyes while the eyes are examined. Problems with vision may, in themselves, contribute to balance and coordination disturbances, or may indicate more serious problems of the nervous system or brain function. **Hearing loss**, fluid in the inner ear, or ear infection might indicate the cause of balance and coordination problems.

Various physical tests may also be used. A patient may be asked to walk a straight line, stand on one foot, or touch a finger to the nose to help assess balance. The patient may be asked to squeeze or push against the doctor's hands, to squat down, to bend over, stand on tiptoes or stand on their heels. Important aspects of these tests include holding positions for a certain number of seconds, successfully repeating movements a certain number of times, and repeating the test accurately with eyes closed. The patient's reflexes may also be tested. For example, the doctor may tap on the

Ear Foundation. 1817 Patterson St., Nashville, TN 37203. (800) 545-4327. < http://www.earfoundation.org > .

Vestibular Disorders Association (VEDA). P.O. Box 4467, Portland, OR 97208-4467. (800) 837-8428 or (503) 229-7705. Fax: (503) 229-8064.

Altha Roberts Edgren

KEY TERMS

Meniere's disease—An abnormality of the inner ear that causes dizziness, ringing in the ears, and hearing loss.

knees, ankles, and elbows with a small rubber mallet to test nervous system functioning. These tests may reveal muscle weakness or nervous system problems that could contribute to incoordination.

Preparation

No special preparation is required prior to administration of balance and coordination tests. The patient may be asked to disrobe and put on an examination gown to make it easier for the doctor to observe muscles and reflex responses.

Aftercare

No special aftercare is generally required, however, some of the tests may cause episodes of dizziness or incoordination. Patients may need to use caution in returning to normal activities if they are experiencing any symptoms of dizziness, lightheadedness, or weakness.

Risks

These simple tests of balance and coordination are generally harmless.

Normal results

Under normal conditions, these test will not cause dizziness, loss of balance, or incoordination.

Abnormal results

The presence of dizziness, lightheadedness, loss of coordination, unusual eye movements, muscle weakness, or impaired reflexes are abnormal results and may indicate the problem causing the loss of balance or incoordination. In some cases, additional testing may be needed to diagnose the cause of balance or coordination problems.

Resources

ORGANIZATIONS

American Academy of Otolaryngology-Head and Neck Surgery, Inc. One Prince St., Alexandria VA 22314-3357. (703) 836-4444. < http://www.entnet.org > .

Balanitis

Definition

Balanitis is an inflammation of the head and foreskin of the penis.

Description

Balanitis generally affects uncircumcised males. These are men who have a foreskin, which is the "hood" of soft skin that partially covers the head of the penis. In balanitis, the head and foreskin become red and inflamed. (In circumcised men, who lack a foreskin, these symptoms only affect the tip of the penis.) The condition often occurs due to the fungus *Candida albicans*, the same organism that causes vaginal yeast infections in women. Balanitis (which is also referred to as balanoposthitis) can be caused by a variety of other fungal or bacterial infections, or may occur due to a sensitivity reaction to common chemical agents.

Uncircumcised men are more at risk for balanitis due to the presence of the foreskin. The snug fit of the foreskin around the top of the penis tends to create a damp, warm environment that encourages the growth of microorganisms. Most of the organisms associated with balanitis are already present on the penis, but in very small numbers. However, if the area between the head and foreskin is not cleansed thoroughly on a regular basis, these organisms can multiply and lead to infection.

Diabetes can increase the risk of developing the condition.

Causes and symptoms

Balanitis is usually a result of poor hygiene—for example, neglecting to bathe for several days. A failure to properly wash (or rinse) the area between the head and foreskin can lead to the development of fungal or bacterial infections that cause the condition. In other cases, balanitis may occur due to an allergic reaction: Some men may be sensitive to chemicals found in harsh soaps, laundry detergents, or contraceptive creams. Men who contract a sexually transmitted disease (STD) such as trichimoniasis may also develop symptoms.

The symptoms of balanitis are limited to the foreskin and head of the penis (in circumcised men, only the head is affected). These include redness, inflammation, **pain**, discharge, sore or itchy skin, and difficulty retracting the foreskin.

Diagnosis

Balanitis is usually diagnosed based on a brief physical examination. This may be conducted by your regular health care provider or by a urologist, the type of doctor who specializes in such disorders. The doctor may take a sample of the discharge (if any) to determine the nature of the possible infection. A urine test may be recommended to evaluate glucose (sugar) levels in the urine. Balanitis treatment is typically covered by medical insurance.

Treatment

The treatment of balanitis depends on the specific cause, which can vary from case to case. Antibiotics are used to treat bacterial infections, while topical antifungals such as clotrimazole can combat balanitis caused by *Candida*. If an allergic reaction is causing symptoms, the goal is to identify the chemical agent responsible. Ointments or creams may be used to ease skin irritation.

No matter what the cause, it is important to thoroughly clean the penis on a daily basis in order to alleviate symptoms. If the condition keeps occurring, or if the inflammation is interfering with urination, **circumcision** may be advised.

Alternative treatment

According to practitioners of alternative medicine, certain herbs may be effective in controlling or preventing yeast infections–a common cause of balanitis. These remedies include garlic, calendula, and goldenseal. Eating yogurt that contains acidophilus may also help to clear up a *Candida* infection.

Prognosis

Most cases go away quickly once the cause is identified and treated. However, regular bouts of balanitis can result in urethral stricture.

Prevention

Proper hygiene is the best way to avoid balanitis. Circumcision is sometimes performed to prevent repeated cases.

Resources

BOOKS

Tierney, Lawrence M., et al. *Current Medical Diagnosis and Treatment.* McGraw-Hill, 2000.

PERIODICALS

Mayser, P. "Mycotic infections of the penis." *Andrologia* 31 Supplement 1 (1999): 13-6.

ORGANIZATIONS

U.S. National Library of Medicine. 8600 Rockville Pike, Bethesda, MD 20894. (888) 346-3656. <http://www.nlm.nih.gov>.

Greg Annussek

Balantidiasis

Definition

Balantidiasis is an infectious disease produced by a single-celled microorganism (protozoan) called *Balantidium coli* that infects the digestive tract. It is primarily a disease of the tropics, although it is also found in cooler, temperate climates. Most persons with balantidiasis do not exhibit any noticeable symptoms (asymptomatic), but a few individuals will develop **diarrhea** with blood and mucus and an inflamed colon (colitis).

Description

Balantidiasis is caused by *Balantidium coli*, a parasitic protozoan that infects the large intestine. *B. coli* is the largest and only protozoan, having cilia or hair-like structures, that is capable of causing disease in

KEY TERMS

Asymptomatic—Persons who carry a disease and are usually capable of transmitting the disease but who do not exhibit symptoms of the disease are said to be asymptomatic.

Biopsy—The removal of a tissue sample for diagnostic purposes.

Ciliated—Covered with short, hair-like protrusions, like *B. coli* and certain other protozoa. The cilia or hairs help the organism to move.

Colitis—An inflammation of the large intestine that occurs in some cases of balantidiasis. It is marked by cramping pain and the passing of bloody mucus.

Protozoan—A single-celled, usually microscopic organism, such as *B. coli*, that is eukaryotic and, therefore, different from bacteria (prokaryotic).

Sigmoidoscopy—A procedure in which a thin, flexible, lighted instrument, called a sigmoidoscope, is used to visually examine the lower part of the large intestine.

humans. Balantidiasis occurs most commonly in areas with poor sanitation and in settings where humans live in close contact with pigs, sheep, or goats.

Causes and symptoms

Balantidiasis is transmitted primarily by eating food or drinking water that has been contaminated by human or animal feces containing *B. coli* cysts. During its life cycle, this organism exists in two very different forms: the infective cyst or capsuled form, which cannot move but can survive outside the human body because of its thick, protective covering; and the disease-producing form, the trophozoite, which although capable of moving, cannot survive once excreted in the feces and, therefore, cannot infect others. In the digestive tract, the cysts are transported to the intestine where the walls of the cysts are broken open by digestive secretions, releasing the mobile trophozoites. Once released within the intestine, the trophozoites multiply by feeding on intestinal bacteria or by invading the lining of the large intestine. Within the lining of the large intestine, the trophozoites secrete a substance that destroys intestinal tissue and creates sores (ulcers) or abscesses. Trophozoites eventually form new cysts that are carried through the digestive tract and excreted in the feces. Under favorable temperature and humidity conditions, the cysts can survive in soil or water for weeks to months, ready to begin the cycle again.

Most individuals with balantidiasis have no noticeable symptoms. Even though these individuals may not feel ill, they are still capable of infecting others by person-to-person contact or by contaminating food or water with cysts that others may ingest, for example, by preparing food with unwashed hands.

The most common symptoms of balantidiasis are chronic diarrhea or severe colitis with abdominal cramps, **pain**, and bloody stools. Complications may include intestinal perforation in which the intestinal wall becomes torn, but the organisms do not spread to other parts of the body in the blood stream.

Diagnosis

Diagnosis of balantidiasis, as with other similar diseases, can be complicated, partly because symptoms may or may not be present. A diagnosis of balantidiasis may be considered when a patient has diarrhea combined with a possible history of recent exposure to **amebiasis** through travel, contact with infected persons, or anal intercourse.

Specifically, a diagnosis of balantidiasis is made by finding *B. coli* cysts or trophozoites in the patient's stools or by finding trophozoites in tissue samples (biopsy) taken from the large bowel. A diagnostic blood test has not yet been developed.

Stool examination

This test involves microscopically examining a stool sample for the presence of cysts and/or trophozoites of *B. coli*.

Sigmoidoscopy

To take a tissue sample from the large intestine, a procedure called a **sigmoidoscopy** is performed. During a sigmoidoscopy, a thin, flexible instrument is used to visually examine the intestinal lining and obtain small tissue specimens.

Treatment

Patients with balantidiasis are treated with prescription medication, typically consisting of a ten day course of either tetracycline or metronidazole. Alternative drugs that have proven effective in treating balantidiasis include iodoquinol or paromomycin.

Prognosis

Although somewhat dependent on the patient's overall health, in general, the prognosis for most patients with balantidiasis is good. Severely infected patients occasionally die as a result of a tear in the intestinal wall (intestinal perforation) and consequent loss of blood.

Prevention

There are no immunization procedures or medications that can be taken prior to potential exposure to prevent balantidiasis. Moreover, people who have had the disease can become reinfected. Prevention requires effective personal and community hygiene. Specific safeguards include the following:

- Purification of drinking water. Water can be purified by filtering, boiling, or treatment with iodine.

- Proper food handling. Measures include protecting food from contamination by flies, cooking food properly, washing one's hands after using the bathroom and before cooking or eating, and avoiding foods that cannot be cooked or peeled when traveling in countries with high rates of balantidiasis.

- Careful disposal of human feces.

- Monitoring the contacts of balantidiasis patients. The stools of family members and sexual partners of infected persons should be tested for the presence of cysts or trophozoites.

Resources

BOOKS

Goldsmith, Robert S. "Infectious Diseases: Protozoal & Helminthic." In *Current Medical Diagnosis and Treatment, 1998*, edited by Stephen McPhee, et al., 37th ed. Stamford: Appleton & Lange, 1997.

Rebecca J. Frey, PhD

Baldness *see* **Alopecia**

Balloon angioplasty *see* **Angioplasty**

Balloon valvuloplasty

Definition

Balloon valvuloplasty is a procedure in which a narrowed heart valve is stretched open using a procedure that does not require open heart surgery.

KEY TERMS

Cardiac catheterization—A technique used to evaluate the heart and fix certain problems. Catheterization is far less invasive than traditional surgery.

Stenosis—The narrowing of any valve, especially one of the heart valves or the opening into the pulmonary artery from the right ventricle.

Valve—Tissue in the passageways between the heart's upper and lower chambers that controls passage of blood and prevents regurgitation.

Purpose

There are four valves in the heart, which are located at the exit of each of the four chambers of the heart. They are called aortic valve, pulmonary valve, mitral valve, and tricuspid valve. The valves open and close to regulate the blood flow from one chamber to the next. They are vital to the efficient functioning of the heart.

In some people the valves are too narrow (a condition called stenosis). Balloon valvuloplasty is performed on children and adults to improve valve function and blood flow by enlarging the valve opening. It is a treatment for aortic, mitral, and pulmonary stenosis. Balloon valvuloplasty has the best results as a treatment for narrowed pulmonary valves. Results in treating narrowing of the mitral valve are generally good. It is more difficult to perform and less successful in treating narrowing of the aortic valve.

Description

Balloon valvuloplasty is a procedure in which a thin tube (catheter) that has a small deflated balloon at the tip is inserted through the skin in the groin area into a blood vessel, and then is threaded up to the opening of the narrowed heart valve. The balloon is inflated, which stretches the valve open. This procedure cures many valve obstructions. It is also called balloon enlargement of a narrowed heart valve.

The procedure is performed in a cardiac catheterization laboratory and takes up to four hours. The patient is usually awake, but is given **local anesthesia** to make the area where the catheter is inserted numb. After the site where the catheter will be inserted is prepared and anesthetized, the cardiologist inserts a catheter into the appropriate blood vessel, then passes a balloon-tipped catheter through the first catheter. Guided by a video monitor and an x ray, the physician slowly threads the catheter into the heart. The deflated balloon is positioned in the valve opening, then is inflated repeatedly. The inflated balloon widens the valve's opening by splitting the valve leaflets apart. Once the valve is widened, the balloon-tipped catheter is removed. The other catheter remains in place for 6 to 12 hours because in some cases the procedure must be repeated.

Preparation

For at least six hours before balloon valvuloplasty, the patient will have to avoid eating or drinking anything. An intravenous line is inserted so that medications can be administered. The patient's groin area is shaved and cleaned with an antiseptic. About an hour before the procedure, the patient is given an oral sedative such as diazepam (Valium).

Aftercare

After balloon valvuloplasty, the patient is sent to the recovery room for several hours, where he or she is monitored for vital signs (such as pulse and breathing) and heart sounds. An electrocardiogram, which is a record of the electrical impulses in the heart, is done. The leg in which the catheter was inserted is temporarily prevented from moving. The skin condition is monitored. The insertion site, which will be covered by a sandbag, is observed for bleeding until the catheter is removed. Intravenous fluids will be given to help eliminate the x-ray dye; intravenous blood thinners or other medications to dilate the coronary arteries may be given. Pain medication is available.

For at least 30 minutes after removal of the catheter, direct pressure is applied to the site of insertion; after this a pressure dressing will be applied. Following discharge from the hospital, the patient can usually resume normal activities. After balloon valvuloplasty lifelong follow-up is necessary because valves sometimes degenerate or narrowing recurs, making surgery necessary.

Risks

Balloon valvuloplasty can have serious complications. For example, the valve can become misshapen so that it doesn't close completely, which makes the condition worse. **Embolism**, where pieces of the valve break off and travel to the brain or the lungs, is another possible risk. If the procedure causes severe damage to the valve leaflets, immediate surgery is required. Less frequent complications are bleeding and hematoma (a local collection of clotted blood) at the puncture site, abnormal heart rhythms, reduced blood flow, heart attack, heart puncture, infection, and circulatory problems.

Resources

ORGANIZATIONS

American Heart Association. 7320 Greenville Ave. Dallas, TX 75231. (214) 373-6300. <http://www.americanheart.org>.

Lori De Milto

Bancroftian filariasis *see* **Elephantiasis**

Bang's disease *see* **Brucellosis**

Barbiturate-induced coma

Definition

A barbiturate-induced **coma**, or barb coma, is a temporary state of unconsciousness brought on by a controlled dose of a barbiturate drug, usually pentobarbital or thiopental.

Purpose

Barbiturate comas are used to protect the brain during major brain surgery, such as the removal of **arteriovenous malformations** or aneurysms. Coma may also be induced to control intracranial **hypertension** caused by brain injury.

Precautions

Barbiturate-induced comas are used when conventional therapy to reduce intracranial hypertension has failed. Barbiturate dosing is geared toward burst suppression–that is, reducing brain activity as measured by **electroencephalography**. This reduction in brain activity has to be balanced against the potential side effects of **barbiturates**, which include allergic reactions and effects on the cardiovascular system.

Description

One of the greatest hazards associated with brain injury is intracranial hypertension. Brain injury may be caused by an accidental **head injury** or a medical condition, such as **stroke**, tumor, or infection. When the brain is injured, fluids accumulate in the brain, causing it to swell. The skull does not allow for the expansion of the brain; in effect, the brain becomes compressed.

If the pressure does not abate, oxygenated blood may not reach all areas of the brain. Also, the brain tissue may be forced against hard, bony edges on the interior of the skull. In either case, the brain tissue may die, causing permanent brain damage or **death**.

Barbiturates reduce the metabolic rate of brain tissue, as well as the cerebral blood flow. With these reductions, the blood vessels in the brain narrow, decreasing the amount of swelling in the brain. With the swelling relieved, the pressure decreases and some or all brain damage may be averted.

Controversy exists, however, over the benefits of using barbiturates to control intracranial hypertension. Some studies have shown that barbiturate-induced coma can reduce intracranial hypertension but does not necessarily prevent brain damage. Furthermore, the reduction in intracranial hypertension may not be sustained.

Preparation

Inducing a barbiturate coma is usually kept in reserve for cases in which conventional treatments for controlling intracranial hypertension have failed. Before coma is induced, intracranial hypertension may be treated by hyperventilation; by facilitation of blood flow from the brain; by decompressive surgical procedures, such as draining excess fluids from under the skull or from the chambers within the brain (ventricles); or by drug therapy, including osmotherapy, diuretic agents, or steroids.

Risks

An estimated 25% of barbiturate-induced comas are accompanied by severe side effects. The side effects of barbiturates, especially the depressive effect on the cardiovascular system, can be too risky for some patients. Other side effects include impaired gastrointestinal motility and impaired immune response and infection. Since barbiturates depress activity in the brain, measurements of brain activity may be unreliable. Careful monitoring of the patient is required to ensure nutritional needs are being met and to guard against complications, such as lung infection, fevers, or deep vein **blood clots**.

Normal results

In many patients who do not respond to conventional therapy, barbiturate-induced coma can achieve the necessary control of intracranial hypertension.

Resources

PERIODICALS

Schwab, Stefan, et al. "Barbiturate Coma in Severe Hemispheric Stroke: Useful or Obsolete?" *Neurology* 48 (1997): 1608.

Julia Barrett

Barbiturate withdrawal *see* **Withdrawal syndromes**

Barbiturates

Definition

Barbiturates are medicines that act on the central nervous system and cause drowsiness and can control seizures.

Purpose

Barbiturates are in the group of medicines known as **central nervous system depressants** (CNS). Also known as sedative-hypnotic drugs, barbiturates make people very relaxed, calm, and sleepy. These drugs are sometimes used to help patients relax before surgery. Some may also be used to control seizures (convulsions). Although barbiturates have been used to treat nervousness and sleep problems, they have generally been replaced by other medicines for these purposes.

These medicines may become habit forming and should not be used to relieve everyday **anxiety** and tension or to treat sleeplessness over long periods.

Description

Barbiturates are available only with a physician's prescription and are sold in capsule, tablet, liquid, and injectable forms. Some commonly used barbiturates are phenobarbital (Barbita) and secobarbital (Seconal).

Recommended dosage

Recommended dosage depends on the type of barbiturate and other factors such as the patient's age and the condition for which the medicine is being taken. Check with the physician who prescribed the drug or the pharmacist who filled the prescription for the correct dosage.

Always take barbiturates exactly as directed. Never take larger or more frequent doses, and do not take the drug for longer than directed. If the medicine does not seem to be working, even after taking it for several weeks, do not increase the dosage. Instead, check with the physician who prescribed the medicine.

Do not stop taking this medicine suddenly without first checking with the physician who prescribed it. It may be necessary to taper down gradually to reduce the chance of withdrawal symptoms. If it is necessary to stop taking the drug, check with the physician for instructions on how to stop.

Precautions

See a physician regularly while taking barbiturates. The physician will check to make sure the medicine is working as it should and will note unwanted side effects.

Because barbiturates work on the central nervous system, they may add to the effects of alcohol and

other drugs that slow the central nervous system, such as **antihistamines**, cold medicine, allergy medicine, sleep aids, medicine for seizures, tranquilizers, some **pain** relievers, and **muscle relaxants**. They may also add to the effects of anesthetics, including those used for dental procedures. The combined effects of barbiturates and alcohol or other CNS depressants (drugs that slow the central nervous system) can be very dangerous, leading to unconsciousness or even **death**. Anyone taking barbiturates should not drink alcohol and should check with his or her physician before taking any medicines classified as CNS depressants.

Taking an overdose of barbiturates or combining barbiturates with alcohol or other central nervous system depressants can cause unconsciousness and even death. Anyone who shows signs of an overdose or a reaction to combining barbiturates with alcohol or other drugs should get emergency medical help immediately. Signs include:

- severe drowsiness
- breathing problems
- slurred speech
- staggering
- slow heartbeat
- severe confusion
- severe weakness

Barbiturates may change the results of certain medical tests. Before having medical tests, anyone taking this medicine should alert the health care professional in charge.

People may feel drowsy, dizzy, lightheaded, or less alert when using these drugs. These effects may even occur the morning after taking a barbiturate at bedtime. Because of these possible effects, anyone who takes these drugs should not drive, use machines or do anything else that might be dangerous until they have found out how the drugs affect them.

Barbiturates may cause physical or mental dependence when taken over long periods. Anyone who shows these signs of dependence should check with his or her physician right away:

- the need to take larger and larger doses of the medicine to get the same effect
- a strong desire to keep taking the medicine
- withdrawal symptoms, such as anxiety, **nausea** or **vomiting**, convulsions, trembling, or sleep problems, when the medicine is stopped

Children may be especially sensitive to barbiturates. This may increase the chance of side effects such as unusual excitement.

Older people may also be more sensitive that others to the effects of this medicine. In older people, barbiturates may be more likely to cause confusion, depression, and unusual excitement. These effects are also more likely in people who are very ill.

Special conditions

People with certain medical conditions or who are taking certain other medicines can have problems if they take barbiturates. Before taking these drugs, be sure to let the physician know about any of these conditions:

ALLERGIES. Anyone who has had unusual reactions to barbiturates in the past should let his or her physician know before taking the drugs again. The physician should also be told about any **allergies** to foods, dyes, preservatives, or other substances.

PREGNANCY. Taking barbiturates during **pregnancy** increases the chance of **birth defects** and may cause other problems such as prolonged labor and withdrawal effects in the baby after birth. Pregnant women who must take barbiturates for serious or life-threatening conditions should thoroughly discuss with their physicians the benefits and risks of taking this medicine.

BREASTFEEDING. Barbiturates pass into breast milk and may cause problems such as drowsiness, breathing problems, or slow heartbeat in nursing babies whose mothers take the medicine. Women who are breastfeeding should check with their physicians before using barbiturates.

OTHER MEDICAL CONDITIONS. Before using barbiturates, people with any of these medical problems should make sure their physicians are aware of their conditions:

- alcohol or drug **abuse**
- depression
- hyperactivity (in children)
- pain
- kidney disease
- liver disease
- diabetes
- overactive thyroid
- underactive adrenal gland
- chronic lung diseases such as **asthma** or **emphysema**
- severe anemia
- porphyria

USE OF CERTAIN MEDICINES. Taking barbiturates with certain other drugs may affect the way the drugs work or may increase the chance of side effects.

Side effects

The most common side effects are **dizziness**, lightheadedness, drowsiness, and clumsiness or unsteadiness. These problems usually go away as the body adjusts to the drug and do not require medical treatment unless they persist or interfere with normal activities.

More serious side effects are not common, but may occur. If any of the following side effects occur, check with the physician who prescribed the medicine immediately:

- **fever**

- muscle or joint pain

- sore throat

- chest pain or tightness in the chest

- wheezing

- skin problems, such as rash, **hives**, or red, thickened, or scaly skin

- bleeding sores on the lips

- sores or painful white spots in the mouth

- swollen eyelids, face, or lips

In addition, check with a physician as soon as possible if confusion, depression, or unusual excitement occur after taking barbiturates.

Patients who take barbiturates for a long time or at high doses may notice side effects for some time after they stop taking the drug. These effects usually appear within 8-16 hours after the patient stops taking the medicine. Check with a physician if these or other troublesome symptoms occur after stopping treatment with barbiturates:

- dizziness, lightheadedness or faintness

- anxiety or restlessness

- **hallucinations**

- vision problems

- nausea and vomiting

- seizures (convulsions)

- muscle twitches or trembling hands

- weakness

- sleep problems, nightmares, or increased dreaming

Other side effects may occur. Anyone who has unusual symptoms during or after treatment with barbiturates should get in touch with his or her physician.

Interactions

Birth control pills may not work properly when taken while barbiturates are being taken. To prevent pregnancy, use additional or additional methods of birth control while taking barbiturates.

Barbiturates may also interact with other medicines. When this happens, the effects of one or both of the drugs may change or the risk of side effects may be greater. Anyone who takes barbiturates should let the physician know all other medicines he or she is taking. Among the drugs that may interact with barbiturates are:

- Other central nervous system (CNS) depressants such as medicine for allergies, colds, hay fever, and asthma; sedatives; tranquilizers; prescription pain medicine; muscle relaxants; medicine for seizures; sleep aids; barbiturates; and anesthetics.

- Blood thinners.

- Adrenocorticoids (cortisone-like medicines).

- Antiseizure medicines such as valproic acid (Depakote and Depakene), and carbamazepine (Tegretol).

The list above does not include every drug that may interact with barbiturates. Be sure to check with a physician or pharmacist before combining barbiturates with any other prescription or nonprescription (over-the-counter) medicine.

Resources

PERIODICALS

Miller, Norman S. "Sedative-Hypnotics: Pharmacology and Use." *Journal of Family Practice* 29 (December 1989): 665.

Nancy Ross-Flanigan

Bariatric surgery

Definition

Bariatric surgery promotes weight loss by changing the digestive system's anatomy, limiting the amount of food that can be eaten and digested.

Purpose

Obesity normally is defined through the use of body mass index (BMI) measurement. Physician offices, obesity associations, nutritionists, and others offer methods for calculating BMI, which is a comparison of height to weight. Those with a BMI of 30 or higher are considered obese. However, at 40 or higher, they are considered severely obese—approximately about 100 pounds overweight for men and 80 pounds overweight for women.

Many people who are obese struggle to lose weight through diet and **exercise** but fail. Only after they have tried other methods of losing weight will they be candidates for bariatric surgery, which today is considered a "last resort" for weight loss. In general, guidelines agree that those with a BMI of 40 or more, or a BMI of 35 to 39.9 and a serious obesity-related

KEY TERMS

Digestive tract—The organs that perform digestion, or changing of food into a form that can be absorbed by the body. They are the esophagus, stomach, small intestine, and large instestine.

Esophagus—A muscular tube about nine inches long that carries food from the throat (pharynx) to the stomach.

health problem, qualify for bariatric surgery. More than 23 million Americans are candidates for bariatric surgery. More than 100,000 of the procedures were performed in 2003 and the number of surgeries performed will probably continue to rise for many years.

Precautions

Bariatric surgery is not for everyone and the surgeon and other physicians will evaluate all medical conditions before allowing a patient to proceed. As a major surgery, there are associated risks and side effects. Women of childbearing age should be aware that rapid weight loss and nutritional deficiency associated with bariatric surgery may be harmful to a developing fetus. It is important that a patient reveal all current medications and conditions during any pre-operative discussions or examinations. Also, the physician will carefully evaluate the patient to ensure that he or she is prepared to make a lifelong commitment to the changes in eating and lifestyle required to make the surgery successful.

Though many studies have shown general safety associated with the major surgeries, they are relatively new and research on long-term effects are not as widespread as they are for many other surgeries and procedures. When choosing a surgeon to perform the operation, patients should check with organizations such as the American Society for Bariatric Surgery for certification. A patient also should ask about the surgeon's experience in performing the particular operation.

Although the number of obese teenagers and resulting bariatric surgeries has increased, some experts are questioning the decision to perform bariatric surgery on teens. There are no specific clinical guidelines for determining a safe age for the procedure, but some physicians agree that bariatric surgery is not appropriate for children younger than

Description

When food is chewed and swallowed, it moves along the digestive tract. In the stomach, a strong acid helps break down food so it can be digested and the body can absorb the food's nutrients and calories. The stomach can hold about three pints of food at one time. As digestion continues, food particles become smaller and move from the stomach into the intestine. The various parts of the small intestine are nearly 20 feet long if laid out straight. Those food particles not digested in the small intestine are stored in the large intestine until they are eliminated as waste.

When a patient has bariatric surgery, this digestive process is altered to help the patient lose weight. There are three main types of bariatric surgery, but only two types are commonly used today. The types are restrictive, malabsorptive, and combined restrictive/malabsorptive.

Restrictive surgery, often referred to as "stomach stapling" uses bands or staples to create a small pouch at the top of the stomach where food enters from the esophagus. This smaller pouch may hold only about 1 ounce of food at first and may stretch to hold about 2-3 ounces. The pouch's lower opening is made small, so that food moves slowly to the lower part of the stomach, adding to the feeling of fullness. The most frequently performed types of restrictive surgeries are vertical banded gastroplasty (VBG), gastric banding, and laparoscopic gastric banding. VBG is used less today in favor of gastric banding, which involves an adjustable hollow band made of silicone rubber.

Laparoscopic gastric banding, or Lap-band, was approved by the U.S. Food and Drug Administration (FDA) in 2001. Sometimes referred to as "minimally invasive" bariatric surgery, the surgeon uses small incisions and a laparoscope, or a small, tubular instrument with a camera attached, to see inside the abdomen and apply the band.

Malabsorptive procedures help patients lose weight by limiting the amount of nutrients and calories the intestine can absorb. Sometimes called intestinal bypasses, they are no longer used in the United States because they have often resulted in severe nutritional deficiencies.

Combined restrictive/malabsorptive operations are the most common bariatric surgeries. They work by restricting both the amount of food the stomach can hold and the amount of calories and nutrients the body absorbs. The most common and successful combined surgery in recent years is called the Roux-en-Y gastric bypass (RGB). In this operation, the surgeon first creates a small pouch at the top of the stomach. Next, a Y-shaped section of the small intestine is connected to the small pouch, allowing food to bypass the lower stomach, the first part of the small intestine (duodenum), and the first portion of the next section of the small intestine (jejunum). It connects into the second half of the jejunum, reducing the amount of calories and nutrients the body absorbs. RGB may be performed with a laparoscope and a series of tiny incisions or with a large abdominal incision.

Procedure times vary, depending on the type of bariatric surgery chosen. However, most patients are in surgery for about one to two hours. Though costs can be as high as $35,000, more insurance companies are beginning to pay for the procedures if they are proven medically necessary. In 2004, the agency that pays for Medicare costs recognized obesity and many of its treatments as a medical cost for the first time, recognizing that obesity leads to many other medical problems.

Preparation

The physician will first make sure that a patient is mentally prepared for the surgery and the commitment to follow-up care that will be required. Patients should have a consultation appointment with the surgeon prior to the procedure to discuss risks and benefits. Pre-operative instructions will be given that will tell the patient specific preparations prior to the surgery. These may include instructions about avoiding food or liquids, certain medications, and other instructions on the day before or the day of the procedure. Patients also may have several laboratory or other diagnostic tests prior to the surgery.

Aftercare

Depending on the type of procedure and any possible complications, patients can expect to stay at the hospital or surgery center for about two to four days following the surgery. Those who have laparoscopic operations typically have shorter hospital stays and speedier recovery times. The physician and nurses will provide instructions for wound care and other follow-up when the patient is discharged from the hospital. Usually, bariatric surgery patients can resume normal activity within about six weeks following surgery, and as little as two weeks after laparoscopic procedures. It

is important for bariatric surgery patients to lose weight at the recommended pace, take **nutritional supplements** as recommended, and attend follow-up visits with physicians and nutritionists.

How a patient complies with instructions from physicians following bariatric surgery is important. Most patients will require lifelong use of nutritional supplements such as multivitamins, calcium, and other vitamin supplements to prevent nutritional deficiencies. Because the stomach is smaller, patients will have to eat small portions of food and often must avoid certain types of food such as sugar.

Risks

The surgeon performing the procedure should discuss its specific risks prior to surgery. Risks for bariatric surgery include infection, **blood clots**, abdominal **hernia**, **gallstones**, nutritional deficiencies, possible nerve complications, and **death**. Death rates have been reported lowest for RGB and VBG, at less than 1% of patients.

Normal results

Weight loss will occur gradually, as patients can eat less food and absorb fewer calories. When patients follow post-operative instructions, they can lead normal lives, eating less food and being careful to limit certain foods that may irritate their new stomach pouches. Most patients will lose 50–60% of their excess weight in the first year or two. With gastric bypass surgery, many can lose up to two-thirds of excess weight by the second postoperative year.

Resources

PERIODICALS

"Gastric Bypass Patients Should Recognize Risk of Nerve Injury Post-surgery." *Life Science Weekly* (Nov. 2, 2004):973.

MacNeil, Jane Saladoff. "Gastric Bypass Beat Medical Care for Moderate Obesity." *Family Practice News* (Jan. 15, 2005):60–61.

Santora, Marc. "Teenagers Turn to Surgery to Shrink Their Stomachs." *The New York Times* (Nov. 26, 2004):B1.

ORGANIZATION

American Obesity Association. 1250 12th St. NW, Suite 300, Washington, DC 20037. 202-776-7711. http://www.obesity.org.

Society of American Gastrointestinal Endoscopic Surgeons. 11300 West Olympic Blvd., Suuite 600, Los Angeles, CA 90064. 310-437-0544. http://www.sages.org.

OTHER

Gastrointestinal Surgery for Severe Obesity Weight-control Information Network, National Institutes of Health, 2004. http://win.niddk.nih.gov/publications/gastric.htm.

Teresa G. Odle

Barium enema

Definition

A barium enema, also known as a lower GI (gastrointestinal) exam, is a test that uses x-ray examination to view the large intestine. There are two types of this test: the single-contrast technique where barium sulfate is injected into the rectum in order to gain a profile view of the large intestine; and the double-contrast (or "air contrast") technique where air is inserted into the rectum.

Purpose

A barium enema may be performed for a variety of reasons, including to aid in the diagnosis of colon and **rectal cancer** (or colorectal **cancer**), and inflammatory disease. Detection of polyps (a benign growth in the tissue lining of the colon and rectum), diverticula (a pouch pushing out from the colon), and structural changes in the large intestine can also be established with this test. The double-contrast barium enema is the best method for detecting small tumors (such as polyps), early inflammatory disease, and bleeding caused by ulcers.

The decision to perform a barium enema is based on a person's history of altered bowel habits. These can include **diarrhea**, **constipation**, any lower abdominal **pain** they are currently exhibiting, blood, mucus, or pus in their stools. It is also recommended that this exam be used every five to 10 years to screen healthy people for colorectal cancer, the second most deadly type of tumor in the United States. Those who have a close relative with colorectal cancer or have had a precancerous polyp are considered to be at an increased risk for the disease and should be screened more frequently to look for abnormalities.

Precautions

While barium enema is an effective screening method in the detection of symptoms and may lead to a timely diagnosis of several diseases, it is not the

---

KEY TERMS

Barium sulfate—A barium compound used during a barium enema to block the passage of x rays during the exam.

Bowel lumen—The space within the intestine.

Colonoscopy—An examination of the upper portion of the rectum performed with a colonoscope or elongated speculum.

Diverticula—A diverticulum of the colon is a sac or pouch in the colon walls which is usually asymptomatic (without symptoms) but may cause difficulty if it becomes inflamed.

Diverticulitis—A condition of the diverticulum of the intestinal tract, especially in the colon, where inflammation may cause distended sacs extending from the colon and pain.

Ulcerative colitis— An ulceration or erosion of the mucosa of the colon.

Proctosigmoidoscopy—A visual examination of the rectum and sigmoid colon using a sigmoidoscope.

---

only method to do this. As of 1997, some studies have shown that the **colonoscopy** procedure performed by experienced gastroenterologists is a more accurate initial diagnostic tool for detecting early signs of colorectal cancer. A colonoscopy is the most accurate way for the physician to examine the entire colon and rectum for polyps. If abnormalities are seen at this time the procedure is accompanied by a biopsy. Some physicians use **sigmoidoscopy** plus a barium enema instead of colonoscopy.

Description

To begin a barium enema, the patient will lie with their back down on a tilting radiographic table in order to have x rays of the abdomen taken. After being assisted to a different position, a well-lubricated rectal tube is inserted through the anus. This tube allows the physician or assistant to slowly administer the barium into the intestine. While this filling process is closely monitored, it is important for the patient to keep the anus tightly contracted against the rectal tube to help maintain its position and prevent the barium from leaking. This step is emphasized to the patient due to the inaccuracy that may be caused if the barium leaks. A rectal balloon may also be inflated to help retain the barium. The table may be tilted or the patient moved to a different position to aid in the filling process.

As the barium fills the intestine, x rays of the abdomen are taken to distinguish significant findings. There are many ways to perform a barium enema. One way is that shortly after filling, the rectal tube is removed and the patient expels as much of the barium as possible. Upon completing this, an additional x ray is taken, and a double-contrast enema may follow. If this is done immediately, a thin film of barium will remain in the intestine, and air is then slowly injected to expand the bowel lumen. Sometimes no x rays will be taken until after the air is injected.

Preparation

In order to conduct the most accurate barium enema test, the patient must follow a prescribed diet and **bowel preparation** instructions prior to the test. This preparation commonly includes restricted intake of diary products and a liquid diet for 24 hours prior to the test, in addition to drinking large amounts of water or clear liquids 12–24 hours before the test. Patients may also be given **laxatives**, and asked to give themselves a cleansing enema.

In addition to the prescribed diet and bowel preparation prior to the test, the patient can expect the following during a barium enema:

- They will be well draped with a gown as they are secured to a tilting x-ray table.

- As the barium or air is injected into the intestine, they may experience cramping pains or the urge to defecate.

- The patient will be instructed to take slow, deep breaths through the mouth to ease any discomfort.

Aftercare

Patients should follow several steps immediately after undergoing a barium enema, including:

- Drink plenty of fluids to help counteract the dehydrating effects of bowel preparation and the test.

- Take time to rest. A barium enema and the bowel preparation taken before it can be exhausting.

- A cleansing enema may be given to eliminate any remaining barium. Lightly colored stools will be prevalent for the next 24–72 hours following the test.

Risks

While a barium enema is considered a safe screening test used on a routine basis, it can cause complications in certain people. The following indications should be kept in mind before a barium enema is performed:

- Those who have a rapid heart rate, severe ulcerative colitis, toxic megacolon, or a presumed perforation in the intestine should not undergo a barium enema.

- The test can be cautiously performed if the patient has a blocked intestine, ulcerative colitis, **diverticulitis**, or severe bloody diarrhea.

- Complications that may be caused by the test include perforation of the colon, water intoxication, barium granulomas (inflamed nodules), and allergic reaction. These are all very rare.

Normal results

When the patient undergoes a single-contrast enema, their intestine is steadily filled with barium to differentiate the colon's markings. A normal result displays uniform filling of the colon. As the barium is expelled, the intestinal walls collapse. A normal result on the x ray after defecation will show the intestinal lining as having a standard, feathery appearance.

Accordingly, the double-contrast enema expands the intestine which is already lined with a thin layer of barium, but with air to display a detailed image of the mucosal pattern. Varying positions taken by the patient allow the barium to collect on the dependent walls of the intestine by way of gravity.

Abnormal results

A barium enema allows abnormalities to appear on an x ray that may aid in the diagnosis of several different conditions. Although most colon cancers occur in the rectosigmoid region, or upper part of the rectum and adjoining portion of the sigmoid colon, and are better detected with a different test called a proctosigmoidoscopy, an enema can identify other early signs of cancer.

Identification of polyps, **diverticulosis**, inflammatory disease, such as diverticulitis and ulcerative colitis is attainable through a barium x ray. Structural changes in the intestine, gastroenteritis, and some cases of acute **appendicitis** may also be apparent by viewing this x ray.

Resources

ORGANIZATIONS

American Cancer Society. 1599 Clifton Rd., NE, Atlanta, GA 30329-4251. (800) 227-2345. < http://www.cancer.org >.

Beth A. Kapes

Barium swallow *see* **Upper GI exam**

Barlow's syndrome *see* **Mitral valve prolapse**

Bartholin's gland cyst

Definition

A Bartholin's gland cyst is a swollen fluid-filled lump that develops from a blockage of one of the Bartholin's glands, which are small glands located on each side of the opening to the vagina. Bartholin's gland cysts and abscesses are commonly found in women of reproductive age, developing in approximately 2% of all women.

Description

The Bartholin's glands are located in the lips of the labia that cover the vaginal opening. The glands (normally the size of a pea) provide moisture for the vulva area. A Bartholin's gland cyst may form in the gland itself or in the duct draining the gland. A cyst normally does not cause pain, grows slowly, and may go away without treatment. It usually ranges in size from 0.4-1.2 in. (1–3 cm), although some may grow much larger.

If infected, a Bartholin's gland cyst can form an **abscess** that will increase in size over several days and is very painful. In order to heal, a Bartholin's gland cyst usually must be drained.

Causes and symptoms

A Bartholin's gland cyst occurs if the duct becomes blocked for any reason, such as infection, injury, or chronic inflammation. Very rarely a cyst is caused by **cancer**, which usually occurs only in women over the age of 40. In many cases, the cause of a Bartholin's gland cyst is unknown.

Symptoms of an uninfected Bartholin's gland cyst include a painless jump on one side of the vulva area (most common symptom) and redness or swelling in the vulva area.

Symptoms of an abscessed Bartholin's gland include:

- **pain** that occurs with walking, sitting, physical activity, or sexual intercourse
- fever and chills
- increased swelling in the vulva area over a two- to four-day period
- drainage from the cyst, normally occurring four to five days after the swelling starts

Abscesses may be caused by sexually transmitted bacteria, such as those causing chlamydial or gonococcal infections, while others are caused by bacteria

normally occurring in the vagina. Over 60 types of bacteria have been found in Bartholin's gland abscesses.

Diagnosis

A Bartholin's gland cyst or abscess is diagnosed by a gynecological **pelvic exam**. If the cyst appears to be infected, a culture is often performed to identify the type of bacteria causing the abscess.

Treatment

Treatment for this condition depends on the size of the cyst, whether it is painful, and whether the cyst is infected.

If the cyst is not infected, treatment options include:

- watchful waiting by the woman and her health care professional
- soaking of the genital area with warm towel compresses
- soaking of the genital area in a sitz bath
- use of non-prescription pain medication to relieve mild discomfort

If the Bartholin's gland is infected, there are several treatments available to treat the abscess, including:

- soaking of the genital area in a sitz bath
- treatment with **antibiotics**
- use of prescription or non-prescription pain medication
- incision and drainage, i.e., cutting into the cyst and draining the fluid (not usually successful, as the cyst often reoccurs)

- placement of a drain (Word catheter) in the cyst for two to four weeks so fluid can drain and prevent reoccurrence of the cyst

- marsupialization

- window operation

- use of a carbon dioxide laser to open the cyst and heat the cyst wall tissue so that the cyst cannot form a sac and reoccur

- incision and drainage, followed by treatment with silver nitrate to burn the cyst wall so the cyst cannot form a sac and reoccur

- removal of the entire Bartholin's gland cyst, if the cyst has reoccurred several times after use of other treatment methods

During surgical treatment, the area will be numbed with a local anesthetic to reduce pain. General anesthesia may be used for treatment of an abscess, as the procedure can be painful.

In a pregnant woman, surgical treatment of cysts that are asymptomatic should be delayed until after delivery to avoid the possibility of excessive bleeding. However, if the Bartholin's gland is infected and must be drained, antibiotics and **local anesthesia** are generally considered safe.

If the cyst is caused by cancer, the gland must be excised, and the woman should be under the care of a gynecologist familiar with the treatment of this type of cancer.

Alternative treatment

If a Bartholin's gland cyst has no or mild symptoms, or has opened on its own to drain, a woman may decide to use watchful waiting, warm sitz baths, and non-prescription pain medication. If symptoms become worse or do not improve, a health care professional should then be consulted.

Infected Bartholin's glands should be evaluated and treated by a health care professional.

Prognosis

A Bartholin's gland cyst should respond to treatment in a few days. If an abscess requires surgery, healing may take days to weeks, depending on the size of the abscess and the type of surgical procedure used. Most of the surgical procedures, except for incision and drainage, should be effective in preventing recurring infections.

Prevention

There are few ways to prevent the formation of Bartholin's gland cysts or abscesses. However, as a Bartholin's gland abscess may be caused by a sexually transmitted disease, the practice of safe sex is recommended. Using good hygiene, i.e., wiping front to back after a bowel movement, is also recommended to prevent bacteria from the bowels from contaminating the vaginal area.

Resources

BOOKS

Toth, P. P. "Management of Bartholin's Gland Duct Cysts and Abscesses." In *Saunders Manual of Medical Practice*. Philadelphia: W.B. Saunders, 2000.

Judith Sims

Bartonella bacilliformis infection *see* **Bartonellosis**

Bartonellosis

Definition

Bartonellosis is an infectious bacterial disease with an acute form (which has a sudden onset and short course) and a chronic form (which has more gradual onset and longer duration). The disease is transmitted by sandflies and occurs in western South America. Characterized by a form of red blood cell deficiency (**hemolytic anemia**) and **fever**, the potentially fatal acute form is called Oroya fever or Carrion's disease. The chronic form is identified by painful **skin lesions**.

Description

The acute form of the disease gets its name from an outbreak that occurred in 1871 near La Oroya, Peru. More than 7,000 people perished. Some survivors later developed a skin disease, called verruga peruana (Peruvian **warts**). These skin lesions were observed prior to the 1871 outbreak–perhaps as far back as the pre-Columbian era–but a connection to Oroya fever was unknown. In 1885, a young medical researcher, Daniel Carrion, inoculated himself with blood from a lesion to study the course of the skin disease. When he became ill with Oroya fever, the connection became apparent. Oroya fever is often called Carrion's disease in honor of his fatal experiment.

KEY TERMS

Acute—Referring to the course of a disease, or a phase of a disease, the short-term experience of prominent symptoms.

Chronic—Referring to the course of a disease, or a phase of a disease, the long-term experience of prominent symptoms.

Erythrocytes—Red blood cells.

Hemolytic anemia—A form of erythrocyte deficiency caused by the destruction of the red blood cells.

Host—The organism that harbors or nourishes another organism (parasite). In bartonellosis, the person infected with *Bartonella basilliformis*.

Vector—An organism, such as insects or rodents, that can transmit disease to humans.

The bacteria, *Bartonella bacilliformis*, was isolated by Alberto Barton in 1909, but wasn't identified as the cause of the fever until 1940. The *Bartonella* genus includes at least 11 bacteria species, four of which cause human diseases, including **cat-scratch disease** and **bacillary angiomatosis**. However, bartonellosis refers exclusively to the disease caused by *B. bacilliformis*. The disease is limited to a small area of the Andes Mountains in western South America; nearly all cases have been in Peru, Colombia, and Ecuador. A large outbreak involving thousands of people occurred in 1940–41, but bartonellosis has since occurred sporadically. Control of sandflies, the only known disease carrier (vector), has been credited with managing the disease.

Causes and symptoms

Bartonellosis is transmitted by the nocturnal sandfly and arises from infection with *B. bacilliformis*. The sandfly, *Lutzomyia verrucarum*, dines on human blood and, in so doing, can inject bacteria into the bloodstream. The sandfly is found only in certain areas of the Peruvian Andes; other, as-yet-unidentified vectors are suspected in Ecuador and Colombia.

Once in the bloodstream, the bacteria latch onto red blood cells (erythrocytes), burrow into the cells, and reproduce. In the process, up to 90% of the host's erythrocytes are destroyed, causing severe hemolytic anemia. The anemia is accompanied by high fever, muscle and joint **pain**, **delirium**, and possibly **coma**.

Two to eight weeks after the acute phase, an infected individual develops verruga peruana. However, individuals may exhibit the characteristic lesions without ever experiencing the acute phase. Left untreated, the lesions may last months or years. These lesions resemble blood-filled blisters, up to 1.6 in (4 cm) in diameter, and appear primarily on the head and limbs. They can be painful to the touch and may bleed or ulcerate.

Diagnosis

Bartonellosis is identified by symptoms and the patient's history, such as recent travel in areas where bartonellosis occurs. Isolation of *B. bacilliformis* from the bloodstream or lesions can confirm the diagnosis.

Treatment

Antibiotics are the mainstay of bartonellosis treatment. The bacteria are susceptible to several antibiotics, including chloramphenicol, **penicillins**, and **aminoglycosides**. Blood transfusions may be necessary to treat the anemia caused by bartonellosis.

Prognosis

Antibiotics have dramatically decreased the fatality associated with bartonellosis. Prior to the development of antibiotics, the fever was fatal in 40% of cases. With antibiotic treatment, that rate has dropped to 8%. Fatalities can result from complications associated with severe anemia and secondary infections. Once the infection is halted, an individual can recover fully.

Prevention

Avoiding sandfly bites is the primary means of prevention. Sandfly eradication programs have been helpful in decreasing the sandfly population, and insect repellant can be effective in preventing sandfly bites.

Resources

BOOKS

Daly, Jennifer S. "Bartonella Species." In *Infectious Diseases*, edited by Sherwood F. Gorbach, John S. Bartlett, and Neil R. Blacklow, 2nd ed. Philadelphia: W. B. Saunders Co., 1998.

Julia Barrett

Basal cell cancer *see* **Skin cancer, non-melanoma**

Basal gastric secretion test *see* **Gastric acid determination**

Battered child syndrome

Definition

Battered child syndrome refers to injuries sustained by a child as a result of physical abuse, usually inflicted by an adult caregiver. Alternative terms include: shaken baby; **shaken baby syndrome**; **child abuse**; and non-accidental trauma (NAT).

Description

Internal injuries, cuts, **burns**, **bruises** and broken or fractured bones are all possible signs of battered child syndrome. Emotional damage to a child is also often the by-product of child **abuse**, which can result in serious behavioral problems such as **substance abuse** or the physical abuse of others. Approximately 14% of children in the United States are physically abused each year, and an estimated 2,000 of those children die as a result of the abuse. Between 1994-1995, 1.1 million cases of child abuse were recorded in the United States; of that number, 55% of the victims were less than a year old.

Causes and symptoms

Battered child syndrome (BCS) is found at every level of society, although the incidence may be higher in low-income households where adult caregivers suffer greater **stress** and social difficulties, without having had the benefit of higher education. The child abuser most often injures a child in the heat of anger, and was often abused as a child himself. The incessant crying of an infant or child may trigger abuse. Symptoms may include a delayed visit to the emergency room with an injured child; an implausible explanation of the cause of a child's injury; bruises that match the shape of a hand, fist or belt; cigarette burns; scald marks; bite marks; black eyes; unconsciousness; bruises around the neck; and a bulging fontanel in infants.

Diagnosis

Battered child syndrome is most often diagnosed by an emergency room physician or pediatrician, or by teachers or social workers. Physical examination will detect bruises, burns, swelling, retinal hemorrhages. X rays, and other imaging techniques, such as MRI or scans may confirm **fractures** or other internal injuries. The presence of injuries at different stages of healing (i.e. having occurred at different times) is nearly always indicative of BCS. Establishing the diagnosis is often hindered by the excessive cautiousness of caregivers or by actual concealment of the true

origin of the childþs injuries, as a result of fear, shame and avoidance or denial mechanisms.

Treatment

Medical treatment for battered child syndrome will vary according to the type of injury incurred. Counseling and the implementation of an intervention plan for the child's parents or guardians is necessary. The child abuser may be incarcerated, and/or the abused child removed from the home to prevent further harm. Reporting child abuse to authorities is mandatory for doctors, teachers, and childcare workers in most states as a way to prevent continued abuse. Both physical and psychological therapy are often recommended as treatment for the abused child.

Prognosis

The prognosis for battered child syndrome will depend on the severity of injury, actions taken by the authorities to ensure the future safety of the injured child, and the willingness of parents or guardians to seek counseling for themselves as well as for the child.

Prevention

Recognizing the potential for child abuse in a situation, and the seeking or offering of intervention and counseling before battered child syndrome occurs is the best way to prevent it. Signs that physical abuse may be forthcoming include parental alcohol or substance abuse; previous abuse of the child or the child's siblings; history of mental or emotional problems in parents; parents abused as children; absence of visible parental love or concern for the child; child's hygiene neglected.

Resources

BOOKS

Lukefahr, James L. *Treatment of Child Abuse.*Baltimore, MD: Johns Hopkins University Press, 2000.

PERIODICALS

Mulryan, Kathleen, "Protecting the Child." *Nursing* (July 2000).

ORGANIZATIONS

Childhelp National Abuse Hotline. (800)422-4453.

Mary Jane Tenerelli, MS

Becker muscular dystrophy *see* **Muscular dystrophy**

Beclomethasone *see* **Corticosteroids**

Bed-wetting

Definition

Bed-wetting is the unintentional (involuntary) discharge of urine during the night. Although most children between the ages of three and five begin to stay dry at night, the age at which children are physically and emotionally ready to maintain complete bladder control varies. Enuresis is a technical term that refers to the continued, usually involuntary, passage of urine during the night or the day after the age at which control is expected.

Description

Most children wet the bed occasionally, and definitions of the age and frequency at which bed-wetting becomes a medical problem vary somewhat. Many researchers consider bed-wetting normal until age 6. About 10% of 6-year-old children wet the bed about once a month. More boys than girls have this problem. The American Psychiatric Association, however, defines enuresis as repeated voiding of urine into the bed or clothes at age five or older. The wetting is usually involuntary but in some cases it is intentional. For a diagnosis of enuresis, wetting must occur twice a week for at least three months with no underlying physiological cause. Enuresis, both nighttime (nocturnal) and daytime (diurnal), at age five affects 7% of boys and 3% of girls. By age 10, it affects 3% of boys and 2% of girls; only 1% of adolescents experience enuresis.

Enuresis is divided into two classes. A child with primary enuresis has never established bladder control. A child with secondary enuresis begins to wet after a prolonged dry period. Some children have both nocturnal and diurnal enuresis.

Causes and symptoms

The causes of bed-wetting are not entirely known. It tends to run in families. Most children with primary

---

KEY TERMS

Acupressure—A technique using pressure to various points on the body to alleviate health problems.

ADH—Antidiuretic hormone, or the hormone that helps to concentrate urine during the night.

Behavior modification—Techniques used to change harmful behavior patterns.

Bladder—The muscular sac or container that stores urine until it is released from the body through the tube that carries urine from the bladder to the outside of the body (urethra).

DDAVP—Desmopressin acetate, a drug used to regulate urine production.

Hypnosis—The technique by which a trained professional relaxes the subject and then asks questions or gives suggestions.

Imipramine hydrochloride—A drug used to increase bladder capacity.

Kidneys—A pair of organs located on each side of the spine in the lower back area. They excrete, or get rid of, urine.

Nocturnal enuresis—Involuntary discharge of urine during the night.

Urinalysis—A urine test.

Urine—The fluid excreted by the kidneys, stored in the bladder, then discharged from the body through the tube that carries urine from the bladder to the outside of the body (urethra).

Void—To empty the bladder.

---

enuresis have a close relative–a parent, aunt, or uncle–who also had the disorder. About 70% of children with two parents who wet the bed will also wet the bed. Twin studies have shown that both of a pair of identical twins experience enuresis more often than both of a pair of fraternal twins.

Sometimes bed-wetting can be caused by a serious medical problem like diabetes, sickle-cell anemia, or epilepsy. **Snoring** and episodes of interrupted breathing during sleep (**sleep apnea**) occasionally contribute to bed-wetting problems. Enlarged adenoids can cause these conditions. Other physiological problems, such as urinary tract infection, severe **constipation**, or **spinal cord injury**, can cause bed-wetting.

Children who wet the bed frequently may have a smaller than normal functional bladder capacity. Functional bladder capacity is the amount of urine a person can hold in the bladder before feeling a strong urge to urinate. When functional capacity is small, the bladder will not hold all the urine produced during the night. Tests have shown that bladder size in these children is normal. Nevertheless, they experience frequent strong urges to urinate. Such children urinate often during the daytime and may wet several times at night. Although a small functional bladder capacity may be caused by a developmental delay, it may also be that the child's habit of voiding frequently slows bladder development.

Parents often report that their bed-wetting child is an extremely sound sleeper and difficult to wake. However, several research studies found that bed-wetting children have normal sleep patterns and that bed-wetting can occur in any stage of sleep.

Recent medical research has found that many children who wet the bed may have a deficiency of an important hormone known as antidiuretic hormone (ADH). ADH helps to concentrate urine during sleep hours, meaning that the urine contains less water and therefore takes up less space. This decreased volume of water usually prevents the child's bladder from overfilling during the night, unless the child drank a lot just before going to bed. Testing of many bed-wetting children has shown that these children do not have the usual increase in ADH during sleep. Children who wet the bed, therefore, often produce more urine during the hours of sleep than their bladders can hold. If they do not wake up, the bladder releases the excess urine and the child wets the bed.

Research demonstrates that in most cases bed-wetting does not indicate that the child has a physical or psychological problem. Children who wet the bed usually have normal-sized bladders and have sleep patterns that are no different from those of non-bed-wetting children. Sometimes emotional **stress**, such as the birth of a sibling, a **death** in the family, or separation from the family, may be associated with the onset of bed-wetting in a previously toilet-trained child. Daytime wetting, however, may indicate that the problem has a physical cause.

While most children have no long-term problems as a result of bed-wetting, some children may develop psychological problems. Low self-esteem may occur when these children, who already feel embarrassed, are further humiliated by angry or frustrated parents who punish them or who are overly aggressive about toilet training. The problem can by aggravated when playmates tease or when social activities such as sleep-away camp are avoided for fear of teasing.

Diagnosis

If a child continues to wet the bed after the age of six, parents may feel the need to seek evaluation and diagnosis by the family doctor or a children's specialist (pediatrician). Typically, before the doctor can make a diagnosis, a thorough medical history is obtained. Then the child receives a **physical examination**, appropriate laboratory tests, including a urine test (**urinalysis**), and, if necessary, radiologic studies (such as x rays).

If the child is healthy and no physical problem is found, which is the case 90% of the time, the doctor may not recommend treatment but rather may provide the parents and the child with reassurance, information, and advice.

Treatment

Occasionally a doctor will determine that the problem is serious enough to require treatment. Standard treatments for bed-wetting include **bladder training** exercises, motivational therapy, drug therapy, psychotherapy, and diet therapy.

Bladder training exercises are based on the theory that those who wet the bed have small functional bladder capacity. Children are told to drink a large quantity of water and to try to prolong the periods between urinations. These exercises are designed to increase bladder capacity but are only successful in resolving bed-wetting in a small number of patients.

In motivational therapy, parents attempt to encourage the child to combat bed-wetting, but the child must want to achieve success. Positive reinforcement, such as praise or rewards for staying dry, can help improve self-image and resolve the condition. Punishment for "wet" nights will hamper the child's self-esteem and compound the problem.

The following motivational techniques are commonly used:

- Behavior modification. This method of therapy is aimed at helping children take responsibility for their nighttime bladder control by teaching new behaviors. For example, children are taught to use the bathroom before bedtime and to avoid drinking fluids after dinner. While behavior modification generally produces good results, it is long-term treatment.

- Alarms. This form of therapy uses a sensor placed in the child's pajamas or in a bed pad. This sensor triggers an alarm that wakes the child at the first sign of wetness. If the child is awakened, he or she can then go to the bathroom and finish urinating. The intention is to condition a response to awaken when the bladder is full. Bed-wetting alarms require the motivation of both parents and children. They are considered the most effective form of treatment now available.

A number of drugs are also used to treat bed-wetting. These medications are usually fast acting; children often respond to them within the first week of treatment. Among the drugs commonly used are a nasal spray of desmopressin acetate (DDAVP), a substance similar to the hormone that helps regulate urine production; and imipramine hydrochloride, a drug that helps to increase bladder capacity. Studies show that imipramine is effective for as many as 50% of patients. However, children often wet the bed again after the drug is discontinued, and it has some side effects. Some bed-wetting with an underlying physical cause can be treated by surgical procedures. These causes include enlarged adenoids that cause sleep apnea, physical defects in the urinary system, or a spinal tumor.

Psychotherapy is indicated when the child exhibits signs of severe emotional distress in response to events such as a death in the family, the birth of a new child, a change in schools, or divorce. Psychotherapy is also indicated if a child shows signs of persistently low self-esteem or depression.

In rare cases, **allergies** or intolerances to certain foods–such as dairy products, citrus products, or chocolate–can cause bed-wetting. When children have food sensitivities, bed-wetting may be helped by discovering the substances that trigger the allergic response and eliminating these substances from the child's diet.

Alternative treatment

A number of alternative treatments are available for bed-wetting.

Massage

According to practitioners of this technique, pressure applied to various points on the body may help alleviate the condition. **Acupressure** or massage, when done by a trained therapist, may also be helpful in bed-wetting caused by a neurologic problem.

Herbal and homeopathic remedies

Some herbal remedies, such as horsetail (*Equisetum arvense*) have also been used to treat bed-wetting. A trained homeopathic practitioner, working at the constitutional level, will seek to rebalance the child's vital force, eliminating the imbalanced behavior of bed-wetting.

Common homeopathic remedies used in this treatment include *Causticum, Lycopodium,* and *Pulsatilla.*

Hypnosis

Hypnosis is another approach that is being used successfully by practitioners trained in this therapy. It trains the child to awaken and go to the bathroom when his or her bladder feels full. Hypnosis is less expensive, less time-consuming, and less dangerous than most approaches; it has virtually no side effects. Recent medical studies show that **hypnotherapy** can work quickly–within four to six sessions.

Prognosis

Occasional bed-wetting is not a disease and it does not have a "cure." If the child has no underlying physical or psychological problem that is causing the bed-wetting, in most cases he or she will outgrow the condition without treatment. About 15% of bedwetters become dry each year after age 6. If bed-wetting is frequent, accompanied by daytime wetting, or falls into the American Psychiatric Association's diagnostic definition of enuresis, a doctor should be consulted. If treatment is indicated, it usually successfully resolves the problem. Marked improvement is seen in about 75% of cases treated with wetness alarms.

Prevention

Although preventing a child from wetting the bed is not always possible, parents can take steps to help the child keep the bed dry at night. These steps include:

- Encouraging and praising the child for staying dry instead of punishing when the child wets.

- Reminding the child to urinate before going to bed, if he or she feels the need.

- Limiting liquid intake at least two hours before bedtime.

Resources

ORGANIZATIONS

Association for the Care of Children's Health (ACCH). 7910 Woodmont Ave., Suite 300, Bethesda, MD 20814. (800) 808-2224.
National Association for Continence. P.O. Box 8310, Spartenburg, SC 29305. (800) 252-3337. < http:// www.nafc.org > .
National Enuresis Society. 7777 Forest Lane, Suite C-737, Dallas, TX 75230-2518. (800) 697-8080. < http:// www.peds.umn.edu/Centers/NES > .

Genevieve Slomski, Ph.D.

Bedsores

Definition

Bedsores are also called decubitus ulcers, pressure ulcers, or pressure sores. These tender or inflamed patches develop when skin covering a weight-bearing part of the body is squeezed between bone and another body part, or a bed, chair, splint, or other hard object.

Description

Each year, about one million people in the United States develop bedsores ranging from mild inflammation to deep **wounds** that involve muscle and bone. This often painful condition usually starts with shiny red skin that quickly blisters and deteriorates into open sores that can harbor life-threatening infection.

Bedsores are not cancerous or contagious. They are most likely to occur in people who must use wheelchairs or who are confined to bed. In 1992, the federal Agency for Health Care Policy and Research reported that bedsores afflict:

- 10% of hospital patients
- 25% of nursing home residents
- 60% of quadriplegics

The Agency also noted that 65% of elderly people hospitalized with broken hips develop bedsores and that doctors fees for treatment of bedsores amounted to $2,900 per person.

Bedsores are most apt to develop on the:

- ankles
- back of the head
- heels
- hips
- knees
- lower back
- shoulder blades
- spine

People over the age of 60 are more likely than younger people to develop bedsores. Risk is also increased by:

- atherosclerosis (hardening of arteries)
- diabetes or other conditions that make skin more susceptible to infection
- diminished sensation or lack of feeling

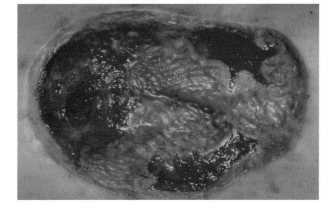

Bedsore. *(Photograph by Michael English, M.D., Custom Medical Stock Photo. Reproduced by permission.)*

- heart problems
- incontinence (inability to control bladder or bowel movements)
- malnutrition
- obesity
- paralysis or immobility
- poor circulation
- prolonged bed rest, especially in unsanitary conditions or with wet or wrinkled sheets
- spinal cord injury

Causes and symptoms

Bedsores most often develop when constant pressure pinches tiny blood vessels that deliver oxygen and nutrients to the skin. When skin is deprived of oxygen and nutrients for as little as an hour, areas of tissue can die and bedsores can form.

Slight rubbing or friction against the skin can cause minor pressure ulcers. They can also develop when a patient stretches or bends blood vessels by slipping into a different position in a bed or chair.

Urine, feces, or other moisture increases the risk of skin infection, and people who are unable to move or recognize internal cues to shift position have a greater than average risk of developing bedsores.

Other risk factors include:

- malnutrition
- anemia (lack of red blood cells)
- diuse atrophy (muscle loss or weakness from lack of use)
- infection

Diagnosis

Bedsores usually follow six stages:

- redness of skin
- redness, swelling, and possible peeling of outer layer of skin
- dead skin, draining wound, and exposed layer of fat
- tissue death through skin and fat, to muscle
- inner fat and muscle death
- destruction of bone, bone, infection, fracture, and blood infection

Treatment

Prompt medical attention can prevent surface pressure sores from deepening into more serious infections. For mild bedsores, treatment involves relieving pressure, keeping the wound clean and moist, and keeping the area around the ulcer clean and dry. **Antiseptics**, harsh soaps, and other skin cleansers can damage new tissue, so a saline solution should be used to cleanse the wound whenever a fresh non-stick dressing is applied.

The patient's doctor may prescribe infection-fighting **antibiotics**, special dressings or drying agents, or lotions or ointments to be applied to the wound in a thin film three or four times a day. Warm whirlpool treatments are sometimes recommended for sores on the arm, hand, foot, or leg.

In a procedure called debriding, a scalpel may be used to remove dead tissue or other debris from the wound. Deep, ulcerated sores that don't respond to other therapy may require skin grafts or **plastic surgery**.

A doctor should be notified whenever a person:

- will be bedridden or immobilized for an extended time
- is very weak or unable to move
- develops bedsores

Immediate medical attention is required whenever:

- skin turns black or becomes inflamed, tender, swollen, or warm to the touch.
- the patient develops a **fever** during treatment.
- the sore contains pus or has a foul-smelling discharge.

With proper treatment, bedsores should begin to heal two to four weeks after treatment begins.

Alternative treatment

Zinc and **vitamins** A, C, E, and B complex help skin repair injuries and stay healthy, but large doses of vitamins or minerals should never be used without a doctor's approval.

A poultice made of equal parts of powdered slippery elm (*Ulmus fulva*), marsh mallow (*Althaea officinalis*), and echinacea (*Echinacea* spp.) blended with a small amount of hot water can relieve minor inflammation. An infection-fighting rinse can be made by diluting two drops of essential tea tree oil (*Melaleuca* spp.) in eight ounces of water. An herbal tea made from the calendula (*Calendula officinalis*) can act as an antiseptic and wound healing agent. Calendula cream can also be used.

Contrasting hot and cold local applications can increase circulation to the area and help flush out waste products, speeding the healing process. The temperatures should be extreme (hot hot and ice cold), yet tolerable to the skin. Hot compresses should be applied for three minutes, followed by 30 seconds of cold compress application, repeating the cycle three times. The cycle should always end with the cold compress.

Prevention

It is usually possible to prevent bedsores from developing or worsening. The patient should be inspected regularly; should bathe or shower every day, using warm water and mild soap; and should avoid cold or dry air. A bedridden patient should be repositioned at least once every two hours while awake. A person who uses a wheelchair should shift his weight every 10 or 15 minutes, or be helped to reposition himself at least once an hour. It is important to lift, rather than drag, a person being repositioned. Bony parts of the body should not be massaged. Even slight friction can remove the top layer of skin and damage blood vessels beneath it.

If the patient is bedridden, sensitive body parts can be protected by:

- sheepskin pads
- special cushions placed on top of a mattress
- a water-filled mattress
- a variable-pressure mattress whose sections can be individually inflated or deflated to redistribute pressure.

Pillows or foam wedges can prevent a bedridden patient's ankles from irritating each other, and pillows placed under the legs from mid-calf to ankle can raise the heels off the bed. Raising the head of the bed slightly and briefly can provide relief, but raising the head of the bed more than 30 degrees can cause the patient to slide, thereby causing damage to skin and tiny blood vessels.

A person who uses a wheelchair should be encouraged to sit up as straight as possible. Pillows behind the head and between the legs can help prevent bedsores, as can a special cushion placed on the chair seat. Donut-shaped cushions should not be used because they restrict blood flow and cause tissues to swell.

Prognosis

Bedsores can usually be cured, but about 60,000 deaths a year are attributed to complications caused by bedsores. Bedsores can be slow to heal. Without proper treatment, they can lead to:

- gangrene (tissue death)

- osteomyelitis (infection of the bone beneath the bedsore)

- sepsis (tissue-destroying bacterial infection)

- other localized or systemic infections that slow the healing process, increase the cost of treatment, lengthen hospital or nursing home stays, or cause death

Resources

ORGANIZATIONS

International Association of Enterstomal Therapy. 27241 La Paz Road, Suite 121, Laguna Niguel, CA 92656. (714) 476-0268.

National Pressure Ulcer Advisory Panel. SUNY at Buffalo, Beck Hall, 3435 Main St., Buffalo, NY 14214. (716) 881-3558. < http://www.npuap.org >.

Maureen Haggerty

Beef tapeworm infection *see* **Tapeworm diseases**

Behavior therapy *see* **Cognitive-behavioral therapy**

Behcet's syndrome

Definition

A group of symptoms that affect a variety of body systems, including musculoskeletal, gastrointestinal, and the central nervous system. These symptoms include ulceration of the mouth or the genital area, **skin lesions**, and inflammation of the uvea (an area around the pupil of the eye).

Description

Behcet's syndrome is a chronic disease that involves multiple body systems. The disease is named for a Turkish dermatologist, Hulusi Behcet, who first reported a patient with recurrent mouth and genital ulcers along with **uveitis** in 1937. The disease occurs worldwide, but is most prevalent in Japan, the Middle East, and in the Mediterranean region. There is a wider prevalence among males than females in a ratio of two to one.

Causes and symptoms

The cause of Behcet's syndrome is unknown. Symptoms include recurring ulcers in the mouth or the genital area, skin lesions, arthritis that affects mainly the knees and ankles, **pain** and irritation in the eyes, and **fever**. The mouth and genital ulcers tend to occur in multiples and can be quite painful. In the mouth, these ulcers are generally found on the tongue, gums, and the inside of the lips or jaws. In the genital area, the ulcers usually occur on the penis and scrotum in males and on the vulva of women. The eye inflammation can lead to blindness.

Diagnosis

Because Behcet's syndrome is a multisystem disease, it is difficult to diagnose. International criteria have been proposed to assist in classifying this disease. There is no one diagnostic feature of this disease, so diagnosis depends on grouping together enough symptoms in order to identify the disease. Symptoms of Behcet's syndrome also occur in other diseases, so it is often necessary to rule out the other diseases before a definitive diagnosis can be reached.

Treatment

Some of the current drugs used to treat Behcet's syndrome include corticosteroids, cyclosporine, azathioprine, chlorambucil, interferon alpha, thalidomide, levamisole and pulse cyclophosphamide.

Prognosis

The prognosis for Behcet's syndrome is generally poor. There has been a documented case of Behcet's lasting for 17 years. Although the disease is considered painful but not fatal, when the central nervous system is involved there is usually severe disability and **death** often occurs. The condition is usually chronic, although there can be remissions during the course of the disease. There is no predictable method to determine which patients will progress into the more serious symptoms, and which might move into remission.

Prevention

There is no known prevention for Behcet's syndrome.

Resources

BOOKS

Ruddy, Shaun. *Kelley's Textbook of Rheumatology.* Philadelphia: W.B. Saunders Company, 2001.

Tierney, Lawrence, et al. *Current Medical Diagnosis and Treatment.* Los Altos: Lange Medical Publications, 2001.

PERIODICALS

Okada, A. A. "Drug Therapy in Behcet's Disease." *OcularImmunology and Inflammation* June 2000: 85-91.

Shed, L. P. "Thalomide Responsiveness in an Infant with Behcet's Syndrome." *Pediatrics* June 1999: 1295-1297.

ORGANIZATIONS

American Behcet's Disease Association. P.O. Box 280240, Memphis, TN 38168-0240. <http://www.behcets.com>.

Behcet's Organization Worldwide, Head Office. P.O. Box 27, Watchet, Somerset TA23 OYJ, United Kingdom. <http://www.behcets.org>.

National Eye Institute. National Institute of Health. Bldg. 31, Rm. 6A32, Bethesda, MD 30892-2510. (800) 869-2020. 2020@nei.nih.gov. <http://www.nei.nih.gov>.

National Organization for Rare Disorders. P.O. Box 8923, New Fairfield, CT 06812-8923. (800) 999-6673. <http://www.rarediseaes.org>.

Kim A. Sharp, M.Ln.

Bejel

Definition

Bejel, also known as endemic **syphilis**, is a chronic but curable disease, seen mostly in children in arid regions. Unlike the better-known venereal syphilis, endemic syphilis is not a sexually transmitted disease.

Description

Bejel has many other names depending on the locality: siti, dichuchwa, njovera, belesh, and skerljevo are some of the names. It is most commonly found in the Middle East (Syria, Saudi Arabia, Iraq), Africa, central Asia, and Australia. Bejel is related to **yaws** and **pinta**, but has different symptoms.

Causes and symptoms

Treponema pallidum, the bacteria that causes bejel, is very closely related to the one that causes the sexually transmitted form of syphilis, but transmission is very different. In bejel, transmission is by direct contact, with broken skin or contaminated hands, or indirectly by sharing drinking vessels and eating utensils. *T. pallidum* is passed on mostly between children living in poverty in very unsanitary environments and with poor hygiene.

The skin, bones, and mucous membranes are affected by bejel. Patches and ulcerated sores are common in the mouth, throat, and nasal passages. Gummy lesions may form, even breaking through the palate. Other findings may include a region of swollen lymph nodes and deep bone **pain** in the legs. Eventually, bones may become deformed.

Diagnosis

T. pallidum can be detected by microscopic study of samples taken from the sores or lymph fluid. However, since antibody tests don't distinguish between the types of syphilis, specific diagnosis of the type of syphilis depends on the patient's history, symptoms, and environment.

Treatment

Large doses of benzathine penicillin G given by injection into the muscle can cure this disease in any stage, although it may take longer and require additional doses in later stages. If penicillin cannot be given, the alternative is tetracycline. Since tetracycline can permanently discolor new teeth still forming, it is usually not prescribed for children unless no viable alternative is available.

Prognosis

Bejel is completely curable with antibiotic treatment.

Endemic disease—An infectious disease that occurs frequently in a specific geographical locale. The disease often occurs in cycles. Influenza is an example of an endemic disease.

Lymph—This is a clear, colorless fluid found in lymph vessels and nodes. The lymph nodes contain organisms that destroy bacteria and other disease causing organisms (also called pathogens).

Syphilis—This disease occurs in two forms. One is a sexually transmitted disease caused by a bacteria. The second form is not sexually transmitted, but passed on by direct contact with the patient or through use of shared food dishes and utensils.

Prevention

The World Health Organization (WHO) has worked with many countries to prevent this and other diseases, and the number of cases has been reduced somewhat. Widespread use of penicillin has been responsible for reducing the number of existing cases, but the only way to eliminate bejel is by improving living and sanitation conditions.

Resources

BOOKS

Fauci, Anthony S., et al., editors. *Harrison's Principles of Internal Medicine*. New York: McGraw-Hill, 1997.

Jill S. Lasker

Benazepril *see* **Angiotensin-converting enzyme inhibitors**

Bence Jones protein test

Definition

Bence Jones proteins are small proteins (light chains of immunoblobulin) found in the urine. Testing for these proteins is done to diagnose and monitor **multiple myeloma** and other similar diseases.

Purpose

Bence Jones proteins are considered the first tumor marker. A tumor marker is a substance, made by the body, that is linked to a certain **cancer**, or malignancy. Bence Jones proteins are made by plasma cells, a type of white blood cell. The presence of these proteins in a person's urine is associated with a malignancy of plasma cells.

Multiple myeloma, a tumor of plasma cells, is the disease most often linked with Bence Jones proteins. The amount of Bence Jones proteins in the urine indicates how much tumor is present. Physicians use Bence Jones proteins testing to diagnose the disease as well as to check how well the disease is responding to treatment.

Other diseases involving cancerous or excessive growth of plasma cells or cells similar to plasma cells can cause Bence Jones proteins in the urine. These diseases include: Waldenström's macroglobulinemia, some lymphomas and leukemias, osteogenic sarcoma, cryoglobulinemia, malignant B-cell disease, **amyloidosis**, light chain disease, and cancer that has spread to bone.

Description

Urine is the best specimen in which to look for Bence Jones proteins. Proteins are usually too large to move through a healthy kidney, from the blood into the urine. Bence Jones proteins are an exception. They are small enough to move quickly and easily through the kidney into the urine.

A routine **urinalysis** will not detect Bence Jones proteins. There are several methods used by laboratories to detect and measure these proteins. The classic Bence Jones reaction involves heating urine to 140 °F (60°C). At this temperature, the Bence Jones proteins will clump. The clumping disappears if the urine is further heated to boiling and reappears when the urine is cooled. Other clumping procedures using salts, acids, and other chemicals are also used to detect these proteins. These types of test will reveal whether or not Bence Jones proteins are present, but not how much is present.

A more complex procedure is done to measure the exact amount of Bence Jones proteins. This procedure–immunoelectrophoresis–is usually done on urine that has been collected for 24-hours.

The test is covered by insurance when medically necessary. Results are usually available within several days.

Preparation

Urine is usually collected throughout a 24-hour time period. A person is given a large container in which to collect the urine. The urine should be refrigerated until it is brought to the laboratory or physician's office.

Normal results

Bence Jones proteins normally are not present in the urine.

Abnormal results

Bence Jones proteins are present in 50–80% of people with multiple myeloma. People with other malignancies also can have a positive Bence Jones proteins test, but less frequently.

Certain nonmalignant diseases, such as **rheumatoid arthritis**, **systemic lupus erythematosus**, and chronic renal insufficiency, can have Bence Jones proteins in the urine. High doses of penicillin or **aspirin** before collecting the urine can give a false positive result.

Resources

BOOKS

Pagana, Kathleen Deska. *Mosby's Manual of Diagnostic and Laboratory Tests.* St. Louis: Mosby, Inc., 1998.

Nancy J. Nordenson

Bender-Gestalt test

Definition

The Bender Visual Motor Gestalt test (or Bender-Gestalt test) is a psychological assessment used to evaluate visual-motor functioning, visual-perceptual skills, neurological impairment, and emotional disturbances in children and adults ages three and older.

Purpose

The Bender-Gestalt is used to evaluate visual-motor maturity and to screen children for developmental delays. The test is also used to assess brain damage and neurological deficits. Individuals who have suffered a traumatic brain injury may be given the Bender-Gestalt as part of a battery of neuropsychological measures, or tests.

The Bender-Gestalt is sometimes used in conjunction with other personality tests to determine the presence of emotional and psychiatric disturbances such as **schizophrenia**.

Precautions

Psychometric testing requires a clinically trained examiner. The Bender Visual Motor Gestalt Test should be administered and interpreted by a trained psychologist or psychiatrist. The Bender-Gestalt should always be employed as only one element of a complete battery of psychological or developmental tests, and should never be used alone as the sole basis for a diagnosis.

Description

The original Bender Visual Motor Gestalt test was developed in 1938 by psychiatrist Lauretta Bender. There are several different versions of the Bender-Gestalt available today (i.e., the Bender-Gestalt test; Modified Version of the Bender-Gestalt test for Preschool and Primary School Children; the Hutt Adaptation of the Bender-Gestalt test; the Bender Visual Motor Gestalt test for Children; the Bender-Gestalt test for Young Children; the Watkins Bender-Gestalt Scoring System; the Canter Background Interference Procedure for the Bender-Gestalt test). All use the same basic test materials, but vary in their scoring and interpretation methods.

The standard Bender Visual Motor Gestalt test consists of nine figures, each on its own 3 x 5 card. An examiner presents each figure to the test subject one at a time and asks the subject to copy it onto a single piece of blank paper. The only instruction given to the subject is that he or she should make the best reproduction of the figure possible. The test is not timed, although standard administration time is typically 10-20 minutes. After testing is complete, the results are scored based on accuracy and organization. Interpretation depends on the form of the test in use. Common features considered in evaluating the drawings are rotation, distortion, symmetry, and perseveration. As an example, a patient with frontal lobe injury may reproduce the same pattern over and over (perserveration).

The Bender-Gestalt can also be administered in a group setting. In group testing, the figures are shown to test subjects with a slide projector, in a test booklet, or on larger versions of the individual test cards. Both the individual and group- administered Bender-Gestalt evaluation may take place in either an outpatient or hospital setting. Patients should check with their insurance plans to determine if these or other mental health services are covered.

Normal results

Children normally improve in this test as they age, but, because of the complexity of the scoring process, results for the Bender-Gestalt should only be interpreted by a clinically trained psychologist or psychiatrist.

Resources

ORGANIZATIONS

American Psychological Association (APA). 750 First St. NE, Washington, DC 20002-4242. (202) 336-5700. < http://www.apa.org > .

ERIC Clearinghouse on Assessment and Evaluation. 1131 Shriver Laboratory (Bldg 075).

Paula Anne Ford-Martin

Bends *see* **Decompression sickness**

Benign *see* **Uterine fibroids**

Benign prostatic hyperplasia *see* **Enlarged prostate**

Benign prostatic hypertrophy *see* **Enlarged prostate**

Benzocaine *see* **Antiseptics**

Benzodiazepines

Definition

Benzodiazepines are medicines that help relieve nervousness, tension, and other symptoms by slowing the central nervous system.

Purpose

Benzodiazepines are a type of **antianxiety drugs**. While **anxiety** is a normal response to stressful situations, some people have unusually high levels of anxiety that can interfere with everyday life. For these people, benzodiazepines can help bring their feelings under control. The medicine can also relieve troubling symptoms of anxiety, such as pounding heartbeat, breathing problems, irritability, **nausea**, and faintness.

Physicians may sometimes prescribe these drugs for other conditions, such as **muscle spasms**, epilepsy and other seizure disorders, **phobias**, **panic disorder**, withdrawal from alcohol, and sleeping problems. However, this medicine should not be used every day for sleep problems that last more than a few days. If used this way, the drug loses its effectiveness within a few weeks.

Description

The family of antianxiety drugs known as benzodiazepines includes alprazolam (Xanax), chlordiazepoxide (Librium), diazepam (Valium), and lorazepam (Ativan). These medicines take effect fairly quickly, starting to work within an hour after they are taken. Benzodiazepines are available only with a physician's prescription and are available in tablet, capsule, liquid, or injectable forms.

Recommended dosage

The recommended dosage depends on the type of benzodiazepine, its strength, and the condition for which it is being taken. Doses may be different for different people. Check with the physician who prescribed the drug or the pharmacist who filled the prescription for the correct dosage.

KEY TERMS

Anxiety—Worry or tension in response to real or imagined stress, danger, or dreaded situations. Physical reactions, such as fast pulse, sweating, trembling, fatigue, and weakness may accompany anxiety.

Asthma—A disease in which the air passages of the lungs become inflamed and narrowed.

Bronchitis—Inflammation of the air passages of the lungs.

Central nervous system—The brain and spinal cord.

Chronic—A word used to describe a long-lasting condition. Chronic conditions often develop gradually and involve slow changes.

Emphysema—An irreversible lung disease in which breathing becomes increasingly difficult.

Epilepsy—A brain disorder with symptoms that include seizures.

Glaucoma—A condition in which pressure in the eye is abnormally high. If not treated, glaucoma may lead to blindness.

Myasthenia gravis—A chronic disease with symptoms that include muscle weakness and sometimes paralysis.

Panic disorder—A disorder in which people have sudden and intense attacks of anxiety in certain situations. Symptoms such as shortness of breath, sweating, dizziness, chest pain, and extreme fear often accompany the attacks.

Phobia—An intense, abnormal, or illogical fear of something specific, such as heights or open spaces.

Porphyria—A disorder in which porphyrins build up in the blood and urine.

Porphyrin—A type of pigment found in living things.

Seizure—A sudden attack, spasm, or convulsion.

Sleep apnea—A condition in which a person temporarily stops breathing during sleep.

Withdrawal symptoms—A group of physical or mental symptoms that may occur when a person suddenly stops using a drug to which he or she has become dependent.

Always take benzodiazepines exactly as directed. Never take larger or more frequent doses, and do not take the drug for longer than directed. If the medicine does not seem to be working, check with the physician who prescribed it. *Do not increase the dose or stop taking the medicine unless the physician says to do so.* Stopping the drug suddenly may cause withdrawal symptoms, especially if it has been taken in large doses or over a long period. People who are taking the medicine for seizure disorders may have seizures if they stop taking it suddenly. If it is necessary to stop taking the medicine, check with a physician for directions on how to stop. The physician may recommend tapering down gradually to reduce the chance of withdrawal symptoms or other problems.

Precautions

Seeing a physician regularly while taking benzodiazepines is important, especially during the first few months of treatment. The physician will check to make sure the medicine is working as it should and will note unwanted side effects.

People who take benzodiazepines to relieve nervousness, tension, or symptoms of panic disorder should check with their physicians every two to three months to make sure they still need to keep taking the medicine.

Patients who are taking benzodiazepines for sleep problems should check with their physicians if they are not sleeping better within 7-10 days. Sleep problems that last longer than this may be a sign of another medical problem.

People who take this medicine to help them sleep may have trouble sleeping when they stop taking the medicine. This effect should last only a few nights.

Some people, especially older people, feel drowsy, dizzy, lightheaded, or less alert when using benzodiazepines. The drugs may also cause clumsiness or unsteadiness. When the medicine is taken at bedtime, these effects may even occur the next morning. Anyone who takes these drugs should not drive, use machines or do anything else that might be dangerous until they have found out how the drugs affect them.

Benzodiazepines may also cause behavior changes in some people, similar to those seen in people who act differently when they drink alcohol. More extreme changes, such as confusion, agitation, and **hallucinations**, also are possible. Anyone who starts having strange or unusual thoughts or behavior while taking this medicine should get in touch with his or her physician.

Because benzodiazepines work on the central nervous system, they may add to the effects of alcohol and other drugs that slow down the central nervous system, such as **antihistamines**, cold medicine, allergy medicine, sleep aids, medicine for seizures, tranquilizers, some **pain** relievers, and **muscle relaxants**. They may also add to the effects of anesthetics, including those used for dental procedures. These effects may last several days after treatment with benzodiazepines ends. *The combined effects of benzodiazepines and alcohol or other CNS depressants (drugs that slow the central nervous system) can be very dangerous, leading to unconsciousness or, rarely, even death.* Anyone taking benzodiazepines should not drink alcohol and should check with his or her physician before using any CNS depressants. *Taking an overdose of benzodiazepines can also cause unconsciousness and possibly death. Anyone who shows signs of an overdose or of the effects of combining benzodiazepines with alcohol or other drugs should get immediate emergency help.* Warning signs include slurred speech or confusion, severe drowsiness, staggering, and profound weakness.

Some benzodiazepines may change the results of certain medical tests. Before having medical tests, anyone taking this medicine should alert the health care professional in charge.

Children are generally more sensitive than adults to the effects of benzodiazepines. This sensitivity may increase the chance of side effects.

Older people are more sensitive than younger adults to the effects of this medicine and may be at greater risk for side effects. Older people who take these drugs to help them sleep may be drowsy during the day. Older people also increase their risk of falling and injuring themselves when they take these drugs.

Special conditions

People with certain medical conditions or who are taking certain other medicines can have problems if they take benzodiazepines. Before taking these drugs, be sure to let the physician know about any of these conditions:

ALLERGIES. Anyone who has had unusual reactions to benzodiazepines or other mood-altering drugs in the past should let his or her physician know before taking the drugs again. The physician should also be told about any **allergies** to foods, dyes, preservatives, or other substances.

PREGNANCY. Some benzodiazepines increase the likelihood of **birth defects**. Using these medicines during **pregnancy** may also cause the baby to become dependent on them and to have withdrawal symptoms after birth. When taken late in pregnancy or around the time of labor and delivery, these drugs can cause other problems in the newborn baby, such as

weakness, breathing problems, slow heartbeat, and body temperature problems.

BREASTFEEDING. Benzodiazepines may pass into breast milk and cause problems in babies whose mothers taken the medicine. These problems include drowsiness, breathing problems, and slow heartbeat. Women who are breastfeeding their babies should not use this medicine without checking with their physicians.

OTHER MEDICAL CONDITIONS. Before using benzodiazepines, people with any of these medical problems should make sure their physicians are aware of their conditions:

- current or past drug or alcohol **abuse**
- depression
- severe mental illness
- epilepsy or other seizure disorders
- swallowing problems
- chronic lung disease such as **emphysema**, **asthma**, or chronic **bronchitis**
- kidney disease
- liver disease
- brain disease
- **glaucoma**
- hyperactivity
- myasthenia gravis
- porphyria
- sleep apnea

USE OF CERTAIN MEDICINES. Taking benzodiazepines with certain other drugs may affect the way the drugs work or may increase the chance of side effects.

Side effects

The most common side effects are **dizziness**, lightheadedness, drowsiness, clumsiness, unsteadiness, and slurred speech. These problems usually go away as the body adjusts to the drug and do not require medical treatment unless they persist or they interfere with normal activities.

More serious side effects are not common, but may occur. If any of the following side effects occur, check with the physician who prescribed the medicine as soon as possible:

- behavior changes
- memory problems
- difficulty concentrating

- confusion
- depression
- seizures (convulsions)
- hallucinations
- sleep problems
- increased nervousness, excitability, or irritability
- involuntary movements of the body, including the eyes
- low blood pressure
- unusual weakness or tiredness
- skin rash or **itching**
- unusual bleeding or bruising
- yellow skin or eyes
- sore throat
- sores in the mouth or throat
- **fever** and chills

Patients who take benzodiazepines for a long time or at high doses may notice side effects for several weeks after they stop taking the drug. They should check with their physicians if these or other troublesome symptoms occur:

- irritability
- nervousness
- sleep problems

Other rare side effects may occur. Anyone who has unusual symptoms during or after treatment with benzodiazepines should get in touch with his or her physician.

Interactions

Benzodiazepines may interact with a variety of other medicines. When this happens, the effects of one or both of the drugs may change or the risk of side effects may be greater. Anyone who takes benzodiazepines should let the physician know all other medicines he or she is taking. Among the drugs that may interact with benzodiazepines are:

- Central nervous system (CNS) depressants such as medicine for allergies, colds, hay fever, and asthma; sedatives; tranquilizers; prescription pain medicine; muscle relaxants; medicine for seizures; sleep aids; **barbiturates**; and anesthetics.

Medicines other than those listed above may interact with benzodiazepines. Be sure to check with a physician or pharmacist before combining benzodiazepines with any other prescription or nonprescription (over-the-counter) medicine.

Resources

OTHER

"Medications." *National Institute of Mental Health Page.* 1995. <http://www.nimh.nih.gov>.

Nancy Ross-Flanigan

Benzoyl peroxide *see* **Antiacne drugs**

Benztropine *see* **Antiparkinson drugs**

Bereavement

Definition

Bereavement refers to the period of mourning and grief following the **death** of a beloved person or animal. The English word *bereavement* comes from an ancient Germanic root word meaning "to rob" or "to seize by violence." *Mourning* is the word that is used to describe the public rituals or symbols of bereavement, such as holding funeral services, wearing black clothing, closing a place of business temporarily, or lowering a flag to half mast. *Grief* refers to one's personal experience of loss; it includes physical symptoms as well as emotional and spiritual reactions to the loss. While public expressions of mourning are usually time-limited, grief is a process that takes most people several months or years to work through.

Description

Bereavement is a highly individual as well as a complex experience. It is increasingly recognized that no two people respond the same way to the losses associated with the death of a loved one. People's reactions to a death are influenced by such factors as ethnic or religious traditions; personal beliefs about life after death; the type of relationship ended by death (relative, friend, colleague, etc.); the cause of death; the person's age at death; whether the death was sudden or expected; and many others. In addition, the death of a loved one inevitably confronts adults (and older adolescents) with the fact that they too will die. As a result of this variety and emotional complexity, most doctors and other counselors advise people to trust their own feelings about bereavement,0 and grieve in the way that seems most helpful to them.

It is also increasingly understood in the early 2000s that people can experience bereavement with regard to other losses. Some examples of these

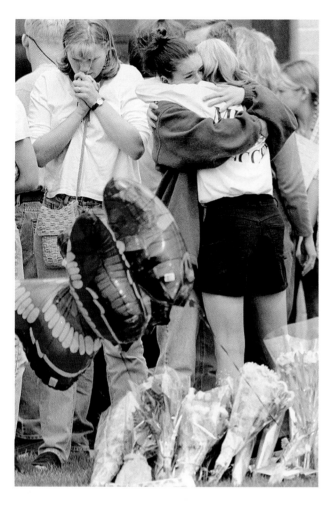

Columbine High School students in Littleton, Colorado, grieving for their slain classmates. *(Photo by David Zalubowski. AP/Wide World Photos. Reproduced by permission.)*

so-called "silent losses" include miscarriages in early **pregnancy**, the death of a child in the womb shortly before birth, or the news that a loved one has Alzheimer's disease or another illness that slowly destroys their personality. In addition, many counselors recognize that bereavement has two dimensions, the actual loss and the symbolic losses. For example, a person whose teenage son or daughter is killed in an accident suffers a series of symbolic losses—knowing that their child will never graduate from high school, get married, or have children—as well as the actual loss of the adolescent to death.

Causes and symptoms

Causes

The immediate cause of bereavement is usually the death of a loved friend or relative. There are a number of situations, however, which can affect or prolong the grief process:

- The relationship with the dead person was a source of **pain** rather than love and support. Examples would include an abusive parent or spouse.

- The person died in military service or in a natural, transportation, or workplace disaster. Bereavement in these cases is often made more difficult by intrusive news reporters as well as **anxiety** over the loved one's possible physical or mental suffering prior to death.

- The person was murdered. Survivors of homicide victims often find the criminal justice system as well as the media frustrating and upsetting.

- The person is missing and presumed dead but their death has not been verified. As a result, friends and relatives may alternate between grief and hope that the person is still alive.

- The person committed **suicide**. Survivors may feel guilt over their inability to foresee or prevent the suicide, shame that the death was self-inflicted, or anger at the person who committed suicide.

- The relationship with the dead person cannot be openly acknowledged. This situation often leads to what is called disenfranchised grief. The most common instances are homosexual or extramarital sexual relationships that have been kept secret for the sake of spouses or other family members.

- The loved one was an animal rather than a human being. Western societies are only beginning to accept that adults as well as children can grieve for a dead animal; many adults still feel that there is "something wrong" about grieving for their pet. The question of euthanasia may be an additional source of sorrow; even when the pet is terminally ill, many people are very uneasy about making the decision to end its life.

Symptoms

Bereavement typically affects a person's physical well-being as well as emotions. Common symptoms of grief include changes in appetite and weight, **fatigue**, **insomnia** and other sleep disturbances, loss of interest in sex, low energy levels, **nausea and vomiting**, chest or throat pain, and **headache**. People who have lost a loved one in traumatic circumstances may have such symptoms of **post-traumatic stress disorder** as an exaggerated startle response, visual or auditory **hallucinations**, or high levels of muscular tension.

Doctors and other counselors have identified four stages or phases in uncomplicated bereavement:

KEY TERMS

Bibliotherapy—The use of books (usually self-help or problem-solving works) to improve one's understanding of personal problems and/or to heal painful feelings.

Biofield healing—A general term for a group of alternative therapies based on the belief that the human body is surrounded by an energy field (or aura) that reflects the condition of the person's body and spirit. Rebalancing or repairing the energy field is thought to bring about healing in mind and body. Reiki, therapeutic touch, polarity balancing, Shen therapy, and certain forms of color therapy are considered forms of biofield healing.

Complicated grief—An abnormal response to bereavement that includes unrelieved yearning for the dead person, the complete loss of previous positive beliefs or worldviews, and a general inability to function.

Disenfranchised grief—Grief that cannot be openly expressed because the death or other loss cannot be publicly acknowledged.

Euthanasia—The act of putting a person or animal to death painlessly or allowing them to die by withholding medical services, usually because of a painful and incurable disease.

Mourning—The public expression of bereavement; it may include funerals and other rituals, special clothing, and symbolic gestures.

Regression—A return to earlier, particularly infantile, patterns of thought and behavior.

Thanatology—The medical, psychological, or legal study of death and dying.

Traumatic grief—Grief resulting from the loss of a loved one in a traumatic situation (natural or transportation disaster, act of terrorism or mass murder, etc.)

- Shock, disbelief, feelings of **numbness**. This initial phase lasts about two weeks, during which the bereaved person finally accepts the reality of the loved one's death.

- Suffering the pain of grief. This phase typically lasts for several months. Some people undergo a mild temporary depression about six months after the loved one's death.

- Adjusting to life without the loved one. In this phase of bereavement, survivors may find themselves taking on the loved one's roles and responsibilities as well as redefining their own identities.

- Moving forward with life, forming new relationships, and having positive expectations of the future. Most people reach this stage within one to two years after the loved one's death.

BEREAVEMENT IN CHILDREN. Children do not experience bereavement in the same way as adolescents and adults. Preschool children usually do not understand death as final and irreversible, and may talk or act as if the dead pet or family member will wake up or come back. Children between the ages of five and nine are better able to understand the finality of death, but they tend to assume it will not affect them or their family. They are likely to be shocked and severely upset by a death in their immediate family. In addition to the physical disturbances that bereaved adults often experience, children sometimes begin to act like infants again (wanting bottle feeding, using baby talk, etc.) This pattern of returning to behaviors characteristic of an earlier life stage is called regression.

TRAUMATIC AND COMPLICATED GRIEF. Since the early 1990s, thanatologists (doctors and other counselors who specialize in issues related to death and dying) have identified two types of grief that do not resolve normally with the passage of time. Traumatic grief is defined as grief resulting from a sudden traumatic event that involves violent suffering, mutilation, and/or multiple deaths; appears to be random or preventable; and often involves the survivor's own brush with death. The symptoms of traumatic grief are similar to those of post-traumatic **stress** disorder (PTSD). Such events as the terrorist attacks of September 11, 2001, the East Asian tsunami of December 2004, and airplane crashes or other transportation disasters may produce traumatic grief in survivors.

In contrast to traumatic grief, complicated grief does not necessarily result from a specific type of event but rather refers to an abnormally intense and prolonged response to bereavement. While most people are able to move through a period of bereavement and recover a sense of purpose and meaning in life, people with complicated grief feel as if their entire worldview has been shattered. They cannot stop thinking of the dead person, long to be with him or her, and may feel that part of them died along with the loved one. They sometimes start acting like the deceased person, mimicking the symptoms of his or her illness, behaving in reckless ways, talking about "joining" the loved one, or refusing to accept the reality of the death. In general they are unable to function normally. Complicated grief should not be regarded as simply a subtype of clinical depression; the two conditions may coexist or overlap in some patients but are nonetheless distinct entities.

Diagnosis

Bereavement is considered a normal response to a death or other loss. A doctor who suspects that a patient is suffering from traumatic or complicated grief, however, may use various psychological inventories or questionnaires to see whether the patient meets the criteria for PTSD, major depression, or **acute stress disorder**. In addition, there are several specific questionnaires to help diagnose complicated grief.

Treatment

Most people do not require formal treatment for bereavement. In the early 2000s, however, many people choose to participate in support groups for recently bereaved people or hospice follow-up programs for relatives of patients who died in that hospice. Bereavement support groups are particularly helpful in guiding members through such common but painful problems as disposing of the dead person's possessions, celebrating holidays without the loved one, coping with anniversaries, etc.

Traumatic grief is usually treated in the same way as post-traumatic stress, with temporary use of medications to control sleep disturbances and anxiety symptoms along with long-term psychotherapy. Those suffering from traumatic grief may also be referred to support groups of people dealing with the same type of sudden and violent loss. Some of these organizations are listed below. Complicated grief is usually managed with a combination of group and individual psychotherapy.

Alternative treatment

Alternative therapies that have been reported to help with the sleep disturbances and other physical symptoms of bereavement include prayer and **meditation**; such movement therapies as **yoga** and **tai chi**; **therapeutic touch**, **Reiki**, and other forms of biofield healing; bibliotherapy and journaling; **music therapy**, **art therapy**, **hydrotherapy**, and **massage therapy**.

Prognosis

Most people move through the stages of the normal grief process within several months to two years, depending on the length and closeness of the relationship. Traumatic grief and complicated grief, however, may take three years or longer to resolve, even with appropriate treatment.

Prevention

Bereavement is considered a normal response to death and loss, which are universal human experiences. It should ordinarily be allowed to run its course; most counselors maintain that trying to stifle or cut short the grief process is more likely to cause emotional problems later on than to prevent them.

Resources

BOOKS

American Psychiatric Association. *Diagnostic and Statistical Manual of Mental Disorders*, 4th edition, text revision. Washington, DC: American Psychiatric Association, 2000.

Dossey, Larry, MD. *Healing Beyond the Body: Medicine and the Infinite Reach of the Mind.* Boston and London: Shambhala, 2001. The chapters on "The Return of Prayer" and "Immortality" are particularly relevant to bereavement.

"Mood Disorders." Section 15, Chapter 189 in *The Merck Manual of Diagnosis and Therapy*, edited by Mark H. Beers, MD, and Robert Berkow, MD. Whitehouse Station, NJ: Merck Research Laboratories, 2005.

PERIODICALS

Bowles, Stephen B., Larry C. James, Diane S. Solursh, et al. "Acute and Post-Traumatic Stress Disorder after Spontaneous Abortion." *American Family Physician* 61 (March 15, 2000): 1689–1696.

Kersting, Karen. "A New Approach to Complicated Grief." *Monitor on Psychology* 35 (November 2004): 51.

Lubit, Roy, MD. "Acute Treatment of Disaster Survivors." *eMedicine*, 17 June 2004. < http://www.emedicine.com/med/topic3540.htm >.

Ogrodniczuk, John S., William E. Piper, Anthony S. Joyce, et al. "Differentiating Symptoms of Complicated Grief and Depression among Psychiatric Outpatients." *Canadian Journal of Psychiatry/Revue canadienne de psychiatrie* 48 (March 2003): 87–93.

ORGANIZATIONS

Alzheimer's Association. 225 North Michigan Avenue, 17th Floor, Chicago, IL 60601-7633. (312) 335-8700. 24-hour hotline: (800) 272-3900. < http://www.alz.org >. This website is an excellent resource for anyone with a loved one suffering from Alzheimer's or another dementing illness.

American Academy of Child and Adolescent Psychiatry. 3615 Wisconsin Avenue, NW, Washington, DC 20016-3007. (202) 966-7300. Fax: (202) 966-2891. < http://www.aacap.org. >.

American Veterinary Medical Association (AVMA). 1931 North Meacham Road, Suite 100, Schaumburg, IL

60173-4360. <http://www.avma.org>. The AVMA website includes links to resources about pet loss.

Dougy Center for Grieving Children and Families. 3909 SE 52nd Avenue, Portland, OR 97206. (866) 775-5683 or (503) 775-5683. Fax: (503) 777-3097. <http://www.grievingchild.org>. Provides age-appropriate support groups, information, and referral services for bereaved children and adolescents.

National Air Disaster Alliance/Foundation (NADA). 2020 Pennsylvania Avenue #315, Washington, DC 20006-1846. (888) 444-NADA. Fax: (336) 643-1394. <http://www.planesafe.org>. NADA was founded in 1995 following the loss of USAir Flight 427 to meet the needs of people who have lost loved ones in air disasters as well as work for better transportation safety standards.

National Hospice and Palliative Care Organization (NHPCO). 1700 Diagonal Road, Suite 625, Alexandria, VA 22314. (703) 837-1500. Fax: (703) 837-1233. <http://www.nho.org>. This website is a good source of information about hospice-based bereavement services and support groups.

National Institute of Mental Health (NIMH). 6001 Executive Boulevard, Room 8184, MSC 9663, Bethesda, MD 20892-9663. (301) 443-4513 or (886) 615-NIMH. <www.nimh.nih.gov.>

Tragedy Assistance Program for Survivors, Inc. (TAPS). National Headquarters, 1621 Connecticut Avenue NW, Suite 300, Washington, DC 20009. (202) 588-TAPS. Hotline: (800) 959-TAPS. <http://www.taps.org>. TAPS provides grief support for those who have lost a loved one serving in the Armed Forces.

OTHER

Alzheimer's Association. *Fact Sheet: About Grief, Mourning and Guilt*. Chicago, IL: Alzheimer's Association, 2004.

American Academy of Child and Adolescent Psychiatry (AACAP). *Children and Grief*. AACAP Facts for Families #8. Washington, DC: AACAP, 2004.

American Academy of Child and Adolescent Psychiatry (AACAP). *When a Pet Dies*. AACAP Facts for Families #78. Washington, DC: AACAP, 2000.

Harper, Linda R., PhD. *Healing after the Loss of Your Pet*. <http://www.bestfriends.org/theanimals/pdfs/allpets/PetLossHarper.pdf>.

National Institute of Mental Health (NIMH). *Mental Health and Mass Violence: Evidence-Based Early Psychological Interventions for Victims/Survivors of Mass Violence*. NIH Publication No. 02-5138. Washington, DC: U. S. Government Printing Office, 2002.

National Organization of Parents of Murdered Children (POMC). *Information Bulletin: Survivors of Homicide Victims*. <http://www.pomc.com/survivor.cfm>.

Rebecca Frey, PhD

Berger's disease *see* **Idiopathic primary renal hematuric/proteinuric syndrome**

Beriberi

Definition

Beriberi is a disease caused by a deficiency of thiamine (vitamin B$_1$) that affects many systems of the body, including the muscles, heart, nerves, and digestive system. Beriberi literally means "I can't, I can't" in Singhalese, which reflects the crippling effect it has on its victims. It is common in parts of southeast Asia, where white rice is the main food. In the United States, beriberi is primarily seen in people with chronic **alcoholism**.

Description

Beriberi puzzled medical experts for years as it ravaged people of all ages in Asia. Doctors thought it was caused by something in food. Not until the early 1900s did scientists discover that rice bran, the outer covering that was removed to create the polished white rice preferred by Asians, actually contained something that prevented the disease. Thiamine was the first vitamin identified. In the 1920s, extracts of rice polishings were used to treat the disease.

In adults, there are different forms of beriberi, classified according to the body systems most affected. Dry beriberi involves the nervous system; wet beriberi affects the heart and circulation. Both types usually occur in the same patient, with one set of symptoms predominating.

A less common form of cardiovascular, or wet beriberi, is known as "shoshin." This condition involves a rapid appearance of symptoms and acute **heart failure**. It is highly fatal and is known to cause sudden **death** in young migrant laborers in Asia whose diet consists of white rice.

Cerebral beriberi, also known as Wernicke-Korsakoff syndrome, usually occurs in chronic alcoholics and affects the central nervous system (brain and spinal cord). It can be caused by a situation that aggravates a chronic thiamine deficiency, like an alcoholic binge or severe **vomiting**.

Infantile beriberi is seen in breastfed infants of thiamine-deficient mothers, who live in developing nations.

Although severe beriberi is uncommon in the United States, less severe thiamine deficiencies do occur. About 25% of all alcoholics admitted to a hospital in the United States show some evidence of thiamine deficiency.

KEY TERMS

B vitamins—This family of vitamins consists of thiamine (B_1), riboflavin (B_2), niacin (B_3), pantothenic acid (B_5), pyridoxine (B_6), biotin, folic acid (B_9), and cobalamin (B_{12}). They are interdependent and involved in converting glucose to energy.

Coenzyme—A substance needed by enzymes to produce many of the reactions in energy and protein metabolism in the body.

Edema—An excess accumulation of fluid in the cells and tissues.

Enzyme—A protein that acts as a catalyst to produce chemical changes in other substances without being changed themselves.

Metabolism—All the physical and chemical changes that take place within an organism.

Peripheral neuropathy—A disease affecting the portion of the nervous system outside the brain and spinal chord. One or more nerves can be involved, causing sensory loss, muscle weakness and shrinkage, and decreased reflexes.

Thiamine pyrophosphate (TPP)—The coenzyme containing thiamine that is essential in converting glucose to energy.

Causes and symptoms

Thiamine is one of the B **vitamins** and plays an important role in energy metabolism and tissue building. It combines with phosphate to form the coenzyme *thiamine pyrophosphate (TPP)*, which is essential in reactions that produce energy from glucose or that convert glucose to fat for storage in the tissues. When there is not enough thiamine in the diet, these basic energy functions are disturbed, leading to problems throughout the body.

Special situations, such as an over-active metabolism, prolonged **fever**, **pregnancy**, and breastfeeding, can increase the body's thiamine requirements and lead to symptoms of deficiency. Extended periods of **diarrhea** or chronic **liver disease** can result in the body's inability to maintain normal levels of many nutrients, including thiamine. Other persons at risk are patients with kidney failure on dialysis and those with severe digestive problems who are unable to absorb nutrients. Alcoholics are susceptible because they may substitute alcohol for food and their frequent intake of alcohol decreases the body's ability to absorb thiamine.

The following systems are most affected by beriberi:

- Gastrointestinal system. When the cells of the smooth muscles in the digestive system and glands do not get enough energy from glucose, they are unable to produce more glucose from the normal digestion of food. There is a loss of appetite, **indigestion**, severe **constipation**, and a lack of hydrochloric acid in the stomach.

- Nervous System. Glucose is essential for the central nervous system to function normally. Early deficiency symptoms are **fatigue**, irritability, and poor memory. If the deficiency continues, there is damage to the peripheral nerves that causes loss of sensation and muscle weakness, which is called **peripheral neuropathy**. The legs are most affected. The toes feel numb and the feet have a burning sensation; the leg muscles become sore and the calf muscles cramp. The individual walks unsteadily and has difficulty getting up from a squatting position. Eventually, the muscles shrink (atrophy) and there is a loss of reflexes in the knees and feet; the feet may hang limp (footdrop).

- Cardiovascular system. There is a rapid heartbeat and sweating. Eventually the heart muscle weakens. Because the smooth muscle in the blood vessels is affected, the arteries and veins relax, causing swelling, known as **edema**, in the legs.

- Musculoskeletal system. There is widespread muscle **pain** caused by the lack of TPP in the muscle tissue.

Infants who are breastfed by a thiamine-deficient mother usually develop symptoms of deficiency between the second and fourth month of life. They are pale, restless, unable to sleep, prone to diarrhea, and have muscle wasting and edema in their arms and legs. They have a characteristic, sometimes silent, cry and develop heart failure and nerve damage.

Diagnosis

A **physical examination** will reveal many of the early symptoms of beriberi, such as fatigue, irritation, **nausea**, constipation, and poor memory, but the deficiency may be difficult to identify. Information about the individual's diet and general health is also needed.

There are many biochemical tests based on thiamine metabolism or the functions of TPP that can detect a thiamine deficiency. Levels of thiamine can be measured in the blood and urine and will be reduced if there is a deficiency. The urine can be collected for 24 hours to measure the level of thiamine excreted. Another reliable test measures the effect of TPP on red blood cell activity since all forms of beriberi affect the metabolism of red blood cells.

An electroencephalogram (EEG), which measures electrical activity in the brain, may be done to rule out other causes of neurologic changes. Observing improvements in the patient after giving thiamine supplements will also confirm the diagnosis.

Treatment

Treatment with thiamine reverses the deficiency in the body and relieves most of the symptoms. Severe thiamine deficiency is treated with high doses of thiamine given by injection into a muscle (intramuscular) or in a solution that goes into a vein (intravenously) for several days. Then smaller doses can be given either by injection or in pill form until the patient recovers. Usually there are other deficiencies in the B vitamins that will also need treatment.

The cardiovascular symptoms of wet beriberi can respond to treatment within a few hours if they are not too severe. Heart failure may require additional treatment with **diuretics** that help eliminate excess fluid and with heart-strengthening drugs like digitalis.

Recovery from peripheral neuropathy and other symptoms of dry beriberi may take longer and patients frequently become discouraged. They should stay active; physical therapy will also help in recovery.

Infantile beriberi is treated by giving thiamine to both the infant and the breast feeding mother until levels are normal.

In Wernicke-Korsakoff syndrome, thiamine should be given intravenously or by injection at first because the intestinal absorption of thiamine is probably impaired and the patient is very ill. Most of the symptoms will be relieved by treatment, though there may be residual memory loss.

Excess thiamine is excreted by the body in the urine, and negative reactions to too much thiamine are rare. Thiamine is unstable in alkali solutions, so it should not be taken with **antacids** or **barbiturates**.

Alternative treatment

Alternative treatments for beriberi deal first with correcting the thiamine deficiency. As in conventional treatments, alternative treatments for beriberi **stress** a diet rich in foods that provide thiamine and other

B vitamins, such as brown rice, whole grains, raw fruits and vegetables, legumes, seeds, nuts, and yogurt. Drinking more than one glass of liquid with a meal should be avoided, since this may wash out the vitamins before they can be absorbed by the body. Thiamine should be taken daily, with the dose depending on the severity of the disease. Additional supplements of B vitamins, a multivitamin and mineral complex, and Vitamin C are also recommended. Other alternative therapies may help relieve the person's symptoms after the thiamine deficiency is corrected.

Prognosis

Beriberi is fatal if not treated and the longer the deficiency exists, the sicker the person becomes. Most of the symptoms can be reversed and full recovery is possible when thiamine levels are returned to normal and maintained with a balanced diet and vitamin supplements as needed.

Prevention

A balanced diet containing all essential nutrients will prevent a thiamine deficiency and the development of beriberi. People who consume large quantities of junk food like soda, pretzels, chips, candy, and high carbohydrate foods made with unenriched flours may be deficient in thiamine and other vital nutrients. They may need to take vitamin supplements and should improve their **diets**.

Dietary Requirements

The body's requirements for thiamine are tied to carbohydrate metabolism and expressed in terms of total intake of calories. The current recommended dietary allowances (RDA) are 0.5 mg for every 1000 calories, with a minimum daily intake of 1 mg even for those who eat fewer than 2,000 calories in a day. The RDA for children and teenagers is the same as for adults: 1.4 mg daily for males over age eleven, and 1.1 mg for females. During pregnancy, an increase to 1.5 mg daily is needed. Because of increased energy needs and the secretion of thiamine in breast milk, breast feeding mothers need 1.5 mg every day. In infants, 0.4 mg is advised.

Food Sources

The best food sources of thiamine are lean pork, beef, liver, brewer's yeast, peas and beans, whole or enriched grains, and breads. The more refined the food, as in white rice, white breads, and some cereals, the lower the thiamine. Many food products are enriched with thiamine, along with riboflavin, niacin, and iron, to prevent dietary deficiency.

During the milling process, rice is polished and all the vitamins in the exterior coating of bran are lost. Boiling the rice before husking preserves the vitamins by distributing them throughout the kernel. Food enrichment programs have eliminated beriberi in Japan and the Phillipines.

Like all B vitamins, thiamine is water soluble, which means it is easily dissolved in water. It will leach out during cooking in water and is destroyed by high heat and overcooking.

Resources

PERIODICALS

Ryan, Ruth, et al. "Beriberi Unexpected." *Psychosomatics* May-June 1997: 191-294.

Karen Ericson, RN

Berry aneurysm *see* **Cerebral aneurysm**

Berylliosis

Definition

Berylliosis is lung inflammation caused by inhaling dust or fumes that contain the metallic element beryllium. Found in rocks, coal, soil, and volcanic dust, beryllium is used in the aerospace industry and in many types of manufacturing. Berylliosis occurs in both acute and chronic forms. In some cases, appearance of the disease may be delayed as much as 20 years after exposure to beryllium.

Description

In the 1930s, scientists discovered that beryllium could make fluorescent light bulbs last longer. During the following decade, the hard, grayish metal was identified as the cause of a potentially debilitating, sometimes deadly disease characterized by **shortness of breath** and inflammation, swelling, and scarring of the lungs.

The manufacture of fluorescent light bulbs is no longer a source of beryllium exposure, but serious health hazards are associated with any work

---

KEY TERMS

Beryllium—A steel-grey, metallic mineral used in the aerospace and nuclear industries and in a variety of manufacturing processes.

Chelation therapy—A treatment using chelating agents, compounds that surround and bind to target substances allowing them to be excreted from the body.

Corticosteroids—A group of anti-inflammatory drugs.

---

environment or process in which beryllium fumes or particles become airborne. Working with pure beryllium, beryllium compounds (e.g. beryllium oxide), or beryllium alloys causes occupational exposure. So do jobs involving:

- electronics
- fiber optics
- manufacturing ceramics, bicycle frames, golf clubs, mirrors, and microwave ovens
- mining
- nuclear weapons and reactors
- reclaiming scrap metal
- space and atomic engineering
- dental and laboratory technology

Beryllium dust and fumes are classified as toxic air pollutants by the Environmental Protection Agency (EPA). It is estimated that 2–6% of workers exposed to these contaminants eventually develop berylliosis.

Causes and symptoms

Coughing, shortness of breath, and weight loss that begin abruptly can be a symptom of acute berylliosis. This condition is caused by beryllium air pollution that inflames the lungs making them rigid; it can affect the eyes and skin as well. People who have acute berylliosis are usually very ill. Most recover, but some die of the disease.

Chronic berylliosis is an allergic reaction to long-term exposure to even low levels of beryllium dust or fumes. A systemic disease that causes formation of abnormal lung tissue and enlargement of the lymph nodes, chronic berylliosis also may affect other parts of the body. The symptoms of chronic berylliosis are largely the same as those seen in acute berylliosis, but they develop more slowly.

Diagnosis

Berylliosis is initially suspected if a patient with symptoms of the disease has a history of beryllium exposure. A **chest x ray** shows characteristic changes in the lungs. However, since these changes can resemble those caused by other lung diseases, further testing may be necessary.

The beryllium lymphocyte proliferation test (BeLPT), a blood test that can detect beryllium sensitivity (i.e. an allergic reaction to beryllium), is used to screen individuals at risk of developing berylliosis. When screening results reveal a high level of sensitivity, BeLPT is performed on cells washed from the lungs. This test is now considered the most definitive diagnostic test for berylliosis.

Treatment

Individuals with beryllium sensitivity or early-stage berylliosis should be transferred from tasks that involve beryllium exposure and regularly examined to determine whether the disease has progressed.

Acute berylliosis is a serious disease that occasionally may be fatal. Ventilators can help patients with acute berylliosis breathe. Prompt corticosteroid therapy is required to lessen lung inflammation.

Chronic beryllium disease is incurable. Corticosteroid therapy is often prescribed, but it is not certain that steroids can alter the progression of the disease, and they have no effect on scarring of lung tissue. Cleansing the lungs of beryllium is a slow process, so long-term therapy may be required. **Chelation therapy** is currently under investigation as a treatment for the disease.

Prognosis

Most patients with acute berylliosis recover fully 7–10 days after treatment begins, and the disease usually causes no after effects.

Patients whose lungs are severely damaged by chronic berylliosis may experience fatal **heart failure** because of the strain placed on the heart.

Prevention

Eliminating exposure to beryllium is the surest way to prevent berylliosis. Screening workers who are exposed to beryllium fumes or dust or who develop an allergic reaction to these substances is an effective way to control symptoms and prevent disease progression.

Resources

ORGANIZATIONS

American Lung Association. 1740 Broadway, New York, NY 10019. (800) 586-4872. < http://www.lungusa.org > .

Beryllium Support Group. P.O. Box 2021, Broomfield, CO 80038-2021. (303) 412-7065. < http://www.dimensional.com/˜mhj > .

Environmental Health Center. 1025 Connecticut Ave., NW, Washington, DC 20036. (202) 293-2270.

Maureen Haggerty

Beryllium pneumonosis *see* **Berylliosis**

Beryllium poisoning *see* **Berylliosis**

Beta-adrenergic blockers *see* **beta blockers**

Beta blockers

Definition

Beta blockers are medicines that affect the body's response to certain nerve impulses. This, in turn, decreases the force and rate of the heart's contractions, which lowers blood pressure and reduces the heart's demand for oxygen.

Purpose

The main use of beta blockers is to treat high blood pressure. Some also are used to relieve the type of chest **pain** called **angina** or to prevent heart attacks in people who already have had one **heart attack**. These drugs may also be prescribed for other conditions, such as migraine, **tremors**, and irregular heartbeat. In eye drop form, they are used to treat certain kinds of **glaucoma**.

Description

Beta blockers, also known as beta-adrenergic blockers, are available only with a physician's prescription. They come in capsule, tablet, liquid, and injectable forms. Some common beta blockers are atenolol (Tenormin), metoprolol (Lopressor), nadolol (Corgard), propranolol (Inderal), and timolol (Blocadren). Timolol and certain other beta blockers are also sold in eye drop form for treating glaucoma.

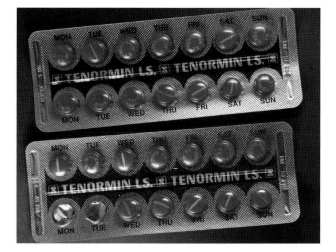

Blister packs of Tenormin LS (atenolol), a type of beta-receptor blocking drug or beta blocker. This type of drug is widely used to treat angina, to lower blood pressure, or to correct abnormal heart rhythms. *(Photograph by Adam Hart-Davis, Photo Researchers, Inc. Reproduced by permission.)*

Eye drops that contain beta blockers include betaxolol (Betoptic), cartelol (Ocupress), and timolol (Timoptic).

Recommended dosage

The recommended dosage depends on the type, strength, and form of beta blocker and the condition for which it is prescribed. The physician who prescribed the drug or the pharmacist who filled the prescription can recommend the correct dosage.

This medicine may take several weeks to noticeably lower blood pressure. Taking it exactly as directed is important.

This medicine should not be stopped without checking with the physician who prescribed it. Some conditions may get worse when patients stop taking beta blockers abruptly. This may also increase the risk of heart attack in some people. Because of these possible effects, it is important to keep enough medicine on hand to get through weekends, holidays, and vacations.

Physicians may recommend that patients check their pulse before and after taking this medicine. If the pulse becomes too slow, circulation problems may result.

Precautions

Seeing a physician regularly while taking beta blockers is important. The physician will check to make sure the medicine is working as it should and will watch for unwanted side effects. People who have high blood pressure often feel perfectly fine. However,

they should continue to see their physicians even when they feel well so that the physician can keep a close watch on their condition. Patients also need to keep taking their medicine even when they feel fine.

Beta blockers will not cure high blood pressure, but will help control the condition. To avoid the serious health problems that high blood pressure can cause, patients may have to take medicine for the rest of their lives. Furthermore, medicine alone may not be enough. Patients with high blood pressure may also need to avoid certain foods and keep their weight under control. The health care professional who is treating the condition can offer advice on what measures may be necessary. Patients being treated for high blood pressure should not change their **diets** without consulting their physicians.

Anyone taking beta blockers for high blood pressure should not take any other prescription or over-the-counter medicine without first checking with his or her physician. Some medicines may increase blood pressure.

Anyone who is taking beta blockers should be sure to tell the health care professional in charge before having any surgical or dental procedures or receiving emergency treatment.

Some beta blockers may change the results of certain medical tests. Before having medical tests, anyone taking this medicine should alert the health care professional in charge.

Some people feel drowsy, dizzy, or lightheaded when taking beta blockers. Anyone who takes these drugs should not drive, use machines or do anything else that might be dangerous until they have found out how the drugs affect them.

Beta blockers may increase sensitivity to cold, especially in older people or people who have poor circulation. Anyone who takes this medicine should dress warmly in cold weather and should be careful not to be exposed to the cold for too long.

People who usually have chest pain when they **exercise** or exert themselves may not have the pain when they are taking beta blockers. This could lead them to be more active than they should be. Anyone taking this medicine should ask his or her physician how much exercise and activity is safe.

Older people may be unusually sensitive to the effects of beta blockers. This may increase the chance of side effects.

Physicians may advise people taking beta blockers to wear or carry medical identification indicating that they are taking this medicine.

Special conditions

People who have certain medical conditions or who are taking certain other medicines may have problems if they take beta blockers. Before taking these drugs, the physician should know about any of these conditions:

ALLERGIES. Anyone who has had unusual reactions to beta blockers in the past should let his or her physician know before taking the drugs again. The physician should also be told about any **allergies** to insect stings, medicines, foods, dyes, preservatives, or other substances. In people with allergies to medicines, foods, or insect stings, beta blockers may make the allergic reactions more severe and harder to treat. Anyone who has an allergic reaction while taking beta blockers should get medical attention right away and should make sure the physician in charge knows that he or she is taking this medicine.

Beta blockers may also cause serious reactions in people who take allergy shots. Anyone taking this medicine should be sure to alert the physician before having any allergy shots.

DIABETES. Beta blockers may make blood sugar levels rise and may hide some symptoms of low blood sugar. Diabetic patients should discuss these possible problems with their physicians.

PREGNANCY. Some studies of beta blockers show that these drugs cause problems in newborns whose mothers use them during **pregnancy**. Other studies do not show such effects. Women who are pregnant or who may become pregnant should check with their physicians about the use of beta blockers.

BREASTFEEDING. Some beta blockers pass into breast milk and may cause breathing problems, slow heartbeat, and low blood pressure in nursing babies whose mothers take the drugs. Women who need to take beta blockers and who want to breastfeed their babies should check with their physicians.

OTHER MEDICAL CONDITIONS. Beta blockers may increase breathing problems or make allergic reactions more severe in people who have allergies, **bronchitis**, or **emphysema**. However, while breathing diseases were once thought to outrule use of beta blockers, new research in 2004 shows that this may have been a large misconception. A clinical trial showed that more than 98% of patients with chronic obstructive pulmonary disease safely used beta blockers. It is advised for patients with emphysema and other serious pulmonary disease to check with a physician and discuss the new findings.

In people with an overactive thyroid, stopping beta blockers suddenly may cause an increase in symptoms. Also, taking this medicine may hide a fast heartbeat, which is one of the symptoms of overactive thyroid.

Effects of these drugs may be greater in people with kidney or **liver disease** because the medicine is cleared from the body more slowly.

Beta blockers may also make the following medical conditions worse:

- Heart or blood vessel disease
- Unusually slow heartbeat (bradycardia)
- Myasthenia gravis (chronic disease causing muscle weakness and possibly **paralysis**)
- Psoriasis (itchy, scaly, red patches of skin)
- Depression (now, or in the past).

Before using beta blockers, people with any of the medical problems listed in this section should make sure their physicians are aware of their conditions.

USE OF CERTAIN MEDICINES. Taking beta blockers with certain other drugs may affect the way the drugs work or may increase the chance of side effects.

Side effects

The most common side effects are **dizziness**, drowsiness, lightheadedness, sleep problems, unusual tiredness or weakness, and decreased sexual ability. In men, this can occur as **impotence** or delayed ejaculation. These problems usually go away as the body adjusts to the drug and do not require medical treatment unless they persist or they interfere with normal activities. On the positive side, research in 2004 showed that use of beta blockers helps reduce risk for boen **fractures**.

More serious side effects are possible. If any of the following side effects occur, the physician who prescribed the medicine should be notified as soon as possible:

- Breathing problems
- Slow heartbeat
- Cold hands and feet
- Swollen ankles, feet, or lower legs
- Mental depression.

Other side effects may occur. Anyone who has unusual symptoms after taking beta blockers should get in touch with his or her physician.

Interactions

Beta blockers may interact with a number of other medicines. When this happens, the effects of one or both of the drugs may change or the risk of side effects may be greater. Anyone who takes beta blockers should let the physician know all other medicines he or she is taking. Among the drugs that may interact with beta blockers are:

- Calcium channel blockers and other blood pressure drugs. Using these drugs with beta blockers may cause unwanted effects on the heart.

- Insulin and diabetes medicines taken by mouth. Beta blockers cause high blood sugar or hide the symptoms of low blood sugar.

- Monoamine oxidase inhibitors (MAO) such as phenelzine (Nardil) or tranylcypromine (Parnate), used to treat conditions including depression and Parkinson's disease. Taking beta blockers at the same time or within two weeks of taking MAO inhibitors may cause severe high blood pressure.

- Airway-opening drugs (**bronchodilators**) such as aminophylline (Somophyllin), dyphylline (Lufyllin) oxtriphylline (Choledyl), or theophylline (Somophyllin-T). When combined with beta blockers, the effects of both the beta blockers and the airway-opening drugs may be lessened.

- **Cocaine**. High blood pressure, fast heartbeat, and heart problems are possible when cocaine and beta blockers are combined. Also, cocaine may interfere with the effects of beta blockers.

- Allergy shots or allergy skin tests. Beta blockers may increase the chance of serious reactions to these medicines.

The list above may not include every drug that interacts with beta blockers. Checking with a physician or pharmacist before combining beta blockers with any other prescription or nonprescription (over-the-counter) medicine is advised.

Resources

PERIODICALS

"Study Reveals Fears Over Beta Blockers in COPD Unfounded." *Pulse* September 13, 2004: 8.
"Use of Beta Blockers Associated With Decreased Risk for Fractures." *Life Science Weekly* September 28, 2004: 944.

Nancy Ross-Flanigan
Teresa G. Odle

Beta-thalassemia *see* **Thalassemia**

Betamethasone *see* **Corticosteroids**

Beta$_2$-microglobulin test

Definition

Beta$_2$-microglobulin is a protein found on the surface of many cells. Testing is done primarily when evaluating a person for certain kinds of **cancer** affecting white blood cells including chronic lymphocytic leukemia, non-Hodgkin's lymphoma, and **multiple myeloma** or **kidney disease**.

Purpose

Beta$_2$-microglobulin is plentiful on the surface of white blood cells. Increased production or destruction of these cells causes Beta$_2$-microglobulin levels in the blood to increase. This increase is seen in people with cancers involving white blood cells, but it is particularly meaningful in people newly diagnosed with multiple myeloma. Multiple myeloma is a malignancy (cancer) of a certain kind of white blood cell, called a plasma cell. At the time of diagnosis, the Beta$_2$-microglobulin levels reflect how advanced the disease is and the likely prognosis for that person.

When kidney disease is suspected, comparing blood and urine levels helps identify where the kidney is damaged. Beta$_2$-microglobulin normally is filtered out of the blood by the kidney's glomeruli (a round mass of capillary loops leading to each kidney tubule), only to be partially reabsorbed back into the blood when it reaches the kidney's tubules. In glomerular kidney disease, the glomeruli can't filter it out of the blood, so levels increase in the blood and decrease in the urine. In tubular kidney disease, the tubules can't reabsorb it back into the blood, so urine levels rise and blood levels fall. After a kidney transplant, increased blood levels may be an early sign of rejection.

KEY TERMS

Beta₂-microglobulin—A protein found on the surface of many cells, particularly white blood cells.

Chronic lymphocytic leukemia—A cancer of the blood cells characterized by large numbers of cancerous, mature white blood cells and enlarged lymph nodes.

Glomerular kidney disease—Disease of the kidney that affects the glomeruli, the part of the kidney that filters certain substances out of the blood.

Muliple myeloma—A malignancy (cancer) of a certain kind of white blood cell, called a plasma cell.

Non-Hodgkin's lymphoma—Cancer that originates in the lymphatic system and typically spreads throughout the body.

Tubular kidney disease—Disease of the kidney that affect the tubules, the part of the kidney that allows certain substances to be reabsorbed back into the blood.

Increased urinary levels are found in people with kidney damage caused by high exposure to the heavy metals cadmium and mercury. Periodic testing of workers exposed to these metals helps to detect beginning kidney damage.

Beta₂-microglobulin levels also rise during infection with some viruses, including cytomegalovirus and human **immunodeficiency** virus (HIV). Studies show that as HIV disease advances, beta₂-microglobulin levels rise.

Description

Testing methods vary, but most involve adding the person's serum–the yellow, liquid part of blood–or urine to one or more substances that bind to beta₂-microglobulin in the serum or urine. The amount of the substance(s) bound to beta₂-microglobulin is measured and the original amount of beta₂-microglobulin is determined.

The test is covered by insurance when medically necessary. Results are usually available the next day.

Preparation

The blood test requires 5 mL of blood. A healthcare worker ties a tourniquet on the person's upper arm, locates a vein in the inner elbow region, and inserts a needle into that vein. Vacuum action draws the blood through the needle into an attached tube. Collection of the sample takes only a few minutes.

Urine may be a single collection or collected throughout a 24-hour time period. The urine should be refrigerated until it is brought to the laboratory and must not become acidic.

Aftercare

Discomfort or bruising may occur at the puncture site or the person may feel dizzy or faint. Pressure to the puncture site until the bleeding stops reduces bruising. Warm packs on the puncture site relieve discomfort.

Normal results

- Serum: less than or equ to 2.7 g/ml
- Urine: less than 1 mg 24 hours 0–160 g/L

Abnormal results

The meaning of an abnormal result varies with the clinical condition of the person tested. In a person with multiple myeloma, a higher level means a poorer prognosis than a lower level. In a person with kidney disease, an increased blood level means the problem is tubular, not glomerular. In a kidney transplant patient, an increase may be a sign of rejection, toxic amounts of antirejection medication, or a viral infection. An increased level in a worker exposed to cadmium or mercury may signal beginning kidney damage and in a person with HIV, advancing disease.

Resources

BOOKS

Lehmann, Craig A. *Saunders Manual of Clinical Laboratory Science*. Philadelphia: W. B. Saunders Co., 1998.

Nancy J. Nordenson

Bile duct infection *see* **Cholangitis**

Bile duct cancer

Definition

Bile duct **cancer**, or cholangiocarcinoma, is a malignant tumor of the bile ducts within the liver (intrahepatic), or leading from the liver to the small

KEY TERMS

Angiography—Radiographic examination of blood vessels after injection with a special dye.

Cholangiography—Radiographic examination of the bile ducts after injection with a special dye.

Computed tomography—Radiographic examination that obtains cross-sectional images of the body.

Jaundice—Yellowish staining of the skin and eyes due to excess bilirubin in the bloodstream.

Lymphatic—Pertaining to lymph, the clear fluid that is collected from tissues, flows through special vessels, and joins the venous circulation.

Metastasis—The spread of cancerous tumor cells from one part of the body to another.

Resection—To surgically remove a part of the body

Stent—Slender hollow catheter or rod placed within a vessel or duct to provide support or maintain patency.

Ultrasound—Radiographic imaging technique utilizing high frequency sound waves.

intestine (extrahepatic). It is a rare tumor with poor outcome for most patients.

Description

Bile is a substance manufactured by the liver that aids in the digestion of food. Bile ducts are channels that carry the bile from the liver to the small intestine. Like the tributaries of a river, the small bile ducts in the liver converge into two large bile ducts called the left and right hepatic ducts. These exit the liver and join to form the common hepatic duct. The gallbladder, which concentrates and stores the bile, empties into the common hepatic duct to form the common bile duct. Finally, this large duct connects to the small intestine where the bile can help digest food. Collectively, this network of bile ducts is called the biliary tract.

Bile duct cancer originates from the cells that line the inner surface of the bile ducts. A tumor may arise anywhere along the biliary tract, either within or outside of the liver. Bile duct tumors are typically slow-growing tumors that spread by local invasion of neighboring structures and by way of lymphatic channels.

Bile duct cancer is an uncommon malignancy. In the United States, approximately one case arises per 100,000 people per year, but it is more common in Southeast Asia. It occurs in men only slightly more often than in women and it is most commonly diagnosed in people in their 50s and 60s. In fact, about 65% of patients with bile duct cancer are over age 65.

Causes and symptoms

A number of risk factors are associated with the development of bile duct cancer:

- Primary sclerosing **cholangitis**. This disease is characterized by extensive scarring of the biliary tract, sometimes associated with inflammatory bowel disease.

- Choledochal cysts. These are abnormal dilatations of the biliary tract that usually form during fetal development. There is evidence that these cysts may rarely arise during adulthood.

- Hepatolithiasis. This is the condition of stone formation within the liver (not including gallbladder stones).

- Liver flukes. Parasitic infection with certain worms is thought to be at least partially responsible for the higher prevalence of bile duct cancer in Southeast Asia.

- Thorotrast. This is a chemical that was previously injected intravenously during certain types of x rays. It is not in use anymore. Exposure to Thorotrast has been implicated in the development of cancer of the liver as well as the bile ducts.

Symptoms

Jaundice is the first symptom in 90% of patients. This occurs when the bile duct tumor causes an obstruction in the normal flow of bile from the liver to the small intestine. Bilirubin, a component of bile, builds up within the liver and is absorbed into the bloodstream in excess amounts. This can be detected in a blood test, but it can also manifest as yellowish discoloring of the skin and eyes. The bilirubin in the bloodstream also makes the urine appear dark. Additionally, the patient may experience generalized **itching** due to the deposition of bile components in the skin. Normally, a portion of the bile is excreted in stool; bile actually gives stool its brown color. But when the biliary tract is obstructed by tumor, the stools may appear pale.

Abdominal **pain**, **fatigue**, weight loss, and poor appetite are less common symptoms. Occasionally, if obstruction of the biliary tract causes the gallbladder to swell enormously yet without causing pain, the physician may be able to feel the gallbladder during a

physical examination. Sometimes the biliary tract can become infected, but this is normally a rare consequence of invasive tests. Infection causes **fever**, chills, and pain in the right upper portion of the abdomen.

Diagnosis

Certain laboratory tests of the blood may aid in the diagnosis. The most important one is the test for elevated bilirubin levels in the bloodstream. Levels of alkaline phosphatase and CA 19-9 may also be elevated.

When symptoms, physical signs, and blood tests point toward an abnormality of the biliary tract, the next step involves radiographic exams. Ultrasound, computed tomography (CT scan), and **magnetic resonance imaging** (MRI) are noninvasive and rapid. In recent years, MRI has become the favored imaging choice for initial diagnosis of cholangiocarcinoma when the exam is available and affordable or covered by insurance. These tests can often detect the actual tumor as well as dilatation of the obstructed biliary tract. If these tests indicate the presence of a tumor, cholangiography is required. This procedure involves injecting dye into the biliary tract to obtain anatomic images of the bile ducts and the tumor. The specialist that performs this test can also insert small tubes, or stents, into a partially obstructed portion of the bile duct to prevent further obstruction by growth of the tumor. This is vitally important since it may be the only intervention that is possible in certain patients. Cholangiography is an invasive test that carries a small risk of infection of the biliary tract. The objective of these radiological tests is to determine the size and location of the tumor, as well as the extent of spread to nearby structures.

The treatment of bile duct tumors is usually not affected by the specific type of cancer cells that comprise the tumor. For this reason, some physicians forego biopsy of the tumor.

Treatment

The treatment is with surgical resection (removal) of the tumor and all involved structures. Unfortunately, sometimes the cancer has already spread too far when the diagnosis is made. Thus, in the treatment of bile duct cancer, the first question to answer is if the tumor may be safely resected by surgery with reasonable benefit to the patient. If the cancer involves certain blood vessels or has spread widely throughout the liver, resection may not be possible. Sometimes further invasive testing is required.

Angiography can determine if the blood vessels are involved. **Laparoscopy** is a surgical procedure that allows the surgeon to directly assess the tumor and nearby lymph nodes without making a large incision in the abdomen. Only about 45% of bile duct cancers are ultimately resectable.

If the tumor is resectable, and the patient is healthy enough to tolerate the operation, the specific type of surgery performed depends on the location of the tumor. For tumors within the liver or high up in the biliary tract, resection of part of the liver may be required. Tumors in the middle portion of the biliary tract can be removed alone. Tumors of the lower end of the biliary tract may require extensive resection of part of the pancreas, small intestine, and stomach to ensure complete resection.

Unfortunately, sometimes the cancer appears resectable by all the radiological and invasive tests, but is found to be unresectable during surgery. In this scenario, a bypass operation can relieve the biliary tract obstruction, but does not remove the tumor itself. This does not produce a cure but it can offer a better quality of life for the patient.

Prognosis

Prognosis depends on the stage and resectability of the tumor. If the patient cannot undergo surgical resection, the survival rate is commonly less than one year. If the tumor is resected, the survival rate improves, with 20% of these patients surviving past five years.

Clinical trials

Studies of new treatments in patients are known as clinical trials. These trials seek to compare the standard method of care with a new method, or the trials may be trying to establish whether one treatment is more beneficial for certain patients than others. Sometimes, a new treatment that is not being offered on a wide scale may be available to patients participating in clinical trials, but participating in the trials may involve some risk. To learn more about clinical trials, patients can call the National Cancer Institute (NCI) at 1-800-4-CANCER or visit the NCI web site for patients at < http://www.cancertrials.nci.nih.gov >.

Prevention

Other than the avoidance of infections caused by liver flukes, there are no known preventions for this cancer.

Resources

BOOKS

Abeloff, Martin D., editor. "Cholangiocarcinoma." In *Clinical Oncology*. 2nd ed. New York: Churchill Livingstone, 2000, pp.1722-1723.

Ahrendt, Steven A., and Henry A. Pitt. "Biliary Tract." In *Sabiston Textbook of Surgery*, edited by Courtney Townsend Jr., 16th ed. Philadelphia: W.B. Saunders Company, 2001, pp. 1076-1111.

PERIODICALS

"COX–2 Promoter Enhances the Efficacy of Cholangiosarcoma Gene Therapy." *Cancer Weekly* (May 20, 2003): 167.

Khan, S.A., et al. "Guidelines for the Diagnosis and Treatment of Cholangiosarcoma: Consensus Document." *Gut* (November 2002): vi1–9.

ORGANIZATIONS

The American Cancer Society. 1-800-ACS 2345. <http://www.cancer.org>.

American Liver Foundation.1425 Pompton Ave., Cedar Grove, NJ 07009. (800) 223-0179. <http://www.liverfoundation.org>.

National Cancer Institute (National Institutes of Health). 9000 Rockville Pike, Bethesda, MD 20892. (800) 422-6237. <http://www.nci.nih.gov>.

Kevin O. Hwang M.D.
Teresa G. Odle

Bile duct atresia *see* **Biliary atresia**

Bile flow obstruction *see* **Cholestasis**

Bilharziasis *see* **Schistosomiasis**

Biliary atresia

Definition

Biliary atresia is the failure of a fetus to develop an adequate pathway for bile to drain from the liver to the intestine.

Description

Biliary atresia is the most common lethal **liver disease** in children, occurring once every 10,000–15,000 live births. Half of all liver transplants are done for this reason.

The normal anatomy of the bile system begins within the liver, where thousands of tiny bile ducts collect bile from liver cells. These ducts merge into larger and larger channels, like streams flowing into rivers, until they all pour into a single duct that empties into the duodenum (first part of the small intestine). Between the liver and the duodenum this duct has a side channel connected to the gall bladder. The gall bladder stores bile and concentrates it, removing much of its water content. Then, when a meal hits the stomach, the gall bladder contracts and empties its contents.

Bile is a mixture of waste chemicals that the liver removes from the circulation and excretes through the biliary system into the intestine. On its way out, bile assists in the digestion of certain nutrients. If bile cannot get out because the channels are absent or blocked, it backs up into the liver and eventually into the rest of the body. The major pigment in bile is a chemical called bilirubin, which is yellow. Bilirubin is a breakdown product of hemoglobin (the red chemical in blood that carries oxygen). If the body accumulates an excess of bilirubin, it turns yellow (jaundiced). Bile also turns the stool brown. Without it, stools are the color of clay.

Causes and symptoms

It is possible that a viral infection is responsible for this disease, but evidence is not yet convincing. The cause remains unknown.

The affected infant will appear normal at birth and during the newborn period. After two weeks the normal **jaundice** of the newborn will not disappear, and the stools will probably be clay-colored. At this point, the condition will come to the attention of a physician. If not, the child's abdomen will begin to swell, and the infant will get progressively more ill. Nearly all untreated children will die of liver failure within two years.

Diagnosis

The persistence of jaundice beyond the second week in a newborn with clay-colored stools is a sure sign of obstruction to the flow of bile. An immediate evaluation that includes blood tests and imaging of the biliary system will confirm the diagnosis.

Treatment

Surgery is the only treatment. Somehow the surgeon must create an adequate pathway for bile to escape the liver into the intestine. The altered anatomy of the biliary system is different in every case, calling upon the surgeon's skill and experience to select and execute the most effective among several options. If the obstruction is only between the gall bladder and

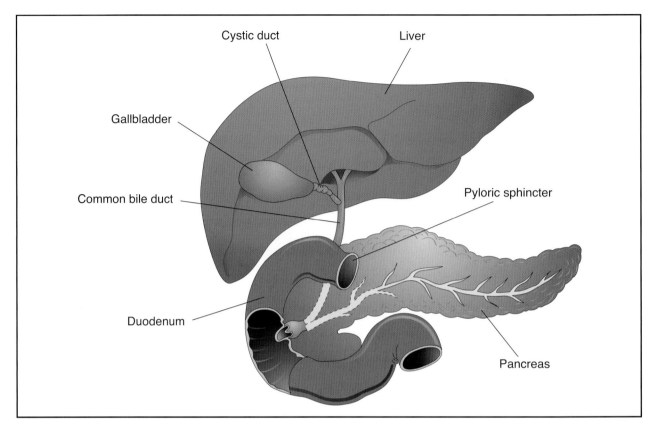

Cystic duct
Liver
Gallbladder
Common bile duct
Pyloric sphincter
Duodenum
Pancreas

Biliary atresia is a congenital condition in which the pathway for bile to drain from the liver to the intestine is undeveloped. It is the most common lethal liver disease in children. *(Illustration by Electronic Illustrators Group).*

KEY TERMS

Duodenum—The first part of the small intestine, beginning at the outlet of the stomach.

Hemoglobin—The red, iron-containing chemical in the blood that carries oxygen to the tissues.

Jaundice—The yellow color taken on by a patient whose liver is unable to excrete bilirubin. A normal condition in the first week of life due to the infant's delayed ability to process certain waste products.

Kernicterus—A potentially lethal disease of newborns caused by excessive accumulation of the bile pigment bilirubin.

the intestine, it is possible to attach a piece of intestine directly to the gall bladder. More likely, the upper biliary system will also be inadequate, and the surgeon will attach a piece of intestine directly to the liver–the Kasai procedure. In its wisdom, the body will discover that the tiny bile ducts in that part of the liver are discharging their bile directly into the intestine. Bile will begin to flow in that direction, and the channels will gradually enlarge. Survival rates for the Kasai procedure are commonly 50% at five years and 15% at 10 years. Persistent disease in the liver gradually destroys the organ.

Prognosis

Before liver transplants became available, even prompt and effective surgery did not cure the whole problem. Biliary drainage can usually be established, but the patients still have a defective biliary system that develops progressive disease and commonly leads to an early **death**. Transplantation now achieves up to 90% one-year survival rates and promises to prevent the chronic disease that used to accompany earlier procedures.

Prevention

The specific cause of this birth defect is unknown, so all that women can do is to practice the many general preventive measures, even before they conceive.

Biliary atresia is a congenital condition in which the pathway for bile to drain from the liver to the intestine is undeveloped. It is the most common lethal liver disease in children.

Resources

BOOKS

Feldman, Mark, et al. "Diseases of the Bile Ducts." *Sleisenger & Fordtran's Gastrointestinal and Liver Disease*. Philadelphia: W. B. Saunders Co., 1998.

J. Ricker Polsdorfer, MD

Biliary duct cancer *see* **Gallbladder cancer**

Biliary tract cancer *see* **Bile duct cancer**

Bilirubin test *see* **Liver function tests**

Binge-eating disorder

Definition

Binge eating disorder (BED) is characterized by a loss of control over eating behaviors. The binge eater consumes unnaturally large amounts of food in a short time period, but unlike a bulimic, does not regularly engage in any inappropriate weight-reducing behaviors (for example, excessive **exercise**, **vomiting**, taking **laxatives**) following the binge episodes.

Description

BED typically strikes individuals sometime between adolescence and the early twenties. Because of the nature of the disorder, most BED patients are overweight or obese. Studies of weight loss programs have shown that an average of 30% of individuals enrolling in these programs report binge eating behavior.

Causes and symptoms

Binge eating episodes may act as a psychological release for excessive emotional **stress**. Other circumstances that may predispose an individual to BED include heredity and affective disorders, such as major depression. BED patients are also more likely to have a comorbid, or co-existing, diagnosis of impulsive behaviors (for example, compulsive buying), **post-traumatic stress disorder** (PTSD), **panic disorder**, or **personality disorders**.

Individuals who develop BED often come from families who put an unnatural emphasis on the

---

importance of food, for example, as a source of comfort in times of emotional distress. As children, BED patients may have been taught to clean their plate regardless of their appetite, or that finishing a meal made them a "good" girl or boy. Cultural attitudes towards beauty and thinness may also be a factor in the BED equation.

During binge episodes, BED patients experience a definite sense of lost control over their eating. They eat quickly and to the point of discomfort even if they aren't hungry. They typically binge alone two or more times a week, and often feel depressed and guilty once the episode has concluded.

Diagnosis

Binge eating disorder is usually diagnosed and treated by a psychiatrist and/or a psychologist. In addition to an interview with the patient, personality and behavioral inventories, such as the **Minnesota Multiphasic Personality Inventory** (MMPI), may be administered as part of the assessment process. One of several clinical inventories, or scales, may also be used to assess depressive symptoms, including the Hamilton Depression Scale (HAM-D) or Beck Depression Inventory (BDI). These tests may be administered in an outpatient or hospital setting.

Treatment

Many BED individuals binge after long intervals of excessive dietary restraint; therapy helps normalize this pattern. The initial goal of BED treatment is to teach the patient to gain control over his eating behavior by focusing on eating regular meals and avoiding snacking. **Cognitive-behavioral therapy**, **group therapy**, or interpersonal psychotherapy may be employed to uncover the emotional motives, distorted thinking, and behavioral patterns behind the binge eating.

Because the prevalence of depression in BED patients is high, psychopharmacological treatment with antidepressants may also be prescribed. Once the binge eating behavior is curbed and depressive symptoms are controlled, the physical symptoms of BED can be addressed. The overweight BED patient may be placed on a moderate exercise program and a nutritionist may be consulted to educate the patient on healthy food choices and strategies for weight loss.

Prognosis

The poor dietary habits and **obesity** that are symptomatic of BED can lead to serious health problems, such as high blood pressure, heart attacks, and diabetes, if left unchecked. BED is a chronic condition that requires ongoing medical and psychological management. To bring long-term relief to the BED patient, it is critical to address the underlying psychological causes behind binge eating behaviors. It appears that up to 50% of BED patients will stop bingeing with cognitive behavioral therapy (CBT).

Resources

ORGANIZATIONS

American Psychiatric Association. 1400 K Street NW, Washington DC 20005. (888) 357-7924. < http://www.psych.org > .

American Psychological Association (APA). 750 First St. NE, Washington, DC 20002-4242. (202) 336-5700. < http://www.apa.org > .

Eating Disorders Awareness and Prevention. 603 Stewart St., Suite 803, Seattle, WA 98101. (206) 382-3587.

National Eating Disorders Organization (NEDO). 6655 South Yale Ave., Tulsa, OK 74136. (918) 481-4044.

Overeaters Anonymous World Service Office. 6075 Zenith Ct. NE, Rio Rancho, NM 87124. (505) 891-2664. < http://www.overeatersanonymous.org > .

Paula Anne Ford-Martin

Biofeedback

Definition

Biofeedback, or applied psychophysiological feedback, is a patient-guided treatment that teaches an individual to control muscle tension, **pain**, body temperature, brain waves, and other bodily functions and processes through relaxation, visualization, and other cognitive control techniques. The name

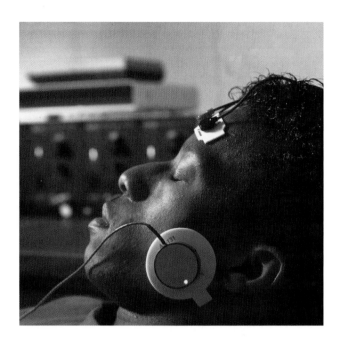

A patient undergoing biofeedback therapy. *(Photo Researchers, Inc. Reproduced by permission.)*

biofeedback refers to the biological signals that are fed back, or returned, to the patient in order for the patient to develop techniques of manipulating them.

Purpose

Biofeedback has been used to successfully treat a number of disorders and their symptoms, including temporomandibular joint disorder (TMJ), chronic pain, **irritable bowel syndrome** (IBS), Raynaud's syndrome, epilepsy, attention-deficit hyperactivity disorder (**ADHD**), migraine headaches, **anxiety**, depression, traumatic brain injury, and **sleep disorders**.

Illnesses that may be triggered at least in part by **stress** are also targeted by biofeedback therapy. Certain types of headaches, high blood pressure, **bruxism** (teeth grinding), **post-traumatic stress disorder**, eating disorders, **substance abuse**, and some **anxiety disorders** may be treated successfully by teaching patients the ability to relax and release both muscle and mental tension. Biofeedback is often just one part of a comprehensive treatment program for some of these disorders.

NASA has used biofeedback techniques to treat astronauts who suffer from severe space sickness, during which the autonomic nervous system is disrupted. Scientists at the University of Tennessee have adapted these techniques to treat individuals suffering from severe **nausea and vomiting** that is also rooted in autonomic nervous system dysfunction.

KEY TERMS

Autonomic nervous system—The part of the nervous system that controls so-called involuntary functions, such as heart rate, salivary gland secretion, respiratory function, and pupil dilation.

Bruxism—Habitual, often unconscious, grinding of the teeth.

Epilepsy—A neurological disorder characterized by the sudden onset of seizures.

Placebo effect—Placebo effect occurs when a treatment or medication with no known therapeutic value (a placebo) is administered to a patient, and the patient's symptoms improve. The patient believes and expects that the treatment is going to work, so it does. The placebo effect is also a factor to some degree in clinically-effective therapies, and explains why patients respond better than others to treatment despite similar symptoms and illnesses.

Raynaud's syndrome—A vascular, or circulatory system, disorder which is characterized by abnormally cold hands and feet. This chilling effect is caused by constriction of the blood vessels in the extremities, and occurs when the hands and feet are exposed to cold weather. Emotional stress can also trigger the cold symptoms.

Schizophrenia—Schizophrenia is a psychotic disorder that causes distortions in perception (delusions and hallucinations), inappropriate moods and behaviors, and disorganized or incoherent speech and behavior.

Temporomandibular joint disorder—Inflammation, irritation, and pain of the jaw caused by improper opening and closing of the temporomandibular joint. Other symptoms include clicking of the jaw and a limited range of motion.

Recent research also indicates that biofeedback may be a useful tool in helping patients with **urinary incontinence** regain bladder control. Individuals learning pelvic-floor muscle strengthening exercises can gain better control over these muscles by using biofeedback. Sensors are placed on the muscles to train the patient where they are and when proper contractions are taking place.

Description

Origins

In 1961, Neal Miller, an experimental psychologist, suggested that autonomic nervous system

responses (for instance, heart rate, blood pressure, gastrointestinal activity, regional blood flow) could be under voluntary control. As a result of his experiments, he showed that such autonomic processes were controllable. This work led to the creation of biofeedback therapy. Willer's work was expanded by other researchers. Thereafter, research performed in the 1970s by UCLA researcher Dr. Barry Sterman established that both cats and monkeys could be trained to control their brain wave patterns. Sterman then used his research techniques on human patients with epilepsy, where he was able to reduce seizures by 60% with the use of biofeedback techniques. Throughout the 1970s, other researchers published reports of their use of biofeedback in the treatment of cardiac **arrhythmias**, headaches, Raynaud's syndrome, and excess stomach acid, and as a tool for teaching deep relaxation. Since the early work of Miller and Sterman, biofeedback has developed into a front-line behavioral treatment for an even wider range of disorders and symptoms.

During biofeedback, special sensors are placed on the body. These sensors measure the bodily function that is causing the patient problem symptoms, such as heart rate, blood pressure, muscle tension (EMG or electromyographic feedback), brain waves (EEC or electroencophalographic feedback), respiration, and body temperature (thermal feedback), and translates the information into a visual and/or audible readout, such as a paper tracing, a light display, or a series of beeps.

While the patient views the instantaneous feedback from the biofeedback monitors, he or she begins to recognize what thoughts, fears, and mental images influence his or her physical reactions. By monitoring this relationship between mind and body, the patient can then use these same thoughts and mental images as subtle cues, as these act as reminders to become deeply relaxed, instead of anxious. These reminders also work to manipulate heart beat, brain wave patterns, body temperature, and other bodily functions. This is achieved through relaxation exercises, mental imagery, and other cognitive therapy techniques.

As the biofeedback response takes place, patients can actually see or hear the results of their efforts instantly through the sensor readout on the biofeedback equipment. Once these techniques are learned and the patient is able to recognize the state of relaxation or visualization necessary to alleviate symptoms, the biofeedback equipment itself is no longer needed. The patient then has a powerful, portable, and self-administered treatment tool to deal with problem symptoms.

Biofeedback that specializes in reading and altering brain waves is sometimes called *neurofeedback*. The brain produces four distinct types of brain waves—delta, theta, alpha, and beta—that all operate at a different frequency. Delta, the slowest frequency wave, is the brain wave pattern associated with sleep. Beta waves, which occur in a normal, waking state, can range from 12-35 Hz. Problems begin to develop when beta wave averages fall in the low end (underarousal) or the high end (overarousal) of that spectrum. Underarousal might be present in conditions such as depression or attention-deficit disorder, and overarousal may be indicative of an anxiety disorder, obsessive compulsive disorder, or excessive stress. Beta wave neurofeedback focuses on normalizing that beta wave pattern to an optimum value of around 14 Hz. A second type of neurofeedback, alpha-theta, focuses on developing the more relaxing alpha (8-13 Hz) and theta waves (4-9 Hz) that are usually associated with deep, meditative states, and has been used with some success in substance **abuse** treatment.

Through brain wave manipulation, neurofeedback can be useful in treating a variety of disorders that are suspected or proven to impact brain wave patterns, such as epilepsy, attention-deficit disorder, migraine headaches, anxiety, depression, traumatic brain injury, and sleep disorders. The equipment used for neurofeedback usually uses a monitor as an output device. The monitor displays specific patterns that the patient attempts to change by producing the appropriate type of brain wave. Or, the monitor may reward the patient for producing the appropriate brain wave by producing a positive reinforcer, or reward. For example, children may be rewarded with a series of successful moves in a displayed video game.

Depending on the type of biofeedback, individuals may need up to 30 sessions with a trained professional to learn the techniques required to control their symptoms on a long-term basis. Therapists usually recommend that their patients practice both biofeedback and relaxation techniques on their own at home.

Preparations

Before initiating biofeedback treatment, the therapist and patient will have an initial consultation to record the patients medical history and treatment background and discuss goals for therapy.

Before a neurofeedback session, an EEG is taken from the patient to determine his or her baseline brain-wave pattern.

Biofeedback typically is performed in a quiet and relaxed atmosphere with comfortable seating for the patient. Depending on the type and goals of biofeedback being performed, one or more sensors will be attached to the patient's body with conductive gel and/or adhesives. These may include:

- Electromyographic (EMG) sensors. EMG sensors measure electrical activity in the muscles, specifically muscle tension. In treating TMJ or bruxism, these sensors would be placed along the muscles of the jaw. Chronic pain might be treated by monitoring electrical energy in other muscle groups.

- Galvanic skin response (GSR) sensors. These are electrodes placed on the fingers that monitor perspiration, or sweat gland, activity. These may also be called skin conductance level (SCL).

- Temperature sensors. Temperature, or thermal, sensors measure body temperature and changes in blood flow.

- Electroencephalography (EEG) sensors. These electrodes are applied to the scalp to measure the electrical activity of the brain, or brain waves.

- Heart rate sensors. A pulse monitor placed on the finger tip can monitor pulse rate.

- Respiratory sensors. Respiratory sensors monitor oxygen intake and carbon dioxide output.

Precautions

Individuals who use a pacemaker or other implantable electrical devices should inform their biofeedback therapist before starting treatments, as certain types of biofeedback sensors have the potential to interfere with these devices.

Biofeedback may not be suitable for some patients. Patients must be willing to take a very active role in the treatment process. And because biofeedback focuses strictly on behavioral change, those patients who wish to gain insight into their symptoms by examining their past might be better served by psychodynamic therapy.

Biofeedback may also be inappropriate for cognitively impaired individuals, such as those patients with organic brain disease or a traumatic brain injury, depending on their levels of functioning.

Patients with specific pain symptoms of unknown origin should undergo a thorough medical examination before starting biofeedback treatments to rule out any serious underlying disease. Once a diagnosis has been made, biofeedback can be used concurrently with conventional treatment.

Biofeedback may only be one component of a comprehensive treatment plan. For illnesses and symptoms that are manifested from an organic disease process, such as **cancer** or diabetes, biofeedback should be an adjunct to (complementary to), and not a replacement for, conventional medical treatment.

Side effects

There are no known side effects to properly administered biofeedback or neurofeedback sessions.

Research and general acceptance

Preliminary research published in late 1999 indicated that neurofeedback may be a promising new tool in the treatment of **schizophrenia**. Researchers reported that schizophrenic patients had used neurofeedback to simulate brain wave patterns that antipsychotic medications produce in the brain. Further research is needed to determine what impact this may have on treatment for schizophrenia.

The use of biofeedback techniques to treat an array of disorders has been extensively described in the medical literature. Controlled studies for some applications are limited, such as for the treatment of menopausal symptoms and premenstrual disorder (PMS). There is also some debate over the effectiveness of biofeedback in ADHD treatment, and the lack of controlled studies on that application. While many therapists, counselors, and mental health professionals have reported great success with treating their ADHD patients with neurofeedback techniques, some critics attribute this positive therapeutic impact to a placebo effect.

There may also be some debate among mental health professionals as to whether biofeedback should be considered a first line treatment for some mental illnesses, and to what degree other treatments, such as medication, should be employed as an adjunct therapy.

Resources

BOOKS

Robbins, Jim. *A Symphony in the Brain: The Evolution of the New Brain Wave Biofeedback.* Boston, MA: Atlantic Monthly Press, 2000.

PERIODICALS

Robbins, Jim. "On the Track with Neurofeedback." *Newsweek* 135, no. 25 (June 2000): 76.

ORGANIZATIONS

Association for Applied Psychotherapy and Biofeedback. 10200 W. 44th Avenue, Suite 304, Wheat Ridge, CO 80033-2840. (303) 422-8436. < http://www.aapb.org > .

Biofeedback Certification Institute of America.10200 W. 44th Avenue, Suite 310, Wheat Ridge, CO 80033. (303) 420-2902.

Paula Anne Ford-Martin

Biopsy *see* **Bone biopsy; Bone marrow aspiration and biopsy; Brain biopsy; Breast biopsy; Cervical conization; CT-guided biopsy; Endometrial biopsy; Joint biopsy; Kidney biopsy; Liver biopsy; Lung biopsy; Lymph node biopsy; Myocardial biopsy; Pleural biopsy; Prostate biopsy; Skin biopsy; Small intestine biopsy; Thyroid biopsy**

Bipolar disorder

Definition

Bipolar, or manic-depressive disorder, is a mood disorder that causes radical emotional changes and mood swings, from manic highs to depressive lows. The majority of bipolar individuals experience alternating episodes of **mania** and depression.

Description

In the United States alone, more than two million people are diagnosed with bipolar disorder. Research shows that as many as 10 million people might be affected by bipolar disorder, which is the sixth-leading cause of disability worldwide. The average age of onset of bipolar disorder is from adolescence through the early twenties. However, because of the complexity of the disorder, a correct diagnosis can be delayed for several years or more. In a survey of bipolar patients conducted by the National Depressive and Manic Depressive Association (MDMDA), one-half of respondents reported visiting three or more professionals before receiving a correct diagnosis, and over one-third reported a wait of ten years or more before they were correctly diagnosed.

Bipolar I disorder is characterized by manic episodes, the "high" of the manic-depressive cycle. A person with bipolar disorder experiencing mania often has feelings of self-importance, elation, talkativeness, increased sociability, and a desire to embark on goal-oriented activities, coupled with the characteristics of irritability, impatience, impulsiveness, hyperactivity,

KEY TERMS

Affective disorder—An emotional disorder involving abnormal highs and/or lows in mood. Now termed mood disorder.

Anticonvulsant medication—A drug used to prevent convulsions or seizures; often prescribed in the treatment of epilepsy. Several anticonvulsant medications have been found effective in the treatment of bipolar disorder.

Antipsychotic medication—A drug used to treat psychotic symptoms, such as delusions or hallucinations, in which patients are unable to distinguish fantasy from reality.

Benzodiazpines—A group of tranquilizers having sedative, hypnotic, antianxiety, amnestic, anticonvulsant, and muscle relaxant effects.

DSM-IV—Diagnostic and Statistical Manual of Mental Disorders, Fourth Edition (DSM-IV). This reference book, published by the American Psychiatric Association, is the diagnostic standard for most mental health professionals in the United States.

ECT—Electroconvulsive therapy sometimes is used to treat depression or mania when pharmaceutical treatment fails.

Hypomania—A milder form of mania which is characteristic of bipolar II disorder.

Mixed mania/mixed state—A mental state in which symptoms of both depression and mania occur simultaneously.

Mania—An elevated or euphoric mood or irritable state that is characteristic of bipolar I disorder.

Neurotransmitter—A chemical in the brain that transmits messages between neurons, or nerve cells. Changes in the levels of certain neurotransmitters, such as serotonin, norepinephrine, and dopamine, are thought to be related to bipolar disorder.

Psychomotor retardation—Slowed mental and physical processes characteristic of a bipolar depressive episode.

patients (for example, depression with the racing thoughts of mania). Also, dysphoric mania is common (mania characterized by anger and irritability).

Bipolar II disorder is characterized by major depressive episodes alternating with episodes of hypomania, a milder form of mania. Bipolar depression may be difficult to distinguish from a unipolar major depressive episode. Patients with bipolar depression tend to have extremely low energy, retarded mental and physical processes, and more profound **fatigue** (for example, hypersomnia; a sleep disorder marked by a need for excessive sleep or sleepiness when awake) than unipolar depressives.

Cyclothymia refers to the cycling of hypomanic episodes with depression that does not reach major depressive proportions. One-third of patients with cyclothymia will develop bipolar I or II disorder later in life.

A phenomenon known as rapid cycling occurs in up to 20% of bipolar I and II patients. In rapid cycling, manic and depressive episodes must alternate frequently; at least four times in 12 months; to meet the diagnostic definition. In some cases of "ultra-rapid cycling," the patient may bounce between manic and depressive states several times within a 24-hour period. This condition is very hard to distinguish from mixed states.

Bipolar NOS is a category for bipolar states that do not clearly fit into the bipolar I, II, or cyclothymia diagnoses.

Causes and symptoms

The source of bipolar disorder has not been clearly defined. Because two-thirds of bipolar patients have a family history of affective or emotional disorders, researchers have searched for a genetic link to the disorder. Several studies have uncovered a number of possible genetic connections to the predisposition for bipolar disorder. A 2003 study found that **schizophrenia** and bipolar disorder could have similar genetic causes that arise from certain problems with genes associated with myelin development in the central nervous system. (Myelin is a white, fat-like substance that forms a sort of layer or sheath around nerve fibers.) Another possible biological cause under investigation is the presence of an excessive calcium build-up in the cells of bipolar patients. Also, dopamine and other neurochemical transmitters appear to be implicated in bipolar disorder and these are under intense investigation.

Over one-half of patients diagnosed with bipolar disorder have a history of **substance abuse**. There is a

and a decreased need for sleep. Usually this manic period is followed by a period of depression, although a few bipolar I individuals may not experience a major depressive episode. Mixed states, where both manic or hypomanic symptoms and depressive symptoms occur at the same time, also occur frequently with bipolar I

high rate of association between **cocaine** abuse and bipolar disorder. Some studies have shown up to 30% of abusers meeting the criteria for bipolar disorder. The emotional and physical highs and lows of cocaine use correspond to the manic depression of the bipolar patient, making the disorder difficult to diagnosis.

For some bipolar patients, manic and depressive episodes coincide with seasonal changes. Depressive episodes are typical during winter and fall, and manic episodes are more probable in the spring and summer months.

Symptoms of bipolar depressive episodes include low energy levels, feelings of despair, difficulty concentrating, extreme fatigue, and psychomotor retardation (slowed mental and physical capabilities). Manic episodes are characterized by feelings of euphoria, lack of inhibitions, racing thoughts, diminished need for sleep, talkativeness, risk taking, and irritability. In extreme cases, mania can induce **hallucinations** and other psychotic symptoms such as grandiose illusions.

Diagnosis

Bipolar disorder usually is diagnosed and treated by a psychiatrist and/or a psychologist with medical assistance. In addition to an interview, several clinical inventories or scales may be used to assess the patient's mental status and determine the presence of bipolar symptoms. These include the Millon Clinical Multiaxial Inventory III (MCMI-III), **Minnesota Multiphasic Personality Inventory** II (**MMPI-2**), the Internal State Scale (ISS), the Self-Report Manic Inventory (SRMI), and the Young Mania Rating Scale (YMRS). The tests are verbal and/or written and are administered in both hospital and outpatient settings.

Psychologists and psychiatrists typically use the criteria listed in the *Diagnostic and Statistical Manual of Mental Disorders, Fourth Edition* (*DSM-IV*) as a guideline for diagnosis of bipolar disorder and other mental illnesses. *DSM-IV* describes a manic episode as an abnormally elevated or irritable mood lasting a period of at least one week that is distinguished by at least three of the mania symptoms: inflated self-esteem, decreased need for sleep, talkativeness, racing thoughts, distractibility, increase in goal-directed activity, or excessive involvement in pleasurable activities that have a high potential for painful consequences. If the mood of the patient is irritable and not elevated, four of the symptoms are required.

Although many clinicians find the criteria too rigid, a hypomanic diagnosis requires a duration

of at least four days with at least three of the symptoms indicated for manic episodes (four if mood is irritable and not elevated). *DSM-IV* notes that unlike manic episodes, hypomanic episodes do not cause a marked impairment in social or occupational functioning, do not require hospitalization, and do not have psychotic features. In addition, because hypomanic episodes are characterized by high energy and goal directed activities and often result in a positive outcome, or are perceived in a positive manner by the patient, bipolar II disorder can go undiagnosed.

Bipolar symptoms often present differently in children and adolescents. Manic episodes in these age groups are typically characterized by more psychotic features than in adults, which may lead to a misdiagnosis of schizophrenia. Children and adolescents also tend toward irritability and aggressiveness instead of elation. Further, symptoms tend to be chronic, or ongoing, rather than acute, or episodic. Bipolar children are easily distracted, impulsive, and hyperactive, which can lead to a misdiagnosis of attention deficit hyperactivity disorder (**ADHD**). Furthermore, their aggression often leads to violence, which may be misdiagnosed as a **conduct disorder**.

Substance abuse, thyroid disease, and use of prescription or over-the-counter medication can mask or mimic the presence of bipolar disorder. In cases of substance abuse, the patient must ordinarily undergo a period of **detoxification** and abstinence before a mood disorder is diagnosed and treatment begins.

Treatment

Treatment of bipolar disorder is usually achieved with medication. A combination of mood stabilizing agents with antidepressants, antipsychotics, and anticonvulsants is used to regulate manic and depressive episodes.

Mood stabilizing agents such as lithium, carbamazepine, and valproate are prescribed to regulate the manic highs and lows of bipolar disorder:

- Lithium (Cibalith-S, Eskalith, Lithane, Lithobid, Lithonate, Lithotabs) is one of the oldest and most frequently prescribed drugs available for the treatment of bipolar mania and depression. Because the drug takes four to ten days to reach a therapeutic level in the bloodstream, it sometimes is prescribed in conjunction with neuroleptics and/or **benzodiazepines** to provide more immediate relief of a manic episode. Lithium also has been shown to be effective in regulating bipolar depression, but is not recommended for mixed mania. Lithium may not be an effective long-term treatment option for rapid cyclers, who typically develop a tolerance for it, or may not respond to it. Possible side effects of the drug include weight gain, thirst, **nausea**, and hand **tremors**. Prolonged lithium use also may cause **hyperthyroidism** (a disease of the thryoid that is marked by heart **palpitations**, nervousness, the presence of **goiter**, sweating, and a wide array of other symptoms.)

- Carbamazepine (Tegretol, Atretol) is an anticonvulsant drug usually prescribed in conjunction with other mood stabilizing agents. The drug often is used to treat bipolar patients who have not responded well to lithium therapy. Blurred vision and abnormal eye movement are two possible side effects of carbamazepine therapy.

- Valproate (divalproex sodium, or Depakote; valproic acid, or Depakene) is one of the few drugs available that has been proven effective in treating rapid cycling bipolar and mixed states patients. Valproate is prescribed alone or in combination with carbamazepine and/or lithium. Stomach cramps, **indigestion**, **diarrhea**, hair loss, appetite loss, nausea, and unusual weight loss or gain are some of the common side effects of valproate. Note: valproate also is approved for the treatment of mania. A 2003 study found that the risk of **death** from **suicide** is about two and one-half times higher in people with bipolar disorder taking divalproex than those taking lithium.

Treating the depression associated with bipolar disorder has proven more challenging. In early 2004, the first drug to treat bipolar administration was approved by the U.S. Food and Drug Administration (FDA). It is called Symbyax, a combination of olanzipine and fluoxetine, the active ingredient in Prozac.

Because antidepressants may stimulate manic episodes in some bipolar patients, their use typically is short-term. **Selective serotonin reuptake inhibitors (SSRIs)** or, less often, **monoamine oxidase inhibitors (MAO inhibitors)** are prescribed for episodes of bipolar depression. **Tricyclic antidepressants** used to treat unipolar depression may trigger rapid cycling in bipolar patients and are, therefore, not a preferred treatment option for bipolar depression.

- SSRIs, such as fluoxetine (Prozac), sertraline (Zoloft), and paroxetine (Paxil), regulate depression by regulating levels of serotonin, a neurotransmitter. **Anxiety**, diarrhea, drowsiness, **headache**, sweating, nausea, sexual problems, and **insomnia** are all possible side effects of SSRIs.

- MAOIs such as tranylcypromine (Parnate) and phenelzine (Nardil) block the action of monoamine oxidase (MAO), an enzyme in the central nervous system. Patients taking MAOIs must cut foods high in tyramine (found in aged cheeses and meats) out of their diet to avoid hypotensive side effects.

- Bupropion (Wellbutrin) is a heterocyclic antidepressant. The exact neurochemical mechanism of the drug is not known, but it has been effective in regulating bipolar depression in some patients. Side effects of bupropion include agitation, anxiety, confusion, tremor, **dry mouth**, fast or irregular heartbeat, headache, and insomnia.

- ECT, or **electroconvulsive therapy**, has a high success rate for treating both unipolar and bipolar depression, and mania. However, because of the convenience of drug treatment and the stigma sometimes attached to ECT therapy, ECT usually is employed after all pharmaceutical treatment options have been explored. ECT is given under anesthesia and patients are given a muscle relaxant medication to prevent convulsions. The treatment consists of a series of electrical pulses that move into the brain through electrodes on the patient's head. Although the exact mechanisms behind the success of ECT therapy are not known, it is believed that this electrical current alters the electrochemical processes of the brain, consequently relieving depression. Headaches, muscle soreness, nausea, and confusion are possible side effects immediately following an ECT procedure. Temporary memory loss has also been reported in ECT patients. In bipolar patients, ECT is often used in conjunction with drug therapy.

Adjunct treatments are used in conjunction with a long-term pharmaceutical treatment plan:

- Long-acting benzodiazepines such as clonazepam (Klonapin) and alprazolam (Xanax) are used for rapid treatment of manic symptoms to calm and sedate patients until mania or hypomania have waned and mood stabilizing agents can take effect. **Sedation** is a common effect, and clumsiness, light-headedness, and slurred speech are other possible side effects of benzodiazepines.

- Neuroleptics such as chlorpromazine (Thorazine) and haloperidol (Haldol) also are used to control mania while a mood stabilizer such as lithium or valproate takes effect. Because neuroleptic side effects can be severe (difficulty in speaking or swallowing, **paralysis** of the eyes, loss of balance control, **muscle spasms**, severe restlessness, stiffness of arms and legs, tremors in fingers and hands, twisting movements of body, and weakness of arms and legs), benzodiazepines are generally preferred over neuroleptics.

- Psychotherapy and counseling. Because bipolar disorder is thought to be biological in nature, therapy is recommended as a companion to, but not a substitute for, pharmaceutical treatment of the disease. Psychotherapy, such as **cognitive-behavioral therapy**, can be a useful tool in helping patients and their families adjust to the disorder, in encouraging compliance to a medication regimen, and in reducing the risk of suicide. Also, educative counseling is recommended for the patient and family. In fact, a 2003 report revealed that people on medication for bipolar disorder had better results if they also participated in family-focused therapy.

Clozapine (Clozaril) is an atypical antipsychotic medication used to control manic episodes in patients who have not responded to typical mood stabilizing agents. The drug has also been a useful prophylactic, or preventative treatment, in some bipolar patients. Common side effects of clozapine include tachycardia (rapid heart rate), hypotension, **constipation**, and weight gain. Agranulocytosis, a potentially serious but reversible condition in which the white blood cells that typically fight infection in the body are destroyed, is a possible side effect of clozapine. Patients treated with the drug should undergo weekly blood tests to monitor white blood cell counts.

Risperidone (Risperdal) is an atypical antipsychotic medication that has been successful in controlling mania when low doses were administered. In early 2004, the FDA approved its use for treating bipolar mania. The side effects of risperidone are mild compared to many other antipsychotics (constipation, coughing, diarrhea, dry mouth, headache, **heartburn**, increased length of sleep and dream activity, nausea, runny nose, **sore throat**, fatigue, and weight gain).

Olanzapine (Zyprexa) is another atypical antipsychotic approved in 2003 for use in combination with lithium or valproate for treatment of acute manic episodes associated with bipolar disorder. Side effects include hypotension (low blood pressure) associated with **dizziness**, rapid heartbeat, and syncope, or low blood pressure to the point of **fainting**.

Lamotrigine (Lamictal, or LTG), an anticonvulsant medication, was found to alleviate manic symptoms in a 1997 trial of 75 bipolar patients. The drug was used in conjunction with divalproex (divalproate) and/or lithium. Possible side effects of lamotrigine include skin rash, dizziness, drowsiness, headache, nausea, and **vomiting**.

Alternative treatment

General recommendations include maintaining a calm environment, avoiding overstimulation, getting plenty of rest, regular **exercise**, and proper diet. Chinese herbs may soften mood swings. **Biofeedback** is effective in helping some patients control symptoms such as irritability, poor self control, racing thoughts, and sleep problems. A diet low in vanadium (a mineral found in meats and other foods) and high in vitamin C may be helpful in reducing depression.

A surprising study in 2004 found that a rarely used combination of magnetic fields used in **magnetic resonance imaging** (MRI) scanning improved the moods of subjects with bipolar disorder. The discovery was made while scientists were using MRI to investigate effectiveness of certain medications. However, they found that a particular type of echo-planar magnetic field led to reports of mood improvement. Further studies may one day lead to a smaller, more convenient use of magnetic treatment.

Prognosis

While most patients will show some positive response to treatment, response varies widely, from full recovery to a complete lack of response to all drug and/or ECT therapy. Drug therapies frequently need adjustment to achieve the maximum benefit for the patient. Bipolar disorder is a chronic recurrent illness in over 90% of those afflicted, and one that requires lifelong observation and treatment after diagnosis. Patients with untreated or inadequately treated bipolar disorder have a suicide rate of 15-25% and a nine-year decrease in life expectancy. With proper treatment, the life expectancy of the bipolar patient will increase by nearly seven years and work productivity increases by ten years.

Prevention

The ongoing medical management of bipolar disorder is critical to preventing relapse, or recurrence, of manic episodes. Even in carefully controlled treatment programs, bipolar patients may experience recurring episodes of the disorder. Patient education in the form of psychotherapy or self-help groups is crucial for training bipolar patients to recognize signs of mania and depression and to take an active part in their treatment program.

Resources

PERIODICALS

"Family-focused Therapy May Reduce Relapse Rate." *Health & Medicine Week* (September 29, 2003): 70.
"FDA Approves Medication for Bipolar Depression." *Drug Week* (January 23, 2004): 320.

"FDA Approves Risperidone for Bipolar Mania." *Psychopharmacology Update* (January 2004): 8.

"Lithium and Risk of Suicide." *The Lancet* (September 20, 2003): 969.

Rossiter, Brian. "Bipolar Disorder." *Med Ad News* (March 2004): 82.

"Schizophrenia and Bipolar Disorder Could Have Similar Genetic Causes." *Genomics & Genetics Weekly* (September 26, 2003): 85.

Sherman, Carl. "Bipolar's Clinical, Financial Impact Widely Missed. (Prevalence May be Greater Than Expected)." *Clinical Psychiatry News* (August 2002): 6.

"Unique Type of MRI Scan Shows Promise in Treating Bipolar Disorder." *AScribe Health News Service* (January 1, 2004).

"Zyprexa." *Formulary* 9 (September 2003): 513.

ORGANIZATIONS

American Psychiatric Association. 1400 K Street NW, Washington DC 20005. (888) 357-7924. <http://www.psych.org>.

National Alliance for the Mentally Ill (NAMI). Colonial Place Three, 2107 Wilson Blvd., Ste. 300, Arlington, VA 22201-3042. (800) 950-6264. <http://www.nami.org>.

National Depressive and Manic-Depressive Association (NDMDA). 730 N. Franklin St., Suite 501, Chicago, IL 60610. (800) 826-3632. <http://www.ndmda.org>.

National Institute of Mental Health. Mental Health Public Inquiries, 5600 Fishers Lane, Room 15C-05, Rockville, MD 20857. (888) 826-9438. <http://www.nimh.nih.gov>.

Paula Anne Ford-Martin
Teresa G. Odle

Bird flu

Definition

Bird flu is an infectious disease caused by strains of the Type A **influenza** viruses that ordinarily only infect birds. Avian influenza A (H5N1) virus infected and caused the deaths of people.

Description

Bird flu, which is also known as avian influenza, was first identified in Italy more than 100 years ago. Avian viruses occur naturally in birds, and can infect birds including chickens, ducks, geese, turkeys, pheasants, quail, and guinea fowl. The avian influenza viruses generally do not infect humans.

Avian viruses are carried around the world by migratory birds. Wild ducks are natural reservoirs of the infection, according to the World Health Organization (WHO). Those wild birds generally don't become ill, but avian flu is extremely contagious and has caused some domesticated birds to become very ill and die. The casualties included chickens, turkeys, and ducks.

Virus suptypes

Reaction to the infection varies among the species because flu viruses are constantly mutating into new strains or subgroups. Low-pathogenic viruses cause few or no symptoms in infected birds. However, some strains can mutate into highly pathogenic avian influenza (HPAI) strains that are extremely infectious and deadly to birds.

The viruses are identified by a series of letters and numbers that refer to two proteins, hemagglutinin (HA) and neuraminidase (NA). There are 16 HA subtypes and nine NA subtypes of influenza A virus. Numerous combinations of the two proteins are possible, and each combination forms a new subtype.

There are 15 different Influenza A subtypes that can infect birds, according to the United States Centers for Disease Control (CDC). In comparison, there are three known subtypes of human flu virus A: H1N1, H1N2, and H3N2. Avian viruses can infect pigs, but people are generally not affected. That changed when there was an outbreak of H5N1 in Hong Kong in 1997.

Deadly outbreaks

The highly pathogenic H5N1 virus was first isolated in terns in South Africa in 1961, and then in Hong Kong in 1997. Hong Kong's avian flu outbreak coincided with 18 cases of severe respiratory disease in people. Those diagnosed with bird flu had close contact with poultry. Six people died, according to WHO. There was "limited transmission" of the virus to health care workers, but they did not become seriously ill.

Medical research showed that the avian virus had jumped from birds to people. Within three days, Hong Kong's poultry population of about 1.5 million birds was destroyed to prevent further infection. There was another H5N1 outbreak in Hong Kong in February of 2003. It affected two members of a family that had recently visited China. One person died, according to the WHO.

In the Netherlands in February of 2003, there was an outbreak of another highly pathogenic avian virus, H7N7. Two months later, a veterinarian died from the virus. It also caused mild illness in 83 people.

In Hong Kong, the avian virus subtype H9N2 caused mild cases of flu in two children in 1999 and one child in the middle of December of 2003, according to WHO. While H9N2 was not highly pathogenic in birds, there was an outbreak of H5N1 in Korea in mid-December of 2003. The next month, there was an outbreak in Vietnam that was followed by outbreaks in other Asian countries.

Human bird flu cases

The World Health Organization tracks bird flu outbreaks and the charts the numbers of human cases that have been confirmed by a laboratory. There were 74 cases and 49 deaths between January of 2004 and March 31, 2005. The flu caused two deaths in Cambodia. In Thailand, 12 of 17 people with bird flu died. In Vietnam, the flu was fatal in 35 of 55 diagnosed cases. Deaths related to the H5N1 viruses have been caused by **pneumonia** and pulmonary complications.

Moreover, the Democratic People's Republic of Korea (North Korea) officially reported the country's first outbreak of avian influenza in poultry on March 27, 2005. Outbreaks occurred at chicken farms, and there were no human cases at that time, according to WHO.

In October 2005, an outbreak of bird flu was reported at a farm near the Mongolian capital of Hohhot in the People's Republic of China. The H5N1 strain of the virus was detected in a parrot located in Britain. The parrot contracted the disease while in quarantine with birds originating in Taiwan. In January 2006, the H5N1 strain was confirmed as the cause of death in at least two cases in Dogubeyazit, Turkey. This case, as well as others documented in countries across Europe, indicate the potential for the disease to spread worldwide.

Preparing for a pandemic

The World Health Organization and nations including the United States are troubled about the deadly consequences that could occur if H5N1 mutated into a new virus subtype that could be transferred from one human to another. That subtype would develop if the avian virus acquired human influenza genes, according to the U.S. Department of Agriculture (USDA). A strain of bird flu spread by human-to-human contact could cause an influenza pandemic.

A pandemic is a worldwide epidemic that is dangerous because people have little or no immunity to the new virus strain. Historically, pandemics occur three to four times during a century when new virus subtypes appear. After World War I, the great influenza pandemic of 1917-1918 caused from 40 to 50 million deaths globally, according to WHO. The flu pandemic of 1968-1969 claimed 1 to 4 million lives.

According to a 2004 WHO report, medical influenza experts agree that another flu pandemic is "inevitable and possibly imminent." In a December 8, 2004 report, WHO warned that the "best case scenario" projection for next pandemic was that the new flu strain would kill from 2 to 7 million people. Moreover, "tens of millions" of people would require medical attention. The appearance of H5N1 signals that the world is moving closer to a pandemic, WHO reported.

The spread of H5N1 to humans increased the likelihood of a new strain emerging that could be transmitted by people. That could create a pandemic. Nations and the World Health Organization are working to prevent a pandemic or cause it to be less deadly. Their strategies include efforts to decrease the spread of flu strains in poultry and the development of vaccines to treat the virus in people.

Causes and symptoms

Avian flu is caused by an influenza virus that birds carry in their intestines. The virus spreads as infected birds excrete saliva, nasal secretions, and feces. Birds vulnerable to the flu become infected when they come into contact with the excretions or surfaces contaminated by the infected matter.

Birds that survive the H5N1 infection can excrete the virus for at least 10 days, according to a WHO report. The strain had proliferated through bird-to-bird contact to flocks on farms and poultry in live bird markets. The virus can also spread in surfaces including manure, bird feed, equipment, vehicles, egg flats, and crates, and the clothing and shoes of people who came into contact with the virus.

A small amount of a highly pathogenic avian influenza virus could be deadly. One gram (0.035 ounces) of contaminated manure could hold enough virus to infect 1 million birds, according to the USDA. From 1997 through the spring of 2005, the viruses primarily infected people in Asia who had contact with infected birds and surfaces.

Bird flu symptoms in people

In early 2005, information about symptoms of H5N1 in humans was based on the 1997 Hong Kong outbreak. People experienced traditional flu symptoms such as a **fever**, **cough**, **sore throat**, and aching muscles. Other symptoms included eye infections (**conjunctivitis**), pneumonia, acute respiratory distress, viral pneumonia, and other severe and life-threatening complications.

Avian flu symptoms in birds

The sudden death of a bird that had not appeared ill is one symptom of the highly pathogenic bird flu. According to the USDA, infected live birds may display one or more of the following symptoms: lack of energy, appetite loss, nasal discharge, coughing, sneezing, a lack of coordination, and **diarrhea**. In addition, the bird may lay fewer eggs or produce eggs that are soft-shelled or misshapen. Furthermore, there may be swelling of the head, eyelids, comb, and wattles. Another symptom is purple discoloration on the combs, wattles, and legs.

If there is an outbreak of the highly pathogenic flu in birds, they are destroyed to prevent the spread of the virus.

Virus mixing vessels

Influenza viruses undergo frequent changes and form new subtypes. In addition, influenza A viruses can trade genetic materials with the viruses of other species. Two different strains trade or merge material, a process known as an antigenic shift. That shift produces a new subtype that is different from the two parent viruses. When the new subtype contains genes from the human virus, a pandemic resulted because there was no immunity to the virus and no vaccine to protect against it.

The genetic shift occurs in a "mixing vessel" that was susceptible to both types of flu. In the past, the shift was thought to be related to people living close to pigs and domestic poultry. Pigs can be infected by avian viruses and mammalian viruses like the human strains, according to WHO. However, research into the H5N1 strain indicates that people can serve as the mixing vessels. As more people become infected with bird flu, the probability increases that humans would serve as the mixing vessel for a new subtype that could be transmitted from one person to another.

Diagnosis

The symptoms of avian flu and human flu are very similar, so laboratory testing is needed to diagnose avian influenza. In addition to diagnosing the individual, testing in 2005 was performed to determine whether the infection was spreading from birds to people or from humans to humans.

Diagnostic tests for human flu are rapid and reliable, according to WHO. The international organization noted that laboratories within WHO's global network have high-security facilities and experienced staff. Test methods include a viral culture that analyses a blood sample and swabbings of the nose or throat. Other testing examines respiratory secretions.

In the United States, the Centers for Disease Control is among the organizations preparing for a possible outbreak of bird flu in humans. In addition to specifics related to diagnosing bird flu, CDC refers healthcare workers to precautions to prevent the spread of flu and other respiratory infections in medical settings.

Precautionary measures include directing people to observe cough etiquette. People with symptoms of respiratory infection should cover their mouths or use facial tissues when coughing or sneezing. After coughing or sneezing, the person should wash their hands with a non-antimicrobial soap and water, alcohol-based hand rub, or antiseptic handwash.

Furthermore, people with flu-like symptoms may be given masks to wear while they are waiting to be examined by medical personnel. The healthcare workers should wear masks in some circumstances. Undoubtedly, they will wear masks when working with people with symptoms of bird flu.

Treatment

As of March of 2005, there was no vaccine to protect people from the H5N1 virus, according to the CDC. However, the U.S. agency and the World Health Organization had isolated seed strains of the virus in order to make a vaccine. Safety tests were scheduled to start in April of 2005 on a vaccine manufactured by Sanofi pasteur, a firm in Swiftwater, Pennsylvania, formerly known as Aventis Pasteur.

On March 23, 2005, the National Institute of Allergy and Infectious Diseases (NIAID) announced that fast-track recruitment had started for volunteers to participate in an investigative study of the vaccine. During the Phase I trial, the trial vaccine will be tested on 450 healthy adults between the ages of 18 to 64, according to NIAID, which is part of the National Institutes of Health.

Studies were to be conducted at University of California at Los Angeles, University of Maryland School of Medicine in Baltimore, and the University of Rochester School of Medicine and Dentistry,

Rochester, New York. If the vaccine is proven safe for adults, there were plans to test it in people in other age groups such as children and the elderly.

Furthermore, research was underway on a vaccine to fight H9N2, another avian flu virus subtype.

Treatment with existing drugs

Existing anti-viral medications may sometimes be effective against avian flu viruses, according to a March 18, 2005, report from CDC. In the United States, four drugs have been approved by the U.S. Food and Drug Administration (FDA) for the treatment and prevention of influenza A viruses.

The medications amantadine (Symmetrel), rimantadine (Flumadine), seltamivir (Tamiflu), and zanamivir (Relenza) were clinically effective in the treatment of influenza A viruses in otherwise healthy adults.

However, avian flu research indicated that the H5N1 virus was resistant to amantadine and rimantadine, according to CCDC. The other two drugs would "probably work," according to CDC. However, studies were needed of the medication's effectiveness.

During the 2004 human flu season in the United States, the Associated Press reported that Relenza cost about $55 for the typical 10-day treatment. Tamiflu cost approximately $66 for the same course of treatment. Insurance frequently covered part of the prescription costs.

For people diagnosed with bird flu, the World Health Organization recommends that patients take Tamiflu twice daily for five days. Treatment should begin as soon as possible. Patients may also receive medication to lower fevers and **antibiotics** to fight secondary infections.

In the spring of 2005, there was no H5N1 vaccine. Countries including the United States were reportedly stockpiling Tamiflu in the event a pandemic erupted. At that time, WHO and CDC recommended the issuing of anti-viral medication as a preventive measure to people working in poultry production. Those people, along with health care workers, would have priority for the medications.

Alternative treatment

In March of 2005, people in South Korea began eating more kimchi to ward off avian flu infection, according to the reports from the British Broadcasting Company and other news organizations. The public turned to the spicy vegetable dish after scientists at

Seoul National University announced that kimchi aided in the recovery of 11 out of 13 infected chickens. The scientists fed the birds an extract of kimchi, a dish made by fermenting cabbage with red peppers, radishes, and large amounts of garlic and ginger. A week later, all but two birds showed signs of recovery.

The researchers acknowledged that their study was unscientific. At that time, they were not sure how or why kimchi was related to the recovery. However, the announcement led people to again regard kimchi as a health remedy. In 2003, interest in kimchi increased when people thought eating it helped prevent **SARS (severe acute respiratory syndrome)**. No scientific confirmation was made between kimchi and SARS prevention.

Prognosis

Bird flu has been fatal to people, and there was concern in 2005 about the virus mutating into a strain that could be transmitted by people. Health organizations and government agencies focused on preventing or reducing the risks of a pandemic caused by bird flu.

In the United States, research was underway on vaccines to fight the flu. Other efforts include the USDA Safety's guidelines for people working with poultry. Strategies included trade restrictions on poultry and poultry products from Asia, according to the USDA. Imported live birds and eggs were quarantined for 30 days. During that time, they were tested for bird flu and exotic Newcastle disease. The United States bans the import of poultry meat from Asia because meat processing plants were not approved by the USDA's Food Safety and Inspection Service.

Prevention

In the spring of 2005, bird flu was primarily a risk for people in the United States who worked with poultry. Potentially vulnerable people included those working with poultry on farms and avian health workers like veterinarians. People working with birds in locations such as commercial poultry facilities, veterinary offices, and live bird markets should wear protective clothing. That equipment includes boots, coveralls, face masks, gloves, and headgear, according to the USDA. If necessary, they should receive anti-viral medications as a safeguard.

Furthermore, poultry producers should implement security measures to prevent the outbreak of a highly pathogenic virus. Those actions include keeping flocks away from wild or migratory birds and providing clothing and disinfectant facilities for employees. Plastic crates should be used at live bird markets because they were easier to clean than wood crates. Cleaning and disinfecting areas were also important for preventing an outbreak.

If necessary birds would be quarantined or destroyed.

Resources

PERIODICALS

Associated Press. "Bird Flu Called Global Human Threat: Asia Outbreak Poses 'Gravest Possible Danger,' U.N. Official Says, Urging Controls." Washington Post. February 24, 2005 [cited March 30, 2005] < http:// www.washingtonpost.com/wp-dyn/articles/A46424-2005Feb23.html >.

ORGANIZATIONS

Centers for Disease Control and Prevention. 1600 Clifton Road, Atlanta, GA 30333. 800-CDC-INFO (232-5636). < http://www.cdc.gov >.

National Institute of Allergy and Infectious Diseases. 6610 Rockledge Drive, MSC 6612, Bethesda, MD 20892-6612. 301-496-5717. < http://www.niaid.nih.gov >.

World Health Organization. Regional Office for the Americas. 525, 23rd Street NW, Washington, DC 20037. 202-974-3000. < http://www.who >.

Highly Pathogenic Avian Influenza. United States Department of Agriculture Animal and Plant Inspection Safety. March 2004 [Cited March 31, 2005]. < http://www.aphis.usda.gov/lpa/pubs/fsheet_faq_notice/fs_ahavianflu.html >.

OTHER

Avian Influenza. World Health Organization. Continuously updated [cited March 31, 2005]. < http://www.who.int/csr/disease/avian_influenza/en/ >.

Avian Flu Index. Centers for Disease Control and Prevention. Continuously updated [cited April 1, 2005]. < http://www.cdc.gov/flu/avian/index.htm >.

Chazan, David. "Korean dish 'may cure bird flu.'" BBC News. March 14, 2005 [cited March 30, 2005]. < http:// news.bbc.co.uk/go/pr/fr/-/2/hi/asia-pacific/4347443.stm >.

Focus on the Flu. National Institute of Allergy and Infectious Diseases. Continuously updated [cited March 31, 2005]. < http://www2.niaid.nih.gov/Newsroom/FocusOn/Flu04/ >.

Liz Swain

Birth control *see* **Diaphragm (birth control); Condom; Contraception**

Birth control pills *see* **Oral contraceptives**

Birth defects

Definition

Birth defects are physical abnormalities that are present at birth; they also are called congenital abnormalities. More than 3,000 have been identified.

Description

Birth defects are found in 2-3% of all newborn infants. This rate doubles in the first year, and reaches 10% by age five, as more defects become evident and can be diagnosed. Almost 20% of deaths in newborns are caused by birth defects.

Abnormalities can occur in any major organ or part of the body. Major defects are structural abnormalities that affect the way a person looks and require medical and/or surgical treatment. Minor defects are abnormalities that do not cause serious health or social problems. When multiple birth defects occur together and have a similar cause, they are called syndromes. If two or more defects tend to appear together but do not share the same cause, they are called associations.

Causes and symptoms

The specific cause of many congenital abnormalities is unknown, but several factors associated with **pregnancy** and delivery can increase the risk of birth defects.

Teratogens

Any substance that can cause abnormal development of the egg in the mother's womb is called a teratogen. In the first two months after conception, the developing organism is called an embryo; developmental stages from two months to birth are called fetal. Growth is rapid, and each body organ has a critical period in which it is especially sensitive to outside influences. About 7% of all congenital defects are caused by exposure to teratogens.

DRUGS. Only a few drugs are known to cause birth defects, but all have the potential to cause harm. For example, in 2003, a study found that use of topical (local) **corticosteroids** in the first trimester of pregnancy may be associated with **cleft lip**. Thalidomide is known to cause defects of the arms and legs; several other types also cause problems.

- Alcohol. Drinking large amounts of alcohol while pregnant causes a cluster of defects called **fetal alcohol syndrome**, which includes **mental retardation**,

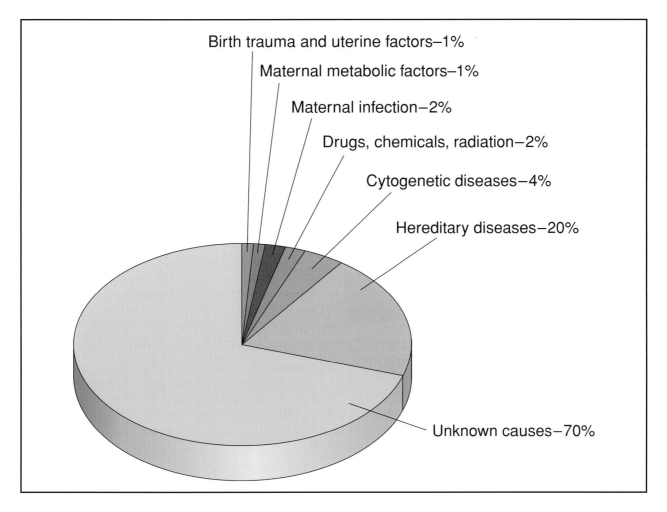

Birth trauma and uterine factors–1%

Maternal metabolic factors–1%

Maternal infection–2%

Drugs, chemicals, radiation–2%

Cytogenetic diseases–4%

Hereditary diseases–20%

Unknown causes–70%

The specific cause of many birth defects is unknown, but several factors associated with pregnancy and delivery can increase the risk of birth defects. These factors include exposure to teratogens, drugs and other chemicals, exposure to radiation, and infections present in the womb. *(Illustration by Electronic Illustrators Group.)*

heart problems, and growth deficiency. In 2004, experts warned that binge drinking early in pregnancy was dangerous even if the woman quit drinking later.

- **Antibiotics**. Certain antibiotics are known tetratogens. Tetracycline affects bone growth and discolors the teeth. Drugs used to treat **tuberculosis** can lead to hearing problems and damage to a nerve in the head (cranial damage).

- Anticonvulsants. Drugs given to prevent seizures can cause serious problems in the developing fetus, including mental retardation and slow growth. Studies in the United Kingdom and Australia have tracked the percentage of birth defects caused by certain antiepileptic drugs.

- Antipsychotic and antianxiety agents. Several drugs given for **anxiety** and mental illness are known to cause specific defects.

- Antineoplastic agents. Drugs given to treat **cancer** can cause major congenital malformations, especially central nervous system defects. They also may be harmful to the health care worker who is giving them while pregnant.

- Hormones. Male hormones may cause masculinization of a female fetus. A synthetic estrogen (DES) given in the 1940s and 1950s caused an increased risk of cancer in the adult female children of the mothers who received the drug.

- Recreational drugs. Drugs such as **LSD** have been associated with arm and leg abnormalities and central nervous system problems in infants. Crack **cocaine** also has been associated with birth defects. Since drug abusers tend to use many drugs and have poor **nutrition** and prenatal care, it is hard to determine the effects of individual drugs.

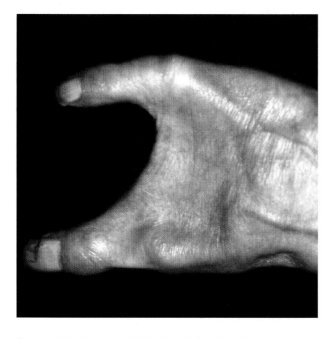

Congenital absence of three fingers. Deformities such as this are usually caused by damage to the developing fetus *in utero.* *(Photograph by Dr. P. Marazzi, Photo Researchers, Inc. Reproduced by permission.)*

CHEMICALS. Environmental chemicals such as fungicides, food additives, and pollutants are suspected of causing birth defects, though this is difficult to prove.

RADIATION. Exposure of the mother to high levels of radiation can cause small skull size (microcephaly), blindness, **spina bifida**, and **cleft palate**. How severe the defect is depends on the duration and timing of the exposure.

INFECTIONS. Three viruses are known to harm a developing baby: **rubella**, cytomegalovirus (CMV), and herpes simplex. *Toxoplasma gondii,* a parasite that can be contracted from undercooked meat, from dirt, or from handling the feces of infected cats, causes serious problems. Untreated **syphilis** in the mother also is harmful.

Genetic factors

A gene is a tiny, invisible unit containing information (DNA) that guides how the body forms and functions. Each individual inherits tens of thousands of genes from each parent, arranged on 46 chromosomes. Genes control all aspects of the body, how it works, and all its unique characteristics, including eye color and body size. Genes are influenced by chemicals and radiation, but sometimes changes in the genes are unexplained accidents. Each child gets half of its

genes from each parent. In each pair of genes one will take precedence (dominant) over the other (recessive) in determining each trait, or characteristic. Birth defects caused by dominant inheritance include a form of dwarfism called **achondroplasia**; **high cholesterol**; Huntington's disease, a progressive nervous system disorder; **Marfan syndrome**, which affects connective tissue; some forms of **glaucoma**, and **polydactyly** (extra fingers or toes).

If both parents carry the same recessive gene, they have a one-in-four chance that the child will inherit the disease. Recessive diseases are severe and may lead to an early **death**. They include sickle cell anemia, a blood disorder that affects blacks, and **Tay-Sachs disease**, which causes mental retardation in people of eastern European Jewish heritage. Two recessive disorders that affect mostly whites are: **cystic fibrosis**, a lung and digestive disorder, and **phenylketonuria** (PKU), a metabolic disorder. If only one parent passes along the genes for the disorder, the normal gene received from the other parent will prevent the disease, but the child will be a carrier. Having the gene is not harmful to the carrier, but there is the 25% chance of the genetic disease showing up in the child of two carriers.

Some disorders are linked to the sex-determining chromosomes passed along by parents. **Hemophilia**, a condition that prevents blood from clotting, and Duchenne **muscular dystrophy**, which causes muscle weakness, are carried on the X chromosome. Genetic defects also can take place when the egg or sperm are forming if the mother or father passes along some faulty gene material. This is more common in older mothers. The most common defect of this kind is **Down syndrome**, a pattern of mental retardation and physical abnormalities, often including heart defects, caused by inheriting three copies of a chromosome rather than the normal pair.

A less understood cause of birth defects results from the interaction of genes from one or both parents plus environmental influences. These defects are thought to include:

- Cleft lip and palate, which are malformations of the mouth.
- Clubfoot, ankle or foot deformities.
- Spina bifida, an open spine caused when the tube that forms the brain and spinal chord does not close properly.
- Water on the brain (**hydrocephalus**), which causes brain damage.
- **Diabetes mellitus**, an abnormality in sugar metabolism that appears later in life.
- Heart defects.
- Some forms of cancer.

A serious illness in the mother, such as an underactive thyroid, or diabetes mellitus, in which her body cannot process sugar, also can cause birth defects in the child. In fact, in 2003, it was shown that babies of diabetic mothers are five times as likely to have structural heart defects as other babies. An abnormal amount of amniotic fluid may indicate or cause birth defects. Amniotic fluid is the liquid that surrounds and protects the unborn child in the uterus. Too little of this fluid can interfere with lung or limb development. Too much amniotic fluid can accumulate if the fetus has a disorder that interferes with swallowing. In 2003, a study linked the mother's weight to risk of birth defects. Obese women were about three times more likely to have an infant with spina bifida or omphalocele (protrusion of part of the intestine through the abdominal wall) than women of average weight. Women who were overweight or classified as obese also were twice as likely to have an infant with a heart defect or multiple birth defects than women classified as average weight.

Diagnosis

If there is a family history of birth defects or if the mother is over 35 years old, then screening tests can be done during pregnancy to gain information about the health of the baby.

- Alpha-fetoprotein test. This is a simple blood test that measures the level of a substance called alpha-fetoprotein that is associated with some major birth defects. An abnormally high or low level may indicate the need for further testing.

- Ultrasound. The use of sound waves to examine the shape, function, and age of the fetus is a common procedure. It also can detect many malformations, such as spina bifida, limb defects, and heart and kidney problems. In 2003, researchers in England announced a new combination of blood tests and ultrasound to detect Down syndrome sooner and more accurately than with the usual blood screenings done at 20 weeks of pregnancy.

- Amniocentesis. This test usually is done between the 13th and 15th weeks of pregnancy. A small sample of amniotic fluid is withdrawn through a thin needle inserted into the mother's abdomen. Chromosomal analysis can rule out Down syndrome and other genetic conditions.

- Chorionic villus sampling (CVS). This test can be done as early as the ninth week of pregnancy to identify chromosome disorders and some genetic conditions. A thin needle is inserted through the abdomen or a slim tube is inserted through the vagina that takes a tiny tissue sample for testing.

If a birth defect is suspected after a baby is born, then confirmation of the diagnosis is very important. The patient's medical records and medical history may hold essential information. A careful **physical examination** and laboratory tests should be done. Special diagnostic tests also can provide genetic information in some cases. In 2003, the March of Dimes, a nonprofit organization, recommended that every baby born in the United States receive, at minimum, screening for the same core group of birth defects including phenylketonuria, **congenital adrenal hyperplasia**, congenital hypothryroidism, biotinidase deficiency, and others. They were concerned that newborn screening varied too much from state to state.

Treatment

Treatment depends on the type of birth defect and how serious it is. When an abnormality has been identified before birth, delivery can be planned at a health care facility that is prepared to offer any special care needed. Some abnormalities can be corrected with surgery. Experimental procedures have been used successfully in correcting some defects, like excessive fluid in the brain (hydrocephalus), even before the baby is born. Early reports have shown success with fetal surgery on spina bifida patients. By operating on these fetuses while still in the womb, surgeons have prevented the need for shunts and improved outcomes at birth for many newborns. However, long-term studies still are needed. Patients with complicated conditions usually need the help of experienced medical and educational specialists with an understanding of the disorder.

Prognosis

The prognosis for a disorder varies with the specific condition.

Prevention

Pregnant women should eat a nutritious diet. Taking **folic acid** supplements before and during pregnancy reduces the risk of having a baby with serious problems of the brain or spinal chord (neural tube defects). It is important to avoid any teratogen that can harm the developing baby, including alcohol and drugs. When there is a family history of congenital defects in either parent, **genetic counseling** and testing can help parents plan for future children. Often, counselors can determine the risk of a genetic condition occurring and the availability of tests for it. Talking to a genetic counselor after a child is born with a defect can provide parents with information about medical management and available community resources.

Resources

PERIODICALS

"Babies of Diabetic Mothers Have Fivefold Increase in Structural Heart Defects." *Diabetes Week* (October 6, 2003): 8.

Bauer, Jeff. "Researchers Link Momós Weight to Babyós Risk of Birth Defects." *RN* (August 2003): 97–102.

"Fetal Alcohol Syndrome Is Still a Threat, Says Publication." *Science Letter* (September 28, 2004): 448.

"Fetal Diagnostic Test Combo Shows Promise." *Health & Medicine Week* (October 27, 2003): 224.

"Fetal Surgery for Spina Bifida Shows Benefits in Leg Function, Fewer Shunts." *Health & Medicine Week* (October 20, 2003): 608.

"March of Dimes Pushes Newborn Screening." *Diagnostics & Imaging Week* (July 31, 2003): 10–11.

"Studies Reveal Risk of Birth Defects from AEDs." *Pharma Marketletter* (September 13, 2004).

"Topical Corticosteroids Use During Pregnancy May Associate With Cleft Lip." *Biotech Week* (September 24, 2003): 190.

ORGANIZATIONS

March of Dimes Birth Defects Foundation. 1275 Mamaroneck Ave., White Plains, NY 10605. (914) 428-7100. resourcecenter@modimes.org. <http://www.modimes.org>.

OTHER

March of Dimes. *Public Health Education Information Sheets.*

Karen Ericson, RN
Teresa G. Odle

▌Birthmarks

Definition

Birthmarks, including angiomas and vascular malformations, are benign (noncancerous) skin growths composed of rapidly growing or poorly formed blood vessels or lymph vessels. Found at birth (congenital) or developing later in life (acquired) anywhere on the body, they range from faint spots to dark swellings covering wide areas.

Description

Skin angiomas, also called vascular (pertaining to vessel) nevi (marks), are composed of blood vessels (hemangiomas) or lymph vessels (lymphangiomas), that lie beneath the skin's surface. Hemangiomas, composed of clusters of cells that line the capillaries, the body's smallest blood vessels, are found on the face and neck (60%), trunk (25%), or the arms and legs (15%). Congenital hemangiomas, 90% of which appear at birth or within the first month of life, grow quickly, and disappear over time. They are found in 1-10% of full-term infants, and 25% of premature infants. About 65% are capillary hemangiomas (strawberry marks), 15% are cavernous (deep) hemangiomas, and the rest are mixtures. Hemangiomas are three times more common in girls. Usually, only one hemangioma is found, in 20% two are found, while fewer than 5% have three or more. Lymphangiomas are skin bumps caused by enlarged lymph vessels anywhere on the body.

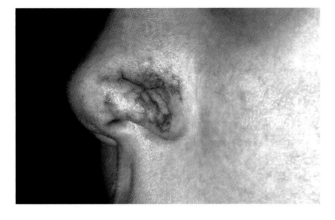

A fading capillary hemangioma on the nose of a child. *(Photograph by Dr. P. Marazzi, Custom Medical Stock Photo. Reproduced by permission.)*

Vascular malformations are poorly formed blood or lymph vessels that appear at birth or later in life. One type, the salmon patch (nevus simplex), a pink mark composed of dilated capillaries, is found on the back of the neck (also called a stork bite) in 40% of newborns, and on the forehead and eyelids (also called an angel's kiss) in 20%. Stork bites are found in 70% of white and 60% of black newborns.

Found in fewer than 1% of newborns, port-wine stains (nevus flammeus), are vascular malformations composed of dilated capillaries in the upper and lower layers of the skin of the face, neck, arms, and legs. Often permanent, these flat pink to red marks develop into dark purple bumpy areas in later life; 85% appear on only one side of the body.

Acquired hemangiomas include spider angiomas (nevus araneus), commonly known as spider veins, and cherry angiomas (senile angiomas or Campbell de Morgan spots). Found around the eyes, cheekbones, arms, and legs, spider angiomas are red marks formed from dilated blood vessels. They occur during **pregnancy** in 70% of white women and 10% of black women, in alcoholics and **liver disease** patients, and in 50% of children. Cherry angiomas, dilated capillaries found mainly on the trunk, appear in the 30s, and multiply with **aging**.

Causes and symptoms

There are no known causes for congenital skin angiomas; they may be related to an inherited weakness of vessel walls. Exposure to estrogen causes spider angiomas in pregnant women or those taking **oral contraceptives**. Spider angiomas tend to run in families, and may be associated with liver disease, sun exposure, and trauma.

Hemangiomas

Hemangiomas first appear as single or multiple, white or pale pink marks, ranging from 2-20 cm (average 2-5 cm) in size. Some are symptomless while others cause **pain** or bleeding, or interfere with normal functioning when they are numerous, enlarged, infected, or ulcerated. Vision is affected by large marks on the eyelids. Spider and cherry angiomas are unsightly but symptomless.

Each type of hemangioma has a characteristic appearance:

• Capillary hemangiomas (strawberry marks). These round, raised marks are bright red and bumpy like a strawberry, and become white or gray when fading.

• Cavernous hemangiomas. These slightly raised, dome-shaped, blue or purple swellings are sometimes associated with lymphangiomas or involve the soft tissues, bone, or digestive tract.

• Spider angiomas. These are symptomless, reddish blue marks formed from blood-filled capillaries radiating around a central arteriole (small artery) in the shape of a spider web.

• Cherry angiomas. These harmless, dilated capillaries appear as tiny, bright red-to-violet colored bumps.

• Lymphangiomas. These dilated lymph vessels form light pink or yellow cysts (fluid-filled sacs) or swellings.

Vascular malformations

These are faint, flat, pink stains that grow as the child grows into larger dark red or purple marks. Some are symptomless but others bleed if enlarged or injured. Disfiguring port-wine stains can cause emotional and social problems. About 5% of port-wine stains on the forehead and eyelids increase eye pressure due to involvement of the eye and surrounding nerves. Abnormalities of the spinal cord, soft tissues, or bone may be associated with severe port-wine stains.

Each type has a characteristic appearance:

- Salmon patches. These symptomless, light red-to-pink marks usually fade with time.

- Port-wine stains. These flat, pink marks progress to raised, dark red-to-purple grape-like lumps distorting the facial features, arms, or legs.

Diagnosis

Patients are treated by pediatricians (doctors who specialize in the care of children), dermatologists (skin disease specialists), plastic surgeons (doctors who specialize in correcting abnormalities of the appearance), and ophthalmologists (eye disease specialists).

Angiomas and vascular malformations are not difficult to diagnose. The doctor takes a complete medical history and performs a **physical examination** including inspection and palpation of the marks. The skin is examined for discoloration, scarring, bleeding, infection, or ulceration. The type, location, size, number, and severity of the marks are recorded. The doctor may empty the mark of blood by gentle pressure. Biopsies or specialized x rays or scans of the abnormal vessels and their surrounding areas may be performed. Patients with port-wine stains near the eye may require **skull x rays**, **computed tomography scans**, and vision and central nervous system tests. Most insurance plans pay for diagnosis and treatment of these conditions.

Treatment

Treatment choices for skin angiomas and vascular malformations depend on their type, location, and severity, and whether they cause symptoms, pain, or disfigurement.

Watchful waiting

No treatment is given, but the mark is regularly examined. This continues until the mark disappears, or requires treatment. This approach is particularly appropriate for the treatment of hemangiomas,

which often do not require treatment, since they eventually shrink by themselves.

Drugs

CORTICOSTEROIDS. Daily doses of the anti-inflammatory drugs prednisone or prednisolone are given for up to 2 months with gradual reduction of the dose. The marks begin to subside within 7-10 days, but may take up to 2 months to fully disappear. If no response is seen in 2 weeks, the drug is discontinued. Treatment may be repeated. Side effects include growth retardation, increased blood pressure and blood sugar, **cataracts**, glandular disorders, and infection. The **corticosteroids** triamcinolone acetate and betamethasone sodium phosphate or acetate are injected directly into the marks with a response usually achieved within a week; additional injections are given in 4-6 weeks. Side effects include tissue damage at the injection site.

INTERFERON ALPHA-2A. This drug reduces cell growth, and is used for vascular marks that affect vision, and that are unresponsive to corticosteroids. Given in daily injections under the skin, a response rate of 50% is achieved after about 7 months. Side effects include **fever**, chills, muscle and joint pain, vision disorders, low white and red blood cell counts, **fatigue**, elevated liver enzymes, **nausea**, blood clotting problems, and nerve damage.

ANTIBIOTICS. Oral or topical (applied to the skin) **antibiotics** are prescribed for infected marks.

Surgery

LASER SURGERY. Lasers create intense heat that destroys abnormal blood vessels beneath the skin, without damaging normal skin. Two types of lasers are used: the flashlamp-pulsed dye laser (FPDL) and the neodymium:YAG (Nd:YAG) laser. The FPDL, used mainly for strawberry marks and port-wine stains, penetrates to a depth of 1.8 mm and causes little scarring, while the Nd:YAG laser penetrates to a depth of 6 mm, and is used to treat deep hemangiomas. **Laser surgery** is not usually painful, but can be uncomfortable. Anesthetic cream is used for FPDL treatment. Treatment with the Nd:YAG laser requires local or **general anesthesia**. Children are usually sedated or anesthetized. Healing occurs within 2 weeks. Side effects include bruising, skin discoloration, swelling, crusting, and minor bleeding.

SURGICAL EXCISION. Under local or general anesthesia, the skin is cut with a surgical instrument, and vascular marks or their **scars** are removed. The cut is repaired with stitches or skin clips.

CRYOSURGERY. Vascular marks are frozen with an extremely cold substance sprayed onto the skin. **Wounds** heal with minimal scarring.

ELECTRODESICCATION. Affected vessels are destroyed with the current from an electric needle.

Other treatments

These include:

- Sclerotherapy. Injection of a special solution causes blood clotting and shrinkage with little scarring. Side effects include stinging, swelling, bruising, scarring, muscle cramping, and allergic reactions. This treatment is used most commonly for spider angiomas.
- Embolization. Material injected into the vessel blocks blood flow which helps control blood loss during or reduces the size of inoperable growths. A serious side effect, **stroke**, can occur if a major blood vessel becomes blocked.
- Make-up. Special brands are designed to cover birthmarks (Covermark or Dermablend).
- Cleaning and compression. Bleeding marks are cleaned with soap and water or hydrogen peroxide, and compressed with a sterile bandage for 5-10 minutes.

Alternative treatment

Alternative treatments for strengthening weak blood vessels include eating high-fiber foods and those containing bioflavonoids, including citrus fruit, blueberries, and cherries, supplementing the diet with vitamin C, and taking the herbs, ginkgo (*Ginkgo biloba*) and bilberry (*Vaccinium myrtillus.*)

Prognosis

The various types of birthmarks have different prognoses:

- Capillary hemangiomas. Fewer than 10% require treatment. Without treatment, 50% disappear by age 5, 70% by age 7, and 90% by age 9. No skin changes are found in half while others have some discoloration, scarring, or wrinkling. From 30-90% respond to oral corticosteroids, and 45% respond to injected corticosteroids; 50% respond to interferon Alpha-2a. About 60% improve after laser surgery.
- Cavernous hemangiomas. Some do not disappear and some are complicated by ulceration or infection. About 75% respond to Nd:YAG laser surgery but have scarring. Severe marks respond to oral corticosteroids, but some require excision.

- Spider angiomas. These fade following **childbirth** and in children, but may recur. About 90% respond to sclerotherapy, electrodesiccation, or laser therapy.
- Cherry angiomas. These are easily removed by electrodesiccation.
- Lymphangiomas. These require surgery.
- Salmon patches. Eyelid marks disappear by 6-12 months of age, and forehead marks fade by age 6; however, 50% of stork bites on the neck persist into adulthood.
- Port-wine stains. Some flat birthmarks are easily covered with make-up. Treatment during infancy or childhood improves results. About 95% of the stains respond to FPDL surgery with minimal scarring; 25% will completely and 70% will partially disappear. For unknown reasons, 5% show no improvement.

Prevention

Congenital hemangiomas or vascular malformations cannot be prevented, but spider angiomas may be prevented by **exercise**, weight control, and a high-fiber diet, as well as avoidance of sun exposure, alcohol drinking, or wearing tight hosiery.

Resources

ORGANIZATIONS

American Academy of Dermatology. 930 N. Meacham Road, P.O. Box 4014, Schaumburg, IL 60168-4014. (847) 330-0230. Fax: (847) 330-0050. < http://www.aad.org > .

American Academy of Pediatrics. 141 Northwest Point Boulevard, Elk Grove Village, IL 60007-1098. (847) 434-4000. < http://www.aap.org > .

Congenital Nevus Support Group. 1400 South Joyce St., Number C-1201, Arlington, VA 22202. (703) 920-3249.

National Congenital Port Wine Stain Foundation. 123 East 63rd St., New York, NY 10021. (516) 867-5137.

Mercedes McLaughlin

Bismuth subsalicylate *see* **Antidiarrheal drugs**

Bites and stings

Definition

Humans can be injured by the bites or stings of many kinds of animals, including mammals such as dogs, cats, and fellow humans; arthropods such as spiders, bees, and wasps; snakes; and marine animals such as jellyfish and stingrays.

Description

Mammals

DOGS. In the United States, where the dog population exceeds 50 million, dogs surpass all other mammals in the number of bites inflicted on humans. However, most dog-bite injuries are minor. A telephone survey of U.S. households conducted in 1994 led researchers to estimate that 3,737,000 dog bites not requiring medical attention occurred in the United States that year, versus 757,000 that required medical treatment. Studies also show that most dog bites are from pets or other dogs known to the bitten person, that males are more likely than females to be bitten, and that children face a greater risk than adults. Each year, about 10-20 Americans, mostly children under 10 years of age, are killed by dogs.

Dog bites result in an estimated 340,000 emergency room visits annually throughout the United States. More than half of the bites seen by emergency departments occur at home. Children under 10 years old, especially boys between 5 and 9 years of age, are more likely than older people to visit an emergency room for bite treatment. Children under 10 years old were also much more liable to be bitten on the face, neck, and head. Nearly all of the injuries suffered by people seeking treatment in emergency rooms were of "low severity," and most were treated and released without being admitted to the hospital or sent to another facility. Many of the bites resulted from people attempting to break up fights between animals.

CATS. Although cats are found in nearly a third of U.S. households, cat bites are far less common than dog bites. According to one study, cats inflict perhaps 400,000 harmful bites in the United States each year. The tissue damage caused by cat bites is usually limited, but they carry a high risk of infection. Whereas the infection rate for dog bite injuries is 15-20%, the infection rate for cat bites is 30-40%.

HUMANS. Bites from mammals other than dogs and cats are uncommon, with one exception—human bites. There are approximately 70,000 human bites each year in the United States. Because the human mouth contains a multitude of potentially harmful microorganisms, human bites are more infectious than those of most other animals.

Arthropods

Arthropods are invertebrates belonging to the phylum Arthropoda, which includes insects, arachnids,

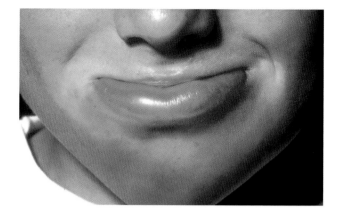

An insect bite caused this person's lower lip to swell. *(Custom Medical Stock Photo. Reproduced by permission.)*

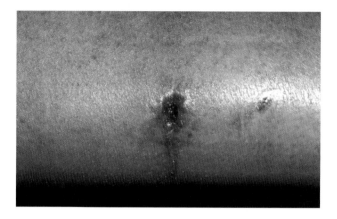

A close-up view of lacerations on the shin of an adult woman inflicted by a Rottweiler dog. *(Custom Medical Stock Photo. Reproduced by permission.)*

crustaceans, and other subgroups. There are more than 700,000 species in all. The list of arthropods that bite or sting humans is extensive and includes lice, bedbugs, fleas, mosquitoes, black flies, ants, chiggers, ticks, centipedes, scorpions, and other species. Spiders, bees, and wasps are the three kinds of arthropod that most often bite people.

SPIDERS. In the United States, only two kinds of venomous spider are truly dangerous: widow spiders and brown (violin or fiddle) spiders. The black widow, which is found in every state but Alaska, is probably the most notorious widow spider. It prefers dark, dry places such as barns, garages, and outhouses, and also lives under rocks and logs. Disturbing a female black widow or its web may provoke a bite. Brown spiders also prefer sheltered places, including clothing, and may bite if disturbed.

BEES AND WASPS. Bees and wasps will sting to defend their nests or if they are disturbed. Species

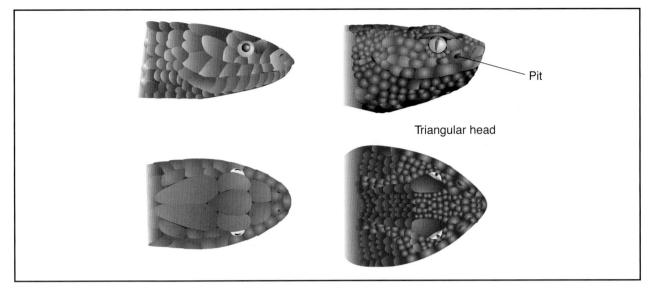

Pit

Triangular head

Profile and top views of typically nonpoisonous and poisonous snakes. Characteristic triangular head and pits on the side of the head are indicative of poisonous pit vipers found in the United States. *(Illustration by Argosy Inc.)*

common to the United States include honeybees, bumblebees, yellow jackets, bald-faced hornets, brown hornets, and paper wasps. Of note are also Africanized bee species, also called "killer bees" that have been found in the United States since 1990. More than 50 Americans die each year after being stung by a bee, wasp, or ant. Almost all of those deaths are the result of allergic reactions, and not of exposure to the venom itself.

Snakes

There are 20 species of venomous snakes in the United States. These snakes are found in every state except Maine, Alaska, and Hawaii. Each year about 8,000 Americans receive a venomous snakebite, but no more than about 15 die, mostly from rattlesnake bites.

The venomous snakes of the United States are divided into two families, the Crotalidae (pit vipers) and the Elapidae. Pit vipers, named after the small heat-sensing pit that lies between each eye and nostril, are responsible for about 99% of the venomous snakebites suffered by Americans. Rattlesnakes, copperheads, and cottonmouths (also called water moccasins) are pit vipers. This family of snakes delivers its venom through two long, hinged fangs in the upper jaw. Some pit vipers carry a potent venom that can threaten the brain and spinal cord. The venom of others, such as the copperheads, is less harmful.

The Elapidae family includes two kinds of venomous coral snakes indigenous to the southern and western states. Because coral snakes are bashful creatures that come out only at night, they almost never

bite humans, and are responsible for approximately 25 bites a year in the United States. Coral snakes also have short fangs and a small mouth, which lowers the risk of a bite actually forcing venom into a person's body. However, their venom is quite poisonous.

Marine animals

Several varieties of marine animal may bite or sting. Jellyfish and stingrays are two kinds that pose a threat to people who live or vacation in coastal communities.

Causes and symptoms

Mammals

DOGS. A typical dog bite results in a laceration, tear, puncture, or crush injury. Bites from large, powerful dogs may even cause **fractures** and dangerous internal injuries. Also, dogs trained to attack may bite repeatedly during a single episode. Infected bites usually cause **pain**, **cellulitis** (inflammation of the connective tissues), and a pus-filled discharge at the wound site within 8-24 hours. Most infections are confined to the wound site, but many of the microorganisms in the mouths of dogs can cause systemic and possibly life-threatening infections. Examples are **bacteremia** and **meningitis**, especially severe in people diagnosed with acquired **immunodeficiency** syndrome (**AIDS**) or other health condition that increases their susceptibility to infection. **Rabies** is rare among pet dogs in the United States, most of which have been vaccinated against the disease. **Tetanus** is also rare but

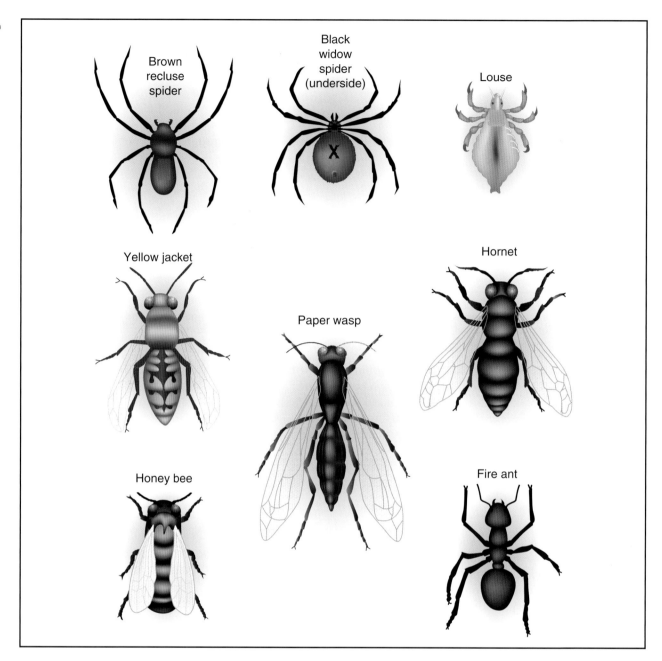

Types of spiders and insects that bite and sting. *(Illustration by Argosy Inc.)*

can be transmitted by a dog bite if the victim is not immunized.

CATS. The mouths of cats and dogs contain many of the same microorganisms. Cat scratches and bites are also capable of transmitting the *Bartonella henselae* bacterium, which can lead to **cat-scratch disease**, an unpleasant but usually not life-threatening illness.

Cat bites are mostly found on the arms and hands. Sharp cat teeth typically leave behind a deep puncture wound that can reach muscles, tendons, and bones,

which are vulnerable to infection because of their comparatively poor blood supply. This is why cat bites are much more likely to become infected than dog bites. Also, people are less inclined to view cat bites as dangerous and requiring immediate attention; the risk that infection has set in by the time a medical professional is consulted is thus greater.

HUMANS. Humans bites result from fights, sexual activity, medical and dental treatment, and seizures. Bites also raise the possibility of spousal or **child abuse**.

KEY TERMS

Anaphylaxis—A life-threatening allergic reaction occurring in persons hypersensitive to bites and stings.

Antibiotics—Substances used against bacteria that cause infection.

Antibodies—Substances created by the body to combat infection.

Antihistamines—Drugs used to treat allergic reactions by acting against a substance called histamine.

Arachnid—Large class of arthropods that includes spiders, scorpions, mites, and ticks. Arachnids have a segmented body divided into two parts, one of which has four pairs of legs but no antennae.

Arachnidism—Poisoning resulting from the bite or sting of an arachnid.

Bacteremia—Bacteria in the blood.

Blood serum—A component of blood.

Immune system—The body system that fights infection and protects the body against foreign invaders and disease.

Killer bees—Hybrids of African bees accidentally introduced into the wild in South and North America in 1956 and first reported in Texas in 1990. They were first imported by Brazilian scientists attempting to create a new hybrid bee to improve honey production.

Lymph nodes—Small, kidney-shaped organs that filter a fluid called lymph and that are part of the body's immune system.

Pus—A thick yellowish or greenish fluid composed of the remains of dead white blood cells, pathogens and decomposed cellular debris.

Children often bite other children, but those bites are hardly ever severe. Human bites are capable of transmitting a wide range of dangerous diseases, including **hepatitis B**, **syphilis**, and **tuberculosis**.

Human bites fall into two categories: occlusional (true) bites and clenched-fist injuries. The former present a lower risk of infection. The latter, which are very infectious and can permanently damage the hand, usually result from a fist hitting teeth during a fight. People often wait before seeking treatment for a clenched-fist injury, with the result that about half of such injuries are infected by the time they are seen by a medical professional.

Arthropods

SPIDERS. As a rule, people rarely see a black widow bite, nor do they feel the bite as it occurs. The first (and possibly only) evidence that a person has been bitten may be a mild swelling of the injured area and two red puncture marks. Within a short time, however, some victims begin to experience severe **muscle cramps** and rigidity of the abdominal muscles. Other possible symptoms include excessive sweating, **nausea**, **vomiting**, headaches, and vertigo as well as breathing, vision, and speech problems.

A brown spider's bite can lead to necrotic arachnidism, in which the tissue in an area of up to several inches around the bite becomes necrotic (dies), producing an open sore that can take months or years to disappear. In most cases, however, the bite simply produces a hard, painful, itchy, and discolored area that heals without treatment in 2-3 days. The bite may also be accompanied by a **fever**, chills, **edema** (an accumulation of excess tissue fluid), **nausea and vomiting**, **dizziness**, muscle and joint pain, and a rash.

BEES AND WASPS. The familiar symptoms of bee and wasp stings include pain, redness, swelling, and itchiness in the area of the sting. Multiple stings can have much more severe consequences, such as **anaphylaxis**, a life-threatening allergic reaction that occurs in hypersensitive persons.

Snakes

Venomous pit viper bites usually begin to swell within 10 minutes and sometimes are painful. Other symptoms include skin blisters and discoloration, weakness, sweating, nausea, faintness, dizziness, bruising, and tender lymph nodes. Severe **poisoning** can also lead to **tingling** in the scalp, fingers, and toes, muscle contractions, an elevated heart rate, rapid breathing, large drops in body temperature and blood pressure, vomiting of blood, and **coma**.

Many pit viper and coral snake bites (20-60%) fail to poison (envenomate) their victim, or introduce only a small amount of venom into the victim's body. The **wounds**, however, can still become infected by the harmful microorganisms that snakes carry in their mouths.

Coral snake bites are painful but may be hard to see. One to seven hours after the bite, a bitten person begins to experience the effects of the venom, which include tingling at the wound site, weakness, nausea, vomiting, excessive salivation, and irrational behavior. Major nerves of the body can become paralyzed for 6-14 days, causing double vision, difficulty swallowing and speaking, **respiratory failure**, and other problems. Six to eight weeks may be needed before normal muscular strength is regained.

Marine animals

JELLYFISH. Jellyfish venom is delivered by barbs called nematocysts, which are located on the creature's tentacles and penetrate the skin of people who brush up against them. Instantly painful and itchy red lesions usually result. The pain can continue up to 48 hours. Severe cases may lead to skin necrosis, **muscle spasms and cramps**, vomiting, nausea, **diarrhea**, headaches, excessive sweating, and other symptoms. In rare instances, cardiorespiratory failure may also occur.

STINGRAYS. Tail spines are the delivery mechanism for stingray venom. Deep puncture wounds result that can cause an infection if pieces of spine become embedded in the wound. A typical stingray injury scenario involves a person who inadvertently steps on a resting stingray and is lashed in the ankle by its tail. Stingray venom produces immediate, excruciating pain that lasts several hours. Sometimes the victim suffers a severe reaction, including vomiting, diarrhea, hemorrhage (bleeding), a drop in blood pressure, and cardiac arrhythmia (disordered heart beat).

Diagnosis

Mammals

DOGS. Gathering information on the circumstances of a dog attack is a crucial part of treatment. Medical professionals need to know when the attack occurred (the chances of infection increase dramatically if the wound has been left untreated for more than eight hours) and what led to the attack (unprovoked attacks are more likely to be associated with rabies). A person's general health must also be assessed, including the tetanus immunization history if any, as well as information concerning possible **allergies** to medication and pre-existing health problems that may increase the risk of infection.

A **physical examination** requires careful scrutiny of the wound, with special attention to possible bone, joint, ligament, muscle, tendon, nerve, or blood-vessel damage caused by deep punctures or severe crush injuries. Serious hand injuries should be evaluated by a specialized surgeon. Most of the time, laboratory tests for identifying the microorganisms in bite wounds are performed if infection is present. X rays and other diagnostic procedures may also be necessary.

CATS. The diagnostic procedures used for dog bites also apply to cat bites.

HUMANS. Testing the blood of a person who has been bitten for immunity to hepatitis B and other diseases is always necessary after a human bite. Ideally, the biter should be tested as well for the presence of transmissible disease. Clenched-fist injuries often require evaluation by a hand surgeon or orthopedist. Because many people will deny having been in a fight, medical professionals usually consider lacerations over the fourth and fifth knuckles—the typical result of a clenched-fist injury—to be evidence of a bite wound. Medical professionals also look for indications of spousal or child **abuse** when evaluating human bites.

Arthropods

SPIDERS. Because bites from widow spiders and brown spiders require different treatments, capturing and identifying the spider helps to establish diagnosis.

Snakes

Diagnosis relies on a physical examination of the victim, information about the circumstances of the bite, and a look at the snake itself (if it can safely be killed and brought in for identification). Blood tests and **urinalysis** supply important data on the victim's condition. Chest x-rays and **electrocardiography** (a procedure for measuring heart activity) may also be necessary.

Treatment

Mammals

DOGS. Minor dog bites can be treated at home. The American Academy of Family Physicians recommends gently washing the wound with soap and water and then applying pressure to the injured area with a clean towel to stop the bleeding. The next step is to apply antibiotic ointment and a sterile bandage to the wound. To reduce swelling and fend off infection, ice should be applied and the injured area kept elevated above the level of the heart. The wound should be cleaned and covered with ointment twice a day until it heals.

Any dog bite that does not stop bleeding after 15 minutes of pressure must be seen by a medical professional. The same is true for bites that are deep or gaping; for bites to the head, hands, or feet; and for bites that may have broken a bone, damaged nerves, or caused a major injury of another kind. Bite victims must also watch for infection. A fever is one sign of infection, as are redness, swelling, warmth, increased tenderness, and pus at the wound site. Diabetics, people with AIDS or **cancer**, individuals who have not had a tetanus shot in five years, and anyone else who has a medical problem that can increase susceptibility to infection should seek medical treatment no matter how minor the bite appears.

Medical treatment of dog bites involves washing the wound with an anti-infective solution. Removal of dead and damaged tissue (under local, regional, or general anesthetic) may be required after the wound has been washed, and any person whose tetanus shots are not up to date should receive a booster injection. Some wounds are left open and allowed to heal on their own, while others require stitches (stitching may be delayed a few days if infection is a concern). Many emergency departments prescribe **antibiotics** for all people with dog bites, but some researchers suggest that antibiotics are usually unnecessary and should be limited to those whose injuries or other health problems make them likely candidates for infection. A follow-up visit after one or two days is generally required for anyone who has received bite treatment.

CATS. Because of the high risk of infection, people who are bitten by a cat should always see a doctor. Cat scratches do not require professional medical treatment unless the wound appears infected or the scratched person has a weakened immune system.

Medical treatment for cat bites generally follows the procedures used for dog bites. Experts advise, however, that cat-bite wounds should always be left open to prevent infection. Persons who have been bitten by cats generally receive antibiotics as a preventive measure.

HUMANS. Human bites should always be examined by a doctor. Such bites are usually treated with antibiotics and left open because of the high risk of infection. A study released in June 2004 showed that routine use of antibiotics for human bites may not be necessary, as physicians try to minimize overuse of antibiotics. Superficial wounds in low-risk areas may no longer need antibiotic treatment, but more serious human bites to high-risk areas such as the hands should be treated with antibiotics to prevent serious infection. A person who has been bitten may also require immunization against hepatitis B and other diseases. Persons who are being treated for a clenched-fist injury will require a daily follow-up examination for 3-5 days.

Arthropods

SPIDERS. No spider bite should be ignored. The antidote for severe widow spider bites is a substance called antivenin, which contains antibodies taken from the blood serum of horses injected with spider venom. Doctors **exercise** caution in using antivenin, however, because it can trigger anaphylactic **shock**, a potentially deadly (though treatable) allergic reaction, and **serum sickness**, an inflammatory response that can give rise to joint pain, a fever, **rashes**, and other unpleasant, though rarely serious, consequences.

An antivenin for brown spider bites exists as well, but it is not yet available in the United States. The drug dapsone, used to treat **leprosy**, can sometimes stop the tissue **death** associated with a brown spider bite. Necrotic areas may need **debridement** (removal of dead and damaged tissue) and skin grafts. Pain medications, **antihistamines**, antibiotics, and tetanus shots are a few of the other treatments that are sometimes necessary after a bite from a brown spider or widow spider.

BEES AND WASPS. Most stings can be treated at home. A stinger that is stuck in the skin can be scraped off with a blade, fingernail, credit card, or piece of paper (using tweezers may push more venom out of the venom sac and into the wound). The area should be cleaned and covered with an ice pack. **Aspirin** and other pain medications, oral antihistamines, and calamine lotion are good for treating minor symptoms. Putting meat tenderizer on the wound has no effect.

Persons who have been stung and experience an allergic reaction, or who are at risk due to their medical history, require immediate medical attention. The danger signs, which usually begin 10 minutes after an individual is stung (though possibly not for several hours), include nausea, faintness, chest pain, abdominal cramps, diarrhea, and difficulty swallowing or breathing.

Snakes

Although most snakes are not venomous, any snakebite should immediately be examined at a hospital. While waiting for emergency help to arrive, the victim should wash the wound site with soap and water, and then keep the injured area still and at a level lower than the heart. Ice should never be used on the wound site nor should attempts be made to suck out the venom. Making a cut at the wound site is also dangerous. It is important to stay calm and wait for emergency medical aid if it can arrive quickly. Otherwise, the victim should proceed directly to a hospital.

When the victim arrives at a hospital, the medical staff must determine whether the bite was inflicted by a venomous snake and, if so, whether envenomation occurred and how much venom the person has received. Patients may develop low blood pressure, abnormal blood clotting, or severe pain, all of which require aggressive treatment. Fortunately, the effects of some snakebites can be counteracted with antivenin. Minor rattlesnake envenomations can be successfully treated without antivenin, as can copper-head and water-moccasin bites. However, coral snake envenomations and the more dangerous rattlesnake envenomations require antivenin, sometimes in large amounts. Other treatment measures include antibiotics to prevent infection and a tetanus booster injection.

Marine animals

JELLYFISH. Vinegar and other acidic substances are used to neutralize jellyfish nematocysts still clinging to the skin, which are then scraped off. Anesthetic ointments, antihistamine creams, and steroid lotions applied to the skin are sometimes beneficial. Other measures may be necessary to counter the many harmful effects of jellyfish stings, which, if severe, require emergency medical care.

STINGRAYS. Stingray wounds should be washed with saltwater and then soaked in very hot water for 30-90 minutes to neutralize the venom. Afterwards, the wound should be examined by a doctor to ensure that no pieces of spine remain.

Alternative treatment

Arthropods

Several alternative self-care approaches are used to treat minor bee, wasp, and other arthropod stings, including **aromatherapy**, **ayurvedic medicine**, **flower remedies**, herbs, homeopathy, and nutritional therapy.

Prognosis

Mammals

Prompt treatment and recognizing that even apparently minor bites can have serious consequences are the keys to a good outcome after a mammal bite. Infected bites can be fatal if neglected. Surgery and hospitalization may be needed for severe bites.

Arthropods

SPIDERS. Even without treatment, adults usually recover from black widow bites after 2-3 days. Those most at risk of dying are very young children, the elderly, and people with high blood pressure. In the case of brown spider bites, the risk of death is greatest for children, though rare.

BEES AND WASPS. The pain and other symptoms of a bee or wasp sting normally fade away after a few hours. People who are allergic to such stings, however,

can experience severe and occasionally fatal anaphylaxis.

Snakes

A snakebite victim's chances of survival are excellent if medical aid is obtained in time. Some bites, however, result in **amputation**, permanent deformity, or loss of function in the injured area.

Marine animals

STINGRAYS. Stingray venom kills its human victims on rare occasions.

Prevention

Mammals

DOGS. The risk of a dog bite injury can be reduced by avoiding sick or stray dogs, staying away from dogfights (people often get bitten when they try to separate the animals), and not behaving in ways that might provoke or upset dogs, such as wrestling with them or bothering them while they are sleeping, eating, or looking after their puppies. Special precautions need to be taken around infants and young children, who must never be left alone with a dog. Pit bulls, rottweilers, and German shepherds (responsible for nearly half of all fatal dog attacks in the United States in 1997-2000) are potentially dangerous pets in households where children live or visit. For all breeds of dog, obedience training as well as spaying or neutering lessen the chances of aggressive behavior.

CATS. Prevention involves warning children to stay away from strange cats and to avoid rough play and other behavior that can anger cats and cause them to bite.

Arthropods

SPIDERS. Common-sense precautions include clearing webs out of garages, outhouses, and other places favored by venomous spiders; keeping one's hands away from places where spiders may be lurking; and, when camping or vacationing, checking clothing, shoes, and sleeping areas.

BEES AND WASPS. When possible, it is advised to avoid the nests of bees and wasps and to not eat sweet food or wear bright clothing, perfumes, or cosmetics that attract bees and wasps.

Emergency medical kits containing self-administrable epinephrine to counter anaphylactic shock are available for allergic people and should be carried by them at all times. People who suspect they are allergic should consult an allergist about shots that can reduce reactions to bee and wasp venom.

Snakes

Snakes should not be kept as pets. Measures such as mowing the lawn, keeping hedges trimmed, and removing brush from the yard also discourages snakes from living close to human dwellings. Tongs should be used to move brush, lumber, and firewood, to avoid exposing one's hands to snakes that might be lying underneath. Similarly, golfers should never use their hands to retrieve golf balls from a water hole, since snakes can be hiding in the rocks and weeds. Caution is also necessary when walking through weedy or grassy areas, and children should be prevented from playing in weedy, vacant lots and other places where snakes may live. Leather boots and long pants offer hikers and campers some protection from bites. Approaching a snake, even a dead one, can be dangerous, for the venom of recently killed snakes may still be active.

Marine animals

JELLYFISH. Prevention of jellyfish stings includes obeying posted warning signs at the beach. Also, jellyfish tentacles may be transparent and up to 120 ft (36.5 m) long, therefore great caution must be exercised whenever a jellyfish is sighted nearby. An over-the-counter cream was being tested at the Stanford University School of Medicine in the summer of 2004. In early tests, it was effective in helping to prevent some jellyfish contact.

STINGRAYS. Shuffling while walking through shallow areas that may be inhabited by stingrays will disturb the water, causing the animal to move before it can be stepped on.

Resources

BOOKS

Holve, Steve. "Envenomations." In *Cecil Textbook of Medicine,* edited by Lee Goldman and J. Claude Bennett, 21st ed. Philadelphia: W. B. Saunders, 2000, pp. 2174-2178.

Sutherland, Struan, and Tibballs, James. *Australian Animal Toxins.* 2nd ed. New York, Oxford Univ Press, 2001.

PERIODICALS

"Cream May Ward Off Jellyfish." *Drug Week* (June 25, 2004): 553.

"Do All Human Bite Wounds Need Antibiotics?" *Emergency Medicine Alert* (June 2004): 3.

Graudins, A., M. Padula, K. Broady, and G. M. Nicholson. "Red-back spider (Latrodectus hasselti) antivenom prevents the toxicity of widow spider venoms." *Annals of Emergency Medicine* 37, no. 2 (2001): 154-160.

Jarvis R. M., M. V. Neufeld, and C. T. Westfall. "Brown recluse spider bite to the eyelid." *Ophthalmology* 107, no. 8 (2000): 1492-1496.

Metry, D. W., and A. A. Hebert. "Insect and arachnid stings, bites, infestations, and repellents." *Pediatric Annals* 29, no. 1 (2000): 39-48.

Sams, H. H., C. A. Dunnick, M. L. Smith, and L. E. King. "Necrotic arachnidism." *Journal of the American Academy of Dermatology* 44, no. 4 (2001): 561-573.

Sams, HH. "Nineteen documented cases of Loxosceles reclusa envenomation." *Journal of the American Academy of Dermatology* 44, no.4 (2001): 603-608.

ORGANIZATIONS

American Academy of Emergency Medicine. 611 East Wells Street, Milwaukee, WI 53202. (800) 884-2236. Fax: (414) 276-3349. < http://www.aaem.org/ > .

American Academy of Family Physicians. 11400 Tomahawk Creek Parkway, Leawood, KS 66211-2672. (913) 906-6000. < http://www.aafp.org/ > . fp@aafp.org.

American Medical Association. 515 N. State Street, Chicago, IL 60610. (312) 464-5000. < http://www.ama-assn.org/ > .

OTHER

City of Phoenix, Arizona. < http://www.ci.phoenix.az.us/ FIRE/bitessna.html > .

Southwestern University School of Medicine. < http:// www.swmed.edu/toxicology/toxlinks.html > .

Toxicology Professional Groups. < http://www.pitt.edu/ ~martint/pages/motoxorg.htm#AAPCC > .

University of Sydney, Australia. < http://www.usyd.edu.au/ su/anaes/spiders.html > .

Vanderbilt University. < http://www.mc.vanderbilt.edu/ clintox/ > .

L. Fleming Fallon Jr., MD, PhD
Teresa G. Odle

Black death *see* **Plague**

Black lung disease

Definition

Black lung disease is the common name for coal workers' pneumoconiosis (CWP) or anthracosis, a lung disease of older workers in the coal industry, caused by inhalation, over many years, of small amounts of coal dust.

Description

The risk of having black lung disease is directly related to the amount of dust inhaled over the

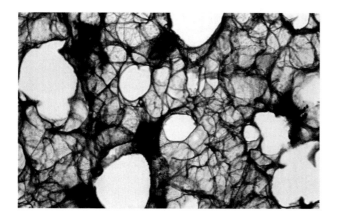

A light micrograph of a human lung containing particles of inspired coal dust (anthracosis). The black masses shown are groups of coal dust particles. *(Photograph by Astrid & Hanns-Frieder Michler, Photo Researchers, Inc. Reproduced by permission.)*

years; the disease typically affects workers over age 50. Its common name comes from the fact that the inhalation of heavy deposits of coal dust makes miners lungs look black instead of a healthy pink. Although people who live in cities often have some black deposits in their lungs from polluted air, coal miners have much more extensive deposits.

In the years since the federal government has regulated dust levels in coal mines, the number of cases of black lung disease has fallen sharply. Since the Federal Coal Mine Health and Safety Act of 1969, average dust levels have fallen from 8.0 mg. per cubic meter to the current standard of 2.0 mg. per cubic meter. The 1969 law also set up a black lung disability benefits program to compensate coal miners who have been disabled by on-the-job dust exposure.

Despite the technology available to control the hazard, however, miners still run the risk of developing this lung disease. The risk is much lower today, however; fewer than 10% of coal miners have any x ray evidence of coal dust deposits. When there is such evidence, it often shows up as only small black spots less than 0.4 in (1 cm). in diameter, and may have been caused by **smoking** rather than coal dust. This condition is called "simple CWP" and does not lead to symptoms or disability.

Causes and symptoms

Since the particles of fine coal dust, which a miner breathes when he is in the mines, cannot be destroyed within the lungs or removed from them, builds up. Eventually, this build-up causes thickening and scarring, making the lungs less efficient in supplying oxygen to the blood.

The primary symptom of the disease is **shortness of breath**, which gradually gets worse as the disease progresses. In severe cases, the patient may develop **cor pulmonale**, an enlargement and strain of the right side of the heart caused by chronic lung disease. This may eventually cause right-sided **heart failure**.

Some patients develop **emphysema** (a disease in which the tiny air sacs in the lungs become damaged, leading to shortness of breath, and respiratory and heart failure) as a complication of black lung disease. Others develop a severe type of black lung disease called progressive massive fibrosis, in which damage continues in the upper parts of the lungs even after exposure to the dust has ended. Scientists aren't sure what causes this serious complication. Some think that it may be due to the breathing of a mixture of coal and silica dust that is found in certain mines. Silica is far more likely to lead to scarring than coal dust alone.

Diagnosis

Black lung disease can be diagnosed by checking a patient's history for exposure to coal dust, followed by a chest x-ray to discover if the characteristic spots in the lungs caused by coal dust are present. A **pulmonary function test** may aid in diagnosis.

X rays can detect black lung disease before it causes any symptoms. If exposure to the dust is stopped at that point, progression of the disease may be prevented.

Treatment

There is no treatment or cure for this condition, although it is possible to treat complications such as lung infections and cor pulmonale. Further exposure to coal dust must be stopped.

Prognosis

Those miners with simple CWP can lead a normal life. However, patients who develop black lung disease at an early age, or who have progressive massive fibrosis, have a higher risk of premature **death**.

Prevention

The only way to prevent black lung disease is to avoid long-term exposure to coal dust. Coal mines may help prevent the condition by lowering coal dust levels and providing protective clothes to coal miners.

A light micrograph of a human lung containing particles of inspired coal dust (anthracosis). The black masses shown are groups of coal dust particles.

Resources

ORGANIZATIONS

Mine Safety and Health Administration. 4015 Wilson Blvd. Arlington, VA 22203. (703) 235-1910. < http:// www.msha.gov > .

Carol A. Turkington

Bladder calculi *see* **Bladder stones**

Bladder cancer

Definition

Bladder **cancer** is a disease in which the cells lining the urinary bladder lose the ability to regulate their growth and start dividing uncontrollably. This abnormal growth results in a mass of cells that form a tumor.

Description

Bladder cancer is the sixth most common cancer in the United States. The American Cancer Society (ACS) estimated that in 2001, approximately 54,300 new cases of bladder cancer would be diagnosed (about 39,200 men and 15,100 women), causing approximately 12,400 deaths. The rates for men of African descent and Hispanic men are similar and are approximately one-half of the rate among white non-Hispanic men. The lowest rate of bladder cancer occurs in the Asian population. Among women, the highest rates also occur in white non-Hispanic females and are approximately twice the rate for Hispanics. Women of African descent have higher rates of bladder cancer than Hispanic women.

The urinary bladder is a hollow muscular organ that stores urine from the kidneys until it is excreted out of the body. Two tubes called the ureters bring the urine from the kidneys to the bladder. The urethra carries the urine from the bladder to the outside of the body.

Bladder cancer has a very high rate of recurrence. Even after superficial tumors are completely removed, there is a 75% chance that new tumors will develop in other areas of the bladder. Hence, patients need frequent and thorough follow-up care.

Causes and symptoms

Although the exact cause of bladder cancer is not known, smokers are twice as likely as nonsmokers to get the disease. Hence, **smoking** is considered the greatest risk factor for bladder cancer. Workers who are exposed to certain chemicals used in the dye industry and in the rubber, leather, textile, and paint industries are believed to be at a higher risk for bladder cancer. The disease also is three times more common in men than in women; caucasians also are at an increased risk. The risk of bladder cancer increases with age. Most cases are found in people who are 50–70 years old. In 2003, studies showed that **hormone replacement therapy** (HRT), a treatment used by many postmenopausal women, significantly increased the risk of bladder and other cancers.

Frequent urinary infections, kidney and **bladder stones**, and other conditions that cause long-term irritation to the bladder may increase the risk of getting bladder cancer. A past history of tumors in the bladder also could increase one's risk of getting other tumors.

One of the first warning signals of bladder cancer is blood in the urine. Sometimes, there is enough blood to change the color of the urine to a yellow-red or a dark red. At other times, the color of the urine appears normal but chemical testing of the urine reveals the presence of blood cells. A change in bladder habits such as painful urination, increased frequency of urination and a feeling of needing to urinate but not being able to do so are some of the signs of possible

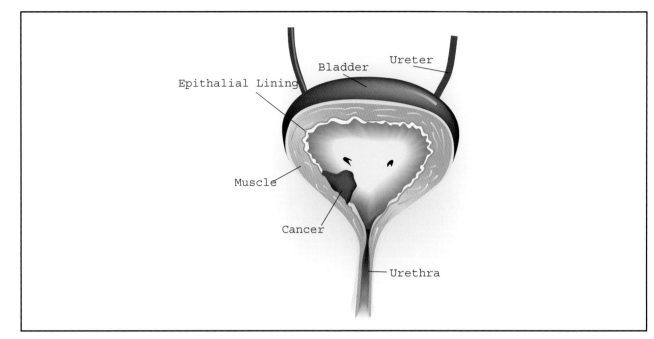

Bladder cancer on the inner lining of the bladder. *(Illustration by Argosy Inc.)*

bladder cancer. All of these symptoms also may be caused by conditions other than cancer, but it is important to see a doctor and have the symptoms evaluated. When detected early and treated appropriately, patients have a very good chance of being cured completely.

Diagnosis

If a doctor has any reason to suspect bladder cancer, several tests can help find out if the disease is present. As a first step, a complete medical history will be taken to check for any risk factors. A thorough **physical examination** will be conducted to assess all the signs and symptoms. Laboratory testing of a urine sample will help to rule out the presence of a bacterial infection. In a urine cytology test, the urine is examined under a microscope to look for any abnormal or cancerous cells. A catheter (tube) can be advanced into the bladder through the urethra, and a salt solution is passed through it to wash the bladder. The solution can then be collected and examined under a microscope to check for the presence of cancerous cells.

A test known as the intravenous pyelogram (IVP) is an x–ray examination that is done after a dye is injected into the blood stream through a vein in the arm. The dye travels through the blood stream and then reaches the kidneys to be excreted. It clearly outlines the kidneys, ureters, bladder, and urethra. Multiple x rays are taken to detect any abnormality in the lining of these organs.

The physician may use a procedure known as a cystoscopy to view the inside of the bladder. A thin hollow lighted tube is introduced into the bladder through the urethra. If any suspicious looking masses are seen, a small piece of the tissue can be removed from it using a pair of biopsy forceps. The tissue is then examined microscopically to verify if cancer is present, and if so, to identify the type of cancer.

If cancer is detected and there is evidence to indicate that it has metastasized (spread) to distant sites in the body, imaging tests such as chest x rays, computed tomography scans (CT), and magnetic resonance imaging (MRI) may be done to determine which organs are affected. Bladder cancer generally tends to spread to the lungs, liver, and bone.

Treatment

Treatment for bladder cancer depends on the stage of the tumor. The patient's medical history, overall health status, and personal preferences also are taken into account when deciding on an appropriate treatment plan. The three standard modes of treatment available for bladder cancer are surgery, **radiation therapy**, and **chemotherapy**. In addition, newer treatment methods such as photodynamic therapy and immunotherapy also are being investigated in clinical trials.

Surgery is considered an option only when the disease is in its early stages. If the tumor is localized to a

Biopsy—The surgical removal and microscopic examination of living tissue for diagnostic purposes.

Chemotherapy—Treatment with anticancer drugs.

Computed tomography (CT) scan—A medical procedure where a series of x rays are taken and put together by a computer in order to form detailed pictures of areas inside the body.

Cystoscopy—A diagnostic procedure where a hollow lighted tube, (cystoscope) is used to look inside the bladder and the urethra.

Electrofulguration—A procedure where a high-energy laser beam is used to burn the cancerous tissue.

Immunotherapy—Treatment of cancer by stimulating the body's immune defense system.

Intravenous pyelogram (IVP)—A procedure where a dye is injected into a vein in the arm. The dye travels through the body and then concentrates in the urine to be excreted. It outlines the kidneys, ureters, and the urinary bladder. An x ray of the pelvic region is then taken and any abnormalities of the urinary tract are revealed.

Magnetic Resonance Imaging (MRI)—A medical procedure used for diagnostic purposes where pictures of areas inside the body can be created using a magnet linked to a computer.

Partial cystectomy—A surgical procedure where the cancerous tissue is removed by cutting out a small piece of the bladder.

Photodynamic therapy—A novel mode of treatment that uses a combination of special light rays and drugs are used to destroy the cancerous cells. First, the drugs, which make cancerous cells more susceptible to the light rays, are introduced into the bladder. Then the light is shone on the bladder to kill the cells.

Radiation therapy—Treatment using high-energy radiation from x-ray machines, cobalt, radium, or other sources.

Radical cystectomy—A surgical procedure that is used when the cancer is in more than one area of the bladder. Along with the bladder, the adjoining organs also are removed. In men, the prostate is removed, while in women, the ovaries, fallopian tubes and uterus may be removed.

Stoma—An artificial opening between two cavities or between a cavity and the surface of the body.

Transurethral resection—A surgical procedure to remove abnormal tissue from the bladder. The technique involves the insertion of an instrument called a cytoscope into the bladder through the urethra, and the tumor is removed through it.

Urostomy—A surgical procedure consisting of cutting the ureters from the bladder and connecting them to an opening (see stoma) on the abdomen, allowing urine to flow into a collection bag.

small area and has not spread to the inner layers of the bladder, then the surgery is done without cutting open the abdomen. A cytoscope is introduced into the bladder through the urethra, and the tumor is removed through it. This procedure is called a transurethral resection (TUR). Passing a high-energy laser beam through the cytoscope and burning the cancer may treat any remaining cancer. This procedure is known as electrofulguration. If the cancer has invaded the walls of the bladder, surgery will be done through an incision in the abdomen. Cancer that is not very large can be removed by partial **cystectomy**, a procedure where a part of the bladder is removed. If the cancer is large or is present in more than one area of the bladder, a radical cystectomy is done. In this operation, the entire bladder and adjoining organs also may be removed. In men, the prostate is removed, while in women, the uterus, ovaries, and fallopian tubes are removed.

If the entire urinary bladder is removed, an alternate place must be created for the urine to be stored before it is excreted out of the body. To do this, a piece of intestine is converted into a small bag and attached to the ureters. This is then connected to an opening (stoma) that is made in the abdominal wall. The procedure is called a urostomy. In some urostomy procedures, the urine from the intestinal sac is routed into a bag that is placed over the stoma in the abdominal wall. The bag is hidden by the clothing and has to be emptied occasionally by the patient. In a different procedure, the urine is collected in the intestinal sac, but there is no bag on the outside of the abdomen. The intestinal sac has to be emptied by the patient, by placing a drainage tube through the stoma.

Radiation therapy that uses high-energy rays to kill cancer cells is generally used after surgery to destroy any remaining cancer cells that may not have been removed during surgery. If the tumor is in a location that makes surgery difficult, or if it is large, radiation may be used before surgery to shrink the tumor. In cases of advanced bladder cancer, radiation therapy is used to ease the symptoms such as **pain**, bleeding, or blockage. Radiation can be delivered by external beam, where a source of radiation that is outside the body focuses the radiation on the area of the tumor. Occasionally, a small pellet of radioactive material may be placed directly into the cancer. This is known as interstitial radiation therapy.

Chemotherapy uses **anticancer drugs** to destroy the cancer cells that may have migrated to distant sites. The drugs are introduced into the bloodstream by injecting them into a vein in the arm or taking them orally in pill form. Generally a combination of drugs is more effective than any single drug in treating bladder cancer. Chemotherapy may be given following surgery to kill any remaining cancer cells. It also may be given even when no remaining cancer cells can be seen. This is called adjuvant chemotherapy. Anticancer drugs, including thiotepa, doxorubicin, and mitomycin, also may be instilled directly into the bladder (intravesicular chemotherapy) to treat superficial tumors. In 2003, the FDA was giving fast track designation to a form of paclitaxel, a common anticancer drug, that was shown effective in treating metastatic or locally advanced bladder cancer.

A 2003 report stated that giving patients with bladder cancer chemotherapy followed by surgery may improve their outcomes. In the study of 307 patients, those with this combination of therapy lived two years longer than those treated with surgery only.

Immunotherapy, or biological therapy, uses the body's own immune cells to fight the disease. To treat superficial bladder cancer, bacille Calmette-Guerin (BCG) may be instilled directly into the bladder. BCG is a weakened (attenuated) strain of the **tuberculosis** bacillus that stimulates the body's immune system to fight the cancer. This therapy has been shown to be effective in controlling superficial bladder cancer.

Photodynamic treatment is a novel mode of treatment that uses special chemicals and light to kill the cancerous cells. First, a drug is introduced into the bladder that makes the cancer cells more susceptible to light. Following that, a special light is shone on the bladder in an attempt to destroy the cancerous cells.

New treatments are continuously being investigated. Scientists have made great strides in gene mapping and research in the twenty-first century. In 2003, a type of **gene therapy** was being tested on patients

with bladder cancer with success, but further enhancements were needed.

Prognosis

When detected in early stages, the prognosis for those with bladder cancer is excellent. At least 94% of people survive five years or more after initial diagnosis. However, if the disease has spread to the nearby tissues, the survival rate drops to 49%. If it has metastasized to distant organs such as the lung and liver, commonly only 6% of patients will survive five years or more. As newer treatment methods are developed, some prognoses improve. For example, neoadjuvant chemotherapy, or giving certain chemotherapy drugs following surgery, may help people live up to 31 months longer than previous treatments allowed.

Prevention

Since the exact causes of bladder cancer are not known, there is no certain way to prevent it. Avoiding risk factors whenever possible is the best alternative.

Since smoking doubles one's risk of getting bladder cancer, avoiding tobacco may prevent at least half the deaths that result from bladder cancer. Taking appropriate safety precautions when working with organic cancer-causing chemicals is another way of preventing the disease. Women should discuss the risks vs. benefits of hormone replacement therapy with their physicians.

If a person has had a history of bladder cancer, or has been exposed to cancer-causing chemicals, he or she is considered to be at an increased risk of getting bladder cancer. Similarly, **kidney stones**, frequent urinary infections, and other conditions that cause long-term irritation to the bladder also increase the chance of getting the disease. In such cases, it is advisable to undergo regular screening tests such as urine cytology, cystoscopy and x rays of the urinary tract, so that bladder cancer can be detected at its early stages and treated appropriately.

Resources

PERIODICALS

Good, Brian. "Battle Against Bladder Cancer." *Men's Health* 18 (December 2003): 32.

Grossman, H. Barton, et al. "Neoadjuvant Chemotherapy Plus Cystectomy Compared With Cystectomy Alone for Locally Advanced Bladder Cancer." *The New England Journal of Medicine* (August 28, 2003): 859.

"HRT Increases Risk of Gallbladder, Breast, Endometrial, and Bladder Cancer." *Women's Health Weekly* (July 17, 2003): 31.

"Intravesical Gene Therapy Appears Safe for Those With Local Bladder Cancer." *Cancer Weekly* (July 8, 2003): 144.

"Tocosol Paclitaxel Receives Expedited Review for Bladder Cancer Indication." *Biotech Week* (November 26, 2003): 443.

ORGANIZATIONS

American Cancer Society. 1599 Clifton Rd., NE, Atlanta, GA 30329-4251. (800) 227-2345. < http://www.cancer.org >.

American Foundation for Urologic Disease. 300 W. Pratt St., Suite 401. Baltimore, MD 21201. Phone: (800)-828-7866.

Cancer Research Institute. 681 Fifth Ave., New York, N.Y. 10022. (800) 992-2623. < http://www.cancerresearch.org >.

National Cancer Institute. Building 31, Room 10A31, 31 Center Drive, MSC 2580, Bethesda, MD 20892-2580. (800) 422-6237. < http://www.nci.nih.gov >.

Oncolink. University of Pennsylvania Cancer Center. < http://cancer.med.upenn.edu >.

OTHER

"Bladder Cancer." National Cancer Institute Page. < http://www.nci.nih.gov >.

Lata Cherath, PhD
Teresa G. Odle

Bladder removal *see* **Cystectomy**

Bladder resection *see* **Transurethral bladder resection**

Bladder stones

Definition

Bladder stones are crystalline masses that form from the **minerals** and proteins, which naturally occur in urine. These types of stones are much less common than **kidney stones**.

Description

Bladder stones can form anywhere in the urinary tract before depositing in the bladder. They begin as tiny granules about the size of a grain of sand, but they can grow to more than an inch in diameter. These stones can block the flow of urine causing **pain** and difficulty with urination. They can also scratch the bladder wall, which may lead to bleeding or infection.

KEY TERMS

Bladder—A small organ that serves as the reservoir for urine prior to its passing from the body during urination.

Prostate gland—A small gland in the male genitals that contributes to the production of seminal fluid.

Urinary tract—The system of organs that produces and expels urine from the body. This system begins at the kidneys, where the urine is formed; passes through the bladder; and, ends at the urethra, where urine is expelled.

Causes and symptoms

While the exact causes of the formation of bladder stones are not completely understood, bladder stones usually occur because of urinary tract infection (UTI), obstruction of the urinary tract, enlargement of the prostate gland in men, or the presence of foreign bodies in the urinary tract. Diet and the amount of fluid intake also appear to be important factors in the development of bladder stones.

Ninety-five percent of all bladder stones occur in men, most of who have an **enlarged prostate** gland or a UTI. These stones are rarely seen in children or in African Americans. People with **gout** may develop bladder stones composed almost entirely of uric acid.

The symptoms of bladder stones may become evident when the wall of the bladder is scratched or when the urinary tract becomes obstructed by the stone. These symptoms include:

- abnormally dark colored urine
- blood in the urine
- difficulty urinating
- frequent urge to urinate
- lower abdominal pain
- pain or discomfort in the penis

Some people with bladder stones also may experience an inability to control urination (**urinary incontinence**).

Diagnosis

The diagnosis of bladder stones is usually made after a **physical examination**, which may include a **rectal examination** to check for enlargement of the prostate gland. Urine tests are then used to determine if there is blood or indications of an UTI in the urine. If bladder stones are suspected, bladder or pelvic x rays may be ordered. Stones that are large enough to cause problems with urinary function are almost always detectable by x ray.

Treatment

Many bladder stones can be passed out of the body in the urine. People with small bladder stones will be asked to increase their fluid intakes to at least six to eight eight-ounce glasses of water per day to increase urinary output. If the stones do not pass after two weeks, or if the patient's symptoms become worse, further medical treatment may be required.

A large bladder stone, or small stone that the patient cannot pass in the urine, may be broken up into smaller stones using ultrasound (shock waves). These smaller stones may then pass in the urine. Stones that cannot be broken into pieces by these methods, or that the patient cannot pass, may have to be surgically removed.

Alternative treatment

Traditional herbal remedies for bladder stones include celery seed and horsetail. Also, because incomplete bladder emptying may cause bladder stones, many patients may benefit from methods and remedies aimed at improving overall bladder function. These include Kegel exercises, which are used to strengthen the muscles involved in urination; herbal supplements (cornsilk, hydrangea, juniper berries, parsley, and uva ursi) used to increase urine flow and flush out sediment from the bladder; and, the consumption of cranberry juice and/or fresh, unsweetened, lemon juice. Cranberry juice helps to control urinary tract infection and contains a chemical that coats the walls of the bladder, making them more resistant to infection. Lemon juice helps to flush out the urinary system.

Prognosis

Most bladder stones can be, and are, passed out of the body in the urine without any permanent damage to the bladder or the rest of the urinary tract. However, most bladder stones arise from an underlying medical condition. Therefore, if this medical condition is not corrected approximately half of all patients will experience a recurrence of bladder stones within five years.

Prevention

Bladder stones may, in some cases, be prevented by the patient receiving prompt medical treatment for an enlarged prostate gland or UTI. The consumption of at least six to eight eight-ounce glasses of water per day and/or the regular consumption of cranberry juice may help to prevent recurrences of bladder stones.

Resources

PERIODICALS

Schwartz, B.F., and M.L. Stoller. "The vesical calculus." *Urologic Clinics of North America* 27 (May 2000): 333-46.

ORGANIZATIONS

American Foundation for Urologic Disease. 1128 North Charles Street, Baltimore, Maryland 21201. (410) 468-1800. Fax: (410) 468-1808. < http://www.afud. org/ > .

OTHER

"Bladder Stones." MEDLINEplus Health Information. May 12, 2001. < http://medlineplus.adam.com/ency/ article/001275.htm > .

Paul A. Johnson, Ed.M.

Bladder training

Definition

Bladder training is a behavioral modification treatment technique for **urinary incontinence** that involves placing a patient on a toileting schedule. The time interval between urination is gradually increased in order to train the patient to remain continent.

Purpose

Bladder training is used to treat urinary urge incontinence. Urge incontinence occurs when an individual feels a sudden need to urinate and cannot control the urge to do so and, as a consequence, involuntarily loses urine before making it to the toilet.

Precautions

Incontinence may be controlled through a number of invasive and non-invasive treatment options, including Kegel exercises, **biofeedback**, bladder training, medication, insertable incontinence devices, and surgery. Each patient should undergo a full diagnostic work-up to determine the type and cause of the incontinence in order to determine the best course of treatment.

Description

Bladder training may be prescribed and implemented by a general physician, urologist, or urogynecologist. A urination schedule is created for the patient. The schedule typically starts out with fairly short intervals between bathroom breaks (e.g., an hour). As soon as the patient is able to consistently remain continent for several days at a certain toileting time interval, the time span is increased. Bladder training continues until the patient regularly achieves continence at a time interval he/she feels comfortable with.

Preparation

A complete evaluation to determine the cause of urinary incontinence is critical to proper treatment. A thorough medical history and **physical examination** should be performed on patients considering bladder training. Diagnostic testing may include x rays, ultrasound, urine tests, and a physical examination of the pelvis. It may include a series of exams called urodynamic testing that measure bladder pressure and capacity and the urinary flow. The patient may also be asked to keep a diary of their urination output and frequency and episodes of incontinence over a period of several days or a week.

Risks

Bladder training may not be successful in all patients with urge incontinence. Patients who demonstrate a strong desire to control their continence and are committed to sticking with a training program tend to have the most success with bladder training.

Normal results

Patients who undergo successful bladder training gain complete or improved control over their urination. In some cases, additional alternate treatment such as biofeedback or pelvic muscle exercises may be recommended to supplement the progress made with bladder training.

Resources

ORGANIZATIONS

American Foundation for Urologic Disease. 1128 North Charles St., Baltimore, MD 21201. (800) 242-2383. < http://www.afud.org >.

National Association for Continence. P.O. Box 8310, Spartanburg, SC 29305-8310. (800) 252-3337. < http://www.nafc.org >.

Paula Anne Ford-Martin

Blastomyces dermatitidis see **Blastomycosis**

Blastomycosis

Definition

Blastomycosis is an infection caused by inhaling microscopic particles (spores) produced by the fungus *Blastomyces dermatitidis*. Blastomycosis may be limited to the lungs or also involve the skin and bones. In its most severe form, the infection can spread throughout the body and involve many organ systems (systemic).

Description

Blastomycosis is a fungal infection caused by *Blastomyces dermatitidis*. Although primarily an airborne disease, farmers and gardeners may become infected from contact with spores in the soil through cuts and scrapes. The fungus that causes the disease is found in moist soil and wood in the southeastern United States, the Mississippi River valley, southern Canada, and Central America. Blastomycosis is also called Gilchrist's disease, Chicago disease, or North American blastomycosis. Another South and Central American disease, paracoccidioidomycosis, is sometimes called South American blastomycosis, but despite the similar name, this disease is substantially different from North American blastomycosis. Canine blastomycosis, a common dog disease, is caused by the same fungus that infects humans. However, people do not get this disease from their dogs except only very rarely through dog bites.

Blastomycosis is a rare disease infecting only about 4 in every 100,000 people. It is at least six times more common in men than in women and tends to more often infect children and individuals in the 30–50 year old age group. People who have

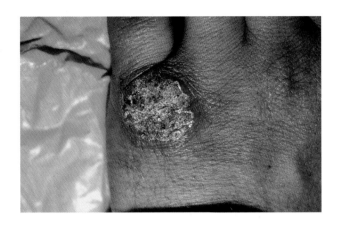

Blastomycosis is usually attributed to contact with yeast-like fungi. *(Custom Medical Stock Photo. Reproduced by permission.)*

diabetes mellitus or who are taking drugs that suppress the immune system (immunocompromised) are more likely to develop blastomycosis. Although people with AIDS can get blastomycosis because of their weakened immune system, blastomycosis has not been one of the more common fungal infections associated with AIDS.

Causes and symptoms

Once inhaled, the spores of *B. dermatitidis* can lodge in the lungs and cause a localized inflammation. This is known as primary pulmonary blastomycosis. The disease does not spread from one person to another. In the early stages, symptoms may include a dry **cough**, **fever**, heavy sweating, fatigue, and a general feeling of ill health. In approximately 25% of blastomycosis cases, only the lungs are affected. As the disease progresses, small lesions form in the lungs causing the air sacs deep within the lungs (alveoli) to break down and form small cavities.

In another 35%, the disease involves both the lungs and the skin. Bumps develop on the skin, gradually becoming small, white, crusted blisters filled with pus. The blisters break open, creating abscesses that do not heal. Approximately 19% of infected people have skin sores without infection in the lungs.

The remaining approximately 20% of the infected population has blastomycosis that has spread or disseminated to other systems of the body. Symptoms may include **pain** and lesions on one or more bones, the male genitalia, and/or parts of the central nervous system. The liver, spleen, lymph nodes, heart, adrenal glands, and digestive system may also be infected.

Diagnosis

A positive diagnosis of blastomycosis is made when the fungus *B. dermatitidis* is identified by direct microscopic examination of body fluids such as sputum and prostate fluid or in tissue samples (biopsies) from the lung or skin. Another way to diagnose blastomycosis is to culture and isolate the fungus from a sample of sputum. Chest x rays are used to assess lung damage, but alone cannot lead to a definitive diagnosis of blastomycosis because any damage caused by other diseases, such as by **pneumonia** or **tuberculosis**, may appear look on the x ray. Because its symptoms vary widely, blastomycosis is often misdiagnosed.

Treatment

Blastomycosis must be treated or it will gradually lead to **death**. Treatment with the fungicidal drug ketoconazole (Nizoral) taken orally is effective in about 75% of patients. Amphotericin B (Fungizone) given intravenously is also very effective, but it has more toxic side effects than ketoconazole. Treatment with amphotericin B usually requires hospitalization, and the patient may also receive other drugs to minimize the its side effects.

Alternative treatment

Alternative treatment for fungal infections focuses on creating an internal environment where the fungus cannot survive. This is accomplished by eating a diet low in dairy products, sugars, including honey and fruit juice, and foods like beer that contain yeast. This is complemented by a diet consisting, in large part, of uncooked and unprocessed foods. Supplements of **vitamins** C, E, A-plus, and B complex may also be useful. *Lactobacillus acidophilus* and *Bifidobacterium* will replenish the good bacteria in the intestines. Some antifungal herbs, like garlic (*Allium sativum*), can be consumed in relatively large doses and for an extended period of time in order to increase effectiveness. A variety of antifungal herbs, such as myrrh (*Commiphora molmol*), tea tree oil (*Melaleuca* spp.), citrus seed extract, pau d'arco tea (*Tabebuia impetiginosa*), and garlic may also be applied directly to the infected skin.

Prognosis

Left untreated, blastomycosis gradually leads to death. When treated, however, patients begin to improve within one week and, with intensive treatment, may be cured within several weeks. The highest rate of recovery is among patients who only have skin lesions. People with the disseminated form of the disease are least likely to be cured and and most likely to suffer a relapse.

Prevention

Because the fungus that causes blastomycosis is airborne and microscopic, the only form of prevention is to avoid visiting areas where it is found in the soil. For many people this is impractical. Since the disease is rare, people who maintain general good health do not need to worry much about infection.

Resources

ORGANIZATIONS

National Organization for Rare Disorders. P.O. Box 8923, New Fairfield, CT 06812-8923. (800) 999-6673. <http://www.rarediseases.org>.

OTHER

"Blastomycosis." Vanderbilt University Medical Center. <http://www.mc.vanterbilt.edu/peds/pid/infect/blastomy.html>.

Tish Davidson, A.M.

Bleeding disorders *see* **Coagulation disorders**

Bleeding time

Definition

Bleeding time is a crude test of hemostasis (the arrest or stopping of bleeding). It indicates how well platelets interact with blood vessel walls to form **blood clots**.

Purpose

Bleeding time is used most often to detect qualitative defects of platelets, such as Von Willebrand's disease. The test helps identify people who have defects in their platelet function. This is the ability of blood to clot following a wound or trauma. Normally, platelets interact with the walls of blood vessels to cause a blood clot. There are many factors in the clotting mechanism, and they are initiated by platelets. The bleeding time test is usually used on patients who have a history of prolonged bleeding after cuts, or who have a family history of bleeding disorders. Also, the bleeding time test is sometimes performed as a preoperative test to determine a patient's likely bleeding response during and after surgery. However, in patients with no history of bleeding problems, or who are not taking anti-inflammatory drugs, the bleeding time test is not usually necessary.

Precautions

Before administering the test, patients should be questioned about what medications they may be taking. Some medications will adversely affect the results of the bleeding time test. These medications include anticoagulants, **diuretics**, **anticancer drugs**, **sulfonamides**, thiazide, **aspirin** and aspirin-containing preparations, and **nonsteroidal anti-inflammatory drugs**. The test may also be affected by anemia (a deficiency in red blood cells). Since the taking of aspirin or related drugs are the most common cause of prolonged bleeding time, no aspirin should be taken two weeks prior to the test.

Description

There are four methods to perform the bleeding test. The Ivy method is the traditional format for this test. In the Ivy method, a blood pressure cuff is placed on the upper arm and inflated to 40 mM Hg. A lancet or scalpel blade is used to make a stab wound on the underside of the forearm. An automatic, spring-loaded blade device is most commonly used to make a standard-sized cut. The area stabbed is selected so that no superficial or visible veins are cut. These veins, because of their size, may have longer bleeding times, especially in people with bleeding defects. The time from when the stab wound is made until all bleeding has stopped is measured and is called the bleeding time. Every 30 seconds, filter paper or a paper towel is used to draw off the blood. The test is finished when bleeding has stopped completely.

The three other methods of performing the bleeding test are the template, modified template, and Duke methods. The template and modified template methods are variations of the Ivy method. A blood pressure cuff is used and the skin on the forearm prepared as in the Ivy method. A template is placed over the area to be stabbed and two incisions are made in the forearm using the template as a location guide. The main difference between the template and the modified method is the length of the cut made.

For the Duke method, a nick is made in an ear lobe or a fingertip is pricked to cause bleeding. As in the Ivy method, the test is timed from the start of bleeding until bleeding is completely stopped. The disadvantage to the Duke method is that the pressure on the blood veins in the stab area is not constant and the results achieved are less reliable. The advantage to the Duke method is that no scar remains after the test. The other methods may result in a tiny, hairline scar where the wound was made. However, this is largely a cosmetic concern.

Preparation

There is no special preparation required of the patient for this test. The area to be stabbed should be wiped clean with an alcohol pad. The alcohol should be left on the skin long enough for it to kill bacteria at the wound site. The alcohol must be removed before stabbing the arm because alcohol will adversely affect the tests results by inhibiting clotting.

Aftercare

If a prolonged bleeding time is caused by unknown factors or diseases, further testing is required to identify the exact cause of the bleeding problem.

Normal results

A normal bleeding time for the Ivy method is less than five minutes from the time of the stab until all bleeding from the wound stops. Some texts extend the normal range to eight minutes. Normal values for the template method range up to eight minutes, while for the modified template methods, up to 10 minutes is considered normal. Normal for the Duke method is three minutes.

Abnormal results

A bleeding time that is longer than normal is an abnormal result. The test should be stopped if the patient hasn't stopped bleeding by 20-30 minutes. Bleeding time is longer when the normal function of platelets is impaired, or there are a lower-than-normal number of platelets in the blood.

A longer-than-normal bleeding time can indicate that one of several defects in hemostasis is present, including severe **thrombocytopenia**, platelet dysfunction, vascular defects, Von Willebrand's disease, or other abnormalities.

Resources

BOOKS

Henry, J. B. *Clinical Diagnosis and Management by Laboratory Methods.* Philadelphia: W. B. Saunders Co., 1996.

John T. Lohr, PhD

Bleeding varices

Definition

Bleeding varices are bleeding, dilated (swollen) veins in the esophagus (gullet), or the upper part of the stomach, caused by **liver disease**.

Description

Engorged veins are called varices (plural of varix). Varices may occur in the lining of the esophagus, the tube that connects the mouth to the stomach, or in the upper part of the stomach. Such varices are called esophageal varices. These varices are fragile and can bleed easily because veins are not designed to handle high internal pressures.

Causes and symptoms

Liver disease often causes an increase in the blood pressure in the main veins that carry blood from the stomach and intestines to the liver (portal veins). As the pressure in the portal veins increases, the veins of the stomach and esophagus swell, until they eventually become varices. Bleeding varices are a life-threatening complication of this increase in blood pressure (portal **hypertension**). The most common cause of bleeding varices is **cirrhosis** of the liver caused by chronic alcohol **abuse** or hepatitis. Bleeding varices occur in approximately one in every 10,000 people.

Symptoms of bleeding varices include:

- vomiting blood, sometimes in massive amounts
- black, tarry stools
- decreased urine output
- excessive thirst
- nausea
- vomiting
- blood in the vomit

If bleeding from the varices is severe, a patient may go into **shock** from the loss of blood, characterized by pallor, a rapid and weak pulse, rapid and shallow respiration, and lowered systemic blood pressure.

Diagnosis

Bleeding varices may be suspected in a patient who has any of the above-mentioned symptoms, and who has either been diagnosed with cirrhosis of the liver or who has a history of prolonged alcohol abuse. The definitive diagnosis is established via a specialized type of endoscopy, namely, **esophagogastroduodeno-scopy** (EGD), a procedure that involves the visual examination of the lining of the esophagus, stomach, and upper duodenum with a flexible fiberoptic endoscope.

Treatment

The objective during treatment of bleeding varices is to stop and/or prevent bleeding and to restore/maintain normal blood circulation throughout the body. Patients with severe bleeding should be treated in intensive care since uncontrolled bleeding can lead to **death**.

Initial treatment of bleeding varices begins with standard resuscitation, including intravenous

---

KEY TERMS

Cirrhosis of the liver—A type of liver disease, most often caused by chronic alcohol abuse. It is characterized by scarring of the liver, which leads to an increase in the blood pressure in the portal veins.

Endoscopy—Medical imaging technique for visualizing the interior of a hollow organ.

Esophagus—The tube in the body which takes food from the mouth to the stomach.

Esophagogastroduodenoscopy (EGD)—An imaging test that involves visually examining the lining of the esophagus, stomach, and upper duodenum with a flexible fiberoptic endoscope.

Portal hypertension—Portal hypertension forces the blood flow backward, causing the portal veins to enlarge and the emergence of bleeding varices across the esophagus and stomach from the pressure in the portal vein. Portal hypertension is most commonly caused by cirrhosis, but can also be seen in portal vein obstruction from unknown causes.

Portal veins—The main veins that carry blood from the stomach and intestines to the liver.

Shock—A state of depression of the vital processes of the body characterized by pallor, a rapid and weak pulse, rapid and shallow respiration, and lowered blood pressure. Shock results from severe trauma, such as crushing injuries, hemorrhage, burns, or major surgery.

Transjugular intrahepatic portosystemic shunt (TIPS)—A transjugular intrahepatic portosystemic shunt (TIPS) is a radiology procedure in which a tubular device is inserted in the middle of the liver to redirect the blood flow.

Varices—A type of varicose vein that develops in veins in the linings of the esophagus and upper stomach when these veins fill with blood and swell due to an increase in blood pressure in the portal veins.

---

fluids and blood transfusions as needed. Definitive treatment is usually endoscopic, with the endoscope used to locate the sites of the bleeding. An instrument, inserted along with the endoscope, is used either to inject these sites with a clotting agent or to tie off the bleeding sites with tiny rubber bands.

Repeated endoscopic treatments (usually four/ six) are generally required to eliminate the varices and to prevent the recurrence of bleeding. These endoscopic techniques are successful in about 90 percent of cases.

Patients who cannot be treated endoscopically may be considered for an alternative procedure called TIPS (transjugular intrahepatic portosystemic shunt). This procedure involves placing a hollow metal tube (shunt) in the liver connecting the portal veins with the hepatic veins (veins that leave the liver and drain to the heart). This shunt lowers the pressure in the portal veins and prevents bleeding and portal hypertension. The TIPS procedure is performed by a radiologist and has become an accepted method for reducing portal vein pressure since 1992. Although the procedure continues to evolve, TIPS can routinely be created in more than 93% of patients.

Medications aimed at controlling bleeding may also be prescribed. These include propanolol, vasopressin, octreotide acetate, and isosorbide mononitrate.

Alternative treatment

Some alternative treatments are aimed at preventing the cirrhosis of the liver that often causes bleeding varices and most are effective. However, once a patient has reached the bleeding varice stage, standard intervention to stop the bleeding is required or the patient may die.

Prognosis

Bleeding varices represent one of the most feared complications of portal hypertension. They contribute to the estimated 32,000 deaths per year attributed to cirrhosis. Half or more of patients who survive episodes of bleeding varices are at risk of renewed esophageal bleeding during the first one to two years. The risk of recurrence can be lowered by endoscopic and drug treatment. Prognosis is usually more related to the underlying liver disease. Approximately 30 to 50 percent of people with bleeding varices will die from this condition within the six weeks of the first bleeding episode.

Prevention

The best way to possibly prevent the development or recurrence of bleeding varices is to eliminate the risk factors for cirrhosis of the liver. The most common cause of cirrhosis is prolonged alcohol abuse, and alcohol consumption must be completely eliminated. People

with **hepatitis B** or **hepatitis C** also have an increased risk of developing cirrhosis of the liver. **Vaccination** against hepatitis B and avoidance of intravenous drug usage reduce the risk of contracting hepatitis.

Resources

BOOKS

Shannon, Joyce Brennfleck, editor. *Liver Disorders Sourcebook*. Detroit, MI: Omnigraphics, Inc., 2000.

PERIODICALS

Burroughs, Andrew K. and David Patch. "Primary prevention of bleeding from esophageal varices." *New England Journal of Medicine* 340 (April 1, 1999): 1033-5.

Hegab, Ahmed M., and Velimir A. Luketic. "Bleeding esophageal varices: How to treat this dreaded complication of portal hypertension." *Postgraduate Medicine* 109 (February 2001): 75-89.

ORGANIZATIONS

American Liver Foundation. 1425 Pompton Ave., Cedar Grove, NJ 07009. (800) 223-0179. < http:// www.liverfoundation.org > .

OTHER

Goff, John. *"Portal hypertensive bleeding."* May 12, 2001. < http://www.nysge.org/PostGrad1999/ Goff_VaricealBleeding.htm > .

Paul A. Johnson, Ed.M.

Blepharitis *see* **Eyelid disorders**

Blepharoplasty

Definition

Blepharoplasty is a cosmetic surgical procedure that removes fat deposits, excess tissue, or muscle from the eyelids to improve the appearance of the eyes.

Purpose

The primary use of blepharoplasty is for improving the cosmetic appearance of the eyes. In some older patients, however, sagging and excess skin surrounding the eyes can be so extensive that it limits the range of vision. In those cases, blepharoplasty serves a more functional purpose.

Precautions

Before performing blepharoplasty, the surgeon will assess whether the patient is a good candidate for the

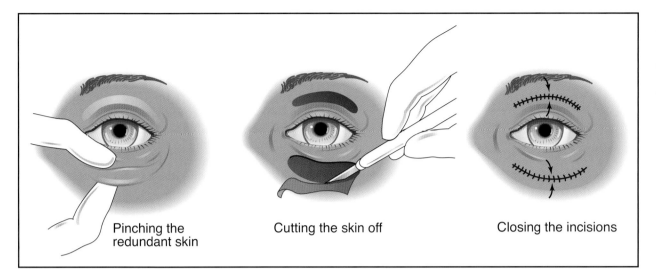

Pinching the redundant skin

Cutting the skin off

Closing the incisions

Blepharoplasty is one of the most common cosmetic surgical procedures. The illustration above depicts a procedure to eliminate dermochalasia, or baggy skin around the eyes. *(Illustration by Electronic Illustrators Group.)*

treatment. A good medical history is important. The surgeon will want to know about any history of thyroid disease, **hypertension**, or eye problems, which may increase the risk of complications.

Description

Blepharoplasty can be performed on the upper or lower eyelid; it can involve the removal of excess skin and fat deposits and the tightening of selected muscles surrounding the eyelids. The goal is to provide a more youthful appearance.

The surgeon will begin by deciding whether excess skin, fat deposits, or muscle looseness are at fault. While the patient is sitting upright, the surgeon will mark on the skin where incisions will be made. Care will be taken to hide the incision lines in the natural skin folds above and below the eye. The patient then receives injections of a local anesthetic to numb the **pain**. Many surgeons also give the patient a sedative intravenously during the procedure.

After a small, crescent-shaped section of eyelid skin is removed, the surgeon will work to tease out small pockets of fat that have collected in the lids. If muscle looseness is also a problem, the surgeon may trim tissue or add a stitch to pull it tighter. Then the incision is closed with stitches.

In some patients, fat deposits in the lower eyelid may be the only or primary problem. Such patients may be good candidates for transconjunctival blepharoplasty. In this procedure the surgeon makes no incision on the surface of the eyelid, but instead enters

from behind to tease out the fat deposits from a small incision. The advantage of this procedure is that there is no visible scar.

Preparation

Prior to surgery, patients meet with their surgeon to discuss the procedure, clarify the results that can be achieved, and discuss the potential problems that might occur. Having realistic expectations is important in any cosmetic procedure. Patients will learn, for example, that although blepharoplasty can improve the appearance of the eyelid, other procedures, such as a chemical peel, will be necessary to reduce the appearance of wrinkles around the eye. Some surgeons prescribe vitamin C and vitamin K for 10 days prior to surgery in the belief that this helps the healing process. Patients are also told to stop **smoking** in the weeks before and after the procedure, and to refrain from alcohol and **aspirin**.

Aftercare

An antibiotic ointment is applied to the line of stitches for several days after surgery. Patients also take an antibiotic several times a day to prevent infection. Ice-cold compresses are applied to the eyes continuously for the first day following surgery, and several times a day for the next week or so, to reduce swelling. Some swelling and discoloration around the eyes is expected with the procedure. Patients should avoid aspirin or alcoholic beverages for one week and should limit their activities, including bending, straining, and lifting. The stitches are removed a few days after surgery. Patients can generally return to their usual activities within a week to 10 days.

Risks

As with any surgical procedure, blepharoplasty can lead to infection and scarring. Good care of the wound following surgery can minimize these risks. In cases where too much skin is removed from the eyelids, the patient may have difficulty closing his eyes. Dry eye syndrome may develop, requiring the use of artificial tears to lubricate the eye. In a rare complication, called retrobulbar hematoma, a pocket of blood forms behind the eyeball.

Normal results

Most patients can expect good results from blepharoplasty, with the removal of excess eyelid skin and fat producing a more youthful appearance. Some swelling and discoloration is expected immediately following the procedure, but this clears in time. Small **scars** will be left where the surgeon has made incisions; but these generally lighten in appearance over several months, and, if placed correctly, will not be readily noticeable.

Abnormal results

As noted, if too much excess skin is removed from the upper eyelid, the patient may be unable to close his eyes completely; another surgery to correct the defect may be required. Similarly, too much skin can be removed from the lower eyelid, allowing too much of the white of the eye (the sclera) to show. In extreme cases, the lower lid may be pulled down too far, revealing the underlying tissue. Called an ectropion, this, too, may require a second, corrective surgery. The eye's ability to make tears may also be compromised, leading to dry eye syndrome. Dry eye syndrome is potentially dangerous; in rare cases it leads to damage to the cornea of the eye and vision loss.

Resources

ORGANIZATIONS

American Society for Dermatologic Surgery. 930 N. Meacham Road, P.O. Box 4014, Schaumburg, IL 60168-4014. (847) 330-9830. < http://www.asds-net.org > .

American Society of Plastic and Reconstructive Surgeons. 44 E. Algonquin Rd., Arlington Heights, IL 60005. (847) 228-9900. < http://www.plasticsurgery.org > .

Richard H. Camer

Blindness *see* **Visual impairment**

Blood-viscosity reducing drugs

Definition

Blood-viscosity reducing drugs are medicines that improve blood flow by making the blood less viscous (sticky).

Purpose

The main use of blood-viscosity reducing drugs is to relieve painful leg cramps caused by poor circulation, a condition called **intermittent claudication**. Physicians also may prescribe this medicine for other conditions, including **stroke**, **impotence**, male **infertility**, **Raynaud's disease**, and nerve and circulation problems caused by diabetes.

Description

Blood-viscosity reducing drugs are available only with a physician's prescription and come in extended-release tablet form. Examples of blood-viscosity reducing drugs are pentoxifylline (Trental) and oxypentifylline.

Recommended dosage

The usual dosage for adults is 400 mg, two to three times a day, with meals. However, the dose may be different for different patients. Check with the physician who prescribed the drug or the pharmacist who filled the prescription for the correct dosage. Dosages for children must be determined by a physician.

Taking an antacid with this medicine may help prevent upset stomach.

Precautions

This medicine may relieve leg **pain** that results from poor circulation, but it should not be considered a substitute for other treatments the physician recommends, such as physical therapy or surgery.

This medicine may take several weeks to produce noticeable results. Be sure to keep taking it as directed, even if it doesn't seem to be helping.

Patients being treated with this medicine should not smoke, as **smoking** may worsen the conditions for which the medicine is prescribed.

Anyone who has had unusual reactions to pentoxifylline, aminophylline, **caffeine**, dyphylline, ethylenediamine (contained in aminophylline), oxtriphylline, theobromine, or theophylline in the past should let his or her physician know before taking a blood-viscosity reducing drug. The physician should also be told about any **allergies** to foods, dyes, preservatives, or other substances.

Women who are pregnant or breastfeeding or who may become pregnant should check with their physicians before using a blood-viscosity reducing drug.

Older people may be especially sensitive to the effects of this medicine, which may increase the chance of side effects.

Before using blood-viscosity reducing drugs, people with any of these medical problems should make sure their physicians are aware of their conditions:

- recent stroke
- any condition in which there is an increased chance of bleeding

- kidney disease
- liver disease

Side effects

Minor discomforts, such as **dizziness**, **headache**, upset stomach, **nausea**, or **vomiting** usually go away as the body adjusts to the drug and do not require medical treatment unless they persist or they interfere with normal activities.

More serious side effects are rare. However, if these or any other unusual or troublesome symptoms occur, check with the physician who prescribed the medicine as soon as possible:

- chest pain
- irregular heartbeat

Interactions

Blood-viscosity reducing drugs may interact with a other medicines, changing the effects of one or both of the drugs or increasing the risk of side effects. Anyone who takes blood-viscosity reducing drugs should let the physician know all other prescription or nonprescription (over-the-counter) medicines he or she is taking. Among the drugs that may interact with blood-viscosity reducing drugs are:

- anticoagulants such as warfarin (Coumadin)(also called blood thinners or clot inhibitors)
- calcium channel blockers such as diltiazem (Cardizem), used to treat high blood pressure
- angiotensin-converting enzyme (ACE) inhibitors such as enalapril (Vasotec), used to treat high blood pressure
- theophylline (Theo-Dur)
- medicines such as cimetidine (Tagamet), taken for ulcers or heartburn

Nancy Ross-Flanigan

Blood clots

Definition

A blood clot is a thickened mass in the blood formed by tiny substances called platelets. Clots form to stop bleeding, such as at the site of cut. But clots should not form when blood is moving through the body; when clots form inside blood vessels or when blood has a tendency to clot too much, serious health problems can occur.

Description

As soon as a blood vessel wall is damaged—by a cut or similar trauma—a series of reactions normally takes place to activate platelets to stop the bleeding. Platelets are the tiny particles in the blood released into the bone marrow that gather together and form a barrier to further bleeding. Several proteins in the body are involved in the platelets clotting process. Chief among these proteins are collagen, thrombin, and von Willebrand factor. Collagen and thrombin help platelets stick together. As platelets gather at the site of injury, they change in shape from round to spiny, releasing proteins and other substances that help catch more platelets and clotting proteins. This enlarges the plug that becomes a blood clot. Formation of blood clots also is called ''coagulation''.

The series of reactions that cause proteins and platelets to create blood clots also are balanced by other reactions that stop the clotting process and dissolve clots after the blood vessel has healed. If this control system fails, minor blood vessel injuries can trigger clotting throughout the body. The tendency to clot too much is called ''hypercoagulation''. Anytime clots form inside blood vessels, they can lead to serious complications.

The formation of a clot in a blood vessels may be called **thrombophlebitis**. The term refers to swelling of one or more veins caused by a blood clot. Although some clots occur in the arms or small, surface blood vessels, most occur in the lower legs. When the blood clot occurs in a deep vein, it is called **deep vein thrombosis**, or DVT. As many as one of every 1,000 Americans develops DVT each year. The danger of DVT comes when pieces of the clot, known as emboli, break off and travel through the bloodstream to an artery.

A blood clot that blocks an artery to the brain can cause a **stroke**. If the clot blocks blood flow to the lungs **pulmonary embolism** can occur. A blood clot that blocks a coronary artery can cause a **heart attack**. Certain people are at higher risk for blood clots than others; surgery, some injuries, **childbirth** and lying or sitting still for extended periods of time put people at higher risk, as do inherited disorders. Once a person has a blood clot, he or she may have to take blood-thinning drugs to prevent clots from recurring. Men

and women are at similar risk for blood clots. A recent study in Austria found that men run a higher risk of recurring blood clots than women, though the reason is unknown.

Causes and symptoms

Many causes can lead to blood clots, some genetic and some environmental. An environmental cause of DVT is prolonged inactivity. For instance, having to sit in a car or airplane for a long period of time decreases blood flow in the lower legs. Recent studies have shown that 1% of air travelers develop blood clots, usually on long flights of five hours or more. However, one study in 2004 found that air travelers developed clots on flights as short as three hours, though they often dissolved naturally and did not lead to complications. Other environmental causes of blood clots include use of **hormone replacement therapy** to ease menopausal symptoms, **oral contraceptives** for birth control, **pregnancy** (and a childbirth within the past six weeks), recent surgery or procedures involving use of a central **venous access** catheter, and **cancer**. **Smoking** also is an important and preventable environmental risk for blood clots.

Some people are born with a higher risk for blood clots. **Hypercoagulation disorders** are genetic conditions. Usually the body doesn t produce enough of the proteins involved in the clotting process, so they cannot do their job to stop the clotting; in other cases, they have an extra protein that causes too much clotting.

There may be no symptoms of blood clots until they grow so large that they block the flow of blood through the vein. Then, symptoms may develop suddenly around the area and include:

- **Pain** or tenderness in the affected area.

- Warmth or redness of the skin in the affected area.

- Sudden swelling in the affected limb.

Additional symptoms may indicate serious complications of blood clots such as pulmonary **embolism**, stroke, and heart attack. If vein swelling or pain are accompanied by high **fever** or **shortness of breath**, rapid pulse, or chest pain, or other symptoms that may indicate stroke, heart attack, or pulmonary embolism, it is advised to go to an emergency room immediately.

Diagnosis

A physician will diagnose blood clots based on patient history and one of several diagnostic imaging exams. The patient's history will help determine possible risk factors that may lead to suspected blood clots. In addition to family history or known genetic disorders, the patient may mention an environmental factor such as recent air travel or use of high-risk mediations.

To help get a picture of suspected clots inside the veins, the first test chosen normally is an ultrasound. Doppler or duplex ultrasound uses sound waves that travel through tissue and reflect back. A computer transforms the sound waves into moving images on the screen that may show the clot, as well as blood flow near the clot and any abnormalities. Ultrasound does not use x rays and is a noninvasive method. Computed tomography (CT) scans also might be used to image the blood vessels. It is similar to x rays, except the images are much like cross-section slices with greater detail that can be computerized and even viewed three-dimensionally. A special dye called a contrast agent may be injected before the exam to help highlight the veins. Magnetic resonance **angiography** uses **magnetic resonance imaging** (MRI) to image the blood vessels. It also may involve injection of a contrast dye. **Venography** is less commonly used, but involves injecting a contrast and using x rays to image the vein.

Treatment

Medicines can help thin blood, making it less likely to clot. The two most common blood thinners are heparin and warfarin. Heparin works right away, keeping blood clots from growing. It usually is injected. In recent years, more physicians have been prescribing low-molecular weight heparin, purified versions of the drug that can be given with less monitoring. Warfarin (coumadin) often is used for long-term treatment of blood clots and is taken orally. Patients must work closely with their physicians to constantly monitor its effects and adjust dose if necessary. Too little warfarin can lead to clotting, but too much can thin the blood so much that causing life-threatening bleeding can occur. The same can be true of low-molecular weight heparin when used on a long-term, at-home basis.

Other treatments for blood clots include injecting clot busting drugs directly into the clot through a catheter, or in rare instances, installation of a filter to block a clot from lodging in the lungs. Sometimes, surgery also is needed to remove a clot blocking a pelvic or abdominal vein or one that is chronic and disabling. A cardiovascular surgeon or interventional radiologist may perform balloon **angioplasty** or insert a stent to open a narrowed or damaged vein. In an emergency situation, a drug called tissue plasminogen activator, or tPA, may be given to immediately dissolve a life-threatening blood clot to the brain or heart. In 2004, the U.S. Food and Drug Administration approved a new, small, corklike device that can be used to remove blood clots from the brains of patients who cannot receive clot-busting drugs.

Alternative treatment

Garlic is thought to lower blood clotting potential. Less evidence suggests onions and cayenne pepper may help keep blood thin. New research from Australia adds tomato juice to the list of potential blood thinners. Subjects who drank a glass of tomato juice a day reduced their risk for DVT, stroke and cardiovascular disease. Research has shown that a natural soy and pine product called pinokinase has been effective in controlling DVT in air travelers. Patients seeking alternative treatments for blood clots should work with certified practitioners and should inform their allopathic provider about their alternative care.

Prognosis

If detected and controlled with medications, blood clots can be safely managed. However, if the clots become dislodged and travel to an artery, they can cause nearly instant **death**. For instance, more than 600,000 people have a pulmonary embolism each year and more than 10% of them die from the embolism, most of them within 30 to 60 minutes after symptoms start.

Prevention

Clots may be avoided by not smoking, and by not using medications that add to the risk. Clotting can be prevented by following physician recommendations concerning medications. Sometimes, physicians will prescribe special support stockings that prevent swelling and reduce chances of DVT. When taking an air flight of six hours or longer, drinking plenty of fluids to avoid **dehydration**, avoiding tight clothing around the waist, and stretching calves every hour can help prevent DVT. It is advised that those on long flights get up and move about once an hour during the flight. If not possible, moving the legs regularly while seated by flexing the ankles, then pressing the feet against the seat in the row ahead or on the floor can help stretch the calves. A physician may advise those at high risk of DVT wear support stockings during the flight or take low-molecular weight heparin two to four hours before departure.

Resources

PERIODICALS

"Air Travel, Especially Long Flights, May Increase the Risk of Blood Clots." *Women's Health Weekly* (Dec. 25, 2003):119.

"In-flight Exercises for a Healthy Trip: Prevent Dangerous Blood Clots With These Three Easy Moves the Next Time You Fly." *Natural Health* (Jan–Feb. 2003):27.

Stephenson, Joan. "FDA Orders Estrogen Safety Warnings: Agency Offers Guidance for HRT Use." *JAMA, The Journal of the American Medical Association* (Feb. 5, 2003):537–539.

"Study Finds One Percent of Air Travelers Develop Injurious Blood Clots." *Heart Disease Weekly* (Jan. 25, 2004):41.

"Tiny Corkscrew Clears Blood Clots." *Hematology Week* (Sept. 6, 2004):99.

ORGANIZATIONS

National Heart, Lung and Blood Institute. P.O. Box 30105, Behtesda, MD 20824-0105. 301-592-8573. www.nhlbi.nih.gov.

Society of Interventional Radiology. 10201 Lee Highway, Suite 500, Fairfax, VA 22030. 703-691-1805. http://www.sirweb.org.

OTHER

Avoid Deep Vein Thrombosis: Keep the Blood Flowing. FDA Web site, 2005. www.fda.gov/fdac/features/2004/604_vein.html.

Teresa G. Odle

Blood count

Definition

One of the most commonly ordered clinical laboratory tests, a blood count, also called a complete blood count (CBC), is a basic evaluation of the cells (red blood cells, white blood cells, and platelets) suspended in the liquid part of the blood (plasma). It involves determining the numbers, concentrations, and conditions of the different types of blood cells.

Purpose

The CBC is a useful screening and diagnostic test that is often done as part of a routine **physical examination**. It can provide valuable information about the blood and blood-forming tissues (especially the bone marrow), as well as other body systems. Abnormal results can indicate the presence of a variety of conditions—including **anemias**, leukemias, and infections—sometimes before the patient experiences symptoms of the disease.

Description

A complete blood count is actually a series of tests in which the numbers of red blood cells, white blood cells, and platelets in a given volume of blood are counted. The CBC also measures the hemoglobin content and the packed cell volume (**hematocrit**) of the red blood cells, assesses the size and shape of the red blood cells, and determines the types and percentages of white blood cells. Components of the complete blood count (hemoglobin, hematocrit, white blood cells, platelets, etc.) can also be tested separately, and are sometimes done that way when a doctor wants to monitor a specific condition, such as the white cell count of a patient diagnosed with leukemia, or the hemoglobin of a patient who has recently received a blood **transfusion**. Because of its value, though, as an indicator of a person's overall health, the CBC package is most frequently ordered.

The blood count is performed relatively inexpensively and quickly. Most laboratories routinely use some type of automated equipment to dilute the blood, sample a measured volume of the diluted suspension, and count the cells in that volume. In addition to counting actual numbers of red cells, white cells, and platelets, the automated cell counters also measure the hemoglobin and calculate the hematocrit and the **red blood cell indices** (measures of the size and hemoglobin content of the red blood cells).

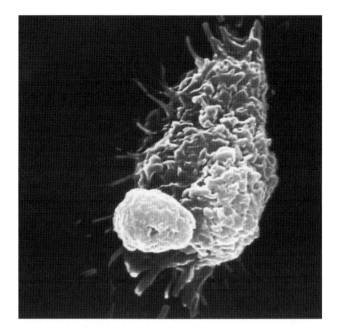

A white blood cell. (Photograph by Institut Pasteur, Phototake NYC. Reproduced by permission.)

Technologists then examine a stained blood smear under the microscope to identify any abnormalities in the appearance of the red blood cells and to report the types and percentages of white blood cells observed.

The red blood cell (RBC) count determines the total number of red cells (erythrocytes) in a sample of blood. The red cells, the most numerous of the cellular elements, carry oxygen from the lungs to the body's tissues. Hemoglobin (Hgb) is the protein-iron compound in the red blood cells that enables them to transport oxygen. Its concentration corresponds closely to the RBC count. Also closely tied to the RBC and hemoglobin values is the hematocrit (Hct), which measures the percentage of red blood cells in the total blood volume. The hematocrit (expressed as percentage points) is normally about three times the hemoglobin concentration (reported as grams per deciliter).

Red blood cell indices provide information about the size and hemoglobin content of the red cells. They are useful in differentiating types of anemias. The indices include four measurements that are calculated using the RBC count, hemoglobin, and hematocrit results. Mean corpuscular volume (MCV) is a measurement of the average size of the red blood cells and indicates whether that is small, large or normal. The red blood cell distribution width

(RDW) is an indication of the variation in RBC size. Mean corpuscular hemoglobin (MCH) measures the average amount (weight) of hemoglobin within a red blood cell. A similar measurement, mean corpuscular hemoglobin concentration (MCHC), expresses the average concentration of hemoglobin in the red blood cells.

The white blood cell (WBC) count determines the total number of white cells (leukocytes) in the blood sample. Fewer in number than the red cells, WBCs are the body's primary means of fighting infection. There are five main types of white cells (neutrophils, lymphocytes, monocytes, eosinophils, and basophils), each of which plays a different role in responding to the presence of foreign organisms in the body. A differential white cell count is done by staining a smear of the patient's blood with a Wright's stain, allowing the different types of white cells to be clearly seen under the microscope. A technologist then counts a minimum of 100 WBCs and reports each type of white cell as a percentage of the total white blood cells counted.

The **platelet count** is an actual count of the number of platelets (thrombocytes) in a given volume of blood. Platelets, the smallest of the cellular elements of blood, are involved in blood clotting. Because platelets can clump together, the automated counting method is subject to a certain level of error and may not be accurate enough for low platelet counts. For this reason, very low platelet levels are often counted manually.

Normal results

Blood count values can vary by age and sex. The normal red blood cell count ranges from 4.2–5.4 million RBCs per microliter of blood for men and 3.6–5.0 million for women. Hemoglobin values range from 14–18 grams per deciliter of blood for men and 12–16 grams for women. The normal hematocrit is 42–54% for men and 36–48% for women. The normal number of white blood cells for both men and women is approximately 4,000–10,000 WBCs per microliter of blood.

Abnormal results

Abnormal blood count results are seen in a variety of conditions. One of the most common is anemias, which are characterized by low RBC counts, hemoglobins, and hematocrits. Infections and leukemias are associated with increased numbers of WBCs.

Resources

BOOKS

Berkow, Robert, ed. *Merck Manual of Medical Information.* Whitehouse Station, NJ: Merck Research Laboratories, 1997.

Henry, J. B. *Clinical Diagnosis and Management by Laboratory Methods.* New York: W. B. Saunders Co., 1996.

Karen A. Boyden

Blood crossmatching *see* **Blood typing and crossmatching**

Blood culture

Definition

A blood culture is done when a person has symptoms of a blood infection, also called **bacteremia**. Blood is drawn from the person one or more times and is tested in a laboratory to find and identify any microorganism present and growing in the blood. If a microorganism is found, more testing is done to determine the **antibiotics** that will be effective in treating the infection.

Purpose

Bacteremia is a serious clinical condition and can lead to **death**. To give the best chance for effective treatment and survival, a blood culture is done as soon as an infection is suspected.

Symptoms of bacteremia are **fever**, chills, mental confusion, **anxiety**, rapid heart beat, hyperventilation, blood clotting problems, and **shock**. These symptoms are especially significant in a person who already has another illness or infection, is hospitalized, or has trouble fighting infections because of a weak immune system. Often, the blood infection results from an infection somewhere else in the body that has now spread.

Additionally, blood cultures are done to find the causes of other infections. These include bacterial **pneumonia** (an infection of the lung), and infectious **endocarditis** (an infection of the inner layer of the heart). Both of these infections leak bacteria into the blood.

After a blood infection has been diagnosed, confirmed by culture, and treated, an additional blood culture may be done to make sure the infection is gone.

Description

Culture strategies

There are many variables involved in performing a blood culture. Before the person's blood is drawn, the physician must make several decisions based on a knowledge of infections and the person's clinical condition and medical history.

Several groups of microorganisms, including bacteria, viruses, mold, and yeast, can cause blood infections. The bacteria group can be further broken down into aerobes and anaerobes. Most aerobes do not need oxygen to live. They can grow with oxygen (aerobic microbes) or without oxygen (anaerobic microbes).

Based on the clinical condition of the patient, the physician determines what group of microorganisms is likely to be causing the infection and then orders one or more specific types of blood culture, including aerobic, anaerobic, viral, or fungal (for yeasts and molds). Each specific type of culture is handled differently by the laboratory. Most blood cultures test for both aerobic and anaerobic microbes. Fungal, viral, and mycobacterial blood cultures can also be done, but are less common.

The physician must also decide how many blood cultures should be done. One culture is rarely enough, but two to three are usually adequate. Four cultures are occasionally required. Some factors influencing this decision are the specific microorganisms the physician expects to find based on the person's symptoms or previous culture results, and whether or not the person has had recent antibiotic therapy.

The time at which the cultures are to be drawn is another decision made by the physician. During most blood infections (called intermittent bacteremia) microorganisms enter the blood at various time intervals. Blood drawn randomly may miss the microorganisms. Since microorganisms enter the blood 30–90 minutes before the person's fever spikes, collecting the culture just after the fever spike offers the best likelihood of finding the microorganism. The second and third cultures may be collected at the same time, but from different places on the person, or spaced at 30-minute or one-hour intervals, as the physician chooses. During continuous bacteremia, such as infective endocarditis, microorganisms are always in the blood and the timing of culture collection is less important. Blood cultures should always be collected before antibiotic treatment has begun.

Laboratory analysis

Bacteria are the most common microorganisms found in blood infections. Laboratory analysis of a bacterial blood culture differs slightly from that of a fungal culture and significantly from that of a viral culture.

Blood is drawn from a person and put directly into a blood culture bottle containing a nutritional broth. After the laboratory receives the blood culture bottle, several processes must be completed:

- provide an environment for the bacteria to grow
- detect the growth when it occurs
- identify the bacteria that grow
- test the bacteria against certain antibiotics to determine which antibiotic will be effective

There are several types of systems, both manual and automated, available to laboratories to carry out these processes.

The broth in the blood culture bottle is the first step in creating an environment in which bacteria will grow. It contains all the nutrients that bacteria need to grow. If the physician expects anaerobic bacteria to grow, oxygen will be kept out of the blood culture bottle; if aerobes are expected, oxygen will be allowed in the bottle.

The bottles are placed in an incubator and kept at body temperature. They are watched daily for signs of growth, including cloudiness or a color change in the broth, gas bubbles, or clumps of bacteria. When there is evidence of growth, the laboratory does a gram stain and a subculture. To do the gram stain, a drop of blood is removed from the bottle and placed on a microscope slide. The blood is allowed to dry and then is stained with purple and red stains and examined under the microscope. If bacteria are seen, the color of stain they picked up (purple or red), their shape (such as round or rectangular), and their size provide valuable clues as to what type of microorganism they are and what antibiotics might work best. To do the subculture, a drop of blood is placed on a culture plate, spread over the surface, and placed in an incubator.

If there is no immediate visible evidence of growth in the bottles, the laboratory looks for bacteria by doing gram stains and subcultures. These steps are repeated daily for the first several days and periodically after that.

When bacteria grows, the laboratory identifies it using biochemical tests and the gram stain. Sensitivity testing, also called antibiotic susceptibility testing, is also done. The bacteria are tested against many different antibiotics to see which antibiotics can effectively kill it.

All information is passed on to the physician as soon as it is known. An early report, known as a preliminary report, is usually available after one day. This report will tell if any bacteria have been found yet, and if so, the results of the gram stain. The next preliminary report may include a description of the bacteria growing on the subculture. The laboratory notifies the physician immediately when an organism is found and as soon as sensitivity tests are complete. Sensitivity tests may be complete before the bacteria is completely identified. The final report may not be available for five to seven days. If bacteria was found, the report will include its complete identification and a list of the antibiotics to which the bacteria is sensitive.

One automated system is considered one of the most important recent technical advances in blood cultures. It is called continuous-monitoring blood culture systems (CMCCS). The instruments automatically monitor the bottles containing the patient blood for evidence of microorganisms, usually every 10 minutes. Many data points are collected daily for each bottle, and fed into a computer for analysis. Sophisticated mathematical calculations can determine when microorganisms have grown. This, combined with more frequent blood tests, make it possible to detect microbial growth earlier. In addition, all CMBCS instruments have the detection system, incubator, and agitation unit in one unit.

Preparation

Ten ml (milliliter) of blood is usually needed for each blood culture bottle. First a healthcare worker locates a vein in the inner elbow region. The area of skin where the blood will be drawn must be disinfected to prevent any microorganisms on a person's skin from entering the blood culture bottle and contaminating it. The area is disinfected by wiping the area with alcohol in a circular fashion, starting with tiny circles at the spot where the needle will puncture the skin and enlarging the size of the circles while wiping away from the puncture site. The same pattern of wiping is repeated using an iodine or iodophor solution. The top of the bottle is disinfected using alcohol. After the person's skin has been disinfected, the healthcare worker draws the blood and about 10 ml of blood is injected into each blood culture bottle. The type of bottles used will vary based on whether the physician is looking for bacteria (aerobes or anaerobes), yeast, mold, or viruses.

Aftercare

Discomfort or bruising may occur at the puncture site or the person may feel dizzy or faint. Pressure to the puncture site until the bleeding stops reduces bruising. Warm packs relieve discomfort.

Normal results

Normal results will be negative. A single negative culture does not rule out a blood infection. False negatives can occur if the person was started on antibiotics before the blood was drawn, if the environment for growth was not right, the timing was off, or for some unknown reason the microorganism just didn't grow. Three negative cultures may be enough to rule out bacteremia in the case of endocarditis.

Abnormal results

The physician's skill in interpreting the culture results and assessing the person's clinical condition is essential in distinguishing a blood culture that is positive because of a true infection from a culture that is positive because it became contaminated. In true bacteremia, the patient's clinical condition should be consistent with a blood infection caused by the microorganism that was found. The microorganism is usually found in more than one culture, it usually grows soon after the bottles are incubated, and it is often the cause of an infection somewhere else in the person's body.

When the culture is positive because of contamination, the patient's clinical condition usually is not consistent with an infection from the identified microorganism. In addition, the microorganism is often one commonly found on skin, it rarely causes infection, it is found in only one bottle, and it may appear after several days of incubation. More than one microorganism often grow in contaminated cultures.

Resources

ORGANIZATIONS

American Society of Microbiology. 1752 N Street N.W., Washington, D.C. 20036. (202) 737-3600. < http:// www.asmusa.org > .

Nancy J. Nordenson

Blood donation and registry

Definition

Blood donation refers to the process of collecting, testing, preparing, and storing blood and blood components. Donors are most commonly unpaid volunteers, but they may also be paid by commercial enterprises. Blood registry refers to the collection and sharing of data about donated blood and ineligible donors.

Purpose

The purpose of the blood collection and distribution system is to help ensure an adequate supply of blood for accident victims, people needing surgery, and people suffering from certain diseases, as well as for medical research.

Sometimes, donors give blood specifically to benefit a particular person. People preparing for elective surgery may donate their own blood to be held and then returned to them during surgery. This is known as autologous blood donation. Directed donor blood has been donated by someone known

KEY TERMS

Apheresis—Extraction of a specific component from donated blood, with the remainder returned to the donor.

Autologous donation—Blood donated for the donor's own use.

Granulocytes—White blood cells.

Plasma—The liquid part of blood.

Platelets—Tiny, disklike elements of plasma that promote clotting.

to the intended recipient, such as a family member or friend.

Each year, more than four million Americans receive blood transfusions involving more than 26 million units of blood (one unit equals 450 milliliters, or about one pint), or an average of about 32,000 units per day. All of that blood must be collected, tested, prepared, stored, and delivered to the appropriate sites. Roughly eight million people in the United States donate blood each year; about half of the total amount needed is provided by the 36 regional blood centers of the American Red Cross.

Whole blood and the various blood components have many uses. Red blood cells, which carry oxygen, are used to treat anemia. Platelets, which play a role in controlling bleeding, are commonly used in the treatment of leukemia and other cancers. Fresh frozen plasma is also used to control bleeding in people deficient in certain clotting factors. Cryoprecipitated AHF, made from fresh frozen plasma, contains a few specific clotting factors.

Precautions

To ensure the safety of the blood supply, a multi-tiered process of donor screening and deferral is employed. This involves donor education, taking a detailed health history of each prospective donor, and giving potential donors a simple **physical examination** (which includes taking a few drops of blood to test for anemia). At any point in the process, a potential donor may be "deferred," or judged ineligible to donate blood. This deferral may be temporary or permanent, depending on the reason. Potential donors are also encouraged to "self-defer," or voluntarily decline to donate, rather than put future blood recipients at risk.

All donated blood is extensively tested before being used. The first step is determining the blood type, which indicates who can receive the blood. Receiving the wrong type of blood can cause **death**. Blood is also screened for any antibodies that could cause complications for recipients. In addition, blood is tested to screen out donors infected with the following diseases: **Hepatitis B** surface antigen ADD, hepatitis B core antibody, **hepatitis C** virus antibody, HIV-1 and HIV-2 antibody, HIV p24 antigen, HTLV-I and HTLV-II antibodies, and **syphilis**. Nucleic Acid Amplification testing is also performed, and other tests may be done if a doctor requests them.

In order to detect the greatest possible number of infections, these screening tests are extremely sensitive. For this reason, however, donors sometimes receive false positive test results. In these cases, more specific confirmatory tests are performed, to help rule out false positive results. Blood found to be abnormal is discarded, and all items coming into direct contact with donors are used only once and then discarded. Donors of infected blood are entered into the Donor Deferral Register, a confidential national data base used to prevent deferred people from donating blood.

In general, blood donors must be at least 17 years old (some states allow younger people to donate blood with their parents' consent), must weigh at least 110 pounds (50 kg), and must be in good health.

Many factors can temporarily or permanently disqualify potential donors. Most of them have to do with having engaged in behaviors that put them at risk of infection or having spent time in certain specified areas. Among these factors are having had a tattoo, having had sex with people in high-risk groups, having had certain diseases, and having been raped.

Description

There are eight different blood types in all—four ABO groups, each of which may be either Rh positive or Rh negative. These types, and their approximate distribution in the U.S. population, are as follows: O+ (38%), O- (7%), A+ (34%), A- (6%), B+ (9%), B- (2%), AB+ (3%), AB- (1%). In an emergency, anyone can safely receive type O red blood cells, and people with this blood type are known as "universal donors." People with type AB blood, known as "universal recipients," can receive any type of red blood cells and can give plasma to all blood types.

Blood donations can be made in community blood centers, at hospitals or in bloodmobiles, which visit schools, churches and workplaces. The actual process of donating whole blood takes about 20 minutes. A sterile needle is inserted into a vein in the donor's arm. The blood flows through plastic tubing into a blood bag. Donors may be asked to clench their fist to encourage blood to flow. Usually, one unit of blood is collected. Afterward, donors are escorted to an observation area, given light refreshments, and allowed to rest.

Plasma, the liquid portion of the blood in which red blood cells, platelets and other elements are suspended, is also collected, often by commercial enterprises that sell it to companies manufacturing clotting factors and other blood products. This is done using a process known as apheresis, in which whole blood is collected, the desired blood component is removed, and the remainder is returned to the donor. Collecting plasma generally takes one to two hours. Apheresis may also be used to collect other blood components, such as platelets and granulocytes.

Preparation

Once whole blood has been collected, it is sent to a lab for testing and processing. Most donated blood is separated into its constituent components, such as red blood cells, platelets, and cryoprecipitate. This enables more than one person to benefit from the same unit of donated blood.

Different blood components vary in how long they can be stored. Red blood cells can be refrigerated for up to 42 days or frozen for as much as 10 years. Platelets, stored at room temperature, may be kept for up to five days. Fresh frozen plasma and cryoprecipitated AHF can be kept for as much as one year.

Aftercare

It generally takes about 24 hours for the donor's body to replenish the lost fluid. Replacing the lost red blood cells, however, may take as much as two months. Whole blood donors must wait a minimum of eight weeks before donating again. Some states place further limits on the frequency and/or total number of times an individual may donate blood within a 12-month period.

Risks

Thanks to the use of a multi-tiered screening system and advances in the effectiveness of screening tests, the transmission of infectious diseases via **transfusion** has been significantly diminished. Nonetheless, there is still a minuscule risk that blood recipients could contract HIV, Hepatitis C or other infections via transfusion. Other diseases that could conceivably be contracted in this way, or that are of particular concern to blood-collection agencies, include **babesiosis**, Chagas disease, HTLV-I and -II, **Creutzfeldt-Jakob disease**, cytomegalovirus, **Lyme disease**, **malaria**, and new variant Creutzfeldt-Jakob disease.

Autologous blood donors run a tiny risk of having the wrong blood returned to them due to clerical error. There is also a faint possibility of bacterial contamination of the autologous blood.

Normal results

For most donors, the process is quick and painless and they leave feeling fine. They may also find satisfaction in knowing that they have contributed to the nation's blood supply and may even have helped save lives.

Abnormal results

Most blood donors suffer no significant aftereffects. Occasionally, however, donors feel faint or dizzy, nauseous, and/or have **pain**, redness, or a bruise where the blood was taken. More serious complications, which rarely occur, include **fainting**, **muscle spasms**, and nerve damage.

Resources

PERIODICALS

McKenna, C. "Blood Minded" *Nursing Times* April 6, 2000: 27-28.

Wagner, H. "Umbilical Cord Blood Banking: Insurance Against Future Diseases?" *USA Today Magazine* (March 2000) : 59-61.

ORGANIZATIONS

American Association of Blood Banks. 8101 Glenbrook Road, Bethesda, MD 20814-2749. (301) 907-6977. < http://www.aabb.org > .

American Red Cross. 430 17th Street NW, Washington, D.C. 20006. < http://www.redcross.org > .

National Blood Data Resource Center. (301) 215-6506. < http://www.nbdrc.org > .

Peter Gregutt

Blood fluke infection *see* **Schistosomiasis**

Blood gas analysis

Definition

Blood gas analysis, also called arterial blood gas (ABG) analysis, is a test which measures the amounts of oxygen and carbon dioxide in the blood, as well as the acidity (pH) of the blood.

Purpose

An ABG analysis evaluates how effectively the lungs are delivering oxygen to the blood and how efficiently they are eliminating carbon dioxide from it. The test also indicates how well the lungs and kidneys are interacting to maintain normal blood pH (acid-base balance). Blood gas studies are usually done to assess respiratory disease and other conditions that may affect the lungs, and to manage patients receiving **oxygen therapy** (respiratory therapy). In addition, the acid-base component of the test provides information on kidney function.

Description

Blood gas analysis is performed on blood from an artery. It measures the partial pressures of oxygen and carbon dioxide in the blood, as well as oxygen content, oxygen saturation, bicarbonate content, and blood pH.

Oxygen in the lungs is carried to the tissues through the bloodstream, but only a small amount of this oxygen can actually dissolve in arterial blood. How much dissolves depends on the partial pressure of the oxygen (the pressure that the gas exerts on the walls of the arteries). Therefore, testing the partial pressure of oxygen is actually measuring how much oxygen the lungs are delivering to the blood. Carbon dioxide is released into the blood as a by-product of cell metabolism. The partial carbon dioxide pressure indicates how well the lungs are eliminating this carbon dioxide.

The remainder of oxygen that is not dissolved in the blood combines with hemoglobin, a protein–iron compound found in the red blood cells. The oxygen content measurement in an ABG analysis indicates how much oxygen is combined with the hemoglobin. A related value is the oxygen saturation, which compares the amount of oxygen actually combined with hemoglobin to the total amount of oxygen that the hemoglobin is capable of combining with.

Carbon dioxide dissolves more readily in the blood than oxygen does, primarily forming bicarbonate and smaller amounts of carbonic acid. When present in

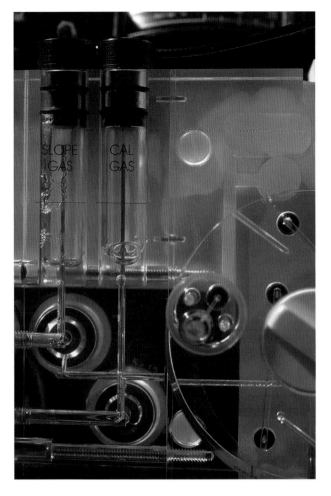

A blood gas analyzer from Corning Corporation. *(Photograph by Hank Morgan, Photo Researchers, Inc. Reproduced by permission.)*

KEY TERMS

Acid-base balance—The condition that exists when the body's carbonic acid-bicarbonate buffer system is in equilibrium, helping to maintain the blood pH at a normal level of 7.35–7.45.

Hemoglobin—A protein—iron compound in red blood cells that functions primarily in carrying oxygen from the lungs to the tissues of the body.

pH—A measure of the acidity of a solution. Normal blood pH ranges from 7.35–7.45.

normal amounts, the ratio of carbonic acid to bicarbonate creates an acid-base balance in the blood, helping to keep the pH at a level where the body's cellular functions are most efficient. The lungs and kidneys both participate in maintaining the carbonic acid-bicarbonate balance. The lungs control the carbonic acid level and the kidneys regulate the bicarbonate. If either organ is not functioning properly, an acid-base imbalance can result. Determination of bicarbonate and pH levels, then, aids in diagnosing the cause of abnormal blood gas values.

The procedure

The blood sample is obtained by arterial puncture (usually in the wrist, although it could be in the groin or arm) or from an arterial line already in place. If a puncture is needed, the skin over the artery is cleaned with an antiseptic. A technician then collects the blood with a small sterile needle attached to a disposable syringe. The patient may feel a brief throbbing or cramping at the site of the puncture. After the blood is drawn, the sample must be transported to the laboratory as soon as possible for analysis.

Preparation

There are no special preparations. Patients have no restrictions on drinking or eating before the test. If the patient is receiving oxygen, the oxygen concentration must remain the same for 20 minutes before the test; if the test is to be taken without oxygen, the gas must be turned off for 20 minutes before the test is taken. The patient should breathe normally during the test.

Aftercare

After the blood has been taken, the technician or the patient applies pressure to the puncture site for 10–15 minutes to stop the bleeding, and then places a dressing over the puncture. The patient should rest quietly while applying the pressure to the puncture site. Health care workers will observe the patient for signs of bleeding or circulation problems

Risks

Risks are very low when the test is done correctly. Risks include bleeding or bruising at the site, or delayed bleeding from the site. Very rarely, there may be a problem with circulation in the puncture area.

Normal results

Normal blood gas values are as follows:

- partial pressure of oxygen (PaO_2): 75–100 mm Hg
- partial pressure of carbon dioxide ($PaCO_2$): 35–45 mm Hg

- oxygen content (O_2CT): 15–23%
- oxygen saturation (SaO_2): 94–100%
- bicarbonate (HCO_3): 22–26 mEq/liter
- pH: 7.35–7.45

Abnormal results

Values that differ from those listed above may indicate respiratory, metabolic, or **kidney disease**. These results also may be abnormal if the patient has experienced trauma that may affect breathing (especially head and neck injuries). Disorders, such as anemia, that affect the oxygen-carrying capacity of blood, can produce an abnormally low oxygen content value.

Resources

BOOKS

Thompson, June, et al. *Mosby's Clinical Nursing.* 4th ed. St. Louis: Mosby, 1997.

Carol A. Turkington

Blood poisoning *see* **Acute lymphangitis**

Blood registry *see* **Blood donation and registry**

Blood removal *see* **Phlebotomy**

Blood sugar tests

Definition

Blood sugar tests include several different tests that measure the amount of sugar (glucose) in a person's blood. These tests are performed either on an empty stomach, or after consuming a meal or pre-measured glucose drink. Blood sugar tests are done primarily to diagnose and evaluate a person with **diabetes mellitus**.

Purpose

The body uses sugar, also called glucose, to supply the energy it needs to function. People get sugar from their diet and from their body tissues. Insulin is made by the pancreas and affects the outer membrane of cells, making it easy for glucose to move from the blood into the cells. When insulin is active, blood glucose levels fall. Sugar from body tissues is stored in the form of glycogen. When glycogen is active, blood glucose levels rise.

After a meal, blood glucose levels rise sharply. The pancreas responds by releasing enough insulin to take care of all the newly added sugar found in the body. The insulin moves the sugar out of the blood and into the cells. Only then does the blood sugar start to level off and begin to fall. A person with diabetes mellitus either does not make enough insulin, or makes insulin that does not work properly. The result is blood sugar that remains high, a condition called hyperglycemia.

Diabetes must be diagnosed as early as possible. If left untreated, it can damage or cause failure of the eyes, kidneys, nerves, heart, blood vessels, and other body organs. **Hypoglycemia**, or low blood sugar, also may be discovered through blood sugar testing. Hypoglycemia is caused by various hormone disorders and **liver disease**, as well as by too much insulin.

Description

There are a variety of ways to measure a person's blood sugar.

Whole blood glucose test

Whole blood glucose testing can be performed by a person in his or her home, and kits are available for this purpose. The person pricks his or her finger (a finger stick) with a sterile sharp blade from the kit. A single drop of blood is placed on a strip in a portable instrument called a glucometer. The glucometer quickly determines the blood sugar and shows the results on a small screen in usually a few seconds.

New technologies for monitoring glucose levels will help diabetics better control their glucose levels. These tests are particularly important for children and adolescents. In mid-2002, the U.S. Food and Drug Administration (FDA) approved a new home test for use by children and adolescents (it had already been approved for adults) called the Cygnus GlucoWatch biographer that helped better detect hypoglycemia. Studies show that more frequent checks are better; new monitors such as this allow for simpler frequent testing. Continuous monitoring was in development in early 2004, as a company called TheraSense, Inc. received preapproval from the FDA for clinical trials on its home continuous glucose monitor. The monitor was designed to provide users with real-time glucose data, alarms for hypoglycemia and hyperglycemia and to show trends in their blood sugar levels.

Fasting plasma glucose test

The **fasting** plasma glucose test is done on an empty stomach. For the eight hours before the test, the person must fast (nothing to eat or drink, except water). The person's blood is drawn from a vein by a health care worker. The blood sample is collected into a tube containing an anticoagulant. Anticoagulants stop the blood from clotting. In the laboratory, the tube of blood spins at high speed within a machine called a centrifuge. The blood cells sink to the bottom and the liquid stays on the top. This straw-colored liquid on the top is the plasma. To measure the glucose, a person's plasma is combined with other substances. From the resulting reaction, the amount of glucose in the plasma is determined.

Oral glucose tolerance test

The oral glucose tolerance test is conducted to see how well the body handles a standard amount of glucose. This test measures the amount of glucose in a person's plasma before and two hours after drinking a large premeasured beverage containing glucose. The person must eat a consistent diet, containing at least 5.25 oz (150g) of carbohydrates each day, for three days before this test. For eight hours before the test, the person must fast. A health care provider draws the first sample of blood at the end of the fast to determine the glucose level at the start of the test. The health care provider then gives the person a beverage containing 2.6oz (75g) of glucose. Two hours later, the person's blood is drawn again. These blood samples are centrifuged and processed in the laboratory. A doctor can then compare the before and after glucose levels to see how well the patient's body processed the sugar.

Two-hour postprandial blood glucose test

The two-hour postprandial blood glucose test measures the amount of glucose in plasma after a person eats a specific meal containing a certain amount of sugar. Although the meal follows a predetermined menu, it is difficult to control many factors associated with this testing method.

Blood sugar tests can be used in a variety of situations including:

- Testing people suspected for diabetes. The American Diabetic Association (ADA) recommends that either a fasting plasma glucose test or an oral glucose tolerance test be used to diagnose diabetes. If the person already has symptoms of diabetes, a blood glucose test without fasting (called a casual plasma glucose test) may be done. If the test result is abnormal, it must be confirmed with another test performed on another day. The two tests can be different or they can be the same, but they must be done on different days. If the second test also is abnormal, the person has diabetes. A two-hour postprandial test is not recommended by the ADA as a test to use for the diagnosis of diabetes. A doctor may order this test, and follow it with the oral glucose tolerance test or the fasting plasma glucose test if the results are abnormal.

• Testing pregnant women. Diabetes that occurs during **pregnancy (gestational diabetes)** is dangerous for both the mother and the baby. Women who may be at risk are screened when they are 24-28 weeks pregnant. A woman is considered at risk if she is older than 25 years, is not at her normal body weight, has a parent or sibling with diabetes, or if she is in an ethnic group that has a high rate of diabetes (Hispanics, Native Americans, Asians, African Americans). The blood sugar test to screen for gestational diabetes is a variation of the oral glucose tolerance test. Fasting is not required. If the result is abnormal, a more complete test is done on another day.

• Testing healthy people. Healthy people without symptoms of diabetes should be screened for diabetes when they are 45 years old and again every three years. Either the fasting plasma glucose or oral glucose tolerance test is used for screening. People in high risk groups should be tested before the age of 45 and tested more frequently.

• Testing of people already diagnosed with diabetes. The ADA recommends that a person with diabetes keep the amount of glucose in the blood at a normal level as much as possible. This can be done by the diabetic person testing his or her own blood at home one or more times a day.

Preparation

Each blood sugar test that uses plasma requires a 5 mL blood sample. A healthcare worker ties a tight band (tourniquet) on the person's upper arm, locates a vein in the inner elbow region, and inserts a needle into the vein. Vacuum action draws the blood through the needle into an attached tube. Collection of the sample takes only a few minutes.

When fasting is required, the person should have nothing to eat or drink (except water) for eight hours before the test and until the test or series of tests is completed. The person should not smoke before or during the testing period because this can temporarily increase the amount of glucose in the blood. Other factors that can cause inaccurate results are a change in diet before the test, illness or surgery two weeks

before the test, certain drugs, and extended bed rest. The doctor may tell a person on insulin or taking pills for diabetes to stop the medication until after the test.

Aftercare

After the test or series of tests is completed (and with the approval of his or her doctor), the person should eat, drink, and take any medications that were stopped for the test.

The patient may feel discomfort when blood is drawn from a vein. Bruising may occur at the puncture site or the person may feel dizzy or faint. Pressure to the puncture site until the bleeding stops will reduce bruising. Warm packs to the puncture site will relieve discomfort.

Risks

If the person experiences weakness, **fainting**, sweating, or any other unusual reaction while fasting or during the test, he or she should immediately tell the person giving the test.

Normal results

Normal results are:

• fasting plasma glucose test less than 120 mg/dL

• oral glucose tolerance test, 2 hours less than 140 mg/dL

For the diabetic person, the ADA recommends an ongoing blood sugar goal of less than or equal to 120 mg/dL.

Abnormal results

These abnormal results indicate diabetes and must be confirmed with repeat testing:

• fasting plasma glucose test less than or equal to 126 mg/dL

• oral glucose tolerance test, 2 hours less than or equal to 200 mg/dL

• casual plasma glucose test (nonfasting, with symptoms) less than or equal to 200 mg/dL

• gestational oral glucose tolerance test, 1 hour less than or equal to 140 mg/dL

Brain damage can occur from glucose levels below 40 mg/dL and **coma** from levels above 470 mg/dL.

A condition known as prediabetes or impaired glucose tolerance, which may lead to Type 2 diabetes, usually is indicated with a reading of 100 mg/dL. Other hormone disorders can cause both hyperglycemia and hypoglycemia. Abnormal results must be interpreted by a doctor who is aware of the person's medical condition and medical history.

Resources

PERIODICALS

"New Guidelines Set Lower Threshold for Precursor to Diabetes." *RN* (January 2004): 17.

Plotnick, Leslie P. "The Next Step in Blood Glucose Monitoring?" *Pediatrics* (April 2003): 885.

"Premarket Approval Application Filed for Continuous Glucose Monitor." *Medical Letter on the CDC & FDA* (January 4, 2004): 26.

ORGANIZATIONS

American Diabetes Association. 1701 North Beauregard Street, Alexandria, VA 22311. (800) 342-2383. < http:// www.diabetes.org > .

Centers for Disease Control and Prevention. 1600 Clifton Rd., NE, Atlanta, GA 30333. (800) 311-3435, (404) 639-3311. < http://www.cdc.gov > .

National Diabetes Information Clearinghouse. 1 Information Way, Bethesda, MD 20892-3560. (800) 860-8747. < http://www.niddk.nih.gov/health/diabetes/ndic.htm > .

Nancy J. Nordenson
Teresa G. Odle

Blood thinners *see* **Anticoagulant and antiplatelet drugs**

Blood transfusion *see* **Transfusion**

Blood typing and crossmatching

Definition

Blood typing is a laboratory test done to determine a person's blood type. If the person needs a blood **transfusion**, another test called crossmatching is done after the blood is typed to find blood from a donor that the person's body will accept.

Purpose

Blood typing and crossmatching are most commonly done to make certain that a person who needs a transfusion will receive blood that matches (is compatible with) his own. People must receive blood of the same blood type, otherwise, a serious, even fatal, transfusion reaction can occur.

Parents who are expecting a baby have their blood typed to diagnose and prevent hemolytic disease of the newborn (HDN), a type of anemia also known as **erythroblastosis fetalis**. Babies who have a blood type different from their mothers are at risk for developing this disease. The disease is serious with certain blood type differences, but is milder with others.

A child inherits factors or genes from each parent that determine his blood type. This fact makes blood typing useful in paternity testing. To determine whether or not the alleged father could be the true father, the blood types of the child, mother, and alleged father are compared.

Legal investigations may require typing of blood or other body fluids, such as semen or saliva, to identify persons involved in crimes or other legal matters.

Description

Blood typing and crossmatching tests are performed in a blood bank laboratory by technologists trained in blood bank and transfusion services. The tests are done on blood, after it has separated into cells and serum (serum is the yellow liquid left after the blood clots.) Costs for both tests are covered by insurance when the tests are determined to be medically necessary.

Blood bank laboratories are usually located in facilities, such as those operated by the American Red Cross, that collect, process, and supply blood that is donated, as well as in facilities, such as most hospitals, that prepare blood for transfusion. These laboratories are regulated by the United States Food and Drug Administration (FDA) and are often inspected and accredited by a professional association such as the American Association of Blood Banks (AABB).

Blood typing and crossmatching tests are based on the reaction between antigens and antibodies. An antigen can be anything that causes the body to launch an attack, known as an immune response, against it. The attack begins when the body builds a special protein, called an antibody, that is uniquely designed to attack and make ineffective (neutralize) the specific antigen that caused the attack. A person's body normally doesn't make antibodies against its own antigens, only against antigens that are foreign to it.

A person's body contains many antigens. The antigens found on the surface of red blood cells are important because they determine a person's blood type. When red blood cells having a certain blood type antigen are mixed with serum containing antibodies against

Frequency (%) Of ABO And Rh Blood Types In U.S. Population						
Racial Group	ABO Blood Type				Rh Blood Type	
	O	A	B	AB	Positive	Negative
Whites	45%	40%	11%	4%	85%	15%
Blacks	49%	27%	20%	4%	90%	10%

that antigen, the antibodies attack and stick to the antigen. In a test tube, this reaction is observed as the formation of clumps of cells (clumping).

When blood is typed, a person's cells and serum are mixed in a test tube with commercially-prepared serum and cells. Clumping tells which antigens or antibodies are present and reveals the person's blood type. When blood is crossmatched, patient serum is mixed with cells from donated blood that might be used for transfusion. Clumping or lack of clumping in the test tube tells whether or not the blood is compatible.

Although there are over 600 known red blood cell antigens, organized into 22 blood group systems, routine blood typing and crossmatching is usually concerned with only two systems: the ABO and Rh blood group systems.

Blood typing

ABO BLOOD GROUP SYSTEM. In 1901, Karl Landsteiner, an Austrian pathologist, randomly combined the serum and red blood cells of his colleagues. From the reactions he observed in test tubes, he discovered the ABO blood group system. This discovery earned him the 1930 Nobel Prize in Medicine.

A person's ABO blood type–A, B, AB, or O–is based on the presence or absence of the A and B antigens on his red blood cells. The A blood type has only the A antigen and the B blood type has only the B antigen. The AB blood type has both A and B antigens, and the O blood type has neither A nor B antigen.

By the time a person is six months old, he naturally will have developed antibodies against the antigens his red blood cells lack. That is, a person with A blood type will have anti-B antibodies, and a person with B blood type will have anti-A antibodies. A person with AB blood type will have neither antibody, but a person with O blood type will have both anti-A and anti-B antibodies. Although the distribution of each of the four ABO blood types varies between racial

groups, O is the most common and AB is the least common.

ABO typing is the first test done on blood when it is tested for transfusion. A person must receive ABO-matched blood. ABO incompatibilities are the major cause of fatal transfusion reactions. ABO antigens are also found on most body organs, so ABO compatibility is also important for organ transplants.

An ABO incompatibility between a pregnant woman and her baby is a minor cause of HDN and usually causes no problem for the baby. The structure of ABO antibodies makes it unlikely they will cross the placenta to attack the baby's red blood cells.

Paternity testing compares the ABO blood types of the child, mother, and alleged father. The alleged father can't be the true father if the child's blood type requires a gene that neither he nor the mother have. For example, a child with blood type B whose mother has blood type O, requires a father with either AB or B blood type; a man with blood type O cannot be the true father.

In some people, ABO antigens can be found in body fluids other than blood, such as saliva and semen. ABO typing of these fluids provides clues in legal investigations.

RH BLOOD GROUP SYSTEM. The Rh, or Rhesus, system was first detected in 1940 by Landsteiner and Wiener when they injected blood from rhesus monkeys into guinea pigs and rabbits. More than 50 antigens have since been discovered belonging to this system, making it the most complex red blood cell antigen system.

In routine blood typing and crossmatching tests, only one of these 50 antigens, the D antigen, also known as the Rh factor or $Rh_o[D]$, is tested for. If the D antigen is present, that person is Rh-positive; if the D antigen is absent, that person is Rh-negative.

Other important antigens in the Rh system are C, c, E, and e. These antigens are not usually tested for in routine blood typing tests. However, testing for the presence of these antigens is useful in paternity testing, and when a technologist tries to identify unexpected

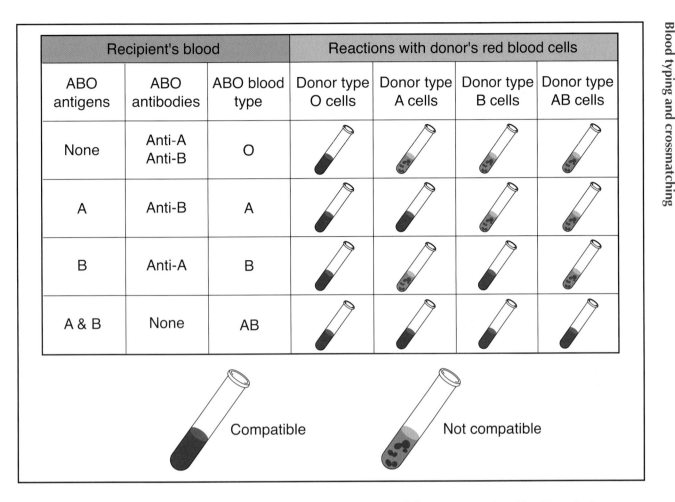

Recipient's blood			Reactions with donor's red blood cells			
ABO antigens	ABO antibodies	ABO blood type	Donor type O cells	Donor type A cells	Donor type B cells	Donor type AB cells
None	Anti-A Anti-B	O				
A	Anti-B	A				
B	Anti-A	B				
A & B	None	AB				

Compatible   Not compatible

Blood typing is a laboratory test done to discover a person's blood type. If the person needs a blood transfusion, cross-matching is done following blood typing to locate donor blood that the person's body will accept. *(Illustration by Electronic Illustrators Group.)*

Rh antibodies or find matching blood for a person with antibodies to one or more of these antigens.

Unlike the ABO system, antibodies to Rh antigens don't develop naturally. They develop only as an immune response after a transfusion or during **pregnancy**.

The incidence of the Rh blood types varies between racial groups, but not as widely as the ABO blood types: 85% of whites and 90% of blacks are Rh-positive; 15% of whites and 10% of blacks are Rh-negative.

In transfusions, the Rh system is next in importance after the ABO system. Most Rh-negative people who receive Rh-positive blood will develop anti-D antibodies. A later transfusion of Rh-positive blood could result in a severe or fatal transfusion reaction.

Rh incompatibility is the most common and severe cause of HDN. This incompatibility can

happen when an Rh-negative woman and an Rh-positive man produce an Rh-positive baby. Cells from the baby can cross the placenta and enter the mother's bloodstream, causing the mother to make anti-D antibodies. Unlike ABO antibodies, the structure of anti-D antibodies makes it likely that they will cross the placenta and enter the baby's bloodstream. There, they can destroy the baby's red blood cells, causing severe or fatal anemia.

The first step in preventing HDN is to find out the Rh types of the expectant parents. If the mother is Rh-negative and the father is Rh-positive, the baby is at risk for developing HDN. The next step is to test the mother's serum to make sure she doesn't already have anti-D antibodies from a previous pregnancy or transfusion. This procedure is similar to blood typing. Finally, the Rh-negative mother is given an injection of Rh Immunoglobulin (RhIg) at 28 weeks of gestation and again after delivery, if the baby is Rh positive.

The RhIg attaches to any Rh-positive cells from the baby in the mother's bloodstream, preventing them from triggering anti-D antibody production in the mother. An Rh-negative woman should also receive RhIg following a **miscarriage**, abortion, or **ectopic pregnancy**.

OTHER BLOOD GROUP SYSTEMS. Several other blood group systems may be involved in HDN and transfusion reactions, although they are much less frequent than ABO and Rh. They are the Duffy, Kell, Kidd, MNS, and P systems. Tests for antigens from these systems are not included in routine blood typing, but they are commonly used in paternity testing.

Like Rh antibodies, antibodies in these systems do not develop naturally, but as an immune response after transfusion or during pregnancy. An antibody screening test is done before a crossmatch to check for unexpected antibodies to antigens in these systems. A person's serum is mixed in a test tube with commercially-prepared cells containing antigens from these systems. If clumping occurs, the antibody is identified.

Crossmatching

Crossmatching is the final step in pretransfusion testing. It is commonly referred to as compatibility testing, or "Type and Cross."

Before blood from a donor and the recipient are crossmatched, both are ABO and Rh typed. In addition, antibody screening is done to look for antibodies to certain Rh, Duffy, MNS, Kell, Kidd, and P system antigens. If an antibody to one of these antigens is found, only blood without that antigen will be compatible in a crossmatch. This sequence must be repeated before each transfusion a person receives.

To begin the crossmatch, blood from a donor with the same ABO and Rh type as the rcipient is selected. In a test tube, serum from the patient is mixed with red blood cells from the donor. If clumping occurs, the blood is not compatible; if clumping does not occur, the blood is compatible. If an unexpected antibody is found in either the patient or the donor, the blood bank does further testing to make sure the blood is compatible.

In an emergency, when there is not enough time for blood typing and crossmatching, O red blood cells may be given, preferably Rh-negative. O blood type is called the universal donor because it has no ABO antigens for a patient's antibodies to attack. In contrast, AB blood type is called the universal recipient because it has no ABO antibodies to attack the antigens on transfused red blood cells. If there is time for blood typing, red blood cells of the recipient type (type specific cells) are given. In either case, the crossmatch is continued, even though the transfusion has begun.

Preparation

To collect the 10 mL blood needed for these tests, a healthcare worker ties a tourniquet above the patient's elbow, locates a vein in the inner elbow region, and inserts a needle into that vein. Vacuum action draws the blood through the needle into an attached tube. Collection of the sample takes only a few minutes.

Blood typing and crossmatching must be done three days or less before a transfusion. A person doesn't need to change diet, medications, or activities before these tests. He should tell his healthcare provider if, during the last three months, he has received a blood transfusion or a plasma substitute, or has had a radiology procedure using intravenous contrast media. These can give false clumping reactions in both typing and crossmatching tests.

Aftercare

The possible side effects of any blood collection are discomfort or bruising at the site where the needle punctured the skin, as well as **dizziness** or **fainting**. Bruising is reduced if pressure is applied with a finger to the puncture site until the bleeding stops. Discomfort is treated with warm packs to the puncture site.

Risks

There are no risks from the blood collection or test procedures. Blood transfusions always have the risk of an unexpected transfusion reaction. A nurse watches a patient for signs of a reaction during the entire transfusion.

Normal results

There is no normal blood type. The desired result of a crossmatch is that compatible donor blood is found. Compatibility testing procedures are designed to provide the safest blood product possible for the recipient, but a compatible crossmatch is no guarantee that an unexpected adverse reaction will not appear during the transfusion.

Abnormal results

Except in an emergency, a person cannot receive a transfusion without a compatible crossmatch result.

Resources

ORGANIZATIONS

American Association of Blood Banks. 8101 Glenbrook Road, Bethesda, MD 20814. (301) 907-6977. < http://www.aabb.org > .

Nancy J. Nordenson

Blood urea nitrogen test

Definition

The blood urea nitrogen (BUN) test measures the level of urea nitrogen in a sample of the patient's blood. Urea is a substance that is formed in the liver when the body breaks down protein. Urea then circulates in the blood in the form of urea nitrogen. In healthy people, most urea nitrogen is filtered out by the kidneys and leaves the body in the urine. If the patient's kidneys are not functioning properly or if the body is using large amounts of protein, the BUN level will rise. If the patient has severe **liver disease**, the BUN will drop.

Purpose

The BUN level may be checked in order to assess or monitor:

- the presence or progression of kidney or liver disease.

- blockage of urine flow.

- mental confusion. Patients with kidney failure are sometimes disoriented and confused.

- abnormal loss of water from the body (**dehydration**).

- recovery from severe **burns**. The body uses larger than normal amounts of protein following serious burns.

Description

The BUN test is performed on a sample of the patient's blood, withdrawn from a vein into a vacuum tube. The procedure, which is called a venipuncture, takes about five minutes.

Preparation

The doctor should check to make sure that the patient is not taking any medications that can affect BUN results. These drugs include the **antibiotics** chloramphenicol, streptomycin, amphotericin B, methicillin, gentamicin, tobramycin, and kanamycin, as well as **diuretics** and **corticosteroids**.

The patient should be advised not to eat large amounts of meat the day before the test.

Aftercare

Aftercare consists of routine care of the area around the venipuncture.

Risks

The primary risk is the possibility of a bruise or swelling in the area of the venipuncture. The patient can apply moist warm compresses.

Normal results

Normal BUN levels are 5-18 mg/dL for children; 7-18 mg/dL for adults; and 8-20 mg/dL in the elderly.

Abnormal results

BUN levels can be too low as well as too high.

Abnormally low BUN

Low levels of BUN may indicate **overhydration**, **malnutrition**, **celiac disease** [a disease characterized by the inability ot tolerate foods containing wheat protein (gluten)], liver damage or disease, or use of corticosteroids. Low BUN may also occur in early **pregnancy**.

Abnormally high BUN

High levels of BUN may indicate **kidney disease** or failure; blockage of the urinary tract by a kidney stone or tumor; a **heart attack** or congestive **heart failure**; dehydration; **fever**; **shock**; or bleeding in the digestive tract. High BUN levels can sometimes occur during late pregnancy or result from eating large amounts of protein-rich foods. A BUN level higher than 100 mg/dL points to severe kidney damage.

Resources

BOOKS

Pagana, Kathleen Deska. *Mosby's Manual of Diagnostic and Laboratory Tests*. St. Louis: Mosby, Inc., 1998.

Rebecca J. Frey, PhD

Blood vessel scan *see* **Doppler ultrasonography**

Body dysmorphic disorder

Definition

Body dysmorphic disorder (BDD) is defined by DSM-IV-TR as a condition marked by excessive preoccupation with an imaginary or minor defect in a facial feature or localized part of the body. The diagnostic criteria specify that the condition must be sufficiently severe to cause a decline in the patient's social, occupational, or educational functioning. The most common cause of this decline is the time lost in obsessing about the "defect"—one study found that 68 percent of patients in a sample of adolescents diagnosed with BDD spent three or more hours every day thinking about the body part or facial feature of concern. DSM-IV assigns BDD to the larger category of **somatoform disorders**, which are disorders characterized by physical complaints that appear to be medical in origin but that cannot be explained in terms of a physical disease, the results of **substance abuse**, or by another mental disorder.

The earliest known case of BDD in the medical literature was reported by an Italian physician named Enrique Morselli in 1886, but the disorder was not defined as a formal diagnostic category until DSM-III-R in 1987. The World Health Organization (WHO) did not add BDD to the International Classification of Diseases (ICD) until 1992. The word *dysmorphic* comes from two Greek words that mean "bad" or "ugly" and "shape" or "form." BDD was previously known as dysmorphophobia.

Description

BDD is characterized by an unusual degree of worry or concern about a specific part of the face or body, rather than the general size or shape of the body. It is distinguished from **anorexia nervosa** and **bulimia nervosa** in that patients with eating disorders are preoccupied with their overall weight and body shape. As many as 50 percent of patients diagnosed with BDD undergo **plastic surgery** to correct their perceived physical defects.

Since the publication of DSM-IV in 1994, some psychiatrists have suggested that there is a subtype of BDD, namely muscle dysmorphia. Muscle dysmorphia is marked by excessive concern with one's muscularity and/or fitness. Persons with muscle dysmorphia spend unusual amounts of time working out in gyms or exercising rather than dieting obsessively or seeking plastic surgery. DSM-IV-TR added references to concern about body build and excessive

KEY TERMS

Body image—A term that refers to a person s inner picture of his or her outward appearance. It has two components: perceptions of the appearance of one's body, and emotional responses to those perceptions.

Delusion—A false belief that is resistant to reason or contrary to actual fact. Common delusions include delusions of persecution, delusions about one s importance (sometimes called delusions of grandeur), or delusions of being controlled by others. In BDD, the delusion is related to the patient's perception of his or her body.

Displacement—A psychological process in which feelings originating from one source are expressed outwardly in terms of concern or preoccupation with an issue or problem that the patient considers more acceptable. In some BDD patients, obsession about the body includes displaced feelings, often related to a history of childhood abuse.

Muscle dysmorphia—A subtype of BDD, described as excessive preoccupation with muscularity and body building to the point of interference with social, educational, or occupational functioning.

Serotonin—A chemical produced by the brain that functions as a neurotransmitter. Low serotonin levels are associated with mood disorders, particularly depression. Medications known as selective serotonin reuptake inhibitors (SSRIs) are used to treat BDD and other disorders characterized by depressed mood.

Somatoform disorders—A group of psychiatric disorders in the DSM-IV-TR classification that are characterized by external physical symptoms or complaints. BDD is classified as a somatoform disorder.

weight lifting to DSM-IV's description of BDD in order to cover muscle dysmorphia.

BDD and muscle dysmorphia can both be described as disorders resulting from the patient's distorted body image. Body image refers to a person's mental picture of his or her outward appearance, including size, shape, and form. It has two major components: how the person perceives their physical appearance, and how they feel about their body. Significant distortions in self-perception can lead to intense dissatisfaction with one's body and dysfunctional behaviors aimed at improving one's

appearance. Some patients with BDD are aware that their concerns are excessive, but others do not have this degree of insight; about 50 percent of patients diagnosed with BDD also meet the criteria for a delusional disorder.

The usual age of onset of BDD is late childhood or early adolescence; the average age of patients diagnosed with the disorder is 17. BDD has a high rate of comorbidity, which means that people diagnosed with the disorder are highly likely to have been diagnosed with another psychiatric disorder—most commonly major depression, social phobia, or **obsessive-compulsive disorder** (OCD). About 29% of patients with BDD eventually try to commit **suicide**.

BDD is thought to affect 1–2 percent of the general population in the United States and Canada, although some doctors think that it is underdiagnosed because it coexists so often with depression and other disorders. In addition, patients are often ashamed of grooming rituals and other behaviors associated with BDD, and may avoid telling their doctor about them. BDD is thought to affect men and women equally; however, there are no reliable data as of the early 2000s regarding racial or ethnic differences in the incidence of the disorder.

Causes and symptoms

Causes

The causes of BDD fall into two major categories, neurobiological and psychosocial.

NEUROBIOLOGICAL CAUSES. Research indicates that patients diagnosed with BDD have serotonin levels that are lower than normal. Serotonin is a neurotransmitter— a chemical produced by the brain that helps to transmit nerve impulses across the junctions between nerve cells. Low serotonin levels are associated with depression and other **mood disorders**.

PSYCHOSOCIAL CAUSES. Another important factor in the development of BDD is the influence of the mass media in developed countries, particularly the role of advertising in spreading images of physically "perfect" men and women. Impressionable children and adolescents absorb the message that anything short of physical perfection is unacceptable. They may then develop distorted perceptions of their own faces and bodies.

A young person's family of origin also has a powerful influence on his or her vulnerability to BDD. Children whose parents are themselves obsessed with appearance, dieting, and/or body building, or who are highly critical of their children's looks, are at greater risk of developing BDD.

An additional factor in some young people is a history of childhood trauma or **abuse**. Buried feelings about the abuse or traumatic incident may emerge in the form of obsession about a part of the face or body. This "reassignment" of emotions from the unacknowledged true cause to another issue is called displacement. For example, an adolescent who frequently felt overwhelmed in childhood by physically abusive parents may develop a preoccupation at the high school level with muscular strength and power.

Symptoms

The central symptom of BDD is excessive concern with a specific facial feature or body part. Research indicates that the features most likely to be the focus of the patient's attention are (in order of frequency) complexion flaws (**acne**, blemishes, **scars**, wrinkles); hair (on the head or the body, too much or too little); and facial features (size, shape, or lack of symmetry). The patient's concerns may, however, involve other body parts, and may shift over time from one feature to another.

Other symptoms of body dysmorphic disorder include:

- Ritualistic behavior. Ritualistic behavior refers to actions that the patient performs to manage **anxiety** and that take up excessive amounts of his or her time. Patients are typically upset if someone or something interferes with or interrupts their ritual. Ritualistic behaviors in BDD may include **exercise** or makeup routines, assuming specific poses or postures in front of a mirror, etc.

- Camouflaging the "problem" feature or body part with makeup, hats, or clothing. Camouflaging appears to be the single most common symptom among patients with BDD; it is reported by 94%.

- Abnormal behavior around mirrors, car bumpers, large windows, or similar reflecting surfaces. A majority of patients diagnosed with BDD frequently check their appearance in mirrors or spend long periods of time doing so. A minority, however, react in the opposite fashion and avoid mirrors whenever possible.

- Frequent requests for reassurance from others about their appearance.

- Frequently comparing one's appearance to others.

- Avoiding activities outside the home, including school and social events.

Diagnosis

The diagnosis of BDD in children or adolescents is often made by physicians in family practice because they are more likely to have developed long-term relationships of trust with young people. At the adult level, it is often specialists in dermatology, **cosmetic dentistry**, or plastic surgery who may suspect that the patient suffers from BDD because of frequent requests for repeated or unnecessary procedures. Reported rates of BDD among dermatology and **cosmetic surgery** patients range between 6 and 15 percent. The diagnosis is made on the basis of the patient's history together with the physician's observations of the patient's overall mood and conversation patterns. People with BDD often come across to others as generally anxious and worried. In addition, the patient's dress or clothing styles may suggest a diagnosis of BDD. It is not unusual, however, for patients with BDD to take offense if their primary care doctor suggests referral to a psychiatrist.

Some physicians may use a self-report questionnaire, such as the Multidimensional Body-Self Relations Questionnaire (MBSRQ) or the short form of the Situational Inventory of Body-Image Dysphoria (SIBID), to evaluate patients during an office visit.

There are no brain imaging studies or laboratory tests as of the early 2000s that can be used to diagnose BDD.

Treatment

The standard course of treatment for body dysmorphic disorder is a combination of medications and psychotherapy. Surgical, dental, or dermatologic treatments have been found to be ineffective.

The medications most frequently prescribed for patients with BDD are the **selective serotonin reuptake inhibitors**, most commonly fluoxetine (Prozac) or sertraline (Zoloft). Other SSRIs that have been used with this group of patients include fluvoxamine (Luvox) and paroxetine (Paxil). In fact, it is the relatively high rate of positive responses to SSRIs among BDD patients that led to the hypothesis that the disorder has a neurobiological component related to serotonin levels in the body. An associated finding is that patients with BDD require higher dosages of **SSRI** medications than patients who are being treated for depression with these drugs.

The most effective approach to psychotherapy with BDD patients is cognitive-behavioral restructuring. Since the disorder is related to **delusions** about one's appearance, cognitive-oriented therapy that challenges inaccurate self-perceptions is more effective than purely supportive approaches. Thought-stopping and relaxation techniques also work well with BDD patients when they are combined with cognitive restructuring.

Some doctors recommend couples therapy or **family therapy** in order to involve the patient s parents, spouse, or partner in his or her treatment. This approach may be particularly helpful if family members are critical of the patient s looks or are reinforcing his or her unrealistic body image.

Alternative treatment

Although no alternative or complementary form of treatment has been recommended specifically for BDD, such herbal remedies for depression as **St. John's wort** have been reported as helping some BDD patients. **Aromatherapy** appears to be a useful aid to relaxation techniques as well as a pleasurable physical experience for BDD patients. **Yoga** has helped some persons with BDD acquire more realistic perceptions of their bodies and to replace obsessions about external appearance with new respect for their body's inner structure and functioning.

Prognosis

As of early 2005, the prognosis of BDD is considered good for patients receiving appropriate treatment. On the other hand, researchers do not know enough about the lifetime course of body dysmorphic disorder to offer detailed statistics. DSM-IV-TR notes that the disorder "has a fairly continuous course, with few symptom-free intervals, although the intensity of symptoms may wax and wane over time."

Prevention

Given the pervasive influence of the mass media in contemporary Western societies, the best preventive strategy involves challenging their unrealistic images of attractive people. Parents, teachers, primary health care professionals, and other adults who work with young people can point out and discuss the pitfalls of trying to look "perfect." In addition, parents or other adults can educate themselves about BDD and its symptoms, and pay attention to any warning signs in their children's dress or behavior.

Resources

BOOKS

American Psychiatric Association. *Diagnostic and Statistical Manual of Mental Disorders*, 4th edition, text revision. Washington, DC: American Psychiatric Association, 2000.

"Body Dysmorphic Disorder," Section 15, Chapter 186 in *The Merck Manual of Diagnosis and Therapy*, edited by Mark H. Beers, MD, and Robert Berkow, MD. Whitehouse Station, NJ: Merck Research Laboratories, 2004.

Johnston, Joni E., Psy D. *Appearance Obsession: Learning to Love the Way You Look*. Deerfield Beach, FL: Health Communications, Inc., 1994.

Rodin, Judith, PhD. *Body Traps: Breaking the Binds That Keep You from Feeling Good About Your Body*. New York: William Morrow, 1992.

PERIODICALS

Arthur, Gary K., MD, and Kim Monnell, DO. "Body Dysmorphic Disorder." *eMedicine*, 3 September 2004. < http://www.emedicine.com/med/topic3124.htm > .

Cafri, G., J. K. Thompson, L. Ricciardelli, et al. "Pursuit of the Muscular Ideal: Physical and Psychological Consequences and Putative Risk Factors." *Clinical Psychology Review* 25 (February 2005): 215–239.

Kirchner, Jeffrey T. "Treatment of Patients with Body Dysmorphic Disorder." *American Family Physician* 61 (March 2000): 1837–1843.

Slaughter, James R. "In Pursuit of Perfection: A Primary Care Physician's Guide to Body Dysmorphic Disorder." *American Family Physician* 60 (October 1999): 569–580.

ORGANIZATIONS

American Academy of Child and Adolescent Psychiatry. 3615 Wisconsin Avenue, NW, Washington, DC 20016-3007. (202) 966-7300. Fax: (202) 966-2891. < www.aacap.org. > .

American Psychiatric Association (APA). 1000 Wilson Boulevard, Suite 1825, Arlington, VA 22209-3901. (800) 368-5777 or (703) 907-7322. Fax: (703) 907-1091. < http://www.psych.org > .

Rebecca Frey, PhD

Body lice *see* **Lice infestation**

Boils

Definition

Boils and carbuncles are bacterial infections of hair follicles and surrounding skin that form pustules (small blister-like swellings containing pus) around the follicle. Boils are sometimes called furuncles. A carbuncle is formed when several furuncles merge to form a single deep **abscess** with several heads or drainage points.

Description

Boils and carbuncles are firm reddish swellings about 0.2–0.4in (5-10 mm) across that are slightly raised above the skin surface. They are sore to the touch. A boil usually has a visible central core of pus; a carbuncle is larger and has several visible heads. Boils occur most commonly on the face, back of the neck, buttocks, upper legs and groin area, armpits, and upper torso. Carbuncles are less common than single boils; they are most likely to form at the back of the neck. Males are more likely to develop carbuncles.

Boils and carbuncles are common problems in the general population, particularly among adolescents and adults. People who are more likely to develop these skin infections include those with:

- diabetes, especially when treated by injected insulin

- alcoholism or drug **abuse**

- poor personal hygiene

- crowded living arrangements

- jobs or hobbies that expose them to greasy or oily substances, especially petroleum products

- allergies or immune system disorders, including HIV infection.

- family members with recurrent skin infections

Causes and symptoms

Boils and carbuncles are caused by *Staphylococcus aureus*, a bacterium that causes an infection in an oil gland or hair follicle. Although the surface of human skin is usually resistant to bacterial infection, *S. aureus* can enter through a break in the skin surface–including breaks caused by needle punctures for insulin or drug injections. Hair follicles that are blocked by greasy creams, petroleum jelly, or similar products are more vulnerable to infection. Bacterial skin infections can be spread by shared cosmetics or washcloths, close human contact, or by contact with pus from a boil or carbuncle.

As the infection develops, an area of inflamed tissue gradually forms a pus-filled swelling or pimple that is painful to touch. As the boil matures, it forms a yellowish head or point. It may either continue to swell until the point bursts open and allows the pus to drain, or it may be gradually reabsorbed into the skin. It takes between one and two weeks for a boil to heal completely after it comes to a head and discharges pus. The bacteria that cause the boil can spread into other areas of the skin or even into the bloodstream if the skin around the boil is injured by squeezing. If the

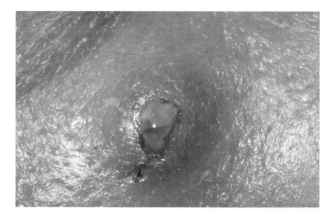

Boils often occur from a bacterial infection in a hair follicle or skin gland. *(Custom Medical Stock Photo. Reproduced by permission.)*

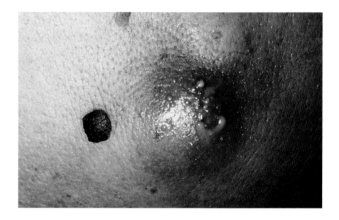

A close-up view of a carbuncle on person's back. *(Photograph by John Watney, Photo Researchers, Inc. Reproduced by permission.)*

infection spreads, the patient will usually develop chills and **fever**, swollen lymph nodes (**lymphadenitis**), and red lines in the skin running outward from the boil.

Furunculosis is a word that is sometimes used to refer to recurrent boils. Many patients have repeated episodes of furunculosis that are difficult to treat because their nasal passages carry colonies of *S. aureus*. These bacterial colonies make it easy for the patient's skin to be reinfected. They are most likely to develop in patients with diabetes, HIV infection, or other immune system disorders.

Carbuncles are formed when the bacteria infect several hair follicles that are close together. Carbunculosis is a word that is sometimes used to refer to the development of carbuncles. The abscesses spread until they merge with each other to form a single large area of infected skin with several pus-filled heads. Patients with carbuncles may also have a low-grade fever or feel generally unwell.

Diagnosis

The diagnosis of boils and carbuncles is usually made by the patient's primary care doctor on the basis of visual examination of the skin. In some cases involving recurrent boils on the face, the doctor may need to consider **acne** as a possible diagnosis, but for the most part boils and carbuncles are not difficult to distinguish from other skin disorders.

Treatment

Patient and family education

Patient education is an important part of the treatment of boils and carbuncles. Patients need to be warned against picking at or squeezing boils because of the danger of spreading the infection into other parts of the skin or bloodstream. It is especially important to avoid squeezing boils around the mouth or nose because infections in these areas can be carried to the brain. Patients should also be advised about keeping the skin clean, washing their hands carefully before and after touching the boil or carbuncle, avoiding the use of greasy cosmetics or creams, and keeping their towels and washcloths separate from those of other family members. Some doctors may recommend an antiseptic soap or gel for washing the infected areas.

If the patient has had several episodes of furunculosis, the doctor may examine family members or close contacts to see if they are carriers of *S. aureus*. In many cases they also need treatment for boils or carbuncles. Skin infections and reinfections involving small groups or clusters of people are being reported more frequently in the United States.

Medications

Boils are usually treated with application of antibiotic creams–usually clindamycin or polymyxin–following the application of hot compresses. The compresses help the infection to come to a head and drain.

Carbuncles and furunculosis are usually treated with oral **antibiotics** as well as antibiotic creams or ointments. The specific medications that are given are usually dicloxacillin (Dynapen) or cephalexin (Keflex). Erythromycin may be given to patients who are allergic to penicillin. The usual course of oral antibiotics is 5-10 days; however, patients with recurrent furunculosis may be given oral antibiotics for longer

periods. Furunculosis is treated with a combination of dicloxacillin and rifampin (Rifadin).

Patients with bacterial colonies in their nasal passages are often given mupirocin (Bactroban) to apply directly to the lining of the nose.

Surgical treatment

Boils and carbuncles that are very large, or that are not draining, may be opened with a sterile needle or surgical knife to allow the pus to drain. The doctor will usually give the patient a local anesthetic if a knife is used; surgical treatment of boils is painful and usually leaves noticeable **scars**.

Alternative treatment

Naturopathic therapy

Naturopathic practitioners usually recommend changes in the patient's diet as well as applying herbal poultices to the infected area. The addition of zinc supplements and vitamin A to the diet is reported to be effective in treating boils. The application of a paste or poultice containing goldenseal (*Hydrastis canadensis*) root is recommended by naturopaths on the grounds that goldenseal helps to kill bacteria and reduce inflammation.

Homeopathy

Homeopaths maintain that taking the proper homeopathic medication in the first stages of a boil or carbuncle will bring about early resolution of the infection and prevent pus formation. The most likely choices are *Belladonna* or *Hepar sulphuris*. If the boil has already formed, *Mercurius vivus* or *Silica* may be recommended to bring the pus to a head.

Western herbal therapies

A variety of herbal remedies can be applied topically to boils to fight infection. These include essential oils of bergamot (*Citrus bergamia*), chamomile (*Matricaria recutita*), lavender (*Lavandula officinalis*), and sage (*Salvia officinalis*), as well as tea tree oil (*Melaleuca* spp.). Herbalists also recommend washing the skin with a mixture of goldenseal and witch hazel. To fight the inflammation associated with boils, herbalists suggest marsh mallow (*Althaea officinalis*) ointment, tinctures (herbal solutions made with alcohol) of blue flag (*Iris versicolor*) or myrrh (*Commiphora molmol*), and slippery elm (*Ulmus fulva*) made into a poultice.

Prognosis

The prognosis for most boils is excellent. Some patients, however, suffer from recurrent carbuncles or furunculosis. In addition, although the spread of infection from boils is relatively unusual, there have been deaths reported from brain infections caused by squeezing boils on the upper lip or in the tissue folds at the base of the nose.

Prevention

There are some precautions that people can take to minimize the risk of developing bacterial skin infections:

- cleanse skin properly with soap and water, and take showers rather than tub baths

- do not share washcloths, towels, or facial cosmetics with others

- cut down on greasy or fatty foods and snacks

- always wash hands before touching the face

- consider using antiseptic soaps and shower gels

- consult a doctor if furunculosis is a persistent problem–it may indicate an underlying disease such as diabetes

Resources

BOOKS

Hacker, Steven M. "Common Bacterial and Fungal Infections of the Integument." In *Current Diagnosis*, edited by Rex B. Conn, et al. Vol 9. Philadelphia: W. B. Saunders Co., 1997.

Rebecca J. Frey, PhD

▌Bone biopsy

Definition

Bone biopsy is the removal of a piece of bone for laboratory examination and analysis.

Purpose

Bone biopsy is used to distinguish between malignant tumors and benign bone disease such as **osteoporosis** and osteomyelitis. This test may be ordered to determine why a patient's bones ache or feel sore, or when a mass or deformity is found on an x ray, CT scan, bone scan, or other diagnostic imaging procedure.

Precautions

The patient's doctor and the surgeon who performs the bone biopsy must be told about any prescription and over-the-counter medications the patient is taking, and about **allergies** or reactions the patient has had to anesthetics or **pain** relievers. Special care must be taken with patients who have experienced bleeding problems.

Description

A bone biopsy involves using a special drill or other surgical instruments to remove bone from the patient's body. The procedure usually lasts about 30 minutes and may be performed in the hospital, a doctor's office, or a surgical center.

A drill biopsy is generally used to obtain a small specimen. After the skin covering the bone has been cleansed with an antiseptic and shaved, the patient is given a local anesthetic. The doctor will not begin the procedure until the anesthetic has numbed the area from which the bone is to be removed, but the patient may feel pressure or mild pain when the needle pierces the bone. The surgeon turns the needle in a half-circle to extract a sample from the core, or innermost part, of the bone. The sample is drawn into the hollow stem of the biopsy needle. The sample is then sent to a laboratory, where it is examined under a microscope.

An open biopsy is used when a larger specimen is needed. After the area covering the bone has been cleansed with an antiseptic and shaved, the patient is given a general anesthetic. After the anesthetic takes effect and the patient is unconscious, the

KEY TERMS

Biopsy—Removal and examination of tissue to determine if cancer is present.

Osteomyelitis—An infection of the bone that is usually treated with antibiotics but sometimes requires surgery.

Osteoporosis—Thinning and loss of bone tissue.

surgeon makes an incision and removes a bone specimen. The specimen is sent to the laboratory for immediate analysis. Results of that analysis may indicate that additional surgery should be performed right away.

Preparation

No special preparation is needed for a drill biopsy, but a patient must fast for at least 12 hours before an open biopsy.

Aftercare

Pain medication will be prescribed after a biopsy, and vital signs will be monitored until they return to normal. Most patients can go home in about an hour. If bone was removed from the spine, the patient may stay in the hospital overnight. The surgical site must be kept clean and dry for 48 hours, and the patient's doctor should be notified if any of these symptoms appear:

- fever
- headache
- pain on movement
- inflammation or pus near the biopsy site
- bleeding through the bandage at the biopsy site

Risks

Risks include bone fracture, injury to nearby tissue, and infection. Bleeding is a rare complication. Factors that increase risk include:

- stress
- obesity
- poor **nutrition**
- chronic illness

- some medications
- mind-altering drugs

Normal results

Normal bone is made up of collagen fibers and bone tissue.

Abnormal results

Bone biopsy can reveal the presence of benign disease, infection, or malignant tumors that have spread to the bone from other parts of the body.

Results of this test are considered reliable, but may be affected by:

- failure to fast before open biopsy
- failure to obtain an adequate specimen
- delayed microscopic examination or laboratory analysis

Resources

ORGANIZATIONS

Cancer Group Institute. 1814 N.E. Miami Gardens Drive, North Miami Beach, FL 33179. (305) 651-5070. < http://www.cancergroup.com/em19.html >.

National Institute of Arthritis and Musculoskeletal and Skin Diseases Information Clearinghouse. National Institutes of Health. 1 AMS Circle, Bethesda, MD 20892-3695. (301) 495-3675.

Maureen Haggerty

Bone break fever *see* **Dengue fever**

Bone cancer *see* **Sarcomas**

Bone densitometry *see* **Bone density test**

Bone density test

Definition

A bone density test, or scan, is designed to check for **osteoporosis**, a disease that occurs when the bones become thin and weak. Osteoporosis happens when the bones lose calcium and other **minerals** that keep them strong. Osteoporosis begins after **menopause** in many women, and worsens after age 65, often resulting in serious **fractures**. These fractures may not only

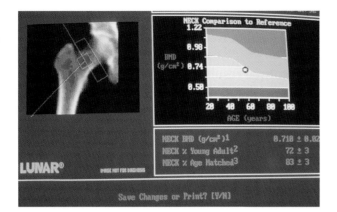

Computer read-out of a bone density scan. *(Photo Researchers. Reproduced by permission.)*

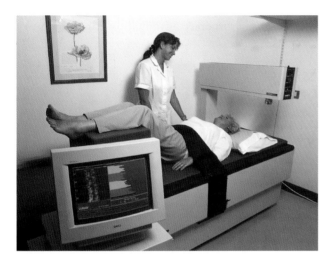

Patient undergoing a bone density scan. *(Photo Researchers. Reproduced by permission.)*

bring disability, but may affect longevity. As many as one-fourth of women who fracture their hip after age 50 die within one year.

Most people today will get a bone density scan from a machine using a technology called Dual Energy X-ray Absorptiometry or DEXA for short. This machine takes a picture of the bones in the spine, hip, total body and wrist, and calculates their density. If a DEXA machine is not available, bone density scans can also be done with dual photon absorptiometry (measuring the spine, hip and total body) and quantitative **computed tomography scans** (measuring the spine). Bone density scanners that use DEXA technology to just measure bone density in the wrist (called pDEXA scans) provide scans at some drugstores. Yet

these tests are not as accurate as those that measure density in the total body, spine or hip–where most fractures occur.

Purpose

A bone density scan measures the strength of an individual's bones and determines the risk of fracture. An observation of any osteoporosis present can be made.

Description

To take a DEXA bone density scan, the patient lies on a bed underneath the scanner, a curving plastic arm that emits x rays. These low-dose x rays form a fan beam that rotates around the patient. During the test, the scanner moves to capture images of the patient's spine, hip or entire body. A computer then compares the patient's bone strength and risk of fracture to that of other people in the United States at the same age and to young people at peak bone density. Bones reach peak density at age 30 and then start to lose mass. The test takes about 20 minutes to do and is painless. The DEXA bone scan costs about $250. Some insurance companies and Medicare cover the cost. pDEXA wrist bone scans in drugstores are available for about $30.

Preparation

The patient puts on a hospital gown and lies on the bed underneath the scanner. Not all doctors routinely schedule this test. If the following factors apply to a patient, they may need a bone density scan and can discuss this with their doctor. The patient:

- is at risk for osteoporosis
- is near menopause
- has broken a bone after a modest trauma
- has a family history of osteoporosis
- uses steroid or antiseizure medications
- has had a period of restricted mobility for more than six months

Risks

The DEXA bone scan exposes the patient to only a small amount of radiation–about one-fiftieth that of a **chest x ray**, or about the amount you get from taking a cross-country airplane flight.

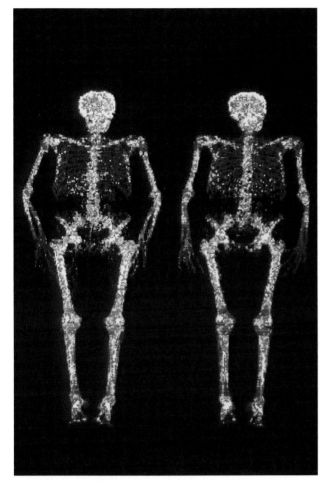

A bone densitometry scan of identical twins. Their bone density is normal and identical to one another. *(Photo Researchers. Reproduced by permission.)*

Normal results

The patient, when compared with people at "young normal bone density" (called the T-score) has the same or denser bones than a healthy 30-year-old. T scores above 1 mean that a patient has a healthy bone mass. Scores from 0 to −1 mean that the patient has borderline bone mass and should repeat the test in two to five years.

Abnormal results

The patient has two to four times the risk of a broken bone as other people in the United States at the same age and those at peak bone density. If a patient's T score ranges from −1 to −2.5 they have low bone mass and are at risk for osteoporosis. A T score below −2.5 means osteoporosis is already evident. These patients should have a repeat bone density scan every year or two.

Calcium—A mineral that helps build bone. After menopause, when women start making less of the bone-protecting hormone estrogen, they may need to increase their intake of calcium.

DEXA bone density scan—A bone density scan that uses a rotating x-ray beam to measure the strength of an individual's bones and his or her fracture risk.

Osteoporosis—A disease that occurs when the bones lose the calcium and structure that keep them strong. It often occurs after menopause (around age 50) in women and in old age in men.

Resources

ORGANIZATIONS

National Osteoporosis Foundation. 1150 17th St., NW, Suite 500, Washington, DC 20036-4603. (800) 223-9994. < http://www.nof.org > .

Barbara Boughton

Bone disorder drugs

Definition

Bone disorder drugs are medicines used to treat diseases that weaken the bones.

Purpose

The drugs described here are used to treat or prevent **osteoporosis** (brittle bone disease) in women past **menopause** as well as older men. They also are used prescribed for Paget's disease, a painful condition that weakens and deforms bones, and they are used to control calcium levels in the blood.

Bone is living tissue. Like other tissue, bone is constantly being broken down and replaced with new material. Normally, there is a balance between the breakdown of old bone and its replacement with new bone. But when something goes wrong with the process, bone disorders may result.

Osteoporosis is a particular concern for women after menopause, as well as for older men. In osteoporosis, the inside of the bones become porous and

KEY TERMS

Estrogen—The main sex hormone that controls normal sexual development in females. During the menstrual cycle, estrogen helps prepare the body for possible pregnancy.

Fracture—A break or crack in a bone.

Hormone—A substance that is produced in one part of the body, then travels through the bloodstream to another part of the body where it has its effect.

Menopause—The stage in a woman's life when the ovaries stop producing egg cells at regular times and menstruation stops.

Osteoporosis—A disease in which bones become very porous and weak. The bones are then more likely to fracture and take longer to heal. The condition is most common in women after menopause but can also occur in older men.

thin. Over time, this condition weakens the bones and makes them more likely to break. Osteoporosis is four times more common in women than in men. This is because women have less bone mass than men, tend to live longer and take in less calcium, and need the female hormone estrogen to keep their bones strong. If men live long enough, they are also at risk of getting osteoporosis later in life. Once total bone mass has peaked–around age 35–all adults start to lose it. In women, the rate of bone loss speeds up during menopause, when estrogen levels fall. Bone loss may also occur if both ovaries are removed by surgery. Ovaries make estrogen. **Hormone replacement therapy** is one approach to preventing osteoporosis. However, not all people can use hormone replacement therapy. Bone disorder drugs are a good alternative for people who already have osteoporosis or who are at risk of developing it. Risk factors include lack of regular **exercise**, early menopause, being underweight, and a strong family history of osteoporosis.

Description

Bone disorder drugs are available only with a physician's prescription and come in tablet, nasal spray, and injectable forms. Commonly used bone disorder drugs are alendronate (Fosamax), calcitonin (Miacalcin, Calcimar), and raloxifene (Evista). Raloxifene belongs to a group of drugs known as selective estrogen receptor modulators (SERMs), which act like estrogen in some parts of the body but not in others. This makes

the drugs less likely to cause some of the harmful effects that estrogen may cause. Unlike estrogen, raloxifene does not increase the risk of **breast cancer**. In fact, research suggests that raloxifene may even reduce that risk.

Recommended dosage

Alendronate

FOR OSTEOPOROSIS. The usual dose is 10 mg once a day. Treatment usually continues over many years.

FOR PAGET'S DISEASE. The usual dose is 40 mg once a day for six months.

This medicine works only when it is taken with a full glass of water first thing in the morning, at least 30 minutes before eating or drinking anything or taking any other medicine. Do not lie down for at least 30 minutes after taking it because the drug can irritate the esophagus, the tube that delivers food form the mouth to the stomach.

Calcitonin

NASAL SPRAY. The usual dose is one spray into the nose once a day. Alternate nostrils, spraying the right nostril one day, the left nostril the next day, and so on.

INJECTABLE. The recommended dosage depends on the condition for which the medicine is prescribed and may be different for different people. Check with the physician who prescribed the medicine or the pharmacist who filled the prescription for the proper dosage.

Raloxifene

The usual dose is one 60-mg tablet daily.

Precautions

Aldendronate

People with low levels of calcium in their blood should not take this medicine. It also is not recommended for women on hormone replacement therapy or for anyone with kidney problems. Before using alendronate, anyone who has digestive or swallowing problems should make sure that his or her physician knows about the condition.

Calcitonin

Calcitonin nasal spray may cause irritation or small sores in the nose. Check with a physician if this becomes very uncomfortable or if there is bleeding from the nose.

The injectable form of calcitonin has caused serious allergic reactions in a few people. The nasal spray is not known to cause such reactions, but the possibility exists. Before starting treatment with calcitonin, the physician who prescribes the drug may order an allergy test to make sure there will not be a problem.

Raloxifene

A rare, but serious side effect of raloxifene is an increased risk of **blood clots** that form in the veins and may break away and travel to the lungs. This is about as likely in women who take raloxifene as it is in women who take estrogen. Because of this possible problem, women with a history of blood clots in their veins should not take raloxifene.

Women who have had breast **cancer** or cancer of the uterus should check with their physicians about whether they can safely use raloxifene.

General precautions for bone disorder drugs

To keep bones strong, the body needs calcium and vitamin D. Dairy products and fish such as salmon, sardines and tuna are good sources of both calcium and vitamin D. People who are taking bone disorder drugs for osteoporosis and who do not get enough of these nutrients in their **diets** should check with their physicians about taking supplements. Other important bone-saving steps are avoiding **smoking** and alcohol and getting enough of the kind of exercise that puts weight on the bones (such as walking or lifting weights).

People who are taking these drugs because they have too much calcium in their blood may need to *limit* the amount of calcium in their diets. Too much calcium may prevent the medicine from working properly. Discuss the proper diet with the physician who prescribed the drug, and do not make any diet changes without the physician's approval.

Anyone who has had unusual reactions to bone disorder drugs in the past should let his or her physician know before taking the drugs again. The physician also should be told about any **allergies** to foods, dyes, preservatives, or other substances.

Women who are pregnant or who may become pregnant and women who are breastfeeding should check with their physicians before using this alendronate or calcitonin. Raloxifene should not be used by women who are pregnant or who may become pregnant. In laboratory studies of rats, raloxifene caused **birth defects**.

Side effects

Aldendronate

Common side effects include **constipation, diarrhea, indigestion, nausea, pain** in the abdomen, and pain in the muscles and bones. These problems usually go away as the body adjusts to the medicine and do not need medical attention unless they continue or they interfere with normal activities.

Calcitonin

The most common side effects of calcitonin nasal spray are nose problems, such as dryness, redness, **itching**, sores, bleeding and general discomfort. These problems should go away as the body adjusts to the medicine, but if they do not or if they are very uncomfortable, check with a physician. Other side effects that should be brought to a physician's attention include **headache**, back pain and joint pain.

Injectable calcitonin may cause minor side effects such as nausea or **vomiting**; diarrhea; stomach pain; loss of appetite; flushing of the face, ears, hands or feet; and discomfort or redness at the place on the body where it is injected. Medical attention is not necessary unless these problems persist or cause unusual discomfort.

Anyone who has a skin rash or **hives** after taking injectable calcitonin should check with a physician as soon as possible.

Raloxifene

Common side effects include hot flashes, leg cramps, **nausea and vomiting**. Women who have these problems while taking raloxifene should check with their physicians.

Interactions

Aldendronate

Taking **aspirin** with alendronate may increase the chance of upset stomach, especially if the dose of alendronate is more than 10 mg per day. If an analgesic is necessary, switch to another drug, such as **acetaminophen** (Tylenol) or use buffered aspirin. Ask a physician or pharmacist for the correct medication to use.

Some calcium supplements, **antacids** and other medicines keep the body from absorbing alendronate. To prevent this problem, do not take any other medicine within 30 minutes of taking alendronate.

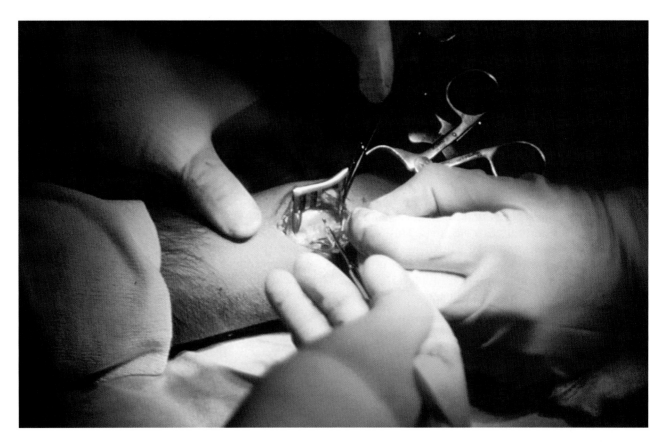

Surgeons harvesting a sample of material for bone grafting. *(Custom Medical Stock Photo, Inc. Reproduced by permission.)*

Calcitonin

Calcitonin may keep certain other drugs for Paget's disease, such as etidronate (Didronel), from working as they should.

Raloxifene

Raloxifene may affect blood clotting. Patients who are taking other drugs that affect blood clotting, such as warfarin (Coumadin), should check with their physicians before using raloxifene.

Resources

ORGANIZATIONS

Foundation For Osteoporosis Research & Education. (888) 266-3015. <http://www.fore.org>.

National Association for the Relief of Paget's Disease. <http://www.demon.co.uk/narpd>.

National Osteoporosis Foundation 1150 17th Street NW Suite 500 Washington, D.C. 20036-4603. <http://www.nof.org>.

Nancy Ross-Flanigan

Bone grafting

Definition

Bone grafting is a surgical procedure by which new bone or a replacement material is placed into spaces between or around broken bone (**fractures**) or holes in bone (defects) to aid in healing.

Purpose

Bone grafting is used to repair bone fractures that are extremely complex, pose a significant risk to the patient, or fail to heal properly. Bone graft is also used to help fusion between vertebrae, correct deformities, or provide structural support for fractures of the spine. In addition to **fracture repair**, bone graft is used to repair defects in bone caused by **birth defects**, traumatic injury, or surgery for bone **cancer**.

Description

Bone is composed of a matrix, mainly made up of a protein called collagen. It is strengthened by

KEY TERMS

Allograft—Tissue for transplantation that is taken from another person.

Autograft—Tissue for transplantation that is taken from the patient.

Hydroxyapatite—A calcium phosphate complex that is the primary mineral component of bone.

Osteoblasts—Bone cells that build new bone tissue.

Osteoclasts—Bone cells that break down and remove bone tissue.

Osteoconduction—Provision of a scaffold for the growth of new bone.

Osteocytes—Bone cells that maintain bone tissue.

Osteogenesis—Growth of new bone.

Osteoinduction—Acceleration of new bone formation by chemical means.

deposits of calcium and phosphate salts, called hydroxyapatite. Within and around this matrix are located the cells of the bones, which are of four types. Osteoblasts produce the bone matrix. Osteocytes are mature osteoblasts and serve to maintain the bone. Osteoclasts break down and remove bone tissue. Bone lining cells cover bone surfaces. Together, these four types of cells are responsible for building the bone matrix, maintaining it, and remodeling the bone as needed.

There are three ways in which a bone graft can help repair a defect. The first is called osteogenesis, the formation of new bone by the cells contained within the graft. The second is osteoinduction, a chemical process in which molecules contained within the graft (bone morphogenetic proteins) convert the patient's cells into cells that are capable of forming bone. The third is osteoconduction, a physical effect by which the matrix of the graft forms a scaffold on which cells in the recipient are able to form new bone.

New bone for grafting can be obtained from other bones in the patient's own body (e.g., hip bones or ribs), called autograft, or from bone taken from other people that is frozen and stored in tissue banks, called allograft. A variety of natural and synthetic replacement materials are also used instead of bone, including collagen (the protein substance of the white fibers of the skin, bone, and connective tissues); polymers, such as silicone and some acrylics; hydroxyapatite; calcium sulfate; and ceramics. A new material, called resorbable

polymeric grafts, is also being studied. These resorbable grafts provide a structure for new bone to grow on; the grafts then slowly dissolve, leaving only the new bone behind.

To place the graft, the surgeon makes an incision in the skin over the bone defect and shapes the bone graft or replacement material to fit into the defect. After the graft is placed into the defect, it is held in place with pins, plates, or screws. The incision is closed with stitches and a splint or cast is used to prevent movement of the bones while healing.

The costs associated with a bone graft vary. These costs include: the surgeon's fee (variable); anesthesiologist's fees (averaging $350 to $400 per hour); hospital charges (averaging $1,500 to $1,800 per day, more for intensive care or private rooms); medication charges ($200 to $400); and additional charges, including an assisting surgeon, treatment of complications, diagnostic procedures (e.g., blood work or x rays), medical supplies, and equipment use. The cost for the graft itself can range from $250 to $900.

This procedure is covered by many third-party insurers; insurance coverage should be explored for each individual case.

Aftercare

The time required for convalescence for fractures or spinal fusion may vary from one to 10 days, and vigorous **exercise** may be limited for up to three months.

Most bone grafts are successful in helping the bone defect to heal. The extent of recovery will depend on the size of the defect and the condition of the bone surrounding the graft at the time of surgery. Severe defects may take some time to heal and may require further attention after the initial graft. In one study of over 1,000 patients who received very large allografts after surgery for bone cancer, researchers found that approximately 85% of the patients were able to return to work or normal physical activities without using crutches. However, about 25% of these patients required a second operation, because the first did not heal properly. Less severe bone defects, though, should heal completely without serious complications.

Risks

The risks for any surgical procedure requiring anesthesia include reactions to the medications and breathing problems. The risks for any surgical procedure include bleeding and infection.

The drawbacks of autografts include: the additional surgical and anesthesia time (typically 30 minutes per procedure) to obtain, or harvest, the bone for grafting; added costs of the additional surgery; **pain** and infection that might occur at the site from which the graft is taken; and the relatively small amount of bone that is available for grafting.

The drawbacks of allografts include: variability between lots, since the bone is harvested from a variety of donors; the bone may take longer to incorporate with the host bone than an autograft would; the graft may be less effective than an autograft; and the possibility of transferring diseases to the patient. Other complications may result from the immune response mounted by the patient's immune system against the grafted bone tissue. With the use anti-rejection agents (drugs to combat rejection of grafted bone tissue) immune rejection is less of a problem.

Resources

ORGANIZATIONS

American Association of Tissue Banks. 1350 Beverly Road, Suite 220-A, McLean, VA 22101. (703) 827-9582.

Lisa Christenson, PhD

Bone growth stimulation

Definition

Bone growth stimulation is the technique of promoting bone growth in difficult to heal **fractures** by applying a low electrical current or ultrasound to the fracture.

Purpose

Bone growth stimulation is done when satisfactory healing is not occurring naturally or when the pace of healing is too slow. This condition is called fracture nonunion, and it occurs more frequently among adults than children, in people with severe or complex fractures, and in people who smoke.

The theory behind applying an electric current to fractures to stimulate healing is based on the fact that the concave side of the bone becomes negatively charged and the convex side is positively charged. It is believed that artificially encouraging this charging with an electric current will speed healing. In 1996, the Food and Drug Administration (FDA) also approved

---

the application of low intensity ultrasound pulses as a treatment for fracture nonunion.

Ultrasound and electromagnetic stimulation are expensive and are used only when healing problems exist for a substantial length of time. Each method must be used for at least three to six months to be effective.

Precautions

Bone growth stimulation cannot be used if the gap between the ends of the fracture is too large.

Description

Electric stimulation can be applied either from the inside of the body (invasively) or from the outside the body (noninvasively). Ultrasound is a noninvasive procedure. The type of stimulation selected depends on the doctor's preference, the type and location of the fracture, and the patient's motivation to comply with the treatment schedule. Treatment can take anywhere from three to six months.

Invasive stimulators

Invasive electric stimulators are either fully or partially implantable. The advantage of these devices is that they apply a direct electric current to the fracture 24 hours a day. The fully implantable stimulator requires little daily attention from the patient. Patients using a semi-implanted stimulator must regulate their own treatment schedule and have to care for the external power pack. The disadvantage of implantable and semi-implantable stimulators is that their implantation is a surgical procedure.

Fully implantable direct current stimulators are installed in a hospital under general or regional anesthesia. Both the stimulator and the power source are implanted. The surgeon makes an incision and places a spiral shaped cathode inside the bone. A wire leads to the power source and a small anode. The power source is a battery pack that is implanted in the nearby muscle. The body transmits electrical current to close the circuit. The incision is then closed. Once in place, the device provides continuous direct electric current for bone growth stimulation.

Partially implanted stimulators use cathode pins that are implanted at the edge of each bone that is fractured. Wires lead to the surface of the skin where a power source and the anode are located. Wires complete the circuit. The external portion of the device is held in place by a cast. This source of stimulation also runs continuously.

Noninvasive stimulators

In the noninvasive stimulator, external electromagnetic coils are placed on either side of the fracture and are held in place by a strap or cuff. Locating the coils correctly is important, and their location relative to the fracture is usually confirmed by x rays.

The coils produce a pulsating electromagnetic field. It is up to the patient to maintain the prescribed treatment schedule. Effective treatment requires stimulation anywhere from three to ten hours each day in periods of no less than one hour.

Ultrasound stimulation is the most recent treatment for stimulating bone growth. A device that generates low intensity pulses of sound is applied to the skin over the fracture. The advantage of this technique is that it is noninvasive and the period of application of the sound pulses can be as short as 20-30 minutes each day. The results of this treatment have been studied less than the effect of electromagnetic stimulation.

Preparation

Bone growth stimulation is done only when healing has failed to occur for many months. Before it is started, x rays are done of the fracture area. If the device is to be implanted, standard preoperative blood and urine tests are done. The patient may meet with an anesthesiologist to discuss any conditions that might affect the administration of anesthesia.

Aftercare

If a noninvasive, pulsating, electromagnetic field device is used, the patient must not put any **stress** or weight on the fracture until it is healed, which is a matter of months in most cases. In all lower limb fractures, regardless of the stimulation method used, the patient can not bear weight on the limb with the fracture until healing is complete. This limits the patient's mobility for many months. Patients have the responsibility for regularly making sure that the

unit works and caring for external devices and the casts that hold them in place.

Risks

Noninvasive devices have few risks associated with them. The main risk associated with implantable devices is the development of infection at the site of implantation.

Normal results

Success in healing a fracture nonunion using bone growth stimulation depends on the type, location, and severity of the fracture and the age and general health of the patient.

Resources

PERIODICALS

Mayo Clinic. "Fractures - Treatment Methods are Tailored to the Break." *Mayo Clinic Health Letter* 14, no. 4 (April 1996): 1-3.

Tish Davidson, A.M.

Bone infection *see* **Osteomyelitis**

Bone marrow aspiration and biopsy

Definition

Bone marrow aspiration, also called bone marrow sampling, is the removal by suction of fluid from the soft, spongy material that lines the inside of most bones. Bone marrow biopsy, or needle biopsy, is the removal of a small piece of bone marrow.

Purpose

Bone marrow aspiration is used to:

• pinpoint the cause of abnormal blood test results

• confirm a diagnosis or check the status of severe anemia (abnormally low numbers of red blood cells in the bloodstream) of unknown cause, or other irregularities in the way blood cells are produced or become mature.

• evaluate abnormalities in the blood's ability to store iron.

• diagnose infection

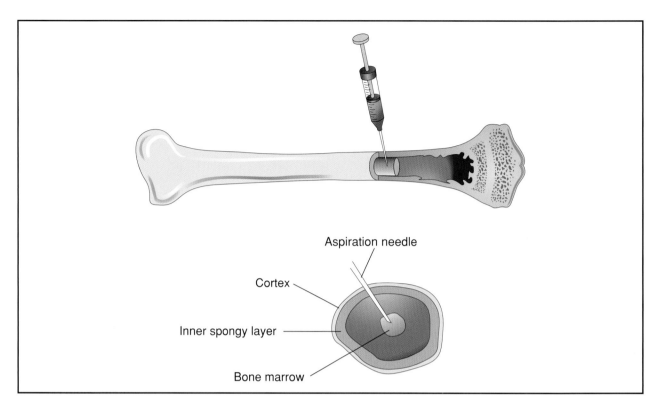

Aspiration needle

Cortex

Inner spongy layer

Bone marrow

In a bone marrow aspiration, a needle is inserted beneath the skin and rotated until it penetrates the cortex, or outer covering of the bone. A small amount of marrow is suctioned out of the bone by a syringe attached to the needle. *(Illustration by Electronic Illustrators Group.)*

Bone marrow biopsy is used to:

- obtain intact bone marrow for laboratory analysis

- diagnose and stage some types of **cancer** or anemia and other blood disorders

- identify the source of an unexplained fever

- diagnose fibrosis of bone marrow or myeloma (a tumor composed of cells normally found in the bone marrow) when bone marrow aspiration has failed to provide an appropriate specimen

Bone marrow aspiration and bone marrow biopsy are also used to gauge the effectiveness of **chemotherapy** and other medical treatments. These procedures are often used together to ensure the availability of the best possible bone marrow specimen.

Precautions

Allergies or previous adverse reactions to medications should be discussed with the doctor. Any current medications, including herbal or nutritional supplements, should be evaluated for the potential to interfere with proper coagulation (clot formation). These would include coumadin, **aspirin**, and other agents used as

blood thinners. Caution should be used when the herbs gingko, ginger, garlic, br ginseng have been utilized as supplements, due to a risk of bleeding.

Pregnancy, lactation (production and secretion of milk), and preexisting platelet or bleeding disorders should be evaluated before either procedure is undertaken.

Description

Bone marrow aspiration and biopsy should be performed by a physician or nurse clinician. Each procedure takes about 20 to 30 minutes and is usually performed on an outpatient basis, but can be done in a hospital if necessary.

The skin covering the biopsy site is cleansed with an antiseptic, and the patient may be given a mild sedative. A local anesthetic is administered. The hematologist or nurse clinician performing the procedure will not begin until the anesthetic has numbed the area from which the specimen is to be extracted. In both adults and children, aspiration and biopsy are most commonly performed on the rear bone of the hip (posterior iliac crest). In adults, sampling from the sternum (breastbone) is sometimes done. The latter location is technically easier, but is somewhat more painful for the patient and presents the risk of heart injury. On rare occasions, a long bone of the leg (tibia) may be used as a sample site for an infant.

In a bone marrow aspiration, a special needle is inserted beneath the skin and rotated until it penetrates the cortex, or outer covering of the bone. At least half a teaspoon of marrow is withdrawn from the bone by a syringe attached to the needle. The patient may experience discomfort when the needle is inserted or when the marrow is aspirated. If more marrow is needed, the needle is repositioned slightly, a new syringe is attached, and a second sample is taken. The samples are transferred from the syringes to slides and vials, then sent to a laboratory for analysis.

Bone marrow biopsy may be performed immediately before or after bone marrow aspiration. The procedure utilizes a special large-bore needle that is used to drill out a core of marrow. In bone marrow biopsy, the needle is inserted, rotated from side to side, withdrawn, and reinserted at a different angle. This procedure is repeated if needed until a small core, about 0.4 inches (1 cm) long, is separated from the bone marrow. The needle is again removed, and a piece of fine wire threaded through its tip transfers the specimen onto sterile gauze. The patient may feel discomfort or pressure when the needle is inserted and experience a brief, pulling sensation when the marrow is withdrawn. Unlike aspiration specimens, which are smeared, these samples contain structurally intact bone marrow. Microscopic examination can show what material its cells contain and how they are alike or different from one another. The bone may either be embedded intact in paraffin (a type of wax), or be decalcified (a process which takes place overnight) for a different type of staining and examination. Each type of preparation has certain advantages.

Preparation

A current history and physical are obtained from the patient, along with proper consent. The patient is generally placed in a prone position (lying face down) for preparation, and local anesthetic, with or without **sedation**, is administered.

Aftercare

After the needle is removed, the biopsy site will be covered with a clean, dry bandage. Pressure is applied to control bleeding. The patient's pulse, breathing, blood pressure, and temperature are monitored until they return to normal, and the patient may be instructed to remain in a supine position (lying face up) for half an hour before getting dressed.

The patient should be able to leave the clinic and resume normal activities immediately. Patients who have received a sedative often feel sleepy for the rest of the day; driving, cooking, and other activities that require clear thinking and quick reactions should therefore be avoided.

The biopsy site should be kept covered and dry for several hours. Walking or taking prescribed **pain** medications usually ease any discomfort felt at the biopsy site, and ice can be used to reduce swelling.

A doctor should be notified if the patient:

- feels severe pain more than 24 hours after the procedure.

- experiences persistent bleeding or notices more than a few drops of blood on the wound dressing.

- has a temperature above 101 °F (38.3 °C). Inflammation and pus at the biopsy site and other signs of infection should also be reported to a doctor without delay.

Risks

Bleeding and discomfort often occur at the biopsy site. Infection and hematoma may also develop. In rare instances, the heart or a major blood vessel is pierced when marrow is extracted from the sternum during bone marrow biopsy. This can lead to severe hemorrhage.

Normal results

Healthy adult bone marrow contains yellow fat cells, connective tissue, and red marrow that produces blood. The bone marrow of a healthy infant is primarily red due to active production of red cells necessary for growth.

Abnormal results

Culture of bone marrow aspirate may yield information about an infectious agent. Microscopic examination of bone marrow can reveal granulomas, **myelofibrosis**, lymphomas, leukemias, or other cancers. Analyzing specimens can help doctors diagnose iron deficiency, vitamin B_{12} deficiency, and folate deficiency, as well as anemia.

Obesity can affect the ease with which a bone marrow biopsy can be done, and the results of either procedure can be affected if the patient has had radiation therapy at the biopsy site.

Maureen Haggerty

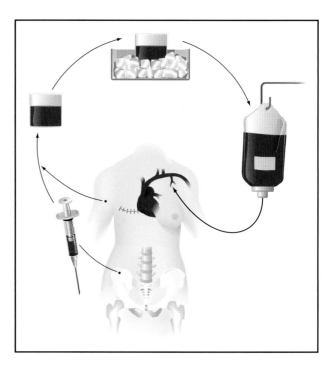

In autologous bone marrow transplantation, stem cells are collected from the patient. Once the patient has undergone chemotherapy, the cells are replaced in the blood via an intravenous catheter. The cells return to the bone marrow and begin producing healthy new cells. *(Illustration by Argosy Inc.)*

Bone marrow transplantation

Definition

The bone marrow—the sponge-like tissue found in the center of certain bones—contains stem cells that are the precursors of white blood cells, red blood cells, and platelets. These blood cells are vital for normal body functions, such as oxygen transport, defense against infection and disease, and clotting. Blood cells have a limited lifespan and are constantly being replaced; therefore, healthy stem cells are vital.

In association with certain diseases, stem cells may produce too many, too few, or otherwise abnormal blood cells. Also, medical treatments may destroy stem cells or alter blood cell production. The resultant blood cell abnormalities can be life threatening.

Bone marrow transplantation involves extracting bone marrow containing normal stem cells from a healthy donor, and transferring it to a recipient whose body cannot manufacture proper quantities of normal blood cells. The goal of the transplant is to rebuild the recipient's blood cells and immune system and hopefully cure the underlying ailment.

Purpose

A person's red blood cells, white blood cells, and platelets may be destroyed or may be abnormal due to disease. Also, certain medical therapies, particularly **chemotherapy** or radiation treatment, may destroy a person's stem cells. The consequence to a person's health is severe. Under normal circumstances, red blood cells carry oxygen throughout the body and remove carbon dioxide from the body's tissues. White blood cells form the cornerstone of the body's immune system and defend it against infection. Platelets limit bleeding by enabling the blood to clot if a blood vessel is damaged.

A bone marrow transplant is used to rebuild the body's capacity to produce these blood cells and bring their numbers to normal levels. Illnesses that may be treated with a bone marrow transplant include both cancerous and noncancerous diseases.

Cancerous diseases may or may not specifically involve blood cells; but, **cancer** treatment can destroy the body's ability to manufacture new blood cells. Bone marrow transplantation may be used in conjunction with additional treatments, such as chemotherapy, for

ABO antigen—Protein molecules located on the surfaces of red blood cells that determine a person's blood type: A, B, or O.

AML—Acute myelogenous leukemia, also called acute myelocytic leukemia. Malignant disorder where myeloid blast cells accumulate in the marrow and bloodstream.

Allogeneic—Referring to bone marrow transplants between two different, genetically dissimilar people.

Anemia—Decreased red cell production which results in deficiency in oxygen-carrying capacity of the blood.

Antigen—A molecule that is capable of provoking an immune response.

Aplastic anemia—A disorder in which the body produces inadequate amounts of red blood cells and hemoglobin due to underdeveloped or missing bone marrow.

Autologous—Referring to bone marrow transplants in which recipients serve as their own donors.

Blank—If an individual has inherited same HLA antigen from both parents, the HLA typing is designated by the shared HLA antigen followed by a "blank"(–).

Blast cells—Blood cells in early stage of cellular development.

Blast crisis—Stage of chronic myelogenous leukemia where large quantities of immature cells are produced by the marrow and is not responsive to treatment.

Bone marrow—A spongy tissue located within flat bones, including the hip and breast bones and the skull. This tissue contains stem cells, the precursors of platelets, red blood cells, and white blood cells.

Bone marrow transplant—Healthy marrow is infused into people who have had high-dose chemotherapy for one of the many forms of leukemias, immunodeficiencies, lymphomas, anemias, metabolic disorders, and sometimes solid tumors.

Chemotherapy—Medical treatment of a disease, particularly cancer, with drugs or other chemicals.

Chronic myelogenous leukemia (CML)—Also called chronic myelocytic leukemia, malignant disorder that involves abnormal accumulation of white cells in the marrow and bloodstream.

Cytomegalovirus (CMV)—Virus that can cause pneumonia in post bone marrow transplant patients.

Conditioning—Process of preparing patient to receive marrow donation, often through the use of chemotherapy and radiation therapy.

Confirmatory typing—Repeat tissue typing to confirm the compatibility of the donor and patient before transplant.

Donor—A healthy person who contributes bone marrow for transplantation.

Graft versus host disease—A life-threatening complication of bone marrow transplants in which the donated marrow causes an immune reaction against the recipient's body.

Histocompatibility—The major histocompatibility determinants are the human leukocyte antigens (HLA) and characterize how well the patient and donor are matched.

HLA (human leuckocyte antigen)—A group of protein molecules located on bone marrow cells that can provoke an immune response. A donor's and a recipient's HLA types should match as closely as possible to prevent the recipient's immune system from attacking the donor's marrow as a foreign material that does not belong in the body.

Hodgkin's disease—A type of cancer involving the lymph nodes and potentially affecting nonlymphatic organs in the later stage.

Immunodeficiency—A disorder in which the immune system is ineffective or disabled either due to acquired or inherited disease.

Leukemia—A type of cancer that affects leukocytes, a particular type of white blood cell. A characteristic symptom is excessive production of immature or otherwise abnormal leukocytes.

Lymphoma—A type of cancer that affects lymph cells and tissues, including certain white blood cells (T cells and B cells), lymph nodes, bone marrow, and the spleen. Abnormal cells (lymphocyte/leukocyte) multiply uncontrollably.

Match—How similar the HLA typing, out of a possible six antigens, is between the donor and the recipient.

Mixed lymphocyte culture (MLC)—Test that measures level of reactivity between donor and recipient lymphocytes.

Neuroblastoma—Solid tumor in children, may be treated by BMT.

Platelets—Fragments of a large precursor cell, a megakaryocyte found in the bone marrow. These fragments adhere to areas of blood vessel damage and release chemical signals that direct the formation of a blood clot.

Recipient—The person who receives the donated blood marrow.

Red blood cells—Cells that carry hemoglobin (the molecule that transports oxygen) and help remove wastes from tissues throughout the body.

Sickle cell anemia—An inherited disorder characterized by a genetic flaw in hemoglobin production. (Hemoglobin is the substance within red blood cells that enables them to transport oxygen.) The hemoglobin that is produced has a kink in its structure that

forces the red blood cells to take on a sickle shape, inhibiting their circulation and causing pain. This disorder primarily affects people of African descent.

Syngeneic—Referring to a bone marrow transplant from one identical twin to the other.

Thalassemia—A group of inherited disorders that affects hemoglobin production. (Hemoglobin is the substance within red blood cells that enables them to transport oxygen.) Because hemoglobin production is impaired, a person with this disorder may suffer mild to severe anemia. Certain types of thalassemia can be fatal.

White blood cells—A group of several cell types that occur in the bloodstream and are essential for a properly functioning immune system.

various types of leukemia, **Hodgkin's disease**, lymphoma, breast and **ovarian cancer**, and other cancers. Noncancerous diseases for which bone marrow transplantation can be a treatment option include **aplastic anemia**, sickle cell anemia, **thalassemia**, and severe **immunodeficiency**.

Precautions

Bone marrow transplants are not for everyone. Transplants are accompanied by a risk of infection, transplant rejection by the recipient's immune system, and other complications. The procedure has a lower success rate the greater the recipient's age. Complications are exacerbated for people whose health is already seriously impaired as in late-stage cancers. Therefore, a person's age or state of health may prohibit use of a bone marrow transplant. The typical cut-off age for a transplant ranges from 40 to 55 years; however, a person's general health is usually the more important factor.

Even in the absence of complications, the transplant and associated treatments are hard on the recipient. Bone marrow transplants are debilitating. A person's ability to withstand the rigors of the transplant is a key consideration in deciding to use this treatment.

Description

Autologous and allogeneic transplants

Two important requirements for a bone marrow transplant are the donor and the recipient. Sometimes, the donor and the recipient may be the same person. This type of transplant is called an autologous

transplant. It is typically used in cases in which a person's bone marrow is generally healthy but will be destroyed due to medical treatment for diseases such as **breast cancer** and Hodgkin's disease. Most bone marrow transplants are autologous. If a person's bone marrow is unsuitable for an autologous transplant, the bone marrow must be derived from another person in an allogeneic transplant.

Allogeneic transplants are more complicated because of proteins called human lymphocyte antigens (HLA) that are on the surface of bone marrow cells. If the donor and the recipient have very dissimilar antigens, the recipient's immune system regards the donor's bone marrow cells as invaders and launches a destructive attack against them. Such an attack negates any benefits offered by the transplant.

HLA matching

There are only five major HLA classes or types—designated HLA–A,–B, –C,–D, and class III—but much variation within the groupings. For example, HLA–A from one individual may be similar to, but not the same as, HLA–A in another individual; such a situation can render a transplant from one to the other impossible.

HLA matching is more likely if the donor and recipient are related, particularly if they are siblings; however, an unrelated donor may be a potential match. Only in rare cases is matching HLA types between two people not an issue: if the recipient has an identical twin. Identical twins carry the same genes; therefore, the same antigens. A bone marrow transplant between identical twins is called a syngeneic transplant.

Peripheral blood stem cell transplants

A relatively recent development in **stem cell transplantation** is the use of peripheral blood cells instead of stem cells from bone marrow. Peripheral blood stem cells (PBSCs) are obtained from circulating blood rather than from bone marrow, but the amount of stem cells found in the peripheral blood is much smaller than the amount of stem cells found in the bone marrow. Peripheral blood stem cells can be used in either autologous or allogeneic transplants. The majority of PBSC transplants are autologous. However, recent clinical studies indicate that PBSCs are being used more frequently than bone marrow for allogeneic bone marrow transplantation.

The advantages of PBSC transplants when compared to bone marrow transplants are: in allogeneic transplantation, haematopoietic and immune recovery are faster with PBSCs which reduces the potential for disease recurrence, primarily graft-versus-host-disease. In autologous transplantation, the use of PBSCs can result in faster **blood count** recoveries. Also, some medical conditions exist in which the recipient cannot accept bone marrow stem cell transplants, but can accept PBSC transplants. Some possible disadvantages to PBSC transplant versus bone marrow transplantation are: so much more fluid volume is necessary to collect enough PBSCs that, at the time of infusing the new stem cells into the recipient, the fluid can collect in the lungs or cause temporary kidney problems. Also, the time commitment for the donor for a PBSC transplant is considerable. When the PBSCs are being collected, several outpatient sessions are needed and each session lasts approximately two–four hours.

The transplant procedure

BONE MARROW TRANSPLANTATION. The bone marrow extraction, or harvest, is the same whether for an autologous or allogeneic transplant. Harvesting is done under **general anesthesia** (i.e., the donor sleeps through the procedure), and discomfort is usually minimal afterwards. Bone marrow is drawn from the iliac crest (the part of the hip bone to either side of the lower back) with a special needle and a syringe. Several punctures are usually necessary to collect the needed amount of bone marrow, approximately 1–2 quarts (0.9–1.91). (This amount is only a small percentage of the total bone marrow and is typically replaced within four weeks.) The donor remains at the hospital for 24–48 hours and can resume normal activities within a few days.

If the bone marrow is meant for an autologous transplant, it is stored at -112 to -320 °F (-80 to -196 °C) until it is needed. Bone marrow for an allogeneic transplant is sometimes treated to remove the donor's T cells (a type of white blood cell) or to remove ABO (blood type) antigens; otherwise, it is transplanted without modification.

The bone marrow is administered to the recipient via a catheter (a narrow, flexible tube) inserted into a large vein in the chest. From the bloodstream, it migrates to the cavities within the bones where bone marrow is normally stored. If the transplant is successful, the bone marrow begins to produce normal blood cells once it is in place, or engrafted.

PERIPHERAL BLOOD STEM CELL TRANSPLANTATION. Before collection for a PBSC transplant, donors receive daily four injections of the drug G-CSF, or filgrastim. (Patients can give it to themselves at home if need be.) These pretreatments stimulate the body to release stem cells into the blood. After these pretreatments, the donors' experience is similar to that of a whole blood donor's experience— PBSC donors' blood is collected at a clinic or hospital as an outpatient procedure. The differences are that several sessions will be needed over days or weeks and the blood is collected in a process called apheresis. The blood travels from one arm into a blood cell separator that removes only the stem cells, and the rest of the blood is returned back to the donor, in the other arm. The cells are then frozen for later use.

The PBSCs are administered to the recipient using the same methods as those used in bone marrow transplantation. As stated, the amount of fluid with PBSCs infused into the recipient's body can be an issue.

Costs

Bone marrow transplantation is an expensive procedure. (Bone marrow donors are volunteers and do not pay for any part of the procedure.) Insurance companies and health maintenance organizations (HMOs) may not cover the costs.

Preparation

A bone marrow transplant recipient can expect to spend four to eight weeks in the hospital. In preparation for receiving the transplant, the recipient undergoes "conditioning"—a preparative regimen in which the bone marrow and abnormal cells are destroyed. Conditioning rids the body of diseased cells and makes room for the marrow to be transplanted. It typically involves chemotherapy and/or radiation treatment, depending on the disease being treated. Unfortunately, this treatment also destroys healthy cells and has many side effects such as extreme weakness, **nausea**, **vomiting**, and **diarrhea**. These side effects may continue for several weeks.

Aftercare

A two- to four-week waiting period follows the marrow transplant before its success can begin to be judged. The marrow recipient is kept in **isolation** during this time to minimize potential infections. The recipient also receives antibiotic medications and blood and platelet transfusions to help fight off infection and prevent excessive bleeding. Further side effects, such as **nausea and vomiting**, can be treated with other medications. Once blood counts are normal and the side effects of the transplant abate, the recipient is taken off **antibiotics** and usually no longer needs blood and platelet transfusions.

Following discharge from the hospital, the recipient is monitored through home visits by nurses or outpatient visits for up to a year. For the first several months out of the hospital, the recipient needs to be careful in avoiding potential infections. For example, contact with other people who may be ill should be avoided or kept to a minimum. Further blood transfusions and medications may be necessary, but barring complications, the recipient can return to normal activities about 6–8 months after the transplant.

Risks

Bone marrow transplants are accompanied by serious and life-threatening risks. Furthermore, they are not always an absolute assurance of a cure for the underlying ailment; a disease may recur in the future. Approximately 30% of people receiving allogeneic transplants do not survive. Autologous transplants have a much better survival rate—nearly 90%—but are not appropriate for all types of ailments requiring a bone marrow transplant. Furthermore, they have a higher failure rate with certain diseases, specifically leukemia.

In the short term, there is the danger of **pneumonia** or other infectious disease, excessive bleeding, or liver disorder caused by blocked blood vessels. The transplant may be rejected by the recipient's immune system, or the donor bone marrow may launch an immune-mediated attack against the recipient's tissues. This complication is called acute graft versus host disease, and it can be a life-threatening condition. Characteristic signs of the disease include **fever**, rash, diarrhea, liver problems, and a compromised immune system.

Approximately 25–50% of bone marrow transplant recipients develop long-term complications. Chronic graft versus host disease symptoms include skin changes such as dryness, altered pigmentation, and thickening; abnormal **liver function tests**; **dry mouth** and eyes; infections; and weight loss. Other long-term complications include **cataracts** (due to radiation treatment), abnormal lung function, hormonal abnormalities resulting in reduced growth or **hypothyroidism**, secondary cancers, and **infertility**.

Normal results

In a successful bone marrow transplant, the donor's marrow migrates to the cavities in the recipient's bones and produces normal numbers of healthy blood cells. Bone marrow transplants can extend a person's life, improve quality of life, and may aid in curing the underlying ailment.

In autologous bone marrow transplantation, stem cells are collected from the patient. Once the patient has undergone chemotherapy, the cells are replaced in the blood via an intravenous catheter. The cells return to the bone marrow and begin producing healthy new cells.

Resources

PERIODICALS

Dreger, P., and N. Schmitz. "Allogeneic transplantation of blood stem cells: coming of age?" *Annals of Hematology* 80, no. 3 (March, 2001): 127-36.

Nuzhat, Iqbal, Donna Salzman, Audrey J. Lazenby, et al. "Diagnosis of Gastrointestinal Graft-Versus-Host Disease." *The American Journal of Gastroenterology* 95 (November, 2000): 3034- 3038.

ORGANIZATIONS

American Society for Blood and Marrow Transplantation (ASBMT). 85 W. Algonquin Road, Suite 550 Arlington Heights, IL 60005. (847) 427-0224. mail@asbmt.org. Founded in 1990, a national professional association that promotes advancement of the field of blood and bone marrow transplantation in clinical practice and research.

Blood & Marrow Transplant Newsletter (Formerly BMT Newsletter). 2900 Skokie Valley Road, Suite B, Highland Park, IL 60035 (847) 433-3313. 1-888-597-7674. help@bmtinfonet.org. < http://www2.bmtnews. org >. Blood & Marrow Transplant Newsletter is a not-for-profit organization that provides publications and support services to bone marrow, peripheral blood stem cell, and cord blood transplant patients and survivors.

BMT Information < http://www.bmtinfo.org/ >. Web site, sponsored by a variety of other bone marrow transplant organizations, lists basic information and resources about bone marrow transplants.

Health Resources and Services Administration. 5600 Fishers Lane, Rm. 14-45, Rockville, MD 20857, 301-443-3376, comments@hrsa.gov. <http://www.hrsa.gov>. HRSA manages contracts for the Organ Procurement and Transplantation Network, Scientific Registry of Transplant Recipients and National Marrow Donor Program and provides public education and technical assistance to increase donation. HRSA also monitors the performance of the nation's transplant centers and provides potential transplant recipients with survival rates and other vital information.

International Bone Marrow Transplant Registry/Autologous Blood and Marrow Transplant Registry N. America. Health Policy Institute, Medical College of Wisconsin. 8701 Watertown Plank Road, P.O. Box 26509, Milwaukee, WI 53226 USA. (414) 456-8325. ibmtr@mcw.edu. Voluntary organizations of more than 400 institutions in 47 countries that submit data on their allogeneic and autologous blood and marrow transplant recipients to the IBMTR/ABMTR Statistical Center at the Medical College of Wisconsin in Milwaukee.

Leukemia & Lymphoma Society, Inc. 1311 Mamaroneck Avenue White Plains, NY 10605. (914) 949-5213. <http://www.leukemia-lymphoma.org/>. National voluntary health agency dedicated to curing leukemia, lymphoma, Hodgkin's disease and myeloma, and to improving the quality of life of patients and their families.

National Marrow Donor Program. Suite 500, 3001 Broadway Street Northeast, Minneapolis, MN 55413-1753. (800) MARROW-2. <http://www.marrow.org>. Founded in 1986, The National Marrow Donor Program (NMDP) is a non-profit international leader in the facilitation of unrelated marrow and blood stem cell transplantation.

National Organ and Tissue Donation Initiative. <http://www.organdonor.gov/>. Created by Health Resources and Services Administration (HRSA) Department of Health and Human Services (DHHS) <http://www.os.dhhs.gov/>. Provides information and resources on organ donation and transplantation issues.

Julia Barrett
Laura Ruth, Ph.D.

Bone nuclear medicine scan

Definition

A bone scan is a diagnostic procedure used to evaluate abnormalities involving bones and joints. A radioactive substance is injected intravenously, and the image of its distribution in the skeletal system is analyzed to detect certain diseases or conditions.

KEY TERMS

Radioisotope—A radioactive, or radiation-emitting form, of an element.

Radionuclide—A substance which emits radiation as it disintegrates.

Purpose

Bone scans are most frequently ordered to check whether a **cancer** that originated elsewhere has spread to the bones. Cancers that begin in the breasts, kidneys, lungs, prostate, thyroid, or urinary bladder are most likely to spread, or metastasize, to the bones. If metastases are found, periodic bone scans may be ordered to see if therapy is effective against a cancer.

Some cancers arise in bone. These are called primary bone cancers. When an abnormality is found on an x ray of a bone, a bone scan may be helpful in deciding if it is a primary bone cancer, or a non-cancerous (benign) condition.

Infection in the bone (**osteomyelitis**) can be detected or confirmed by a bone scan, often days or weeks before an x ray would reveal it. Bone scans are useful in diagnosing early arthritic changes, and monitoring both the progression of the disease and the effectiveness of treatment. Unexplained **pain** may be evaluated with a bone scan, because it can demonstrate **fractures** that are difficult to detect on x ray. Bone scans can be used to see if artificial joints have loosened or become infected. Suspected **child abuse** may be evaluated with a bone scan, due to its ability to show an overall pattern of repeated trauma. Abnormalities caused by altered circulation to the bone may be diagnosed with a bone scan.

Precautions

Women who are pregnant or breastfeeding should not have this test. A patient who is unable to remain still for an extended period of time may require **sedation** for a bone scan.

Description

This test is performed in a radiology facility, either in a hospital department or an outpatient x-ray center. The patient usually sits or lies down while a radioactive substance is injected through a vein in the arm. For a bone scan, the radionuclide used is specifically chosen to accumulate in the bone. The patient then waits from three to four hours, for the substance to collect within the skeletal system. During this time, he or she will be instructed to drink several glasses of water. Patients are free to get up and move around as they desire during this waiting time, and should urinate frequently. Just before the scanning begins, the patient should empty his or her bladder again. This ensures that a lot of radioactive material is not concentrated in the urinary bladder, which could obscure part of the pelvic bones.

During the scan, the patient lies on his or her back on a table, but may be repositioned to the stomach or side during the study. It is important for the patient not to move, except when directed to by the technologist.

The radionuclide scanner, sometimes called a gamma camera, or scintillation camera, is positioned against the body part to be examined. Either the camera, the table, or both, may change position during the study. For a total body bone scan, the patient is scanned from head to foot, over a period of 30-60 minutes. Patients should experience no discomfort from this examination.

A special kind of bone scan, called a SPECT (Single Photon Emission Computed Tomography) scan may be added, to study a particular part of the body in more detail. Suspected diseases of the hips, lower back, or jaw are often evaluated using this study. It usually takes an additional 30-45 minutes. The camera circles completely around the area in question or multiple cameras are used to create a cross-sectional image. This helps pinpoint the location of the abnormality being evaluated.

The bone scan might be done in phases. The procedure is the same, except the scanning takes place immediately after the radioactive substance is injected, then again at set intervals to image how the radioactive tracer pools and distributes in the body and bone. For example, a two-phase bone scan for osteomyelitis may involve a scan about five minutes after injection, then about three hours later.

Preparation

Some specialized blood studies should be drawn before this study is begun. Jewelry or metallic objects need to be removed. No other special physical preparation is required.

The patient should understand that there is no danger of radioactive exposure to themselves or others, as only small amounts of the radioisotope are used. The total dose of radiation absorbed is minimal, often less than the amount received from ordinary x rays. The radionuclide scanner does not emit any radiation at all, but detects and records it from the patient.

Aftercare

Fluids are encouraged after the scan to aid in the excretion of the radioisotope. It is almost completely eliminated from the body within 24 hours. However, since increased airport security methods resulting from the September 11, 2001 attacks, isolated cases of people who have had recent diagnostic nuclear medicine procedures setting off airport security systems have occurred. One state's Homeland Security Department has warned people having nuclear medicine procedures and flying soon afterward to bring adequate documentation of the procedure along to the airport.

Normal results

The normal appearance of the scan will vary according to the patient's age. In general, a uniform concentration of radionuclide uptake is present in all bones in a normal scan.

Abnormal results

A high concentration of radionuclide occurs in areas of increased bone activity. These regions appear brighter and may be referred to as "hot spots." They may indicate healing fractures, tumors, infections, or other processes that trigger new bone formation. Lower concentrations of radionuclide may be called "cold spots." Poor blood flow to an area of bone, or bone destruction from a tumor may produce a cold spot.

The bone scan is a very sensitive test and can detect subtle conditions more readily than other studies. However, it is not a very specific examination, and often cannot distinguish exactly what disease process is causing an abnormality. Results need to be correlated with the patient's medical history, and other radiologic and laboratory studies to make a definite diagnosis.

Resources

PERIODICALS

Frank, John. "Introduction to Imaging: Bone and Joint." *Student BMJ* March 2004: 101–105.
Gebhart, Fred. "Nuclear Medicine Creating Patient Travel Problems." *Drug Topics* July 28, 2004: 11.

Ellen S. Weber, MSN
Teresa G. Odle

Bone tumor *see* **Sarcomas**

Bone x rays

Definition

Bone x rays are a diagnostic test in which ionizing radiation passing through the bones being examined enables an image to be produced on film.

Purpose

Bone x rays are ordered to detect disease or injury to the bone such as broken bones, tumors, and other problems. They can determine bone density, texture, erosion, and changes in bone relationships. Bone x rays also evaluate the joints for diseases such as **osteoarthritis**.

Precautions

Precautions should be taken to protect patients from unnecessary exposure to radiation. Patients should be shielded with lead aprons as much as possible. Women of childbearing age who could be pregnant should not have x rays of their trunk or pelvic regions. The fetus is especially at risk during the first trimester of **pregnancy**. Women who are pregnant should not have x rays of their pelvic region, lumbar spine, and abdomen unless absolutely necessary. If other types of x rays are necessary, a lead apron should be used to shield the abdominal and pelvic regions.

Description

X rays are a common diagnostic test in which a form of energy called x-ray radiation penetrates the patient's body. In bone x rays, electrical current passes through an x-ray tube and produces a beam of ionizing radiation that passes through the bone(s) being examined. This produces a picture of the inside of the body on film. The physician reads the developed x ray on a wall-mounted light box.

Digital x rays are a new type of x ray in which conventional equipment is used to take the x ray but the image is produced via computer. In a digital x ray, the image is created on a reusable plate. After being read by a laser reader, the information is sent in digital form to a storage unit connected to a computer network from which the radiologist reads the image. An electronic report can then be sent to the patient's physician.

Problems with bones that x rays can detect result from injury or from disease caused by a malfunction in the patient's bone chemistry. Bone injuries, especially broken bones (**fractures**), are common and can be accurately diagnosed by bone x rays. X rays are

> ### KEY TERMS
>
> **Arthritis**—A disease of the joints that arises from wear and tear, age and less often from inflammation.
>
> **Osteogenesis imperfecta**—Also called brittle bones, this is a condition present at birth in which bones are abnormally fragile, brittle and break easily.
>
> **Osteomalacia**—A disease in which bones gradually soften and bend.
>
> **Osteomyelitis**—An infection of the bone marrow and the bone.
>
> **Osteoporosis**—A disease that occurs primarily in post-menopausal women in which the amount of bone is reduced or skeletal tissue wastes away.
>
> **Paget's disease**—A disease, whose cause is unknown, which is generally found in older people. Symptoms include bone pain, bowed legs, curves spine, and broken bones. Another name for this disease is osteitis deformans.

especially helpful in diagnosing simple and incomplete fractures that can't be detected during a **physical examination**. X rays can also be used to check for bone position in a fracture. Some bone diseases can be definitively diagnosed with bone x rays while others require additional tests.

Osteoporosis, a common bone disease, can be detected in bone x rays but other tests are then ordered to determine the extent of the disease. For osteomalacia and **rickets**, a blood test and x rays of the affected bone are usually definitive; in some cases a **bone biopsy** (microscopic analysis of a small amount of tissue) is also done. In a rare bone disease called Paget's disease, x rays may be used in conjunction with bone, blood, and urine tests to make a diagnosis. In another rare bone disease, fibrous dysplasia, bone x rays or a bone biopsy (microscopic analysis of a small amount of tissue) are used to confirm the diagnosis. Bone x rays are definitive in diagnosing **osteogenesis imperfecta**. For **osteomyelitis**, bone x rays are used in conjunction with a blood test, bone scan, or needle biopsy to make the diagnosis. For arthritis, x rays of the bone are occasionally used in conjunction with blood tests. For bone tumors, bone x rays are helpful but they may not be definitive.

Bone x rays are performed by a technologist, and interpreted by a radiologist. They are taken in a physician's office, radiology department, outpatient clinic, or diagnostic clinic. Bone x rays generally take less than

10 minutes. There is no **pain** or discomfort associated with the test, but some people find it difficult to remain still. The results are often available in minutes.

During the test, the patient lies on a table. The technologist taking the x ray will check the patient's positioning and place the x-ray machine over the part of the body being examined. After asking the patient to remain motionless, he or she steps out of the area and presses a button to take the picture.

Preparation

The patient is asked to remove clothing, jewelry, and any other metal objects from the area being x rayed. If appropriate, a lead shield will be placed over other body parts to minimize exposure to radiation.

Aftercare

The patient can immediately resume normal activities.

Risks

The human body contains some natural radiation and is also exposed to radiation in the environment. There is a slight risk from exposure to radiation during bone x rays, however, the amount of radiation is small and the risk of harm is very low. If reproductive organs are exposed to radiation, genetic alterations may occur. Excessive or repeated doses of radiation can cause changes in other types of body tissue. No radiation remains in the body after the x ray.

Normal results

Normal bones show no fractures, **dislocations**, or other abnormalities.

Abnormal results

Results that indicate the presence of bone injury or disease differ in appearance according to the nature of the injury/disease. For example, fractures show up as clear breaks in the bones, while osteoporotic bone has the same shape as a normal bone on an x ray but is less dense. Even though a bone x ray may not show definite results, it often is the first imaging choice, to be followed up by another imaging technique such as **magnetic resonance imaging** (MRI). Bone x rays are still the easiest was to show a typical bone fracture and to check on healing of broken bones.

Resources

PERIODICALS

Frank, John. "Introduction to Imaging: Bone and Joint." *Student BMJ* (March 2004): 101–105.

Lori De Milto
Teresa G. Odle

Borderline personality disorder *see* **Personality disorders**

Bordetella pertussis infection *see* **Whooping cough**

Borrelia burgdorferi infection *see* **Lyme disease**

Botanical medicine *see* **Herbalism, western**

Botox injections *see* **Botulinum toxin injections**

Botulinum toxin injections

Definition

Botulinum is a bacterium (*Clostridium botulinum*) that produces seven different toxins that can cause **botulism** and is also medically used to block muscle contractions.

Purpose

Botulinum toxin (Botox) injection is used in conditions of excessive and inappropriate muscle contraction, spasticity (persistent states of muscle contraction), sphincter contraction, eye-movement disorders, tics and **tremors**, and cosmetically to treat facial lines and wrinkles. The FDA approved Botox for treating excessive underarm sweating in 2004.

Botox has also been used in the treatment of chronic muscle tension and migraine headaches. The relief is likely due to the decrease in localized **muscle spasms**, as no direct effect of Botox on the sensory nerves has been established. Researchers in New Zealand were testing Botox as means to help improve movement in children with a form of **cerebral palsy** called hemiplegia in 2004. The application of the therapy seems to be growing continuously beyond its more popularly known cosmetic uses.

Precautions

Botulinum toxin is produced from the bacterium that causes **food poisoning** in humans. High doses of the toxin can be fatal; however, doses administered therapeutically are so small that harmful effects are uncommon.

Description

The number of potential applications for botulinum toxin extends to every muscle group. The first therapeutic use of Botox was in the treatment of **strabismus** (eyes are unable to direct toward the same object) and since then it has been used to treat a variety of involuntary muscle contractions or disorders. Its cosmetic use is the result of treatment for facial spasms where smoothing of facial lines was reported by patients. In general, 90% of injections for facial spasms are resolved satisfactorily.

Toxin type A has a duration of effect that lasts approximately three months and is the therapeutic agent of choice for most conditions.

Preparation

The dosage of Botox must be monitored and adjusted, with multiple injections showing a lower incidence of complications versus administration by one larger dose.

Risks

In over 30 years of therapeutic use in humans, botulinum toxin has proven to be remarkably safe. Difficulties associated with administration of toxin are: different patients may experience different effects at the same dose, patients new to the treatment may experience exaggerated effects at subsequent visits and/or neighboring muscles may become activated at subsequent treatments. Patients should ask about their provider s experience with injecting Botox before proceeding with the procedure.

Additional side effects may include excessive muscle weakness at the injection site or adjacent muscles. These effects typically resolve quickly. Occasionally, patients report flu-like symptoms but they are usually self-limited.

A certain percentage of patients may also experience resistance to the toxin. The presence of circulating antibodies to the toxin is presumed to be the primary reason for resistance to Botox injections. Patients who have little reaction to Botox 'A' may benefit from injections using one of the other six serotypes. Using the smallest effective dose limits the likelihood of immunoresistance in unresponsive patients.

Normal results

The anticipated outcome of Botox injections is relaxation of the target muscle tissue. The pharmacological effects of botulinum toxin are typically isolated to local areas and do not result in tissue destruction or prolonged **paralysis**. Varying the dose can deliver a precise amount of toxin to achieve graded degrees of paralysis for the desired level of response.

Abnormal results

Most side effects, such as weakness in the injected muscle or overall muscle soreness, will go away quickly. Some patients have received too much of the substance when having Botox for cosmetic purposes and have been unhappy with the results. Physicians and patients should discuss the procedure and the amount to be used. Many clinicians believe that it is best to err on the side of low dosage with a return trip for more, rather than too high a dosage that might result in unwanted cosmetic effects.

Resources

BOOKS

Blitzer, A., W. J. Binder, J. Brian Boyd, and Alastair Carruthers. *Management of Facial Lines and Wrinkles*. Philadelphia: Lippincott Williams & Wilkins, 1999.

Brin, M.F. *Botulinum Toxin Therapy: Basic Science and Overview of Other Therapeutic Applications*. Department of Neurology, Movement Disorders Program, The Mount Sinai Medical Center, New York, New York 10029.

PERIODICALS

"Another Botox Use." *Dermatology Times* (October 2004): 24.

Franklin, Deeanna. "Separate Fact from Fiction With Botox Techniques, Safety." *Skin & Allergy News* (August 2004): 41.

Johnson, Kate. "FDA Approves Botox for Severe Underarm Sweating." *Family Practice News* (September 1, 2004): 13.

OTHER

Blitzer A and L. Sulica. "Botulinum toxin: basic science and clinical uses in otolaryngology." New York Center for Voice and Swallowing Disorders, St. Luke's Roosevelt Hospital Center.

Bonny McClain, DC
Teresa G. Odle

Botulism

Definition

Botulism is caused by botulinum toxin, a natural poison produced by certain bacteria in the *Clostridium* genus. Exposure to the botulinum toxin occurs mostly from eating contaminated food, or in infants, from certain clostridia growing in the intestine. Botulinum toxin blocks motor nerves' ability to release acetylcholine, the neurotransmitter that relays nerve signals to muscles, and flaccid **paralysis** occurs. As botulism progresses, the muscles that control the airway and breathing fail.

Description

Botulism occurs rarely, but it causes concern because of its high fatality rate. Clinical descriptions of botulism possibly reach as far back in history as ancient Rome and Greece. However, the relationship between contaminated food and botulism wasn't defined until the late 1700s. In 1793 the German physician, Justinius Kerner, deduced that a substance in spoiled sausages, which he called *wurstgift* (German for sausage poison), caused botulism. The toxin's origin and identity remained elusive until Emile von Ermengem, a Belgian professor, isolated *Clostridium botulinum* in 1895 and identified it as the poison source.

Three types of botulism have been identified: food-borne, wound, and infant botulism. The main difference between types hinges on the route of exposure to the toxin. In the United States, there are approximately 110 cases of botulism reported annually. Food-borne botulism accounts for 25% of all botulism cases and usually can be traced to eating contaminated home-preserved food. Infant botulism accounts for 72% of all cases, but the recovery rate is good (about 98%) with proper treatment. From 1990 to 2000, 263 cases of food-borne cases were reported in the United States, most of them in Alaska. Though most were related to home canning, two restaurant-associated outbreaks affected 25 people.

Though domestic **food poisoning** is a problem world-wide, there has been a growing concern regarding the use of botulism toxin in biological warfare and terrorist acts. The Iraqi government admitted in 1995 that it had loaded 11,200 liters of botulinum toxin into SCUD missiles during the Gulf War. Luckily, these special missiles were never used. As of 1999, there were 17 countries known to be developing biological weapons, including the culture of botulism toxins.

Causes and symptoms

Toxin produced by the bacterium *Clostridium botulinum* is the main culprit in botulism. Other members of the *clostridium* genus can produce botulinum toxin, namely *C. argentinense*, *C. butyricum*, and *C. baratii*, but they are minor sources. To grow, these bacteria require a low-acid, oxygen-free environment that is warm (40-120 °F or 4.4–48.8 °C) and moist. Lacking these conditions, the bacteria transform themselves into spores that, like plant seeds, can remain dormant for years. Clostridia and their spores exist all over the world, especially in soil and aquatic sediments. They do not threaten human or animal health until the spores encounter an environment that favors growth. The spores then germinate, and the growing bacteria produce the deadly botulism toxin.

Scientists have discovered that clostridia can produce at least seven types of botulism toxin, identified as A, B, C, D, E, F, and G. Humans are usually affected by A, B, E, and very rarely F. Domesticated animals such as dogs, cattle, and mink are affected by botulism C toxin, which also affects birds and has caused massive die-offs in domestic bird flocks and wild waterfowl. Botulism D toxin can cause illness in cattle, and horses succumb to botulism A, B, and C toxin. There have been no confirmed human or animal botulism cases linked to the G toxin.

In humans, botulinum toxin latches onto specific proteins in nerve endings and irreversibly destroys them. These proteins control the release of acetylcholine, a neurotransmitter that stimulates muscle cells. With acetylcholine release blocked, nerves are not able to stimulate muscles. Ironically, botulinum toxin has found a beneficial niche in the world of medicine due to this

KEY TERMS

Acetylcholine—A chemical released by nerve cells to signal other cells.

Antitoxin—A substance that inactivates a poison (e.g., toxin) and protects the body from being injured by it.

CT scan—The abbreviated term for computed or computerized axial tomography. The test may involve injecting a radioactive contrast into the body. Computers are used to scan for radiation and create cross-sectional images of internal organs.

Electromyographic test—A medical test which determines if a muscle's response to electrical stimuli. The test results allow medical personnel to assess how nerves to the muscle are functioning.

Flaccid paralysis—Paralysis characterized by limp, unresponsive muscles.

Lumbar puncture—A procedure in which a small amount of cerebrospinal fluid is removed from the lower spine. Examination of this fluid helps diagnose certain illnesses.

MRI—The abbreviated term for magnetic resonance imaging. MRI uses a large circular magnet and radio waves to generate signals from atoms in the body. These signals are used to construct images of internal structures.

Neurotransmitter—A chemical found in nerves that relays nerve signals to other cells. Acetylcholine is a neurotransmitter.

Sepsis—The presence of infection-causing organisms or associated toxins in the blood or within body tissues.

Spores—A state of "suspended animation" that some bacteria can adopt when conditions are not ideal for growth. Spores are analogous to plant seeds and can germinate into growing bacteria when conditions are right.

Toxin—A poisonous substance produced by a microorganism, plant, or animal.

Tracheostomy—The procedure used to open a hole in the neck to the trachea, or windpipe. It is sometimes used in conjunction with a respirator.

action. Certain medical disorders are characterized by involuntary and uncontrollable muscle contractions. Medical researchers have discovered that injecting a strictly controlled dose of botulinum toxin into affected muscles inhibits excessive muscle contractions. The muscle is partially paralyzed and normal movement is retained. This is commonly referred to as Botox injection.

The three types of human botulism include the following symptoms:

- Food-borne. Food that has been improperly preserved or stored can harbor botulinum toxin-producing clostridia. Botulism symptoms typically appear within 18-36 hours of eating contaminated food, with extremes of four hours to eight days. Initial symptoms include blurred or double vision and difficulty swallowing and speaking. Possible gastrointestinal problems include **constipation**, **nausea**, and **vomiting**. As botulism progresses, the victim experiences weakness or paralysis, starting with the head muscles and progressing down the body. Breathing becomes increasingly difficult. Without medical care, **respiratory failure** and **death** are very likely.

- Infant. Infant botulism was first described in 1976. Unlike adults, infants younger than 12 months are vulnerable to *C. botulinum* colonizing the intestine. Infants ingest spores in honey or simply by swallowing spore-containing dust. The spores germinate in the large intestine and, as the bacteria grow, they produce botulinum toxin that is absorbed into the infant's body. The first symptoms include constipation, lethargy, and poor feeding. As infant botulism progresses, sucking and swallowing (thus eating) become difficult. A nursing mother will often notice breast engorgement as the first sign of her infant's illness. The baby suffers overall weakness and cannot control head movements. Because of the flaccid paralysis of the muscles, the baby appears "floppy." Breathing is impaired, and death from respiratory failure is a very real danger.

- Wound. Confirmed cases of wound botulism have been linked to trauma such as severe crush injuries to the extremities, surgery, and illegal drug use. Wound botulism occurs when clostridia colonize an infected wound and produce botulinum toxin. The symptoms usually appear four to 18 days after an injury occurs and are similar to food-borne botulism, although gastrointestinal symptoms may be absent.

Diagnosis

Diagnosis of botulism can be tricky because symptoms mimic those presented by other diseases. Botulism may be confused with Guillain-Barre syndrome, **myasthenia gravis**, drug reactions, **stroke**, or nervous system infection, intoxications (e.g. carbon monoxide or atropine), or **shellfish poisoning**. **Sepsis** is the most common initial diagnosis for infant botulism. **Failure to thrive** may also be suspected. Some reports have linked infant botulism to 5-15% of **sudden infant death syndrome** (SIDS, crib death) cases. Laboratory tests are used for definitive diagnosis, but if botulism seems likely, treatment starts immediately.

While waiting for laboratory results, doctors ask about recently consumed food and work to dismiss other disease possibilities. A **physical examination** is done with an emphasis on the nervous system. As part of this examination, CT scans, MRIs, electromyographic tests, or lumbar punctures may be ordered. Laboratory tests involve testing a suspected food and/or the patient's serum, feces, or other specimens for traces of botulinum toxin or clostridia.

Treatment

Drugs

Adults with botulism are treated with an antitoxin derived from horse serum that is distributed by the Centers for Disease Control and Prevention. The antitoxin (effective against toxin types A, B, and E) inactivates only the botulinum toxin that is unattached to nerve endings. Early injection of antitoxin (usually within 24 hours of onset of symptoms) can preserve nerve endings, prevent progression of the disease, and reduce mortality.

Infants, however, cannot receive the antitoxin used for adults. For them, human botulism immune globulin (BIG) is available in the United States through the Infant Botulism Treatment and Prevention Program in Berkeley, California. BIG neutralizes toxin types A, B, C, D, and E before they can bind to nerves. This antitoxin can provide protection against A and B toxins for approximately four months. Though many infants recover with supportive care, BIG cuts hospital stay in half, and therefore reduces hospital costs by 50% as well.

Aside from antitoxin, no drugs are used to treat botulism. **Antibiotics** are not effective for preventing or treating botulism. In fact, antibiotic use is discouraged for infants because dying bacteria could potentially release more toxin into a baby's system. Antibiotics can be used, however, to treat secondary respiratory tract and other infections.

Respiratory support

Treatment for infants usually involves intensive respiratory support and tube feeding for weeks or even months. Once an infant can breathe unaided, physical therapy is initiated to help the child relearn how to suck and swallow. A respirator is often required to help adult patients breathe, and a tracheostomy may also be necessary.

Surgery

Surgery may be necessary to clean an infected wound and remove the source of the bacteria that is producing the toxin. Antimicrobial therapy may be necessary.

Gastric lavage

When botulism is caused by food, it often is necessary to flush the gastrointestinal tract (gastric lavage). Often cathartic agents or **enemas** are used. It is important to avoid products that contain magnesium, since magnesium enhances the effect of the toxin.

Prognosis

With medical intervention, botulism victims can recover completely, though slowly. It takes weeks to months to recover from botulism, and severe cases can take years before a total recovery is attained. Recovery depends on the nerve endings building new proteins to replace those destroyed by botulinum toxin.

Prevention

Vaccines against botulism do not exist to prevent infant botulism or other forms of the disease. However, scientists announced in 2004 that they had successfully vaccinated mice and ducks against type C and D, which may help lead to vaccines for humans. Food safety is the surest prevention for botulism. Botulinum toxin cannot be seen, smelled, or tasted, so the wisest course is to discard any food that seems spoiled *without tasting it*. Home canners must be diligent about using sterile equipment and following U.S. Department of Agriculture canning guidelines. If any part of a canned food container is rusty or bulging, the food should not be eaten. Infant botulism is difficult to prevent, because controlling what goes into an infant's mouth is often beyond control, especially in regard to spores in the air. One concrete preventive is to never feed honey to infants younger than 12 months since it is one known source of botulism spores. As infants begin eating solid foods, the same food precautions should be followed as for adults.

Resources

PERIODICALS

Cadou, Stephanie G. "Diagnosing Infant Botulism." *The Nurse Practitioner* 26, no.3 (March 2001): 76.

Shapiro, Roger L. and David L. Swerdlow. "Botulism: Keys to Prompt Recognition and Therapy." *Consultant* (April 1999): 1021–1024.

Sobel, Jeremy, et al. "Foodborne Botulism in the United States, 1990–2000." *Emerging Infectious Diseases* (September 2004): 1606–1612.

"Vaccination With Botulinum Neurotoxin Fragments Prevents Botuism." *Obesity, Fitness & Wellness Week* (August 7, 2004): 117.

Janie F. Franz
Teresa G. Odle

Bovine spongiform encephalopathy *see*
Creutzfeldt-Jakob disease

Bowel incontinence *see* **Fecal incontinence**

Bowel preparation

Definition

Bowel preparation is a procedure usually undertaken before a diagnostic procedure or treatment can be initiated for certain colorectal diseases. Bowel preparation is a cleansing of the intestines from fecal matter and secretions.

Purpose

The ultimate goal of bowel preparation is to empty and cleanse the bowel for a diagnostic procedure (using x rays to detect a disease process in the intestines) or for surgical intervention (such as removal of polyps, **cancer**, or narrowing of the intestinal diameter). **Colonoscopy** is an effective treatment procedure for polyps (a growing mass of tissue). This procedure enables the doctor to visualize the entire large bowel. During a colonoscopy, polyps can be cauterized (applying an electric current which incinerates the polyp). The procedure can be both diagnostic and therapeutic. A **sigmoidoscopy** scope is a flexible tube that allows clinicians to view the sigmoid colon (the part of the large intestine before the rectum). This procedure is important for detection of colorectal cancer. It is safe, quick to perform (usually 30–45 minutes in about 90% of cases), and an effective diagnostic tool for evaluation of:

- rectal bleeding
- other abnormalities detected by imaging studies
- removal of polyps
- biopsy
- evaluation of chronic **diarrhea** or inflammatory bowel disease
- recurrences of colorectal cancer or polyps

- relieving a twisted bowel
- foreign body removal
- treating bleeding lesions
- preventive surveillance of cancer in patients with a positive family history of colon cancer

Precautions

Antibiotic **prophylaxis** is not routinely recommended. In some cases of prosthetic heart valves, **antibiotics** can be prescribed. Evidence exists that evacuation of intestinal waste products in conjunction with antibiotics before (prophylactic) the procedure reduces the possibility of **sepsis** (infection which spreads from the primary site to blood).

Description

The bowel is emptied of any contents for such procedures as **barium enema** (introducing a compound containing barium to promote better visualization of intestines during x rays) or colonoscopy. Preparation of the bowel distally—from the rectum—is necessary for such diagnostic procedures as sigmoidoscopy. Bowel emptying is done through taking oral laxative solutions that speed up the excretion of the contents of the lower bowel together with restrictions on solid food intake.

A newer type of imaging study may eventually make current laxative methods of bowel preparation obsolete. According to a group of researchers in the United Kingdom, computed tomography (CT) colonography (sometimes called virtual colonoscopy) has shown itself to be as accurate in diagnosing colorectal tumors as optical colonoscopy. CT colonography allows a radiologist to examine the colon and nearby organs in less than 30 seconds.

Preparation

Bowel preparation for visualization of the colon is performed to ensure the procedure will be accurate and complete. There are several effective cleansing preparations including polyethylene glycol solution (Colyte), sodium phosphate solution (Phospho-Soda), magnesium citrate with bisacodyl tablets, and castor oil with bisacodyl tablets. One of these preparations should be administered starting at 4:00 p.m. the day before the procedure. Patients are usually asked to avoid solid foods for about 36 hours before diagnostic procedures. Such clear liquids as vegetable or beef broth, apple or white grape juice, soda pop or fruit-flavored gelatin are permitted, although some doctors ask patients to avoid red-colored beverages or gelatin flavors on the grounds that the red food coloring in these products may make bleeding more difficult to detect.

In most cases, patients may continue to take other prescription medications at the usual times while they are restricted to clear liquids. It is a good idea, however, to check with the doctor beforehand.

Aftercare

Patients should have a friend or relative to drive them home after the procedure, as the combination of a period of dietary restriction, frequent bowel movements, and the procedure itself leaves most people feeling tired and slightly weak. Many doctors advise patients to postpone vigorous physical activity or work requiring mental concentration until the day after the procedure. Patients can resume eating solid foods as soon as they get home.

Some patients may notice a small amount of blood on toilet tissue or underwear following a colonoscopy or other examination of the lower digestive tract. Spotting is not cause for concern; however, patients who have steady or heavy bleeding from the rectum should call their doctor as soon as possible.

Risks

The current standard of care dictates that patients receive antibiotic prophylaxis if they are at increased risk of developing an infection. High-risk patients include those with cardiac diseases or patients with prostheses.

Bowel preparation can be stressful for some patients, particularly those with pre-existing nutritional problems associated with cancer treatment or malabsorption. In addition, many patients find the various oral solutions unpleasant to the taste and difficult to swallow for that reason. According to one British study, oral solutions flavored with lemon are more acceptable to patients than unflavored forms. Both Colyte and Phospho-Soda are available with flavoring added; patients may wish to ask their pharmacist for these specific products. Mild **nausea**, **vomiting**, stomach cramps, intestinal gas, **dry mouth**, and increased thirst are common side effects of these products. Some patients are helped by taking an electrolyte

supplement along with oral sodium phosphate solution to lower the risk of **dehydration**.

Some people may have severe allergic reactions to commonly used oral **laxatives** used for bowel preparation. Patients who develop **hives**, swelling of the face or hands, swelling or **tingling** in the throat or mouth, difficulty breathing, or tightness in the chest should call their doctor *at once*. This type of reaction is a medical emergency.

Normal results

Absence of anatomical changes or abnormalities in the intestines would result in normal diagnosis.

Abnormal results

Polyps can be treated with electrocautery. A biopsy is taken of any suspicious polyps and further analyzed. Sigmoidoscopy can detect masses, bleeding, and ulcerative disease.

Resources

BOOKS

Tierney, Lawrence M., et al, editors. *Current Medical Diagnosis and Treatment 2001*. 40th ed. New York: McGraw-Hill, 2001.
Wilson, Billie A., Margaret T. Shannon, and Carolyn L. Stang. *Nurses Drug Guide 2000*. Stamford, CT: Appleton & Lange, 2000.

PERIODICALS

Bulmer, Frances M. "Bowel Preparation for Rectal and Colonic Investigation." *Nursing Standard* 14 (February 2000): 32–35.
Burling, D., S. Taylor, and S. Halligan. "Computerized Tomography Colonography." *Expert Review of Anticancer Therapy* 4 (August 2004): 615–625.
Tjandra, J. J., and P. Tagkalidis. "Carbohydrate-Electrolyte (E-Lyte) Solution Enhances Bowel Preparation with Oral Fleet Phospho-Soda." *Diseases of the Colon and Rectum* 47 (July 2004): 1181–1186.

ORGANIZATIONS

American College of Gastroenterology. 4900 B South 31st Street, Arlington, VA 22206. (703) 820-7400. < http://www.acg.gi.org/ct_html > .
American Society of Health-System Pharmacists (ASHP). 7272 Wisconsin Avenue, Bethesda, MD 20814. (301) 657-3000. < http://www.ashp.org > .
United States Food and Drug Administration (FDA). 5600 Fishers Lane, Rockville, MD 20857-0001. (888) INFO-FDA. < http://www.fda.gov > .

Laith Farid Gulli, M.D.
Bilal Nasser, M.Sc.
Rebecca J. Frey, PhD

Bowel resection

Definition

A bowel resection is a surgical procedure in which a part of the large or small intestine is removed.

Purpose

Bowel resection may be performed to treat various disorders of the intestine, including **cancer**, obstruction, inflammatory bowel disease, ruptured diverticulum, **ischemia** (compromised blood supply), or traumatic injury.

Description

The preferred type of bowel resection involves removal of the diseased portion of intestine, and surgically re-joining the remaining ends. In this procedure, the continuity of the bowel is maintained and normal passage of stool is preserved. When deemed necessary by the surgeon, the diseased portion of the bowel may be removed, and the functioning end of the intestine may be brought out onto the surface of the abdomen, forming an temporary or permanent **ostomy**. Use of the large intestine to form the ostomy results in a **colostomy**; use of small intestine to form the ostomy results in an ileostomy.

Preparation

As with any surgical procedure, the patient will be required to sign a consent form after the procedure is explained thoroughly. Blood and urine studies, along with various x rays and an electrocardiogram (EKG) may be ordered as the doctor deems necessary. In order to empty and cleanse the bowel, the patient may be placed on a low residue diet for several days prior to surgery. A liquid diet may be ordered for at least the day before surgery, with nothing taken by mouth after midnight. A series of **enemas** and/or oral preparations (GoLytely or Colyte), may be ordered to empty the bowel of stool. Oral anti-infectives (neomycin, erythromycin, or kanamycin sulfate) may be ordered to decrease bacteria in the intestine and help prevent post-operative infection. A nasogastric tube is inserted through the nose into the stomach on the day of surgery or during surgery. This removes the gastric secretions and prevents **nausea and vomiting**. A urinary catheter (thin tube inserted into the bladder) may also be inserted to keep the bladder empty during surgery, giving more space in the surgical field and decreasing chances of accidental injury.

KEY TERMS

Diverticulum—Small tubes or pouches that project off the wall of the intestine, visible as opaque on an x ray after the patient has swallowed a contrast (dye) substance.

Embolism—Blockage of a blood vessel by any small piece of material traveling in the blood. The emboli may be caused by germs, air, blood clots, or fat.

Ischemia—A compromise in blood supply to body tissues that causes tissue damage or death.

Ostomy—A surgically-created opening in the abdomen for elimination of waste products (urine or stool).

Aftercare

Post-operative care for the patient who has had a bowel resection, as with those who have had any major surgery, involves monitoring of blood pressure, pulse, respirations, and temperature. Breathing tends to be shallow because of the effect of anesthesia and the patient's reluctance to breathe deeply and experience **pain** that is caused by the abdominal incision. The patient is instructed how to support the operative site during deep breathing and coughing, and is given pain medication as necessary. Fluid intake and output is measured, and the operative site is observed for color and amount of wound drainage. The nasogastric tube will remain in place, attached to low intermittent suction until bowel activity resumes. Fluids and electrolytes are infused intravenously until the patient's diet can gradually be resumed, beginning with liquids and advancing to a regular diet as tolerated. The patient is generally out of bed approximately eight to 24 hours after surgery. Postoperative weight loss follows almost all bowel resections. Weight and strength are slowly regained over a period of months.

Risks

Potential complications of this abdominal surgery include:

- excessive bleeding

- surgical wound infection

- incisional **hernia** (An organ projects through the muscle wall that surrounds it. The hernia occurs through the surgical scar.)

- thrombophlebitis (inflammation and blood clot to veins in the legs)

- pneumonia
- pulmonary **embolism** (blood clot or air bubble in the lungs' blood supply)

Normal results

Complete healing is expected without complications after bowel resection. The period of time required for recovery from the surgery may vary depending of the patient's overall health status prior to surgery.

Abnormal results

The doctor should be made aware of any of the following problems after surgery:

- increased pain, swelling, redness, drainage, or bleeding in the surgical area
- headache, muscle aches, **dizziness**, fever
- increased abdominal pain or swelling, **constipation**, **nausea** or **vomiting**, rectal bleeding, or black, tarry stools

Resources

ORGANIZATIONS

United Ostomy Association, Inc. (UOA). 19772 MacArthur Blvd., Suite 200, Irvine, CA 92612-2405. (800) 826-0826. < http://www.uoa.org > .

Wound Ostomy and Continence Nurses Society. 1550 South Coast Highway, Suite #201.

Kathleen D. Wright, RN

Bowel surgery with ostomy *see* **Colostomy**

Bowel training

Definition

Bowel training helps to reestablish normal bowel movements in persons who suffer from **constipation**, **diarrhea**, incontinence, or irregularity. Healthy bowel activity is considered one or two movements of moderate size every day.

Purpose

Many people for many reasons have irregular bowel function. In some cases, the irregularity lasts beyond the condition that caused it. The bowels by themselves develop bad habits that can be retrained with suitable exercises and education. Normal bowel

---

KEY TERMS

Defecate—To pass feces (stool) out of the rectum through the anus.

Diverticulitis—Infection of outpouchings in the large bowel.

Fecal impaction—Obstruction of the rectum by a large mass of feces (stool).

Hiatal hernia—Part of the stomach displaced through the diaphragm into the chest.

---

habits not only improve the quality of life, they help prevent several common diseases–for example, **diverticulitis** and fecal impaction. Gall stones, **appendicitis**, **colon cancer**, hiatal **hernia**, diabetes, and heart disease have also been related to the quality of bowel movements and the foods that affect them.

- One of the most common causes of constipation is the laxative habit. Repeated artificial stimulation of the bowels destroys their natural emptying reflex, so that they will no longer move without artificial stimulants. The laxative habit begins innocently enough with the correct belief that bowels should move every day, however, **laxatives** will cause the evacuation of several days worth of stool in a single movement. Impatient for stool to reaccumulate for the necessary few days, the patient takes another laxative, and the cycle begins.

- The other major cause of constipation is a diet with insufficient bulk or roughage. The bowel works more smoothly the more contents it has. Western **diets** of highly refined foods have eliminated most of the residue from food. The result is that most food is absorbed, leaving little to pass through and be excreted as feces.

- Constipation occurs acutely with impaction–the presence in the rectum of a mass of feces too large to pass. Fecal impaction is usually the result of poor bowel habits, a diet with too little liquid and roughage, and inadequate physical activity.

- Diarrhea, whether acute or chronic, can disrupt the bowel's normal rhythm and lead to irregularity.

- Several diseases of the nervous system affect bowel reflexes.

Description

Bowel training reestablishes the bowel's normal reflexes by repeating a routine until it becomes a habit.

Naturally the patient must be able and willing to cooperate. Some patients are so convinced they need daily laxatives that they are afraid to do without them. It takes time for a changed diet to effect the bowels and for the bowel to regain its normal rhythm. Trust and patience are necessary.

After gaining the patient's cooperation, the next step is to optimize the diet. Healthy bowel movements require ingestion of a large amount of liquids and bulk foods. The patient should drink two to three quarts of liquids every day, with liberal inclusion of prune juice and perhaps coffee for their natural laxative effect. Bulk comes from unrefined foods. Oat bran, wheat bran, brown rice, green vegetables, apples, and pears are a few examples of high residue foods. Many patients will benefit from adding bulk preparations of psyllium. Constipating foods like bananas and cheese should be avoided until a natural rhythm is well established.

To assure that stools are soft enough to pass easily, it is a good idea to add a pure stool softener like DOSS (dioctyl sodium sulfosuccinate), two to four per day as needed. DOSS also helps prevent impaction.

There is usually a time of day when bowel movements are more likely to occur. In anticipation of this time, the patient should participate in activities that stimulate a normal bowel movement. Walking, eating unrefined foods, and drinking prune juice or coffee, encourage natural evacuation. It is acceptable to use lubricants such as glycerine suppositories or oil **enemas** at this time. For severe constipation, water enemas may be needed to initiate a movement.

It is also important for the patient to recognize the urge to defecate and to respond right away to that urge. The longer stool sits in the rectum, the more water the rectum will absorb from it, making it harder and more difficult to pass.

Normal results

With patience and diligence, normal bowel habits and the health that comes with them will return in most patients.

Resources

BOOKS

Barker, L. Randol, et al., eds. *Principles of Ambulatory Medicine*. Baltimore: William & Wilkins, 1994.

J. Ricker Polsdorfer, MD

Braces *see* **Immobilization**

Brachytherapy *see* **Radioactive implants**

Brain abscess

Definition

Brain **abscess** is a bacterial infection within the brain.

Description

The brain is usually well insulated from infection by bacteria, protected by the skull, the meninges (tissue layers surrounding the brain), the immune system, and the highly regulated barrier between the bloodstream and the brain. Under certain circumstances, however, bacteria can invade the brain and cause a localized infection called an abscess. Brain abscess is relatively rare, accounting for 1 in 10,000 hospital admissions. Single abscess occurs in 75% of cases, and the remainder of cases involve multiple abscesses. If not treated, brain abscess is almost always fatal.

Causes and symptoms

One-half of all brain abscesses are caused by the spread of bacteria from a nearby infection. Sources of bacteria include:

- middle ear infections (**otitis media**) or infections in the bony spaces in front of the middle ear (**mastoiditis**)
- sinus infections
- an abscessed tooth.

Other sources of bacteria include lung infections, abdominal infection, infection of the heart's lining (**endocarditis**) penetrating heart wounds, and neurosurgery.

Acquired Immune Deficiency Syndrome (**AIDS**) or the presence of another immune deficiency greatly increases the risk of brain abscess. Approximately 25% of cases have no detectable cause of infection.

Brain abscess can be caused by a variety of organisms, many of them related to ear and sinus infections. Many times brain abscess cases are caused by two or more bacteria. In 30–60% of cases, the bacteria combination includes streptococci, microorganisms that can live without oxygen (anaerobes), and enterobacteria. A small number of cases are caused by yeast, fungi, and single-cell organisms (protozoa).

The symptoms of brain abscess often develop slowly, usually within a period of about two weeks. The most common symptoms are:

- headache
- neurologic symptoms related to the specific part of the brain that is infected

- altered mental status
- seizures

Diagnosis

Diagnosis of brain abscess is performed by using a computed tomography scan (CT) or a **magnetic resonance imaging** (MRI) scan to determine the site of infection. Tissue removal (biopsy) is usually performed as well. A biopsy is performed to determine the type of bacterium involved. Biopsies can also be used to rule out tumor or other noninfectious localized lesions, which may look the same on the scans.

Other tests are performed to determine the source of the infection. These tests include blood cultures, x rays of the chest, and a physical exam of the ears, sinuses, and teeth. A test for human **immunodeficiency** virus (HIV) is usually also performed.

Treatment

Treatment for brain abscess begins with intravenous **antibiotics**, chosen to match the infecting bacterium if known, or to cover a wide spectrum of possibilities if not. Treatment usually continues for six to eight weeks.

Aspiration surgery is almost always done to drain the abscess. In this procedure, a needle is guided to the infected site by CT scan, and fluid is removed (aspirated) from the abscess. Aspiration may be repeated several times until the bacteria are completely killed or removed. Surgical removal of infected or dead tissue may be needed in some cases. For patients with many sites of infection, aspiration or surgical removal is not done because of the increased difficulty and risk of the procedure. For these patients, antibiotic therapy alone is used. Steroid treatment is controversial, but may be indicated in some cases.

Prognosis

Even with prompt treatment, brain abscess is fatal in about 20% of cases. About half of those who survive have some residual neurological problems, including seizures in many patients.

There are several reasons why patients with brain abscess can have a poor prognosis. The illness may not be diagnosed correctly or an accurate diagnosis may take additional time. The patient may receive an antibiotic that does not match the infecting organism. Sometimes the infection may not be limited to a definite area in the brain, making diagnosis and treatment difficult. The small number of cases caused by fungal infection may take additional time to diagnose. A patient may also have a poor prognosis because there is more than one abscess, the location of the abscess may be deep within the brain, or the infection may have moved into many locations within the brain. Severe complications can result from brain abscess, including comma and brain rupture. In 80-100% of cases involving brain rupture, the patient dies.

Prevention

Brain abscess may be preventable by prompt and aggressive treatment of the infections which give rise to it, especially sinus and ear infections.

Resources

BOOKS

Fauci, Anthony S., et al., editors. *Harrison's Principles of Internal Medicine.* New York: McGraw-Hill, 1997.

Richard Robinson

Brain aneurysm *see* **Cerebral aneurysm**

Brain biopsy

Definition

A brain biopsy is the removal of a small piece of brain tissue for the diagnosis of abnormalities of the brain, such as **Alzheimer's disease**, tumors, infection, or inflammation.

Purpose

By examining the tissue sample under a microscope, the biopsy sample provides doctors with the information necessary to guide diagnosis and treatment.

KEY TERMS

Alzheimer's disease—A progressive, neurodegenerative disease characterized by loss of function and death of nerve cells in several areas of the brain, leading to loss of mental functions such as memory and learning.

Computed axial tomography (CT)—Computed axial tomography (CT) is a x-ray technique that has the ability to image soft tissue, bone, and blood vessels.

Cortex—The thin convoluted surface of the brain comprised primarily of cell bodies of neurons.

MRI—Magnetic resonance imaging is an imaging technique that uses radiowaves, magnetic fields, and computer analysis to visualize body tissue and structures.

Stereotactic brain needle biopsy—In this procedure a computer uses information from a CT or MRI to create a three-dimensional map of the operation site to better guide the needle to perform the biopsy.

Precautions

Imaging of the brain is performed to determine the precise positioning of the needle to enter the brain.

Description

When an abnormality of the brain is suspected, Stereotactic (probing in three dimensions) brain needle biopsy is performed and guided precisely by a computer system to avoid serious complications. A small hole is drilled into the skull, and a needle is inserted into the brain tissue guided by computer-assisted imaging techniques (CT or MRI scans). Historically, the patient's head was held in a rigid frame to direct the probe into the brain; however since the early nineties, it has been possible to perform these biopsies without the frame. Since the frame was attached to the skull with screws, this advancement is less invasive and better tolerated by the patient. The doctor (pathologist) prepares the sample for analysis and studies it further under a microscope.

Preparation

A CT or MRI brain scan is done to find the position where the biopsy will be performed. Prior to the biopsy, the patient is placed under **general anesthesia**.

Aftercare

The patient is monitored in the recovery room for several hours and is usually required to spend a few days in the hospital since general anesthesia is required.

Risks

The procedure is invasive and includes risks associated with anesthesia and surgery. Brain injury may occur due to removal of brain tissue. The resulting scar, left on the brain has the potential to trigger seizures.

Normal results

After examining the brain tissue directly, no abnormalities are detected.

Abnormal results

Various brain abnormalities can be diagnosed by microscopic analysis of the tissue sample. The pathologist (a physician trained in how disease affects the body's tissues) looks for abnormal growth, changes in cell membranes, and/or abnormal collections of cells. In Alzheimer's disease, the cortex of the brain contains abnormal collections of plaques. If infection is suspected, the infectious organism can be cultured from the tissue and identified. Classification of tumors is also possible after biopsy.

Resources

ORGANIZATIONS

Alzheimer's Association. 919 North Michigan Ave., Suite 1100 Chicago, IL 60611-1676.(800) 272-3900 < http://www.alz.org > .

American Brain Tumor Association. 2720 River Road, Suite 146, Des Plaines, IL 60018-4110. (800) 886-2282. < http://www.abta.org > .

National Institute of Neurological Disorders and Stroke, NIH Neurological Institute. P.O. Box 5801 Bethesda, MD 20824. (800) 352-9424. < http://www.ninds.nih.gov/index.htm > .

Bonny McClain, MS

Brain circulation scan *see* **Transcranial Doppler ultrasonography**

Brain infection *see* **Encephalitis**

Brain injury *see* **Head injury**

Brain surgery *see* **Craniotomy**

Brain tumor

Definition

A brain tumor is an abnormal growth of tissue in the brain. Unlike other tumors, brain tumors spread by local extension and rarely metastasize (spread) outside the brain. A benign brain tumor is composed of non-cancerous cells and does not metastasize beyond the part of the brain where it originates. A brain tumor is considered malignant if it contains **cancer** cells, or if it is composed of harmless cells located in an area where it suppresses one or more vital functions.

Description

Each year, more than 17,000 brain tumors are diagnosed in the United States. About half of all primary brain tumors are benign, but in life-threatening locations. The rest are malignant and invasive.

Benign brain tumors

Benign brain tumors, composed of harmless cells, have clearly defined borders, can usually be completely removed, and are unlikely to recur. Benign brain tumors do not infiltrate nearby tissues but can cause severe **pain**, permanent brain damage, and **death**. Benign brain tumors sometimes become malignant.

Malignant brain tumors

Malignant brain tumors do not have distinct borders. They tend to grow rapidly, increasing pressure within the brain (IICP) and can spread in the brain or spinal cord beyond the point where they originate. It is highly unusual for malignant brain tumors to spread beyond the central nervous system (CNS).

Primary brain tumors

Primary brain tumors originate in the brain. They represent about 1% of all cancers and 2.5% of all cancer deaths.

Metastatic or secondary brain tumors

Approximately 25% of all cancer patients develop secondary or metastatic brain tumors when cancer cells spread from another part of the body to the brain. Secondary brain tumors are most apt to occur in patients who have:

- breast cancer.
- colon cancer.

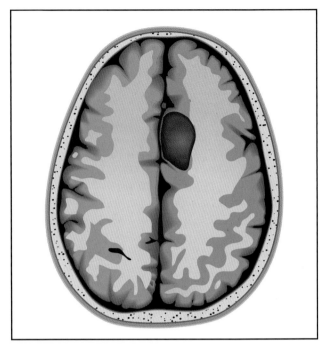

A scan of a brain with a tumor located in the central right portion of the brain. *(Illustration by Argosy Inc.)*

- kidney cancer.
- lung cancer.
- melanoma (cancer) of the skin. These metastatic brain tumors can develop on any part of the brain or spinal cord.
- cancer within the nasal passages and/or throat that follow the nerve pathways into the skull, and metastasize to the brain.

Who gets brain tumors

Brain tumors can develop at any age, but are most common in children between the ages of 3-12, and in adults aged 55-65. Primary brain cancer is the second most common cause of cancer death between birth and the age of 34, and the fourth most common cause of cancer death in men aged 35-54. Primary tumors of the brain and central nervous system are often associated with HIV infection. Men and caucasians have a higher risk of developing brain tumors. Other risk factors being studied include children with a history of previous radiation treatment to the head for cancer; parents with certain cancers (nervous system, salivary gland, colon); having an older father; having well-educated parents; occupational exposure to vinyl chloride, lead, and pesticides; history of epilepsy; history of certain genetic conditions (tuberous sclerosis, **neurofibromatosis**, von Hippel Lindau, **familial polyposis**, Osler-Weber-Rendu, Li-Fraumeni).

Naming and grading brain tumors

The name of a brain tumor describes where it originates, how it grows, and what kind of cells it contains. A tumor in an adult is also graded or staged according to:

- how malignant it is
- how rapidly it is growing and how likely it is to invade other tissues
- how closely its cells resemble normal cells. (The more abnormal a tumor cell looks, the faster it is likely to grow)

Low-grade brain tumors usually have well-defined borders. Some low-grade brain tumors form or are enclosed (encapsulated) in cysts. Low-grade brain tumors grow slowly, if at all. They may spread throughout the brain, but rarely metastasize to other parts of the body.

Mid-grade and high-grade tumors grow more rapidly than low-grade tumors. Described as "truly malignant," these tumors usually infiltrate healthy tissue. The growth pattern makes it difficult to remove the entire tumor, and these tumors recur more often than low-grade tumors.

A single brain tumor can contain several different types of cells. The tumor's grade is determined by the highest-grade (most malignant) cell detected under a microscope, even if most of the cells in the tumor are less malignant. An infiltrating tumor is a tumor of any grade that grows into surrounding tissue.

Types of brain tumors

Glioma is the term used to refer to the most prevalent primary brain tumors. Gliomas arise from glial tissue, which supports and nourishes cells that send messages from the brain to other parts of the body. These tumors may be either malignant or benign. Astrocytomas, ependymomas, and mixed gliomas are three of the most common gliomas.

ASTROCYTOMAS. Named for the star-like shape of their cells, astrocytomas can develop on any part of the brain or spinal cord. Non-infiltrating astrocytomas grow slowly, and rarely spread to nearby tissue. Mild-to-moderately anaplastic astrocytomas with well-differentiated borders do not grow as slowly as non-infiltrating astrocytomas, and they do spread to surrounding tissues.

Anaplastic astrocytomas, which are also called Grade III astrocytomas, look more abnormal and grow more rapidly than non-infiltrating or mild-to-moderately anaplastic tumors.

Grade IV astrocytomas are also called glioblastoma multiforme (GBM) tumors. Accounting for 30% of all primary brain tumors, GBMs are the most common brain tumors in middle-aged adults. GBMs are the most malignant of all brain tumors. Because they contain a greater mixture of cells than any other brain tumor, they are the most difficult to treat.

EPENDYMOMAS. Also called ependymal tumors, ependymomas account for 9% of all gliomas, and 5% of all intracranial tumors. These tumors, which are most common in children and adolescents, begin in the very thin membranes that help form cerebrospinal fluid (CSF) and line the brain cavities (ventricles) that contain it.

Ependymomas are usually benign, have well-differentiated borders, resemble normal cells, and grow very slowly. The cells of anaplastic (malignant) ependymomas look abnormal and grow more rapidly than the cells of benign tumors.

MIXED GLIOMAS. These heterogeneous tumors contain elements of astrocytomas and ependymomas and/or oligodendrogliomas. These are rare tumors that usually occur in middle-aged adults, grow slowly, and do not usually spread beyond the part of the brain where they originate. Mixed gliomas behave like tumors composed of the highest-grade cells they contain.

Non-glial brain tumors

The most common brain tumors that do not develop from glial cells are medulloblastomas, meningiomas, and Schwannomas.

MEDULLOBLASTOMAS. Scientists once thought medulloblastomas (MDLs) developed from glial cells. These fast-growing, malignant tumors are now believed to originate in developing cells not normally present in the body after birth. They are sometimes called primitive neurodectal tumors (PNET).

MDL tumors are most common in children and are more common in boys than in girls. Only 30% of MDL tumors occur in adults. MDL tumors usually originate in the cerebellum (the part of the brain that controls coordination and some muscle activity), and are often carried to other parts of the brain by cerebrospinal fluid. MDL tumors rarely metastasize beyond the brain and spinal cord.

MENINGIOMAS. Meningiomas, which represent more than 20% of all primary brain tumors, originate in the membranes that enclose the brain and spinal cord (meninges). These tumors are usually benign and most often occur in women aged 30-50 years old. Meningiomas grow so slowly that the brain can sometimes become accustomed to their presence. Meningiomas compress, rather than invade, brain tissue and may grow to be quite large before any symptoms appear.

SCHWANNOMAS. Schwannomas originate in the Schwann cells. These cells produce myelin, material that protects the acoustic nerve, which controls hearing. These benign tumors are twice as common in women as in men, and are most often diagnosed in patients between the ages 30-60.

Schwannomas grow very slowly, and many people adapt to the slight **hearing loss** and balance problems that are the tumors' earliest symptoms. A pear-shaped Schwannoma can cause sudden or gradual loss of hearing in an ear. As the tumor progresses, it can press on the nerves that control movement and feeling in the face, and cause headaches and facial **numbness** or **tingling**. The patient may have trouble walking, swallowing, or controlling eye movements, and the sense of taste can be affected. A Schwannoma that grows large enough to press on the brainstem can be deadly.

CHILDHOOD BRAIN TUMORS. Brain tumors that occur in children are described as supratentorial (in the upper part of the brain) or infratentorial (in the lowest part of the brain). Astrocytomas and ependymomas are common supratentorial tumors. Infratentorial tumors include medulloblastomas, astrocytomas, and ependymomas.

Causes and symptoms

The cause of primary brain tumors is unknown, but people who work with rubber and certain chemicals have a greater-than-average risk of developing them. There is no evidence that **head injury** causes brain tumors, but researchers are trying to determine the relationship, if any, between brain tumors and viruses, family history, and long-term exposure to electromagnetic fields.

Symptoms do not usually appear until the tumor grows large enough to displace, damage, or destroy delicate brain tissue. When that happens, the patient may experience:

- headaches that become increasingly painful and are most painful when lying down
- nausea and **vomiting** or sudden attacks of vomiting not accompanied by nausea
- seizures
- dizziness, loss of coordination or balance
- personality changes
- sudden loss of vision
- memory loss
- speech problems
- sensory changes
- mental impairment
- weakness or **paralysis** on one side of the body

A doctor should be notified whenever a patient experiences one or more of the symptoms.

Diagnosis

Although brain tumor symptoms resemble those of many other illnesses, the presence of a brain tumor may be indicated by:

- persistent headaches with vomiting or convulsions
- progressive deterioration of sight, speech, hearing, touch; or deterioration in the ability to use an arm, hand, foot, or leg

When a patient experiences one or more of the above symptoms, a primary care physician will perform a complete **physical examination**, take a detailed medical history, and conduct a basic neurologic examination to evaluate:

- balance and coordination
- abstract thinking and memory
- eye movements
- hearing, touch, and sense of smell
- reflexes

- control of facial muscles and movements of the head and tongue

- awareness

If the results of these examinations suggest a patient may have a brain tumor, a neurologist recommends some or all of these additional diagnostic tests:

- computed tomography scan (CT scan) to reveal brain abnormalities

- magnetic resonance imaging (MRI) to detect tumors beneath the bones of the skull

- complex imaging techniques such as **Positron emission tomography** (**PET** scan), Single photon emission tomography (SPECT scan)

- electroencephalography (EEG) to measure electrical activity in the brain

- magnetoencephalography (MEG scan) to measure the magnetic fields produced by nerve cells and their electric currents

- x rays to reveal any distortion in the bones of the skull

- angiography to outline a tumor and the blood vessels that lead to it

- a brain scan to identify and record the location of abnormal cells in the brain

- radionuclide brain scintigraphy to view the capillaries feeding the tumor after highlighting them with a radioactive substance

- myelography (x ray of the spine) to detect a spinal cord tumor

- a lumbar puncture (spinal tap) to obtain spinal fluid, which may contain tumor cells.

- digital holography to view a complete three-dimensional map of the tumor and surrounding brain structures

Interpreting these images and results of laboratory analysis allows neurologists to determine whether a tumor is present, but microscopic examination of tumor tissue (biopsy) is the only way to identify the kind of cells it contains.

Treatment

Brain tumors are treated by multidisciplinary teams of highly skilled specialists whose decisions are based on:

- results of diagnostic tests

- tumor size, position, and growth pattern

- the patient's health history and current medical status

- the wishes of the patient and his family

Surgery

Surgery is the treatment of choice for accessible brain tumors, which can be removed without causing serious neurologic damage. The procedure most often performed is a **craniotomy**, but the goals of any type of brain tumor surgery include:

- removing as much of the tumor as possible (called debulking the tumor)

- removing tumor tissue for microscopic analysis

- allowing neurosurgeons to see exactly how the tumor is situated and how it is growing

- creating an entry channel for **chemotherapy** drugs and forms of radiation that are implanted in the brain

Depending on the type of brain tumor, its location, and its size, a number of different techniques may be used to surgically remove it. Surgical techniques include:

- classic operation

- laser microsurgery (uses high temperatures to vaporize tumor cells

- ultrasonic aspiration (uses ultrasound waves to break up the tumor into smaller bits which can be "vacuumed" out

Before undergoing brain surgery, patients are often given:

- steroids to reduce swelling of brain tissue

- anticonvulsant medications to prevent or control seizures

- radiation treatments to reduce tumor size

Patients whose benign brain tumors can be completely removed may not require any additional treatment, but periodic physical and neurologic examinations and CT or MRI scans are sometimes recommended to determine whether the tumor has returned. Because surgeons cannot be sure that every bit of an infiltrating or metastasizing tumor has been removed, radiation and chemotherapy are used to eradicate cells that may have escaped the scalpel.

If a tumor cannot be completely removed, removing a portion of it (debulking) can alleviate the patient's symptoms, enhance the sense of well-being, and increase the effectiveness of other treatments.

Radiation therapy

External radiotherapy, generally delivered on an outpatient basis, directs radiation to the tumor and the area around it. Implant **radiation therapy** involves placing tiny pieces of radioactive material in the brain. Left in place permanently, or for a short time, these radioactive pellets release measured doses of radiation each day. This technique is called brachytherapy. Patients are usually hospitalized during the several days the pellets are most active.

Stereoactic radiosurgery involves fitting the patient with a frame to stabilize the head, using imaging techniques to determine the exact location of tumor cells, and using a sophisticated instrument to administer radiation precisely to that point. Instruments used for delivery of radiation include the gamma knife, adapted linear accelerator (LINAC), and cyclotron.

A variety of drugs may also be given during radiation therapy, to protect brain cells from the effects of radiation (radioprotective drugs), to increase the sensitivity of tumor cells to radiation (radiosensitizers), or to boost radiation's effects (radioenhancers).

Chemotherapy

One or more cancer-killing drugs may be taken by mouth or injected into a blood vessel, muscle, or the cerebrospinal fluid. Chemotherapy may be used with radiation and surgery as part of a patient's initial treatment, or used alone to treat tumors that recur in the same place or in another part of the body. The usual chemotherapy regimen for a brain tumor is a combination approach, most commonly using procarbazine, CCNU, and vincristine.

New methods of delivering chemotherapy are being used as well. These include:

- interstitial chemotherapy is performed at the time of surgery. A chemotherapy-soaked wafer is placed in the cavity left after tumor removal.
- Intrathecal chemotherapy instills the medications right into the spinal fluid.
- Intraarterial chemotherapy uses tiny catheter tubes to delivery high-dose chemotherapy directly into the arteries of the brain.
- Potentially toxic chemotherapy drugs can be wrapped in special biologic envelopes called liposomes, to allow the drugs to be delivered to the tumor without adversely affecting other healthy tissues along the way.
- Electrochemotherapy uses electric voltage to transport chemotherapy agents into the brain.

When a young child has a brain tumor, chemotherapy is often used to eliminate or delay the need for radiation.

Other treatments

If a brain tumor cannot be cured, treatment is designed to make the patient as comfortable as possible and preserve as much of his neurologic functioning as possible. The patient's doctor may prescribe:

- analgesics to relieve pain
- anticancer drugs to limit tumor growth
- anticonvulsants to control seizures
- steroids to reduce swelling of brain tissue

Potential therapies

Scientists are studying ways to empower chemotherapy drugs to penetrate the blood-brain barrier (which protects the CNS by separating the brain from blood circulating throughout the body), and attack cancer cells that have infiltrated tissue inside it. Agents under investigation include both mannitol and substances called receptor-mediated permeabilizers

Brain tumor researchers are also investigating:

- Less invasive surgical procedures.
- Monoclonal antibodies, which pair antibodies with radioactive substances. The antibodies are directed to find and attach to tumor cells, at which time the radioactive substance kills the tumor cell.
- Interleukin and interferon, which are substances produced naturally by the human immune system which seem to kill tumor cells. Scientists seek to produce these substances in the laboratory and incorporate their use in brain tumor treatment.
- T-lymphocytes, which are also produced normally by the human immune system, and are being used to inject directly into the tumor location during surgery and to infuse into the bloodstream after surgery, in the hopes that they will boost the immune system's ability to fight tumor cells.
- Tumor vaccines, which use elements of tumor cells to stimulate the patient's immune system.
- Methods of incorporating chemotherapy drugs into tumor cells to reduce the need for radiation.
- Laboratory techniques that enable physicians to select the chemotherapy drugs most likely to kill particular types of tumors.

- Gene therapy in which genetically engineered material is transported to tumor cells by viruses that infect tumor cells and convert them to normal cells, stop their growth, or kill them.

Alternative treatment

Alternative treatments have not been shown to cure brain tumors and should never be substituted for conventional therapy. However, complementary therapies (used with, not instead of, standard treatments) can help some patients cope with the **stress** of their illness and side effects of their treatment.

Massage, **meditation**, and **reflexology** help some patients relax; while **yoga** is said to soothe the body, spirit, and mind. **Hydrotherapy** uses ice, liquid, and steam to improve circulation and relieve pain. **Therapeutic touch** practitioners say they can relieve pain and other symptoms by moving their hands in slow, rhythmic motions several inches above the patient's body.

Botanical therapies, homeopathic treatment, **traditional Chinese medicine** treatments, nutritional focuses on diet and supplements, and **detoxification** can also be incorporated as complementary therapies.

Prognosis

The patient's prognosis depends on where the tumor is located, what type of cells it contains, the size of the tumor, and the effect its already had on adjacent brain structures. A patient whose tumor is discovered early and removed completely may make a full recovery, but the surgery itself can harm or destroy normal brain tissue and cause:

- problems with thought, speech, and coordination
- seizures
- weakness
- personality changes.

Although these post-operative problems may initially be more severe than the symptoms produced by the tumor, they will probably diminish or disappear in time.

Occupational therapy can teach patients and their families new ways to approach daily tasks. Physical therapy can benefit patients who have difficulty keeping their balance, expressing their thoughts, speaking, or swallowing. Children may need special tutors before and after returning to school. For patients who have incurable brain tumors, hospice care may be available.

Hospices provide a supportive environment and help patients manage pain and remain comfortable.

Consequences of radiation therapy

Cells killed by radiation can cluster in the brain, resembling tumors. They can cause headaches, seizures, and memory loss. Children treated with radiation may lose some of their eyesight and develop learning problems. Radiation damage to the pituitary gland can hinder normal growth and development.

Consequences of chemotherapy

Some drugs used to treat brain tumors can cause kidney damage and temporary or permanent tingling in the fingers and ringing in the ears.

Inoperable tumors

Brain tumors that cannot be removed may cause irreversible brain damage and death.

Prevention

The cause of primary brain tumors has not been determined, so there is no known way to prevent them.

The best way to prevent secondary or metastatic brain tumors is to eliminate such risk factors as:

- poor **nutrition** and a low-fiber diet; since these contribute to development of intestinal cancers
- smoking, which causes lung cancer
- excessive use of alcohol, which is associated with liver cancer
- excessive exposure to the sun, which can cause melanoma (a deadly form of skin cancer).

Monthly self-examinations of the breasts and testicles can detect breast and **testicular cancer** at their earliest, most curable stages.

Resources

ORGANIZATIONS

American Brain Tumor Association. 2770 River Road, Des Plaines, IL 60018. (847) 827-9918, (800) 886-2289. <http:/www.abta.org>.

Brain Tumor Foundation for Children, Inc. 2231 Perimeter Park Drive, Suite 9, Atlanta, GA 30341. (404) 454-5554.

Brain Tumor Information Services. Box 405, Room J341, University of Chicago Hospitals, 5841 S. Maryland Avenue, Chicago, IL 60637. (312) 684-1400.

MedHelp International. 6300 N. Wickham, Suite 130, Box 188, Melbourne, FL 32940. (407) 253-9048. < http://www.medhlp.netusa.net >.

National Brain Tumor Foundation. 785 Market Street, #1600, San Francisco, CA 94103. < http://www.oncolink.penn.edu/psychosocial >.

OTHER

Adult Brain Tumor. May 2001. < http://cancernet.nci.nih.gov/clinpdq/pif/Adult_brain_tumor_Patient.html >.

Brain Tumor, Primary. Nidus Information Services, Well Connected, 2001.

"Brain Tumors," Abeloff: Clinical Oncology, 2nd ed. Churchill Livingstone, Inc., 2000.

"Brain Tumors," Goldman: Cecil Textbook of Medicine. 21st ed. W. B. Saunders Company, 2000.

Childhood Brain Tumor. May 2001. < http://cancernet.nci.nih.gov/clinpdq/pif/Childhood_brain_tumor_Patient.html >.

Question: What is a Gamma Knife? April 13, 2001. < http://oncolink.upenn.edu/specialty/med_phys/gamma.html >.

Rosalyn Carson-DeWitt, MD

Breast-feeding *see* **Lactation**

Breast biopsy

Definition

A breast biopsy is removal of breast tissue for examination by a pathologist. This can be accomplished surgically, or by withdrawing tissue through a needle.

Purpose

A biopsy is recommended when a significant abnormality is found, either on **physical examination** and/or by an imaging test. Examples of abnormality can include a breast lump felt during physical self examination or tissue changes noticed from a mammogram test. Before a biopsy is performed, it is important to make sure that the threat of **cancer** cannot be disproved or ruled out by a simpler, less invasive examination. A lump may be obviously harmless when examined by ultrasound. If this is not decisive, the presence of cancer or a variety of benign breast conditions can be determined using a biopsy.

Precautions

The type of biopsy recommended should be considered. This will depend on whether the area can be

felt, how well it can be seen on mammogram or ultrasound, and how suspicious it feels or appears. Specialized equipment is needed for different types of biopsy and availability may vary. Generally, needle biopsy is less invasive than surgical biopsy. It is appropriate for most, but not all situations. However, some surgeons feel it is far less accurate.

Description

Surgical biopsy

If an abnormality is not felt during a self examination, there are signs that indicate the need for medical attention. These include:

- severe breast **pain**
- changes in the size of a breast or the nipple
- changes in the shape of both breast or nipple
- pitting, dumpling or redness of the breast skin
- nipple redness, irritation, or inversion
- changes in the pattern of veins visible on the surface of the breast
- some types of nipple discharge

If the abnormality is not felt, a needle localization must be done before the actual surgery. After local anesthetic is administered, a fine wire is placed in the area of concern. Either x ray or ultrasound guidance is used. The patient is awake and usually sitting up.

There are two types of breast biopsy considered here, excisional and incisional. An excisional biopsy is a surgical procedure, where the entire area of concern and some surrounding tissue is removed. It is usually done as an outpatient procedure, in a hospital or free standing surgery center. The patient may be awake, and is sometimes given medication to make her drowsy. The area to be operated on is numbed with local anesthetic. Infrequently, **general anesthesia** is used.

An excisional biopsy itself usually takes under one hour. The total amount of time spent at the facility

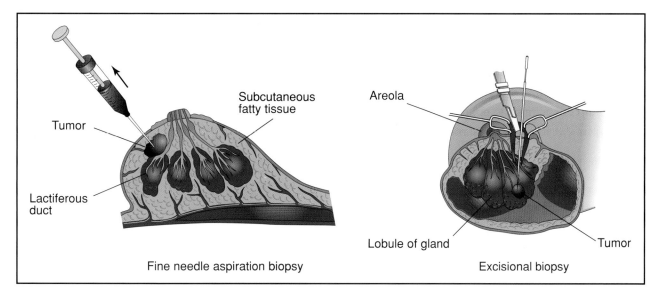

Tumor

Subcutaneous
fatty tissue

Areola

Lactiferous
duct

Lobule of gland

Tumor

Fine needle aspiration biopsy

Excisional biopsy

A fine needle aspiration biopsy uses a very thin needle to withdraw fluid and cells from the breast to be examined. An excisional biopsy is a surgical procedure in which the entire area of concern and some surrounding tissue is removed for analysis. *(Illustration by Electronic Illustrators Group.)*

depends on the type of anesthesia used, whether a needle localization was done, and the extent of the surgery.

If a mass is very large, an incisional biopsy may be performed. In this case only a portion of the area is removed and sent for analysis. The procedure is the same as an excisional biopsy in other respects.

Needle biopsy

A needle biopsy removes part of the suspicious area for examination. There are two types, aspiration biopsy (using a fine needle), and large core needle biopsy. Either of these may be called a percutaneous needle biopsy. Percutaneous refers to a procedure done through the skin.

A fine needle aspiration biopsy uses a very thin needle to withdraw fluid and cells that can be studied. It can be done in a doctor's office, clinic, or hospital. Local anesthetic may be used, but is sometimes withheld, as it may be more painful than the biopsy needle. The area to place the needle may be located by touch. No specialized equipment is needed. However, using ultrasound guidance enables the physician to feel and see the lesion at the same time. The actual withdrawing of fluid and cells can be visualized as it occurs. This helps ensure that the specimen is taken from the right place.

A large core needle biopsy uses a larger diameter needle to remove small pieces of tissue, about the size of a grain of rice. It can be done in a clinic or hospital that has the appropriate facilities. Local anesthetic is

routinely used. Ultrasound or x ray is used for guidance of a large core needle biopsy.

If the suspicious area is seen best with x ray, a stereotactic device is used. This means that x rays are taken from several angles. This information is fed into a computer, which analyzes the data and guides the needle to the correct place. The patient may be sitting up, or she may be lying on her stomach, with her breast positioned through an opening in the table. The breast is held firmly, but comfortably between a plastic paddle and a metal plate, similar to those used for mammograms (a set of x rays taken of the front and side of the breast). X rays may be taken before, during, and after the tissue is drawn into the needle, to confirm that the correct spot is biopsied. This procedure may also be referred to as a stereotactic core biopsy, or a mammotomy.

Ultrasound is used to guide needle placement for some lesions. The patient lies on her back or side. After the area is numbed, sterile gel is applied. The physician places a transducer, an instrument about the size of an electric shaver, over the skin. This produces an image from the reflection of sound waves. A special needle, usually in a spring loaded device, is used to obtain the tissue. The procedure is observed on a monitor as it is happening.

Preparation

A surgical breast biopsy may require the patient to have nothing to eat or drink for a period of time before the operation. This will typically be from midnight the night before, if general anesthesia is planned. No food restrictions are necessary for needle biopsy. It is advisable to eat lightly before the procedure. This is especially important if the patient will be lying on her stomach for a stereotactic biopsy.

Aftercare

After a surgical biopsy, the incision will be closed with stitches, and covered with a bandage. The bandage can usually be removed in one or two days. Stitches are taken out approximately one week afterward. Depending on the extent of the operation, normal activities can be resumed in approximately one to three days. Vigorous **exercise** may be limited for one to three weeks.

The skin opening for a needle biopsy is minimal. It may be closed with thin, clear tape, called a steri strip, or covered with a bandaid and a small gauze bandage. The patient can return to her usual routine immediately after the biopsy. Strenuous activity or heavy lifting is not recommended for 24 hours. Any bandages can be removed one or two days after the biopsy.

Risks

Infection is always a possibility when the skin is broken, although this rarely occurs. Redness, swelling, or severe pain at the biopsy site would indicate a possible infection. Another possible consequence of a breast biopsy is a hematoma. This is a collection of blood at the biopsy site. It is usually absorbed naturally by the body. If it is very large and uncomfortable, it may need to be drained. A surgical breast biopsy may produce a visible scar on the breast. Sometimes this may make future mammograms harder to interpret accurately.

A false negative pathology report is another risk. This means that no cancer was found when a cancer was present. The incidence of this varies with the biopsy technique. In general, fine needle aspiration biopsies have the highest rate of false negative results, but there may be variation in results between facilities.

Normal results

A normal pathology report indicates no malignancy is present. The tissue sample may be further classified as a benign breast condition, such as tumor of the breast (**fibroadenoma**) or connective tissue that resembles fiber (fibrosis). Studies have demonstrated that approximately 80% of all breast biopsies result in a benign pathology report.

Abnormal results

An abnormal pathology report indicates a cancer is present. If a fine needle aspiration biopsy was performed, the pathologist has viewed individual cells under a microscope to see if they appear cancerous. Large core needle biopsy and surgical biopsy will be able to give more information. This includes the type of cancer, whether it has invaded surrounding tissue, and how likely it is to spread quickly. There are some conditions which are not malignant but indicate high risk for future development of **breast cancer**. If these are identified, more frequent monitoring of the area may be recommended.

Resources

ORGANIZATIONS

American Cancer Society. 1599 Clifton Rd., NE, Atlanta, GA 30329-4251. (800) 227-2345. < http:// www.cancer.org > .

National Cancer Institute. Building 31, Room 10A31, 31 Center Drive, MSC 2580, Bethesda, MD 20892-2580. (800) 422-6237. < http://www.nci.nih.gov > .

Ellen S. Weber, MSN

Breast cancer

Definition

Breast **cancer** is caused by the development of malignant cells in the breast. The malignant cells originate in the lining of the milk glands or ducts of the breast (ductal epithelium), defining this malignancy as a cancer. Cancer cells are characterized by uncontrolled division leading to abnormal growth and the ability of these cells to invade normal tissue locally or to spread throughout the body, in a process called metastasis.

Description

Breast cancer arises in the milk-producing glands of the breast tissue. Groups of glands in normal breast tissue are called lobules. The products of these glands are secreted into a ductal system that leads to the nipple. Depending on where in the glandular or ductal unit of the breast the cancer arises, it will develop certain characteristics that are used to sub-classify breast cancer into types. The pathologist will denote the subtype at the time of evaluation with the microscope. Ductal carcinoma

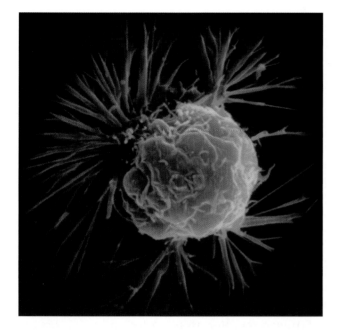

A **breast cancer cell.** *(Phototake NYC. Reproduced by permission.)*

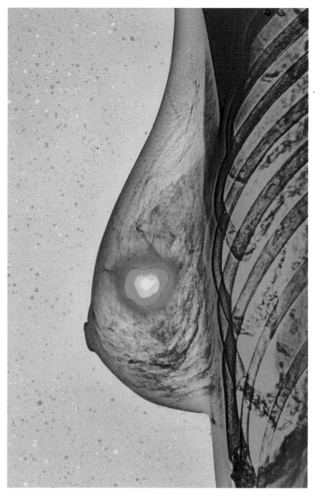

Mammogram indicating a tumor in the center of the breast. *(Chris Bjornberg, Photo Researchers. Reproduced by permission.)*

begins in the ducts, lobular carcinoma has a pattern involving the lobules or glands. The more important classification is related to the evaluated tumor's capability to invade, as this characteristic defines the disease as a true cancer. The stage before invasive cancer is called *in situ*, meaning that the early malignancy has not yet become capable of invasion. Thus, ductal carcinoma in situ is considered a minimal breast cancer.

How breast cancer spreads

The primary tumor begins in the breast itself but once it becomes invasive, it may progress beyond the breast to the regional lymph nodes or travel (metastasize) to other organ systems in the body and become systemic in nature. Lymph is the clear, protein-rich fluid that bathes the cells throughout the body. Lymph will work its way back to the bloodstream via small channels known as lymphatics. Along the way, the lymph is filtered through cellular stations known as nodes, thus they are called lymph nodes. Nearly all organs in the body have a primary lymph node group filtering fluid that comes from that organ. In the breast, the primary lymph nodes are under the armpit, or axilla. Classically, the primary tumor begins in the breast and the first place to which it is likely to spread is the regional lymph nodes. Cancer, as it invades in its place of origin, may also work its way into blood vessels. If cancer gets into the blood vessels, the blood

vessels provide yet another route for the cancer to spread to other organs of the body.

Breast cancer follows this classic progression though it often becomes systemic or widespread early in the course of the disease. By the time one can feel a lump in the breast it is often 0.4 inches, or one centimeter, in size and contains roughly a million cells. It is estimated that a tumor of this size may take one to five years to develop. During that time, the cancer may metastasize, or spread by lymphatics or blood to areas elsewhere in the body.

When primary breast cancer spreads, it may first go to the axillary nodes. If this occurs, regional metastasis exists. If it proceeds elsewhere either by lymphatic or blood-borne spread, the patient develops systemic metastasis that may involve a number of other organs in the body. Favorite sites of systemic involvement for breast cancer are the lung, bones, liver, and the skin

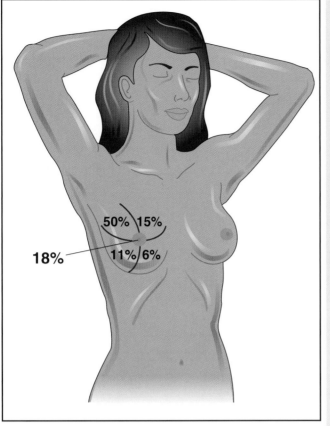

This illustration shows the frequency of breast cancer developing in the four quadrants of the breast and the nipple. *(Illustration by Electronic Illustrators Group.)*

and soft tissue. As it turns out, the presence of, and the actual number of, regional lymph nodes containing cancer remains the single best indicator of whether or not the cancer has become widely metastatic. Because tests to discover metastasis in other organs may not be sensitive enough to reveal minute deposits, the evaluation of the axilla for regional metastasis becomes very important in making treatment decisions for this disease.

If breast cancer spreads to other major organs of the body, its presence will compromise the function of those organs. **Death** is the result of extreme compromise of vital organ function.

Demographics

Every woman is at risk for breast cancer. If she lives to be 85, there is a one out of nine chance that she will develop the condition sometime during her life. As a woman ages, her risk of developing breast cancer rises dramatically regardless of her family history. The

KEY TERMS

Adjuvant therapy—Treatment involving radiation, chemotherapy (drug treatment), or hormone therapy, or a combination of all three given after the primary treatment for the possibility of residual microscopic disease.

Aneuploid—An abnormal number of chromosomes in a cell.

Aspiration biopsy—The removal of cells in fluid or tissue from a mass or cyst using a needle for microscopic examination and diagnosis.

Benign—Not malignant, noncancerous.

Biopsy—A procedure in which suspicious tissue is removed and examined by a pathologist for cancer or other disease. For breast biopsies, the tissue may be obtained by open surgery, or through a needle.

Estrogen-receptor assay—A test to see if a breast cancer needs estrogen to grow.

Hormones—Chemicals produced by glands in the body that circulate in the blood and control the actions of cells and organs. Estrogens are hormones that affect breast cancer growth.

Hormone therapy—Treating cancers by changing the hormone balance of the body, instead of by using cell-killing drugs.

Lumpectomy—A surgical procedure in which only the cancerous tumor in the breast is removed, together with a rim of normal tissue.

Lymph nodes—Small, bean-shaped masses of tissue scattered along the lymphatic system that act as filters and immune monitors, removing fluids, bacteria, or cancer cells that travel through the lymph system. Breast cancer cells in the lymph nodes under the arm or in the chest are a sign that the cancer has spread, and that it might recur.

Malignant—Cancerous.

Mammography—X-ray imaging of the breast that can often detect lesions in the tissue too small or too deep to be felt.

Oncogene—A gene that has to do with regulation of cancer growth. An abnormality can produce cancer.

breast cancer risk of a 25-year-old woman is only one out of 19,608; by age 45, it is one in 93. In fact, less than 5% of cases are discovered before age 35 and the majority of all breast cancers are found in women over age 50.

In 2002, 200,000 new cases of breast cancer were diagnosed. About 45,000 women die of breast cancer each year, accounting for 16% of deaths caused by cancer in women. However, deaths from breast cancer are declining in recent years, a reflection of earlier diagnosis from screening mammograms and improving therapies.

Causes and symptoms

There are a number of risk factors for the development of breast cancer, including:

- family history of breast cancer in mother or sister

- early onset of menstruation and late **menopause**

- reproductive history: women who had no children or have children after age 30 and women who have never breastfed have increased risk

- history of abnormal breast biopsies

Though these are recognized risk factors, it is important to note that more than 70% of women who get breast cancer have no known risk factors. Having several risk factors may boost a woman's chances of developing breast cancer, but the interplay of predisposing factors is complex. In addition to those accepted factors listed above, some studies suggest that high-fat **diets**, **obesity**, or the use of alcohol may contribute to the risk profile. Another factor that contributes to a woman's risk profile is **hormone replacement therapy** (HRT).

HRT provides significant relief of menopausal symptoms, prevention of **osteoporosis**, and possibly protection from cardiovascular disease and **stroke**. While physicians have long known a small increased risk for breast cancer was linked to use of HRT, a landmark study released in 2003 proved the risk was greater than thought. The Women's Health Initiative found that even relatively short-term use of estrogen plus progestin is associated with increased risk of breast cancer, diagnosis at a more advanced stage of the disease, and a higher number of abnormal mammograms. The longer a woman used HRT, the more her risk increased.

Of all the risk factors listed above, family history is the most important. In *The Biological Basis of Cancer*, the authors estimate that about half of all familial breast cancer cases (families in which there is a high breast cancer frequency) have mutations affecting the genes BRCA-1 or BRCA-2. In 2003, scientists discovered a third gene called EMSY. However, breast cancer due to heredity is only a small proportion of breast cancer cases; only 5%–10% of all breast cancer

cases will be women who inherited a susceptibility through their genes. Nevertheless, when the family history is strong for development of breast cancer, a woman's risk is increased.

Not all lumps detected in the breast are cancerous. Fibrocystic changes in the breast are extremely common. Also known as **fibrocystic condition of the breast**, fibrocystic changes are a leading cause of noncancerous lumps in the breast. Fibrocystic changes also cause symptoms of **pain**, swelling, or discharge and may become evident to the patient or physician as a lump that is either solid or filled with fluid. Complete diagnostic evaluation of any significant breast abnormality is mandatory because though women commonly develop fibrocystic changes, breast cancer is common also, and the signs and symptoms of fibrocystic changes overlap with those of breast cancer. Certain benign changes in the breast may now be linked to increased risk for breast cancer.

Diagnosis

The diagnosis of breast cancer is accomplished by the biopsy of any suspicious lump or mammographic abnormality that has been identified. (A biopsy is the removal of tissue for examination by a pathologist. A mammogram is a low-dose, 2-view, x-ray examination of the breast.) The patient may be prompted to visit her doctor upon finding a lump in a breast, or she may have noticed skin dimpling, nipple retraction, or discharge from the nipple. A patient may not have noticed a symptom or abnormality, and a lump was detected by a screening mammogram.

When a patient has no signs or symptoms

Screening involves the evaluation of women who have no symptoms or signs of a breast problem. **Mammography** has been helpful in detecting breast cancer that cannot be identified on **physical examination**. However, 10%–13% of breast cancer does not show up on mammography, and a similar number of patients with breast cancer have an abnormal mammogram and a normal physical examination. These figures emphasize the need for examination as part of the screening process.

Screening

It is recommended that women get into the habit of doing monthly breast self examinations to detect any lump at an early stage. If an uncertainty or a lump is found, evaluation by an experienced physician and a mammogram is recommended. The American Cancer Society (ACS) has made recommendations for the use of mammography on a screening basis. In 2003, the ACS updated its guidelines concerning screening mammograms. The most notable change was that women should begin annual screening at age 40 instead of age 50. (in the past, the ACS, recommended beginning mammograms at age 40, but only ever one or two years instead of annually.) Women at higher risk for breast cancer should benefit from beginning screenings at earlier ages and at more frequent intervals.

Because of the greater awareness of breast cancer in recent years, screening evaluations by examinations and mammography are performed much more frequently than in the past. The result is that the number of breast cancers diagnosed increased, but the disease is being diagnosed at an earlier stage than previously. The earlier the stage of disease at the time it is discovered, the better the long-term outcome (prognosis) becomes.

When a patient has physical signs or symptoms

A common finding that leads to diagnosis is the presence of a lump within the breast. Skin dimpling, nipple retraction, or discharge from the nipple are less frequent initial findings prompting biopsy. Though bloody nipple discharge is distressing, it is most often caused by benign disease. Skin dimpling or nipple retraction in the presence of an underlying breast mass on examination is a more advanced finding. Actual skin involvement, with **edema** or ulceration of the skin, are late findings.

The presence of a breast lump is a common sign of breast cancer. If the lump is suspicious and the patient has not had a mammogram by this point, a study should be done on both breasts prior to anything else so that the original characteristics of the lesion can be studied. The opposite breast should also be evaluated mammographically to determine if other problems exist that were undetected by physical examination.

Whether an abnormal screening mammogram or one of the signs mentioned above followed by a mammogram prompted suspicion, the diagnosis is established by obtaining tissue by biopsy of the area. There are different types of biopsy, each utilized with its own indication. If signs of widespread metastasis are already present, biopsy of the metastasis itself may establish diagnosis.

Biopsy

Depending on the situation, different types of biopsy may be performed. The types include incisional and excisional biopsies. In an incisional biopsy, the physician takes a sample of tissue, and in excisional biopsy, the mass is removed. Fine needle aspiration biopsy and core needle biopsy are kinds of incisional biopsies.

FINE NEEDLE ASPIRATION BIOPSY. In a fine needle aspiration biopsy, a fine-gauge needle may be passed into the lesion and cells from the area suctioned into the needle can be quickly prepared for microscopic evaluation (cytology). (The patient experiencing nipple discharge also can have a sample taken of the discharge for cytological evaluation.) Fine needle aspiration is a simple procedure that can be done under **local anesthesia**, and will tell if the lesion is a fluid-filled cyst or whether it is solid. The sample obtained will yield much diagnostic information. Fine needle aspiration biopsy is an excellent technique when the lump is palpable and the physician can easily hit the target with the needle. If the lesion is a simple cyst, the fluid will be evacuated and the mass will disappear. If it is solid, the diagnosis may be obtained. Care must be taken, however, because if the mass is solid and the specimen is non-malignant, a complete removal of the lesion may be appropriate to be sure.

CORE NEEDLE BIOPSY. Core needle biopsies also are obtained simply under local anesthesia. The larger piece of tissue obtained with its preserved architecture may be helpful in confirming the diagnosis short of open surgical removal. An open surgical incisional biopsy is rarely needed for diagnosis because of the needle techniques. If there remains question as to diagnosis, a complete open surgical biopsy may be required.

EXCISIONAL BIOPSY. When performed, the excisional (complete removal) biopsy is a minimal outpatient procedure often done under local anesthesia.

NON-PALPABLE LESIONS. As screening increases, non-palpable lesions demonstrated only by mammography are becoming more common. The use of x rays and computers to guide the needle for biopsy or to place markers for the surgeon performing the excisional biopsy are commonly employed. Some benign lesions can be fully removed by multiple directed core biopsies. These techniques are very appealing because they are minimally invasive; however, the physician needs to be careful to obtain a good sample.

Other tests

If a lesion is not palpable and has simple cystic characteristics on mammography, ultrasound may be utilized both to determine that it is a cyst and to guide its evacuation. Ultrasound may also be used in some cases to guide fine needle or core biopsies of the breast.

Computed tomography (CT) scans have only rare in the evaluation of breast lesions. **Magnetic resonance** imaging (MRI) has been used more often in recent years to follow up on suspicious findings from mammograms or for certain patients.

Treatment

Staging

Once diagnosis is established and before treatment is rendered, more tests are done to determine if the cancer has spread beyond the breast. These tests include a **chest x ray** and **blood count** with **liver function tests**. Along with the liver function measured by the blood sample, the level of alkaline phosphatase, an enzyme from bone, is also determined. A radionuclear bone scan may be ordered. This test looks at the places in the body to which breast cancer usually metastasizes. A CT scan also may be ordered. The physician will do a careful examination of the axillae to assess likelihood of regional metastasis. Sometimes, the physician removed all of the axillary lymph nodes to assess breast cancer stage. However, recent studies show great success with sentinel **lymph node biopsy**. This technique removes the sentinel lymph node, or that lymph node that receives fluid drainage first from the area where the cancer is located. If this node is free of cancer, staging can be assigned accordingly. This method saves women the discomfort and side effects associated with removing additional lymph nodes in her armpit.

Using the results of these studies, clinical stage is defined for the patient. This helps define treatment protocol and prognosis. After surgical treatment, the final, or pathologic, stage is defined as the true axillary lymph node status is known. Detailed staging criteria are available from the American Joint Commission on Cancer Manual and are generalized here:

- Stage 1—The cancer is no larger than 2 cm (0.8 in) and no cancer cells are found in the lymph nodes.
- Stage 2—The cancer is between 2 cm and 5 cm, and the cancer has spread to the lymph nodes.
- Stage 3A—Tumor is larger than 5 cm (2 in) or is smaller than 5 cm, but has spread to the lymph nodes, which have grown into each other.
- Stage 3B—Cancer has spread to tissues near the breast, (local invasion), or to lymph nodes inside the chest wall, along the breastbone.
- Stage 4—Cancer has spread to skin and lymph nodes beyond the axilla or to other organs of the body.

Treatment

Surgery, radiation, and **chemotherapy** are all utilized in the treatment of breast cancer. Depending on the stage, they will be used in different combinations or sequences to effect an appropriate strategy for the type and stage of the disease being treated.

SURGERY. Historically, surgical removal of the entire breast and axillary contents along with the muscles down to the chest wall was performed as the lone therapy, (radical **mastectomy**). In the last 25 years, as it has been appreciated that breast cancer often spreads early, surgery remains a primary option but other therapies have risen in importance. Recent studies have suggested that breast conserving treatment improves the quality of life.

Today, surgical treatment is best thought of as a combination of removal of the primary tumor and staging of the axillary lymph nodes. A modified radical mastectomy involves removing the whole breast along with the entire axillary contents but not the muscles of the chest wall.

If the tumor is less than 1.5 (4 cm) in size and located so that it can be removed without destroying the reasonable cosmetic appearance of the residual breast, just the primary tumor and a rim of normal tissue will be removed. The axillary nodes will still be removed for staging purposes, usually through a separate incision. Because of the risk of recurrence in the remaining breast tissue, **radiation therapy** is used to lessen the chance of local recurrence. This type of primary therapy is known as **lumpectomy**, (or segmental mastectomy), and axillary dissection.

Sentinel lymph node biopsy, a technique for identifying which nodes in the axilla drain the tumor, has been developed to provide selective sampling and further lessen the degree of surgical trauma the patient experiences.

When patients are selected appropriately based on the preoperative clinical stage, all of these surgical approaches have been shown to produce similar results. In planning primary surgical therapy, it is imperative that the operation is tailored to fit the clinical circumstance of the patient.

The pathologic stage is determined after surgical treatment absolutely defines the local parameters. In addition to stage, there are other tests that are very necessary to aid in decisions regarding treatment such as adjuvant therapies. Adjuvant therapies are treatments utilized after the primary treatment to help ensure that no microscopic disease exists and to help prolong patients' survival time.

RADIATION THERAPY. Like surgical therapy, radiation therapy is a local modality—it treats the tissue exposed to radiation and not the rest of the body.

Radiation is usually given post-operatively after surgical **wounds** have healed. The pathologic stage of the primary tumor is now known and this aids in treatment planning. The extent of the local surgery also influences the planning. Radiation may not be needed at all after modified radical mastectomy for stage I disease, but is almost always utilized when breast-preserving surgery is performed. If the tumor was extensive or if multiple nodes were involved, the field of tissue exposed will vary accordingly. Radiation is utilized as an adjunct to surgical therapy and is considered important to gaining local control of the tumor. The use of radiation therapy does not affect decisions for adjuvant treatment. In the past, radiation was used as an alternative to surgery on occasion. However, now that breast-preserving surgical protocols have been developed, primary radiation treatment of the tumor is no longer performed. Radiation also has an important role in the treatment of the patient with disseminated disease, particularly if it involves the skeleton. Radiation therapy can affect pain control and prevention of fracture in this circumstance.

DRUG THERAPY. Many breast cancers, particularly those originating in post-menopausal women, are responsive to hormones. These cancers have receptors on their cells for estrogen and progesterone. Part of primary tumor assessment after removal of the tumor is the evaluation for the presence of these estrogen and progesterone receptors. If they are present on the cancer cells, altering the hormone status of the patient will inhibit tumor growth and have a positive impact on survival. The drug tamoxifen binds up these receptors on the cancer cells so that the hormones can't have an effect and, in so doing, inhibits tumor growth. If the patient has these receptors present, tamoxifen is commonly prescribed for five years as an adjunct to primary treatment. Adjuvant hormonal therapy with tamoxifen has few side effects but they have to be kept in mind, particularly the need for yearly evaluation of the uterus. Other agents directed at altering hormone environment are under study. Because of these agents, there is rarely any need for surgical removal of hormone-producing glands, such as the ovary or adrenal, that was sometimes necessary in the past.

In late 2003, cancer experts were beginning to recommend a new group of drugs called aromatase inhibitors (Arimidex, common name anastrozole, or more recently Femara and Novartis, common name letrozole). New guidelines also recommend letrozole following five years of tamoxifen therapy. These drugs fight breast cancer differently, but early research shows they fight it as effectively and with fewer side effects.

Shortly after the modified radical mastectomy replaced the radical mastectomy as primary surgical treatment, survival after local treatment in stage II breast cancer was improved by the addition of chemotherapy. Adjuvant chemotherapy for an interval of four to six months is now standard treatment for patients with stage II disease. The addition of systemic therapy to local treatment in patients who have no evidence of disease is performed on the basis that some patients have metastases that are not currently demonstrable because they are microscopic. By treating the whole patient early, before widespread disease is diagnosed, the adjuvant treatment improves survival rates from roughly 60% for stage II to about 75% at five years after treatment. The standard regimen of cytoxan, methotrexate, and 5-flourouracil, (CMF), is given for six months and is well tolerated. The regimen of cytoxan, adriamycin (doxorubicin), and 5-floururacil, (CAF), is a bit more toxic but only requires four months. (Adriamycin and cytoxin may also be used alone, without the fluorouracil.) The two methods are about equivalent in results. Adjuvant hormonal therapy may be added to the adjuvant chemotherapy as they work through different routes.

The encouraging results from adjuvant therapy in stage II disease have led to the study of similar therapy in stage I disease. The results are not as dramatic, but they are real. Currently, stage I disease is divided into categories a, b, and c on the basis of tumor size. Stage Ia is less than a centimeter in diameter. Adjuvant hormonal or chemotherapy is now commonly recommended for stage Ib and Ic patients. The toxicity of the treatment must be weighed individually for the patient as patients with stage I disease have a survivorship of over 80% without adjuvant chemotherapy.

If patients are diagnosed with stage IV disease or, in spite of treatment, progress to a state of widespread disease, systemic chemotherapy is utilized in a more aggressive fashion. In addition to the adriamycin-containing regimens, the taxols (docetaxel and paclitaxel) have been found to be effective in inducing remission.

On the basis of prognostic factors such as total number of involved nodes over 10, aneuploid DNA with a high synthesis value, or aggressive findings on microscopic evaluation, some patients with stage II or III disease can be predicted to do poorly. If their performance status allows, they can be considered for treatment with highly aggressive chemotherapy. The toxicity is such that bone marrow failure will result. To get around this anticipated side effect of the aggressive therapy, either the patients will be transplanted with their own stem cells, (the cells that will give rise to new marrow), or a traditional **bone marrow transplantation** will be required. This therapy can be a high-risk procedure for patients. It is given with known risk to patients predicted to do poorly and only if it is felt they can tolerate it. Most patients who receive this therapy receive it as part of a clinical trial. At present, it is unclear that such aggressive therapy can be justified.

For patients who are diagnosed with advanced local disease, surgery may be preceded with chemotherapy and radiation therapy. The disease locally regresses allowing traditional surgical treatment to those who could not receive it otherwise. Chemotherapy and sometimes radiation therapy will continue after the surgery. The regimens of this type are referred to as neo-adjuvant therapy. This has been proven to be effective in stage III disease. Neo-adjuvant therapy is now being studied in patients with large tumors that are stage II in an effort to be able to offer breast preservation to these patients.

A drug known as Herceptin (trastuzumab), a monoclonal antibody, is now being used in the treatment of those with systemic disease. The product of the Human Epidermal Growth Factor 2 gene, (HER-2) is overexpressed in 25%–30% of breast cancers. Herceptin binds to the HER-2 receptors on the cancer, resulting in the arrest of growth of these cells.

Prognosis

The prognosis for breast cancer depends on the type and stage of cancer. Over 80% of stage I patients are cured by current therapies. Stage II patients survive overall about 70% of the time, those with more extensive lymph nodal involvement doing worse than those with disease confined to the breast. About 40% of stage III patients survive five years, and about 20% of stage IV patients do so. In 2003, research showed that young women who choose breast-conserving surgery are at higher risk for local recurrence and should receive indefinite follow-up care from their physicians.

Prevention

The use of tamoxifen and other agents which alter the hormone status of the patient are under study. The National Surgical Adjuvant Breast and Bowel Project (NSABP) with support from the National Cancer Institute began a study in 1992 (called the Breast Cancer Prevention Trial, or BCPT) studying the use of tamoxifen as a breast cancer preventative for high-risk women. The results yielded from the study showed that tamoxifen significantly reduced breast cancer risk, and the U.S. Food and Drug Administration approved the use of tamoxifen to reduce breast cancer risk for high-risk patients in 1998. Another NSABP study, known as STAR, is seeking to understand if another drug, raloxifene, is as effective as tamoxifen in reducing breast cancer risk in high-risk patients. That study was begun in 1999, and participants were to be monitored for five years.

And, while most breast cancer can't be prevented, it can be diagnosed from a mammogram at an early stage when it is most treatable. The results of awareness and routine screening have allowed earlier diagnosis, which results in a better prognosis for those discovered.

Resources

BOOKS

Abelhoff, Armitage, Lichter, and Niederhuber. *Clinical Oncology Library*. Philadelphia: Churchill Livingstone 1999.

Schwartz, Spencer, Galloway, Shires, Daly, and Fischer. *Principles of Surgery*. New York: McGraw Hill, 1999.

PERIODICALS

"Early Detection Saves Lives." *Women's Health Weekly* (November 14, 2003): 13.

Esteva and Hortobagyi. "Adjuvant Systemic Therapy for Primary Breast Cancer." *Surgical Clinics of North America* 79, no. 5 (October 1999): 1075-1090.

"HRT Linked to Higher Breast Cancer Risk, Later Diagnosis, Abnormal Mammograms." *Women's Health Weekly* (July 17, 2003): 2.

Margolese, R. G., M. D. "Surgical Considerations For Invasive Breast Cancer." *Surgical Clinics of North America* 79, no. 5 (October 1999): 1031-1046.

Munster and Hudis. "Adjuvant Therapy for Resectable Breast Cancer." *Hematology Oncology Clinics of North America* 13, no. 2 (April 1999): 391-413.

"New Human Breast and Ovarian Cancer Gene Described." *Biotech Week* (December 31, 2003): 89.

Pennachio, Dorothy L. "Letrozole Improves Breast Cancer Outlook." *Patient Care* (December 2003): 4.

"Quality of Life Seems to be Better After Conservative Treatment of Breast Cancer." *Women's Health Weekly* (July 17, 2003): 22.

"Revised Guidelines Show Changes for Breast Cancer Treatment." *Biotech Week* (December 24, 2003): 296.

"Sentinel Lymph Node Biopsy is Accurate for Staging." *Women's Health Weekly* (June 5, 2003): 4.

Shuster, et al. "Multidisciplinary Care For Patients With Breast Cancer." *Surgical Clinics of North America* 80, no. 2 (April 2000): 505-533.

Smith, Robert A., et al. "American Cancer Society Guidelines for Breast Cancer Screening: Update 2003." *Cancer* (May-June 2003): 141.

ORGANIZATIONS

American Cancer Society. 1599 Clifton Road NE, Atlanta, GA 30329. (800)ACS-2345. < http://www.cancer.org > .

Cancer Care, Inc. 275 Seventh Ave., New York, NY 10001.(800) 813-HOPE. < http://www.cancercare.org > .

Cancer Information Service of the NCI. 9000 Rockville Pike, Building 31, Suite 10A18, Bethesda, MD 20892. 1-800-4-CANCER. < http://wwwicic.nci.nih.gov > .

National Alliance of Breast Cancer Organizations. 9 East 37th St., 10th floor, New York, NY 10016. (888) 80-NABCO.

National Coalition for Cancer Survivorship. 1010 Wayne Ave., 5th Floor, Silver Spring, MD 20910. (301) 650-8868.

National Women's Health Resource Center. 120 Albany St., Suite 820, New Brunswick, NJ 08901. (877) 986-9472. < http://www.healthywomen.org > .

OTHER

Breast Cancer Online. < http://www.bco.org/ > .

National Alliance of Breast Cancer Organizations. < http://www.nabco.org/ > .

National Cancer Institute. < http://rex.nci.nih.gov/PATIENTS/INFO_PEOPL_DOC.html > .

Richard A. McCartney, M.D.
Teresa G. Odle

Breast enlargement *see* **Breast implants**

Breast implants

Definition

Breast implantation is a surgical procedure for enlarging the breast. Breast-shaped sacks made of a silicone outer shell and filled with silicone gel or saline (salt water), called implants, are used.

Purpose

Breast implantation is usually performed to make normal breasts larger for cosmetic purposes. Sometimes a woman having a **breast reconstruction** after a **mastectomy** will need the opposite breast enlarged to make the breasts more symmetric. Breasts that are very unequal in size due to trauma or congenital deformity may also be corrected with an enlargement procedure.

Precautions

A woman in poor health or with a severe chronic disease is not a good candidate for this procedure.

Description

A cosmetic breast enlargement is usually an outpatient procedure. It may be done under local or

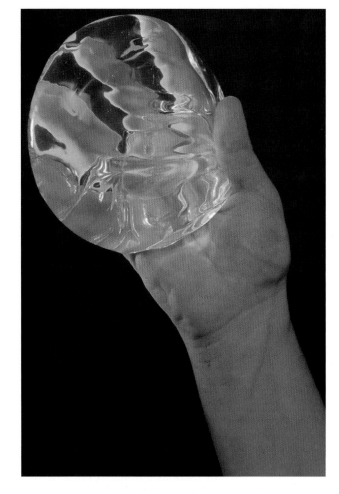

A silicone breast implant. *(Photograph by Dale O'Dell, The Stock Market. Reproduced by permission.)*

general anesthesia, depending on patient and physician preference. The incision is made through the armpit, under the breast, or around the areola (the darkened area around the nipple). These techniques create the most inconspicuous **scars**. The implant is placed between the breast tissue and underlying chest muscle, or under the chest muscle. The operation takes approximately one to two hours. The cost of a cosmetic procedure is rarely covered by insurance. However, if enlargement is part of breast reconstruction after a mastectomy, health plans may pay for some or all of it. The surgeon's fee ranges from $2,700-$4,200 and up. The procedure may also be called breast augmentation or augmentation mammaplasty.

Preparation

Before the surgery is performed, the woman should have a clear understanding of what her new

650

breasts will look like. She and her physician should agree about the desired final result. Many surgeons find it helpful to have the patient review before and after pictures, to clarify expectations.

Aftercare

Driving and normal activities may be restricted for up to one week. Stitches are usually removed in seven to 10 days. Typically, a woman can resume all routines, including vigorous **exercise**, in about three weeks. The scars will be red for approximately one month, but will fade to their final appearance within one or two years.

Risks

Risks which are common to any surgical procedure include bleeding, infection, anesthesia reaction, or unexpected scarring. A breast enlargement may also result in decreased sensation in the breast, or interference with breast-feeding. Implants can also make it more difficult to read and interpret mammograms, possibly delaying **breast cancer** detection. Also, the implant itself can rupture and leak, or become displaced. A thick scar that normally forms around the implant, called a capsule, can become very hard. This is called capsular contracture, and may result in **pain** and/or an altered appearance of the breast. The older the implant, the greater the chances that these problems will occur.

There has been intermittent publicity about possible health risks from breast implants. Most concerns have focused on silicone gel-filled implants. As of 1992, the Food and Drug Administration (FDA) restricted the use of this type of implant, and ordered further studies. Today only saline-filled implants are used for cosmetic breast surgery. Recent studies have shown no evidence long-term health risks from silicone implants. However, research on the possible links between these implants and autoimmune or connective tissue diseases is continuing.

Normal results

Breasts of expected size and appearance would be the normal results of this surgery.

Resources

ORGANIZATIONS

American Society of Plastic and Reconstructive Surgeons. 44 E. Algonquin Rd., Arlington Heights, IL 60005. (847) 228-9900. < http://www.plasticsurgery.org > .

Ellen S. Weber, MSN

Breast infection *see* **Mastitis**

Breast radiography *see* **Mammography**

Breast reconstruction

Definition

Breast reconstruction is a series of surgical procedures performed to recreate a breast. Reconstructions are commonly done after one or both breasts are removed as a treatment for **breast cancer**. Also, a breast may need to be refashioned for other reasons, such as trauma or abnormalities that occur during breast development.

Purpose

Many authorities consider reconstruction an integral part of the therapy for breast **cancer**. A breast that appears natural offers a sense of wholeness and normalcy, which can aid in the psychological recovery from breast cancer. It eliminates the need for an external prosthesis (false breast), which many women find physically uncomfortable as well as inconvenient.

Precautions

Not all women are good candidates for breast reconstruction. Overall poor physical health, or specific problems such as cigarette **smoking**, **obesity**, high blood pressure, or diabetes, will increase the chance of complications. Also, a difficult and/or prolonged recovery period or failure of the reconstruction may be a result. A woman's physical ability to cope with major surgery and recuperation also need to be considered.

Description

Breast reconstruction is done in two stages, with the ultimate goal of creating a breast which looks and feels as natural as possible. It is important to remember that while a good result may mimic a normal breast closely, there will inevitably be **scars** and loss of sensation. The reconstructed breast cannot be exactly like the original.

The first step is to form a structure called a breast mound. This can be accomplished using artificial materials called **breast implants**, or by using tissues from other parts of the woman's body. The second

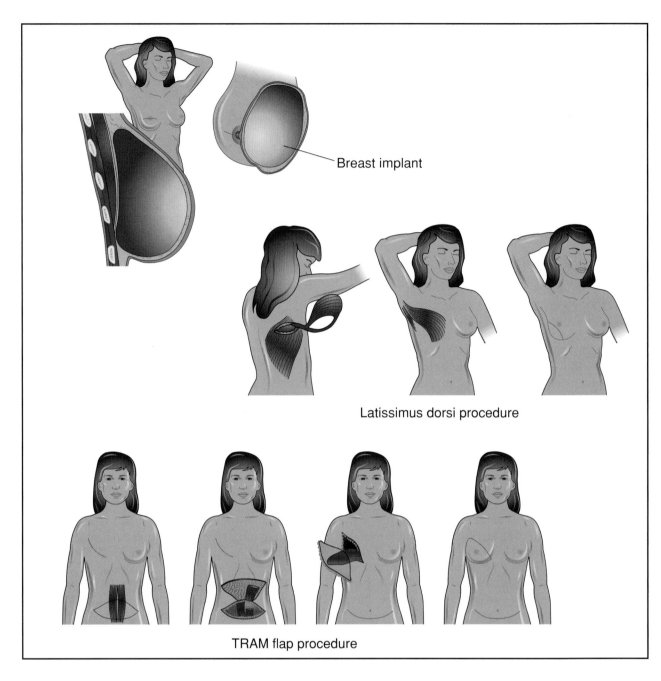

Breast implant

Latissimus dorsi procedure

TRAM flap procedure

Breast reconstruction surgery may be performed by inserting an artificial substance, or implant, to replace breast tissue. Autologous reconstruction, in which a woman's own tissues are used, includes the latissimus dorsi flap, where skin and muscle taken from the back is rotated around to the breast area, and the TRAM flap, in which abdominal fat and muscle are tunneled under the skin to the breast area. *(Illustration by Electronic Illustrators Group.)*

step involves creating a balance between the newly constructed breast and the breast on the opposite side. The nipple and areolar complex (darker area around the nipple) are recreated. This is usually done several months after the mound is created, to allow swelling to go down. Other procedures may be necessary, such as lifting the opposite breast (mastopexy),

or making it larger or smaller to match the reconstructed breast.

Timing, immediate or delayed reconstruction

While immediate reconstruction (IR) is not recommended for women with breast cancer who need to undergo other, more important treatments, breast

KEY TERMS

Autologous—From the same person. An autologous breast reconstruction uses the woman's own tissues. An autologous blood transfusion is blood removed then transfused back to the same person at a later time.

Capsular contracture—Thick scar tissue around a breast implant, which may tighten and cause discomfort and/or firmness.

Flap—A section of tissue moved from one area of the body to another.

Free flap—A section of tissue detached from its blood supply, moved to another part of the body, and reattached by microsurgery to a new blood supply.

Mastopexy—Surgical procedure to lift up a breast. May be used on opposite breast to achieve symmetrical appearance with a reconstructed breast.

Pedicle flap—Also called an attached flap. A section of tissue, with its blood supply intact, which is maneuvered to another part of the body.

reconstruction can be done almost anytime. It even can be done during the same procedure as the **mastectomy**, or it can be delayed. There are psychological benefits to IR. The ability to return to normal activities and routines is often enhanced when reconstruction follows immediately after mastectomy. A better appearance may result from IR. There is less skin removal, often resulting in a shorter scar. The surgeon is better able to preserve the normal boundaries of the breast, so it is easier to match the opposite breast more closely.

The cost of IR is generally lower than the cost of delayed reconstruction (DR). There is one fewer operation and hospital stay. Surgeon's fees may be lower for a combined procedure than for two separate surgeries.

There are disadvantages of IR as well. The surgery itself is longer, causing more time under anesthesia. Post-operative **pain** and recovery time will be greater than for mastectomy alone.

Other authorities contend that delayed reconstruction (DR) offers different physical and psychological advantages. The initial mastectomy procedure alone takes less time, and has a shorter recovery period and less pain than mastectomy and IR. The patient has more time to adjust to her diagnosis and recover from additional therapy. She is better able to research her options, and to formulate realistic goals for

reconstruction. Some **reconstructive surgery** requires blood transfusions. With DR, the patient can donate her own blood ahead of time (autologous **transfusion**), and/or arrange to have family and friends donate blood for her use (directed donation).

The psychological **stress** of living without a breast is a disadvantage of DR. The extra procedure DR entails results in higher costs. Although initial recovery is faster, an additional recuperation period is required after the delayed operation.

Type of reconstruction

There are two basic choices for breast reconstruction. The breast tissue can be replaced with an implant or the breast is created using some of the woman's own tissues (autologous reconstruction).

ARTIFICIAL IMPLANTS. In general, implant procedures take less time, and are less expensive than autologous ones. Implants are breast shaped pouches. They are made of silicone outer shells, which may be smooth or textured. The inside may contain silicone gel, saline (salt water), or a combination of both.

An implant may be a fixed volume type, which cannot change its size. Implants that have the capacity to be filled after insertion are called tissue expanders. These may be temporary or permanent.

The initial procedure for any implant insertion uses the mastectomy incision to make a pocket of tissue, usually underneath the chest wall muscle. In DR, the mastectomy scar may be re opened and used for this purpose, or a more cosmetic incision may be made. The implant is inserted into the pocket, the skin is stretched as needed and stitched closed.

If there is inadequate tissue to achieve the desired size, or a naturally sagging breast is desired, a tissue expander is used. It resembles a partially deflated balloon, with an attached valve or port through which saline can be injected. After the initial surgical incision is healed, the woman returns to the doctor's office, on a weekly or bi-weekly basis, to have small amounts of saline injected. Injections can continue for about six to eight weeks, until the preferred size is obtained. In some cases it may be overfilled, and later partially deflated to allow for a more pliable, natural result. A temporary tissue expander will be removed after several months and replaced with a permanent implant.

IR surgery using an implant takes approximately two to three hours, and usually requires up to a three day hospital stay. Implant insertion surgery, as part of DR, takes one to two hours and can sometimes be done as an outpatient, or it or it may entail overnight hospitalization.

AUTOLOGUS RECONSTRUCTION. Attached flap and free flap are two types of surgery where a woman's tissue is used in reconstruction. An attached flap uses skin, muscle, and fat, leaving blood vessels attached to their original source of blood. The flap is maneuvered to the reconstruction site, keeping its original blood supply for nourishment. This may also be known as a pedicle flap. The second kind of surgery is called a free flap. This also uses skin, muscle, and fat, but severs the blood vessels, and attaches them to other vessels where the new breast is to be created. The surgeon uses a microscope to accomplish this delicate task of sewing blood vessels together. Sometimes the term microsurgery is used to refer to free flap procedures. Either type of surgery may also be called a myocutaneous flap, referring to the skin and muscle used.

The skin and muscle used in autologous reconstruction can come from one of several possible places on the body, including the abdomen (TRAM flap or "tummy tuck"), the back (latissimus dorsi flap), or the buttocks (gluteus maximus free flap).

Finishing the reconstruction

Other procedures may be necessary to achieve the goal of symmetrical breasts. It may be necessary to make the opposite breast larger (augmentation), smaller (reduction), or higher (mastopexy). These, or any other refinements should be completed before the creation of a nipple and areola. Tissue to form the new nipple may come from the reconstructed breast itself, the opposite breast, or a more distant donor site, such as the inner thigh or behind the ear. The nipple and areolar construction is usually an outpatient procedure. A final step, often done in the doctor's office, is tattooing the new nipple and areola, to match the color of the opposite nipple and areola as closely as possible.

Insurance

Insurance coverage for breast reconstruction varies widely. Some policies will allow procedures on the affected breast, but refuse to pay for alterations to the opposite breast. Other plans may cover the cost of an external prosthesis, or reconstructive surgery, but not both. As of January 1998, 25 states had different laws regarding required insurance coverage for post mastectomy reconstruction.

Implants may pose additional insurance concerns. Some companies will withdraw coverage for women with implants, or add a disclaimer for future implant-related problems. Careful reading of insurance policies, including checking on the need for pre-approval and/or a second opinion, is strongly recommended.

Preparation

Routine preoperative preparations, such as taking nothing to eat or drink the night before surgery are needed for reconstructive procedures. Blood transfusions are often necessary for autologous reconstructive surgeries. The patient may donate her own blood, and/or have family and friends donate several weeks before the surgery.

Emotional preparation is also important. Breast reconstruction will not resolve a psychological problem the woman had before mastectomy, nor make an unstable relationship strong. An expectation of physical perfection is unrealistic. A woman who cites any of these reasons for reconstruction shows that she has not been adequately informed or prepared. Complete understanding of the benefits and limitations of this surgery is necessary for a satisfactory result.

Aftercare

The length of the hospital stay, recovery period, and frequency of visits to the doctor after surgery varies considerably with the different kinds of reconstruction. In general, autologous procedures require longer hospitalization and recovery time than implant procedures. Bandages and drainage tubes remain in place for at least a day for all surgeries. Microsurgical or free flaps are most closely monitored in the first day or two after surgery. The circulation to the breast may be checked as often as every hour. Complete breast reconstruction requires at least one additional surgery to create a nipple and areola. Scars may remain red and raised for a month or longer. The true, final appearance of the breasts will not be visible for at least one year.

Risks

Some women have reported various types of autoimmune related connective-tissue disorders, which they attribute to their implants–usually involving silicone gel implants. Lawsuits have been filed against the manufacturers of implants. Food and Drug Administration guidelines, issued in 1992, now limit their use to women who need to replace an existing silicone gel-filled implant, have had surgery for breast cancer, or have a medical condition which results in serious breast abnormality. In addition, patients must sign a consent form which details the potential risks of silicone gel-filled implants, and become enrolled in a long range study. Saline filled implants are permitted for all uses, although manufacturers must collect data on possible risks.

The FDA issued a status report on Breast Implant Safety in 1995, and revised it in March 1997. It noted that studies so far have not shown a serious increase in the risk of recognized autoimmune diseases in women with silicone gel-filled breast implants. It also addressed concerns about other complications and emphasized the need for further study of this issue.

There are a number of risks common to any surgical procedure such as bleeding, infection, anesthesia reaction, or unexpected scarring. Hematoma (accumulation of blood at the surgical site), or seroma (collection of fluid at the surgical site) can delay healing if not drained. Any breast reconstruction also poses a risk of asymmetry and/or the need for unplanned surgical revision. Persistent pain is another potential complication possible with all types of breast reconstruction.

Implants have some unique problems that may develop. A thick scar, also called a capsule, forms around the implant, as part of the body's normal reaction to a foreign substance. Capsular contracture occurs when the scar becomes firm or hardened. This may cause pain and/or change the texture and appearance of the breast. Implants can rupture and leak, deflate, or become displaced. The chances of capsular contracture or rupture increase with the age of the implant. These complications can usually be remedied with outpatient surgery to loosen the capsule or remove and/or replace the implant as needed. There is some evidence that using implants with textured surfaces may decrease the incidence of these problems. An implant tends to remain firm indefinitely. It will not grow larger or smaller as the woman's weight changes. Asymmetry can develop if a woman gains or loses a large amount of weight.

The autologous procedures all carry a risk of flap failure–loss of blood supply to the tissue forming the new breast. If a large portion of the flap develops inadequate blood supply, another reconstructive technique may be necessary. TRAM flap procedures can result in decreased muscle tone and weakness in the abdomen and/or abdominal **hernia**. Arm weakness may occur after latissimus dorsi flap surgery.

Normal results

A normal result of breast reconstruction depends on the woman's goals and expectations. It will not be the same as the breast it replaces. In general, it should be similar in size and shape to the opposite breast, but will have less sensation and be less mobile than a natural breast. A reconstruction using implants will usually be firmer and rounder than the other breast. It may feel cooler to touch, depending on the amount of tissue over it. Scars are unavoidable, but should be as unobtrusive as possible.

Breast reconstruction surgery may be performed by inserting an artificial substance, or implant, to replace breast tissue. Autologous reconstruction, in which a woman's own tissues are used, includes the latissimus dorsi flap, where skin and muscle taken from the back is rotated around to the breast area, and the TRAM flap, in which abdominal fat and muscle are tunneled under the skin to the breast area.

Resources

ORGANIZATIONS

American Cancer Society. 1599 Clifton Rd., NE, Atlanta, GA 30329-4251. (800) 227-2345. < http://www.cancer.org > .

American Society of Plastic and Reconstructive Surgeons. 44 E. Algonquin Rd., Arlington Heights, IL 60005. (847) 228-9900. < http://www.plasticsurgery.org > .

Ellen S. Weber, MSN

Breast reduction

Definition

Breast reduction is a surgical procedure performed in order to decrease the size of the breasts.

Purpose

Women with very large breasts (macromastia or mammary hyperplasia) seek breast reduction for relief of **pain** in the back, shoulder, and neck. They may also feel uncomfortable about their breast size and have difficulty finding clothing that will fit properly. Additionally, breast reduction may be needed after **reconstructive surgery** following the surgical removal of cancerous breast tissue (**mastectomy**), to make the breasts more symmetric.

Men who have enlarged breasts (**gynecomastia**) may also be candidates for breast reduction. However, excessive alcohol intake, **smokingmarijuana**, or using anabolic steroids may cause gynecomastia, and surgery is not recommended for men who continue to use these products.

Precautions

Breast reduction is not recommended for women whose breasts are not fully developed or who plan to breast feed.

Description

Breast reduction may also be called reduction mammaplasty. It is most often done in the hospital, under general anesthetic. However, studies have suggested that an outpatient procedure, using local anesthetic and mild **sedation** may be appropriate for some patients. The operation takes approximately two to four hours. The most commonly made incision encircles the areola (darkened area around the nipple) and extends downward and around the underside of the breast. This produces the least conspicuous scar. The excess tissue, fat, and skin are removed, and the nipple and areola are repositioned. In certain cases, **liposuction** (fat suctioning) is used to remove extra fat from the armpit area. A hospital stay of up to three days may be needed for recovery.

If deemed medically necessary, breast reduction is covered by some insurance plans. However, a specified amount of breast tissue may need to be removed in order to qualify for coverage. Surgeon's fees range from $4,800-$6,500 and up.

Preparation

Consultation between surgeon and patient is important to ensure that the woman understands and agrees with the expected final results of the procedure. Measurements and photographs may be taken. Many doctors also recommend a mammogram before the operation, to make sure there is no **cancer**.

Aftercare

After the surgery, an elastic bandage or special supportive bra is placed over gauze bandages and drainage tubes. The bandages and tubes are removed in a day or two. The bra will need to be worn around the clock for several weeks. Stitches are removed one to three weeks after the operation. Normal activities, including sexual relations may be restricted for several weeks. **Scars** will typically remain red, and perhaps lumpy for up to several months, but will gradually fade and become less noticeable. It may take up to a year before the breasts achieve their final position and size.

Risks

Risks common to any operation include bleeding, infection, anesthesia reactions, or unexpected scarring. Breast reduction may result in decreased feeling in the breasts or nipples and/or impaired ability to breastfeed. When healing is complete, the breasts may be slightly uneven, or the nipples may be asymmetric.

Normal results

Smaller breast size should be achieved, and with that, the accompanying pain and discomfort should be alleviated.

Resources

ORGANIZATIONS

American Society of Plastic and Reconstructive Surgeons. 44 E. Algonquin Rd., Arlington Heights, IL 60005. (847) 228-9900. < http://www.plasticsurgery.org >.

Ellen S. Weber, MSN

Breast self-examination

Definition

A breast self-examination (BSE) is an inspection by a woman of her breasts to detect **breast cancer**.

Purpose

A BSE is one of three tests the American **Cancer** Society recommends to help detect breast cancer in its earliest stages. By regularly examining her own breasts, a woman is more likely to find any changes that may have occurred. The best time to perform a BSE is about a week after a woman's period ends, when her breasts are not tender or swollen. If her periods are not regular, a BSE should be completed on the same day every month. A BSE should also be regularly completed by women who are pregnant, breastfeeding, or have **breast implants**. By combining a BSE with a **mammography** and clinical breast examination, a woman is offered the best opportunity for reducing chances of **death** from breast cancer through early detection. Close to 90% of breast cancers are found through a BSE. The American Cancer Society recommends that beginning at the age of 20, women complete a BSE each month by feeling for lumps or anything suspicious, as well as looking at their breasts carefully in a mirror for any changes in contour, swelling, dimpling, puckering of the skin, or changes in the nipple.

Description

To complete a monthly BSE:

- When lying down, place a pillow under the right shoulder and position the right arm behind the head. Using the finger pads of the three middle fingers on the left hand, check the entire breast area. Use small circles and follow an up-and-down pattern while pressing firmly enough to know how the breast feels from month to month. This exam should then be repeated on the left breast using the finger pads of the right hand with the pillow under the left shoulder.

- When standing before a mirror, any changes in the shape or look of the breasts should be checked. In order to look for any skin or nipple changes such as dimpling or nipple discharge, the arms should first be placed at the sides and then overhead. Hands are then placed firmly on hips to flex chest muscles, and then the body should be bent forward.

- When taking a shower, the right arm should be raised. By using soapy hands and fingers flat the right breast and outer part of the breast can be examined. The same small circles and up-and-down pattern used when lying down should be used in an upright position. Repeat on the left breast.

Preparation

Before beginning a monthly BSE, a woman's breasts should be completely exposed.

Normal results

Each woman's breasts has their own normal look and feel. By completing a BSE each month, a woman can determine what is normal for her and check for changes that may arise. A regular pattern of lumpiness in the breasts is normal.

Abnormal results

If any changes are noticed during a monthly BSE, such as a new, hard lump in the breast or underarms, a doctor should examine the area immediately. Other trouble signs that should not be ignored include:

- change in breast size or shape
- dimpling or puckering of the skin
- redness, swelling, or warmth that does not go away
- a **pain** in one area that does not vary with a woman's monthly cycle
- a nipple that pulls in
- discharge from the nipple that begins suddenly and appears only in one breast
- one nipple that has an itchy, sore, or scaling area

Resources

BOOKS

Altman, Roberta, and Michael J. Sarg. "Breast Self-examination." *The Cancer Dictionary*. Checkmark Books, 2000.

ORGANIZATIONS

American Cancer Society. 1599 Clifton Road NE, Atlanta, GA 30329. (800)ACS-2345. < http:// www.cancer.org > .

Komen Foundation. 5005 LBJ Freeway, Suite 250, Dallas, TX 75244. (972) 855-1600. < http://www.komen.org > .

OTHER

"How to do a Breast Self-Exam." Women.com. May 5, 2001. < http://www.women.com > .

Beth A. Kapes

Breast sonogram *see* **Breast ultrasound**

Breast ultrasound

Definition

Breast ultrasound (or sonography) is an imaging technique for diagnosing breast disease, such as **cancer**. It uses harmless, high frequency sound waves to form an image (sonogram). The sound waves pass through the breast and bounce back or echo from various tissues to form a picture of the internal structures. It is not invasive and involves no radiation.

Purpose

Breast ultrasound may be used in several ways. The most common application is to investigate a specific area of the breast where a problem is suspected. A palpable lump and/or a lump or density

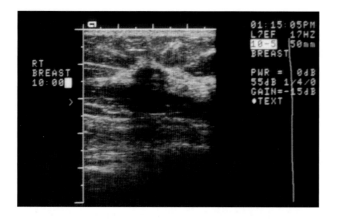

A breast ultrasound image. *(Custom Medical Stock Photo. Reproduced by permission.)*

Cyst—A thin-walled, fluid-filled benign structure in the breast.

Ductal carcinoma—A type of cancer that accounts for as much as 80% of breast cancers. These tumors feel bigger than they look on ultrasound or mammogram.

Fibroadenoma—A benign breast growth made up of fibrous tissue. It is the most common mass in women under 35 years of age, and is found in both breasts in 3% of cases.

Infiltrating lobular carcinoma—A type of cancer that accounts for 8% to 10% of breast cancers. In breasts that are especially dense, ultrasound can be useful in identifying these masses.

Microcalcifications—Tiny flecks that are too small to be felt. They are important markers of cancer that show up on ultrasound and mammogram.

Mucinous (colloid) carcinoma—A type of cancer that accounts for 1% to 2% of breast cancers. Resembles medullary carcinoma in ultrasound and mammogram, but usually affects older women.

Nonpalpable—Cannot be felt by hand. In cancer, growths that are nonpalpable are too small to be felt, but may be seen on ultrasound or mammogram.

Papillary carcinoma—A type of breast cancer that primarily occurs in older women. On ultrasound, this type of tumor may look like a solid or complex mass, or it may show up as solid tissue protruding into a cyst.

Tubular carcinoma—A type of cancer that accounts for approximately 1% to 2% of breast cancers. Can appear small on ultrasound or mammogram.

discovered by x-ray imaging (mammogram) can be further evaluated by ultrasound. It is especially helpful in distinguishing between a fluid-filled cyst and a solid mass. It also can identify small lesions that are too tiny to be felt.

Breast ultrasound is often the first study performed to evaluate masses in women under 35 whose mammograms can be difficult to interpret due to the density of their breast tissue. In 2003, a new study found that ultrasound was more accurate than **mammography** at diagnosing **breast cancer** in women under age 45. However, mammography still works as a screening tool, with breast ultrasound as the follow-up examination. Another study in that year found that combining ultrasound with **magnetic resonance imaging** (MRI) direction greatly improved diagnostic decisions about breast cancer lesions. The lesions detected by MRI could also be localized using ultrasound needle guidance for follow-up biopsy.

The lack of radiation used with ultrasound makes it ideal for studying breast abnormalities in women who are pregnant. Assessing **breast implants** for leakage or rupture is another use for ultrasound. Breast inflammation, where pockets of infection or abscesses may form, can be diagnosed and monitored by ultrasound.

Thickened and swollen breast skin may be a sign of inflammatory breast cancer. Ultrasound can sometimes identify a cancerous growth within the breast causing the thickened skin. These cases are usually followed by a core biopsy guided by ultrasound.

Breast ultrasound is employed to observe and guide a needle for several interventional procedures. These include cyst aspiration, fine needle aspiration, large core needle biopsy (as a first step in determining

treatment for a lesion that is likely to be cancerous), and needle localization in surgical **breast biopsy**. Biopsies guided by ultrasound have distinct advantages. Patients usually find that the procedure is less traumatic and more comfortable than surgical biopsies. Ultrasound is known for its accuracy in determining how far a cancerous growth extends into the surrounding tissue in lesions that cannot be felt. Biopsies guided by ultrasound are generally less costly than surgical biopsies. Additionally, if the abnormality that requires biopsy can be seen on both a mammogram and ultrasound, an ultrasound-guided biopsy is often more comfortable for the patient as no compression is necessary.

Description

Ultrasound can be done in a doctor's office or another outpatient setting, such as a hospital or imaging center.

The patient removes her clothing from the waist up and puts on a hospital gown, open in the front. She lies on her back or side on an examining table. A gel that enhances sound transmission is spread over the area to be examined. The technologist then places a transducer, an instrument about the size of an electric shaver, against the skin. The images from reflected sound waves appear on a monitor screen.

A physician called a radiologist interprets the images obtained from ultrasound imaging. In 2003, it was reported that new computer-aided diagnosis (CAD) technology that had recently been widely added to mammography may help improve ultrasound as well. The CAD system uses computer algorithms applied to a three-dimensional ultrasound image to assign scores to mass characteristics. Though the technology will not replace human observation and judgment, it may soon be added to support the radiologist's interpretation.

A good ultrasound study is difficult to obtain if the patient is unable to remain quietly in one position. **Obesity** may hinder clear viewing of internal structures, and the accuracy of an ultrasound study is highly dependent on the skill of the person performing the examination. The images recorded vary with the angle and pressure of the transducer and the equipment settings. The examination may take from 30 to 45 minutes. Most insurance plans cover the cost of an ultrasound examination.

Normal results

An ultrasound examination may reveal either normal tissue or a benign condition such as a cyst. Ultrasound can confidently diagnose a benign structure that has certain characteristics of a simple cyst. In the case of a simple cyst with no symptoms, additional treatment beyond continued observation is usually not needed.

Abnormal results

A potentially malignant mass can be identified by breast ultrasound. Abnormal results fall into the following categories: benign fibrous nodule, complex cyst, suspicious lesion, and lesion highly suggestive of cancer. In cases where ultrasound shows the presence of a complex cyst or fibrous nodule, a biopsy is justified because 10% to 15% of these growths are malignant. Lesions falling into the last two categories (suspicious or highly suggestive of cancer) have a higher chance of being cancerous, and should be investigated further, either by biopsy or surgery.

Breast cancers such as the following may be identified on ultrasound: ductal carcinoma, infiltrating lobular carcinoma, medullary carcinoma, mucinous (colloid) carcinoma, tubular carcinoma, and papillary carcinoma. On ultrasound, the shape of a lesion and the type of edges it has can sometimes indicate if it is benign or cancerous, but there are exceptions. For example, benign fibroadenomas are usually oval, and some cancers can be similarly shaped. Cancerous tumors usually have jagged edges, but some benign growths can have these edges as well. Ultrasound is not a definitive test. Tissue diagnosis is often required.

Resources

PERIODICALS

"CAD Software Improves Breast Ultrasound, Digital Mammograms." *Cancer Weekly* (December 23, 2003): 13.

Rubin, Eva, et al. "Reducing the Cost of Diagnosis of Breast Carcinoma: Impact of Ultrasound and Imaging–Guided Biopsies on a Clinical Breast Practice." *Cancer* 91 (January 2001): 324-31.

Smith, LaNette F., et al. "Intraoperative Ultrasound–guided Breast Biopsy." *The American Journal of Surgery* 180 (December 2000): 419-23.

Trevino, Merlino. "MR-directed US Provides Economical Breast Diagnosis — Ultrasound Characterizes Indeterminate Lesions Already Found by MRI." *Diagnostic Imaging* (April 1, 2003): 59.

Velez, Nitzet, et al. "Diagnostic and Interventional Ultrasound for Breast Disease." *The American Journal of Surgery* 180 (October 2000): 284-7.

Ellen S. Weber, MSN
Teresa G. Odle

Breast x ray *see* **Mammography**

Breech birth

Definition

Breech birth is the delivery of a fetus (unborn baby) hind end first. Between 3-4% of fetuses will start labor in the breech position, which is a potentially dangerous situation.

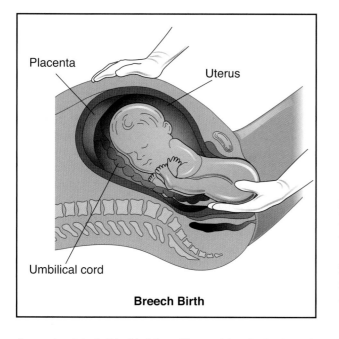

Placenta

Uterus

Umbilical cord

Breech Birth

Approximately 3-4% of babies will start labor in the breech (buttocks first) position. While this is a potentially dangerous situation, many full-term babies can be safely delivered from the breech position. (Illustration by Electronic Illustrators Group.)

Description

Throughout most of **pregnancy**, the developing fetus is completely free to move around within the uterus. Between 32-36 weeks, it becomes so large that movement is restricted. It is much harder for the fetus to turn over, so whatever position it has assumed by this point is likely to be the same position that he or she will be in when labor begins.

For reasons that are not fully understood, almost all unborn babies settle into a head down position. The fetus is upside down in the uterus, and the head will lead the way during the birth process.

Unfortunately, some fetuses do not cooperate. Most of these are in the breech position. The buttocks lead the way out of the uterus, and the legs are folded in front of the body (frank breech). Delivery from the breech position poses far more risks than delivery head first (vertex position).

The biggest part of the fetus's body is usually its head. If the head fits through the mother's pelvis, then the rest of the fetus's body should slip out fairly easily. If the fetus is born bottom first, it is possible that the body will fit through the mother's pelvis, but the baby's head will get stuck at the level of the chin. This condition, known as a trapped head, is very dangerous.

When the baby's head comes first, it has a chance to "mold" during labor. The bones of the baby's skull are not yet fastened together the way they are in a child or adult's skull, meaning that the bones of the baby's skull can move. During the long hours of labor the skull can change shape to fit through the pelvis more easily, which is why many babies are born with a "cone head". If the baby is born from the breech position, the skull does not have a chance to change shape to fit the pelvis, and it is even more likely to get stuck.

If the baby's head gets trapped, the possibility of injury is high. Once the baby's body is born, the umbilical cord usually stops pulsating (just as it would during a normal delivery). This cuts off the oxygen supply from the mother to the baby. If the baby's head is still inside the uterus the baby cannot yet breathe on its own. Therefore, it is essential to deliver the baby as quickly as possible.

The life saving attempts to deliver the baby's head can cause injury to the baby's neck or head resulting in permanent handicaps. In extreme cases, if the baby cannot be delivered within a few minutes, the baby might die. Obviously, it is critical to avoid a breech delivery with a trapped head.

Of course, many babies are safely delivered from the breech position. There are certain factors that make a breech delivery more likely to be successful: if ultrasound (a technique that uses sound waves to visualize the fetus) shows that the fetus is in the frank breech position, the fetus's head is tucked on its chest, and the fetus is not big, it is less likely that its head will get stuck.

Among breech babies born after the full nine-month term, smaller babies usually do better. This is not true for premature babies. Premature babies are more likely to have a trapped head because the body of a premature baby is usually much smaller than his or her head. Premature babies are generally not delivered from the breech position.

The risks of vaginal breech delivery can be avoided by delivering the baby through a surgical procedure (**cesarean section**, also known as c-section). For the past twenty years, cesarean section has been recommended when the fetus is breech. More recently, many providers have offered the option of version, attempting to turn the fetus within the uterus to a head first position before labor begins.

Version is based on a very simple idea. If a fetus in the breech position does a somersault, it will end up head down. During a version, the obstetrician tries to make the fetus do a somersault.

A version should only be done in a hospital, with an ultrasound machine used to guide the obstetrician in turning the fetus. The fetus should be monitored with a fetal monitor before and after the version. Some obstetricians give the mother an injection of medication to relax the mother's uterus and prevent any contractions.

During the procedure, the obstetrician places his or her hands on the mother's abdomen to feel the location of the unborn baby's buttocks and head. The buttocks are lifted up slightly and the doctor pushes on the baby's head to encourage him to perform a somersault. It may take several tries before the fetus cooperates, but over half will eventually turn.

A version is not appropriate for every fetus who is in the breech position at the end of pregnancy. It can only be tried if there is one fetus in the uterus, if the placenta is not lying in front of the fetus, and if the umbilical cord does not appear to be wrapped around the fetus at any point.

Causes and symptoms

The cause of breech birth is not known. There are generally no identifiable symptoms. However, some women can tell the position of the fetus by where they feel the fetus kicking. Most women cannot tell what position the fetus is in at any given moment.

Diagnosis

A health care provider can often tell the position of the fetus by feeling it through the wall of the mother's abdomen. Another clue to the position is the location where the heartbeat is heard best. If the fetus's heartbeat is best heard below the level of the mother's navel, it is likely to be positioned head first. On the other hand, if the heartbeat is best heard above the level of the navel, it is likely to be breech.

The only way to really be sure, however, is to do an ultrasound exam. Using this technique it is very easy to tell the position of the fetus.

Treatment

If a fetus is in the breech position in the last weeks of pregnancy, there are three possible courses of action: Cesarean section, attempted version, or vaginal breech delivery.

Cesarean section is the most common way to deliver a breech baby. This surgical procedure carries more risk for the mother, but many women prefer to take the risk of surgery on themselves rather than let the baby face the risks of breech delivery.

Version is gaining in popularity. Version is a medical procedure in which the obstetrician tries to turn the breech fetus to the head first position. Version is successful more than 50% of the time. However, some babies who are successfully turned will turn back to the breech position after the procedure is done.

Some women choose breech vaginal delivery. This should only be attempted if ultrasound shows that the fetus is in a favorable breech position. Most babies will do very well during a breech delivery, but it is always possible that the fetus will be injured, perhaps seriously.

Prevention

There is no way to prevent a fetus from settling into the breech position at the end of pregnancy. A woman who has had one breech fetus is more likely than average to have another.

Resources

BOOKS

Cunningham, F. Gary, et al., editors. "Techniques for Breech Delivery." In *Williams Obstetrics.* 20th ed. Stamford: Appleton & Lange, 1997.

Amy B. Tuteur, MD

Breech presentation *see* **Breech birth**

Brill-Zinsser disease *see* **Typhus**

Brittle bone disease *see* **Osteogenesis imperfecta**

Broken nose *see* **Nasal trauma**

Bronchiectasis

Definition

Bronchiectasis is a condition in which an area of the bronchial tubes is permanently and abnormally widened (dilated), with accompanying infection.

Description

The bronchial tubes are the networks of branching tubes which deliver air to the tiny sacs of the lungs (alveoli). In bronchiectasis, the diameter of the bronchi is unusually large. Examination of the walls of the

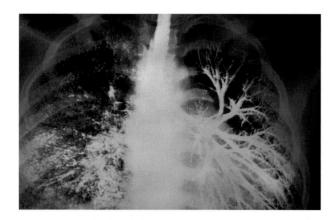

Colorized bronchogram of lungs—right tree has almost no structure caused by chronic inflammation. *(Mehau Kulyk, Photo Researchers. Reproduced by permission.)*

bronchial tubes reveals destruction of the normal structural elements, with replacement by scar tissue. Pus collects within the bronchi, and the normal flow of oxygen into the lungs, and carbon dioxide out of the lungs (air exchange) is impaired. The bronchi show signs of inflammation, with swelling and invasion by a variety of immune cells. The inflamed areas show signs of increased growth of blood vessels. The area of the lung which should be served by a diseased bronchial tube is also prone to inflammation and infection.

Causes and symptoms

Prior to the widespread use of immunizations, bronchiectasis was often the result of a serious infection with either **measles** or **whooping cough**. Currently, viruses that cause **influenza** (flu) or influenza-like syndromes, as well as a number of bacteria may precede the development of bronchiectasis. Patients who have been infected with **tuberculosis** or the virus which causes **AIDS** (HIV or human **immunodeficiency** virus) also have an increased chance of bronchiectasis.

A number of pre-existing conditions may cause an individual to be more susceptible than normal to infection, with increased risk of bronchiectasis developing. These conditions include disorders of cilia, and immune disorders.

Cilia are the tiny hairs which usually line the bronchial tubes. Cilia wave constantly, sweeping the bronchial tubes clean of bacterial or viral invaders, and cleaning away excess secretions (mucus, sputum) which may be produced by the bronchi. When these cilia are abnormal or absent at birth, various bacterial or viral invaders may remain in the respiratory tract, multiply, and cause serious infections.

Immune disorders include decreased production of certain immune chemicals (immunoglobulins) which usually serve to fight off infection by bacterial or viral invasion. When these immunoglobulins are not produced in large enough quantity, bacterial and viral invaders are not effectively killed off, and infection occurs.

Other causes of bronchiectasis include an abnormally blocked (obstructed) airway. This can be due to tumor growth within the bronchial tube, or due to a child accidentally inhaling a small object which then blocks off the bronchial tube. People with the disease called **cystic fibrosis** (CF) often have their bronchial tubes obstructed by the thick, sticky mucus which is a hallmark of CF. Toxic exposures (breathing ammonia, for example) can harm the bronchi, and lead to bronchiectasis. An extreme allergic response of the immune system to the presence of certain fungi (especially one called *Aspergillus*) can also damage the bronchial tubes enough to result in bronchiectasis.

Symptoms of bronchiectasis include constant **cough** and the production of infected sputum (sputum is a mixture of mucus and pus), which may be bloody. In some cases, there may be **wheezing** and **shortness of breath**. The constant, low-level of infection may flare, resulting in increased production of sputum, worsening of the cough, and **fever**. The area of the lung served by the affected bronchial tube may become severely infected, resulting in **pneumonia**.

Diagnosis

Chest x ray may reveal evidence of bronchiectasis, and CT scans are particularly good at revealing the thick, dilated bronchial walls of bronchiectasis. Sputum will need to be collected and cultured (grown in a laboratory dish), in order to examine it microscopically for the specific type of organism responsible for infection. A careful search for other underlying diseases is important, looking in particular for ciliary abnormalities, cystic fibrosis, or immunoglobulin deficiencies.

Treatment

Treatment should involve efforts to resolve any underlying disorder. Infections will require **antibiotics**, obstruction may require the removal of a foreign object or tumor. Medications are available to help thin the sputum, so that it can be more effectively coughed up. Rhythmic clapping on the chest and back, while the patient assumes a number of positions (head down, primarily), may help the lungs to drain more effectively. This is called **chest physical therapy**, or percussion and postural drainage.

When a particular area of the lung is constantly and severely infected, surgery may be needed to remove it. When bleeding occurs from irritated bronchial tubes and overgrown bronchial blood vessels, surgery may be required either to remove an area of the bronchial tube, or to inject the bleeding blood vessel with a material to stop the bleeding.

In some patients, bronchiectasis eventually leads to a constantly low level of blood oxygen, despite other treatments. These patients usually have an associated increase in the size of the right side of their hearts, along with a decrease in the heart's ability to pump blood through the lungs. Some patients with extremely severe symptoms and disability have been treated with **lung transplantation**.

Prognosis

Prognosis varies widely, depending on how widespread or focal the bronchiectasis, and the presence of other underlying disorders.

Resources

ORGANIZATIONS

American Lung Association. 1740 Broadway, New York, NY 10019. (800) 586-4872. < http://www.lungusa.org >.

Rosalyn Carson-DeWitt, MD

Bronchiolitis

Definition

Bronchiolitis is an acute viral infection of the small air passages of the lungs called the bronchioles.

Description

Bronchiolitis is extremely common. It occurs most often in children between the ages of two and 24 months, with peak infection occurring between three and six months of age. About 25% of infants have bronchiolitis during their first year, and 95% have had the disease by their second birthday. In temperate climates, bronchiolitis peaks from winter to late spring. In subtropical climates, the disease peaks from October to February.

Children who attend daycare or who live in crowded conditions and those who are exposed to second-hand smoke at home are more likely to develop bronchiolitis. Premature infants and children born with heart and lung defects or HIV/AIDS are more likely to have severe, life-threatening infections. Bronchiolitis occurs more often in boys than girls, with boys being hospitalized at 1.5 times the rate of girls. Bronchiolitis is a significant cause of respiratory disease worldwide. The World Health Organization (WHO) has funded research to develop a vaccine against the disease, but thus attempts have been unsuccessful.

Causes and symptoms

Bronchiolitis is caused by several different viruses. The most common of these is respiratory syncytial virus (RVS), which is responsible for about 100,000 hospitalizations of children under age four each year. Two subtypes of RSV have been identified, one of which causes most of the severe bronchiolitis infections. In addition, bronchiolitis can be caused by **influenza**, parainfluenza, and adenoviruses, all of which are common from fall through spring. These viruses are spread in tiny drops of fluid from an infected person's nose and mouth through direct contact, such as shaking hands, or kissing. The viruses can also live several hours on countertops, toys, or used tissues and easily infect people who handle contaminated items. The time from infection to the appearance of symptoms varies from two to seven days.

Bronchiolitis affects individuals differently depending on their age. In adults, older children, and some infants, bronchiolitis viruses causes symptoms similar to a mild cold—runny nose, stuffy head, and mild **cough**. The lungs are not involved, and these symptoms clear up without any medical treatment. In some children under age two, the cold-like upper respiratory symptoms worsen after a day or two. The lung tissue begins to swell and produce mucus, and the cells lining the bronchioles begin to slough off into the air passages. As the airways narrow from swelling, and mucus accumulation, breathing becomes difficult, and the child makes a **wheezing** or whistling sound with each breath. Lung involvement can occur quite rapidly.

The most common signs of bronchiolitis involve the infant's struggle to breathe. The child may take 50–60 breaths per minute and may develop brief periods when they stop breathing (apnea) and begin to turn blue (**cyanosis**). This occurs most often in babies who were born very prematurely or who are under six weeks of age and babies with congenital heart and lung problems and compromised immune systems. Babies may also stop eating, because it is becomes difficult for them to swallow and breathe at the same time. They may have a low **fever**, cough, and **vomiting**.

Diagnosis

Bronchiolitis is usually diagnosed through a **physical examination** by a pediatrician or family physician. The physician often finds an increased heart rate, rapid, labored breathing, and crackles in the lungs when the child inhales. Signs of ear infection (**otitis media**) and throat infection (pharyngitis) are sometimes present.

Although laboratory tests are available that can within in a few hours confirm the presence of RSV, these tests are not routinely necessary. The oxygen level in the blood may be measured through pulse oximetry in babies who are having difficulty breathing. Inadequate oxygen in the blood is an indication that hospitalization is necessary. Chest x-rays may be done on severely ill children to rule out other conditions.

Treatment

The degree of respiratory distress determines treatment. Individuals with mild symptoms are treated as if they have a cold with rest, fluids, and a cool air humidifier. Babies who are struggling to breath may hospitalized and given supplemental humidified oxygen. Their breathing will be monitored and if necessary fluids will be given intravenously to prevent **dehydration**. Occasionally infants need mechanical ventilation to fill and empty the lungs until the airways open.

Those children with compromised immune systems from diseases such as congenital HIV/AIDS and transplant patients are at highest risk for severe infections, serious complications, and **death**. Children with congenital heart and lung disorders are also at higher risk, as are infants under six weeks old. These high risk children may be admitted to pediatric intensive care units and treated with ribvarin (Virazole), a drug that keeps the virus from reproducing. This drug is reserved for the most critical cases.

Alternative treatment

Although there are alternative treatments for cold symptoms, such as **echinacea** and zinc, parents should consult their health practitioner about the appropriateness of using these treatments in very young children.

Prognosis

The majority of children who get bronchiolitis, even severe infections, recover without complications in one to two weeks, although **fatigue** and a light cough may linger longer. About 60% of people develop only cold-like symptoms without lung involvement. However, the disease accounts for about 100,000 pediatric hospitalizations and 4,500 deaths each year. Deaths usually occur because medical care is not sought soon enough.

Although many viral illnesses, like chicken pox, can be contracted only once, after which individuals develop immunity, people can get bronchiolitis multiple times. However, after the first infection, the symptoms are usually mild.

Prevention

The viruses that cause bronchiolitis spread very easily, making prevention difficult. Common sense measures such as frequent hand washing and keeping children away from crowds and sick individuals are only partially effective. Certain very high risk babies can be treated during the peak virus season with monthly injections of antiviral immunoglobulins to protect against RSV infection. These injections cost several thousand dollars per child per season and are reserved for children whose life could be at risk if they became infected. Antiviral immunoglobulins are used only for prevention and are not effective as a treatment once the infection has been acquired.

Resources

OTHER

"Bronchitis." *Medline Plus Medical Encyclopedia* 19 January 2005 [cited 16 February 2005]. <http://www.nlm.nih. gov/medlineplus/ency/article/000975.htm>.

DeNicola, Lucian K. and Michael Gayle. *Bronchiolitis*, 17 July 2003 [cited 16 February 2005]. <http://www.eme dicine.com/ped/topic287.htm>.

Kirlov, Leonard R. *Respiratory Syncytial Virus Infection*, 24 November 2004 [cited 16 February 2005]. <http:// www.emedicine.com/ped/topic2706.htm>.

Louden, Mark. *Pediatrics, Bronchiolitis*, 21 May 2001 [cited 16 February 2005]. <http://www.emedicine.com/ emerg/topic365.htm>.

"Respiratory Syncytial Virus (RSV)." *Medline Plus Medical Encyclopedia* 19 January 2005 [cited 16 February 2005]. <http://www.nlm.nih.gov/medlineplus/ency/article/ 001564.htm>

Tish Davidson, A. M.

> ## KEY TERMS
>
> **Acute**—Disease or condition characterized by the rapid onset of severe symptoms.
>
> **Bronchi**—The larger air tubes of the lung that bring air in from the trachea.
>
> **Chronic**—Disease or condition characterized by slow onset over a long period of time.
>
> **Chronic obstructive pulmonary disease (COPD)**— A term used to describe chronic lung diseases, like chronic bronchitis, emphysema, and asthma.
>
> **Emphysema**—One of the several diseases called chronic obstructive pulmonary diseases, emphysema involves the destruction of air sac walls to form abnormally large air sacs that have reduced gas exchange ability and that tend to retain air within the lungs. Symptoms include labored breathing, the inability to forcefully blow air out of the lungs, and an increased susceptibility to respiratory tract infections.

Bronchitis

Definition

Bronchitis is an inflammation of the air passages between the nose and the lungs, including the windpipe or trachea and the larger air tubes of the lung that bring air in from the trachea (bronchi). Bronchitis can either be of brief duration (acute) or have a long course (chronic). Acute bronchitis is usually caused by a viral infection, but can also be caused by a bacterial infection and can heal without complications. Chronic bronchitis is a sign of serious lung disease that may be slowed but cannot be cured.

Description

Although acute and chronic bronchitis are both inflammations of the air passages, their causes and treatments are different. Acute bronchitis is most prevalent in winter. It usually follows a viral infection, such as a cold or the flu, and can be accompanied by a secondary bacterial infection. Acute bronchitis resolves within two weeks, although the **cough** may persist longer. Acute bronchitis, like any upper airway inflammatory process, can increase a person's likelihood of developing **pneumonia**.

Anyone can get acute bronchitis, but infants, young children, and the elderly are more likely to get the disease because people in these age groups generally have weaker immune systems. Smokers and people with heart or other lung diseases are also at higher risk of developing acute bronchitis. Individuals exposed to chemical fumes or high levels of air pollution also have a greater chance of developing acute bronchitis.

Chronic bronchitis is a major cause of disability and **death** in the United States. The American Lung Association estimates that about 14 million Americans suffer from the disease. Like acute bronchitis, chronic bronchitis is an inflammation of airways accompanied by coughing and spitting up of phlegm. In chronic bronchitis, these symptoms are present for at least three months in each of two consecutive years.

Chronic bronchitis is caused by inhaling bronchial irritants, especially cigarette smoke. Until recently, more men than women developed chronic bronchitis, but as the number of women who smoke has increased, so has their rate of chronic bronchitis. Because this disease progresses slowly, middle-aged and older people are more likely to be diagnosed with chronic bronchitis.

Chronic bronchitis is one of a group of diseases that fall under the name chronic obstructive pulmonary disease (COPD). Other diseases in this category include **emphysema** and chronic asthmatic bronchitis. Chronic bronchitis may progress to emphysema, or both diseases may be present together.

Causes and symptoms

Acute bronchitis

Acute bronchitis usually begins with the symptoms of a cold, such as a runny nose, sneezing, and dry cough. However, the cough soon becomes deep and painful. Coughing brings up a greenish yellow phlegm or sputum. These symptoms may be accompanied by a **fever** of up to 102 °F (38.8 °C). **Wheezing** after coughing is common.

In uncomplicated acute bronchitis, the fever and most other symptoms, except the cough, disappear after three to five days. Coughing may continue for several weeks. Acute bronchitis is often complicated by a bacterial infection, in which case the fever and a general feeling of illness persist. To be cured, the bacterial infection should be treated with **antibiotics**.

Chronic bronchitis

Chronic bronchitis is caused by inhaling respiratory tract irritants. The most common irritant is cigarette smoke. The American Lung Association estimates that 80-90% of COPD cases are caused by **smoking**. Other irritants include chemical fumes, air pollution, and environmental irritants, such as mold or dust.

Chronic bronchitis develops slowly over time. The cells that line the respiratory system contain fine, hairlike outgrowths from the cell called cilia. Normally, the cilia of many cells beat rhythmically to move mucus along the airways. When smoke or other irritants are inhaled, the cilia become paralyzed or snap off. When this occurs, the cilia are no longer able to move mucus, and the airways become inflamed, narrowed, and clogged. This leads to difficulty breathing and can progress to the life-threatening disease emphysema.

A mild cough, sometimes called smokers' cough, is usually the first visible sign of chronic bronchitis. Coughing brings up phlegm, although the amount varies considerably from person to person. Wheezing and **shortness of breath** may accompany the cough. Diagnostic tests show a decrease in lung function. As the disease advances, breathing becomes difficult and activity decreases. The body does not get enough oxygen, leading to changes in the composition of the blood.

Diagnosis

Initial diagnosis of bronchitis is based on observing the patient's symptoms and health history. The physician will listen to the patient's chest with a stethoscope for specific sounds that indicate lung inflammation, such as moist rales and crackling, and wheezing, that indicates airway narrowing. Moist rales is a bubbling sound heard with a stethoscope that is caused by fluid secretion in the bronchial tubes.

A **sputum culture** may be performed, particularly if the sputum is green or has blood in it, to determine whether a bacterial infection is present and to identify the disease-causing organism so that an appropriate antibiotic can be selected. Normally, the patient will be asked to cough deeply, then spit the material that comes up from the lungs (sputum) into a cup. This sample is then grown in the laboratory to determine which organisms are present. The results are available in two to three days, except for tests for **tuberculosis**, which can take as long as two months.

Occasionally, in diagnosing a chronic lung disorder, the sample of sputum is collected using a procedure called a **bronchoscopy**. In this procedure, the patient is given a local anesthetic, and a tube is passed into the airways to collect a sputum sample.

A **pulmonary function test** is important in diagnosing chronic bronchitis and other variations of COPD. This test uses an instrument called a spirometer to measure the volume of air entering and leaving the lungs. The test is done in the doctor's office and is painless. It involves breathing into the spirometer mouthpiece either normally or forcefully. Volumes less than 80% of the normal values indicate an obstructive lung disease.

To better determine what type of obstructive lung disease a patient has, the doctor may do a **chest x ray**, electrocardiogram (ECG), and blood tests. An electrocardiogram is an instrument that is used to measure the electrical activity of the heart and is useful in the diagnosis of heart conditions. Other tests may be used to measure how effectively oxygen and carbon dioxide are exchanged in the lungs.

Treatment

Acute bronchitis

When no secondary infection is present, acute bronchitis is treated in the same way as the **common cold**. Home care includes drinking plenty of fluids, resting, not smoking, increasing moisture in the air with a cool mist humidifier, and taking **acetaminophen** (Datril, Tylenol, Panadol) for fever and **pain**. **Aspirin** should not be given to children because of its association with the serious illness, **Reye's syndrome**.

Expectorant cough medicines, unlike cough suppressants, do not stop the cough. Instead they are used to thin the mucus in the lungs, making it easier to cough up. This type of cough medicine may be helpful to individuals suffering from bronchitis. People who are unsure about what type of medications are in over-the-counter cough syrups should ask their pharmacist for an explanation.

If a secondary bacterial infection is present, the infection is treated with an antibiotic. Patients need to take the entire amount of antibiotic prescribed. Stopping the antibiotic early can lead to a return of the infection. Tetracycline or ampicillin are often used to treat adults. Other possibilities include trimethoprim/ sulfamethoxazole (Bactrim or Septra) and the newer erythromycin-like drugs, such as azithromycin (Zithromax) and clarithromycin (Biaxin). Children under age eight are usually given amoxicillin (Amoxil, Pentamox, Sumox, Trimox), because tetracycline discolors permanent teeth that have not yet come in.

Chronic bronchitis

The treatment of chronic bronchitis is complex and depends on the stage of chronic bronchitis and whether other health problems are present. Lifestyle changes, such as quitting smoking and avoiding secondhand smoke or polluted air, are an important first step. Controlled **exercise** performed on a regular basis is also important.

Drug therapy begins with **bronchodilators**. These drugs relax the muscles of the bronchial tubes and allow increased air flow. They can be taken by mouth or inhaled using a nebulizer. A nebulizer is a device that delivers a regulated flow of medication into the airways. Common bronchodilators include albuterol (Ventolin, Proventil, Apo-Salvent) and metaproterenol (Alupent, Orciprenaline, Metaprel, Dey-Dose).

Anti-inflammatory medications are added to reduce swelling of the airway tissue. **Corticosteroids**, such as prednisone, can be taken orally or intravenously. Other steroids are inhaled. Long-term steroid use can have serious side effects. Other drugs, such as ipratropium (Atrovent), are given to reduce the quantity of mucus produced.

As the disease progresses, the patient may need supplemental oxygen. Complications of COPD are many and often require hospitalization in the latter stages of the disease.

Alternative treatment

Alternative practitioners focus on prevention by eating a healthy diet that strengthens the immune system and practicing **stress** management. Bronchitis can become serious if it progresses to pneumonia, therefore, antibiotics may be required. In addition, however, there are a multitude of botanical and herbal medicines that can be formulated to treat bronchitis. Some examples include inhaling eucalyptus or other essential oils in warm steam. Herbalists recommend a tea made of mullein (*Verbascum thapsus*), coltsfoot (*Tussilago farfara*), and anise seed (*Pimpinella anisum*). **Homeopathic medicine** and **traditional Chinese medicine** may also be very useful for bronchitis, and **hydrotherapy** can contribute to cleaning the chest and stimulating immune response.

Prognosis

When treated, acute bronchitis normally resolves in one to two weeks without complications, although a cough may continue for several more weeks. The progression of chronic bronchitis, on the other hand, may be slowed, and an initial improvement in symptoms may be achieved. Unfortunately, however, there is no cure for chronic bronchitis, and the disease can often lead to or coexist with emphysema. Taken together, all forms of COPD are a leading cause of death.

Prevention

The best way to prevent bronchitis is not to begin smoking or to stop smoking. Smokers are ten times more likely to die of COPD than non-smokers. Smokers who stop show improvement in lung function. Other preventative steps include avoiding chemical and environmental irritants, such as air pollution, and maintaining good overall health. Immunizations against certain types of pneumonia (as well as **influenza**) are an important preventative measure for anyone with lung or immune system diseases.

Resources

ORGANIZATIONS

American Lung Association. 1740 Broadway, New York, NY 10019. (800) 586-4872. < http:// www.lungusa.org > .

National Heart, Lung and Blood Institute. P.O. Box 30105, Bethesda, MD 20824-0105. (301) 251-1222. < http:// www.nhlbi.nih.gov > .

National Jewish Center for Immunology and Respiratory Medicine. 1400 Jackson St., Denver, CO 80206. (800) 222-5864. < http://www.nationaljewish.org/ main.html > .

Tish Davidson, A.M.

Bronchodilators

Definition

Bronchodilators are medicines that help open the bronchial tubes (airways) of the lungs, allowing more air to flow through them.

Purpose

People with **asthma** have trouble breathing, because their airways are inflamed and become narrowed. Normally, air moves smoothly from the mouth and nose through the airways and into the tiny air sacs of the lungs as a person breathes in. Breathing out (exhaling) happens automatically when the person stops breathing in. In a person with asthma, breathing in (inhaling) is not a problem. Incoming air can slide around the blockage, because the act of breathing in makes the airways expand. The problem comes when the person with asthma tries to breathe out. The air can no longer get past the blockage, and it remains trapped in the lungs. The person can then only take shallow breaths. Bronchodilators work by relaxing the smooth muscles that line the airways. This makes the airways open wider and allows air to leave the lungs. These drugs also are used to relieve breathing problems associated with **emphysema**, chronic **bronchitis**, and other lung diseases.

Description

Some bronchodilators are inhaled, using a nebulizer or an inhalation aerosol. Others are taken as injections or by mouth. Most are available only by prescription, but a few, such as ephedrine, can be bought without a physician's prescription. Examples of bronchodilators are albuterol (Proventil, Ventolin), epinephrine (Primatene), ipratropium (Atrovent), metaproterenol (Alupent, Metaprel), and terbutaline (Brethine).

Recommended dosage

The recommended dosage depends on the type of bronchodilator and may be different for different patients. The physician who prescribed the drug or the pharmacist who filled the prescription can recommend correct dosage.

Precautions

Bronchodilators come with patient instructions that must be carefully read before using the medicine. If there is any confusion about how to use the

medicine, patients should check with the physician or pharmacist. These medicines must be used exactly as directed. Taking larger than recommended doses or using the medicine too often can lead to serious side effects and even **death**.

If symptoms do not improve or if they get worse after using a bronchodilator, the patient should call a physician right away.

Although some bronchodilators are available without a physician's prescription, these medicines should not be used unless a physician has diagnosed the patient's condition as asthma.

Research shows that frequent bronchodilator use over time can tighten airway muscles in some people. Some physicians advise patients to consider controlling asthma with anti-inflammatory drugs including inhaled steroids such as beclomethasone dipropionate (Beclovent, Vanceril), flunisolide (AeroBid) or triamcinolone acetonide (Azmacort). A 2004 Canadian study has questioned a standard practice of increasing steroids after asthma attacks or worsened symptoms. Also, research in 2004 showed that people with asthma who worked closely with their physicians to self-manage their asthma had fewer attacks, which reduces the need for bronchodilators. Carefully managing asthma also reduces visits to the emergency department and hospitalizations.

Persons with diabetes should be aware that the bronchodilator epinephrine may raise their blood sugar levels.

Patients who are using an aerosol bronchodilator and an aerosol form of either ipratropium or a corticosteroid such as beclomethasone dipropionate (Beclovent, Vanceril) should use the bronchodilator first, then wait 5 minutes before using the other medicine. A physician should be consulted before using any other inhaled medications or other asthma medicines. The physician must determine the proper amount of time between doses.

Some bronchodilator products contain sulfites that trigger an allergic reaction in certain people. Anyone who has a sulfite allergy should read the label carefully or check with a physician or pharmacist before using a bronchodilator. Call a physician immediately if any of these signs of an allergic reaction to sulfite occur:

- bluish coloration of the skin
- flushed or red face or skin
- faintness
- severe **dizziness**
- increased **wheezing** or other breathing problems
- skin rash, **hives**, or **itching**
- swelling of the face, lips, or eyelids

Special conditions

People with certain medical conditions or who are taking certain other medicines can have problems if they use bronchodilators. Before using these drugs, a physician should be made aware of any of these conditions:

ALLERGIES. Anyone who has had unusual reactions to any bronchodilator or an inhaled form of any other drug in the past should let his or her physician know before taking the drugs again. The physician should also be told about any **allergies** to foods, dyes, preservatives, or other substances.

Patients who are allergic to soybeans, soy lecithin, peanuts, or drugs based on atropine should not use the bronchodilator ipratropium (Atrovent).

PREGNANCY. In studies of laboratory animals, some bronchodilators cause **birth defects** or **miscarriage** when the animals are given doses many times the usual human dose. Whether these drugs cause such problems in humans in unknown. Any woman who is pregnant or plans to become pregnant should check with her physician before using a bronchodilator.

BREASTFEEDING. Some bronchodilators pass into breast milk. Breastfeeding mothers should check with their physicians before using bronchodilators.

OTHER MEDICAL CONDITIONS. Before using bronchodilators, people with any of these medical problems should make sure their physicians are aware of their conditions:

- glaucoma
- brain damage
- convulsions (seizures)—recently or anytime in the past
- mental illness
- parkinson's disease
- diabetes
- heart or blood vessel diseases
- rapid or irregular heartbeat
- high blood pressure
- overactive thyroid
- enlarged prostate
- obstruction of the neck of the bladder

USE OF CERTAIN MEDICINES. Using bronchodilators with certain other drugs may affect the way the drugs work or may increase the chance of side effects.

Side effects

Some patients have a dry or irritated throat or a **dry mouth** after using bronchodilators. To help prevent these problems, gargling and rinsing the mouth or taking a sip of water after each dose.

The most common side effects are nervousness or restlessness and trembling. These problems usually go away as the body adjusts to the drug and do not require medical treatment. Less common side effects, such as bad taste in the mouth, coughing, dizziness or lightheadedness, drowsiness, **headache**, sweating, fast or pounding heartbeat, **muscle cramps** or twitches, **nausea**, **vomiting**, **diarrhea**, sleep problems and weakness also may occur and do not need medical attention unless they do not go away or they interfere with normal activities.

More serious side effects are not common, but may occur. If any of the following side effects occur, the physician who prescribed the medicine should be contacted as soon as possible:

- chest **pain** or discomfort
- irregular or fluttery heartbeat
- unusual bruising
- hives or rash
- swelling

- wheezing or other breathing problems

- numbness in the hands or feet

- blurred vision

Other side effects are possible. Anyone who has unusual symptoms after using a bronchodilator should get in touch with his or her physician.

Interactions

Bronchodilators may interact with a number of other medicines. When this happens, the effects of one or both of the drugs may change or the risk of side effects may be greater. Anyone who takes these drugs should let the physician know all other medicines he or she is taking. Among the drugs that may interact with bronchodilators are:

- monoamine oxidase inhibitors (MAO inhibitors) such as phenelzine (Nardil) and tranylcypromine (Parnate), used to treat depression

- other bronchodilators

- tricyclic antidepressants such as amitriptyline (Elavil) and imipramine (Tofranil)

- beta blockers such as propranolol (Inderal) and atenolol (Tenormin), used to control high blood pressure

- digitalis medicines, used to treat heart conditions, such as digoxin (Lanoxin)

- drugs, such as certain **diuretics** (water pills), that lower potassium levels

- ergoloid mesylates such as Hydergine, used to treat symptoms of **Alzheimer's disease** or multiple small stokes

- ergotamine (Cafergot, Ergostat, and other brands), used to treat migraine and cluster headaches

- the antidepressant maprotiline (Ludiomil).

The list above does not include every drug that may interact with bronchodilators. Be sure to check with a physician or pharmacist before combining bronchodilators with any other prescription or non-prescription (over-the-counter) medicine.

Resources

PERIODICALS

"Study Calls Standard Asthma Management Into Doubt." *Doctor* July 15, 2004: 4.

"What's New in: Asthma and Allergic Rhinitis." *Pulse* September 20, 2004: 50.

"Wheezing? Check Your Inhaler." *Prevention* September 2004: 34.

ORGANIZATIONS

American Academy of Allergy, Asthma, and Immunology. 611 East Wells St., Milwaukee, WI 53202. (800) 822-2762. <http://www.aaaai.org>.

Asthma and Allergy Foundation of America. 1233 20th Street, NW, Suite 402, Washington, DC 20036. (800) 727-8462. <http://www.aafa.org>.

National Heart, Lung and Blood Institute. P.O. Box 30105, Bethesda, MD 20824-0105. (301) 251-1222. <http://www.nhlbi.nih.gov>.

Nancy Ross-Flanigan
Teresa G. Odle

Bronchoscopy

Definition

Bronchoscopy is a procedure in which a cylindrical fiberoptic scope is inserted into the airways. This scope contains a viewing device that allows the visual examination of the lower airways.

Purpose

During a bronchoscopy, a physician can visually examine the lower airways, including the larynx, trachea, bronchi, and bronchioles. The procedure is used to examine the mucosal surface of the airways for abnormalities that might be associated with a variety of lung diseases. Its use includes the visualization of airway obstructions such as a tumor, or the collection of specimens for the diagnosis of **cancer** originating in the bronchi of the lungs (bronchogenic cancer). It can also be used to collect specimens for culture to diagnose infectious diseases such as **tuberculosis**. The type of specimens collected can include sputum (composed of saliva and discharges from the respiratory passages), tissue samples from the bronchi or bronchioles, or cells collected from washing the lining of the bronchi or bronchioles. The instrument used in bronchoscopy, a bronchoscope, is a slender cylindrical instrument containing a light and an eyepiece. There are two types of bronchoscopes, a rigid tube that is sometimes referred to as an open-tube or ventilating bronchoscope, and a more flexible fiberoptic tube. This tube contains four smaller passages—two for light to pass through, one for seeing through and one that can accommodate medical instruments that may be used for biopsy or suctioning, or that medication can be passed through.

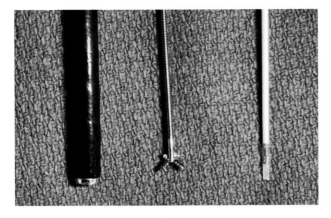

Instruments used in bronchoscopy procedures. *(Custom Medical Stock Photo. Reproduced by permission.)*

Bronchoscopy may be used for the following purposes:

- to diagnose cancer, tuberculosis, lung infection, or other lung disease

- to examine an inherited deformity of the lungs

- to remove a foreign body in the lungs, such as a mucus plug, tumor, or excessive secretions

- to remove tissue samples, also known as biopsy, to test for cancer cells, help with staging the advancement of the lung cancer, or to treat a tumor with laser therapy

- to allow examination of a suspected tumor, obstruction, secretion, bleeding, or foreign body in the airways

- to determine the cause of a persistent **cough**, **wheezing**, or a cough that includes blood in the sputum

- to evaluate the effectiveness of lung cancer treatments

Precautions

Patients not breathing adequately on their own due to severe **respiratory failure** may require mechanical ventilation prior to bronchoscopy. It may not be appropriate to perform bronchoscopy on patients with an unstable heart condition. All patients must be constantly monitored while undergoing a bronchoscopy so that any abnormal reactions can be dealt with immediately.

Description

There are two types of bronchoscopes, a rigid tube and a fiberoptic tube. Because of its flexibility, the fiberoptic tube is usually preferred. However, if the purpose of the procedure is to remove a foreign body caught in the windpipe or lungs of a child, the more rigid tube must be used because of its larger size. The patient will either lie face-up on his/her back or sit upright in a chair. Medication to decrease secretions, lessen **anxiety**, and relax the patient are often given prior to the procedure. While breathing through the nose, anesthesia is sprayed into the mouth or nose to numb it. It will take one to two minutes for the anesthesia to take effect. Once this happens, the bronchoscope will be put into the patient's mouth or nose and moved down into the throat. While the bronchoscope is moving down the throat, additional anesthesia is put into the bronchoscope to numb the lower parts of the airways. Using the eyepiece, the physician then observes the trachea and bronchi, and the mucosal lining of these passageways, looking for any abnormalities that may be present.

If the purpose of the bronchoscopy is to take tissue samples or biopsy, forceps or a bronchial brush are used to obtain cells. If the purpose is to identify an infectious agent, a bronchoalveolar lavage (BAL) can be used to gather fluid for culture purposes. Also, if any foreign matter is found in the airways, it can be removed.

Another procedure using bronchoscopy is called fluorescence bronchoscopy. This can be used to detect precancerous cells present in the airways. By using a fluorescent light in the bronchoscope, precancerous tissue will appear dark red, while healthy tissue will appear green. This technique can help detect lung cancer at an early stage, so that treatment can be started early.

Alternative procedures

Depending upon the purpose of the bronchoscopy, alternatives might include a computed tomography scan (CT) or no procedure at all. Bronchoscopy is often performed to investigate an abnormality that shows up on a **chest x ray** or CT scan. If the purpose is to obtain biopsy specimens, one option is to perform surgery, which carries greater risks. Another option is percutaneous (through the skin) biopsy guided by computed tomography.

Preparation

The doctor should be informed of any **allergies** and all the medications that the patient is currently taking. The doctor may instruct the patient not to take medications like **aspirin** or anti-inflammatory drugs, which interfere with clotting, for a period of time prior to the procedure. The patient needs to fast for 6 to 12 hours prior to the procedure and refrain from drinking any liquids the day of the procedure. The bronchoscopy takes about 45 to 60 minutes, with results usually available in one day. Prior to the bronchoscopy, several tests may be done, including a chest x ray and blood work. Sometimes a bronchoscopy is done under **general anesthesia**. Patients usually have an intravenous (IV) line in the arm. Most likely, the procedure will be done under **local anesthesia**, which is sprayed into the nose or mouth. This is necessary to decrease the gag reflex. A sedative may also be used to help the patient relax. It is important that the patient understands that at no time will the airway be blocked and that oxygen can be supplied through the bronchoscope. A signed consent form is necessary for this procedure.

Aftercare

After the bronchoscopy, the patient will be monitored for vital signs such as heart rate, blood pressure, and breathing, while resting in bed. Sometimes patients have an abnormal reaction to anesthesia. All saliva should be spit into a basin so that it can be examined for the presence of blood. If a biopsy was taken, the patient should not cough or clear the throat as this might dislodge any blood clot that has formed and cause bleeding. No food or drink should be consumed for about two hours after the procedure or until the anesthesia wears off. Diet is gradually progressed from ice chips and clear liquids to the patient's regular diet. There will also be a temporary **sore throat** and hoarseness that may last for a few days.

Risks

Minor side effects arise from the bronchoscope causing abrasion of the lining of the airways. This results in some swelling and inflammation, as well as hoarseness caused from abrading the vocal cords. If this abrasion is more serious, it can lead to respiratory

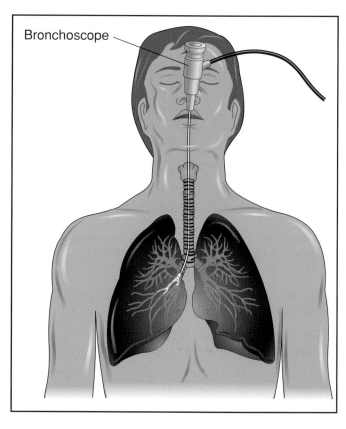

Bronchoscopy is a procedure in which a hollow, flexible tube is inserted into the airways, allowing the physician to visually examine the lower airways, including the larynx, trachea, bronchi, and bronchioles. It can also be used to collect specimens for bacteriological culture to diagnose infectious diseases such as tuberculosis. *(Illustration by Electronic Illustrators Group.)*

difficulty or bleeding of the airway lining. A more serious risk involved in having a bronchoscopy performed is the occurrence of a **pneumothorax**, due to puncturing of the lungs, which allows air to escape into the space between the lung and the chest wall. These risks are greater with the use of a rigid bronchoscope than with a fiberoptic bronchoscope. If a rigid tube is used, there is also a risk of chipped teeth.

Normal results

Normal tracheal appearance consists of smooth muscle with C-shaped rings of cartilage at regular intervals. The trachea and the bronchi are lined with a mucous membrane.

Abnormal results

Abnormal bronchoscopy findings may involve abnormalities of the bronchial wall such as inflammation, swelling, ulceration, or anatomical abnormalities. The bronchoscopy may also reveal the presence of abnormal substances in the trachea and bronchi. If samples are taken, the results could indicate cancer, disease-causing agents or other lung disease. Other abnormalities include constriction or narrowing (stenosis), compression, dilation of vessels, or abnormal branching of the bronchi. Abnormal substances that might be found in the airways include blood, secretions, or mucous plugs. Any abnormalities are discussed with the patient.

Cindy L. Jones, Ph.D.

Brucellosis

Definition

Brucellosis is a bacterial disease caused by members of the *Brucella* genus that can infect humans but primarily infects livestock. Symptoms of the disease include intermittent **fever**, sweating, chills, aches, and mental depression. The disease can become chronic and recur, particularly if untreated.

Description

Also known as undulant fever, Malta fever, Gibraltar fever, Bang's disease, or Mediterranean fever, brucellosis is most likely to occur among those individuals who regularly work with livestock. The disease originated in domestic livestock but was passed on to wild animal species, including the elk and buffalo of the western United States. In humans, brucellosis continues to be spread via unpasteurized milk obtained from infected cows or through contact with the discharges of cattle and goats during **miscarriage**. In areas of the world where milk is not pasteurized, for example in Latin America and the Mediterranean, the disease is still contracted by ingesting unpasteurized dairy products. However, in the United States, the widespread pasteurization of milk and nearly complete eradication of the infection from cattle has reduced the number of human cases from 6,500 in 1940 to about 70 in 1994.

Causes and symptoms

The disease is caused by several different species of parasitic bacteria of the genus Brucella. *B. abortus* is found in cattle and can cause cows to abort their fetuses. *B. suis* is most often found in hogs and is more deadly when contracted by humans than the organism found in cattle. *B. melitensis* is found in goats and sheep and causes the most severe illness in humans. *B. rangiferi* infects reindeer and caribou, and *B. canis* is found in dogs.

A human contracts the disease by coming into contact with an infected animal and either allowing the bacteria to enter a cut, breathing in the bacteria, or by consuming unpasteurized milk or fresh goat cheese obtained from a contaminated animal. In the United States, the disease is primarily confined to slaughterhouse workers.

Scientists do not agree about whether brucellosis can be transmitted from one person to another, although some people have been infected from a tainted blood **transfusion** or bone marrow transplant. Newborn babies have also contracted the illness from their mothers during birth. Currently, it is believed that brucellosis can also be transmitted sexually.

The disease is not usually fatal, but the intermittent fevers (a source of its nickname, "undulant fever") can be exhausting. Symptoms usually appear between five days and a month after exposure and begin with a single bout of high fever accompanied by shivering, aching, and drenching sweats that last for a few days. Other symptoms may include **headache**, poor appetite, backache, weakness, and depression. Mental depression can be so severe that the patient may become suicidal.

In rare, untreated cases, the disease can become so severe that it leads to fatal complications, such as **pneumonia** or bacterial **meningitis**. *B. melitensis* can cause miscarriages, especially during the first three months of **pregnancy**. The condition can also occur in a chronic form, in which symptoms recur over a period of months or years.

Diagnosis

Brucellosis is usually diagnosed by detecting one or more *Brucella* species in blood or urine samples. The bacteria may be positively identified using biochemical methods or using a technique whereby, if present in the sample, the brucellosis bacteria are made to fluoresce. Brucellosis may also be diagnosed by culturing and isolating the bacteria from one of the above samples. Blood samples will also indicate elevated antibody levels or increased amounts of a protein produced directly in response to infection with brucellosis bacteria.

Treatment

Prolonged treatment with **antibiotics**, including **tetracyclines** (with streptomycin), co-trimoxazole, and **sulfonamides**, is effective. Bed rest is also imperative. In the chronic form of brucellosis, the symptoms may recur, requiring a second course of treatment.

Prognosis

Early diagnosis and prompt treatment is essential to prevent chronic infection. Untreated, the disease may linger for years, but it is rarely fatal. Relapses may also occur.

Prevention

There is no human vaccine for brucellosis, but humans can be protected by controlling the disease in livestock. After checking to make sure an animal is not already infected, and destroying those that are, all livestock should be immunized. Butchers and those who work in slaughterhouses should wear protective glasses and clothing, and protect broken skin from infection.

Some experts suggest that a person with the disease refrain from engaging in unprotected sex until free of the disease. The sexual partners of an infected person should also be closely monitored for signs of infection.

Resources

ORGANIZATIONS
Centers for Disease Control and Prevention. 1600 Clifton Rd., NE, Atlanta, GA 30333. (800) 311-3435, (404) 639-3311. < http://www.cdc.gov > .

OTHER
"Bacterial Diseases." Healthtouch Online Page. < http:www.healthtouch.com > .

Centers for Disease Control. < http://www.cdc.gov/nccdphp/ddt/ddthome.htm > .

Carol A. Turkington

Brugian filariasis *see* **Elephantiasis**

Bruises

Definition

Bruises, or ecchymoses, are a discoloration and tenderness of the skin or mucous membranes due to the leakage of blood from an injured blood vessel into the tissues. Pupura refers to bruising as the result of a disease condition. A very small bruise is called a petechia. These often appear as many tiny red dots clustered together, and could indicate a serious problem.

Description

Bruises change colors over time in a predictable pattern, so that it is possible to estimate when an injury occurred by the color of the bruise. Initially, a bruise will be reddish, the color of the blood under the skin. After one to two days, the red blood cells begin to break down, and the bruise will darken to a blue or purplish color. This fades to green at about day six. Around the eighth or ninth day, the skin over the bruised area will have a brown or yellowish appearance, and it will gradually diminish back to its normal color.

Long periods of standing will cause the blood that collects in a bruise to seep through the tissues. Bruises are actually made of little pools of blood, so the blood in one place may flow downhill after awhile and appear in another. For instance, bruising in the back of the abdomen may eventually appear in the groin; bruising in the thigh or the knee will work its way down to the ankle.

Causes and symptoms

Healthy people may develop bruises from any injury that doesn't break through the skin. Vigorous **exercise** may also cause bruises due to bringing about small tears in blood vessels walls. In a condition known as purpura simplex, there is a tendency to bruise easily due to an increased fragility of the blood vessels. Bruises also develop easily in the elderly, because the skin and blood vessels have a tendency to become thinner and more fragile with **aging**, and there is an increased use of medications that interfere with

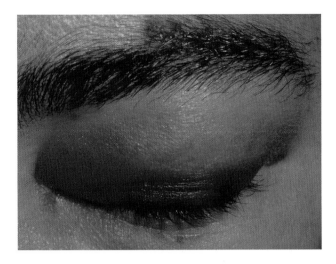

A close-up view of woman's bruised left eye. *(Custom Medical Stock Photo. Reproduced by permission.)*

the blood clotting system. In the condition known as purpura senilis, the elderly develop bruises from minimal contact that may take up to several months to completely heal.

The use of nonsteroidal anti-inflammatories such as ibuprofen (Advil) and naproxen (Aleve) may lead to increased bruising. **Aspirin**, antidepressants, **asthma** medications, and cortisone medications also have this effect. The anti-clotting medications also known as blood thinners, especially the drug Warfarin (Coumadin), may be the cause of particularly severe bruising.

Sometimes bruises are connected with more serious illnesses. There are a number of diseases that cause excessive bleeding or bleeding from injuries too slight to have consequences in healthy people. An abnormal tendency to bleed may be due to hereditary bleeding disorders, certain prescription medications, diseases of the blood such as leukemia, and diseases that increase the fragility of blood vessels. If there are large areas of bruising or bruises develop very easily, this may herald a problem. Other causes that should be ruled out include **liver disease**, **alcoholism**, drug **addiction**, and acquired immune deficiency syndrome (**AIDS**). Bruising that occurs around the navel may indicate dangerous internal bleeding; bruising behind the ear, called Battle's sign, may be due to a skull fracture; and raised bruises may point to autoimmune disease.

Diagnosis

Bruising is usually a minor problem, which does not require a medical diagnosis. However, faced with extensive bruising, bruising with no apparent cause, or bruising in certain locations, a physician will pursue an evaluation that will include a number of blood tests. If the area of the bruise becomes hard, an x ray may be required.

Treatment

A bruise by itself needs no medical treatment. It is often recommended that ice packs be applied on and off during the first 24 hours of injury to reduce the bruising. After that, heat, especially moist heat, is recommended to increase the circulation and the healing of the injured tissues. Rest, elevation of the effected part, and compression with a bandage will also retard the accumulation of blood. Rarely, if a bruise is so large that the body cannot completely absorb it or if the site becomes infected, it may have to be surgically removed.

Alternative treatment

Several types of topical applications are usually recommend to speed healing and to reduce the **pain** associated with bruises. Vitamin K cream can be applied directly to the site of injury. Astringent herbs such as witch hazel, *Hamamelis virginiana*, can be used. This will tighten the tissues and therefore diminish the bruising. The homeopathic remedy, *Arnica montana*, can be applied as a cream or gel to unbroken skin.

Oral homeopathic remedies may reduce bruising, pain, and swelling as well. *Arnica montana*, at 30 ml (1 oz), taken one to two times per day is highly recommended. For ledum, 30 ml (1 oz) one to two times per day is also useful.

Prognosis

The blood under the skin which causes the discoloration of bruising should be totally reabsorbed by the body in three weeks or less. At that time, the skin color should completely return to normal.

Sometimes, a bruise may become solid and increase in size instead of dissolving. This may indicate blood trapped in the tissues, which may be need to be drained. This is referred to as a hematoma. Less commonly, the body may develop calcium deposits at the injury site in a process called heterotopic ossification.

Prevention

Vitamin K promotes normal clotting in the blood, and therefore may help reduce the tendency to bruise easily. Green leafy vegetables, alfalfa, broccoli, seaweed, and fish liver oils are dietary sources of vitamin K. Other good foods to eat would be those containing bioflavonoids, such as reddish-blue berries. These can assist in strengthening the connective tissue, which will decrease the spread of blood and bruising. Zinc and vitamin C supplements are also recommended for this.

Resources

BOOKS

Editors of Prevention Magazine Health Books, editors. *The Doctors Book of Home Remedies*. Prevention Health Books, 2000.

Patience Paradox

Bruton's agammaglobulinemia *see* **X-linked agammaglobulinemia**

Bruxism

Definition

Bruxism is the habit of clenching and grinding the teeth. It most often occurs at night during sleep, but it may also occur during the day. It is an unconscious behavior, perhaps performed to release **anxiety**, aggression, or anger.

Description

Bruxism is one of the oldest disorders known, and approximately one in four adults experiences it. Most people are not aware of it before their teeth have been damaged.

Causes and symptoms

While bruxism is typically associated with **stress**, it may also be triggered by abnormal occlusion (the way the upper and lower teeth fit together), or crooked or missing teeth.

Symptoms of bruxism include: dull headaches; sore and tired facial muscles; earaches; sensitive teeth; and locking, popping, and clicking of the jaw.

During a dental examination, a dentist may recognize damage resulting from bruxism, including: enamel loss from the chewing surfaces of teeth; flattened tooth surfaces; loosened teeth; and fractured teeth and fillings. Left untreated, bruxism may lead to tooth loss and jaw dysfunction.

KEY TERMS

Enamel—The hard outermost surface of a tooth.

High spot—An area of a tooth or restoration that feels abnormal or uncomfortable because it hits its opposing tooth before other teeth meet.

Night guard—A removable, custom-fitted plastic appliance that fits between the upper and lower teeth to prevent them from grinding against each other.

Occlusion—The way upper and lower teeth fit together during biting and chewing.

Rolfing—Based on the belief that proper alignment of various parts of the body is necessary for physical and mental health, rolfing uses deep tissue massage and movement exercises in an attempt to bring the body into correct alignment.

Temporomandibular joint (TMJ)—The jaw joint formed by the mandible (lower jaw bone) moving against the temporal bone of the skull.

Diagnosis

Medical and dental histories and examinations are necessary to differentiate bruxism from other conditions that may cause similar **pain**, such as ear infections, dental infections, and temporomandibular joint (TMJ) dysfunction. However, uncommonly worn-down teeth strongly suggest a diagnosis of bruxism.

Treatment

To prevent further damage to the teeth, bruxism is treated by placing a removable, custom-fitted plastic appliance called a night guard between the upper and lower teeth. Although the clenching and grinding behavior may continue, the teeth wear away the plastic instead of each other.

In some cases, abnormal occlusion may be adjusted and high spots removed so that the teeth fit together in a more comfortable position. Missing teeth may be replaced and crooked teeth may be straightened with orthodontic treatment to eliminate possible underlying causes of bruxism. In cases where jaw muscles are very tight, a dentist may prescribe **muscle relaxants**.

Alternative treatment

Stress management and behavior modification techniques may be useful to break the habit of

---

clenching and teeth grinding. Tight jaw muscles may be relaxed by applying warm compresses to the sides of the face. Herbal muscle relaxants also can be helpful. **Massage therapy** and deep tissue realignment, including **rolfing**, can assist in releasing the clenching pattern. This is a more permanent alternative treatment for bruxism.

Prognosis

Bruxism may cause permanent damage to teeth and chronic jaw pain unless properly diagnosed and promptly treated. The behavior may be eliminated if its underlying causes are found and addressed.

Prevention

Increased awareness in patients prone to anxiety, aggression, or anger may prevent the habit of bruxism from developing.

Resources

ORGANIZATIONS

Academy of General Dentistry. Suite 1200, 211 East Chicago Ave., Chicago, IL 60611.(312) 440-4300. <http://www.agd.org>.

American Dental Association. 211 E. Chicago Ave., Chicago, IL 60611. (312) 440-2500. <http://www.ada.org>.

Bethany Thivierge

Bubonic plague *see* **Plague**

Budd-Chiari syndrome

Definition

Budd-Chiari syndrome is a rare problem that results from blood clotting in the veins flowing out of the liver (hepatic veins). The high pressure of blood in these veins leads to an enlarged liver, and to an accumulation of fluid in the abdomen, called **ascites**.

Description

The liver, the largest internal organ in the human body, is responsible for many vital physiologic processes. Blood flow through the liver nourishes the liver, carries in substances that the liver will process, and carries away substances that the liver has produced. When blood cannot flow out freely from the liver, blood pressure rises in the veins of the liver,

---

KEY TERMS

Ascites—Accumulation of fluid in the abdomen.

Biopsy—Surgical removal of a tiny bit of tissue for examination under the microscope.

Catheter—A tubular surgical instrument.

Phlebitis—Inflammation of a vein.

Polycythemia vera—An excess number of red blood cells in the blood.

Sickle cell anemia—An inherited disease in which red blood cells take an unusual shape, leading to circulation problems.

---

leading to **blood clots** within the liver. Also, some of the blood plasma can leak through the walls of the veins and accumulate within the abdomen (ascites).

Causes and symptoms

The major symptoms include **pain** in the upper right-hand portion of the abdomen and a build-up of fluid in the abdomen. In the United States, blood disorders are the most common causes. Among these disorders are **polycythemia vera** (an increase in the number of red blood cells), and sickle cell anemia. In parts of the world where **liver cancer** is common, a form of liver **cancer** is the most frequent cause.

Other causes sometimes include:

- certain infections
- use of **oral contraceptives**
- body changes in **pregnancy** and the postpartum period
- phlebitis (inflammation of a vein)
- injury to the abdomen
- membranous webs (especially in Asia)

Diagnosis

Diagnosis of Budd-Chiari syndrome can be made by an internist (a specialist in diseases of the internal organs), a gastroenterologist (a specialist in the diseases of the digestive system), or a general surgeon. On **physical examination**, the doctor will note that the liver is larger than normal. Often an ultrasound scan of the liver will show abnormalities in the size of the liver, an abnormal pattern of the veins in the liver, and other abnormalities. A CT scan will often show similar abnormalities.

Once these abnormalities are confirmed, the key test is called hepatic vein catheterization. In this test, a narrow tube is snaked through the body until it reaches the hepatic veins. An instrument at the tip of the catheter can measure the pressure within each segment of the hepatic vein.

In some cases, a tiny amount of radioactive material is injected into a patient, and then an abnormal pattern of radioactivity in the liver can be revealed. In other cases, a **liver biopsy** enables a physician to examine cells from the liver itself. Cells damaged by Budd-Chiari syndrome have a characteristic appearance easily identifiable to a physician.

Treatment

Surgery

Most patients with Budd-Chiari syndrome must have surgery. A surgeon will re-route blood flow around the clotted hepatic vein into a large vein called the vena cava. The exact technique will depend on the specific location of the clots and other factors. In certain patients, other surgical techniques may be used. For patients who otherwise would have less than six months to live, **liver transplantation** is sometimes performed.

In a few patients, a "balloon catheter" can open the blocked blood vessels, without the need for major surgery.

Drugs

Sometimes, anti-clotting drugs such as urokinase can be used for patients with a sudden onset of clotting in the veins of the liver. These drugs do not seem to work when the clots have become established.

Prognosis

If surgery is done before permanent liver damage sets in, long-term survival is possible. In these cases, damaged liver cells can actually recover. If patients are already very sick with **liver disease**, the surgery may not be as helpful.

Prevention

The best approach to prevention is to carefully control the blood disorders that can lead to Budd-Chiari syndrome.

Resources

BOOKS

Gadacz, Thomas R., and John L. Cameron. "Budd-Chiari Syndrome and Surgery of the Hepatic Vasculature." In *Shackelford's Surgery of the Alimentary Tract*, edited by J.G. Turcotte, 3rd ed. Vol. 3. Philadelphia: W. B. Saunders Co., 1991.

Richard H. Lampert

Buerger's disease

Definition

Buerger's disease is an inflammation of the arteries, veins, and nerves in the legs, principally, leading to restricted blood flow. Left untreated, Buerger's disease can lead to **gangrene** of the affected areas. Buerger's disease is also known as thromboangitis obliterans.

Causes and symptoms

The exact cause of Buerger's disease is not known. It is seen most often in young to middle-aged men (ages 20-40) who are heavy smokers of cigarettes. Cases of this disease in non-smokers are very rare, hence, cigarette **smoking** is considered a causative factor. Approximately 40% of the patients have a history of inflammation of a vein (phlebitis), which may play a role in the development of Buerger's disease. The disease is mainly seen in the legs of affected persons, but may also appear in their arms. Early symptoms include decrease in the blood supply (arterial **ischemia**) and superficial (near the skin surface) phlebitis. The main symptom is **pain** in the affected areas. Onset of the disease is gradual and first occurs in the feet or hands. Inflammation occurs in small and medium-sized arteries and veins near the surface of the limb. In advanced cases, blood vessels in other parts of the body may be affected. There is a progressive decrease in the blood flow to the affected areas. The pulse in arteries of the feet is weak or undetectable. The lack of blood flow can lead to gangrene, which is decay of tissue due to restricted blood supply. A cold sensitivity in the hands, similar to that seen in **Raynaud's disease**, can develop. In this case, the hands turn color–white, blue, and then red–when exposed to the cold.

Diagnosis

Diagnosis is usually made from the clinical symptoms. Patients frequently complain of **numbness, tingling**, or burning sensations in the affected area before evidence of vascular inflammation becomes apparent.

KEY TERMS

Gangrene—A decay of the tissue in a part of the body that experiences restricted blood flow.

Inflammation—A local reaction to irritation, injury, or infection characterized by pain, swelling, redness, and occasional loss of function.

Ischemia—A decrease in the blood supply to an area of the body caused by obstruction or constriction of blood vessels.

Phlebitis—Inflammation of a vein.

Treatment

There is no effective medication or surgery for this disease. Patients must stop smoking to halt further development of the symptoms. **Vasodilators**, drugs that increase the diameter of the blood vessels, can be administered, but may not be effective. Exposure of affected areas to heat or cold should be avoided. Trauma to the feet and other affected areas should be avoided and infections must be treated promptly.

Prognosis

The disease is progressive in patients who do not stop smoking. Areas with gangrene must be removed surgically.

Prevention

Smoking is the only known causative agent for this disease and should be avoided.

Resources

BOOKS

Berkow, R., editor. *The Merck Manual.* 17th ed. Rahway, NJ: Merck and Co., 1997.

John T. Lohr, PhD

Bulging eyes *see* **Exophthalmos**

Bulimia nervosa

Definition

Bulimia nervosa is a serious and sometimes life-threatening eating disorder affecting mainly young

KEY TERMS

Binge—To consume large amounts of food uncontrollably within a short time period.

Diuretic—A drug that promotes the formation and excretion of urine.

Neurotransmitters—Certain brain chemicals that may function abnormally in acutely ill bulimic patients.

Obsessive-compulsive disorder (OCD)—A disorder that may accompany bulimia, characterized by the tendency to perform repetitive acts or rituals in order to relieve anxiety.

Purge—To rid the body of food and calories, commonly by vomiting or using laxatives.

women. People with bulimia, known as bulimics, consume large amounts of food (binge) and then try to rid themselves of the food and calories (purge) by **fasting**, excessive **exercise**, **vomiting**, or using **laxatives**. The behavior often serves to reduce **stress** and relieve **anxiety**. Because bulimia results from an excessive concern with weight control and self-image, and is often accompanied by depression, it is also considered a psychiatric illness.

Description

Bulimia nervosa is a serious health problem for over two million adolescent girls and young women in the United States. The bingeing and purging activity associated with this disorder can cause severe damage, even **death**, although the risk of death is not as high as for **anorexia nervosa**, an eating disorder that leads to excessive weight loss.

Binge eating may in rare instances cause the stomach to rupture. In the case of purging, **heart failure** can result due to loss of vital **minerals** such as potassium. Vomiting causes other serious problems, including acid-related scarring of the fingers (if used to induce vomiting) and damage to tooth enamel. In addition, the tube that brings food from the mouth to the stomach (the esophagus) often becomes inflamed and salivary glands can become swollen. Irregular menstrual periods can also result, and interest in sex may diminish.

Most bulimics find it difficult to stop their behavior without professional help. Many typically recognize that the behavior is not normal, but feel out of control. Some bulimics struggle with other compulsive, risky

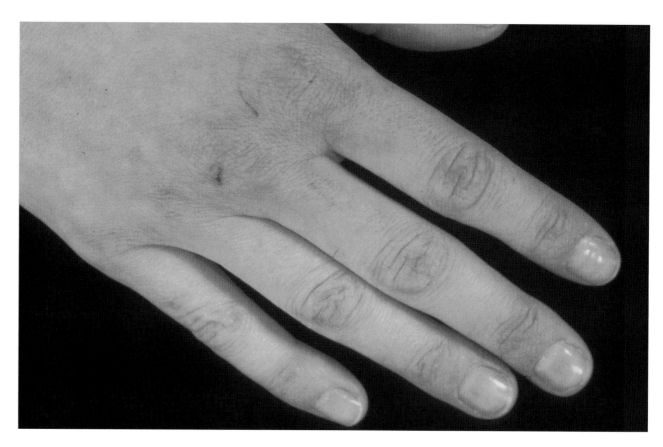

The cuts on the knuckles shown in this photograph are due to the teeth breaking the skin during self-induced vomiting.
(B. Bodine/Custom Medical Stock Photo, Inc. Reproduced by permission.)

behaviors such as drug and alcohol **abuse**. Many also suffer from other psychiatric illnesses, including clinical depression, anxiety, and **obsessive-compulsive disorder** (OCD).

Most bulimics are females in their teens or early 20s. Males account for only 5-10% of all cases. People of all races develop the disorder, but most of those diagnosed are white.

Bulimic behavior is often carried out in secrecy, accompanied by feelings of guilt or shame. Outwardly, many people with bulimia appear healthy and successful, while inside they have feelings of helplessness and low self-esteem.

Causes and symptoms

Causes

The cause of bulimia is unknown. Researchers believe that it may be caused by a combination of genetic and environmental factors. Bulimia tends to run in families. Research shows that certain brain chemicals, known as neurotransmitters, may function abnormally in acutely ill bulimia patients. Scientists also believe there may be a link between bulimia and other psychiatric problems, such as depression and OCD. Environmental influences include participation in work or sports that emphasize thinness, such as modeling, dancing, or gymnastics. Family pressures also may play a role. One study found that mothers who are extremely concerned about their daughters' physical attractiveness and weight may help to cause bulimia. In addition, girls with eating disorders tend to have fathers and brothers who criticize their weight.

Symptoms

According to the American Anorexia/Bulimia Association, Inc., warning signs of bulimia include:

- eating large amounts of food uncontrollably (bingeing)
- vomiting, abusing laxatives or **diuretics**, or engaging in fasting, dieting, or vigorous exercise (purging)
- preoccupation with body weight
- using the bathroom frequently after meals

- depression or mood swings
- irregular menstrual periods
- onset of dental problems, swollen cheeks or glands, **heartburn** or bloating

Diagnosis

Bulimia is treated most successfully when diagnosed early. But because the bulimic may deny there is a problem, getting medical help is often delayed. A complete **physical examination** in order to rule out other illnesses is the first step to diagnosis.

According to the American Psychiatric Association, a diagnosis of bulimia requires that a person have all of the following symptoms:

- recurrent episodes of binge eating (minimum average of two binge-eating episodes a week for at least three months)
- a feeling of lack of control over eating during the binges
- regular use of one or more of the following to prevent weight gain: self-induced vomiting, use of laxatives or diuretics, strict dieting or fasting, or vigorous exercise
- persistent over-concern with body shape and weight

Treatment

Early treatment is important otherwise bulimia may become chronic, with serious health consequences. A comprehensive treatment plan is called for in order to address the complex interaction of physical and psychological problems in bulimia. A combination of drug and behavioral therapies is commonly used.

Behavioral approaches include individual psychotherapy, **group therapy**, and **family therapy**. **Cognitive-behavioral therapy**, which teaches patients how to change abnormal thoughts and behavior, is also used. **Nutrition** counseling and self-help groups are often helpful.

Antidepressants commonly used to treat bulimia include desipramine (Norpramin), imipramine (Tofranil), and fluoxetine (Prozac). These medications also may treat any co-existing depression.

In addition to professional treatment, family support plays an important role in helping the bulimic person. Encouragement and caring can provide the support needed to convince the sick person to get help, stay with treatment, or try again after a failure. Family members can help locate resources, such as eating disorder clinics in local hospitals or treatment programs in colleges designed for students.

Alternative treatment

Light therapy–exposure to bright, artificial light– may be useful in reducing bulimic episodes, especially during the dark winter months. Some feel that massage may prove helpful, putting people in touch with the reality of their own bodies and correcting misconceptions of body image. **Hypnotherapy** may help resolve unconscious issues that contribute to bulimic behavior.

Prognosis

Bulimia may become chronic and lead to serious health problems, including seizures, irregular heartbeat, and thin bones. In rare cases, it may be fatal.

Timely therapy and medication can effectively manage the disorder and help the bulimic look forward to a normal, productive, and fulfilling life.

Prevention

There is no known method to prevent bulimia.

Resources

ORGANIZATIONS

American Anorexia/Bulimia Association, Inc. 293 Central Park West, Suite IR, New York, NY 10024. (212) 501-8351.

Anorexia Nervosa and Related Eating Disorders, Inc. P.O. Box 5102, Eugene, OR 97405. (541) 344-1144.

Center for the Study of Anorexia and Bulimia. 1 W. 91st St., New York, NY 10024. (212) 595-3449.

Eating Disorder Awareness. & Prevention, Inc., 603 Stewart St., Suite 803, Seattle, WA 98101. (206) 382-3587.

National Association of Anorexia Nervosa and Associated Disorders. Box 7, Highland Park, IL 60035. (708) 831-3438.

National Eating Disorders Organization (NEDO). 6655 South Yale Ave, Tulsa, OK 74136. (918) 481-4044.

Jennifer Lamb

Bulla *see* **Skin lesions**

Bumetanide *see* **Diuretics**

BUN *see* **Blood urea nitrogen test**

Bundle branch block

Definition

Bundle branch block (BBB) is a disruption in the normal flow of electrical pulses that drive the heart beat.

Description

Bundle branch block belongs to a group of heart problems called intraventricular conduction defects (IVCD). There are two bundle branches, right and left. The right bundle carries nerve impulses that cause contraction of the right ventricle (the lower chamber of the heart) and the left bundle carries nerve impulses that cause contraction of the left ventricle. The two bundles initially are together at a junction called the bundle of His. Nerve impulses come through the sinus node of the heart to the bundle of His and then move into the right and left bundle branches. Bundle branch block is a slowing or interruption of nerve impulses. A problem may exist in any of the three bundles.

Patients with BBB are generally without symptoms unless the disease is severe enough to cause a complete infranodal A-V block and very slow heart rate. In patients with right bundle branch block (RBBB), the nerve impulse is conducted slowly or not at all. The right ventricle finally receives the impulse through muscle-to-muscle spread, outside the regular nerve pathway. This mechanism of impulse transmission is slow and results in a delayed contraction of the right ventricle. There are several types of left bundle branch block (LBBB), each producing its own characteristic mechanism of failure. In each case, the nerve impulse is blocked or delayed. Patients with LBBB may have left ventricular disease or **cardiomyopathy**.

Causes and symptoms

Left bundle branch block usually happens as a consequence of other diseases such as arteriosclerosis, **rheumatic fever**, **congenital heart disease**, **myocarditis**, myocardial infarction, metastatic heart tumors, or other invasions of the heart tissue. Right bundle branch block happens less often from underlying heart disease.

Diagnosis

Detection of BBB usually takes place during a normal **physical examination**. The block shows up as a widening of the second heart sound. Confirmation

---

KEY TERMS

Electrocardiogram—The pattern of the heart's electrical impulses that indicate the order and condition of the heart's components.

QRS—A pattern seen in an electrocardiogram that indicates the pulses in a heart beat and their duration. Variations from a normal QRS pattern indicate heart disease.

---

of BBB is obtained by electrocardiogram (ECG). The pattern seen in the electrocardiogram indicates pulses in a heart beat and their duration. A QRS duration of greater than 110 milliseconds is a diagnostic indication of BBB. There is a unique ECG pattern for blocks in each of the three bundles.

Treatment

There is no specific therapy for BBB. Patients are usually treated for associated heart diseases.

Prognosis

The prognosis of blockage in any of the three bundle branches depends on the prognosis of the associated heart disease. The associated diseases determine the outcome of the patient's health. Occasionally, disruptions in bundle branches lead to complete infranodal A-V block, a more serious blockage of nerve impulses. Approximately 2% of patients with BBB develop infranodal A-V blockage and these patients often require artificial **pacemakers**.

Resources

BOOKS

Alexander, R. W., R. C. Schlant, and V. Fuster, editors. *The Heart*. 9th ed. New York: McGraw-Hill, 1998.

John T. Lohr, PhD

Bunion

Definition

A bunion is an abnormal enlargement of the joint (the first metatarsophalangeal joint, or MTPJ) at the base of the great or big toe (hallux). It is caused

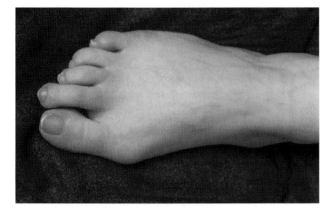

Woman's right foot with bunion on big toe. *(Photograph by Wedgworth, Custom Medical Stock Photo. Reproduced by permission.)*

by inflammation and usually results from chronic irritation and pressure from poorly fitting footwear.

Description

A displacement of two major bones of the foot (hallux valgus) causes bunions, although not everyone with this displacement will develop the joint swelling and bone overgrowth that characterize a bunion. One of the bones involved is called the first metatarsal bone. This bone is long and slender, with the big toe attached on one end and the other end connected to foot bones closer to the ankle. This foot bone is displaced in the direction of the four other metatarsals connected with the toes. The other bone involved is the big toe itself, which is displaced toward the smaller toes. As the big toe continues to move toward the smaller toes, it may become displaced under or over the second toe. The displacement of these two foot bones causes a projection of bone on the inside portion of the forefoot. The skin over this projection often becomes inflamed from rubbing against the shoe, and a callus may form.

The joint contains a small sac (bursa) filled with fluid that cushions the bones and helps the joint to move smoothly. When a bunion forms, this sac becomes inflamed and thickened. The swelling in the joint causes additional **pain** and pressure in the toe.

Causes and symptoms

Bunions may form as a result of abnormal motion of the foot during walking or running. One common example of an abnormal movement is an excessive amount of **stress** placed upon the inside of the foot. This leads to friction and irritation of the involved

structures. Age has also been noted as a factor in developing bunions, in part because the underlying bone displacement worsens over time unless corrective measures are taken.

Wearing improperly fitting shoes, especially those with a narrow toe box and excessive heel height, often causes the formation of a bunion. This forefoot deformity is seen more often in women than men. The higher frequency in females may be related to the strong link between footwear fashion and bunions. In fact, in a recent survey of more than 350 women, nearly 90% wore shoes that were at least one size too small or too narrow.

Because genetic factors can predispose people to the hallux valgus bone displacement, a strong family history of bunions can increase the likelihood of developing this foot disorder. Various arthritic conditions and several genetic and neuromuscular diseases, such as **Down syndrome** and **Marfan syndrome**, cause muscle imbalances that can create bunions from displacement of the first metatarsal and big toe. Other possible causes of bunions are leg-length discrepancies, with the bunion present on the longer leg, and trauma occurring to the joint of the big toe.

Symptoms of bunions include the common signs of inflammation such as redness, swelling, and pain. The discomfort is primarily located along the inside of the foot just behind the big toe. Because of friction, a callus may develop over the bunion. If an overlapping of the toes is allowed, additional rubbing and pain occurs. Inflammation of this area causes a decrease in motion with associated discomfort in the joint between the big toe and the first metatarsal. If allowed to worsen, the skin over the bunion may break down causing an ulcer, which also presents a problem of potential infection. (Foot ulcers can be particularly dangerous for people with diabetes, who may have trouble feeling the ulcer forming and healing if it becomes infected.)

Diagnosis

A thorough medical history and physical exam by a physician is always necessary for the proper diagnosis of bunions and other foot conditions. X rays can help confirm the diagnosis by showing the bone displacement, joint swelling, and, in some cases, the overgrowth of bone that characterizes bunions. Doctors will also consider the possibility that the joint pain is caused by or complicated by arthritis (which causes destruction of the cartilage of the joint), **gout** (which causes the accumulation of uric acid crystals in the joint), tiny **fractures** of a bone in the foot (stress fractures), or infection and may order additional tests to rule out these possibilities.

Treatment

Conservative

The first step in treating a bunion is to remove as much pressure from the area as possible. People with bunions should wear shoes that have enough room in the toe box to accommodate the bunion and avoid high-heeled shoes and tight-fitting socks or stockings. Dressings and pads help protect the bunion from additional shoe pressure. The application of splints or customized shoe inserts (orthotics) to correct the alignment of the big toe joint is effective for many bunions. Most patients are instructed to rest or choose exercises that put less stress on their feet, at least until the misalignment is corrected. In some cases, physicians also use steroid injections with local anesthetic around the bunion to reduce inflammation.

Surgery

If conservative treatment is not successful, surgical removal of the bunion may be necessary to correct the deformity. This procedure is called a bunionectomy, and there are many variations on the operation, which is usually performed by a surgeon who specializes in treating bone conditions (orthopedics) or by one who specializes in treating the foot (podiatry). Surgeons consider the angle of the bone misalignment, the condition of the bursa, and the strength of the bones when they choose which procedure to use. Most bunionectomies involve the removal of a section of bone and the insertion of pins to rejoin the bone. Sometimes the surgeons may move ligaments (which connect bone to bone in the joint) or tendons (which connect bone to muscle) in order to realign the bones. After this procedure, the bones and other tissues are held in place while they heal by compression dressings or a short cast. The individual must refrain from vigorous **exercise** for six weeks.

Alternative treatment

Deep friction massage techniques by a physical or massage therapist can be helpful to increase circulation, reduce inflammation, and prevent soft tissue build up. Physical therapy also provides useful approaches such as ultrasound to help retard or reverse the formation of the bunion. Various taping techniques can be useful to realign the toe and decrease friction and rubbing that may be present. The homeopathic tissue salt *Calcarea phosphorica* can be useful in balancing the bone formation/remodeling.

Prognosis

Often modifications in footwear allow a good prognosis without surgery. If surgery is necessary, complete healing without complications requires approximately four to six weeks. Even after surgery corrects the bone misalignment, patients are usually instructed to continue wearing low-heeled, roomy shoes to prevent the bunion from reforming.

Prevention

Prevention begins with proper foot wear. Shoes with a wide and deep toe box are best. High-heeled shoes should not be worn for long periods of time. If a bunion is present and becomes inflamed, the foot should be elevated with the application of an ice pack over the painful area for not more than 20 minutes every other hour. If pain and swelling continue, a podiatrist or physician should be contacted.

Resources

ORGANIZATIONS

American Orthopedic Foot and Ankle Society. 222 South Prospect, Park Ridge, IL 60068.

American Podiatry Medical Association. 9312 Old Georgetown Road, Bethesda, MD 20814.

OTHER

Griffith, H. Winter. "Complete Guide to Symptoms, Illness & Surgery." ThriveOnline. < http://thriveonline.oxygen.com > .

Jeffrey P. Larson, RPT

Burkitt's lymphoma *see* **Malignant lymphomas**

Burns

Definition

Burns are injuries to tissues caused by heat, friction, electricity, radiation, or chemicals.

Description

Burns are characterized by degree, based on the severity of the tissue damage. A first-degree burn causes redness and swelling in the outermost layers of skin (epidermis). A second-degree burn involves redness, swelling and blistering, and the damage may extend beneath the epidermis to deeper layers of skin (dermis). A third-degree burn, also called a full-thickness burn, destroys the entire depth of skin, causing significant scarring. Damage also may extend to the underlying fat, muscle, or bone.

The severity of the burn is also judged by the amount of body surface area (BSA) involved. Health care workers use the "rule of nines" to determine the percentage of BSA affected in patients more than 9 years old: each arm with its hand is 9% of BSA; each leg with its foot is 18%; the front of the torso is 18%; the back of the torso, including the buttocks, is 18%; the head and neck are 9%; and the genital area (perineum) is 1%. This rule cannot be applied to a young child's body proportions, so BSA is estimated using the palm of the patient's hand as a measure of 1% area.

The severity of the burn will determine not only the type of treatment, but also where the burn patient should receive treatment. Minor burns may be treated at home or in a doctor's office. These are defined as first- or second-degree burns covering less than 15% of an adult's body or less than 10% of a child's body, or a third-degree burn on less than 2% BSA. Moderate burns should be treated at a hospital. These are defined as first- or second-degree burns covering 15%-25% of an adult's body or 10%-20% of a child's body, or a third-degree burn on 2%-10% BSA. Critical, or major, burns are the most serious and should be treated in a specialized burn unit of a hospital. These are defined as first- or second-degree burns covering more than 25% of an adult's body or more than 20% of a child's body, or a third-degree burn on more than 10% BSA. In addition, burns involving the hands, feet, face, eyes, ears, or genitals are considered critical. Other factors influence the level of treatment needed, including associated injuries such as bone **fractures** and **smoke inhalation**, presence of a chronic disease, or a history of being abused. Also,

children and the elderly are more vulnerable to complications from burn injuries and require more intensive care.

Causes and symptoms

Burns may be caused by even a brief encounter with heat greater than 120°F (49°C). The source of this heat may be the sun (causing a **sunburn**), hot liquids, steam, fire, electricity, friction (causing rug burns and rope burns), and chemicals (causing a caustic burn upon contact).

Signs of a burn are localized redness, swelling, and **pain**. A severe burn will also blister. The skin may also peel, appear white or charred, and feel numb. A burn may trigger a **headache** and **fever**. Extensive burns may induce **shock**, the symptoms of which are faintness, weakness, rapid pulse and breathing, pale and clammy skin, and bluish lips and fingernails.

Diagnosis

A physician will diagnose a burn based upon visual examination, and will also ask the patient or family members questions to determine the best treatment. He or she may also check for smoke inhalation, **carbon monoxide poisoning**, cyanide **poisoning**, other event-related trauma, or, if suspected, further evidence of **child abuse**.

Treatment

Burn treatment consists of relieving pain, preventing infection, and maintaining body fluids, electrolytes, and calorie intake while the body heals. Treatment of chemical or electrical burns is slightly different from the treatment of thermal burns but the objectives are the same.

Thermal burn treatment

The first act of thermal burn treatment is to stop the burning process. This may be accomplished by letting cool water run over the burned area or by soaking it in cool (not cold) water. Ice should never be applied to the burn. Cool (not cold) wet compresses may provide some pain relief when applied to small areas of first- and second-degree burns. Butter, shortening, or similar salve should never be applied to the burn since it prevents heat from escaping and drives the burning process deeper into the skin.

If the burn is minor, it may be cleaned gently with soap and water. Blisters should not be broken. If the skin of the burned area is unbroken and it is not likely to be further irritated by pressure or friction, the burn

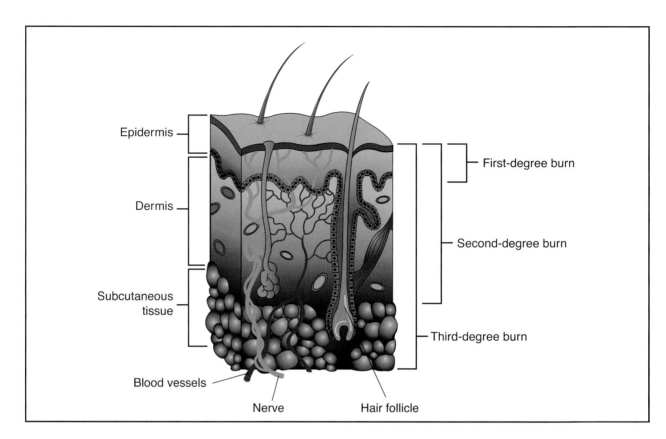

Epidermis

Dermis

Subcutaneous
tissue

Blood vessels

Nerve

Hair follicle

First-degree burn

Second-degree burn

Third-degree burn

There are three classifications of burns: first-degree, second-degree, and third-degree burns. *(Illustration by Electronic Illustrators Group.)*

Classification Of Burns

First-Degree (Minor)	The burned area is painful. The outer skin is reddened. Slight swelling is present.
Second-Degree (Moderate)	The burned area is painful. The underskin is affected. Blisters may form. The area may have a wet, shiny appearance because of exposed tissue.
Third-Degree (Critical)	The burned area is insensitive due to the destruction of nerve endings. Skin is destroyed. Muscle tissues and bone underneath may be damaged. The area may be charred, white, or grayish in color.

should be left exposed to the air to promote healing. If the skin is broken or apt to be disturbed, the burned area should be coated lightly with an antibacterial ointment and covered with a sterile bandage. **Aspirin, acetaminophen** (Tylenol), or ibuprofen (Advil) may be taken to ease pain and relieve inflammation. A doctor should be consulted if these signs of infection appear: increased warmth, redness, pain, or swelling; pus or similar drainage from the wound; swollen lymph nodes; or red streaks spreading away from the burn.

In situations where a person has received moderate or critical burns, lifesaving measures take precedence over burn treatment and emergency medical assistance must be called. A person with serious burns may stop breathing, and artificial respiration (also called mouth-to-mouth resuscitation or rescue breathing) should be administered immediately. Also, a person with burns covering more than 12% BSA is likely to go into shock; this condition may be prevented by laying the person flat and elevating the feet about 12 in (30 cm). Burned arms and hands should also be raised higher than the person's heart.

In rescues, a blanket may be used to smother any flames as the person is removed from danger. The person whose clothing is on fire should "stop, drop, and roll" or be assisted in lying flat on the ground and rolling to put out the fire. Afterwards, only burnt clothing that comes off easily should be removed; any clothing embedded in the burn should not be disturbed. Removing any smoldering apparel and covering the person with a light, cool, wet cloth, such as a sheet but not a blanket or towel, will stop the burning process.

KEY TERMS

Debridement—The surgical removal of dead tissue.

Dermis—The basal layer of skin; it contains blood and lymphatic vessels, nerves, glands, and hair follicles.

Epidermis—The outer portion of skin, made up of four or five superficial layers.

Shock—An abnormal condition resulting from low blood volume due to hemorrhage or dehydration. Signs of shock include rapid pulse and breathing, and cool, moist, pale skin.

At the hospital, the staff will provide further medical treatment. A tube to aid breathing may be inserted if the patient's airways or lungs have been damaged, as can happen during an explosion or a fire in a enclosed space. Also, because burns dramatically deplete the body of fluids, replacement fluids are administered intravenously. The patient is also given **antibiotics** intravenously to prevent infection, and he or she may also receive a **tetanus** shot, depending on his or her immunization history. Once the burned area is cleaned and treated with antibiotic cream or ointment, it is covered in sterile bandages, which are changed two to three times a day. Surgical removal of dead tissue (**debridement**) also takes place. As the burns heal, thick, taut scabs (eschar) form, which the doctor may have to cut to improve blood flow to the more elastic healthy tissue beneath. The patient will also undergo physical and occupational therapy to keep the burned areas from becoming inflexible and to minimize scarring.

In cases where the skin has been so damaged that it cannot properly heal, a skin graft is usually performed. A skin graft involves taking a piece of skin from an unburned portion of the patient's body (autograft) and transplanting it to the burned area. When doctors cannot immediately use the patient's own skin, a temporary graft is performed using the skin of a human donor (allograft), either alive or dead, or the skin of an animal (xenograft), usually that of a pig.

The burn victim also may be placed in a **hyperbaric chamber**, if one is available. In a hyperbaric chamber (which can be a specialized room or enclosed space), the patient is exposed to pure oxygen under high pressure, which can aid in healing. However, for this therapy to be effective, the patient must be placed in a chamber within 24 hours of being burned.

Chemical burn treatment

Burns from liquid chemicals must be rinsed with cool water for at least 15 minutes to stop the burning process. Any burn to the eye must be similarly flushed with water. In cases of burns from dry chemicals such as lime, the powder should be completely brushed away before the area is washed. Any clothing which may have absorbed the chemical should be removed. The burn should then be loosely covered with a sterile gauze pad and the person taken to the hospital for further treatment. A physician may be able to neutralize the offending chemical with another before treating the burn like a thermal burn of similar severity.

Electrical burn treatment

Before electrical burns are treated at the site of the accident, the power source must be disconnected if possible and the victim moved away from it to keep the person giving aid from being electrocuted. Lifesaving measures again take priority over burn treatment, so breathing must be checked and assisted if necessary. Electrical burns should be loosely covered with sterile gauze pads and the person taken to the hospital for further treatment.

Alternative treatment

In addition to the excellent treatment of burns provided by traditional medicine, some alternative approaches may be helpful as well. (Major burns should always be treated by a medical practitioner.) The homeopathic remedies *Cantharis* and *Causticum* can assist in burn healing. A number of botanical remedies, applied topically, can also help burns heal. These include aloe (*Aloe barbadensis*), oil of St.-John's-wort (*Hypericum perforatum*), calendula (*Calendula officinalis*), comfrey (*Symphytum officinale*), and tea tree oil (*Melaleuca* spp.). Supplementing the diet with vitamin C, vitamin E, and zinc also is beneficial for wound healing.

Prognosis

The prognosis is dependent upon the degree of the burn, the amount of body surface covered, whether critical body parts were affected, any additional injuries or complications like infection, and the promptness of medical treatment. Minor burns may heal in five to 10 days with no scarring. Moderate burns may heal in 10-14 days and may leave scarring. Critical or major burns take more than 14 days to heal and will leave significant scarring. Scar tissue may limit mobility and functionality, but physical therapy may overcome these limitations. In some cases, additional surgery may be advisable to remove scar tissue and restore appearance.

Prevention

Burns are commonly received in residential fires. Properly placed and working smoke detectors in combination with rapid evacuation plans will minimize a person's exposure to smoke and flames in the event of a fire. Children must be taught never to play with matches, lighters, fireworks, gasoline, and cleaning fluids.

Burns by scalding with hot water or other liquids may be prevented by setting the water heater thermostat no higher than 120 °F (49 °C), checking the temperature of bath water before getting into the tub, and turning pot handles on the stove out of the reach of children. Care should be used when removing covers from pans of steaming foods and when uncovering or opening foods heated in a microwave oven.

Thermal burns are often received from electrical appliances. Care should be exercised around stoves, space heaters, irons, and curling irons.

Sunburns may be avoided by the liberal use of a sunscreen containing either an opaque active ingredient such as zinc oxide or titanium dioxide or a nonopaque active ingredient such as PABA (para-aminobenzoic acid) or benzophenone. Hats, loose clothing, and umbrellas also provide protection, especially between 10 A.M. and 3 P.M. when the most damaging ultraviolet rays are present in direct sunlight.

Electrical burns may be prevented by covering unused electrical outlets with safety plugs and keeping electrical cords away from infants and toddlers who might chew on them. Persons should also seek shelter indoors during a thunderstorm to avoid being struck by lightning.

Chemical burns may be prevented by wearing protective clothing, including gloves and eyeshields. Chemical agents should always be used according to the manufacturer's instructions and properly stored when not in use.

Resources

ORGANIZATIONS

Shriners Hospitals for Children. 2900 Rocky Point Drive, Tampa, FL 33607-1435. (813) 281-0300. < http://www.shrinershq.org > .

OTHER

HealthAnswers.com. < http://www.healthanswers.com > .

Bethany Thivierge

Bursitis

Definition

Bursitis is the painful inflammation of the bursa, a padlike sac found in areas subject to friction. Bursae cushion the movement between the bones, tendons and muscles near the joints. Bursitis is most often caused by repetitive movement and is known by several common names including weaver's bottom, clergyman's knee, and miner's elbow, depending on the affected individual's occupation and area of injury.

Description

There are over 150 bursae in the human body. Usually bursae are present from birth, but they may form in response to repeated pressure. Each sac contains a small amount of *synovial fluid,* a clear liquid that acts as a lubricant. Inflammation causes **pain** on movement. The most common site for bursitis to occur is the shoulder (subdeltoid), but it also is seen in the elbows (olecranon), hips (trochanteric), knees, heels (Achilles), and toes. The affected area may be referred to as "frozen," because movement is so limited. In the knee there are four bursae, and all can become inflamed with overuse.

Causes and symptoms

The most common cause of bursitis is repeated physical activity, but it can flare up for no known reason. It can also be caused by trauma, **rheumatoid arthritis**, **gout**, and acute or chronic infection.

Pain and tenderness are common symptoms. If the affected joint is close to the skin, as with the shoulder, knee, elbow, or Achilles tendon, swelling and redness are seen and the area may feel warm to the touch. The bursae around the hip joint are deeper, and swelling is not obvious. Movement may be limited and is painful. In the shoulder, it may be difficult to raise the arm out from the side of the body. Putting on a jacket or combing the hair becomes a troublesome activity.

KEY TERMS

Arthritis—Inflammation of a joint that may lead to changes in the joint's structure. It causes pain and swelling. Rheumatoid arthritis is a chronic disease that leads to crippling deformities.

Diabetes mellitus—A metabolic disease caused by a deficiency of insulin, which is essential to process carbohydrates in the body.

Gout—A hereditary metabolic disease that is a form of arthritis and causes inflammation of the joints. It is more common in men.

Inflammation—The reaction of tissue to injury.

Kinesiology—The science or study of movement.

In acute bursitis symptoms appear suddenly; with chronic bursitis, pain, tenderness, and limited movement reappear after **exercise** or strain.

Diagnosis

When a patient has pain in a joint, a careful **physical examination** is needed to determine what type of movement is affected and if there is any swelling present. Bursitis will not show up on x-rays, although sometimes there are also calcium deposits in the joint that can be seen. Inserting a thin needle into the affected bursa and removing (aspirating) some of the synovial fluid for examination can confirm the diagnosis. In most cases, the fluid will not be clear. It can be tested for the presence of microorganisms, which would indicate an infection, and crystals, which could indicate gout. In instances where the diagnosis is difficult, a local anesthetic (a drug that numbs the area) is injected into the painful spot. If the discomfort stops temporarily, then bursitis is probably the correct diagnosis.

Treatment

Conservative treatment of bursitis is usually effective. The application of heat, rest, and **immobilization** of the affected joint area is the first step. A sling can be used for a shoulder injury; a cane is helpful for hip problems. The patient can take **nonsteroidal anti-inflammatory drugs** (NSAIDs) like **aspirin**, ibuprofen, and naproxen. They can be obtained without a prescription and relieve the pain and inflammation. Once the pain decreases, exercises of the affected area can

begin. If the nearby muscles have become weak because of the disease or prolonged immobility, then exercises to build strength and improve movement are best. A doctor or physical therapist can prescribe an effective regimen.

If the bursitis is related to an inflammatory condition like arthritis or gout, then management of that disease is needed to control the bursitis.

When bursitis does not respond to conservative treatment, an injection into the joint of a long-acting corticosteroid preparation, like prednisone, can bring immediate and lasting relief. A corticosteroid is a hormonal substance that is the most effective drug for reducing inflammation. The drug is mixed with a local anesthetic and works on the joint within five minutes. Usually one injection is all that is needed.

Surgery to remove the damaged bursa may be performed in extreme cases.

If the bursitis is caused by an infection, then additional treatment is needed. *Septic* bursitis is caused by the presence of a pus-forming organism, usually *staphylococcus aureus*. This is confirmed by examining a sample of the fluid in the bursa and requires treatment with **antibiotics** taken by mouth, injected into a muscle or into a vein (intravenously). The bursa will also need to be drained by needle two or three times over the first week of treatment. When a patient has such a serious infection, there may be underlying causes. There could be undiscovered diabetes, or an inefficient immune system caused by human **immunodeficiency** virus infection (HIV).

Alternative treatment

Alternative treatments take into consideration the role of diet in causing bursitis. The faulty use of calcium by the body, magnesium deficiency, and **food allergies** may have a role. Diet changes and vitamin supplements may be helpful. The use of herbs, homeopathy, **aromatherapy**, and **hydrotherapy** can help relieve symptoms. Ginger is useful in reducing inflammation. **Acupuncture** has been proven effective in treating hip and shoulder pain caused by bursitis and other conditions. Other therapies that deal effectively with musculoskeletal problems (relating to the muscles and skeleton), may also be helpful, such as body work, **magnetic field therapy**, **naturopathic medicine**, **chiropractic**, and **applied kinesiology**.

Prognosis

Bursitis usually responds well to treatment, but it may develop into a chronic condition if the underlying cause is not corrected.

Prevention

Aggravating factors should be eliminated to prevent bursitis. Overexercising or the repetition of a movement that triggers the condition should be avoided. Doing exercises to strengthen the muscles around the joint will also help. When doing repetitive tasks, frequent breaks should be taken and the activity should be alternated with others using different parts of the body. To cushion the joints, it is a good idea to use cushioned chairs when sitting and foam kneeling pads for the knees. Leaning on the elbows, kneeling or sitting on a hard surface for a long period of time should be avoided. Not wearing high heels can help prevent bursitis in the heel, as can changing to new running shoes as soon as the old ones are worn out.

Resources

OTHER

"Bursitis." HealthAnswers.com. 1998. < http://www.healthanswers.com >.

Karen Ericson, RN

Bypass surgery *see* **Coronary artery bypass graft surgery**

Byssinosis

Definition

Byssinosis is a chronic, asthma-like narrowing of the airways. Also called brown lung disease, byssinosis results from inhaling particles of cotton, flax, hemp, or jute.

Description

Although inhaling cotton dust was identified as a source of respiratory disease more than 300 years ago, byssinosis has been recognized as an occupational hazard for textile workers for less than 50 years. More than 800,000 workers in the cotton, flax, and rope-making industries are exposed in the workplace to airborne particles that can cause byssinosis. Only workers in mills that manufacture yarn, thread, or fabric have a significant risk of dying of this disease.

In the United States, byssinosis is almost completely limited to workers who handle unprocessed cotton. More than 35,000 textile workers have been disabled by byssinosis and 183 died between 1979 and 1992. Most of the people whose deaths were due to byssinosis lived in the textile-producing regions of North and South Carolina.

Causes and symptoms

As many as 25% of workers with byssinosis have symptoms that continue or recur throughout the workweek. More severe breathing problems seem to result both from exposure to high levels of dust and from longer dust exposure. Workers who also smoke cigarettes suffer the most severe impairment.

Diagnosis

Tests that detect decreasing lung capacity during the workday are used to diagnose byssinosis. Obstructive patterns are likely in patients who have had recurrent symptoms for more than 10 years.

Treatment

Therapy for early-stage byssinosis focuses on reversing airway narrowing. **Antihistamines** may be prescribed to reduce tightness in the chest. **Bronchodilators** (drugs used to relax breathing passages and improve air flow) may be used with an inhaler or taken in tablet form. Reducing exposure is essential. Any worker who has symptoms of byssinosis or who has trouble breathing should transfer to a less-contaminated area.

Prognosis

Smoking, impaired lung function, and a history of respiratory allergy increase a textile worker's risk of developing byssinosis. Prolonged exposure makes patients wheeze more often and can cause chronic **bronchitis**. It does not lead to permanently disabling lung disease.

Prevention

Eliminating exposure to textile dust is the surest way to prevent byssinosis. Using exhaust hoods, improving ventilation, and employing wetting procedures are very successful methods of controlling dust levels to prevent byssinosis. Protective equipment required during certain procedures also prevents exposure to levels of contamination that exceed the current United States standard for cotton dust exposure.

Resources

ORGANIZATIONS

American Lung Association. 1740 Broadway, New York, NY 10019. (800) 586-4872. <http://www.lungusa.org>.

Centers for Disease Control and Prevention. 1600 Clifton Rd., NE, Atlanta, GA 30333. (800) 311-3435, (404) 639-3311. <http://www.cdc.gov>

Maureen Haggerty